Advanced Physiology and Pathophysiology

Nancy C. Tkacs, PhD, RN, received her BSN and MSN degrees from the University of Pennsylvania School of Nursing and her PhD in physiology with a focus in neuroscience from Loyola University of Chicago Graduate School at the Stritch School of Medicine. She completed postdoctoral training in neuroendocrinology in the laboratory of Dr. William F. (Fran) Ganong at University of California San Francisco. Dr. Tkacs conducted preclinical research on neuroendocrine responses to physiological stressors in rodent models, particularly pertaining to the diabetes complication hypoglycemia unawareness. Dr. Tkacs has been teaching pathophysiology for advanced nursing practice for over 25 years, drawing on her knowledge of organ systems physiology and pathophysiology to provide a strong basic science foundation for advanced nursing practice. As a master's-prepared nurse with a doctorate in physiology, she is able to build a bridge between physiology concepts and the pathophysiology of disease. Students learn how findings from the history and physical and diagnostic test results relate to the underlying disease process at the cell and organ level. She taught advanced pathophysiology and neuroscience courses at the University of Medicine and Dentistry of New Jersey and the New Jersey Medical School; she taught advanced pathophysiology and pathogenesis of mental health disorders courses at the University of Pennsylvania; and she directed and taught advanced pathophysiology and advanced pharmacology online courses at the University of Southern California. She also served as assistant dean for Diversity and Inclusivity at the University of Pennsylvania School of Nursing.

Linda L. Herrmann, PhD, RN, AGACNP-BC, GNP-BC, ACHPN, FAANP, is a clinical assistant professor and nurse practitioner with expertise in gerontology, neuroscience, and palliative care. Dr. Herrmann's clinical and research interests are acute neurological injury in older adults, dementia, stroke, caregivers, palliative care of patients with neurological diseases, and transitional care of older adults. Dr. Hermann teaches advanced pathophysiology and aging at the graduate level. Her research also explores innovative pedagogy using virtual reality and mixed reality to teach advanced pathophysiology and advanced nurse practitioner courses in acute care and aging. Dr. Herrmann earned her BSN, MSN, and PhD from the University of Pennsylvania School of Nursing under the mentoring of Neville E. Strumpf, PhD, RN. She was a John A. Hartford predoctoral scholar and is currently a Fellow of the Hartford Institute for Geriatric Nursing and a Fellow of the American Association of Nurse Practitioners. She is a nationally recognized expert in neuroscience, aging, and advanced pathophysiology; and is known internationally for expertise in patient safety in hospital and clinic settings in Africa.

Randall L. Johnson, PhD, RN, is an associate professor of nursing at the University of Tennessee Health Science Center. He is also a pediatric critical care nurse practitioner. Dr. Johnson has clinical experience in pediatric medical–surgical nursing and pediatric intensive care and trauma. His research interests are in clinical care of hospital-acquired infection reduction. Dr. Johnson has taught pathophysiology in both undergraduate and graduate degree programs. He has also taught various pediatric and pharmacology courses through the course of his academic career. Dr. Johnson earned his BSN from Cedarville University, his MSN from the University of Pennsylvania, and his PhD from the University of Central Florida. Dr. Johnson has held academic appointments since 1999 and has served in a leadership capacity in academics.

Advanced Physiology and Pathophysiology

ESSENTIALS FOR CLINICAL PRACTICE

Nancy C. Tkacs, PhD, RN

Linda L. Herrmann, PhD, RN, AGACNP-BC, GNP-BC, ACHPN, FAANP

Randall L. Johnson, PhD, RN

SPRINGER PUBLISHING COMPANY

Springer Publishing Company, LLC
11 West 42nd Street, New York, NY 10036
www.springerpub.com
connect.springerpub.com/

Acquisitions Editor: Suzanne Toppy
Developmental Editor: Donna Frassetto
Compositor: diacriTech

ISBN: 978-0-8261-7707-0
ebook ISBN: 978-0-8261-7708-7
DOI: 10.1891/9780826177087

Qualified instructors may request supplements by emailing textbook@springerpub.com
Instructor's Manual: 978-0-8261-7726-1
Instructor's Test Bank: 978-0-8261-7728-5
Instructor's PowerPoints: 978-0-8261-7727-8
Instructor's Image Bank: 978-0-8261-7729-2

20 21 22 23 / 5 4 3 2 1

The author and the publisher of this Work have made every effort to use sources believed to be reliable to provide information that is accurate and compatible with the standards generally accepted at the time of publication. Because medical science is continually advancing, our knowledge base continues to expand. Therefore, as new information becomes available, changes in procedures become necessary. We recommend that the reader always consult current research and specific institutional policies before performing any clinical procedure or delivering any medication. The author and publisher shall not be liable for any special, consequential, or exemplary damages resulting, in whole or in part, from the readers' use of, or reliance on, the information contained in this book. The publisher has no responsibility for the persistence or accuracy of URLs for external or third-party Internet websites referred to in this publication and does not guarantee that any content on such websites is, or will remain, accurate or appropriate.

Library of Congress Control Number: 2019919432

Publisher's Note: **New and used products purchased from third-party sellers are not guaranteed for quality, authenticity, or access to any included digital components.**

Printed in the United States of America.

We dedicate the book to our students who have asked such great questions through the years. You inspire us to do all we can to provide detailed, yet understandable explanations of the pathophysiological phenomena underlying advanced clinical practice.

CONTENTS

1. THE FOUNDATIONAL CONCEPTS OF CLINICAL PRACTICE   1

Nancy C. Tkacs, Linda L. Herrmann, Randall L. Johnson, and Loretta A. Sernekos

2. CHEMICAL AND BIOCHEMICAL FOUNDATIONS   9

Gioia Petrighi Polidori

3. MOLECULAR BIOLOGY, GENETICS, AND GENETIC DISEASES   37

Sheila A. Alexander and Michael J. Groves

4. CELL PHYSIOLOGY AND PATHOPHYSIOLOGY   73

Nancy C. Tkacs, Fruzsina K. Johnson, Robert A. Johnson, and Spencer A. Rhodes

5. INFECTIOUS DISEASE   113

Ross S. Johnson, Jennifer Bailey, and Roseann Velez

7. NEOPLASIA   215

*Kolbrun (Kolla) Kristjansdottir, Thomas M. Bodenstine,
and Sandhya Noronha*

14. LIVER   509

Jennifer Andres, Adam Diamond, Kimberly A. Miller,
Nicole E. Omecene, and Dusty Lisi

15. NERVOUS SYSTEM   541

Nancy C. Tkacs, Peggy A. Compton, and Kara Pavone

17. ENDOCRINE SYSTEM   663

*Christine Yedinak, Carolina R. Hurtado, Angela M. Leung,
Meredith Annon, Hanne S. Harbison, Diane L. Spatz, Gioia
Petrighi Polidori, and Victoria Fischer*

CASE STUDIES

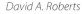

FOREWORD

Dr. Tkacs and I "met" when she emailed me about an error she spotted in my physiology textbook. Perhaps a surprising start to a warm friendship, but I was immediately taken by Dr. Tkacs's thorough understanding of a tricky topic and I wrote back to express gratitude to her for taking the time to improve my book. Thus began our correspondence on matters of physiology teaching. I was thrilled to learn that she was writing a physiology and pathophysiology book for advanced practitioners, as it was clear that she has the gift for explaining difficult topics.

Students in advanced practice programs face the monumental challenge of applying knowledge of pathophysiology to clinical practice. To do this, the student must first have solid command of the principles of physiology, translate those principles to the pathophysiology of diseases, and then translate them again to the clinical setting. Each step must be undergirded by a firm understanding of the "whys" of the physiologic mechanisms.

Dr. Tkacs's book guides the student through those "whys"—in a step-wise fashion that is logical and systematic. The physiology of each system is presented at the appropriate level, in an easily accessible book that is complemented by clear tables and figures. Throughout, she provides relevant examples and metaphors to help the student visualize and relate to complex pathophysiologic mechanisms. Thought-provoking questions challenge the student and offer practice for long-term retention. Equations—which are inescapable in physiology—are explained in words to make them less daunting to the student; every equation is also presented in the context of its pathophysiological application. Pathophysiology and case studies are integrated throughout the text, serving to link the physiology with clinical practice and treatment.

Dr. Tkacs's credentials ideally qualify her to write a pathophysiology book for advanced practice students. Her credibility derives from the depth of her graduate and postgraduate training in nursing and physiology and her many years of experience in the trenches teaching advanced practice students. In other words, she is the "real deal" author—a serious, practicing physiologist *and* an educator with vast experience, who can translate her depth of knowledge at the appropriate level for her students.

I heartily recommend Dr. Tkacs's exceptional book and wish you well on your pathophysiology journey with her.

Linda S. Costanzo, PhD
Professor of Physiology and Biophysics
Virginia Commonwealth University
School of Medicine

ACKNOWLEDGMENTS

The editors gratefully acknowledge:

- Our authors and reviewers for generously sharing their time and expertise to help us realize our vision for this book
- Suzanne Toppy for her support and encouragement from the inception of this project
- Donna Frassetto for her superb and meticulous work as developmental editor
- Joanne Jay, Cindy Yoo, and all of the team members within Springer Publishing Company and associates who contributed to this project
- Our families and friends without whose support this would not have been possible

CONTRIBUTORS

Stacy M. Alabastro, MS, AGACNP-BC, RN, SCRN
Nurse Practitioner
Critical Care Medicine
Memorial Sloan Kettering Cancer Center
New York, New York
Chapter 17: Endocrine System

Sheila A. Alexander, BSN, PhD, FCCM
Associate Professor
University of Pittsburgh School of Nursing
Pittsburgh, Pennsylvania
Chapter 3: Molecular Biology, Genetics, and Genetic Diseases

Jennifer Andres, PharmD, BCPS
Clinical Associate Professor of Pharmacy Practice
Temple University School of Pharmacy
Philadelphia, Pennsylvania
Chapter 14: Liver

Meredith Annon, MSN, CNM, WHNP-BC
Women's Health Nurse Practitioner
The Hospital of the University of Pennsylvania
Philadelphia, Pennsylvania
Chapter 17: Endocrine System

Melissa Assaf, DNP, CPNP-PC, APN-Genetics
Pediatric Nurse Practitioner
Advanced Practice Nurse in Genetics
Banner Children's Specialists, Child Neurology
Scottsdale, Arizona
Chapter 15: Nervous System

Patrick C. Auth, PhD, PA-C
Clinical Professor
Philadelphia, Pennsylvania
Chapter 8: Blood and Clotting

Jennifer Bailey, PharmD, BCPS, AAHIVP
Assistant Professor
Department of Clinical and Administrative Sciences
School of Pharmacy
Notre Dame of Maryland University
Baltimore, Maryland
Chapter 5: Infectious Disease

Nicholas A. Barker, PharmD, BCCCP
Clinical Pharmacy Specialist, Cardiology
Emory Saint Joseph's Hospital
Atlanta, Georgia
Chapter 11: Lungs

Thomas M. Bodenstine, PhD
Assistant Professor
Biochemistry and Molecular Genetics Department
Midwestern University
Downers Grove, Illinois
Chapter 7: Neoplasia

Alyssa Bondy, PA-C, MMS, EMT-B
Physician Assistant
Department of Internal Medicine
New York Presbyterian Weill Cornell Medicine
New York, New York
Chapter 5: Infectious Disease

Stephanie L. Carper, MSN, APRN, CPNP-PC
Nurse Practitioner
Rainbow Pediatric Center
Jacksonville, Florida
Chapter 8: Blood and Clotting

CASE STUDY CONTRIBUTORS

Melissa Assaf, DNP, CPNP-PC, APN-Genetics
Pediatric Nurse Practitioner
Advanced Practice Nurse in Genetics
Banner Children's Specialists, Child Neurology
Glendale, Arizona
Perseverance Research Center
Scottsdale, Arizona
Case Study 15.2: A Child With a Seizure Disorder

Beth Boyer, PA-C, MS
Physician Assistant, Hematology/Oncology
Mayo Clinic
Jacksonville, Florida
Case Study 7.1: A Patient With Breast Cancer

Stephanie L. Carper, MSN, APRN, CPNP-PC
Nurse Practitioner
Rainbow Pediatric Center
Jacksonville, Florida
*Case Study 5.2: A Child With Hand, Foot, and Mouth
    Disease*
Case Study 11.1: A Child With Asthma

Amanda Chaney, DNP, APRN, FNP-BC, FAANP
Transplant Nurse Practitioner/Chair, Advanced
    Practice Provider Subcommittee
Mayo Clinic
Jacksonville, Florida
Case Study 13.1: A Patient With Peptic Ulcer Disease
Case Study 13.2: A Teenage Boy With Celiac Disease
*Case Study 14.1: A Patient With Hepatitis A Virus
    Infection*
*Case Study 14.2: A Patient With Nonalcoholic Fatty
    Liver Disease*

Jane S. Davis, CRNP, DNP
Division of Nephrology
University of Alabama at Birmingham
Birmingham, Alabama
Case Study 12.1: A Patient With Chronic Kidney Disease
Case Study 12.2: A Patient With a Kidney Stone

Colleen Diering, DNP, APRN
Advanced Practice Provider, Neurology
Mayo Clinic
Jacksonville, Florida
Case Study 15.1: A Teenage Girl With Migraine

Katherine Edwards, PA-C
Advanced Practice Provider, Neurology
Mayo Clinic
Jacksonville, Florida
Case Study 15.2: A Child With a Seizure Disorder

Linda W. Good, MD
Family Practice Physician
Mt. Airy Family Practice
Philadelphia, Pennsylvania
Case Study 6.1: A Patient With Allergic Rhinitis
Case Study 10.3: A Patient With Atrial Fibrillation
Case Study 11.2: A Patient With Chronic Bronchitis
Case Study 15.3: A Patient With Depression
Case Study 17.1: A Patient With Graves Disease

Lisa Rathman, MSN, CRNP, CHFN
Lead Nurse Practitioner
The Heart Group of Lancaster General Health/PENN
    Medicine Heart Failure Program
Lancaster, Pennsylvania
*Case Study 10.1: A Patient With Heart Failure
    Symptoms*

David A. Roberts, MSPAS, PA-C
Heart and Vascular Center of West Tennessee
Jackson, Tennessee
Case Study 9.1: A Patient With Hypertension
Case Study 9.2: A Patient With Edema
Case Study 10.2: A Patient With Angina

Allison Rusgo, MPH, PA-C
Assistant Clinical Professor
Physician Assistant Program
Drexel University
Philadelphia, Pennsylvania
Case Study 8.1: A Patient With Pernicious Anemia
Case Study 8.2: A Patient With a Deep Venous
   Thrombosis
Case Study 16.1: A Patient With a Sprained Ankle
Case Study 16.2: A Patient With Acute Gouty
   Arthritis

Nancy C. Tkacs, PhD, RN
Associate Professor Emerita
University of Pennsylvania School of Nursing
Philadelphia, Pennsylvania
Case Study 17.2: A Patient With Hyperparathyroidism

Kimberly K. Trout, PhD, CNM, APRN, FAAN
Assistant Professor of Women's Health
University of Pennsylvania School of Nursing
Philadelphia, Pennsylvania
Case Study 17.3: A Patient With Gestational Diabetes

Sampath Wijesinghe, DHSc, MS, MPAS, AAHIVS,
   PA-C
Principal Faculty and Clinical Site Director,
   Central Valley
MSPA Program, School of Medicine
Stanford University
Stanford, California
Case Study 5.1: A Patient With Acute HIV Infection

Michelle Zappas, DNP, FNP-BC
Clinical Associate Professor
School of Social Work, Department of Nursing
University of Southern California
Los Angeles, California
Case Study 8.2: A Patient With a Deep Venous
   Thrombosis
Case Study 9.1: A Patient With Hypertension
Case Study 9.2: A Patient With Edema
Case Study 13.1: A Patient With Peptic Ulcer Disease
Case Study 13.2: A Teenage Boy With Celiac Disease
Case Study 14.1: A Patient With Hepatitis A Virus
   Infection
Case Study 14.2: A Patient With Nonalcoholic Fatty
   Liver Disease
Case Study 15.1: A Teenage Girl With Migraine
Case Study 16.1: A Patient With a Sprained Ankle
Case Study 16.2: A Patient With Acute Gouty
   Arthritis

Kim Zuber, PA-C, DFAAPA
Executive Director
American Academy of Nephrology PAs
St. Petersburg, Florida
Case Study 12.1: A Patient With Chronic Kidney
   Disease
Case Study 12.2: A Patient With a Kidney Stone

REVIEWERS

Rebecca Baldwin
Physician Assistant Student
Drexel University
Philadelphia, Pennsylvania

Joseph Boullata, PharmD, RPh, CNS-S, FASPEN, FACN
Clinical Professor
Department of Nutrition Sciences
Drexel University

Patrick Brown, MSPAS, PA-C
Assistant Professor of Clinical Medicine
Bethel University
Paris, Tennessee

Rachel Cloutier, MS, RN, ACNP-BC
Clinical Instructor
School of Nursing
Virginia Commonwealth University
Richmond, Virginia

Lisa Connor, PhD
School of Biological Sciences
Victoria University of Wellington
Wellington, New Zealand

Margaret Eckert-Norton, RN, PhD, FNP-BC, CDE, CNE
Associate Professor
St. Joseph's College/SUNY Downstate
Brooklyn, New York

Desiree Fleck, PhD, ACNP-BC, CPNP-BC
Nurse Practitioner
The Children's Hospital of Philadelphia
Lecturer
University of Pennsylvania School of Nursing
Philadelphia, Pennsylvania

Cecilia Follin, PhD
Associate Professor
Lund University
Lund, Sweden

Lynda A. Frassetto, MD, FASN
Professor Emerita of Medicine and Nephrology
University of California, San Francisco
San Francisco, California

Ranjodh S. Gill, MD, FACP
Professor
Department of Internal Medicine
Division of Endocrinology, Diabetes, & Metabolism
Virginia Commonwealth University
VA Medical Center
Richmond, Virginia

Lexy Kristen Green
Acute Care Nurse Practitioner Student
New York University
Rory Meyers College of Nursing
New York, New York

Lisa M. Harrison-Bernard, PhD, FAHA, FASN, FAPS
Associate Professor
Department of Physiology
Louisiana State University School of Medicine
New Orleans, Louisiana

Jonathan Howard, MD
Associate Professor of Neurology and Psychiatry and
    Clerkship Director
Clinical Neurological Sciences
NYU Langone Medical Center
New York, New York

Tracie Kirkland, DNP, ANP-BC, CPNP
Clinical Assistant Professor
Suzanne Dworak-Peck School of Social Work
Department of Nursing
University of Southern California
Los Angeles, California

Kathryn Evans Kreider, DNP, APRN, FNP-BC
Associate Professor
Duke University School of Nursing
Durham, North Carolina

Mary Ann Lafferty-DellaValle, PhD
Practice Professor (Retired)
University of Pennsylvania School of Nursing
Philadelphia, Pennsylvania

Laura Gunder McClary, DHSc, MHE, PA-C
Professor, Doctor of Medical Science
Rocky Mountain University of Health Professions
Provo, Utah

Amanda Miller
Physician Assistant Student
Midwestern University
Downers Grove, Illinois

Lynn M. Oswald, PhD, MSN, RN
Associate Professor
Department of Family and Community Health
University of Maryland School of Nursing
Baltimore, Maryland

Sherry Pikul, MSN, APRN, FNP-C
Family Nurse Practitioner
Bozeman Creek Family Health
Bozeman, Montana

David A. Roberts, MSPAS, PA-C
Assistant Professor
Bethel University
Paris, Tennessee

Loretta A. Sernekos, PhD, MSN, AGPCNP-BC, PMHNP-BC, CNE
Senior Lecturer
University of Pennsylvania School of Nursing
Philadelphia, Pennsylvania

Dexter F. Speck, PhD
Professor of Physiology
University of Kentucky College of Medicine
Lexington, Kentucky

Ignacio Valencia, MD
Professor of Pediatrics
Drexel University College of Medicine
Philadelphia, Pennsylvania

William F. Wright, DO, MPH
Division of Infectious Diseases
Department of Medicine
Johns Hopkins School of Medicine
Baltimore, Maryland

Michael Zychowicz, DNP, ANP, ONP, FAAN, FAANP
Professor and Director, MSN Program
Duke University School of Nursing
Durham, North Carolina

HOW TO USE THIS BOOK

Physiology and pathophysiology are subjects that are loved by some students even as they scare others! These disciplines cover challenging topics that, while necessary for success in future clinical courses, can be seen as a painful rite of passage or as an enlightening journey to clinical competence. The features of the book were developed by master pathophysiology teachers and clinician faculty members with the goal of helping students to synthesize complex content and extend that synthesis to clinical application. The following features, recognizable by their easy-to-find design elements, appear consistently in the chapters to help reinforce the physiologic and pathophysiologic concepts discussed in this book.

THE CLINICAL CONTEXT

Each chapter begins with a short introduction that sets the stage for the content's relevance to clinical practice. This section introduces the common disease states of that organ system, briefly highlighting their incidence and prevalence.

THOUGHT QUESTIONS

In each chapter, major subtopics conclude with questions to improve student mastery of information. These open-ended questions require students to pause and reflect on the section they have just read, to recall important facts, and often to use higher-level thinking to synthesize and apply what they have learned. Answers are provided in the online student supplement on Springer Publishing Company Connect™ to encourage self-instruction, immediate feedback, and remediation.

Thought Question

2. What are some ways in which chemical bonding contributes to essential body functions?

PEDIATRIC CONSIDERATIONS

These sections briefly review prenatal and postnatal development as it relates to physiology and pathophysiology. Congenital malformations and genetic conditions generally present at birth or in the pediatric population. Additionally, children metabolize therapeutic agents differently than adults—critical information to understand when treating children. All the system chapters as well

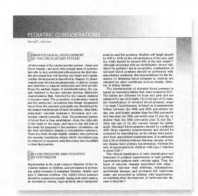

as Chapter 3, Molecular Biology, Genetics, and Genetic Diseases, provide an in-depth look at the most common conditions, genetic disorders, and important treatment considerations related to this patient population.

GERONTOLOGICAL CONSIDERATIONS

Understanding how aging affects organ systems is imperative in providing competent patient care. Healthy aging is inevitably associated with certain trends in organ function, for example, reduced liver biotransformation of drugs, decreased renal glomerular filtration, and other alterations that must be considered when assessing disease and planning management in older adults. Additionally, certain diseases are more prevalent in older adults, and phenomena such as frailty and complex comorbidities become more common with aging. All of these considerations factor into the special care that must be taken when providing clinical care to older adults. This section appears in all system chapters as well as in Chapter 4, Cell Physiology and Pathophysiology.

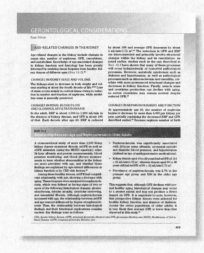

CASE STUDY 9.1: A Patient With Hypertension

Patient Complaint: *"I was here a couple of weeks ago for a checkup. The nurse said my blood pressure was high. She gave me a machine, and I have been taking my pressures at home since then. I was told to come back today. I feel fine."*

History of Present Illness/Review of Systems: A 43-year-old African American man presents to the office for a blood pressure recheck. On his two previous visits to the office, his blood pressure was 142/88 mm Hg and 154/92 mm Hg, respectively. After the most recent visit, he was sent home with a blood pressure cuff to perform at-home blood pressure monitoring. The results of his home blood pressure readings reveal a mean systolic blood pressure that is 130 mm Hg or higher, and a diastolic pressure that is 80 mm Hg or higher. From the home readings, white coat hypertension is ruled out and he is diagnosed with essential hypertension. The review of systems finds no chest pain or shortness of breath. Right knee pain and stiffness are noted, but all other findings are negative.

Past Medical/Family History: The patient's past medical history is significant for obesity and osteoarthritis of his knees. He works a desk job and is sedentary most days. He frequently consumes fast food for convenience. His family history is significant for prostate cancer, hypertension, and hyperlipidemia on his father's side, and hypertension, hyperlipidemia, and type 2 diabetes mellitus on his mother's side. He currently takes naproxen, 500 mg twice a day as needed, for knee pain.

Physical Examination: You observe a well-appearing obese man in no acute distress. His body mass index

CBC, complete blood count; TSH, thyroid-stimulating hormone.

(BMI) is 31 kg/m². *General appearance:* The patient is alert and oriented. Funduscopic examination is negative for hemorrhage, papilledema, cotton wool spots, arteriolar narrowing, and arteriovenous nicking. Neck is supple, with no carotid bruits, thyromegaly, or nodules. Cardiovascular examination reveals regular rate and rhythm, with no murmurs, thrills, or gallops. Lungs are clear to auscultation bilaterally. Abdomen is soft, nontender, and nondistended, with no renal masses or aortic or renal artery bruits. Extremities reveal no edema bilaterally, and peripheral pulses are normal. Neurological examination is grossly intact, with no focal weakness.

Laboratory and Diagnostic Findings: You perform baseline tests, including electrolytes and serum creatinine, fasting glucose, urinalysis, CBC, TSH, and lipids; obtain an ECG; and initiate amlodipine, 5 mg by mouth daily. You set a follow-up appointment in 2 weeks to check on this patient's blood pressure and review the laboratory results.

CASE STUDY 9.1 QUESTIONS
- *Amlodipine is a calcium channel blocker. What site of blood pressure regulation does this medication work on, and why does it help?*
- *What vasodilating mediator may be reduced in a patient taking naproxen, a nonsteroidal anti-inflammatory drug?*
- *Long-standing blood pressure control is mediated by endocrine and renal function. Describe the hormones involved and how they contribute to blood pressure control.*

CASE STUDIES

In each system chapter, one to three case studies help students apply concepts learned from the chapter to a patient scenario, setting the stage for the Bridge to Clinical Practice. Focusing primarily on common disorders managed in a primary care setting, the case studies detail a patient complaint, history and system review, physical examination, and laboratory/diagnostic findings. Application-based open-ended questions guide students through the underlying pathophysiology of the patient's condition. Answers to the case study questions are found in the online student supplement on Springer Publishing Company Connect™.

BRIDGE TO CLINICAL PRACTICE

This unique feature is designed to help students transition from the basic pathophysiology covered in the chapter to the implications for the clinical role. For each system this section provides a succinct summary of system-specific aspects of the history and physical examination, the most common laboratory tests and diagnostic tools, major drug classes used for disorders of that system, and other commonly used non-pharmacologic modalities that students will encounter as they transition into clinical settings.

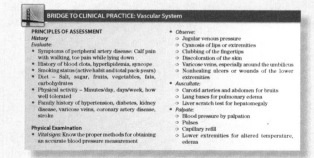

BRIDGE TO CLINICAL PRACTICE: Vascular System

PRINCIPLES OF ASSESSMENT
History
Evaluate:
- Symptoms of peripheral artery disease: Calf pain with walking, toe pain while lying down
- History of blood clots, hyperlipidemia, syncope
- Smoking status (active habit and total pack-years)
- Diet – Salt, sugar, fruits, vegetables, fats, carbohydrates
- Physical activity – Minutes/day, days/week, how well tolerated
- Family history of hypertension, diabetes, kidney disease, varicose veins, coronary artery disease, stroke

Physical Examination
- *Vital signs:* Know the proper methods for obtaining an accurate blood pressure measurement

- *Observe:*
  - Jugular venous pressure
  - Cyanosis of lips or extremities
  - Clubbing of the fingertips
  - Discoloration of the skin
  - Varicose veins, especially around the umbilicus
  - Nonhealing ulcers or wounds of the lower extremities
- *Auscultate:*
  - Carotid arteries and abdomen for bruits
  - Lung bases for pulmonary edema
  - Liver scratch test for hepatomegaly
- *Palpate:*
  - Blood pressure by palpation
  - Pulses
  - Capillary refill
  - Lower extremities for altered temperature, edema

KEY POINTS

This feature highlights the important takeaways for which students should be able to demonstrate an understanding at the conclusion of each chapter. These points are not intended as a comprehensive summary of the chapter; instead, they capture the main ideas conveyed throughout the chapter in short bullet points that students can reflect upon as they assess their mastery of the content.

KEY POINTS

- The kidney has several functions that contribute to homeostasis, but the primary role of the kidney is to maintain fluid and electrolyte balance over a wide range of body states and varying intake of water, electrolytes, and nutrients.
- The kidney has several endocrine roles, including production of erythropoietin, which stimulates red blood cell production, activation of vitamin D, and production of renin.
- The body is 50% to 60% water, depending on sex, age, and body composition, and the kidneys regulate the amount of body water as well as its composition.
- The functional unit of the kidney is the nephron, and each kidney contains about 1 million nephrons. There is considerable functional

reserve; therefore, someone with healthy kidney function can donate a kidney and still maintain normal kidney function.
- The kidney receives a far greater blood flow (20% of cardiac output) than its size and weight (~0.5% of body weight) would dictate. High RBF enables a high rate of glomerular filtration (referred to as the GFR).
- The high rate of glomerular filtration is enabled by two principal factors:
  o Net filtration pressure in glomerular capillaries is much higher than in other capillary beds, primarily because of a high glomerular capillary hydrostatic pressure.
  o Glomerular capillary permeability is much higher than in other capillary beds, with a three-layer structure that promotes a high rate of fluid movement while restricting filtration of proteins.

KEY DISORDERS

All disorders reviewed in this book are highlighted within the text to facilitate quick identification and discovery. These disorders are also listed in the List of Disorders to help students locate content rapidly. Highlighted disorders appear throughout each chapter, in the main discussion as well as in the pediatric and geriatric consideration sections.

As noted in the chapter introduction, kidney disease encompasses several entities, including acute kidney injury (AKI), which is often, but not always, reversible, and chronic kidney disease (CKD), which tends to progress through several stages until ending at stage 5 (also known as end-stage renal disease [ESRD]). The definitions of these terms and stages usually depend on laboratory assessments of kidney function, evaluation of the history and physical findings, and presence of comorbidities. For the CKD-ESRD continuum, global prevalence is estimated at 13.4%. Prevalence by stage was determined based on the eGFR and ACR (Table 12.3). CKD staging has evolved to include consideration of both eGFR and ACR, as some individuals have eGFR within the normal range but demonstrate renal impairment in the form of excessive urinary albumin excretion.[13]

the airway; second, bronchial smooth muscle contraction is able to narrow the collapsible airway.

MECHANISMS OF LUNG PROTECTION

Inspiration of 5 to 8 L of air each minute of the day represents a large risk of exposure of the delicate airways to environmental toxins, particulate matter, and pathogens such as bacteria and viruses. The lungs are well protected from larger particles by the mucociliary escalator mechanism described earlier. Epithelial cells of the mucosa are tightly joined and prevent movement of pathogens across that surface lining. Nonspecific defenses such as lysozyme, defensins, and antimicrobial peptides attack many pathogens. Mucosal dendritic cells phagocytose and present antigen to T lymphocytes, activating the adaptive immune system to produce secretory immunoglobulin isotype A (IgA). IgA provides protection against specific invaders by intercepting incoming pathogens and marking them for phagocytosis and destruction. At the level of

alveoli, the final small particles that arrive are phagocytosed by resident alveolar macrophages, in addition to being neutralized by IgG. Once activated, alveolar macrophages secrete cytokines that recruit additional monocytes, neutrophils, and lymphocytes to assist in host defense. Natural killer cells are present in the alveoli and can contribute to a rapid response to invading pathogens. Finally, protective antimicrobial proteins are also components of the surfactant that lines the alveoli.

Cystic Fibrosis: A Genetic Disorder That Compromises Lung Protection

Cystic fibrosis (CF) is a common autosomal recessive genetic disorder among certain populations. The prevalence of CF is highest in people of northern European ancestral descent. CF is screened for at birth in the United States, and neonatal screening results indicate a prevalence of 1:3,500 infants who are Caucasian, 1:7,000 infants who are Latinx, and 1:17,000 in those of African

GENETIC CONDITIONS

As the fields of molecular biology and genetics provide ever more understanding of the genetic basis of disease and disease risk factors, the book uses an easily identifiable icon next to all genetic conditions described throughout the text for quick reference and discovery. These disorders are also included among the key disorders found in the List of Disorders.

SHARE YOUR FEEDBACK AND FOLLOW DR. TKACS ON TWITTER

The editors would like to hear your feedback on this first edition. If you would like to share your thoughts on potential additions, corrections, or updates that you believe should be incorporated into this book, please contact Nancy Tkacs at tkacs@nursing.upenn.edu.

You can also follow Dr. Tkacs on Twitter: @DrTkacsPatho.

INSTRUCTOR RESOURCES

Advanced Physiology and Pathophysiology: Essentials for Clinical Practice includes a robust ancillary package that qualified instructors may obtain by emailing textbook@springerpub.com

Instructor's Manual
- Chapter Outline
- Chapter Summary
- Objectives
- Connecting the Dots (Tips and Pointers for Faculty on How to Approach the Content of the Chapter With Their Students)
- Key Points
- Thought Questions and Suggested Answers
- Case Studies Suggested Answers
- Discussion Questions
- Assignment Suggestions (Individual and Group) and Suggested Answers
- Additional Resources

Chapter-Based PowerPoint Presentations

Test Bank
- Multiple Choice Questions With Rationales
- Essay Questions and Suggested Answers

Image Bank

THE FOUNDATIONAL CONCEPTS OF CLINICAL PRACTICE

Nancy C. Tkacs, Linda L. Herrmann, Randall L. Johnson, and Loretta A. Sernekos

PATHOPHYSIOLOGY AND THE PROCESS OF CLINICAL DECISION-MAKING

Clinicians' ability to correctly identify disease processes and develop management plans with their patients relies on a deep knowledge of the pathophysiology of disease. This book was developed to meet that clinical need. Physiology seeks to understand the mechanisms of body function, and pathophysiology seeks to understand the mechanisms of altered body function due to pathological states. People, whether patients or clinicians, often fail to appreciate the fine-tuned machine that is the human body until they experience alterations in function that lead to signs and symptoms of disease. Pathophysiology can be viewed with the same lens: Studying the manifestations of body function *loss* can illuminate the exquisite and intricate functions of our organs that we do not even think about when we are healthy. For every physiological function, there is a pathophysiological consequence when that normal function goes awry. Clinicians-in-training are well positioned to reinforce their knowledge of normal physiological principles when they are presented as the context for disease development, as we have in this book.

In disease states, one or more normal homeostatic mechanisms malfunction, and the organism increasingly relies on compensatory mechanisms to maintain homeostasis. The clinician must know the principles of normal function, the alteration of these functions during disease states, and the benefits and risks of compensatory mechanisms. In addition, one cannot study physiology and pathophysiology in isolation: To understand the complex mechanisms of body function requires application of fundamental principles from chemistry, genetics, cell biology, and other basic sciences.

The data gathered during the clinical encounter include details from the history and physical examination, comprising both subjective and objective findings; results of laboratory studies; results of imaging studies; and other measurements. The clinician must then evaluate these data, consider the differential diagnosis, and formulate a plan. At each step, knowledge of pathophysiology is integral to the process. The aims of this book are to:

- Provide a foundation of core *principles* of physiology for each system and organ discussed
- Link the pathophysiology of common and selected less common disorders to those core principles
- Alternate discussion of each core principle with the clinical applications, sequencing the content to emphasize the application of those core principles and mechanisms
- Present in-depth life span considerations for each organ and system as developed by geriatric and pediatric content experts who
  - Emphasize developmental aspects of organ functions and their relationships to disorders commonly encountered in infants and children
  - Describe organ and system alterations of normal healthy aging and their relationships to disorders commonly encountered in older adults
- Provide a bridge between pathophysiology and concurrent or later coursework on health history and physical assessment, diagnostic tools and laboratory testing, pharmacology, and nonpharmacologic management strategies

- Offer an interdisciplinary perspective on the intricacies of the body's systems in both a normal and a diseased state, with an author team comprising experienced clinicians and educators: nurses and nurse practitioners, physician assistants, dietitians, doctors of pharmacy, physicians, and basic scientists

At the same time, we endeavored to avoid redundancy with topics covered more extensively in other courses in the graduate curriculum of advanced practitioners. The book does not have a freestanding chapter on the skin, for example. The most common skin disorders have unique presentations that are well described in physical assessment books and clinical lectures on dermatology. We feel that these disorders are best covered in textbooks associated with those topics. Rather than devoting a lengthy chapter to this topic, the mechanisms of selected skin disorders are covered within the context of infectious disease (Chapter 5, Infectious Disease) and immune and leukocyte function (Chapter 6, The Immune System and Leukocyte Function), which are the primary origins of many skin disorders and consistent with our approach of discussing disease in the context of alterations of existing physiological principles and mechanisms.

Similarly, we have selected certain common and uncommon disorders for discussion in the book because of their educational value and the way they illustrate an underlying principle of function. In many curricula, the pathophysiology course spans only one semester, making it impossible to describe an exhaustive list of diseases in detail. While this book explores a wide range of disorders, our approach aims to provide mastery of concepts, vocabulary, and diagnostic evaluation strategies that students can use throughout their remaining clinical semesters to broaden their knowledge of diseases they encounter. Each principle-focused segment ends with *Thought Questions* to immediately engage the students in reflection and analysis of their level of mastery of that chunk of content. Chapters conclude with *Key Points* to return students to the *big picture* of function and dysfunction for the chapter's main topics. We sincerely hope that this approach produces a resource that students will actually read and keep reading as a companion to their subsequent coursework.

BUILDING FROM A BASIC SCIENCE FOUNDATION: CHAPTERS 2 TO 4

Physiological and pathophysiological processes are carried out at the level of chemistry, biochemistry and biophysics, and molecular and cellular biology. Owing to the rapid pace of scientific discovery in these fields, our knowledge can never be complete, and independent practitioners must make a commitment to lifelong learning. A clear understanding of important concepts and terminology from these disciplines contributes to the ability of clinicians to continually update their knowledge as science advances.

Examples of clinical applications of these disciplines are highlighted here. They underscore the importance of the basic sciences for clinical decision-making, diagnosis, and management, as well as for understanding new research and clinical innovations. Chapters 2 to 4 provide brief reviews of chemistry, biochemistry, molecular biology and genetics, and cell biology that cover principles and terminology of these disciplines that are used in all subsequent chapters. These chapters could be the basis for a short online review course or for self-study to increase students' success and satisfaction in their graduate pathophysiology coursework.

CHEMISTRY (CHAPTER 2)

All body functions can ultimately be described in terms of chemical interactions. The body's chemistry begins at the level of single atoms, including many of the electrolytes. Sodium, chloride, potassium, calcium, and hydrogen ions must be kept within a normal range of concentration in both the intracellular and extracellular fluid. Ion imbalance can lead to cardiac arrhythmias, paresthesias, and acidosis. Minerals, including those present in small amounts (trace minerals), are required for proper function of many enzymes. Iron is the site of oxygen binding within hemoglobin and myoglobin molecules, and iodine is required for thyroid hormone synthesis. The chemistry of the body has an undisputed role in health and disease.

Atoms combine through ionic and covalent bonds to form molecules. In addition to the previously listed elements, key atoms that make up the molecules of the body are carbon, hydrogen, oxygen, nitrogen, phosphorus, and sulfur. Molecular oxygen (O_2) is needed by all cells for synthesis of adenosine triphosphate (ATP) and other energy sources. This role of oxygen comes with a cost, in that oxidative metabolism generates oxygen-derived free radicals that can damage cell components.

The most abundant molecule in the body is water, and the polar nature of water's molecular structure is a major determinant of physiological function. The aqueous environment of the body's extracellular and intracellular fluids creates the shape and interactions of proteins, lipids, and carbohydrates to sustain life. The nonpolar, hydrophobic molecular nature of fatty acids underlies the function of the plasma membrane as a barrier between intracellular and extracellular fluids. With a hydrophobic fatty acid core, the plasma membrane defines the cell, the smallest unit of biological function.

Solubility, diffusion, equilibrium reactions, and many other core concepts of atomic and molecular function will appear throughout this book.

BIOCHEMISTRY (CHAPTER 2)

The biomolecules—carbohydrates, lipids, proteins, and nucleic acids—are the workhorses of cell and organ function. Abnormalities in metabolism, such as phenylketonuria, result in abnormally high levels of certain biomolecules and abnormally low levels of others, transforming function in devastating ways. Nutritional deficiencies (iron-deficiency anemia) and excesses (obesity) underlie many disease processes and may be preventable or readily treatable, once recognized.

MOLECULAR BIOLOGY AND GENETICS (CHAPTER 3)

The human genome project was completed in 2003, and was followed by additional haplotype mapping studies to identify common variant alleles and single-nucleotide polymorphisms (SNPs). The impact of these developments on clinical practice is profound and far reaching. Understanding heredity, single gene disorders, penetrance, expressivity, and the impact of human gene variants on disease risk is integral to clinicians entering independent practice. Common genetic disorders and variants are discussed in this book, and each chapter features one or more highlighted genetic disorders. Some less common genetic disorders are included because they illustrate important concepts in genetic disease.

The consequences of many genetic disorders are detectable in the perinatal period, as described in the *Pediatric Considerations* section of this chapter. Prenatal genetic screening and diagnosis are discussed here, along with genetic disorders identified after birth. Newborn screening programs continually expand their targets—identifying genetic and biochemical abnormalities in enzymes and other biomolecules within a few days after birth, allowing early intervention and management that prevents or lessens long-term disability.

CELL BIOLOGY (CHAPTER 4)

As molecular biology knowledge has expanded, so too has knowledge of cell biology. Membrane transport proteins and membrane-bound receptors are the targets of many drug classes in common use, and new subtypes of these membrane proteins continue to be discovered. Knowledge of intracellular signaling cascades involved in immune function and neoplastic transformation is growing rapidly, leading to better tools for management of autoimmunity, hypersensitivity, and cancer.

A fundamental understanding of the impact of aging at cellular, tissue, organ, and systemic levels is crucial in order for clinicians to tailor individualized age-appropriate interventions, given the demographics on aging domestically and abroad. By 2060, 23% of U.S. residents will be aged 65 and older, an increase from 16% in 2018.[1] In 2015, the number of persons aged 60 and older worldwide was 900 million; this is expected to increase to 2 billion people by 2050.[2] Knowledge of the pathophysiological underpinnings of age-related changes, both normal and abnormal, is paramount when considering changes in implicit body regulatory mechanisms, metabolism, and nutrition; selecting pharmacotherapy; and critically analyzing the interplay of systemic manifestations of disease, clinical data, and patient presentation. Hypotheses of aging at the cellular level are described in the *Gerontological Considerations* section of Chapter 4.

ADVANCED PHYSIOLOGY AND PATHOPHYSIOLOGY: CHAPTERS 5 TO 17

After introducing the building blocks of physiological and pathophysiological function, the book transitions, first to an overview of infectious disease mechanisms with exemplar organisms, then to a system-by-system walkthrough of the body, reviewing principles of function and their clinical applications. An example of the book's sequencing approach is shown in **Figure 1.1**, which visually maps how foundational principles and concepts relating to the lung are linked with specific pulmonary disorders. Selected disorders receive an in-depth discussion, and learners are introduced to principles of dysfunction related to each mechanism that can be generalized to many other disorders. We believe that this approach best serves the short-term goal of providing knowledge of pathophysiology of specific diseases, and the long-term goal of mastering pharmacological and clinical applications. These clinically related chapters also feature specific sections on *Pediatric* and *Gerontological Considerations, Case Studies*, and a unique *Bridge to Clinical Practice* segment that briefly summarizes principles of assessment, diagnostic tools and laboratory evaluation, and major drug classes pertinent to the chapter's main topic.

INFECTIOUS DISEASE (CHAPTER 5)

In keeping with our emphasis on principles and concepts, this chapter begins with an overview of the interactions between humans and microbes, and concepts such as infection versus colonization, pathogen virulence, and host characteristics that determine infection severity. A brief review of characteristics of bacteria, viruses, protozoa, fungi, and yeasts is provided, followed by clinical concepts of pathogen identification strategies, drug resistance, and antimicrobial stewardship. This chapter concludes with snapshots of the structure and function of selected microbes commonly encountered in clinical settings in the United States or globally. Selected infectious diseases are further discussed in the relevant organ systems chapters; for example, pneumonia in Chapter 11, Lungs, and infectious diarrheas in Chapter 13, Gastrointestinal Tract.

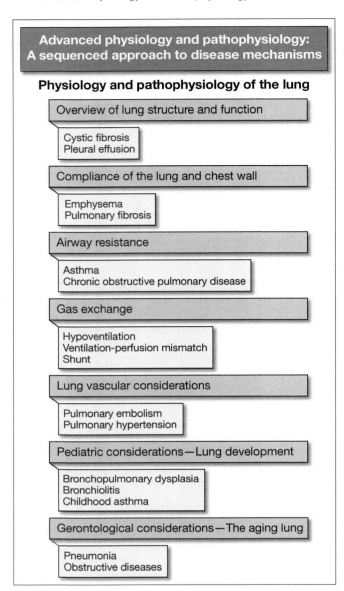

FIGURE 1.1 The organization and sequence of topics in Chapter 11, Lungs, focusing on the lungs, illustrate the overarching approach used throughout this book. Main principles and concepts in organ function (*shown in blue boxes*) are immediately followed by descriptions of disorders linked to pathophysiology of those principles and concepts (*shown in beige boxes*).

THE IMMUNE SYSTEM AND LEUKOCYTE FUNCTION (CHAPTER 6)

Knowledge of immunology continues to grow exponentially, and identification of lymphocyte subsets, cytokines, and other members of the immune system's "cast of characters" continues to provide new targets for biologic drugs. At the same time, innate immunity (inflammation) continues to cause a great deal of morbidity and mortality, wreaking havoc in the blood vessels

of patients with atherosclerosis, the adipose tissue of persons with obesity and metabolic syndrome, and the joints of patients with rheumatoid arthritis. This chapter explores the latest concepts of innate and adaptive immunity; details the pathophysiology of hypersensitivity, autoimmunity, and immunodeficiency; and builds the foundation for understanding the pharmacology of biological therapies for immune-related disorders. The waxing and waning of immune function across the life span, and implications for care of both children and older adults, are placed in that context.

NEOPLASIA (CHAPTER 7)

This chapter focuses on the principles underlying a cell's movement into the cell cycle and cell division— the critical event that is inappropriately activated in cells that have undergone neoplastic transformation. Characteristics of cancer cells are described, with emphasis on the implications for current and projected treatments of certain cancers. The discussion of genetic and viral causes of cancer highlights the critical role of genotyping in cancer care. The most common cancers of children are described, as well as specific aspects of cancer pathophysiology in older adults.

BLOOD AND CLOTTING (CHAPTER 8)

This chapter builds on the content of Chapter 6, The Immune System and Leukocyte Function, by focusing on red blood cells in health and disease and the processes of blood clotting. The concept of anemia and the principles underlying the different forms of anemia provide the foundation for developing differential diagnoses in patients with suspected anemia based on clinical manifestations and diagnostic findings. The process of hemostasis is described, focusing on the complementary roles of platelets and coagulation factors, as well as relevant laboratory assessments. This underpins the subsequent discussion of pathophysiological and genetic causes of states of excess clotting and excess bleeding. Life span considerations include the unique changes in red blood cell size and number in the perinatal period, and the bone marrow–related changes of older adults.

CIRCULATION (CHAPTER 9)

The circulatory system receives the output of the heart and channels the blood flow through a series of tubes that diverge and narrow as they proceed outward to the tissues, and then converge and enlarge as they return to the heart. Although some aspects of this flow are true for all segments of the circulation, structural and biophysical characteristics of each segment determine the pathophysiological vulnerabilities of each. The large muscular arteries move blood rapidly and efficiently to various body sites but are prone to atherosclerosis, as well as hypertrophy and aneurysm. The arterioles provide vascular resistance that helps to maintain organ perfusion pressures—they are the site of blood pressure control by neural and humoral mediators, and their dysfunction is associated with hypertension and shock. The capillaries exchange essential substances with the tissues, and are also the locus of physiological and pathophysiological edema formation. The veins are low-pressure storage vessels that are vulnerable to gravitational influences, varicosities, and coagulability. Hypertension can occur in children as well as adults, and recognizing this disorder depends on knowledge of age-related population norms. Older adults have additional clinical concerns related to vascular stiffness due to age-related collagen deposition in vessel walls.

HEART (CHAPTER 10)

The heart is an autonomously functioning pump, ejecting a volume of blood (stroke volume) with each beat into the circulation for delivery to the body. Heart function is critically dependent on electrical automaticity of pacemaker cells and rapid action potential propagation that produces coordinated chamber contractions. Cardiac cells have unique action potentials that can be vulnerable to abnormal cardiac beats and rhythms (arrhythmias). These electrical signals are linked to calcium entry that initiates the mechanical steps of contraction—the pumping action of the heart. The mechanical properties of the heart determine the stroke volume—the amount of blood pumped with each beat, at rest and during exercise, to meet the body's need for oxygen delivery and carbon dioxide removal. Ischemic heart disease results in both electrical and mechanical dysfunction. Recently, research has begun to illuminate how the pathophysiology and presentation of ischemic heart disease differ in men and women, and clinical practice is beginning to change accordingly.

Heart failure can result from ischemic heart disease, among other causes, and is a chronic, progressive loss of pumping capacity that ultimately limits physical activity and can result in death. Structural cardiac disorders range from valve diseases in children and adults to malformations arising during embryonic and fetal development. Many of these are managed surgically, albeit with varying degrees of success depending on severity. Cardiac changes during healthy aging generally do not result in activity limitations; however, many disorders, such as atrial fibrillation, show increased prevalence with aging.

LUNGS (CHAPTER 11)

The lungs interface with the environment, bringing in atmospheric air during inspiration, and expelling mixed airway and alveolar air during expiration. Thus, the airways—the diverging and narrowing tubes that lead to the alveoli—are exposed to pollutants, irritants, and pathogens. Several mechanisms, including antimicrobial and mucociliary responses, protect the airways from these damaging substances. The lungs' delicate structure is encased in a more rigid thoracic chamber, surrounded by the chest wall (ribs, sternum, associated muscles and lining), and bounded below by the diaphragm. The ability of inspiratory muscles (diaphragm and others) to inflate the lungs depends on compliance of the lungs and the chest wall, and pathophysiological changes in either component can alter the amount of effort required for inspiration. The airways are the site of airway resistance that must be overcome to generate inspiratory and expiratory airflow. Airway diameter can be pathologically altered in a variety of disease processes, leading to acute or chronic obstructive disease.

Gas exchange occurs in the alveoli and depends on lung mechanics (for ventilation) as well as blood flow (for perfusion) in taking up oxygen and releasing carbon dioxide. Diseases may alter blood oxygenation (and carbon dioxide removal) through their effects on ventilation, perfusion, or the diffusion barrier of the alveolar wall. The lungs receive all of the blood flow of the right heart, a low-pressure system that perfuses the millions of alveolar capillaries for gas exchange. Abnormalities of lung blood flow can lead to secondary heart disease, lung fluid accumulation, and acutely impaired oxygenation. Much of the alveolar development occurs postnatally, and preterm birth is associated with persistent lung pathology. In older adults, pneumonia is a common occurrence, related in part to decreased protective mechanisms.

KIDNEYS (CHAPTER 12)

The kidneys are highly vascular organs that filter the blood, removing wastes for excretion and returning the rest of the blood to the vascular system. The functional units of the kidneys are nephrons, each composed of a glomerulus and a tubule. In a two-step process, the glomeruli receive blood for filtration and release an ultrafiltrate of plasma into the tubules, which then process the filtrate and greatly reduce its volume, leading to the final step of urine production. The extremely high blood flow and capillary permeability of the glomeruli relative to other vascular beds make them vulnerable to damage by hypertension, diabetic hyperglycemia, antibodies, and complement components. The tubules are transport membranes that return most of the glomerular filtrate to the circulation, while secreting substances destined for clearance, including many drugs. Tubules can be damaged by many filtered and secreted substances, including proteins such as myoglobin and certain medications. Hypotension and hypovolemia can also lead to tubular necrosis in the renal medulla, which receives relatively low blood flow and is prone to hypoxia. Acute kidney injury may resolve, but compromised function may progress to chronic kidney injury and end-stage renal disease. At both ends of the life span, childhood and older age, the kidneys are more vulnerable to damage owing to decreased number or function of nephrons.

GASTROINTESTINAL TRACT (CHAPTER 13)

Similar to the circulatory system, the basic structure of the gastrointestinal tract is a generalized tube with a series of segments that are specialized in structure and function. Similar to the respiratory tract, the gut is exposed to environmental toxins—in this case, a wide variety of ingested foods and beverages, as well as pathogens. In addition to a sequential description of structure, function, and disorders of the esophagus, stomach, and small and large intestines, this chapter emphasizes general concepts of gut control by neurotransmitters and hormones that are the basis for many of the drugs used to manage gastrointestinal disorders. The abundant and intricate immune system of the gut plays a role in development of immune responses in early life and is protective against ingested pathogens, but also is implicated in inflammatory bowel disease. Life span considerations include structural disorders as well as common infectious diarrheas of children, and structural disorders of older adults, including greater occurrence of reflux and diverticular disease.

LIVER (CHAPTER 14)

This book places a substantial emphasis on the physiology and pathophysiology of the liver, providing a critical foundation for clinicians who will be responsible for prescribing medications. We have dedicated a chapter solely to this organ rather than including it in the gastrointestinal tract chapter because drug-induced liver injury is extremely common, and prescribers must appreciate the role of the liver in drug metabolism and excretion. Understanding the metabolic functions of the liver is also key to appreciating its significance in diabetes, the metabolic syndrome, and nonalcoholic fatty liver disease—a disorder with steadily increasing prevalence in the developed world. Infectious hepatitis is common in the United States and globally; an understanding of the patterns of dysfunction and laboratory assessment of different subtypes of hepatitis is critical for advanced practice. Individuals at both ends of the life span are more vulnerable to liver injury—children, because of the relative immaturity of many of the drug-metabolizing enzymes, and older adults, because of reduced liver mass and blood flow.

NERVOUS SYSTEM (CHAPTER 15)

The nervous system is arguably the most complex body system, with both physiological and behavioral components, all of which make up the *whole person* cared for by clinicians. To provide a strong foundation of knowledge for practitioners with prescriptive privileges, this chapter focuses in detail on concepts of neurotransmission and functions of major neurotransmitters. In primary care, a clinician can expect to spend a significant portion of each day interacting with patients who are trying to manage anxiety, depression, pain, or substance use disorders. Antidepressants, anxiolytics, analgesics, and nonpharmacologic modalities are widely prescribed. Although our knowledge of exact mechanisms of many neurological and affective disorders is incomplete, this chapter presents current hypotheses, concepts, and vocabulary. Knowledge of the long-term effects of adverse childhood experiences and other contributing factors can help clinicians explain the biological basis of these disorders to patients experiencing mental health challenges. Having this understanding also helps the clinician to reduce stigma and promote adherence to management approaches.

The section on sensory function and dysfunction emphasizes pain, as this is a major patient complaint. Motor disorders are very common and must be carefully evaluated and described, so they are given expanded coverage in this chapter. The major disorders of brain function in children include epilepsy and developmental delay, as well as headache and concussion. Cerebrovascular structural changes in older adults increase risk of subdural hematomas, and functional losses can accompany cognitive dysfunction as well as neurodegenerative disorders. Neurovascular disorders are also emphasized in the *Gerontological Considerations* section of this chapter.

MUSCULOSKELETAL SYSTEM (CHAPTER 16)

The musculoskeletal system is responsible for the structure of the body and the ability to have purposeful movements. This chapter begins with a review of structure and function of bones, with an emphasis on the remodeling process of dynamic bone maintenance. A discussion of fractures and the fracture healing process follows. The structure and function of joints are described, emphasizing synovial joints and the manifestations of sprains and strains. Particular emphasis is placed on the knee, and the associated ligament and meniscal injuries. This chapter also discusses other common structural and functional disorders, such as herniated disc disease and cumulative trauma disorders. Developmental disorders and sports injuries in children, as well as genetic conditions of muscles and bones, are the focus of the *Pediatric Considerations* section. Disorders in older adults include general principles of sarcopenia and frailty, as well as osteoporosis, osteoarthritis, and Parkinson-associated Pisa syndrome.

ENDOCRINE SYSTEM (CHAPTER 17)

The book concludes with the longest chapter, focusing on the endocrine system. This is the third integrative system of the body, along with the nervous and immune systems. Found in many locations throughout the body, endocrine glands and cells secrete hormones that act locally and also travel through the circulation to alter the activities of target cells in other organs. General concepts of endocrine signaling are described first, focusing on cellular mechanisms of hormone action, hormone control axes, feedback mechanisms, and temporal regulation of hormone secretion. An important principle of endocrine pathophysiology is that the most common sources of dysfunction fall into three major categories: pathological increases of hormone levels (which are often produced by hormone-secreting tumor cells), pathological decreases of hormone levels (which can be caused by autoimmune destruction of hormone-secreting cells), and insensitivity of target tissues to hormone actions (some of which have genetic causes).

Following the introduction, this chapter content is divided into six major sections that group key content blocks. The initial section provides an overview of the endocrine system. Following this overview begins a more in-depth look at the various parts of the endocrine system. The section covering hypothalamus and pituitary glands provides an in-depth overview of these structures—as sources of direct-acting hormones (oxytocin, vasopressin, growth hormone, and prolactin) and master regulators of other endocrine glands and tissues. The focus then turns to those glands, with separate sections covering adrenals, thyroid, and female and male gonads. The final section of this chapter opens with a review of metabolic physiology that prepares students for detailed coverage of pancreatic hormones and diabetes mellitus. This section begins with an extensive discussion of the hormone insulin, including its mechanisms of signaling and cellular actions, followed by descriptions of the hormones that oppose the actions of insulin. Included are extensive discussions of type 1 and type 2 diabetes, as well as other types of diabetes and related conditions of dysregulated metabolism. Reflecting the unique organization of this chapter, *Pediatric and Gerontological Considerations* and *Key Points* appear at the end of each main section rather than at the end of this chapter. Bridge to Clinical practice segments appear in the sections on the thyroid gland and metabolism and diabetes, as management of these disorders is common in primary care settings.

CONNECTING THE DOTS

As this content overview has emphasized, the conceptually driven organization of this book, linking principles with their clinical applications, aims to reinforce the unique aspects of each organ or system's function and the ways in which alterations of these functions contribute to disease. The rationale for this approach was derived from clinical practice and refined through teaching pathophysiology courses at an advanced level for over 25 years. Having mastered the concepts and vocabulary of function for each system in this way, the reader will best be prepared for later or concurrent courses in pharmacology, clinical diagnosis, and management.

The ability to *connect the dots* between pathophysiological principles and clinical applications is a major emphasis in this book. This knowledge can provide a rational basis for clinical decision-making and can make it easier to generalize knowledge to new pathological conditions encountered in practice. Knowledge of these core principles assists in learning the strategies and medications used to manage disease states, ultimately facilitating safe and effective advanced patient care.

PATHOPHYSIOLOGY AND THE INDEPENDENT CLINICIAN

The ultimate goal of graduate education in healthcare practice is to prepare to deliver the highest and safest care possible. This entails knowing not only what signs and symptoms are associated with a certain disorder but *why* they are associated. Knowing about compensatory mechanisms for impaired oxygen delivery, for example, helps the clinician immediately recognize that a patient presenting with dyspnea and tachypnea is likely hypoxemic, even before applying a pulse oximeter or listening to the lungs. Knowing about the oxygen-carrying capacity of hemoglobin helps the clinician put iron-deficiency anemia at the top of the differential diagnosis list when a patient presents with fatigue, dyspnea on exertion, and pallor.

Knowledge of pathophysiology also directs the logical choice of diagnostic tests. This is something that all novice clinicians struggle with. Which blood test(s) should be ordered? Does this patient need imaging and, if so, which type of imaging will yield the most diagnostically relevant information? One may know to order a complete blood count for suspected anemia, but what other tests will be informative and narrow the differential diagnosis? When the results are obtained, how should they be interpreted? The answers to many of these questions are clearer when there is a strong grounding in pathophysiology. Likewise, the knowledge of normal and abnormal physiology is essential for understanding which medications are the logical choices and *why*—and equally if not more importantly, why certain medications should *not* be used in people with certain disease states.

Knowledge of core principles emphasized in this book will make it easier to generalize knowledge to new pathological conditions encountered in practice. Novice clinicians should anticipate that they cannot possibly graduate with knowledge of every disease and disorder. There will be times when their patients are diagnosed—usually by a specialist—with a disease they have never heard of or one that was only briefly touched on in their training. A strong foundation in pathophysiology makes it possible to read an online update or journal article about a disease, to understand what normal function is altered, and by extension, how the abnormal state is treated.

Finally, patients and their families expect clinicians to be able to explain and interpret for them what is going on in their particular disease state. Understanding the pathophysiology of a disease is essential to being able to explain the disease in ways your patients will understand. It also helps patients *own* their disease. With knowledge of what is going on and why certain tests are ordered or why certain medications are prescribed, patients are more likely to take responsibility for those aspects of their illness that they can influence. A clinician can order many tests and prescribe many medications, but ultimately the patient must go get the tests and take the medications. The more successful the clinician is in patient teaching, the greater the likelihood that the patient will feel a partnership with the clinician in the journey to wellness. A deep understanding of pathophysiology facilitates clear explanations tailored to the patient's level of understanding.

REFERENCES

1. Population Reference Bureau. Fact sheet, aging in the United States. https://www.prb.org/aging-unitedstates-fact-sheet. Published July 15, 2019. Accessed August 26, 2019.
2. World Health Organization. Fact sheet: Ageing and health. https://www.who.int/news-room/fact-sheets/detail/ageing-and-health. Published February 5, 2018. Accessed August 26, 2019.

CHEMICAL AND BIOCHEMICAL FOUNDATIONS

Gioia Petrighi Polidori

THE CLINICAL CONTEXT

Physiological and pathophysiological processes are carried out at the molecular level of chemistry and biochemistry; thus, it is of paramount importance that healthcare providers have a clear understanding of key concepts from general, organic, and biological chemistry. A simple clinical example illustrates the chemical underpinnings of pathological conditions.

A child born in an uncomplicated home birth in March is brought to the family physician in December of that year because of stunted growth and delayed behavioral development. During a physical examination, the child is noted to have pale skin and light blue eyes, inability to sit up unassisted, decreased muscle tone, and microcephaly. A urine sample has a mousy odor, and biochemical tests confirm a diagnosis of phenylketonuria (PKU).

- What is PKU?
- What is hyperphenylalaninemia?
- How does this condition lead to these signs?

This chapter builds the chemical and biochemical foundations necessary to understand pathophysiological processes, such as PKU, by explaining basic concepts about atoms, molecules, and the structure and interactions of the biomolecules that make up the body. The pathophysiological basis of many conditions often comes down to the shapes and interactions of these atoms and molecules. The complex structure and processes of the body begin at the level of atoms: Atoms bond together to form small molecules, and small molecules such as sugars, fatty acids, amino acids, and nucleotides bond to form complex macromolecules. These large molecules—carbohydrates, lipids, proteins, and nucleic acids—form the structures and do the work of cells, the next unit of body organization.

CHEMICAL FOUNDATIONS OF LIFE

ATOMIC STRUCTURE

Matter is anything that has mass and occupies space. Liquids, solids, and gases are all examples of matter, and atoms are their building blocks. A substance that consists of only one type of atom is called an element. Although 118 elements are recognized, our bodies are made up almost entirely of just four: carbon, oxygen, hydrogen, and nitrogen. Twenty other elements are found in lesser or trace amounts in the body, including calcium, phosphorus, sulfur, sodium, potassium, chlorine, magnesium, iron, copper, and zinc. Each element is characterized by unique physical, chemical, and biological properties that depend on the structure of its atoms.

The atom can be structurally divided into two regions: a nucleus made of protons (p^+) and neutrons (n^0), and a cloud of electrons (e^-) that orbit around the nucleus. As the names imply, protons have a positive charge, whereas neutrons do not have a charge. Taken together these particles give the nucleus a net positive charge. Because electrons have a negative charge, they are attracted to the nucleus and orbit around it. Overall,

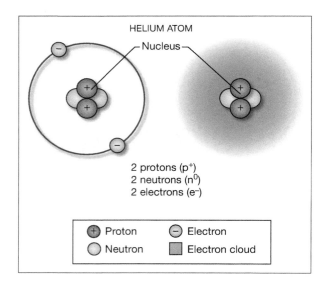

FIGURE 2.1 Two models of the structure of a helium atom: planetary model (left) and orbital model (right).

atoms are electrically neutral because the number of protons equals the number of electrons.

Atoms are usually represented in one of two ways: the planetary model or the orbital model (**Figure 2.1**). Although the former representation is useful for illustration purposes, it incorrectly depicts electrons orbiting around the nucleus in fairly fixed and predictable trajectories, much like planets in the solar system (see **Figure 2.1a**). This representation oversimplifies the complex and unpredictable behavior of electrons. A more plausible model depicts electrons in orbitals, which are areas where electrons are more likely to be found. As electrons are more likely to be found within a space near the nucleus, they create a negatively charged cloud, as represented in **Figure 2.1b**.

THE PERIODIC TABLE AND FAMILIES OF ELEMENTS

Elements are classified according to their atomic structure in the periodic table (**Figure 2.2**). In this table, each element has a specific symbol, which is a one- or two-letter abbreviation. For instance, the symbol for carbon is C, and the symbol for sodium is Na. The atomic number is the number of protons in a nucleus, and it is used to arrange elements in the periodic table.

The list of elements begins at the top left corner of the table and continues in a series of horizontal rows. Hydrogen, which only contains one proton, is followed by helium, which contains two protons, and then lithium, with three protons, and so on. In the table, the atomic number of the element is indicated above its symbol, and the average mass of the atoms is indicated below. A *period* is the name given

to a horizontal row of elements in the periodic table. This arrangement also places elements in 18 vertical groups. For instance, hydrogen, lithium, sodium, potassium, rubidium, and cesium all belong to the first group. Likewise, helium, neon, and argon are the first three elements of group 18.

As **Figure 2.2** illustrates, there is yet another method of organizing groups of elements in the periodic table. Elements that follow a predictable behavior when making bonds are found in groups 1 and 2, and 13 to 18. These main-group elements are thus further labeled as groups 1A through 8A. The remaining groups, which do not follow the same rules, are the transition metals, lanthanides, and actinides, which are labeled as groups 1B through 8B.

ELECTRON SHELLS AND CHEMICAL REACTIVITY

In an atom, electrons are arranged on different energy levels, called shells. Lower energy levels are closer to the nucleus and are occupied by electrons first; higher energy levels are farther from the nucleus and are only occupied with electrons if the inner shells are already full. In the periodic table, elements are assigned to a specific row, or period, according to the number of shells present in the atoms. For instance, hydrogen has one shell and can be found in the first period of the periodic table. Sodium, with three shells, is found in the third period of the table.

Because electrons have a negative charge, they have a tendency to repel each other. This repulsion, together with the attraction of the protons in the nucleus, determines the number of electrons that can occupy each orbital. The first electron shell is the smallest and only allows up to two electrons, but higher shells found in elements with higher atomic numbers allow up to eight electrons. Returning to the earlier example, we know that hydrogen has one electron and one shell; therefore, the electron occupies the only shell. However, potassium has an atomic number of 19, which means that it has 19 protons in the nucleus and an equal number of electrons. These electrons are distributed as follows: The first two electrons occupy the first shell, the second shell contains eight electrons, the third shell contains eight more electrons, and the fourth and last shell hosts the remaining electron ($2 + 8 + 8 + 1 = 19$ electrons). Potassium has four electron shells and thus belongs to the fourth period of the periodic table.

The electrons found in the outermost shell (valence electrons) determine the reactivity of an atom as they can interact with other atoms and form chemical bonds. The number of valence electrons in main-group elements is equal to the group number. For instance, both hydrogen and potassium, which belong to the first group, have one electron in the valence shell and use it to interact with other atoms. Carbon belongs to

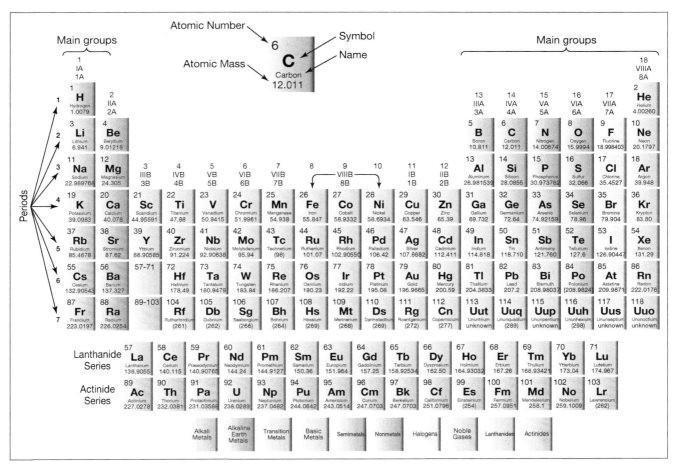

FIGURE 2.2 The periodic table of the elements.

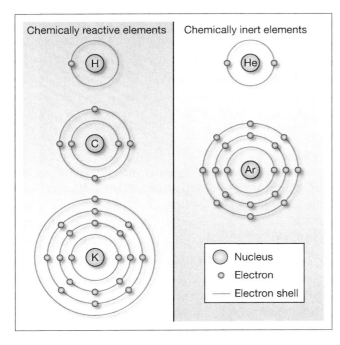

FIGURE 2.3 Electron shells in chemically reactive and inert elements. Hydrogen and helium have one and two electrons, respectively, and follow the duet rule. Carbon, potassium, and argon are examples of elements that follow the octet rule.

the fourth group and has four valence electrons. This means that a carbon atom uses these four electrons to interact with other atoms (**Figure 2.3**).

The octet rule has long been regarded as a simple rule to determine the reactivity of a given element. This rule states that atoms strive to occupy their valence shell by collecting eight electrons in this energy level. In fact, elements with eight valence electrons, such as argon, are very stable and tend not to interact with other atoms as they already fulfill the octet rule. These elements, found in group 8A, are known as noble or inert gases. Small atoms are an exception to the octet rule. Those with atomic numbers of 5 or lower do not have enough protons to hold eight electrons and instead follow the duet rule, which states that hydrogen, helium, and lithium need only two electrons to be stable—this is the number of electrons that the innermost shell can hold (see **Figure 2.3**). Atoms that do not have a full valence shell strive to fulfill the octet rule and thus are more reactive. Two examples are potassium and carbon. Based on their atomic structures, these atoms may form different types of chemical bonds by releasing, acquiring, or sharing electrons.

Thought Questions

1. What are the major and minor elements that make up the body?

2. How many electrons are in the outer (valence) shell of the major elements?

3. How many members of group 4A are in the group of elements that make up the body?

ION FORMATION AND ROLES IN THE BODY

Sodium is assigned atomic number 11 as it has 11 protons and 11 electrons. The electrons in an atom of sodium are organized into three shells: two in the lowest energy level, eight in the middle level, and the remaining electron in the valence shell. In order for a sodium atom to fulfill the octet rule, it is easier for it to lose one electron than to gain seven. In this case, when sodium releases one electron, the completely filled middle shell becomes its valence shell and the atom achieves stability but loses its neutrality. It is now positively charged.

On the other hand, elements that belong to the seventh group of the periodic table have a strong tendency to acquire an extra electron and fulfill the octet rule. For instance, chlorine has atomic number 17, with 17 protons and 17 electrons distributed among three shells: two in the first shell, eight in the middle shell, and seven in the valence shell. Because chlorine needs only one electron to fulfill the octet rule, it is a good electron acceptor, becoming negatively charged. Therefore, if an atom of sodium donates an electron to an atom of chlorine, both atoms fulfill the octet rule with eight electrons in the outermost shell, and they are stable (**Figure 2.4**). After the electron transfer, sodium is left with 11 protons and 10 electrons, resulting in a net positive charge. Similarly, once chlorine acquires the extra electron, it has a complete outer shell, and it becomes negatively charged. Atoms that have an overall charge are called ions. Negatively charged atoms are called anions and positively charged atoms are called cations.

An ionic bond is a chemical bond that is formed when one atom donates one or two electrons to another atom. This electron transfer leads to the formation of a cation and an anion that remain in close contact due to the attraction between their opposite charges, and results in an ionic compound such as table salt, sodium chloride. Sodium and chloride, as well as several other ions, play critical roles in body functions.

Water constitutes 70% of body weight, and most ionic compounds in the body are found dissolved in water (**Figure 2.5**). The polarity of water molecules (see section Chemical Patterns in Physiology and Pathophysiology, later in this chapter) is responsible for forming a hydration shell around individual anions and cations, thus breaking the ionic bond and dissolving the newly released ions (see **Figure 2.5a** and **b**).

All ions are electrolytes because they can conduct an electric current in solution. Ions in the body are abundant in the aqueous solutions found inside and outside cells. These ions are differentially distributed between the intracellular compartment (cytosol) and the extracellular compartment, which is composed of interstitial fluid and plasma. Ions such as sodium, chloride, and bicarbonate have higher concentrations in the extracellular space whereas potassium, phosphate, and protein anions are highly concentrated intracellularly (**Figure 2.6**). This differential distribution of ions also contributes to the generation of a membrane potential: cells have an overall positive charge on the external side of cell membranes and a negative charge on the internal side. In excitable cells, such as cardiomyocytes and neurons, alterations of these charges may cause an action potential.

ACIDS AND BASES

Biological acids and bases can form ions in the aqueous solutions of the body. One definition of acids depicts them as molecules that release protons (hydrogen ions, H^+) when placed in an aqueous solution. The process of dissolving the acid involves water molecules binding the protons, forming hydronium ions (H_3O^+). **Figure 2.5c**

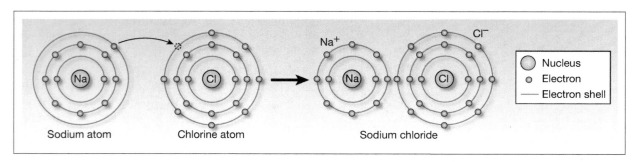

FIGURE 2.4 Formation of the ionic bond between sodium and chlorine, producing sodium chloride.

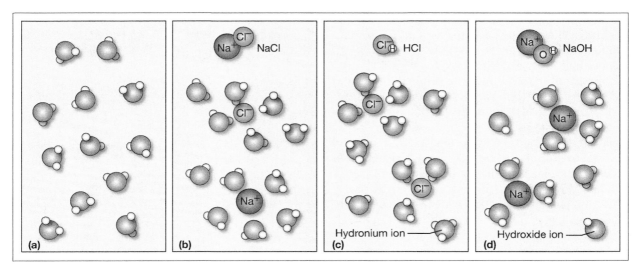

FIGURE 2.5 Ion formation of common body compounds. **(a)** Organization of water molecules; **(b)** ionization of sodium chloride (NaCl) in water; **(c)** ionization of hydrochloric acid (HCl) in water; and **(d)**, ionization of sodium hydroxide (NaOH) in water.

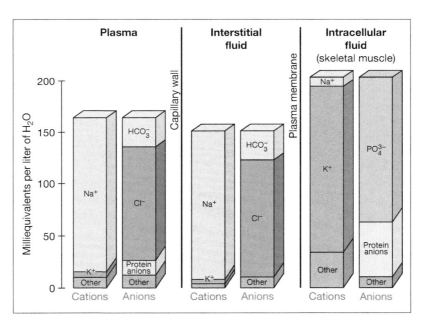

FIGURE 2.6 Differential distribution of ions in the intracellular and extracellular space.

illustrates the dissociation of hydrochloric acid (HCl) in an aqueous solution. Many other substances release protons when placed in water; for example, carbonic acid (H_2CO_3) and phosphoric acid (H_3PO_4). Although all these molecules are acids, they do not all behave in exactly the same way. Acids are classified based on their tendency to lose protons. Strong acids have a greater tendency to release protons than do weak acids. For instance, hydrochloric acid is considered a strong acid as its ionization in water is virtually complete, meaning that all molecules are separated into protons and anions. Conversely, carbonic acid and phosphoric acid are only partly ionized in aqueous solutions and

thus are considered weak acids. Once acids are dissolved in water, the ions formed can conduct electricity and therefore are electrolytes, just like other ionic compounds. Apart from HCl formed in the process of gastric acid secretion, most acids in the body are weak acids.

A base is a compound that can dissociate, releasing a hydroxide ion (OH⁻) and a cation. Bases can also accept a proton, becoming positively charged; thus, bases can be defined as proton acceptors. **Figure 2.5d** illustrates the behavior of a strong base, sodium hydroxide (NaOH), in aqueous solutions. Dissociation of sodium from the hydroxide ion provides a free hydroxide that is capable of neutralizing acid. Bicarbonate ion (HCO_3^-)

is the base that plays a major physiological role in pH homeostasis as part of the carbonic acid buffer system. One homeostatic role of bicarbonate ions relates to gastrointestinal function. Bicarbonate is produced by the pancreas and released into the duodenum to neutralize the acidity of the chyme that comes from the stomach. Pancreatic bicarbonate secretion is necessary because, while the stomach is usually well protected from acidity, the small intestine is not. Acid-induced damage can result in gastric and duodenal irritation and ulcer formation. Just like acids, bases can be classified depending on their ability to dissociate in water, and physiological bases are generally relatively weak. In addition to bicarbonate, ammonia is an important base that contributes to physiological pH regulation.

The concentration of hydrogen ions in a solution can be expressed in terms of the pH. The pH of a solution is defined as the negative logarithm of the proton concentration in moles per liter (mol/L). At the extremes of pH range, a 1 M solution of hydrochloric acid has a pH of 0 whereas a 1 M solution of sodium hydroxide has a pH of 14. Distilled water has a neutral pH of 7, with equal amounts of hydrogen and hydroxide ions. A solution that has a pH below 7 is considered to be acidic, and a solution with a pH above 7 is considered to be basic or alkaline.

Maintenance of acid–base homeostasis is of paramount importance in the human body. In fact, the normal pH of the blood is between 7.35 and 7.45. Homeostasis of pH in the body is maintained by the renal and respiratory systems, together with chemical buffers (**Figure 2.7**). A buffer is a solution that resists pH changes. The bicarbonate–carbonic acid buffer system can accommodate more than 80% of the excess ions produced in, or lost by, the body. The reactions of this buffer system are represented in **Figure 2.7a**. Carbonic acid (H_2CO_3) is a weak acid that is formed by the addition of water to carbon dioxide, or by the addition of hydrogen ion to bicarbonate ion. As circulating bicarbonate reacts with excess hydrogen ion, the equilibrium is shifted toward H_2CO_3, which readily dissociates into H_2O and CO_2. As the CO_2 level rises, an increase in respiratory rate can rid the body of this potential source of acid. A typical example of this phenomenon is the Kussmaul breathing observed in patients with diabetic ketoacidosis. Similarly, the carbonic acid buffer can accommodate for the presence of excess base by shifting the balance of the buffer toward the right of the equation, increasing the production of H^+ and HCO_3^-. The HCO_3^- ions can then be excreted by the kidneys as needed to maintain physiological pH.

Proteins can also buffer body pH because amino acids are made of an amino group, which is a base, and a carboxylic acid group. Therefore, proteins can neutralize either excess acid or excess base (**Figure 2.7b**). Although the amino acids have weak acid and weak base constituents, the relative abundance of plasma

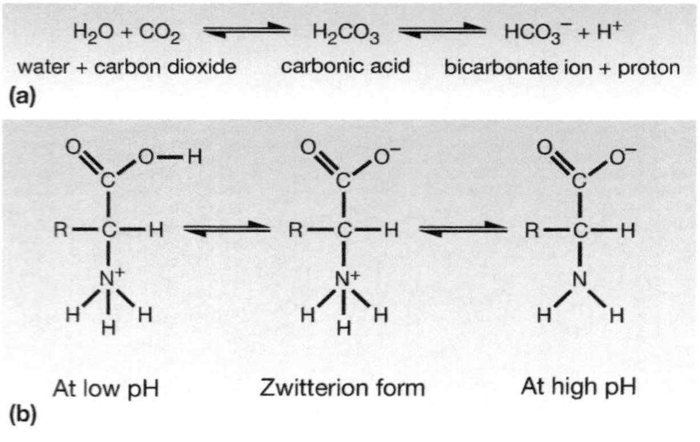

FIGURE 2.7 Buffer systems that maintain acid–base homeostasis. (**a**) The carbonic acid–bicarbonate buffer and (**b**) amino acid as a buffer.
Cl^-, chloride ion; HCO_3^-, bicarbonate ion; K^+, potassium ion; Na^+, sodium ion; PO_4^{3-}, phosphate ion.

proteins in the circulation make this a significant contributor to physiological pH buffering along with the bicarbonate–carbonic acid system.

COVALENT BOND STRUCTURE AND FORMATION

Ionic bonds are not the only strategy that atoms use to fulfill the octet rule. Another strategy involves the sharing, rather than the exchange, of electrons. When electrons occupy a single orbital that is common to two atoms, they form a covalent bond. This bond may allow both atoms to occupy their valence shells and have a stable electron configuration. **Figure 2.8** depicts examples of covalent bonds. As previously noted, carbon has four electrons in the valence shell and therefore needs four more to fulfill the octet rule. Hydrogen has only one electron, and needs another one to be stable. Thus, one atom of carbon can interact with four atoms of hydrogen in such a way that the carbon atom shares one electron with each one of the four hydrogen atoms and each hydrogen atom shares one electron with the carbon atom. This sharing results in a carbon atom with eight electrons in the valence shell and four hydrogen atoms with two electrons each. The bonds formed between the carbon atom and each one of the hydrogen atoms are called single covalent bonds, and the resulting compound is a molecule.

Depending on the atoms involved, several pairs of electrons can be shared between two atoms, leading to multiple bonds. For instance, when two oxygen atoms interact, each atom shares two of its electrons with the other atom, thus forming a double bond. Oxygen belongs to the sixth group of the periodic table and, in fact, it contains six electrons in the outermost shell. In molecular oxygen (O_2), each atom has its six electrons plus two additional electrons that come from the

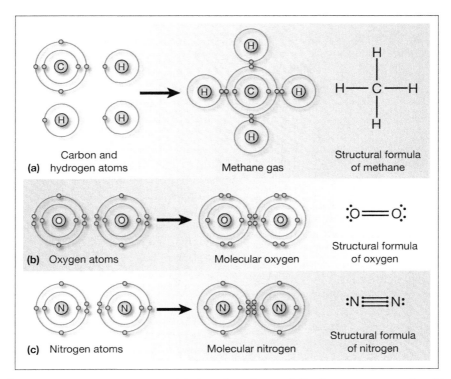

FIGURE 2.8 Covalent bond formation. **(a)** A single carbon and 4 hydrogen atoms can bond together to form methane. **(b)** Two oxygen atoms can be joined by a double bond, forming molecular oxygen. **(c)** Two nitrogen atoms can be joined by a triple bond, forming molecular nitrogen.

other oxygen atom. This allows both oxygen atoms to fulfill the octet rule. The two electrons shared between bonding atoms are called a bonding pair, and each pair of electrons that is not contributing to the formation of a bond is called a lone pair. Therefore, in molecular oxygen, each atom has two bonding pairs and two lone pairs. Nitrogen, which has five valence electrons, needs three more to reach stability and fulfill the octet rule. Therefore, two nitrogen atoms can share three pairs of electrons to form a triple bond. In molecular nitrogen, each nitrogen atom also has one lone pair (N_2). When double or triple bonds are formed, the molecule becomes planar, as multiple bonds between two atoms limit the movement of the two atoms involved. **Figure 2.8** also shows the structural formula of these compounds on the right. This is a geometric representation of the structure of a molecule, with lines representing covalent bonds and dots representing electrons.

Thought Questions

4. What are the ways in which the duet or octet rule can be satisfied for an atom with an incomplete valence shell?

5. What are the main ions found in the body, and where are they found? Are they in the extracellular fluid or intracellular fluid?

CHEMICAL PATTERNS IN PHYSIOLOGY AND PATHOPHYSIOLOGY

NONPOLAR VERSUS POLAR COVALENT BONDS

Electronegativity is defined as the tendency of an element to attract a bonding pair of electrons. Electronegativity depends on the number of protons in the nucleus; thus, an element with more protons will be more electronegative than an element with fewer protons, within a given period of the periodic table. Because elements that have a higher proton number also have a higher group number, electronegativity increases across a period in the periodic table. For instance, oxygen (with a main-group number of 6A) is more electronegative than carbon (main-group number 4A). Contrarily, atoms that belong to the first or second group, such as hydrogen or beryllium, have a greater tendency to release valence electrons and are less electronegative. For this reason, they are sometimes referred to as being electropositive.

When a covalent bond is formed between an atom that has higher electronegativity and an atom that has lower electronegativity, electrons spend more time in the vicinity of the electronegative atom. This in turn confers a partial negative charge (referred to as delta negative: δ^-) around the electronegative atom and a partial positive charge (delta positive: δ^+) around the other atom. The development of a positive pole and a negative pole creates a polar bond, and the polarity

TABLE 2.1 Bond Types and Electronegativity

Bond Type	Electronegativity Difference	Example
Nonpolar covalent	0–0.4	O_2
Polar covalent	0.4–2.0	H_2O
Ionic	>2.0	NaCl

of that bond depends on the electronegativity difference between the two elements participating in the bond. As shown in **Table 2.1**, two elements with a large electronegativity difference form an ionic bond (e.g., NaCl). Two elements with similar electronegativity form a nonpolar covalent bond (e.g., O_2). Lastly, two elements with a moderate electronegativity difference form a polar covalent bond (e.g., H_2O). The polar nature of the water molecule is a critical feature of water as the solvent of both intracellular and extracellular fluids.

Applying the concept of polar and nonpolar covalent bonds to common biomolecules described later in this chapter, hexose sugars that are rich in hydroxyl (–OH) groups, have many polar regions due to the electropositive hydrogen atoms bound to electronegative oxygen atoms. Nucleotide bases have polar regions due to electropositive nitrogen or oxygen atoms bound to neutral carbon or electronegative hydrogen atoms—these elements contribute to hydrogen bonds holding together complementary base pairs in double-stranded DNA. For this reason, sugars and nucleotides tend to be polar molecules, with partial charges in the bonds connecting oxygen or nitrogen atoms to hydrogens. On the other hand, fatty acids that make up triglycerides and phospholipids have long stretches consisting entirely of nonpolar covalent carbon–hydrogen (C–H) bonds, making these molecular regions nonpolar.

MOLECULAR GEOMETRY

In a molecule, the repulsion forces operating among electron groups, such as lone pairs or bonding pairs, determine the molecular geometry (**Figure 2.9**). Consider a molecule that has three atoms connected by two bonding pairs, with no lone pairs. Because the electrons that constitute bonding pairs are negatively charged, they will repel each other, creating a linear geometry. A common biological molecule that illustrates linear geometry is carbon dioxide (CO_2). Its electron groups form two double bonds that repel each other, and no lone pairs are present, as shown in **Figure 2.9a**.

Repulsion forces in molecules with four electron groups determine tetrahedral geometry. For instance, methane has four identical single C–H bonds with 109.5-degree angles between them, forming a perfect tetrahedron (**Figure 2.9b**). The presence of different types of electron groups (bonding pairs versus lone pairs) causes a distortion in the molecular geometry. This is the case in a water molecule (H_2O). Here, the oxygen atom has two lone pairs and two bonding pairs that make single bonds with two hydrogen atoms. Because the repulsion between the two lone pairs is greater than the repulsion between the bonding pairs, the molecule acquires a bent shape in which the H–O–H bond angle is 104.5 degrees instead of 109.5 degrees (**Figure 2.9c**).

MOLECULAR PROPERTIES OF WATER

In water molecules, the bonds between oxygen and hydrogen atoms are polar; hence, electrostatic attraction forces develop between the slightly negative charge on oxygen atoms and the slightly positive charge on the hydrogen atoms in neighboring molecules. This attraction is also called a hydrogen bond (see **Figure 2.10**). Each water molecule can make up to four hydrogen bonds with neighboring water molecules and is subject to pulling forces in different directions. However, on the surface of a liquid, the molecules can make fewer hydrogen bonds; thus, each molecule is more strongly

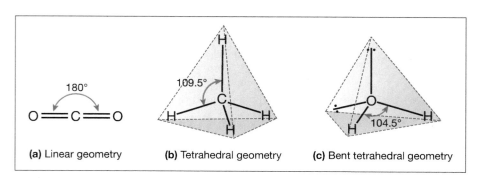

(a) Linear geometry **(b)** Tetrahedral geometry **(c)** Bent tetrahedral geometry

FIGURE 2.9 Molecular geometry. Solid black lines show the electron groups; dotted lines outline the tetrahedron. **(a)** Carbon dioxide, **(b)** methane, and **(c)** water.

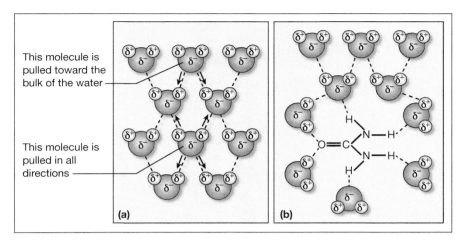

FIGURE 2.10 Hydrogen bonds (**a**) among water molecules and (**b**) when urea is dissolved in water.

pulled toward the bulk of the liquid. In this way, hydrogen bonds are responsible for creating the cohesiveness that pulls water molecules close together, leading to the surface tension that characterizes water. Indeed, this surface tension allows water to form drops and allows a needle or an insect to gently or temporarily float on water. Overall, hydrogen bonds are weaker than ionic or covalent bonds. However, since the body is mostly water, and solutes are dissolved in aqueous intracellular or extracellular solution, hydrogen bonding contributes greatly to the stabilization of small and large molecules, including proteins and nucleic acids.

HYDROGEN BONDING AND AQUEOUS SOLUTIONS OF POLAR MOLECULES AND IONS

Hydrogen bonds also form between other polar molecules. More precisely, these bonds form between an electronegative atom (with a slight negative charge, δ^-) and a hydrogen atom that is bound to another electronegative atom (and thus with a slight positive charge, δ^+). **Figure 2.10** illustrates what happens when a molecule can form hydrogen bonds with water, using the example of the dissolved form of urea. Urea is a molecule produced by the liver from ammonia (a toxic compound generated from amino acid metabolism). Urea is polar, containing oxygen and hydrogen atoms that can form hydrogen bonds with water molecules. Because the interactions between water and urea are stronger than the intermolecular attractions among molecules of urea, the formation of hydrogen bonds allows urea to be easily dissolved in water. Soluble urea can be readily excreted by the kidneys, effectively removing ammonia from the body. Hydrogen bonds also stabilize large molecules, such as the double helix of DNA or three-dimensional structures in proteins, as described later in "Protein Folding" and "The Principle of Complementary Base Pairing."

Because of its polar nature, water is also an excellent solvent for ionic compounds. As **Figure 2.5** illustrates, acids, bases, and ionic compounds dissociate in aqueous solutions, releasing anions and cations, which in turn interact with water molecules to maximize electrostatic interactions. In fact, water molecules rearrange to form a hydration shell surrounding the ions according to their polarity. Hydration shells also develop surrounding large charged molecules, such as proteins in intracellular fluid or plasma. Taken together, all these properties make water not only an exceptional solvent but also the major transport medium in the body, capable of carrying nutrients, respiratory gases, electrolytes, hormones, and waste products.

HYDROPHOBICITY AND HYDROPHILICITY

Polar and ionic compounds that readily dissolve in water are referred to as hydrophilic, or water loving. On the other hand, nonpolar molecules are unable to interact through hydrogen bonding or ionic interactions. Instead, they tend to aggregate with other nonpolar molecules, minimizing the exposure to water molecules. Therefore, nonpolar compounds are called hydrophobic, or water fearing, and the interactions that hold nonpolar molecules together are called hydrophobic interactions. This phenomenon can be easily illustrated by the immiscibility of water and oil. Hydrocarbon chains, such as those found in triglycerides (the major form of energy storage in the body), are the typical examples of hydrophobic molecules and require special packaging in order to be transported in aqueous solutions, such as the blood.

Hydrophobic interactions are also particularly important in determining the three-dimensional structure of macromolecules. An example of this phenomenon is the aggregation of phospholipids to form biological membranes in the body. Phospholipids are

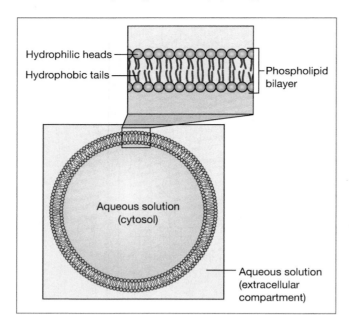

FIGURE 2.11 A biological membrane. A phospholipid bilayer separates two aqueous solutions.

amphipathic molecules because they contain two hydrophobic tails and a polar hydrophilic head. When phospholipids are placed in aqueous solutions, they rearrange to hide their hydrophobic chains away from the water while exposing the polar heads toward the solution. This leads to the formation of a phospholipid bilayer that separates two aqueous solutions—the extracellular space outside and the cytosol inside—while the hydrophobic chains are facing toward the inside of the membrane (**Figure 2.11**).

Biological gases, such as molecular oxygen and carbon dioxide, are nonpolar and thus poorly soluble in aqueous solutions. To obviate this problem, the body has dedicated systems facilitating their transport. Oxygen is transported and stored bound to specialized proteins hemoglobin and myoglobin. Carbon dioxide combines with water and is transported as carbonic acid and bicarbonate ion (see **Figure 2.7a**), which are both hydrophilic and thus soluble in aqueous solutions. Some carbon dioxide also is carried by hemoglobin, particularly in venous blood.

Thought Questions

6. What are the similarities and differences between ionic, nonpolar, and polar molecules?

7. Can you draw and label a water molecule, showing the special properties that make it an excellent solvent for body solutions?

ORGANIC CHEMISTRY FOUNDATIONS

CARBON-BASED MOLECULES

Carbon compounds are the focus of organic chemistry, and are the principal building blocks of the body. Because of the chemical properties of carbon, this exceptional element can form very stable bonds with itself and with hydrogen atoms, leading to the formation of molecular chains and rings that can be assembled into an enormous number of organic compounds. The more than 12 million compounds on which all living organisms are based are predominantly made up of carbon, hydrogen, oxygen, and nitrogen. As illustrated in **Figure 2.3**, carbon has four electrons in the valence shell and thus is able to make combinations of single, double, or triple covalent bonds. Organic molecules can contain polar or nonpolar functional groups that determine their solubility in water. Some of the specific arrangements that occur repeatedly in the body are named and described next.

MAJOR ORGANIC FUNCTIONAL GROUPS

Six molecules that contain common functional groups are shown in **Figure 2.12**. A methyl group consists of a carbon bound to three hydrogens. The fourth binding site of the carbon is bound to a larger molecule. A typical example of a methyl group can be found in the amino acid alanine. **Figure 2.12a** shows the chemical structure of a methyl group and the structure of alanine. Addition of one or more methyl groups adds a nonpolar/hydrophobic region to the larger structure.

A hydroxyl group consists of an attached oxygen bound to hydrogen (**Figure 2.12b**). Addition of one or more hydroxyl groups makes a larger structure more polar and hydrophilic. A carbonyl group is a functional group in which a carbon atom is double bonded to an oxygen atom. Molecules that contain a carbonyl group are called aldehydes or ketones depending on the location of the carbonyl group in the molecule. In the former, the carbon is bound to another carbon atom and to a hydrogen atom. In the latter, the carbon is bound to two other carbon atoms. Carbohydrates are found in the form of aldehydes and ketones; **Figure 2.12** illustrates the structure of two carbohydrates—ribose (**Figure 2.12b**, containing an aldehyde) and ribulose (**Figure 2.12c**, containing a ketone).

Another common organic functional group is the carboxyl group (**Figure 2.12a**). In a carboxyl group, the carbon is double bonded to one oxygen, and has a single bond to the oxygen of a hydroxyl group. Carboxyl groups behave as acids because they can release the proton from the hydroxyl group; thus, they are also called carboxylic acids. A carboxylic acid group is present in all amino acids, and in fact the name *amino acid* refers to the fact that the molecule contains a carboxylic acid and an amino group.

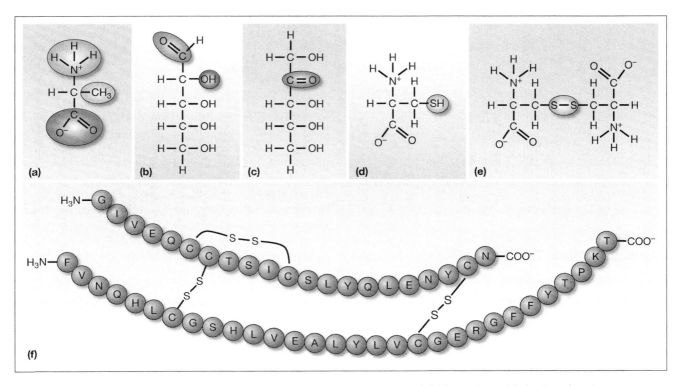

FIGURE 2.12 Molecules that contain common functional groups. (**a**) The amino acid alanine, showing a methyl group in yellow, the amino group in blue, and the carboxylic group in red, in its zwitterionic form. (**b**) A ribose molecule, showing the aldehyde group in green and a hydroxyl group in purple. (**c**) A ribulose molecule, showing the ketone highlighted in blue. (**d**) The amino acid cysteine, with its thiol group shown in orange. (**e**) The formation of a disulfide bond (in orange) linking two cysteines. (**f**) The amino acid sequence of insulin, showing the disulfide bonds that hold the two chains of the protein together.

Amino groups are functional groups that contain a basic nitrogen atom with two hydrogens (**Figure 2.12a**). The suffix *-amine* and the prefix *amino-* are two ways to describe a functional group containing nitrogen. Amines are called primary when the nitrogen is bound to one carbon, secondary when it is bound to two carbons, and tertiary when it is bound to three carbons. Primary amines can function as bases, accepting an additional proton.

Another functional group that plays a pivotal role in the body is the thiol group. This is composed of a sulfur (S) atom bound to a hydrogen atom in an organic compound (**Figure 2.12d**). This substituent of organic compounds will be referred to as thiol or sulfhydryl. The presence of a thiol group on the amino acid cysteine gives the molecule the ability to form disulfide bonds by losing the hydrogen atoms and forming a covalent bond between the sulfur atoms of two amino acids (**Figure 2.12e**). Disulfide bonds are extremely common in the body, as they can link together two protein chains. **Figure 2.12f** shows the structure of insulin and the disulfide bonds that link cysteines (C in the diagram), forming one intrachain and two interchain disulfide bonds that create the shape of this protein hormone.

MAJOR BIOCHEMICAL REACTION TYPES

Biochemical reactions in the body can be classified into three main categories: synthesis, decomposition, and exchange reactions (**Figure 2.13**). Synthesis reactions entail the binding of molecules, also called monomers, to form more complex structures. Many synthesis reactions are anabolic, in that they are occurring in the context of building up fuel stores after a meal. In the body, glucose is stored in the liver and muscle in its polymeric form called glycogen. The reactions that combine glucose molecules to form glycogen are synthesis reactions and take place in the fed state when glucose is available. On the other hand, decomposition reactions take place when a single compound is broken down into two or more components. Most decomposition reactions are catabolic. In the fasting state, when glucose availability is decreased, the body performs decomposition reactions to break down glycogen and release glucose (**Figure 2.13a**).

Exchange reactions entail the transfer of an atom or group between two molecules. Phosphorylation reactions are a typical example of exchange reactions as they entail the transfer of a phosphate or phosphoryl

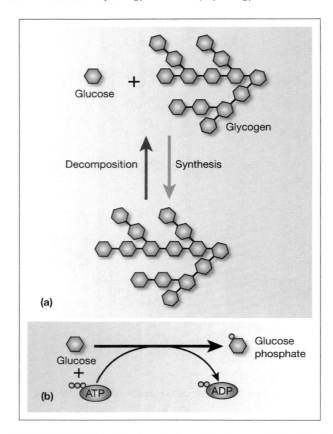

FIGURE 2.13 Major biochemical reaction types. **(a)** Synthesis and decomposition reactions that convert glucose to glycogen and vice versa. **(b)** Exchange reaction entailing glucose phosphorylation.
ADP, adenosine diphosphate; ATP, adenosine triphosphate.

group ($-PO_3^{2-}$) from a donor, often adenosine triphosphate (ATP), to an acceptor molecule that could be a protein or a carbohydrate. Phosphorylation reactions have a plethora of different functions in the body. For instance, when glucose enters a cell, it is immediately phosphorylated, giving rise to glucose phosphate in an exchange reaction in which ATP is converted into adenosine diphosphate (ADP; **Figure 2.13b**). This reaction allows cells to accumulate glucose in the cytoplasm because phosphorylated glucose is unable to leave the cell. The release of a phosphoryl group from ATP is also used to provide energy to propel reactions that would otherwise be energetically unfavorable. An example is the splitting of ATP by the transport protein sodium–potassium ATPase, which moves sodium against its concentration gradient from the inside of the cell to the outside of the cell and moves potassium against its concentration gradient from the outside of the cell to the inside. Additionally, the phosphorylation of specific protein residues is used to regulate protein function.

BIOMOLECULES BUILD FROM SMALL TO LARGE

CARBOHYDRATES
Carbohydrate Molecular Formulas

Together with proteins, lipids, and nucleic acids, carbohydrates are one of the four major classes of biological macromolecules. Monomers of carbohydrates are called monosaccharides and are classified based on the number of carbon atoms they contain: trioses, tetroses, pentoses, hexoses, and heptoses are carbohydrates with three, four, five, six, or seven carbon atoms, respectively. Hexoses are the most common sugars; an example is glucose, which is central to human metabolic processes.

Because carbohydrates contain chiral carbons, which are carbon atoms bound to four different substituents, they can exist in two different forms called enantiomers: L (for Latin *laevus*, left) or D (for Latin *dexter*, right). D- and L-forms of carbohydrates have the chiral carbon oriented in such a way that one enantiomer is the mirror image of the other. In nature, D-forms of carbohydrates are the most prevalent. **Figure 2.14** shows D-glucose and L-glucose. Additionally, a hexose may be present in its linear form or may cyclize, leading to the development of hexagonal or pentagonal structures. **Figure 2.14** illustrates the common cyclic form of hexoses, such as galactose and fructose, as well as pentoses, such as ribose and deoxyribose. Because fructose and galactose have the same molecular formula as glucose but display a different structural organization of the constituent groups, they are called isomers of glucose.

Another carbohydrate that has a major role in the body is the pentose ribose. This is the building block for nucleic acids and it is found in two main forms: ribose in RNA and deoxyribose in DNA. The two forms have identical structures, but the deoxyribose lacks one oxygen (**Figure 2.14**).

Disaccharides are made from two monosaccharides bound together by covalent bonds. As **Figure 2.15** illustrates, during the synthesis reaction that produces a disaccharide from two monosaccharides, a molecule of water is removed (dehydration reaction) while the opposite reaction adds a molecule of water to break the disaccharide into two monosaccharides. This is called a hydrolysis reaction. Three disaccharides deserve specific consideration: maltose, sucrose, and lactose. Maltose is made of two molecules of glucose bound together; in the body it is formed during digestion when polymeric chains of glucose (e.g., dietary starches) are broken down. Sucrose is made of one molecule of glucose bound to one molecule of fructose; it is the main component of common table sugar. Lactose (milk sugar) is made of glucose and galactose. During

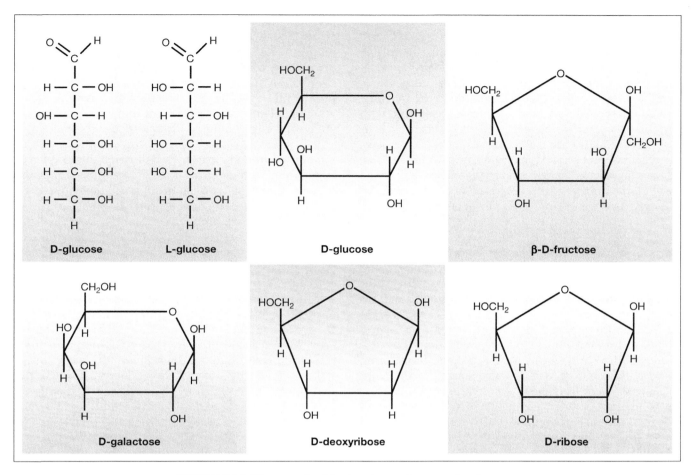

FIGURE 2.14 Monosaccharide structure: D-forms and L-glucose.

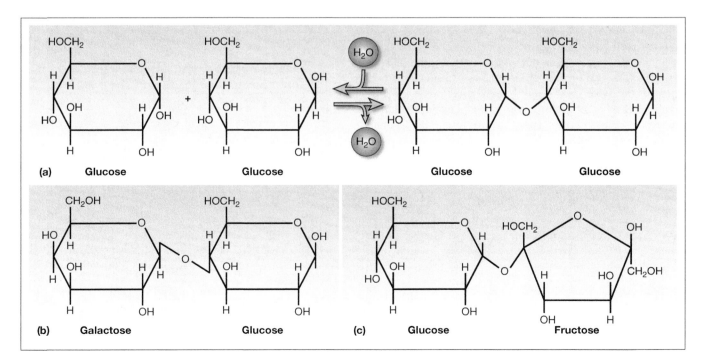

FIGURE 2.15 Monosaccharides and disaccharides. (**a**) Two molecules of glucose form the disaccharide maltose. (**b**) Lactose is formed when a molecule of glucose binds to galactose, and (**c**) sucrose is formed when a molecule of glucose binds to fructose.

digestion of milk and dairy products, lactose is broken down into its monomers, which are then assimilated. The enzyme lactase is responsible for this hydrolysis reaction; individuals who lack the ability to produce lactase during adulthood suffer from lactose intolerance, and the persistence of the disaccharide in the intestine causes the typical signs and symptoms associated with the condition (abdominal pain, bloating, diarrhea, etc.).

Polysaccharides are long chains of monosaccharides. As previously mentioned, glucose is stored in the form of the polysaccharide glycogen in the muscle and in the liver. Starch could be considered the plant equivalent of glycogen as it is also a polymeric form of glucose.

Hydrophilic Nature of Carbohydrates

Carbohydrates are aldehydes or ketones that contain several hydroxyl groups. In aqueous solutions, these groups can easily form hydrogen bonds with water molecules and because such polar interactions are greater than the interactions among carbohydrate molecules, they readily dissolve in water. This hydrophilicity of carbohydrates is a great advantage because it allows them to be easily solubilized and transported in aqueous solutions, such as the plasma or the cytoplasm. However, it makes carbohydrates poorly soluble in hydrophobic environments such as membranes. For this reason, carbohydrates are unable to cross the hydrophobic portion of biological membranes and require specific transporters to enter or exit cells.

Functions of Carbohydrates

Glucose has a central role in metabolic processes as all cells in the body can use it as an energy source. Certain cell types or organs, like the brain, rely almost completely on glucose availability to perform their functions and, in fact, the maintenance of a constant glucose concentration in the blood (glycemia) is of pivotal importance in the body. Excessively high or excessively low levels of glucose in the blood (hyperglycemia and hypoglycemia, respectively) have immediate pathological consequences. Carbohydrates are also used to modify components of cell membranes. Proteins modified by the addition of carbohydrates are termed *glycoproteins*; lipids modified by the addition of carbohydrates are termed *glycolipids*. Glycoproteins and glycolipids are abundant in the plasma membrane, forming a *glycocalyx*—a sugary membrane coat. These molecules play diverse roles in the body: they provide support or attachment sites, transport other molecules, and mediate hormonal signaling or host–pathogen interactions.

ABO blood groups are an interesting example of membrane-bound carbohydrates responsible for distinguishing self from non-self, and thus regulating immune functions. These groups are determined by the presence of carbohydrate residues that are found on the surface membrane of red blood cells in the form of glycoproteins or glycolipids. The sequence of oligosaccharides determines whether the antigen is A, B, or O. **Figure 2.16** illustrates sphingolipids bound to A, B, or O groups. Individuals with blood type A have a modified form of galactose, *N*-acetylgalactosamine, at the end of the glycolipid, whereas those with type B express galactose instead. Individuals with blood type AB express both types of glycolipids on their red blood cells, and those with blood type O express neither galactose nor *N*-acetylgalactosamine at the end of the glycolipid or glycoprotein. Transfusion reactions, sometimes fatal, arise when blood is not correctly matched between donor and recipient. For example, recipients with type O blood have antibodies to both A and B antigens; therefore, they cannot be transfused with blood from donors who are type A, type B, or type AB.

Thought Questions

8. **What features of carbohydrate molecules contribute to their tendency to be polar and hydrophilic?**

9. **How many biological functions of carbohydrates can you identify?**

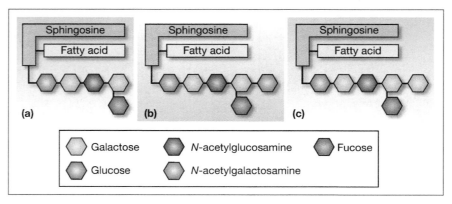

FIGURE 2.16 Blood groups: **(a)** O antigen, **(b)** A antigen, and **(c)** B antigen.

LIPIDS

Types of Lipids

Lipids are a diverse group of biological molecules that have a common feature: their insolubility in aqueous solutions (**Figures 2.17** and **2.18**). Fatty acids and their derivatives constitute the main form of lipids and are present in fats and oils. As the name implies, fatty acids are made of a hydrophobic portion, which is a nonpolar hydrocarbon chain, and a terminal carboxylic acid portion (**Figure 2.17**). Fatty acids are classified into short-, medium-, long-, and very long-chain fatty acids depending on the length of their hydrocarbon chain. The most abundant fatty acid in the body is palmitic acid: a long-chain fatty acid of 16 carbons. At physiological pH, palmitic acid spontaneously loses its proton and thus is present as an anion, referred to as palmitate, as shown in **Figure 2.17a**. The carboxylic end of a fatty acid can easily react with other molecules to form more complex lipids. This is the case for triglycerides, also known as triacylglycerols. Triglycerides are composed of three fatty acids joined to a glycerol molecule. **Figure 2.17b** illustrates the (dehydration) reaction of triglyceride synthesis, starting from three fatty acids and yielding one triglyceride. Triglycerides are nonpolar, hydrophobic, and insoluble in water. In adipocytes (fat cells), triglycerides coalesce into fat droplets that make up the bulk of the cytoplasm.

Phospholipids are common lipids in which a glycerol molecule is bound to two fatty acids and to a highly polar or charged group via binding of a phosphate group (see **Figures 2.17c** and **2.18**). Molecules such as phospholipids that contain a polar and a nonpolar region are called amphipathic. In phospholipids, this characteristic is the basis for their major biological role in forming cell membranes. In aqueous solutions, they spontaneously aggregate to form bilayers. Phospholipids are one of the most abundant classes of lipids in the body as they are the main constituent of plasma membranes. The phospholipid phosphatidylcholine, also known as lecithin, has choline as its polar group (**Figure 2.17c**). Choline can be synthesized from the amino acid methionine, but humans also need to acquire it from the diet; thus, it is considered a quasivitamin. Another very abundant phospholipid is phosphatidylethanolamine, which is structurally similar to phosphatidylcholine. Phosphatidylcholine and phosphatidylethanolamine are the two major components of biological membranes. Some biological membranes, particularly in the brain, also contain sphingolipids such as sphingomyelin. These are amphipathic molecules built from fatty acids and a polar group attached to the amino acid serine, rather than glycerol (**Figure 2.18a**).

Steroids are another class of lipids, with cholesterol and its derivatives as the major forms in the human body. Cholesterol is made of a short hydrocarbon chain connected to four hydrocarbon rings fused to form a planar structure. Most of the cholesterol molecule is nonpolar and hydrophobic. However, there is a hydroxyl group on the first carbon ring

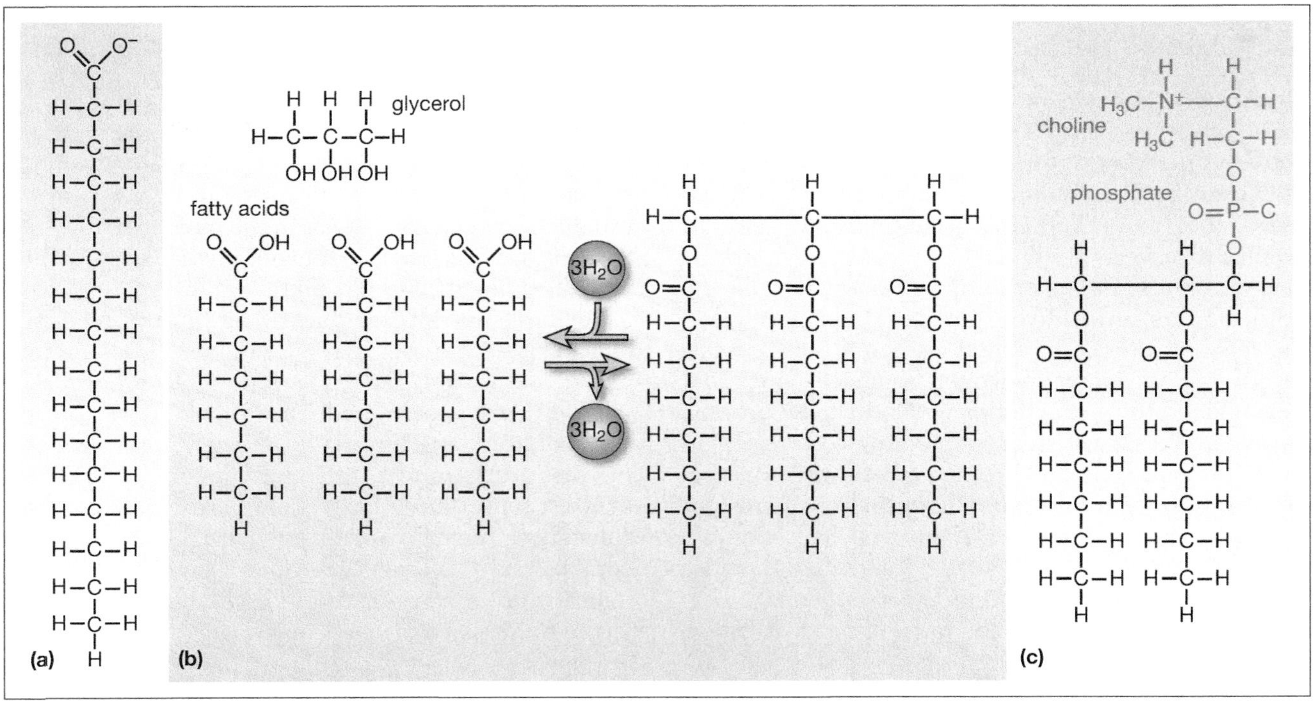

FIGURE 2.17 Lipid structure. (**a**) Palmitate, (**b**) triglycerides formed when three fatty acids are bound to glycerol, and (**c**) phosphatidylcholine.

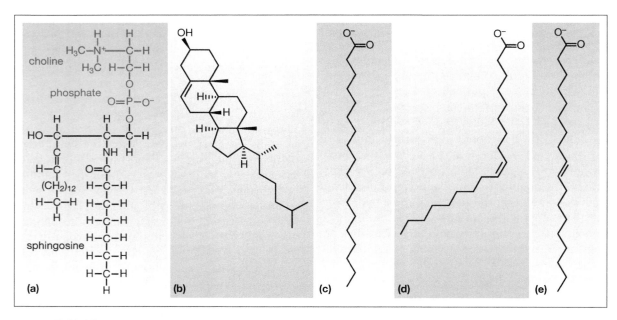

FIGURE 2.18 Lipid configuration, showing single and double bonds, and *cis* and *trans* configurations. (**a**) Sphingomyelin; (**b**) cholesterol; (**c**) stearate, a saturated fatty acid; (**d**) *cis*-oleate, an unsaturated fatty acid in *cis* configuration; and (**e**) *trans*-oleate, an unsaturated fatty acid in *trans* configuration.

that makes this part of the molecule polar; thus, cholesterol is overall amphipathic (**Figure 2.18b**). Physiological roles of cholesterol and its derivatives include contributing to plasma membrane structure, formation of steroid hormones, and formation of bile salts that function in gastrointestinal digestion and absorption of fats.

Structure and Function of Lipids

Fatty Acids and Derivatives

Lipids are a very diverse class of biological molecules that perform many body functions. Because of their low solubility in aqueous solutions, fatty acids are transported in the blood bound noncovalently to the serum protein albumin. Fatty acids have different configurations based on the bonds between the carbon atoms in the hydrocarbon chain. Saturated fatty acids are those in which carbon atoms are saturated with as many hydrogen atoms as possible, thus making only single bonds with adjacent carbons. **Figure 2.18c** shows stearate, a saturated fatty acid that contains 18 carbon atoms (C18). In this figure, carbons are omitted for simplicity and each straight line represents a single bond between two carbons. For comparison, in **Figures 2.18d** and **2.18e**, a double line represents a double bond between two carbons. Unsaturated fatty acids have fewer hydrogens because they contain at least one carbon to carbon double bond. Some carbons form one double bond and two single bonds: one with the next carbon in the chain and the other with a hydrogen. Therefore, in unsaturated fatty acids not all carbons are saturated with two hydrogen atoms. The carbons that form a double bond may assume two possible configurations: *cis* or *trans*. The double bond within the fatty acid is in *cis* configuration when the hydrogens bound to adjacent carbons are on the same side of the molecule, while it is in *trans* configuration when the bound hydrogens are on opposite sides of the molecule (see **Figures 2.18d** and **2.18e**).

Biological membranes contain both saturated and unsaturated fatty acids. When saturated fatty acids predominate, they can be tightly packed, increasing the rigidity of the membrane. Conversely, because unsaturated fatty acids have a kink in the molecule, they tend to occupy more space, leading to a membrane that has increased fluidity and flexibility.

A simple observation may better illustrate this principle. Consider butter and oil. The former is of animal origin, and roughly 60% of its fatty acids are saturated while 40% are unsaturated. The latter is of plant origin, and roughly 80% of its fatty acids are unsaturated while the rest are saturated. At room temperature, the fatty acids in butter are tightly packed, resulting in a solid substance. The unsaturated fatty acids in oil, however, confer fluidity and make the substance liquid at room temperature. Because unsaturated fatty acids are subject to oxidation and can become rancid, the process of artificial partial hydrogenation was developed. This process lengthens the shelf life of oils by converting some *cis* double bonds into single bonds and some other *cis* double bonds into *trans* double bonds. Unfortunately, there is now compelling evidence that dietary intake of *trans* fatty acids (also called *trans* fats) increases the risk of developing cardiovascular disease by raising the levels of so-called *bad* cholesterol (low-density lipoprotein [LDL]). In light of these findings, the Food and Drug Administration (FDA) in 2018 recommended banning the use of partially hydrogenated oils, which are the main source of *trans* fatty acids.[1] Food manufacturers are required to completely remove them from food products by 2020.

Triglycerides are the major form of energy storage as the hydrocarbon chains can undergo catabolic reactions that release large amounts of energy. Triglycerides are mainly stored in adipose tissue, where lipase enzymes catalyze the reaction that releases fatty acids and glycerol so that they can be exported to tissues and organs that need energy.

Eicosanoids

Certain lipid components of biological membranes, such as arachidonic acid, may be released and converted into paracrine hormones, substances that act near their production site. Arachidonic acid is a 20-carbon unsaturated fatty acid containing four *cis* double bonds that give it a hairpin shape. It is the precursor for many lipid molecules that participate in inflammation and other homeostatic responses, such as thromboxane, prostaglandins, and leukotrienes. These molecules are collectively called eicosanoids, from the Greek word for 20. Eicosanoids are involved in physiological processes such as inflammation, control of blood flow and pressure, and reproductive functions. Understanding their structure and synthesis led to the development of nonsteroidal anti-inflammatory drugs (NSAIDs), which inhibit cyclooxygenases, the enzymes that catalyze an early step in the conversion of arachidonate to prostaglandins and thromboxane (see **Figure 2.19**). This mechanism allows aspirin and ibuprofen to decrease pain, fever, and inflammatory responses in general.

Another membrane lipid component that has a key role in the body is phosphatidylinositol-4,5-bisphosphate (PIP$_2$). This compound is cleaved into diacylglycerol (DAG) and inositol-1,4,5-trisphosphate (IP$_3$) by the enzyme phospholipase C. DAG and IP$_3$ are two second messengers that mediate the signaling cascade activated by norepinephrine at α-adrenergic receptors and other neurotransmitters and hormones.

Cholesterol and Derivatives

Cholesterol (see **Figure 2.18b**) is an amphipathic molecule and therefore, when placed in a biological membrane, it spontaneously orients itself with the polar hydroxyl group facing aqueous solutions and the hydrophobic component toward the internal part of the membrane. Although phospholipids are the main lipids making up the cell membrane, cholesterol is inserted in

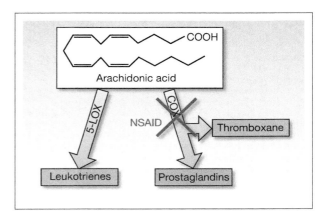

FIGURE 2.19 Formation of inflammatory mediators from arachidonic acid follows two pathways: COX, which is blocked by NSAIDs, and 5-LOX.
5-LOX, 5-lipoxygenase; COX, cyclooxygenase NSAID, nonsteroidal anti-inflammatory drug.

smaller amounts and is important at stabilizing membrane fluidity for normal function of membrane proteins. Cholesterol is also the precursor for all steroid hormones: androgens, estrogens, progestins, glucocorticoids, and mineralocorticoids. These hormones regulate various functions in the body, ranging from the development of sexual characteristics to electrolyte balance. Because all these hormones are hydrophobic in nature, their mode of action is fundamentally different from that of protein hormones. Finally, cholesterol is the precursor for bile acids made by the liver. Bile acids are secreted into the bile, traveling to the gastrointestinal tract where they play major roles in the digestion and absorption of dietary lipids.

Lipoproteins

Cholesterol and triglycerides are not soluble in aqueous blood plasma, so they are transported in the blood packaged as particles called lipoproteins. As the name implies, these substances have a core made of lipids and an outer coat made up of phospholipids and a form of protein called apolipoproteins. In such aggregates, apolipoproteins have a two-fold role: to coat and solubilize the lipids and to regulate lipid exchange between blood and tissues. Based on their composition and associated density, role, and origin, lipoproteins are classified into several categories—chylomicrons, very low density lipoproteins (VLDLs), intermediate-density lipoproteins (IDLs), LDLs, and high-density lipoproteins (HDLs)—as summarized in **Table 2.2**.

Chylomicrons are formed in intestinal cells as the last step in digestion and absorption of dietary fats (**Figure 2.20**). They enter the circulatory system via the lymphatic circulation bearing apolipoprotein B-48, after which they acquire apolipoproteins C and E from HDL. Chylomicrons consist mostly of triglycerides;

Lipoprotein	Source	Diameter (nm)	Density (g/mL)	Main Component	Apolipoproteins
Chylomicron	Intestine	100–500	<0.9	Triglycerides	A-1, B-48, C-II, E
VLDL	Liver	30–90	0.9–1.0	Triglycerides	B-100, C-II, E
IDL	VLDL	25–30	~1.0	Triglycerides, cholesterol	B-100, C-II, E
LDL	VLDL/IDL	20–25	~1.0	Cholesterol	B-100
HDL	Intestine and liver	5–15	>1.0	Cholesterol, phospholipids, and proteins	A-1, C-II, E

TABLE 2.2 Lipoproteins

HDL, high-density lipoprotein; IDL, intermediate-density lipoprotein; LDL, low-density lipoprotein; VLDL, very low density lipoprotein.

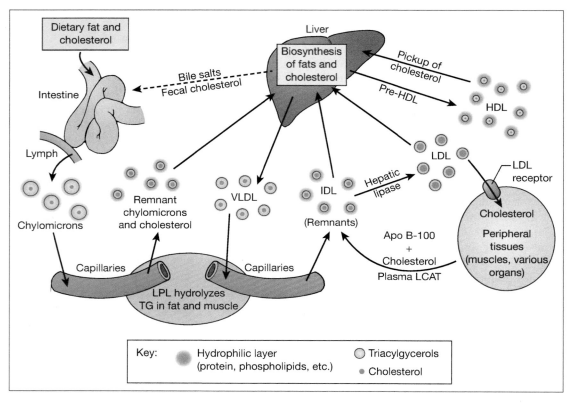

FIGURE 2.20 Lipoprotein metabolism.
Apo B-100, apolipoprotein B-100; HDL, high-density lipoprotein; IDL, intermediate-density lipoprotein; LCAT, lecithin–cholesterol acyltransferase; LDL, low-density lipoprotein; LPL, lipoprotein lipase; TG, triglyceride; VLDL, very low density lipoprotein.

they also contain phospholipids such as phosphatidylcholine, cholesterol, and very little protein. Because of their high fat content, these particles are very large and have the lowest density of all lipoproteins. The main role of chylomicrons is to deliver triglycerides to the tissues in the body, particularly to muscle and fat tissue. Because chylomicrons carry lipids from dietary sources, this pathway of lipid delivery is referred to as the exogenous pathway. Once these particles have

released the majority of their triglyceride content, what remains, called chylomicron remnants, is cleared by the liver.

After digestion and absorption of a meal, the liver produces and packages triglyceride-rich VLDLs coated with apolipoprotein B-100 (Apo B-100), which are also responsible for delivering triglycerides to the tissue. HDL also transfers additional apolipoproteins to VLDL in the circulation. Because VLDL carries lipids produced by the liver, this pathway of lipid delivery is referred to as the endogenous pathway. The particles that are left after VLDLs release triglycerides to peripheral cells are called IDLs. The liver is responsible for clearing some IDL particles while other IDL particles are converted to LDL by hepatic lipase. At this point, LDL particles are mostly made of cholesterol, and their main purpose is to release cholesterol to cells throughout the body before being cleared by the liver. Individuals who have a high dietary intake of cholesterol and saturated fat accumulate excessive amounts of LDLs in the circulation, which eventually migrate into arterial walls promoting atherogenesis and the development of atherosclerosis.

HDL particles have the highest density of all lipoproteins as they contain a large amount of proteins. They also contain the highest phospholipid content, as well as some cholesterol, and very little triglyceride. HDL particles are synthesized in the liver and intestine to be released into the circulation, where they are responsible for transferring apolipoproteins to nascent chylomicrons and VLDL, and collecting cholesterol from IDL and chylomicron remnants. Clinically, low HDL levels are markers of increased cardiovascular risk (**Figure 2.20**).

There are many apolipoproteins; each is found on certain lipoproteins and performs a specific role in body lipid cycling. Mutations in apolipoprotein genes or alterations in gene expression can lead to dyslipidemias, as illustrated by the following examples. Apolipoprotein C-II (Apo C-II) is present in chylomicron and VLDL particles. Its interaction with lipoprotein lipase (LPL) is necessary for the hydrolysis of triglycerides and delivery of fatty acids to tissues, such as adipose tissue. Certain genetic mutations in the genes that code for either Apo C-II or LPL impair triglyceride delivery to tissues, causing chylomicrons and VLDL to accumulate in circulation. This condition is called familial chylomicronemia syndrome.

Apo B-100 is an apolipoprotein required for LDL particles to deliver cholesterol to tissues. Mutations in the gene that codes for Apo B-100 cause familial forms of hypercholesterolemia that are usually associated with normal triglyceride levels. This mutation is often inherited in a dominant fashion, in which only one copy of the mutated gene is needed to cause the disorder. Because of the role of Apo B-100, elevated levels of this apolipoprotein in the blood are associated with a higher risk of atherosclerosis. Apolipoprotein A-1 (Apo A-1) is a structural apolipoprotein for HDL particles and is necessary for returning cholesterol from peripheral tissues to the liver. Low levels of Apo A-1 are detrimental because they impair the body's ability to clear cholesterol.

Thought Questions

10. Can you identify three lipoproteins and identify a major function that each type serves in the body?

11. Why are lipoproteins required for transport of lipids throughout the body?

12. Why might a person need to have a laboratory assay to determine their lipoprotein levels?

AMINO ACIDS AND PROTEINS

Amino Acid Structures and Organic Functional Groups

Proteins perform an exceptional variety of functions in the body: they form enzymes, support structures, antibodies, hormones, membrane transporters, and more. This variety arises from their unique sequences and modifications of only 20 ubiquitous monomers: the amino acids. Amino acids are assigned a three-letter abbreviation and a one-letter symbol; for example, leucine is abbreviated Leu and identified by the symbol L (**Figure 2.21**). The backbone of all amino acids is characterized by a central carbon, also called the α-carbon, bound to an amino group, a carboxylic group, a hydrogen atom, and a unique side chain: the R group (see **Figure 2.21**). The fact that every amino acid has a carboxyl group and an amino group means that individual amino acids are generally polar and hydrophilic. They also contribute to pH buffering, as previously noted. In addition to these general properties, each R group has distinctive chemical characteristics, and the unique sequence of amino acids determines a protein's shape, and therefore its biological functions. **Figure 2.21** shows the amino acids grouped into the following types based on their R group structures: nonpolar, uncharged polar, acidic, basic, and polar with hydroxyl groups.

Amino Acid Classes and Their Properties

Nonpolar Amino Acids

The first class of amino acids has nonpolar, hydrophobic R groups. These amino acids are glycine, alanine, valine, leucine, isoleucine, methionine, proline, tryptophan, and phenylalanine. The simplest amino acid is glycine, which has a hydrogen atom as its R group. Because of its structure, the R group in glycine does not contribute significantly to the development of hydrophobic interactions; thus, glycine is often classified separately from other nonpolar amino acids. Alanine is another simple amino acid as it has a methyl group as a

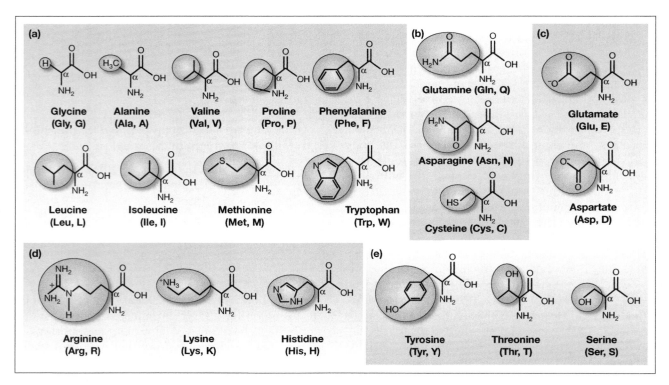

FIGURE 2.21 Major amino acid groups classified based on their R groups (in yellow). **(a)** Nonpolar, hydrophobic; **(b)** uncharged polar; **(c)** negatively charged, acidic; **(d)** positively charged, basic; and **(e)** hydroxylic.

side chain. Three slightly larger amino acids are valine, isoleucine, and leucine. Although the hydrocarbon chain in valine has three carbons, isoleucine and leucine are both made of four carbons that are arranged in different ways. These chains confer hydrophobicity to the molecule.

Methionine contains a sulfur group that is slightly more polarizable than hydrocarbon chains, yet it is predominantly hydrophobic and thus often considered part of the nonpolar amino acids. Proline is unusual as the hydrocarbon group is arranged to form a five-membered ring that includes the amino group. The remaining two nonpolar amino acids are tryptophan and phenylalanine. These are also called aromatic amino acids as they contain aromatic rings: cyclic hydrocarbon chains that are stabilized by resonance and assume a planar configuration. Tryptophan is made of two ring structures that contain a single nitrogen. Because tryptophan is capable of participating in hydrophobic interactions, it is usually classified as nonpolar. Phenylalanine is formed when alanine is bound to a phenyl group, which is a six-membered aromatic ring.

Uncharged Polar Amino Acids
The second class of amino acids contains three uncharged polar amino acids: cysteine, asparagine, and glutamine. Cysteine was introduced earlier in the foundational discussion of organic chemistry as it contains a thiol group that allows it to form disulfide bonds and contribute significantly to the development of three-dimensional structures in proteins, as illustrated in the example of insulin (see **Figure 2.12f**). The remaining two amino acids in this group are the amides of the acidic amino acids, which have a polar structure that makes them hydrophilic.

Acidic Amino Acids
The amino acids with an acidic R group, aspartic acid and glutamic acid, are the third class of amino acids. Both contain a carboxylic acid and thus at pH 7 they dissociate into the proton and anion, referred to as aspartate and glutamate. The negative charge further contributes to the hydrophilic nature of these amino acids.

Basic Amino Acids
The fourth class of amino acids, comprising lysine, arginine, and histidine, contains basic groups. All these amino acids contain one or more amino groups that can act as a proton acceptor and become positively charged.

Uncharged Polar Amino Acids With a Hydroxyl Group
Lastly, there are three amino acids with a hydroxyl group: serine, threonine, and tyrosine. These are polar

and uncharged, yet they are discussed separately to emphasize their special role in cell signaling. As previously mentioned, kinases are enzymes that can transfer a phosphate group from a molecule, usually ATP, to an acceptor. When the acceptor is a protein, phosphorylation usually takes place on hydroxyl groups of serine, threonine, and sometimes tyrosine. The hydrogen of the hydroxyl is displaced by the phosphate group in this reaction. Common signaling cascades in cells, such as those activated by neurotransmitters and hormones, involve serine/threonine kinases and this modification of protein activity by phosphorylation is a common pathway of cell adaptation to maintain homeostasis. Tyrosine kinases contribute to cell signaling by growth factors, cytokines, and the hormone insulin, and can be implicated in neoplastic transformation that leads to cancer.

Specific Amino Acid Functions

Although amino acids are primarily used as building blocks for protein synthesis, individual amino acids can also serve specific functions in the body. First, amino acids can be used as energy sources. These amino acids are classified based on their ability to be converted into either ketone bodies (ketogenic amino acids) or intermediates of glucose metabolism (glucogenic amino acids). During times of fasting, these metabolic pathways are able to supply some of the body's energy needs.

Second, some amino acids have additional roles as precursors of key hormones and neurotransmitters. For instance, tyrosine is the precursor for the pigment melanin and the thyroid hormones thyroxine (T_4) and triiodothyronine (T_3), as well as for the synthesis of the catecholamine neurotransmitters and hormones dopamine, norepinephrine, and epinephrine. Tryptophan is the precursor to serotonin and melatonin and to the coenzyme nicotinamide adenine dinucleotide (NAD), which is necessary for metabolic functions. Histidine is the precursor to histamine, which serves as an inflammatory mediator, a local mediator, and a neurotransmitter. Glycine is the monomer that is used to produce porphyrins, the precursors of heme, the prosthetic group of hemoglobin. The amino acid glutamate is also a neurotransmitter and the precursor to gamma-aminobutyric acid (GABA), another neurotransmitter.

Peptide Bond Formation

Proteins are linear polymers of amino acids joined by peptide bonds (**Figure 2.22**). When the carboxylic group of one amino acid is bound to the amino group of the neighboring amino acid, a hydroxyl group and a proton are released in the form of water in a dehydration reaction (**Figure 2.22a**). Two amino acids bound together by a peptide bond are called a dipeptide, and the term *peptide* usually refers to a short chain of less than 30 amino acids. Peptide bond formation takes place during protein synthesis.

The amino acid sequence of a protein is termed the primary structure, and this sequence profoundly affects the final three-dimensional protein configuration. Proteins are made of hundreds and, in some cases, even thousands of amino acids, which are numbered starting from the amino terminus, the end of the protein molecule containing a free amino group. This convention is used when describing genetic mutations. For instance, sickle cell anemia develops in individuals who carry a mutation of the gene coding for the β-globin protein. Owing to a change in the gene's base sequence, the sixth amino acid of the β-globin protein is a valine, rather than the normal glutamic acid. This is referred to by the single-letter abbreviations and position as an E6V (glutamic acid in the sixth position is replaced by valine), leading to the formation of hemoglobin S. The consequences of this substitution are discussed in Chapter 8, Blood and Clotting.

Protein Folding

During protein synthesis, certain amino acid sequences favor the formation of secondary structures stabilized by hydrogen bonds between the amino group of one peptide bond and the carbonyl group of a nearby peptide bond. The two common motifs that are stable secondary structures of peptide chains are the α-helix and the β-sheet. In an α-helix, the peptide is coiled to form a single right-handed helix in which hydrogen bonds run parallel to the main axis of the helix (see **Figure 2.22b**). The carbonyl groups point in one direction of the helix while the amino groups point in the opposite direction. Another very common secondary motif is the β-sheet, also called β-pleated sheet. In this case, hydrogen bonds are formed between different sequences of amino acids that lie parallel to each other to form a sheet. The amino acid sequences may be oriented in the same direction, giving rise to a parallel configuration, or in the opposite direction, giving rise to an antiparallel configuration (see **Figure 2.22c**). In both cases, the hydrogen bonds remain on the same plane.

Secondary structures of large proteins are further assembled to form a tertiary structure. **Figure 2.22d** shows the representation of the protein angiogenin. Here β-sheets are represented by the blue arrows, while α-helices are in red. The process of folding and consolidating the α-helices and β-sheets of proteins and their connecting loops is a critical event for proper function. This process is assisted by chaperone proteins in the endoplasmic reticulum that manage the assembly of the final protein into the proper form and eliminate incorrect folding. Proper folding is such an important requirement for these complex structures that the endoplasmic reticulum has a detection system for improperly folded proteins. The unfolded protein response (UPR) is capable of stopping all protein production by cells and either restoring normal function

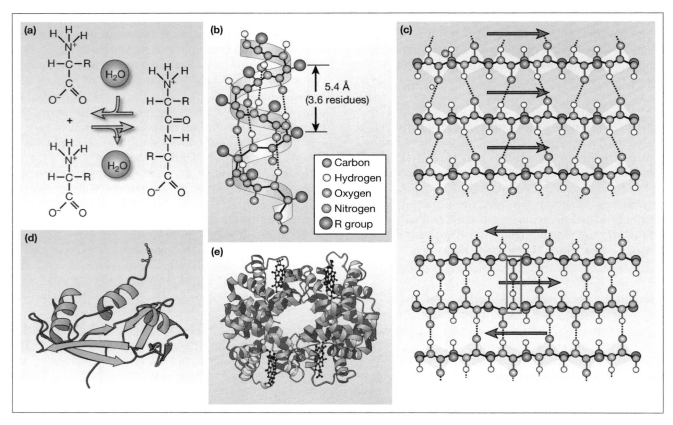

FIGURE 2.22 Protein structure: **(a)** peptide bond formation. Protein folding: **(b)** α-helix, **(c)** β-sheet in parallel configuration on the top and antiparallel configuration at the bottom, **(d)** structure of angiogenin (red = α-helices; blue arrows = β-sheets), and **(e)** structure of hemoglobin (gray = heme; blue = α-globin; red = β-globin).

or inducing apoptosis (programmed cell death) when protein misfolding is detected.

Much of the folding that occurs in formation of the tertiary structure of the protein is stabilized by interactions between amino acid side chains (R groups). A key determinant is the hydrophobic interactions between nonpolar R groups. Protein folding of intracellular and secreted globular proteins functions to position the hydrophobic regions in the inner core of the protein, while exposing the hydrophilic regions as a coat facing the aqueous environment of the intracellular fluid. This common strategy is known as stabilization by hydrophobic interactions (**Figure 2.23**). Additional stabilization comes from the attraction between charged amino acid residues, such as attractions between negatively charged glutamate and aspartate side chains and positively charged arginine, lysine, or histidine.

The structure of some proteins is complete at the tertiary level, and such proteins are called monomeric. Other proteins have an additional level of organization: a quaternary structure. In these cases, the functional unit is made of two or more proteins leading to the formation of a multimeric protein. For instance, dimers, trimers, and tetramers are made by assembling two,

three, and four protein subunits, respectively. An example is the oxygen-carrying protein hemoglobin, which is a tetrameric protein as it is made of four subunits. Each subunit consists of a globin protein and a heme, a nonprotein prosthetic group. The heme, represented in gray in **Figure 2.22e**, is a form of porphyrin that contains an iron atom in its center that is responsible for oxygen binding. There are two types of globin subunits in hemoglobin—α-globin and β-globin—represented in **Figure 2.22e** by blue and red, respectively. Because there are four subunits, each hemoglobin molecule can bind up to four oxygen molecules.

Protein Functions

Proteins perform an impressive number and variety of body functions: they allow movement, provide structural support, and work as hormones, enzymes, transporters, and more. Proteins such as myosin are able to convert the chemical energy stored in ATP into mechanical energy that is used for many types of cell and body movements. Other proteins are structural components that shape and support tissues and organs, such as the ground substance of connective tissue that is made of proteoglycans: proteins bound to

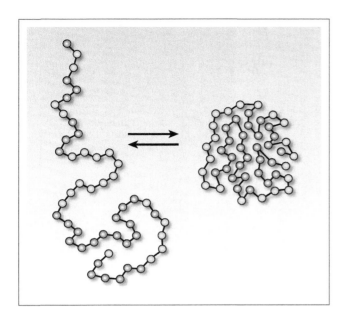

FIGURE 2.23 Hydrophobic attraction influences protein folding. Red circles indicate hydrophobic amino acids, and yellow circles indicate hydrophilic amino acids. After synthesis of the linear protein chain, it folds, bringing hydrophobic R groups to the core, and hydrophilic R groups form a surrounding shell. This conformation is stable in the aqueous environment of the intracellular or extracellular fluid.

named by adding the suffix *-ase* to the reaction they catalyze. For instance, glycogen synthase is the enzyme that combines glucose molecules to form glycogen. Many physiological reactions depend on the transfer of a phosphate group to a target molecule. The transferase enzymes catalyzing this phosphorylation reaction are called kinases and are a major focus of cellular physiology and pathophysiology.

Thought Questions

13. Can you name three different amino acids that are associated with specific body functions and identify those functions?

14. How does hydrogen bonding contribute to secondary protein structures?

15. What are some hydrophobic amino acids that might be found in the core of a folded protein?

16. What are some hydrophilic amino acids that might be found on the outside of a folded protein?

carbohydrate residues. Other proteins confer unique properties to the tissues. For example, elastin confers elasticity to walls of the alveoli in the lungs, allowing the elastic recoil that drives expiration. Collagen confers tensile strength to bones and connective tissues. Without collagen and other organic components, bones would be made of brittle hydroxyapatite crystals.

Protein hormones are synthesized by endocrine glands and released into the circulation, traveling to target cells, where they act by binding to membrane receptor proteins. Membrane receptors activate multistep signal transduction pathways inside the cell. Such pathways allow cells to finely regulate, amplify, and activate downstream targets. Plasma proteins include carriers needed to bind or transport hydrophobic compounds, or to carry substances with high affinity, as hemoglobin carries oxygen.

Other proteins are transmembrane transporters that allow the movement of water-soluble molecules across biological membranes. Ion channels and ion pumps are also integral membrane proteins that allow the movement of ions from one side of the membrane to the other, either according to their concentration gradient or using energy sources, respectively.

Enzymes are proteins that catalyze biochemical reactions. More than 6,000 enzymes are thought to be encoded by the human genome. Enzymes are often

NUCLEOTIDES AND NUCLEIC ACIDS
Structure of Bases, Nucleosides, and Nucleotides

Nucleic acids such as DNA and RNA are linear polymers of nucleotides, which in turn are made of a nitrogenous base, a pentose sugar, and one or more phosphate groups. Nitrogenous bases are classified into two categories: pyrimidines and purines (**Figure 2.24**). The former consists of a six-membered aromatic ring that contains two atoms of nitrogen. The latter is made of a pyrimidine interconnected with a five-membered aromatic ring containing two additional nitrogen atoms. The three pyrimidine bases are cytosine (C), uracil (U), and thymine (T). The two purine bases are adenine (A) and guanine (G). These bases share a similar general structure and are synthesized from a common progenitor.

When a nitrogenous base is bound to a pentose sugar, it is called a nucleoside, and when this is further bound to a phosphate, the resulting molecule is called a nucleotide. The specific names of the nucleosides and nucleotides are modified from the name of the bases. For instance, when adenine is bound to a sugar and to one phosphate, it is called adenosine monophosphate (AMP). If the adenosine is bound to two phosphate groups, it takes the name ADP, and if the phosphate groups are three, ATP. **Table 2.3** summarizes the nomenclature for the bases and nucleotides.

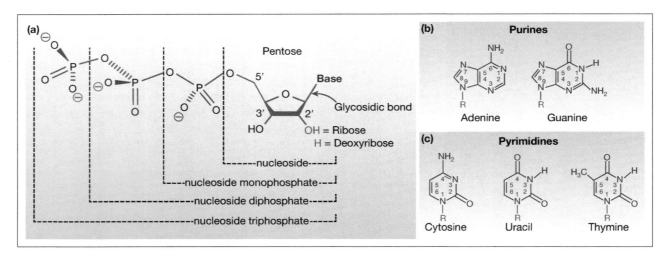

FIGURE 2.24 **(a)** A nucleotide is made up of a nitrogenous base either **(b)** purine or **(c)** pyrimidine, a ribose sugar, and one or more phosphates. The combination of base and sugar is referred to as a nucleoside. Note the two possible forms of the sugar based on the bond at the number 2 carbon. When this is a hydroxyl, it is ribose, when it is a hydrogen, it is deoxyribose. Ribonucleotides are used to synthesize RNA; deoxyribonucleotides are used to synthesize DNA.

TABLE 2.3 Nomenclature of Nitrogenous Bases

Class	Base	Symbols	Nucleoside With Ribose	Nucleoside With Deoxyribose	Nucleotide With Ribose	Nucleotide With Deoxyribose
Purines	Adenine	Ade, A	Adenosine	Deoxyadenosine	Adenosine phosphate	Deoxyadenosine phosphate
	Guanine	Gua, G	Guanosine	Deoxyguanosine	Guanosine phosphate	Deoxyguanosine phosphate
Pyrimidines	Cytosine	Cyt, C	Cytidine	Deoxycytidine	Cytidine phosphate	Deoxycytidine phosphate
	Uracil	Ura, U	Uridine	N/A	Uridine phosphate	N/A
	Thymine	Thy, T	N/A	Thymidine	N/A	Deoxythymidine phosphate

N/A, not applicable.

Individual Nucleotide Contributions to Cell Energy Transfers and Cell Signaling

ATP is the primary energy currency in the body. The phosphate groups are bound by high-energy bonds; thus, the release of a phosphoryl group from ATP is used to supply energy for many cellular functions and enzyme reactions. Note that neither the pentose nor the base is involved in these energy transfers.

Nucleotides also play a pivotal role in cell signaling cascades. Cyclic versions of both AMP and guanosine monophosphate (GMP) serve as intracellular second messengers. Historically, the first of these to be described was cyclic AMP (cAMP; see **Figure 2.25**). cAMP is formed when ATP undergoes a reaction that converts it into a ring structure. This reaction is catalyzed by adenylyl cyclase and is often activated in response to a ligand-receptor interaction on the plasma membrane. cAMP acts as an intracellular second messenger, turning on a signaling cascade, often through the activation of downstream kinases. Like cAMP, cyclic GMP can also serve as an intracellular second messenger. Finally, guanosine triphosphate (GTP) plays a key role in signal transduction as its hydrolysis to guanosine diphosphate (GDP) provides a timing switch for many membrane

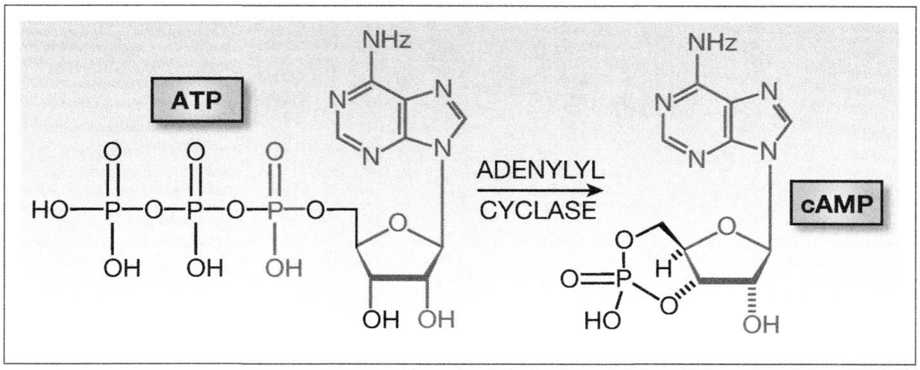

FIGURE 2.25 ATP serves as the main energy supply for cells. It is also the precursor of the second messenger, cAMP.
ATP, adenosine triphosphate; cAMP, cyclic adenosine monophosphate.

receptors. For this reason, many receptors in this category are referred to as G protein–coupled receptors.

Structural and Functional Aspects of RNA and DNA

Deoxyribonucleic acid (DNA) and ribonucleic acid (RNA) are the biomolecules responsible for genetic inheritance (DNA) and for ongoing cell function through protein synthesis (RNA). The human genome is made up of approximately 3 billion DNA base pairs of nucleotides arranged on 23 pairs of chromosomes, for a total of 46 chromosomes within the nucleus of each cell. DNA is produced by the enzyme DNA polymerase, which catalyzes the serial addition of deoxynucleotides to create the linear molecule. This process is called replication. RNA is produced by the enzyme RNA polymerase, which catalyzes the serial addition of ribonucleotides. This process is called transcription. These large molecules have a high degree of similarity in chemical structure but have significant differences as well. Bonds between the phosphate group of a nucleotide and the ribose sugar of an adjacent nucleotide form the nucleic acid backbone. In this structure, the bases project from the backbone.

The linear structures of DNA and RNA are similar in that they have a polarity that is based on the ability of oxygen atoms on the 3′ and 5′ carbons of the deoxyribose or ribose sugar to be the sites of synthesis reactions (**Figure 2.26**). Synthesis of either DNA or RNA occurs in the 5′ to 3′ direction, with the phosphate group of new nucleotides added onto the free 3′ end of the growing chain. Double-stranded DNA consists of two antiparallel strands such that the 5′ end of one strand aligns with the 3′ end of the opposite strand (**Figure 2.27**).

DNA and RNA also differ in composition and structural organization, as well as in function and cellular location. Compared with the ribose sugar of RNA

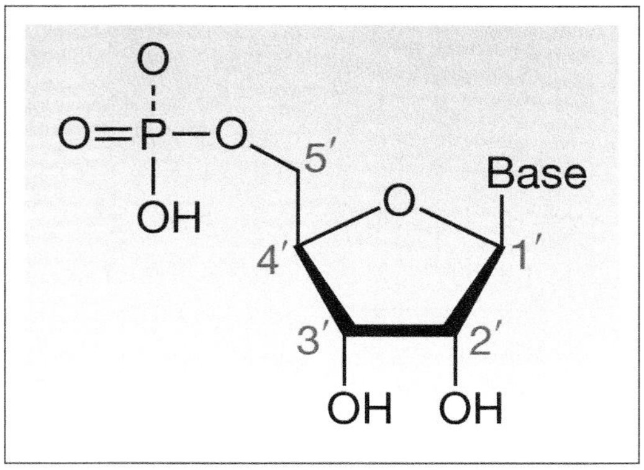

FIGURE 2.26 The carbons of the ribose (shown here) or deoxyribose sugar are numbered from 1′ (one prime) to 5′. Phosphate groups are attached to the 5′ carbon. Polymerization of nucleotides during DNA or RNA synthesis occurs by bonding the phosphate group of the incoming nucleotide to the 3′ end of the chain.

nucleotides, the deoxyribose of DNA lacks one oxygen atom (see **Figure 2.24**). Another difference between DNA and RNA is that cytosine and thymine are the pyrimidines found in DNA whereas cytosine and uracil are found in RNA. In DNA, two strands are connected through hydrogen bonds between complementary bases (see **Figure 2.27**), with the resulting molecular structure resembling a double helix. RNA, on the other hand, is synthesized as a single strand. RNA can assume different shapes; for example, messenger RNA is generally a linear molecule, whereas transfer RNA has a looped structure.

Functionally, DNA acts as a repository of genetic information in cells as it stores all the information necessary to produce proteins—information that is completely duplicated before a cell can divide by the process of

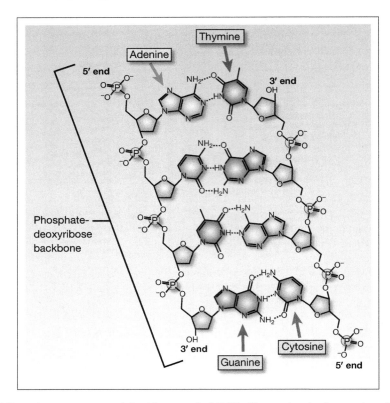

FIGURE 2.27 A short segment of double-stranded DNA illustrating hydrogen bonding between complementary bases adenine and thymine (joined by two hydrogen bonds), and guanine and cytosine (joined by three hydrogen bonds). This alignment is favored by the antiparallel arrangement of the sugar phosphate backbones: The 5′ to 3′ orientation of one strand lines up against the 3′ to 5′ orientation of the complementary strand.

mitosis, which then passes identical genetic information on to both daughter cells. In addition, half of a parent's genome is passed on to offspring through the meiotic division of germ cells, producing egg and sperm. RNA has the major role of transporting the information stored in DNA to the ribosomes where protein synthesis occurs.

The Principle of Complementary Base-Pairing

The bases on one strand of the DNA make hydrogen bonds with the bases on the other strand. Each purine bonds with a pyrimidine: guanine always makes three hydrogen bonds with cytosine, and adenine always makes two hydrogen bonds with thymine. Although individual hydrogen bonds lack strength, the billions of hydrogen bonds holding together the antiparallel strands of DNA give it extraordinary structural stability. During the process of gene transcription, the double-stranded DNA separates, allowing access to transcription factors and to the RNA polymerase, which catalyzes the production of a messenger RNA. This product is synthesized using DNA as a template to establish the nucleotide sequence and synthesize a complementary RNA sequence.

 Thought Questions

17. What are some of the roles individual nucleotides play in cell function?

18. Which DNA base pairs participate in complementary base-pairing through hydrogen bond formation?

CONCLUSION: PHENYLKETONURIA REVISITED

This chapter lays the foundations for understanding the molecular underpinning of human disease. The opening clinical example describes PKU, a disease that is inherited in an autosomal-recessive fashion. In autosomal-recessive disorders, individuals who inherit two copies of the disease-conferring gene develop the disease. Patients with PKU carry a

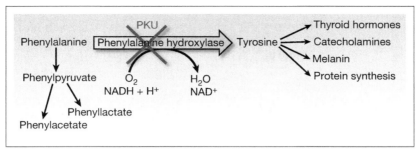

FIGURE 2.28 Phenylalanine metabolism.

mutation in the gene coding for the enzyme phenylalanine hydroxylase. This enzyme is responsible for adding a hydroxyl group to phenylalanine, thereby converting it into tyrosine.

Patients with PKU develop hyperphenylalaninemia, which means they accumulate high levels of the amino acid phenylalanine. At the same time, patients may not have enough tyrosine; thus, all the metabolites downstream from this amino acid may be decreased. This explains the hypopigmentation seen in the child described in the opening example. Melanin is produced from tyrosine. The excess phenylalanine is shunted into a secondary metabolic pathway that would normally have a minor role. This pathway converts phenylalanine into phenylpyruvate and then into phenylacetone phenylacetate and phenyllactate. These metabolites accumulate in the blood and are excreted in the urine; phenylacetone phenylacetate is responsible for the mousy odor of the child's urine.

Newborn screening for PKU became widely available in the 1960s in the United States and many other countries.[2] In fact, it was one of the first disorders in the class of *inborn errors of metabolism* to be identified and screened. Early intervention is key to improving outcomes, as infants maintained on a low-protein/low-phenylalanine diet can avoid many of the cognitive delays that occurred in infants prior to screening. People with PKU are normally treated with a strict dietary regimen that limits intake of foods containing phenylalanine to prevent hyperphenylalaninemia and the associated mental retardation. The mechanisms whereby hyperphenylalaninemia causes mental retardation are still being elucidated. As the opening clinical example highlights, disease pathogenesis often is caused by events that take place at the level of the genes, with repercussions for metabolic pathways. **Figure 2.28** illustrates this process in PKU.

KEY POINTS

- The body is composed of molecules that are made by chemical bonds between individual atoms. Properties of atoms depend on their atomic weight and structure. The nucleus of an atom is made up of protons and neutrons with a surrounding shell of electrons. Electrons are arranged in orbitals, and atomic properties depend on the extent to which the outermost orbital shell (the valence shell) is occupied by electrons.
- Biomolecules are formed when covalent bonds are made between atoms and molecules, building up from simple to very complex macromolecular structures.
- The elements found in highest amounts in biomolecules are carbon, hydrogen, oxygen, and nitrogen. Several other elements are found in lesser amounts. Elements that are stabilized by

losing or gaining electrons are called ions, and several ions have distinct biological roles.
- Covalent bonds in biomolecules can be characterized as nonpolar or polar. In nonpolar bonds, there is a relatively equal sharing of electrons between the two bonding atoms. In polar bonds, one atom exerts a greater attraction on the shared electrons than the other atom. Because of the unequal sharing, partial charges develop within the molecule such that one atom carries a partial negative charge (referred to as δ^-) and the other a partial positive charge (referred to as δ^+). In biomolecules, structures containing only carbon and hydrogen are nonpolar, whereas structures containing hydrogen bonded to oxygen or nitrogen are often polar.
- Water is the most abundant molecule in the body, and it is the polar solvent of the extracellular and the intracellular fluid. Substances that

are charged (ions) or polar are soluble in water and are referred to as hydrophilic. Substances that are nonpolar are not soluble in water and are referred to as hydrophobic.

- Biomolecules found in the body consist of carbons bonded to hydrogen, oxygen, nitrogen, phosphorus, sulfur, and other atoms to lesser degrees.
- Carbohydrates consist only of carbon, hydrogen, and oxygen. These are polar molecules and include simple sugars (monosaccharides), most containing five to six carbons. The most abundant carbohydrate is glucose, used as the primary energy source for many tissues, and stored in the form of glycogen.
- Lipid molecules contain regions that are very hydrophobic, consisting of carbons bonded to hydrogen. Major body lipids are triglycerides, which represent a major body energy store; phospholipids, which make up cell plasma membranes; and cholesterol, which contributes to plasma membrane structure and is the basis for synthesis of bile acids and steroid hormones.
- Amino acids contain carbon, hydrogen, oxygen, nitrogen, and sulfur. Individual amino acids have properties conferred by their unique side chains. Amino acids are the building blocks of proteins—chains of amino acids linked by peptide bonds. Proteins are the most structurally diverse biomolecules in the body and serve innumerable structural and functional roles.
- Nucleotides contain carbon, hydrogen, oxygen, nitrogen, and phosphorus and serve several roles in cell function, most notably the critical cell energy compound ATP. Nucleotides are the building blocks of the nucleic acids DNA and RNA.

REFERENCES

1. U.S. Food and Drug Administration. Final determination regarding partially hydrogenated oils. https://www.fda.gov/Food/IngredientsPackagingLabeling/FoodAdditivesIngredients/ucm449162.htm. Published May 14, 2018. Accessed August 10, 2018.
2. NIH Consensus Development Program. *Phenylketonuria: Screening and Management.* 2000;17(3):1–27. https://consensus.nih.gov/2000/2000phenylketonuria113html.htm. Accessed August 10, 2018.

SUGGESTED RESOURCE

Marieb EN, Hoehn K. Chemistry comes alive. In: Marieb EN, Hoehn K, eds. *Human Anatomy & Physiology.* 11th ed. Boston, MA: Pearson Education; 2019:23–59.

3

MOLECULAR BIOLOGY, GENETICS, AND GENETIC DISEASES

Sheila A. Alexander and Michael J. Groves

THE CLINICAL CONTEXT

We begin Chapter 3 where Chapter 2 ended, with phenylketonuria (PKU)—a genetic disease inherited in an autosomal dominant fashion. What is a genetic disease? What is the significance of a pattern of inheritance? The ability to rapidly sequence DNA, to understand the heritability and impact of DNA changes (mutations) on health and homeostasis, and to appreciate the many factors regulating gene expression has greatly expanded our understanding of molecular biology and genetics.

Current research studies are investigating the ways in which genetic variability contributes to well-known, but rare, single gene disorders such as cystic fibrosis and PKU, as well as the more common multifactorial disorders such as atherosclerosis and type 2 diabetes mellitus. Research is also being conducted to identify genetic variability impacting healthcare interventions, including the evidence-based treatment of genetic disorders, genetics-based treatment of both rare and common diseases, and pharmacogenomics. Each area of exploration continues to expand in complexity, but this chapter discusses some fundamental concepts to support a clear understanding of basic principles in genetics, genomics, and epigenetics.

INFORMATION TRANSMISSION WITHIN CELLS AND BETWEEN CELL AND HUMAN GENERATIONS

There are two primary roles for the nucleic acids DNA and RNA in eukaryotic cells. On a minute-to-minute basis, cells synthesize proteins based on the processes of gene transcription and messenger RNA (mRNA) translation. These proteins are often unique to cell type and are tightly linked to structure and function of differentiated cells. On the other hand, cells age and must be replaced with new cells that are specialized to take up the structure and function of their precursors. Furthermore, generation of descendants requires that cells be duplicated many times over in the process of sexual reproduction, fertilization, and embryogenesis. Meiosis produces gametes (germ cells) that are haploid, with only one copy of each chromosome and containing only half of the genetic information from each parent. In fertilization, two haploid germ cells combine, producing the normal diploid cell with two copies of each chromosome. This method of reproduction adds to overall genetic diversity by bringing together information from two genetically different parents. DNA contains the cell's genetic information in a very stable, double-stranded molecule that can be faithfully replicated and used to produce daughter cells with the identical information present in the parent cell. DNA also provides the template for transcription of RNA needed for new protein synthesis by translation (**Figure 3.1**).

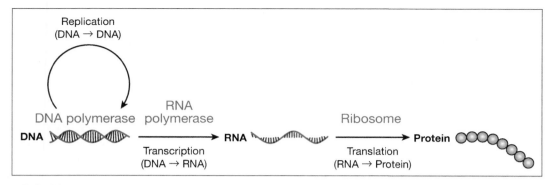

FIGURE 3.1 Nucleic acid functions. The role of nucleic acids in the transmission of genetic information and instructing protein synthesis. DNA is replicated prior to cell division, providing daughter cells with identical genetic information. The genes found in DNA are the instructions transcribed into RNA and used as a template for translation of proteins.

At various steps in the processes of germ cell formation and cell reproduction, changes in DNA sequence can occur. When such variations—also known as *mutations*—occur, cell programs often detect and correct them. However, over evolutionary time, some mutations turned out to be beneficial in certain environments, and they were retained. Others were small changes in a single base, termed *single nucleotide polymorphisms*, and they had little biological impact, so they were also retained. Although the human genome project found that humans have genomes that are 99.9% identical, the remaining 0.1% accounts for differences such as body features, disease susceptibility or resistance, and a multitude of other aspects of human function in health and disease. Gene mapping studies continue to determine these associations with the goal of providing ever more precise personalized health care.

DNA STRUCTURE

Continuing the thread of small molecules building to macromolecules, as described in Chapter 2, Chemical and Biochemical Foundations, DNA is a polymer of nucleotides and consists of a series of bases attached to a sugar–phosphate backbone, making up a strand with the bases projecting away from the backbone. Of the four DNA bases, two are larger purines (adenine, guanine) and two are smaller pyrimidines (cytosine, thymine). DNA is a double-stranded molecule held together by hydrogen bonds between complementary bases projecting from each backbone. The backbones have a polarity based on the free ends of the chain, one of which is a phosphate attached to the 5′ (five prime) carbon of the ribose sugar, and the other of which is a hydroxyl attached to the 3′ carbon of the ribose sugar. For correct base pairing and hydrogen bond formation, the backbones of double-stranded DNA are antiparallel to each other, with the 5′ end of one strand opposite to the 3′ end of the complementary strand.

When properly aligned, adenine makes two hydrogen bonds with its complementary base thymine, while cytosine makes three hydrogen bonds with its complementary base guanine (**Figure 3.2**). The comparative weakness of these hydrogen bonds allows the strands of DNA to separate and rejoin with relative ease during the replication process as well as the transcription portion of protein synthesis. Based on the complementary base pairing, the strand twists during formation, assuming the famous double helical structure.

In human cells, the DNA is found in 46 chromosomes—two copies each of 22 autosomes (1–22) and two sex chromosomes, XX (in females) and XY (in males). The more than 3 billion base pairs (bp) of DNA are distributed in chromosomes ranging from the longest, chromosome 1 (almost 250 million bp) to the shortest, chromosome 21 (54 million bp).[1] Mitochondria have their own DNA, about 16,000 bp worth.

These long DNA strands could be subject to tangling and breaking if not organized in some fashion. The first level of DNA organization involves wrapping around small protein balls called *histones*. Histones serve as an anchor around which DNA can coil but are also active structures in DNA replication, transcription, and translation. As histones wrap around the DNA, the entire structure further coils. Prior to mitosis, chromosomes appear in their most tightly packaged form (**Figure 3.3**).

The 46 chromosomes of each individual form that individual's genome. Among the approximately 20,000 to 25,000 genes in each person's genome are large sections that contain noncoding regions. These regions, which lack protein-encoding genes, were originally thought to be areas of "junk DNA." However, ongoing investigations are finding that these regions can impact gene expression or RNA and protein stability.

Although there is considerable standardization of the base sequence across the human population, there is also variability in that sequence, with up to 0.6% of the genome varying between individuals. These differences

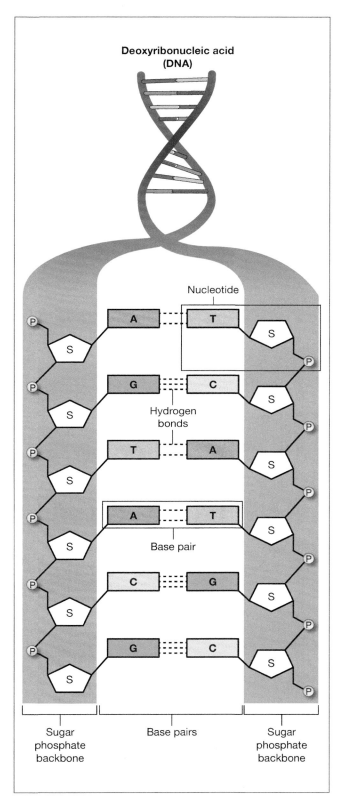

Deoxyribonucleic acid (DNA)

Nucleotide

Hydrogen bonds

Base pair

Sugar phosphate backbone

Base pairs

Sugar phosphate backbone

FIGURE 3.2 DNA structure. DNA is a double-stranded molecule twisted into a helix and held together by complementary base pairing. Hydrogen bonds hold together complementary adenine–thymine (A–T) pairs (two hydrogen bonds) and cytosine–guanine (C–G) pairs (three hydrogen bonds).

account for our uniqueness as individuals. Additionally, while we share over 99% of our genes with one another, we also share about 98% with chimpanzees, 92% with mice, 90% with cats, 85% with zebrafish, and 84% with dogs.

MOLECULAR BIOLOGY OF THE CELL AND DNA REPLICATION

The Cell Cycle

The cells of the body are divided into somatic cells and gametes. Somatic cells divide in a process called *mitosis*, the endpoint of which is the creation of two daughter cells that are genetically identical to the parent cell. The parent cell and the two daughter cells each have 46 chromosomes, which is referred to as the diploid, or $2n$, state. The sex cells divide through meiosis, a process that is similar to mitosis but occurs in two separate stages termed *meiosis I* and *meiosis II*. The endpoint of meiosis is the creation of four daughter cells that have been reduced to the haploid state ($1n$) of 23 chromosomes each. When fertilization occurs, the resulting cell then returns to the diploid state and contains 23 chromosomes from the male and 23 chromosomes from the female.

The cell cycle consists of four stages beginning immediately after a cell divides (**Figure 3.4**). The first three stages are collectively referred to as the interphase and include the G_1 or gap 1 phase, the S or synthesis phase, and the G_2 or gap 2 phase. During the G_1 phase the newly divided cell grows, synthesizes additional organelles, and engages in whatever the function of that cell might be. Some cell types have limited or no ability to divide once they have differentiated (including many neurons and muscle cells). They are then considered to be in a G_0 state. The G_1 checkpoint is a point of delay until appropriate signals indicate that the cell can proceed. With these signals, including availability of needed DNA precursors and synthetic enzymes, the G_1 checkpoint permits the cell to enter the S phase. During the S phase, all of the DNA is copied in the process of replication. After DNA replication, the cell enters the G_2 phase. During this phase, the cell continues to grow and perform its essential function as it also prepares for cellular division or the mitotic or M phase. The G_2 checkpoint ensures that the cell's DNA has replicated correctly and enzymatically fixes any errors in replication that may have occurred. When the verification and repair process is successfully completed, the cell proceeds to the M phase. If the DNA has become too damaged and cannot be repaired, the cell is stimulated to undergo apoptosis and is destroyed.

Mitosis

Mitosis proceeds in four stages, ending in two identical daughter cells (**Figure 3.5**). During prophase, the chromosomes condense and appear in paired sets referred

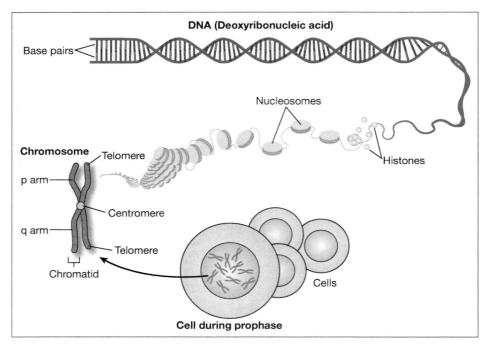

FIGURE 3.3 DNA packing. DNA strands are compacted by winding around histone proteins. Further condensation can be achieved by further coiling and packing, as occurs after DNA replication and before mitosis, when chromosomes appear in their most condensed form. p arm refers to the short arm of the chromosome, q arm refers to the long arm.

to as sister chromatids. Spindle fibers form and attach to the kinetochores of the chromatids, and the nuclear envelope disintegrates. Prophase is followed by metaphase during which the sister chromatids align along the equator of the cell and the attachment of the spindle fibers is checked. During anaphase, the spindles pull back from the cell equator; hence, sister chromatids separate and migrate toward the poles of the cell. In telophase, the nuclear envelope re-forms around the

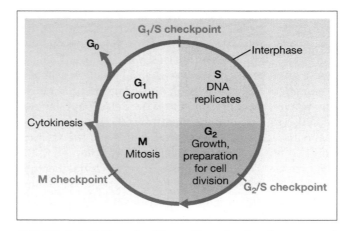

FIGURE 3.4 Cell cycle. The cell cycle showing gap and mitotic phases.

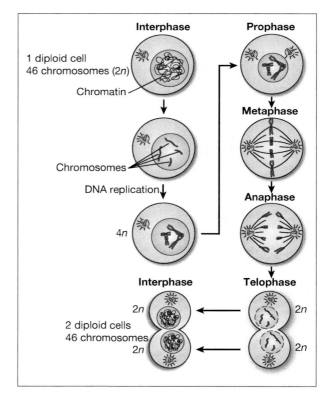

FIGURE 3.5 Mitosis. The steps in mitosis; two representative homologous chromosomes are shown.

chromosomes at each pole and the chromosomes begin to decondense into chromatin. Telophase is immediately followed by cytokinesis during which the plasma membrane invaginates and completes division, surrounding the two new cells, each having a nearly equal portion of the parent cell's cytoplasm.

Meiosis

Meiosis occurs in two stages, meiosis I and meiosis II, and each stage includes the same phases as in mitosis: prophase, metaphase, anaphase, and telophase (**Figure 3.6** and **Box 3.1**). In males, the progression through both stages is continuous and spermatogenesis

---

BOX 3.1
Steps in Meiosis

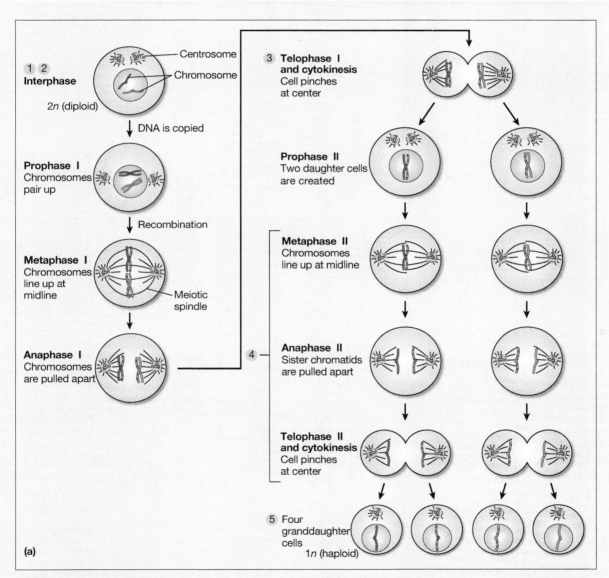

FIGURE 3.6 (a) Steps in meiosis.

1. During phase G_1, the cell readies itself for S phase. The representative chromosome pair shown consists of one chromosome inherited from mother and one chromosome inherited from father.

2. DNA is copied, similar to S phase of mitosis. The duplicated homologous chromosomes (sister chromatids) are adjacent, and because of their similarities, crossing over can occur with segments swapped between a maternal

(continued)

BOX 3.1 (*continued*)
Steps in Meiosis

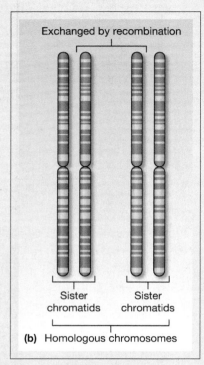

Exchanged by recombination

Sister chromatids

Sister chromatids

(b) Homologous chromosomes

FIGURE 3.6 (b) Recombination. Recombination of portions of homologous chromosomes can occur before the first meiotic division.

and paternal version (**Figure 3.6b**) of the chromosome. This process of homologous recombination increases genetic diversity.

3. At telophase I and cytokinesis, the new versions of the chromosome pairs are separated into daughter cells.

4. A second cell division occurs for each daughter cell. This reduces the chromosome number to 1, with a random chance of the gamete having:

   ○ A paternal chromosome
   ○ A maternal chromosome
   ○ A chromosome that has some combination of maternal and paternal contributed segments

5. Mature eggs and sperm have 23 chromosomes and are termed *haploid*. When fertilization occurs, the resulting zygote has 46 chromosomes (diploid) and cell division (embryogenesis) begins.

occurs from early puberty through late adulthood. In females, meiosis begins during the first 6 months of fetal development and is interrupted at prophase of meiosis I. At the time of ovulation, each oocyte completes meiosis I and again stops during prophase of meiosis II. When an oocyte is fertilized, that cell rapidly completes meiosis II. The process of meiosis is not completed in oocytes that fail to be released during ovulation or are not fertilized.

The principal function of meiosis is reductive in nature (see **Box 3.1**). The product of meiosis in males is four mature spermatids. In females, each meiotic division results in a large oocyte in which most of the cytoplasm is reserved and a second cell with virtually no cytoplasm. This smaller cell is referred to as a polar body and it is unable to engage in reproduction. During the female reproductive years, approximately 400 primary oocytes will mature and become ova.

DNA Replication

Replication of DNA takes place during the S phase of the cell cycle, and there is no difference in the

replication process in somatic cells or gametes. The ability of DNA to replicate depends on the unwinding of the double helix, the presence of the raw materials to make new strands (free nucleotides), and the activity of enzymes that construct the new strands of DNA. Replication does not occur in a linear fashion but rather occurs simultaneously at multiple points along the length of the DNA molecule. The simultaneous replication process permits the strand to replicate very rapidly, given the billions of base pairs that need to be lined up and joined. This multisite replication also requires the connecting or ligation of DNA segments as well as the action of topoisomerases, which work to prevent supercoiling of the DNA helix.

As noted earlier, at either end of the backbone of a DNA molecule, there is a phosphate bonded to the deoxyribose 5′ carbon on one end and a hydroxyl bonded to the deoxyribose 3′ carbon on the other end. On the opposite strand, the ends are reversed. In essence, the two strands of DNA run in opposite directions, referred to as antiparallel orientation.

By convention, the 5′ end of the upper strand is presented on the left with the complementary 3′ end of the lower strand on the left. An example of a short section of DNA is presented here:

5′-ATTCGCGATTGC-3′
3′-TAAGCGCTAACG-5′

Note that the 5′ and 3′ ends are arranged in a "head-to-toe" orientation and that the upper and lower strands are complementary. These conditions dictate the process by which DNA is replicated.

The replication process begins with DNA helicase unwinding the double helix of DNA. As the DNA unwinds, the downstream portion of the molecule is subject to supercoiling, which may result in the coils looping back on each other and either breaking the molecule or halting the process of unwinding. DNA topoisomerases have the task of cutting the DNA molecule at precise locations. This allows the coils to unwind by passing through each other. The topoisomerases then reattach the nucleotides and the process of unwinding and replication can safely continue.

DNA must be constructed beginning with a 5′ end and adding nucleotides sequentially to the 3′ end. Therefore, the template strand is "read" beginning at the 3′ end. Primase creates RNA primers that are necessary to begin replication. DNA polymerase binds to the primer and builds a new strand of DNA that is complementary to the existing strand. The two strands of the original DNA molecule, once separated, are referred to as either the leading strand or the lagging strand. The leading strand has the 3′ position of the phosphate molecule free while the lagging strand has the 5′ position free. On the leading strand, DNA replication proceeds uninterrupted, in a continuous process, reading the existing strand from the 3′ end and building the new strand from the 5′ prime end (**Figure 3.7**).

Construction of the lagging strand is somewhat more complex. The process of reading the lagging strand is discontinuous. The lagging strand is a complementary image of the leading strand with the 3′ and 5′ ends of the lagging strand reversed. Still, DNA polymerase can only read the DNA from the 3′ end. On the lagging strand, primase lays down a primer a short distance from the end of the strand. DNA polymerase reads the strand from the 3′ end and builds the new strand from the 5′ end. When the end of the strand is reached, primase travels farther down the strand and creates a new primer. Reading and building of the new strand begins again, proceeding in the 3′ to 5′ direction. When the newly constructed strand meets the prior segment, the primer is removed, and DNA ligase connects the two segments. These segments are called *Okazaki fragments*. When the process is complete, the result is two identical DNA molecules each having one original strand and one replicated strand. This mode of synthesis is referred to as semiconservative because the template strand is conserved from the original molecule, now bonded to the newly synthesized complementary strand.

Exonucleolytic Proofreading

Essential to the successful replication of DNA is the ability to repair the infrequent errors that occur during this process. DNA polymerases are responsible for the process of DNA repair during the replication process. These enzymes proofread the sequence of nucleotides and, when an error is located, excise the incorrect nucleotide and replace it with the correct one. During the initial process of replication, approximately one error occurs in every 100,000 replicated nucleotides. DNA repair mechanisms, proofreading and nucleotide selection, reduce this error rate to approximately one in 10 million nucleotides during the replication process. Postreplication corrective processes further reduce this error rate to about one error per 1 billion nucleotides (**Figure 3.8**).

RNA FUNCTION AND PROTEIN SYNTHESIS

The principal function of most genes is to produce one or more proteins. The synthesis of proteins includes several steps and uses a different nucleic acid to do this work. RNA is essential to the process of protein synthesis. The steps in this process include transcription of a gene or a portion of a gene into pre-mRNA, post-transcriptional processing to create mRNA, transport of the mRNA out of the cell nucleus, translation of the mRNA into a polypeptide chain of amino acids, and finally, post-translational processing to create a finished, functional protein.

There are several types of RNAs, serving different cell functions. Globally, differences exist between RNA and DNA. First, the sugar ribose replaces deoxyribose in the RNA molecule. RNA is usually a single-stranded molecule in contrast to the double-stranded DNA. DNA is a linear molecule that becomes coiled, whereas some RNAs assume different shapes. In RNA, the pyrimidine base uracil replaces the thymine found in DNA. DNA is found in the nucleus and mitochondria and functions as the major control of cell heredity, as well as the template for protein production. RNA is found in the cytoplasm and also in the nucleus—many forms have been identified, and their functions are still being explored. Some of the best-understood RNAs are listed in **Box 3.2**. Finally, RNA is a much less stable molecule than DNA; mRNA, in particular, degrades quickly under certain conditions. It tends to serve its purpose, such as in protein synthesis, and then is degraded by enzymes back down into its component nucleotides.

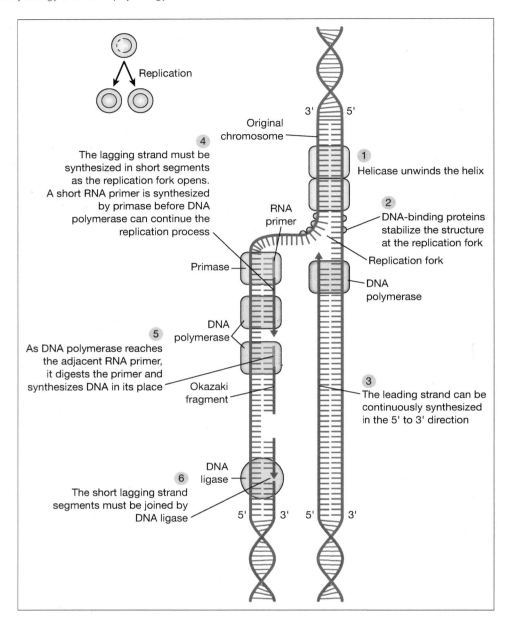

FIGURE 3.7 DNA replication. Replication begins when double strands separate at replication origin sites. With the actions of several proteins and enzymes, including DNA polymerase, each existing strand serves as a template for the synthesis of a new antiparallel strand. The sequence of the new strand lines up complementary bases to the template strand, allowing re-formation of the double-stranded structure as replication ends.

Transcription

In order for transcription to occur there must be a DNA template that gives start, sequence, and stop instructions to the RNA polymerase that manages the process. The gene is the DNA template and consists of three parts: (a) a promoter region, (b) the coding region, and (c) the terminator region. The promoter region instructs RNA polymerase where to begin transcription as well as which strand of DNA is to be transcribed. Generally, the promoter region is not translated into part of the amino acid chain. The coding region is that portion of the gene that will give rise to the polypeptide chain and the eventual protein. The terminator region instructs the RNA polymerase where to stop transcribing, and this region is usually transcribed into the pre-RNA.

The process of transcribing the strand of RNA is similar to replication of DNA. RNA polymerase adds complementary nucleotides to the growing RNA strand, substituting uracil for thymine (**Figures 3.9** and **3.10**).

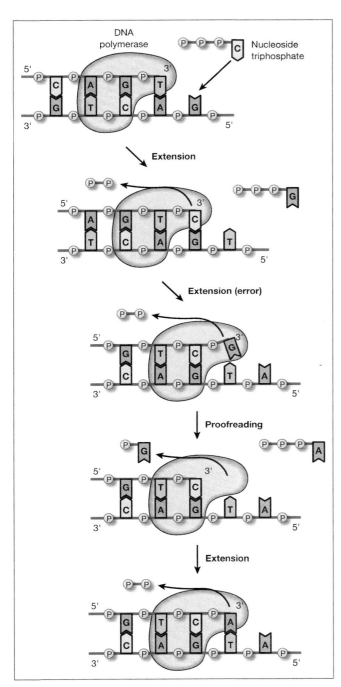

FIGURE 3.8 Proofreading. Proofreading during DNA replication is able to identify mismatched bases and remove them before moving further down the strand. This greatly reduces spontaneous mutation formation.

The strand of DNA being copied is referred to as the *template strand* and the other strand of DNA as the *nontemplate strand*. Because of the complementary nature of DNA and RNA, the RNA molecule will be the same sequence of nucleotides as the nontemplate strand—with the exception of uracil being substituted for thymine in the RNA. Once the entire strand of

pre-RNA is transcribed, the molecule must undergo post-transcriptional processing before it is ready for use.

Post-Transcriptional Processing

Genes contain regions that code for the amino acid sequence that produces a protein and regions that do not code for amino acids. The coding regions are referred to as *exons* (expressed regions), whereas the noncoding regions are called *introns*. Although introns are noncoding, they are not inert. Introns play essential roles in the regulation of gene expression and mRNA transport. An essential step in the processing of pre-RNA is the removal of introns from the molecule. Once the introns have been removed, what is left are the coding exons. The human genome contains somewhere between 20,000 and 25,000 genes and yet is capable of producing several hundred thousand different proteins. One mechanism that makes this possible is the alternate splicing of exons during post-transcription processing. In alternate splicing, different proteins are produced by splicing together different combination of exons (**Figures 3.10** and **3.11**).

Once the introns have been excised and the required exons spliced together, a 5′ cap is added to one end of the molecule and a poly-A tail to the other. The 5′ cap is used as an anchor for the ribosome to attach to the mRNA to begin the process of translation. Very often the DNA molecule is transcribed much farther down the sequence than is necessary to create the required mRNA. During post-transcriptional processing, these extra nucleotides are cleaved from the pre-RNA and a sequence of adenine bases is added to the end of the pre-RNA. This poly-A tail may be as long as 250 adenine bases. The tail adds to the stability of the mRNA molecule, extending the time it takes before the molecule is degraded by enzymes in the cytoplasm. Post-transcriptional processing results in a mature mRNA molecule that is now ready to move to the cytoplasm and begin the next stage of protein synthesis, translation.

Regulation of Transcription

Gene expression and thus protein production within individual cells is determined in part by the type of cell. For example, β cells in the pancreas express the insulin gene to produce the hormone insulin, while renal proximal tubule cells produce the many membrane protein transporters responsible for reabsorption of glomerular filtrate. Of the 20,000 or so genes capable of producing 60,000 to 70,000 proteins in the body, each tissue and cell type has its own expression profile. This is partly regulated by epigenetic changes to the chromosomes discussed later, and also by varying levels of transcription factors. Certain genes are always being transcribed (e.g., the genes for albumin and clotting factors are always produced by liver

BOX 3.2
Examples of RNAs

- **mRNA (*messenger RNA*)**
  Transcribed from a gene within the chromatin and used as the template for protein synthesis

- **tRNA (*transfer RNA*)**
  A carrier molecule able to recognize triplet codons of mRNA and carrying an amino acid to contribute to a growing protein chain

- **rRNA (*ribosomal RNA*)**
  Large protein/RNA complexes comprising small and large ribosomal subunits—the site of protein synthesis

- **snRNA (*small nuclear RNA*)**
  Splicing of pre-mRNA as one component of a spliceosome complex

- **siRNA (*small interfering RNA*) and miRNA (*micro-RNA*)**
  Short segments of RNA complementary to cellular mRNAs
  Capable of binding to mRNA and accelerating its degradation, reducing expression of the associated protein
  Can be used as a form of genetic therapy

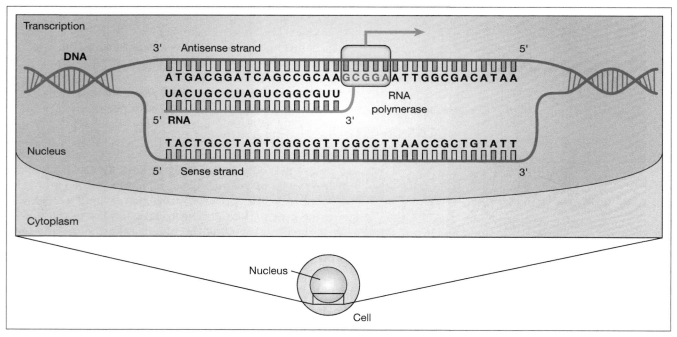

FIGURE 3.9 Transcription. In transcription, RNA polymerase synthesizes a complementary RNA strand to a gene—a DNA segment coding for a protein. The result is a pre-mRNA molecule complementary to the length of the gene.
pre-mRNA, pre-messenger RNA.

cells), whereas others wait on specific signals (B lymphocytes must be stimulated by their specific antigen and by factors from helper T lymphocytes before synthesizing and secreting the antibodies that target that specific antigen). Much physiology at the cellular level is conducted by altered gene expression patterns to maintain homeostasis, as directed by many hormones and other cell signaling molecules.

Translation

Translation is the mechanism by which the sequence of nucleotides in mRNA is interpreted and a chain of amino acids is produced. During this phase of protein synthesis, two additional types of RNA are introduced to the process. Ribosomes are factories made of ribosomal RNA (rRNA) and proteins. These complexes read the mRNA message and synthesize protein chains

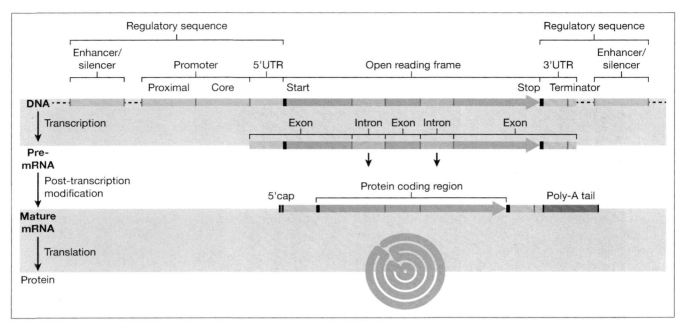

FIGURE 3.10 Post-transcriptional processing. The pre-mRNA is shortened by spliceosomes that remove introns, and polymerases that rejoin the exons that will ultimately be expressed. A 5′ cap and poly-A tail are added before the mature mRNA moves to the cytoplasm.
pre-mRNA, pre-messenger RNA; UTR, untranslated region.

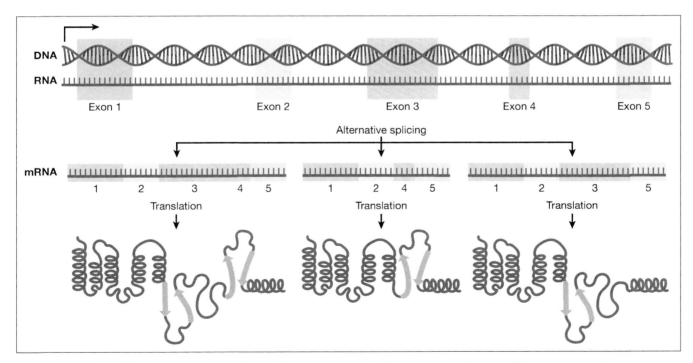

FIGURE 3.11 Alternative splicing. Multiple exons coded for by a gene allow for different potential protein products to be translated, in a mix-and-match fashion.
mRNA, messenger RNA.
Source: Courtesy of the Human Genome Institute.

based on that message. Transfer RNA (tRNA) carries amino acids, one by one, to the ribosome where each amino acid is added to the growing polypeptide chain (**Figure 3.12**). In order for this process to work, the tRNA must have a mechanism for recognizing which amino acid is to be delivered to the ribosome, and the ribosome must have some way of knowing when to begin and end translation.

The Genetic Code and Reading Frame

During the process of translation, the mRNA molecule is read as a series of three nucleotide units called *codons* (**Figure 3.13**). The four available RNA bases—adenine, uracil, guanine, and cytosine—can combine any order, giving 64 possible combinations of three bases. Given that there are 20 amino acids, it stands to reason that more than one codon will code for the same amino acid (**Figure 3.14**). Three of these codons serve as stop codons, which signal the ribosome to cease translation. The stop codons are UAA, UAG, and UGA. A single codon, AUG, serves as the start codon and signals the beginning of translation. The AUG codon codes for the amino

acid methionine, which is the beginning amino acid for virtually all human proteins, although it is often removed during post-translational processing. This reading frame is subject to disruption via several of the genetic mutation mechanisms discussed later.

The Ribosome

The ribosome is a complex structure containing a variety of proteins as well as thousands of nucleotides in the form of rRNA. The structure is composed of a large ribosomal unit and a small ribosomal unit that work together to clamp around the mRNA and construct the polypeptide chain of amino acids. The ribosome is also a very plentiful structure with a single cell having as many as 20,000 or more ribosomes.

Translation Processes

To initiate translation, the ribosome attaches to the 5′ cap of the mRNA and travels down the mRNA molecule until the AUG start codon is encountered. The tRNA with the anticodon UAC aligns with the codon and leaves its methionine to begin the peptide sequence. The mRNA continues to pass through the ribosome, and the tRNA

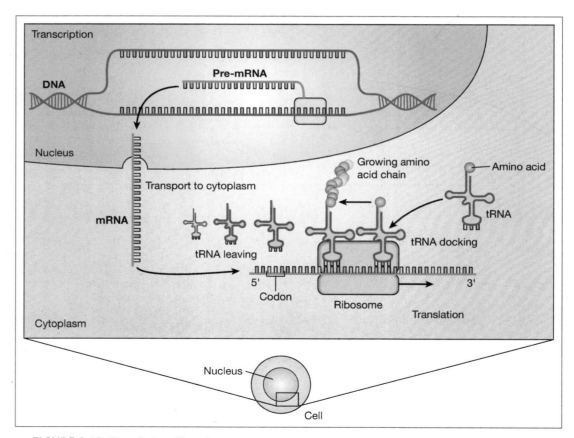

FIGURE 3.12 Translation. Translation occurs in the cytoplasm, when small and large ribosomal subunits attach to the mRNA. The ribosome moves along the mRNA, with tRNAs binding briefly to bring individual amino acids to be added to a growing polypeptide chain, then exiting.
mRNA, messenger RNA; tRNA, transfer RNA.

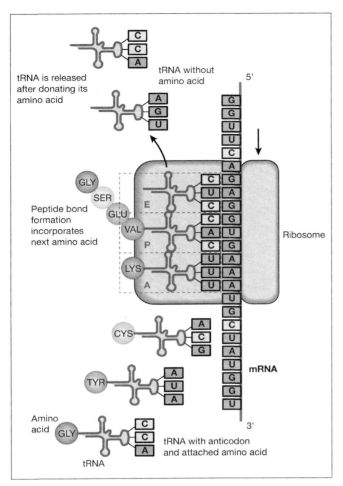

FIGURE 3.13 Ribosome function in translation. The ribosome slides along the mRNA, with the growing peptide chain coming out the opposite side. Amino acid–carrying tRNAs enter at the A site, then move to the P site, where a peptide bond is formed between that amino acid and the growing peptide chain. As the tRNA reaches the E site, it exits. The genetic code is based on the codon recognized by each complementary tRNA, specifying the sequence of amino acids of the protein.
CYS, cysteine; GLU, glutamate; GLY, glycine; LYS, lysine; mRNA, messenger RNA; SER, serine; tRNA, transfer RNA; TYR, tyrosine; VAL, valine.

molecule carrying the next appropriate amino acid enters the ribosome. The tRNA briefly binds with the mRNA, and a peptide bond is formed between the amino acid carried by the tRNA and the amino acid that precedes it in the chain. Once the peptide bond is formed, the tRNA is released from the mRNA and exits the ribosome. This part of the translation process is referred to as *elongation* and is characterized by a growing chain of amino acids trailing from the ribosome. When the ribosome reaches a stop codon, the large and small subunits of the ribosome detach from the mRNA and the amino acid chain is released into the cytoplasm.

Post-Translational Processing

As in transcription, the initial product undergoes additional modifications before a functional protein has reached its final form. Post-translational processes can include folding of the polypeptide chain into a three-dimensional shape, as described in Chapter 2, Chemical and Biochemical Foundations, combining the emerging protein with other polypeptides to create quaternary structures, and sometimes removing some of the amino acids from the chain. The folding process may occur either during or after translation and is often facilitated by chaperone proteins. Phosphate, carboxyl, methyl, and carbohydrate groups may be added to alter the function of the resulting protein. Some proteins include a sequence of amino acids called a *signal sequence* that is used to direct the protein to a particular cellular compartment; this sequence may be removed once the protein reaches that site.

Thought Questions

1. Why are spontaneously occurring sequence variations, such as single nucleotide polymorphisms and mutations, biologically useful?

2. What steps lead from reading a DNA sequence coding for a protein (a gene) to production of the final protein?

CONCEPTS IN GENETICS AND GENOMICS

CHROMOSOME TERMINOLOGY

As previously described, the human genome normally has 46 chromosomes—two copies each of autosomes 1 to 22, and two sex chromosomes, either XX or XY (Figure 3.15). The two copies of each chromosome are termed homologous chromosomes, and an individual's genome is made up of two homologous copies of each autosome plus two sex chromosomes. Within each of the chromosome pairs, one chromosome was contributed by the egg at the time of fertilization, and one was contributed by the sperm. These are referred to as the maternal and paternal chromosomes, respectively. Each chromosome has a centromere, a region that will become the connection point between sister chromatids during mitosis. At the end of the S phase of the cell cycle, the centromeric connection between sister chromatids appears as a constricted region. This becomes the attachment point to spindle fibers that pull the chromatids to opposite poles of the dividing cell.

		Second base of codon								
		U		**C**		**A**		**G**		
	U	UUU	Phenylalanine (Phe)	UCU	Serine (Ser)	UAU	Tyrosine (Tyr)	UGU	Cysteine (Cys)	U
		UUC	Phenylalanine (Phe)	UCC	Serine (Ser)	UAC	Tyrosine (Tyr)	UGC	Cysteine (Cys)	C
		UUA	Leucine (Leu)	UCA	Serine (Ser)	UAA	STOP codon	UGA	STOP codon	A
		UUG	Leucine (Leu)	UCG	Serine (Ser)	UAG	STOP codon	UGG	Tryptophan (Trp)	G
	C	CUU	Leucine (Leu)	CCU	Proline (Pro)	CAU	Histidine (His)	CGU	Arginine (Arg)	U
		CUC	Leucine (Leu)	CCC	Proline (Pro)	CAC	Histidine His)	CGC	Arginine (Arg)	C
		CUA	Leucine (Leu)	CCA	Proline (Pro)	CAA	Glutamine (Gin)	CGA	Arginine (Arg)	A
First base of codon		CUG	Leucine (Leu)	CCG	Proline (Pro)	CAG	Glutamine (Gin)	CGG	Arginine (Arg)	G
	A	AUU	Isoleucine (Ile)	ACU	Threonine (Thr)	AAU	Asparagine (Asn)	AGU	Serine (Ser)	U
		AUC	Isoleucine (Ile)	ACC	Threonine (Thr)	AAC	Asparagine (Asn)	AGC	Serine (Ser)	C
		AUA	Isoleucine (Ile)	ACA	Threonine (Thr)	AAA	Lysine (Lys)	AGA	Arginine (Arg)	A
		AUG	Methionine (met) START codon	ACG	Threonine (Thr)	AAG	Lysine (Lys)	AGG	Arginine (Arg)	G
	G	GUU	Valine (Val)	GCU	Alanine (Ala)	GAU	Aspartic acid (Asp)	GGU	Glycine (Gly)	U
		GUC	Valine (Val)	GCC	Alanine (Ala)	GAC	Aspartic acid (Asp)	GGC	Glycine (Gly)	C
		GUA	Valine (Val)	GCA	Alanine (Ala)	GAA	Glutamic acid (Glu)	GGA	Glycine (Gly)	A
		GUG	Valine (Val)	GCG	Alanine (Ala)	GAG	Glutamic acid (Glu)	GGG	Glycine (Gly)	G

FIGURE 3.14 The genetic code. Each amino acid has at least one, and usually more than one, triplet codon that corresponds to a mitochondrial RNA sequence. Within the ribosome, a complementary transfer RNA carrying the appropriate amino acid will bind to this codon so the amino acid can be incorporated into the growing polypeptide chain. Because many amino acids have more than one codon, a single base substitution in a gene may not result in an incorrect amino acid in a protein product. A, adenine; C, cytosine; G, guanine; U, uracil.

GENE TERMINOLOGY

Distributed along the chromosomes are the genes, the sections of DNA that code for protein production via transcription and translation. Genetic science uses a standard system to identify the location of a gene within the genome:

- The gene locus (plural: loci) is indicated by a short-hand nomenclature that includes the chromosome, the arm of the chromosome, and the gene's location within that chromosome.
- The arms of the chromosomes are the portions of the chromosome located either above or below the centromere. The long arm is indicated by the letter "q" and the short arm by the letter "p."
- The remaining numbers refer to the region, band, and sub-band in which the gene is located based on the characteristic pattern of banding created by Giemsa staining.

If a single locus is indicated, it is generally taken to refer to the starting point of the gene. A range may be indicated, giving the starting and end points for the gene. Also, the starting point may be given along with the number of base pairs contained in the gene. For example, the gene associated with the huntingtin protein altered in Huntington disease is located at 4p16.3. This indicates that the *HTT* gene is located at the tip of the short arm of chromosome 4, position 3 within band 16.

There are two copies of each gene—one on the maternal chromosome and one on the paternal chromosome. These copies may be identical, or they may have slight or large differences. Each of these gene versions is called an *allele*. A person may be homozygous at a given gene locus, with the maternal and paternal alleles of the gene being identical, or a person may be heterozygous, with two different alleles at that locus. An allele version associated with normal gene structure and function is often referred to as the "wild-type" version while a version that does not function normally is often referred to as having a mutation.

GENE VARIATIONS

As noted earlier, despite the greater than 99.4% similarity of genetic information among humans, there are also substantial variations. The source of these variations are small changes in stretches of DNA that can be anywhere from 1 to about 2,000 bp long. These have developed over the millennia of human evolution and are found both in coding regions of genes and in noncoding regions between genes. Patterns of these variations

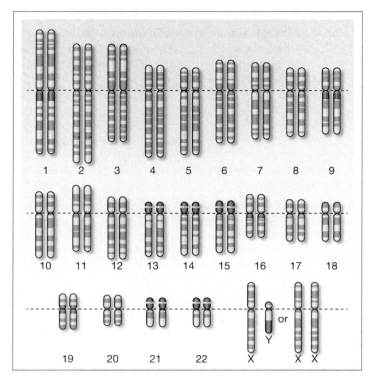

FIGURE 3.15 Homologous chromosomes. An individual's genome is contained in 46 chromosomes, consisting of 22 pairs of autosomes (1–22) and two sex chromosomes, either XX or XY. The chromosomes of each pair are termed homologous chromosomes and have similar banding patterns when treated with a Giemsa stain. The dashed lines indicate the position of the centromere, and the chromosomes are aligned with p arms above the dashed line and q arms below.

diverged with human migrations and give scientists (and direct-to-consumer ancestry testing companies) the ability to predict continent and general region of ancestral origin. All of these variations resulted from spontaneous or induced changes in so-called germline DNA—the DNA found in gametes that can be transmitted to progeny and propagated through generations.

The term *genetic mutation* has sometimes been used to describe all changes in DNA sequence, but the term *genetic variation* is also coming into use as a general way of describing the vast, yet subtle, variability that makes up the human genome. Another related term is *polymorphism*—this implies a position or chromosomal region that has been identified through genome sequencing to be quite variable among individuals. This variability can be seen at a single base (also known as a *single nucleotide polymorphism* [SNP, pronounced "snip"]). More commonly, DNA sequences as short as two bases and as long as hundreds of bases are repeated varying numbers of times in sequenced genomes. The term *variable number tandem repeats* is used to describe these forms of variability. Most of these changes cannot be directly linked to disease-causing variations in proteins, although some of them give clues as to someone's risk for developing a disease.

For the purposes of this book, we focus on genetic mutations that are known to cause diseases (monogenic diseases), while acknowledging that the most common human diseases are complex and polygenic in origin. Genetic mutations can occur spontaneously, but also arise as a consequence of chemical- or radiation-induced damage. The damage may be in the form of reactive oxygen species, chemical mutagens from environmental or occupational exposures, radiation (as in sun exposure affecting the skin), or failure of cell protective strategies. Mutations may impact the final protein product in a quantitative or qualitative manner. They may result in functional differences in the protein product, increased or decreased amount of protein produced, or no differences at all. When a mutation increases the activity of the protein made, it is called a *gain-of-function mutation*. When a mutation decreases the activity of the protein made, it is called a *loss-of-function mutation*. Some mutations are inherited (germline mutations that come from the parental gametes), whereas others are acquired over a lifetime.

Assessment for the presence of one or more mutations could involve whole genome sequencing to determine an individual's entire DNA sequence. More commonly, however, nucleic acid amplification and hybridization techniques are used to evaluate specific genes of interest. These technical approaches are discussed later in the chapter. DNA sequencing informs investigators about an individual's *genotype*—the unique sequence of nucleotides in his or her genes. If a mutation alters protein expression and body attributes and functions, it is said to alter the *phenotype*—the physical expression associated with the trait (straight or curly hair, eye color) or disorder.

Single Nucleotide Polymorphisms

A change in a single base pair in a chromosome is a very common event and gives rise to SNPs that are present in about one of every 1,000 bases. SNPs are found in coding and noncoding regions, exons and introns alike, and their identification has helped geneticists map population-wide descendance patterns related to continent and region of origin (as used by publicly available genetic ancestry services). Most SNPs are found between rather than within genes. The alterations in noncoding regions may still have an impact on human functioning, as they may affect gene splicing, mRNA stability, and transcription. Global databases of SNPs are maintained and continually added to, and knowledge of the role of specific SNPs in gene expression, disease risk, and pharmacogenomics continues to grow.

Synonymous SNPs are those that reside in the coding region of a gene but do not affect the amino acid sequence of the protein product. Nonsynonymous SNPs are those that reside in the coding region of a gene and change the amino acid sequence of the protein, often impacting the structure or function. Most SNPs have no effect on human health, but some SNPs increase disease risk, directly cause disease, or alter protein function. For example, in clinical practice, the anticoagulant drug warfarin was long known to have very variable clinical outcomes, with prolongation of the international normalized ratio (INR)—the desired outcome— showing an unpredictable response to warfarin dose. Pharmacogenomics studies found that there are two major alleles of the gene coding for target protein VKORC1 (vitamin K epoxide reductase complex) that affect its sensitivity to warfarin. Furthermore, CYP2C9, the enzyme that metabolizes warfarin, has three different alleles, each of which has a different level of activity. A large clinical trial found six different levels of warfarin responsiveness based on genotype, from above-average warfarin sensitivity (33% of patients, requiring a lower dose and frequent monitoring of prothrombin time) to below-average warfarin sensitivity (25% of patients, who may require a higher dose), with only 30% expected to have a "normal" response to warfarin.[2]

Another example of a common polymorphism associated with disease risk is that of the apolipoprotein E (APOE) associated with plasma lipoproteins. There are three variants of the APOE allele—APOE-2, APOE-3, and APOE4—with APOE-3 being the most common.

Individuals may be either homozygous for one of these or heterozygous, with two different alleles. Having one APOE4 allele is associated with greater risk of developing Alzheimer disease, and being homozygous for the APOE4 allele is associated with four to ten times the risk of developing Alzheimer disease.

Combinations of SNPs are used in genome-wide association studies to identify genomic regions that are different in two populations; for example, individuals with or without ischemic stroke or type 2 diabetes mellitus. There is a significant amount of ongoing research aimed at identifying panels of SNPs that may predict risk of common multifactorial diseases.

Point Mutations in Coding Regions

Point mutations that occur specifically within coding regions are named based on their effect on protein expression (**Figure 3.16**). The examples shown are to be compared with the wild-type sequence (**Figure 3.16a**).

- *Silent* mutations do not result in any amino acid change in the final protein, generally due to the redundancy within the genetic code (**Figure 3.16b**). These mutations do not cause disease.
- *Missense* mutations cause a change in one amino acid of the protein's primary sequence (**Figure 3.16c**). Some missense mutations are conservative, substituting an amino acid from within the same class (e.g., a hydrophobic valine may be added in place of a hydrophobic leucine). Other missense mutations substitute an amino acid with completely different properties than the original, as is the case with the sickle cell mutation, which substitutes a valine (hydrophobic amino acid) for a glutamate (charged, hydrophilic amino acid), with major clinical consequences.
- *Nonsense* mutations insert a premature stop codon, terminating protein synthesis before the full protein is completed and thereby blocking that cell from making usable protein (**Figure 3.16d**).

Additional examples of disease-causing mutations are described throughout the book, marked with the genetics icon seen here. The human gene mutation database and other studies have determined that missense mutations are by far the most common source of pathogenic mutations, followed by small deletions, and then nonsense mutations.[3]

Deletion or Insertion Mutations

Removal or addition of extra base pairs changes the actual number of base pairs in a coding or noncoding DNA sequence. If this occurs in a coding region, it may affect the amino acid sequence. The sequence ATCTTT, with complimentary strand TAGAAA, is the normal sequence for a segment of the cystic fibrosis

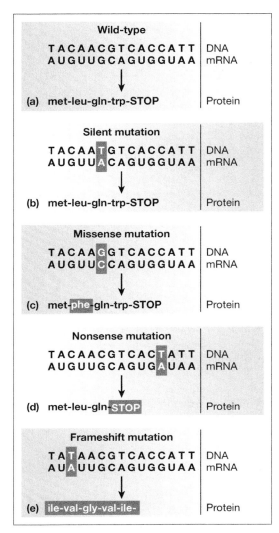

FIGURE 3.16 Point mutations. The effect of change of a single nucleotide on the resulting amino acid sequence is depicted. **(a)** *Wild-type* (no mutation)—gene and peptide sequence in the absence of a mutation, the default version, **(b)** *silent*—base change from C to T at position 6 does not alter the amino acid sequence, **(c)** *missense*—base change from C to G at position 6 changes the second amino acid from leucine to phenylalanine, **(d)** *nonsense*—base change from C to T at position 12 adds a stop codon and truncates the peptide prematurely, and **(e)** *frameshift*—insertion of a T after position 2 shifts the reading frame and changes all of the amino acids in the peptide.
gln, glutamine; gly, glycine; leu, leucine; met, methionine; mRNA, messenger RNA; phe, phenylalanine; trp, tryptophan; val, valine.

transmembrane conductance regulator (*CFTR*) gene and codes for isoleucine (position 507) and phenyl-alanine (position 508). A relatively small deletion of the C–G pair and two T–A pairs (in red) changes that sequence to …ATT… at position 507, which is translated into isoleucine; however, the next codon is lost, so phenylalanine is missing from the protein

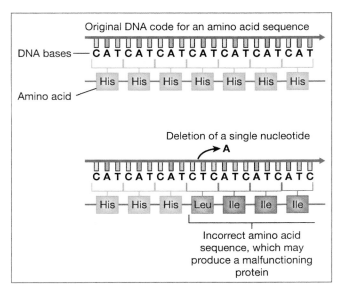

FIGURE 3.17 Deletion mutation. Similar to the insertion mutation of **Figure 3.16e**, loss of a single nucleotide changes the triplet sequence that constitutes a gene's reading frame. In this example, the amino acid sequence is normal up to the point of the deletion, after which the reading frame shifts and the gene will code for incorrect amino acids until a stop codon is reached.
His, histidine; Ile, isoleucine; Leu, leucine.

sequence. This specific example results in a misfolded CFTR protein that cannot insert into the cell membrane and is degraded. If an individual has two copies of this mutation, or one copy of this mutation and another within the *CFTR* gene, that person will have cystic fibrosis.

Frameshift Mutations

Deletion or insertion of one or more bases, *not* divisible by 3, in a coding DNA sequence changes the reading frame for transcription, producing a frameshift mutation (**Figures 3.16e** and **3.17**). The sequence beyond the insertion, or deletion, will have different codons and often results in a different amino acid sequence in the resulting protein, as well as length variations—shorter or longer than the original protein. Frameshift mutations have been implicated in Tay–Sachs disease,[4] Crohn disease,[5,6] and some forms of cancer.[7–9]

Trinucleotide Repeats and Other Copy Number Variants

Trinucleotide repeats are places in the DNA sequence where three nucleotides repeat more than once. Common trinucleotides that reside in the genome include CAG and CGG. Repeats of trinucleotides lengthen the gene and have variable impact on the gene product and hence health of the individual. Trinucleotide repeats associated with disease often increase in number during meiosis, a process known as *expansion*.

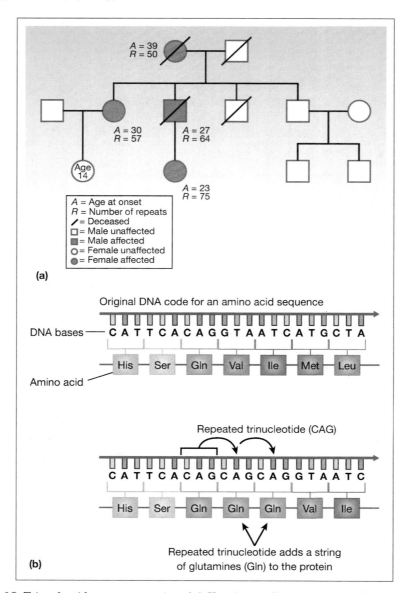

FIGURE 3.18 Trinucleotide repeat mutation. **(a)** Huntington disease is caused by an expansion of the triplet "CAG" repeated several times within the sequence of the gene. The pedigree indicates an autosomal dominant pattern with two children of an affected mother also manifesting the disease. The mother's disease onset was at age 39 years, and she had 50 copies of the repeat (normal genotype is 10–35 repeats at this locus). A daughter had onset at age 30 years and 57 repeats; a son had 64 repeats and onset at age 27 years. A granddaughter had 75 repeats and onset at age 23 years. This is termed *genetic anticipation,* as the number of repeats expands and the age of onset gets younger with subsequent generations. **(b)** *Top*—original gene sequence of CAG coding for one glutamine. *Bottom*—expansion of the CAG repeat, coding for additional glutamines in the translated protein. His, histidine; Ile, isoleucine; Leu, leucine; Met, methionine; Ser, serine; Val, valine.
Source: (b) Courtesy of the National Library of Medicine.

Huntington disease, an adult-onset, fatal neurodegenerative disease, is caused by excess trinucleotide repeats in the gene coding for huntingtin protein. Individuals with Huntington disease have over 35 to 40 CAG repeats, as opposed to the normal number of 17 to 20 CAG repeats. Because CAG codes for glutamine, the translated protein has a longer stretch of glutamines than normal. Over time, the mutant huntingtin protein accumulates, damaging neurons and causing neurodegeneration. Huntington disease manifests in individuals at around age 35 to 45 years and is characterized by uncontrollable chorea (brief twitching, nonpurposeful movements that occur sporadically), which progresses to greater motor dysfunction as well as cognitive loss and psychiatric manifestations. Huntington disease and other trinucleotide repeat diseases exhibit genetic anticipation, in which each generation tends to have a worse phenotype and earlier presentation (**Figure 3.18**). Other trinucleotide repeat disorders include fragile X syndrome, juvenile myoclonic epilepsy, myotonic dystrophy, spinocerebellar ataxia, and Friedreich ataxia.

Copy Number Variants

Copy number variants are polymorphisms in which short sequences of nucleotides within the DNA are repeated, either in or near a gene. These are inherited or spontaneous variations and may or may not be disease related. Similar to the Huntington disease CAG repeats, in other disorders larger sections of the DNA sequence, even whole genes, repeat or are deleted. Copy number variants have been associated with some types of dementia, Parkinson disease, autism, and schizophrenia.

INHERITANCE: MENDELIAN AND NON-MENDELIAN

Inheritance is how genes—and hence genetic-related diseases, conditions, and traits—are passed down through generations. Knowledge of inheritance patterns is helpful in determining the risk for single gene disorders and, increasingly, for some complex disorders.

Mendelian Inheritance

The principles of Mendelian inheritance derive from the work of the monk Gregor Mendel, who recorded observations while growing garden peas and tracking select characteristics such as smooth versus wrinkled skin among the offspring of parent plants. These patterns are based on each individual having two alleles for each gene and on the strength of the genes influencing a trait. Single gene traits and disorders due to genes on the numbered chromosomes are inherited in a Mendelian

pattern. Mendelian inheritance includes autosomal dominant and autosomal recessive inheritance patterns, which relate to the autosomes—chromosomes 1 to 22—that occur in homologous pairs. Different patterns of inheritance are associated with the X chromosome, as they differ between genetic males and females.

Autosomal Dominant Disorders

In the autosomal dominant pattern of inheritance, only one copy of the abnormal gene is required for the phenotype to present in the individual. When a person has one nonmutated copy of the gene, body functions are disrupted as a result of the abnormal allele, and having a heterozygous genotype is associated with development of the disease phenotype. Characteristics of autosomal dominant inheritance include the following:

- Sexes are equally likely to be affected and to transmit the gene.
- An affected person will have at least one affected parent.
- Numbers of affected individuals in a pedigree are higher than would be expected for autosomal recessive and sex-linked inheritance patterns (**Figure 3.19**).

If one parent has the disorder, there is a 50% chance he or she will pass on the abnormal copy of the gene to each offspring. If the other parent does not have the disorder or the gene, that parent can only pass on the normal copy of the gene. Risk of offspring inheriting the gene and having the disorder is entirely dependent upon the affected parent's genetic contribution with each pregnancy. A Punnett square is often used to diagram possible genotypes of offspring based on parental genotypes (**Figure 3.20**).

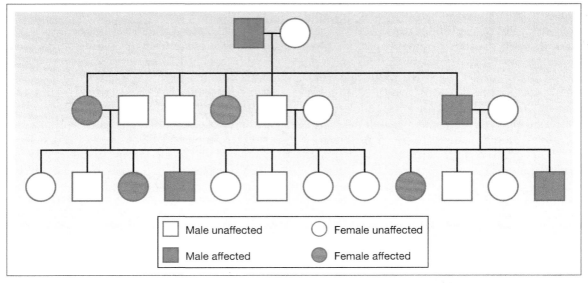

☐ Male unaffected	◯ Female unaffected
◼ Male affected	● Female affected

FIGURE 3.19 Autosomal dominant pedigree. Notable features include the presence of the phenotype (*filled symbols*) in every generation and equal probability of males and females being affected.

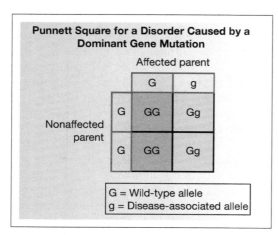

FIGURE 3.20 A Punnett square is a way of estimating probability of a particular phenotype being expressed in offspring, given known genotypes of the parents. This square diagrams a given disorder (dominant) caused by mutation within a given gene, where G is the "normal" allele and g is the "disease" allele. Affected parent has the genotype Gg for the risk gene, whereas the nonaffected parent has only the normal version of the genes, genotype GG. If the affected parent donates the normal gene, the offspring does not have the gene or disorder. If the affected parent donates the disease allele, the offspring does have the gene and disorder.

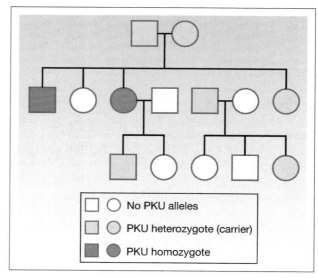

FIGURE 3.21 Autosomal recessive pedigree. Notable features include the relatively small numbers of individuals with the phenotype (*solid filled symbols*) and greater number of individuals who are heterozygous and are carriers (*lightly shaded symbols*).
PKU, phenylketonuria.

Although most autosomal dominant mutations are inherited, in some cases the mutation occurs randomly. Random mutations resulting in disease in offspring are called *de novo mutations*. Diseases with an autosomal dominant inheritance pattern include Huntington disease, familial hypercholesterolemia, Marfan syndrome, and neurofibromatosis.

Autosomal Recessive Disorders

In autosomal recessive disorders, both alleles must be the mutated version (the individuals must be homozygous for the mutation) in order to develop the phenotype. In this case, one normal copy of the gene makes enough protein to carry out that protein's function in the body. Individuals who are heterozygous do not express the phenotype, whereas individuals who are homozygous for the mutation do express it. Disorders with an autosomal recessive inheritance pattern may not present in every generation; thus they appear to "skip" a generation (**Figure 3.21**). Characteristics of autosomal recessive inheritance include the following:

- Affected individuals are usually born to unaffected carriers.
- Both sexes are equally affected.
- Overall, there are fewer affected individuals in a family pedigree.

For genes with an autosomal recessive inheritance pattern, persons with one copy of the mutated gene are known as *carriers* because they carry the gene and can pass it on to their offspring. During mating, the risk of an offspring having an autosomal recessive disorder requires that both parents carry a copy of the mutated gene (**Figure 3.22**).

- If one parent is a carrier and the other is not affected (i.e., does not have the disorder) and is not a carrier, with each pregnancy there is a 50% chance that their offspring will be carriers (**Figure 3.22a**).
- If both parents are carriers but neither has the disorder, there is a 25% chance with each pregnancy that the offspring will have the disorder, a 50% chance their offspring will be a carrier, and a 25% chance the offspring will be a nonaffected noncarrier (**Figure 3.22b**).
- If an affected individual mates with a nonaffected, noncarrier person, all of the offspring will be carriers but none will be affected or nonaffected noncarriers. The nonaffected, noncarrier parent only has the nonmutated gene to donate and the affected parent only has the mutated gene to donate, so the offspring has one copy of each parent's gene (**Figure 3.22c**).
- If an affected individual mates with a carrier, with each pregnancy there is a 50% chance their offspring will be affected and a 50% chance the offspring will

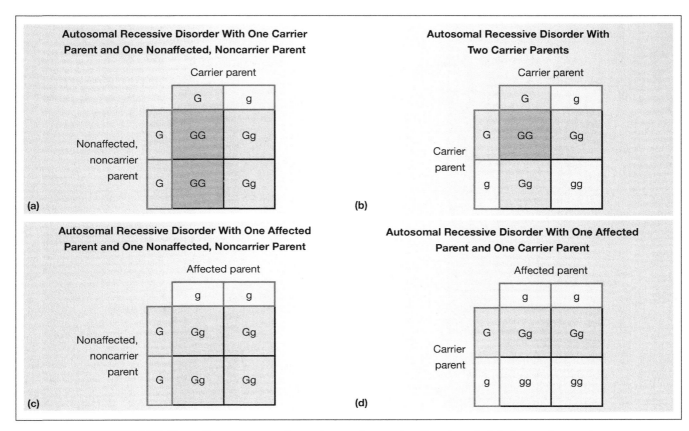

FIGURE 3.22 Punnett square examples: autosomal recessive disorders. **(a)** Autosomal recessive disorder with one carrier parent (genotype Gg) and one nonaffected, noncarrier parent (genotype GG). "G" represents the wild-type or nonmutated version of the gene, whereas "g" represents the mutated version. None of their children will develop the disorder (genotype gg). With each pregnancy, there is a 50% chance the offspring will be a carrier (genotype Gg) and 50% chance the offspring will be a nonaffected noncarrier (genotype GG). **(b)** Autosomal recessive disorder with two carrier parents (genotype Gg). With each pregnancy, there is a 50% chance the offspring will be a carrier (genotype Gg), a 25% chance the offspring will be a noncarrier, nonaffected (genotype GG), and a 25% chance the offspring will be affected with the disorder (genotype gg). **(c)** Autosomal recessive disorder with one affected parent and one nonaffected, noncarrier parent. Given each parent only has one version of the gene to give (G or g), none of the children will be affected but all will be carriers. **(d)** Autosomal recessive disorder with one affected parent and one carrier parent. The affected parent will always donate the mutated gene and the carrier parent has a 50% chance of donating the mutated gene.

be a carrier (**Figure 3.22d**). In this scenario, there is no chance of the offspring being a nonaffected non-carrier because the affected parent always donates a mutated gene.

If two affected individuals mate, all children will have two copies of the mutated gene and be affected because the parents only have a mutated gene to donate. Some examples of diseases with an autosomal recessive inheritance pattern are cystic fibrosis, PKU, sickle cell anemia, and Tay–Sachs disease.

Non-Mendelian Inheritance

X-Linked Dominant Inheritance

This pattern is seen when a gene on the X chromosome exerts dominance, so only one copy is needed to exhibit the trait or disorder. The inheritance pattern is different from the autosomal dominant pattern because there are not always two copies of the X chromosome—biological males have one X and one Y chromosome, whereas biological females have two X chromosomes. As such, there are sex-related differences in inheritance risk (**Figure 3.23**).

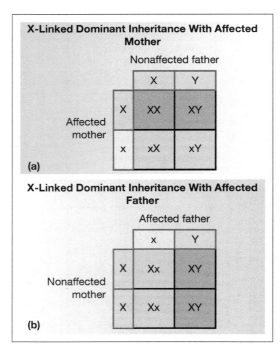

FIGURE 3.23 Punnett square examples: X-linked dominant inheritance. **(a)** X-linked dominant inheritance with female affected. X is the normal gene on the X chromosome, x is the mutated gene on the X chromosome. Father is nonaffected and does not possess the mutated gene (karyotype 46 XY) and the mother has the disorder and gene (karyotype 46 Xx). There is a 50% chance of either offspring (male or female) having the mutated gene and the disorder. **(b)** X-linked dominant inheritance with affected father. X is the normal gene, x is the mutated gene. Father is affected and possesses the mutated gene. Mother is nonaffected and does not possess the mutated gene. Because the father contributes the Y chromosome to his sons, none of them will be carriers or affected. Because the father contributes the X chromosome to all his daughters, they will all receive the mutated gene (x) and be affected.

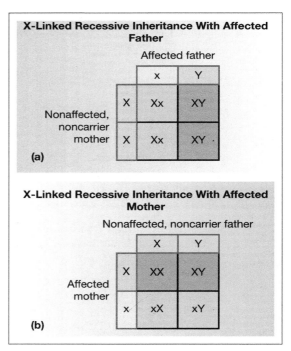

FIGURE 3.24 Punnett square examples: X-linked recessive inheritance. **(a)** X-linked recessive inheritance with affected father. In this case, the mother contributes an X chromosome with a nonmutated gene to all children. The father donates the X chromosome with the mutated gene (x) to all female offspring and the normal Y chromosome to all male offspring. **(b)** X-linked recessive inheritance with affected mother. The father contributes a normal X chromosome to all female offspring and a normal Y chromosome to all male offspring. Daughters will have a 50% chance of having a normal genotype or being a carrier. Sons have a 50% chance of having a normal genotype or being affected, because they have only one X chromosome.

- A heterozygous mother will have the phenotype of the disorder, and there is a 50% chance she will pass it on to each of her offspring regardless of sex (**Figure 3.23a**).
- If the father has the disorder, there is a 50% chance he will pass it on to his female offspring, but no chance he will pass it on to his male offspring because he donates the Y chromosome (**Figure 3.23b**). Some disorders with an X-linked dominant inheritance pattern include Rett syndrome, fragile X syndrome, and X-linked hypophosphatemia (vitamin D–resistant rickets).

X-Linked Recessive Inheritance

In this inheritance pattern, one copy of the normal gene on the X chromosome is sufficient to prevent the disease from expressing. All males inheriting the abnormal gene on the X chromosome will be affected as they have no other X chromosome to make that protein. The risk to offspring is variable based on which parent has the trait or disease (**Figure 3.24a** and **b**). If the father is affected, all female offspring will be carriers but his sons will not have the disorder. If the mother is affected, 50% of male offspring will have the disorder while 50% of all female offspring will be carriers. Some examples of diseases with X-linked recessive inheritance patterns are hemophilia A, glucose-6-phosphate dehydrogenase (G6PD) deficiency, and Duchenne muscular dystrophy.

Mitochondrial Inheritance

Mitochondria contain their own DNA apart from the nuclear DNA. Mitochondrial DNA is in circular form and includes genes coding for some proteins of the Krebs cycle and oxidative phosphorylation, and hence adenosine triphosphate (ATP) production. Although some proteins used by the mitochondria for energy production are imported from the cytosol, several are made within the mitochondria. Variability within the mitochondrial DNA leads to variable energy production, and there are known variants that lead to poor energy production and drive energy failure in cells with high needs, such as neurons and the lens cells of the eye.

Sperm have few or no mitochondria, whereas eggs have the usual cellular complement of mitochondria. For this reason, all mitochondrial DNA comes from the mother. There is mitochondrial variability within cells, because within any individual's cells there are multiple mitochondria with different DNA. The concept of multiple versions of DNA, and mitochondrial DNA in this case, in the same individual and even within a single cell is known as *heteroplasmy*. The presence of a large number of mitochondria with mutated or faulty DNA in an individual can cause disease.

Leber hereditary optic neuropathy (LHON) is the best known of the mitochondrial disorders. Individuals with LHON have no phenotype at birth or throughout childhood. At 20 to 30 years of age, they begin to have a loss of vision in one eye, which rapidly progresses to blindness and then loss of vision and blindness in the other eye. In early-onset disease, children begin to lose vision as early as the toddler years, although these cases are less common. If the mother is a carrier, she will pass on some of this mutated DNA to her children. There is variability in the heteroplasmy of each egg, and hence each offspring. Some children may have high percentage of faulty DNA and develop LHON; others have low to no faulty DNA and do not develop the disease. A male with LHON will not pass it on to any of his children because the sperm contributes little to no mitochondrial DNA.

PHENOTYPIC VARIABILITY IN GENETIC DISORDERS: PENETRANCE AND EXPRESSIVITY

Penetrance

The presence of a gene mutation does not necessarily cause the phenotype of a disease. Penetrance refers to the percentage of individuals with a mutation who actually develop the related phenotype. Cystic fibrosis is 100% penetrant, and therefore, every individual who has a mutation of the *CFTR* gene will have the disease. Some mutations have variable penetrance whereby individuals who have the disease-related genotype do not have the associated phenotype. Reduced penetrance is driven by several mechanisms including mutation type, variations in gene expression of different alleles, epigenetic factors, gene–environment interaction, allele dose, age, sex, modifier genes, copy number variants, and variability in related genes. Reduced penetrance can occur in both

autosomal dominant and autosomal recessive disorders. Examples include subtypes of retinitis pigmentosa, long QT syndrome, hemochromatosis, and deafness.

Expressivity

Expressivity is defined as variability in the expression of the phenotype for individuals with the same genotype. Variable expressivity is caused by genetic variability in other genes that impact the condition or disease-causing mutation, epigenetic factors such as micro-RNA stability, and sometimes environment. Although cystic fibrosis is 100% penetrant, it has variable expressivity. The signs and symptoms may differ in terms of pathology and severity depending on which specific *CFTR* mutations are present or other genetic variability, alternative RNA splicing, or other modifier. Phenylketonuria (PKU), mentioned at the start of this chapter, is an excellent example of a disease in which penetrance is modified by gene–environment interaction. Although PKU is 100% penetrant, modification of diet to maintain low phenylalanine intake thwarts the most severe phenotype, severe developmental delay, and intellectual disability. Many single gene disorders are not modifiable by environmental influence, but others are quite modifiable. Complex disorders in which genes interact with one another and with the environment can exhibit variable penetrance and expressivity.

Examples of Single Gene and Multifactorial Diseases

Examples of both single gene and polygenic/multifactorial disorders can illustrate the genomic/genetic principles discussed. The underlying genetic disease mechanisms are presented along with phenotypic features.

Marfan Syndrome
Marfan syndrome is most often inherited as an autosomal dominant condition, although approximately 25% of cases are due to sporadic mutations. As an autosomal dominant condition, Marfan syndrome occurs equally in males and females and tends to occur in every generation in affected families. Families in which unaffected parents have an affected child are most likely to be cases of sporadic (de novo) mutation.

Marfan syndrome is due to mutation of the *FBN1* gene, which is located at 15q21.1. This gene codes for the protein fibrillin-1, which is involved in the formation of microfibrils necessary for the proper development of connective tissue. The disorder also results in the excess activation of transforming growth factor beta (TGF-β), which further destabilizes the connective tissue. More than 1,300 possible mutations have been identified, most of which are missense mutations resulting in a change in a single amino acid in the protein.

The pathophysiological alterations associated with the mutations cause the phenotypic features of Marfan syndrome, which include tall stature, aortic dilation and dissection, scoliosis, joint hypermobility, arachnodactyly, pectus excavatum or pectus carinatum, and mitral valve prolapse. There is wide clinical variation in symptomatology, although Marfan syndrome appears to exhibit 100% penetrance. The disorder shows no ethnic, racial, or gender preference and has an incidence of one in approximately 10,000 people. Marfan syndrome is the leading cause of aortic aneurysm in people younger than age 40 years.

Treatment of the disorder is based on frequent monitoring, particularly of the size of the aortic root as well as the rate of increase in size. The use of β-adrenergic blockade may slow the rate of enlargement, and grafting of the aorta may be necessary. Treatment may also be necessary for mitral valve regurgitation and dislocated ocular lenses (ectopia lentis) as well as other complications.

Hereditary Breast and Ovarian Cancer

Mutations in the *BRCA1* and *BRCA2* genes form the genetic basis for one monogenic form of **hereditary breast and ovarian cancer**. Although mutations in *BRCA1* and *BRCA2* genes impart a heightened lifetime risk for breast or ovarian cancer, the percentages of all breast or ovarian cancers caused by these mutations remains relatively small—5% to 10% of breast cancers and 10% to 25% of ovarian cancers. The balance of these cancers are caused by sporadic mutations that are generally multifactorial.

BRCA1 is found at 17q12-21, and more than 900 mutations have been identified in this gene. *BRCA2* is found at 13q12-13 and is subject to a similar number of mutations. An affected individual receives one mutated allele from one parent, which increases the risk of developing cancer; but both alleles must be mutated for cancer to develop. What is inherited is the predisposition to develop cancer rather than cancer itself. Whether the individual with a mutated allele ultimately develops cancer or not depends on a spontaneous mutation occurring in the nonmutated allele, as described in Chapter 7, Neoplasia. Although risk estimates depend on the specific mutation and continue to evolve with additional studies, the lifetime breast cancer risk for women with a *BRCA1* mutation is 55% to 65%, with a 40% risk of ovarian cancer. A *BRCA2* mutation imparts a breast cancer risk of slightly less than 50%, with a 15% risk of ovarian cancer. The lifetime *BRCA*-associated risk of breast cancer in men is 7%, with a 20% risk of prostate cancer. In addition to increasing lifetime risk of cancer, individuals with these mutations also tend to develop cancer at an earlier age.

Coronary Artery Disease

Coronary artery disease (CAD) is an example of a multifactorial disorder and illustrates the complexity of understanding the genetic contribution to common or chronic illnesses. Multifactorial disorders result from some combination of genetic, environmental, and lifestyle causes. Often multiple genes contribute to the genetic component of the disorder, and it is difficult and time consuming to identify all of the contributory genes and to parse out the contribution of each gene to the overall phenotype. Genes associated with multifactorial disorders may number in the hundreds and may either directly affect the phenotype or affect other genes associated with the disorder.

CAD is a progressive disorder resulting from the accumulation of atherosclerotic plaque in the coronary arteries and associated inflammation. Numerous risk factors, including hypertension, hyperlipidemia, diabetes, obesity, and smoking, are well known. Monogenic disorders of lipid metabolism contribute to earlier onset of CAD and include familial hypercholesterolemia, familial defective apolipoprotein A, and others. Genome-wide association studies, more fully discussed later, have identified multiple candidate genes associated with CAD phenotypes.

In addition to directly affecting the phenotype, genes may also moderate the individual's response to treatment, particularly drug therapy. For example, the *SLCO1B1* gene affects the risk of development of myopathy with the use of statins, and different alleles of the gene coding CYP2C19 affect the metabolism of the drug clopidogrel. Patients may be high, normal, or low metabolizers of this and other drugs, and this status moderates both drug efficacy and dosing.

Major Depressive Disorder

Major depressive disorder (MDD) is a mood disorder that is associated with high morbidity and mortality rates. Risk of MDD is as much as three-fold higher in people with first-degree relatives with MDD. Women are affected nearly twice as often as men, and non-Hispanic Whites are affected at a higher rate than other racial or ethnic groups. Twin studies have shown the incidence to be in the 35% to 40% range, and that percentage is higher in women than in men. In mood disorders, more generally, higher heritability was found as severity of the disorders increased. Studies focusing on adopted children found that the incidence of mood disorders in adoptees more closely matches that in the biological parents than that in the adoptive parents. This finding lends credence to the existence of a genetic component to these disorders, although there is currently no definitively identified gene or set of genes that are associated with MDD.

It is likely that there are genetic determinants of drug response in MDD, as is the case with other disorders. The cytochrome P450 class of drugs appears to have an effect on the metabolism of drugs used to treat MDD, and genetic testing may assist in both drug selection and dosing.

Thought Questions

3. Is it possible for a deletion mutation to also be a frameshift mutation? Could you diagram an example in which a deletion mutation would not be a frameshift mutation?

4. In general, which inheritance pattern is associated with a pedigree showing the greatest number of affected individuals?

5. How might you modify your answer if you had additional information about gene penetrance in a given disorder?

TECHNICAL APPROACHES IN GENETICS AND GENOMICS

Advances in the techniques and tools of genetic science are quickly multiplying and provide several avenues for assessment of clients. Other techniques have been used for decades but maintain their usefulness and applicability to genetic assessment. Several of these technologies and practices are explored here, but this list is by no means exhaustive.

FAMILY HISTORY AND PEDIGREE ANALYSIS

The family history and the resulting genetic pedigree remain an important part of the clinician's analysis regarding genetic risk. The history/pedigree has often been referred to as the first genetic test because of its power in identifying the direction and scope of further testing. The analysis of the family history assists in the identification of genetic risk and genetic red flags. Although not generally a diagnostic tool, the family history guides clinicians in identifying candidates for carrier testing or other more diagnostic assessments. The family history is, of course, a recognized part of the initial assessment for any new patient and so may not necessarily be first performed with any specific genetic ends in mind. Consequently, the history should be both far reaching and specific and include as much detail about each family member as is available.

From a genetic perspective, the family history may be limited in usefulness by several barriers. The relatively small size of nuclear families, particularly in the Western developed nations, allows recessive disorders to "hide" for generations and then suddenly reappear as if out of nowhere. The family history is also limited by poor family record-keeping, geographically dispersed families whose members may have lost touch with each other, and a lack of specific knowledge about family members.

Obtaining the History

The clinician should plan for adequate time to take the history, which should be obtained from the most knowledgeable family member available. Having the patient or responsible family member complete an initial form before the first visit has the benefit of stimulating recall of pertinent information, as well as allowing the individual to consult with living relatives regarding their health histories. Family photographs may be useful in identifying dysmorphologies indicative of genetic syndromes. The client should be requested to bring copies of these photographs to the clinician. Digital images may be more helpful as they can be enlarged with ease for more accurate assessment.

If the purpose of taking the history is to determine the genetic risk for the offspring of a mating couple, histories about both families may have genetic relevance. Taking this type of history can quickly become a large and complex task. The scope of this type of assessment may need to be narrower and more focused on a particular risk of interest. These bi-familial pedigrees can be large and unwieldy, so the purpose of the assessment should be carefully considered.

Genetic Red Flags

Red flags are diseases or characteristics of diseases that lead the clinician to reasonably conclude the higher likelihood of a strong genetic component to the disease. Whelan and colleagues provide a useful approach to thinking systematically as one assesses patients for the presence of red flags.[10] "Family GENES" is suggested as a mnemonic to aid the clinician in identifying potential red flags (**Box 3.3**).

KARYOTYPING

Karyotyping is a method of depicting, through a standardized presentation, the set of chromosomes for an individual (**Figure 3.25**). Although this is an older genetic technology, it remains useful in identifying chromosomal structural abnormalities. The chromosomes are arranged first by size and then by the location of the centromere. In the resulting karyogram, the autosomes are arranged from 1 to 22, followed by the sex chromosomes.

In order to construct a karyotype, the laboratory stimulates cells to enter the cell cycle, then stops the cycle during metaphase. The arrested cells are then exposed to a hypotonic solution, which releases the chromosomes from the cell. Next, the Giemsa stain that gives the chromosomes their characteristic banding is applied. The chromosome set is then photographed and arranged in the standard order, enabling the study of any abnormalities.

Through karyotyping it is possible to identify errors in both chromosome number and chromosome structure. *Aneuploidy* is the general term describing any

---

BOX 3.3
Genetic Red Flags: Family GENES*

Family

Multiple family members are affected across multiple generations. But note that lack of a family history does not rule out genetic causes.

G—Groups of anomalies

The presence of multiple anomalies increases the probability of an underlying genetic syndrome. Several anomalies clustered together should raise the index of suspicion and may warrant referral of the patient to a geneticist or genetic counselor. The cluster of anomalies will likely not be diagnostic, as many genetic disorders have similar dysmorphic findings, and further testing may be necessary.

E—Early or extreme presentation of illnesses

Onset of diseases at an earlier-than-expected age or in the uncharacteristic sex likely indicates a genetic basis for the disease. Breast cancer occurring in women before the age of 60 or breast cancer in males is one such occurrence. Early onset of cardiovascular disease is another

example. Cardiovascular disease in males before age 60 or women before age 65 should lead the clinician to consider a more thorough genetic assessment.

N—Neurodevelopmental delay or neurodegenerative diseases

Neurodevelopmental delay in infants and children should prompt consideration of a genetic disorder, particularly when the delay is found in combination with other red flags such as congenital dysmorphologies.

E—Exceptional pathology

Among these pathologies would be finding in either organs or structures of paired or bilateral organs. Another example of exceptional pathology would be to find several different cancers in the same patient simultaneously.

S—Surprising laboratory values

An example would be extremely high lipid levels in a young, otherwise healthy person.

*Mnemonic developed by the Red Flags Working Group of the Genetics in Primary Care (GPC) project.
Source: From Whelan AJ, Ball S, Best L, et al. Genetic red flags: clues to thinking genetically in primary care practice: *Clinics in Office Practice. Prim Care.* 2004;31:497–508. doi:10.1016/j.pop.2004.04.010.

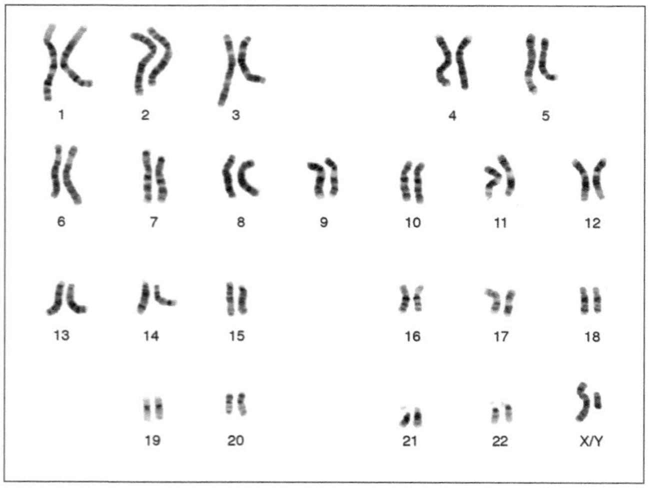

FIGURE 3.25 A karyotype is a method of aligning and marking a complete set of chromosomes from a subject. In this male (XY) karyotype, the individual chromosomes have undergone Giemsa staining, making it easy to distinguish between individual chromosomes, particularly those of similar size. By convention, autosomes are numbered 1 to 22, based on their length.
Source: National Human Genome Research Institute.

chromosomal number other than the normal set of 46 chromosomes. In describing aneuploid states, the suffix "-somy" refers to the aneuploidy of a single chromosome, whereas the suffix "-ploidy" refers to the entire set of chromosomes. Thus, if an individual has trisomy 21 (Down syndrome), three copies of chromosome 21 are present. If an individual has triploidy, there are three copies of all chromosomes.

In addition to determining aneuploid states, the karyotype is able to reveal structural abnormalities such as balanced or unbalanced translocations, inversions, or deletions.

HYBRIDIZATION ARRAYS AND GENE CHIPS

Hybridization arrays, or DNA microarrays, take advantage of the principle of hydrogen bonding between complementary strands of DNA. This method requires knowledge of the exact nucleotide sequence of genes or DNA sequences of interest. A gene chip is a device that holds small segments of DNA in an array on a slide. The DNA segments located on the chip are synthesized based on the known sequence of clinically relevant genes, and are referred to as *probes*. The chip is exposed to a sample of DNA from the patient. The patient's DNA is treated with enzymes to break it down into small segments prior to the hybridization step. The patient's DNA will hybridize to spots on the gene chip that have the complementary base sequence, while failing to hybridize to spots that do not contain a complementary strand (**Figure 3.26**).

This strategy can be used to quickly assess large segments of a patient's DNA or RNA. RNA measurements allow the determination of gene expression and are particularly useful in cancer diagnosis and treatment. Samples of a patient's tissues from a tumor biopsy and an adjacent region that is tumor free can

demonstrate the changes in gene expression associated with the tumor, allowing chemotherapy to be targeted to the particular stage of tumor development.

Gene chips have wide applications in diagnosis and treatment. Some are specialized for use in pathogen identification in infectious disease; others are used for SNP detection and pharmacogenomic screening to identify individuals who may have altered drug-metabolizing enzymes.

WHOLE GENOME SEQUENCING

Whole genome sequencing (WGS), as the name implies, determines the complete DNA sequence for a given individual. Until recently, the cost of WGS, and the time

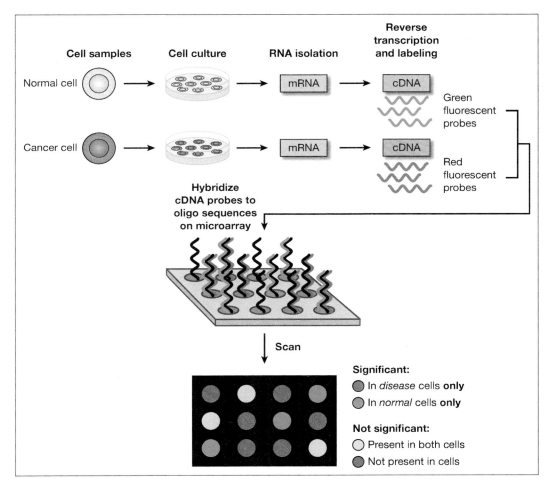

FIGURE 3.26 DNA hybridization microarray. How does cancer alter gene expression in cells? Hybridization technology is one method aiming to answer that question. Synthetic DNA sequences (probes) are constructed to be complementary to a desired group of gene transcripts. Messenger RNAs (mRNAs) from a biopsy sample of a tumor and a sample from noncancerous tissue from the patient with cancer are isolated, converted to complementary DNA (cDNA) using a reverse transcriptase enzyme, and labeled. Small volumes of each set of cDNAs are added to each spot on the gene chip. Analysis detects transcripts that are not found in any cells, those that are found in all cells, and those that are uniquely found in tumor or nontumor cells.

involved, has limited its use to research applications. As the cost of WGS decreases and the time to complete the sequence shortens, clinical or commercial applications for WGS will become more feasible.

Sequencing a DNA molecule one base at a time from beginning to end is obviously exceedingly time consuming. In shotgun sequencing, the genome is first cut into randomly sized short segments. Thousands of these shorter segments are sequenced and then reassembled by using their overlapping regions. Research and development are ongoing to develop ever-faster sequencing technology that will ultimately allow for the commercialization of WGS.

RESEARCH APPROACHES

Genetic research can often resemble a trek through the forest at night without a flashlight or the search for the proverbial needle in the haystack. The most difficult question can be where to begin the search. Several research approaches that can be used to begin the journey are considered here.

Genome-Wide Association Studies

A genome-wide association study (GWAS) can be a useful tool to begin exploration of a trait or disease of interest. In a GWAS, hundreds or thousands of genomes are separated into two groups. The "experimental" or "case" group is affected by the trait or disease of interest, whereas the "control" group is not. The genomes are evaluated looking for SNPs that the affected group have in common in statistically significant greater numbers than the control group. The identified SNPs are then said to be associated with the disease or trait. It is not possible from a GWAS to determine if the associated region or adjacent genes are causative or otherwise affect the disease without further exploration and testing.

Candidate Gene Association Studies

Candidate genes are those for which the researcher has evidence to support the contention that the particular genes may be involved in a given disease. Candidate genes are selected in a variety of ways. The researchers might use the results of other studies such as a GWAS to identify reasonable candidates. Genes may be identified through a literature search or by data-mining one of a number of databases. Further work identifies SNPs associated with the disease, locating regions of the DNA worthy of further analysis. These studies further narrow the field of disease-associated genes in an attempt to find genes with a significant effect on some aspect of the disease.

Pathway Analysis

One of the criticisms of both GWAS and candidate gene studies is that they tend to identify large numbers of "associated" genes for which there is little to no knowledge about the effect on the disease. Pathway analysis seeks to understand how the genes identified in these other studies work together in networks to affect disease processes. Using the gene expression analysis discussed earlier, pathway analysis looks for a significant relationship between the biological pathway and a disease phenotype.

DIRECT-TO-CONSUMER TESTING

Direct-to-consumer (DTC) biomedical testing is not a new concept. Appearing relatively recently on that landscape is the growing market for DTC genetic testing. In DTC testing, the consumer works directly with the vendor providing the test and the results. Most often no intervening healthcare provider is required to guide or educate the consumer about the test itself or the interpretation of the results. DTC genetic tests include disease or health testing, trait testing, and ancestry or genealogy testing.

Ancestry testing uses a DNA sample, most frequently a saliva sample that will contain cells of the buccal mucosa, to look for SNPs associated with various geographic, ethnic, and ancestral groups. These tests are done by comparing the new sample to people of known genealogy. Trait testing identifies a variety of physical traits such as cleft chin, dimples, or eye color. Health testing may include carrier status for a variety of diseases such as the presence of risk alleles for traits such as *BRCA1/BRCA2* genes, Parkinson disease, late-onset Alzheimer disease, and others. Unfortunately, the databases for most DTC genetic tests are often limited in breadth of racial and ethnic diversity, which can skew the data they report.

Other limitations of DTC genetic testing include the inability of most companies to test for all gene variants that have been associated with a given disorder and the unavailability for most vendors of in-person support mechanisms. Clinicians should be aware of the potential for patients to arrive at the clinic, genetic information in hand, seeking counseling, education, or explanation of their genetic information and test results. Many laypeople may also not be fully cognizant that genetic testing is different from other biomedical testing. When genetic tests are performed on one member of a family, those tests are being performed on most or all of the members of that family. Other members of the family may not be interested in knowing their genetic information and the potential for disruption of family relationships is present. Failure of genetic DTC testing companies to fully explain the ramifications of genetic testing and to educate their clients well regarding test interpretation raises significant social and ethical questions. It is likely that appropriate regulation of this testing environment will struggle to keep pace with the growing number of vendors of these tests.

EPIGENETICS

Epigenetics is a term that has undergone several changes in meaning and has evolved to mean the study of heritable changes that do not involve alterations in the DNA sequence.[11] These mechanisms impact how and when a gene is transcribed. Major mechanisms of epigenetic modification include histone modification, DNA methylation, and noncoding RNA expression.[12,13] Epigenetic mechanisms are heritable, but they are also modifiable by environmental and interpersonal factors. There is additional variability in epigenetic changes over the life span and specific to each tissue of an individual.

Transgenerational epigenetic inheritance, often referred to as simply epigenetic inheritance, is the transmission of non-DNA sequence genetic control information from one generation to the next. Genomic imprinting is an epigenetic process whereby DNA methylation and histone methylation patterns are established in the germline of the parent and in that way are passed down to the child and then maintained during mitotic cell divisions.

Histone modification is a well-studied epigenetic mechanism. Acetylation and deacetylation of histones has been well described. Histone acetylation appears to make the DNA in that region more accessible to transcription factors and promotes gene expression. Deacetylation has the opposite effect such that hypoacetylation decreases transcription. Addition of methyl groups (methylation) to histones can also alter, and specifically decrease, transcription.

Methylation of the DNA is another well-studied epigenetic mechanism. The addition of a methyl group to the DNA sequence occurs primarily at *CpG islands*—sites in the DNA strand where a cytosine (C) is found immediately adjacent to a guanine (G) in the 3′ direction. CpG islands are common in promoter regions, and methylation at these sites can repress transcription of that gene. DNA methylation stabilizes chromatin; hence, hypomethylation increases the possibility of DNA damage and dysfunctional repair. Global hypomethylation is found in many cancers, including breast, cervical, thyroid, lung, prostate, bladder, stomach, esophagus, colon, and liver cancer. Hypomethylation of promotor regions upregulates proto-oncogene activity, allowing cancer cells to grow unregulated, and metastasize. Hypermethylation of other CpG islands for other genes, including tumor suppressor genes, facilitates the avoidance of apoptosis, and modifies cell cycle, differentiation, and DNA repair activities. T-cell genome-wide DNA hypomethylation has been noted in individuals with lupus.[14,15] DNA hypomethylation of select genes, such as catechol-*O*-methyltransferase, has been linked to schizophrenia.[16,17]

Epigenetic mechanisms are influenced by environmental chemical exposure, drugs, aging, and diet. Many genes are silenced during development (in utero or childhood) by methylation, whereas others are "turned on" by demethylation. As we age, there is a general hypomethylation pattern across the genome; however, there are some gene-specific CpG island hypermethylation sites. It has been hypothesized that hypomethylation promotes overexpression of proto-oncogenes,[18,19] contributing to increased risk of cancer and other genes that increase risk for autoimmune diseases.

Thought Questions

6. How does the principle of complementary base pairing contribute to DNA sequence analysis using hybridization arrays?

7. How does epigenetic modification of DNA compare with mutation of DNA, in terms of the processes and molecules involved?

Theresa Kyle

Genetic disorders and birth defects combined are the greatest cause of infant mortality in the United States.[20] Advances in prenatal screening and diagnosis include ever more detailed information about the fetal genome, allowing for planning to improve outcomes. Early postnatal genetic testing can now rapidly identify mutations in neonates who appear to have abnormal development and function at birth. This knowledge can shape care, although many conditions cannot be cured.

PRENATAL IDENTIFICATION OF GENETIC DISORDERS

Although many genetic disorders may be identified prenatally, it is not possible to identify all fetal abnormalities before birth. The purpose of screening for and identifying genetic disorders prenatally is to dispel parental anxiety and to allow for preparation prior to birth if a disorder is identified. Additionally, if a disorder is identified, it is possible in some instances to provide fetal treatment. Particular tests are recommended at specific time points throughout pregnancy and may be used for screening purposes or to yield a diagnosis.

PRENATAL SCREENING TESTS

Screening tests are used to determine risk for particular birth defects and chromosomal abnormalities.

An abnormal result indicates the possibility of a problem needing further diagnostic testing. Tests commonly used to screen fetal genetic anomalies are assessment of cell-free DNA (cfDNA) of fetal origin, fetal nuchal translucency (FNT), and maternal serum markers of key fetal and placental proteins.

Circulating cfDNA of fetal origin is found in maternal plasma, composing approximately 3% to 13% of the total cell-free maternal DNA after 9 weeks of gestation.[21] FNT describes the sonographic appearance of a collection of fluid under the skin behind the fetal neck. Four maternal serum markers are routinely measured:

- α-Fetoprotein—fetal-specific globulin, synthesized by the yolk sac, liver, and gastrointestinal tract of the fetus
- Estriol—an estrogen produced by the placenta and the fetus
- β-Human chorionic gonadotropin—a hormone produced within the placenta
- Inhibin A—a protein produced by the ovaries and placenta

Table 3.1 outlines the recommended timing for completing these tests and relevance of the test results for assessment of genetic disorders.

TABLE 3.1 Tests Used to Screen for Genetic Disorders

Test	Timing	Considerations
cfDNA	9 weeks of gestation, or later	Screens for common trisomies and sex chromosome composition
FNT	11 to 13 weeks + 6 days of gestation	Increased thickness (>2.5 mm) of FNT may be associated with trisomy 13, 18, or 21; Turner syndrome; major heart or great artery defects; skeletal dysplasia; or other genetic syndromes
MSAFP	15 to 18 weeks of gestation	Decreased level indicates possible aneuploidy such as Down syndrome, trisomy 18, or Turner syndrome; increased level indicates possible neural tube defect, abdominal wall defect, liver or kidney issue, or multiple gestation
Quadruple marker test or quad screen (MSAFP, estriol, β-hCG, inhibin A)	15 to 18 weeks of gestation	Decreased MSAFP, with low estriol, elevated hCG, and elevated inhibin A, indicates possible Down syndrome; decreased MSAFP, with low estriol and low hCG, indicates possible trisomy 18

cfDNA, cell-free DNA; FNT, fetal nuchal translucency; hCG, human chorionic gonadotropin; MSAFP, maternal serum α-fetoprotein.
Source: Data from Latendresse G, Deneris A. An update on current prenatal testing options: first trimester and noninvasive prenatal testing. *J Midwifery Womens Health.* 2015;60:24–36.

TABLE 3.2 Tests Used to Diagnose Genetic Disorders

Test	Timing	Considerations
Amniocentesis	15 to 20 weeks of gestation	Enables karotyping, chromosome analysis, DNA markers, and identification of inborn errors of metabolism
Chorionic villus sampling	10 to 12 weeks of gestation	Enables karotyping and identification of numerous genetic disorders such as Down syndrome, phenylketonuria, Duchenne muscular dystrophy, sickle cell anemia
Percutaneous umbilical blood sampling	>16 weeks of gestation	Enables karotyping and identification of inherited blood disorders, isoimmunization

PRENATAL DIAGNOSTIC TESTS

Other prenatal tests are completed for the purpose of diagnosing or ruling out a genetic disorder (Table 3.2). Chorionic villus sampling, amniocentesis, and percutaneous umbilical blood sampling may be performed for chromosome analysis. In chorionic villus sampling, a small piece of tissue is removed from the placenta (fetal portion). Amniocentesis allows needle aspiration of amniotic fluid. Percutaneous umbilical blood sampling is achieved by ultrasound-guided aspiration of blood from the umbilical cord. Although these procedures may diagnose chromosomal abnormalities, they pose a higher risk to the fetus than do the screening tests.

Finally, in cases of in vitro fertilization (IVF), embryos may be tested for genetic alterations preimplantation in order to prevent inheritable genetic diseases.

GENETIC DISORDERS IDENTIFIED AFTER BIRTH

CHROMOSOMAL DISORDERS

Chromosomal disorders often result from an error in cell division in the first meiotic division (meiotic disjunction). Structural alterations may occur such as deletion, inversion, or translocation of a chromosome. The most common and clinically significant type of chromosomal disorder is aneuploidy (an abnormal chromosome number). Aneuploidy may be identified in the prenatal period by karyotyping via chorionic villus sampling, amniocentesis, or percutaneous umbilical blood sampling.[22] These disorders are also often identified soon after birth based on physical findings and subsequent chromosomal analysis, or later in life. Table 3.3 provides information related to the more commonly encountered disorders of chromosome number.

DISORDERS IDENTIFIED BY NEWBORN SCREENING

Newborn screening tests vary by state, but common genetic disorders tested at birth include several inborn errors of metabolism (in the categories of organic acid disorders, fatty acid oxidation disorders, and amino acid disorders, including PKU); endocrine disorders (primary congenital hypothyroidism, congenital adrenal hyperplasia); blood disorders (sickle cell disease and β-thalassemia); and other relatively common single gene disorders (cystic fibrosis, classic galactosemia, severe combined immunodeficiencies, and X-linked adrenoleukodystrophy).

Single Gene Disorders

Single gene disorders follow Mendelian inheritance patterns and result from a mutated or defective allele at a single gene location. The pattern of transmission may be determined with a family genetic history.[23] For those disorders not included in newborn screening, prenatal or postnatal testing may be chosen for infants known to be at risk by reason of ethnicity (e.g., evaluation for Tay–Sachs disease in an infant with Ashkenazi ancestry). PKU, introduced in Chapter 2, Chemical and Biochemical Foundations, is an example of an inborn error of metabolism in a single gene, with autosomal recessive inheritance. PKU is particularly interesting from a genetics perspective in that hundreds of different mutations of the phenylalanine hydroxylase (PAH) gene exist, producing phenotypes of varying severity. Several splicing, nonsense, and insertion/deletion (indel) combinations cause a complete loss of PAH function and the potential for a very severe phenotype. On the other hand, several missense and indel mutations lead to variant PAH protein and some normal activity that improves with treatment using the PAH cofactor tetrahydrobiopterin. The importance of newborn screening for PKU is that immediate adoption of a low-phenylalanine diet prevents many of the phenotypic manifestations from developing.[24]

Indications for Neonatal Genetic Diagnostic Testing

Given the high incidence of genetic disorders presenting in infancy and the greater availability of genetic testing, it is likely that genetic evaluation will be used more extensively in the future. Infants with craniofacial dysmorphism; congenital anomalies; disorders affecting the heart, kidneys, or liver; growth

TABLE 3.3 Disorders in Chromosome Number

Disorder	Chromosome Number Abnormality	Clinical Manifestations	Long-Term Effects or Prognosis
Down syndrome (trisomy 21)	Three copies of chromosome 21 instead of two	More frequent with maternal age >35 years; infants have hypotonia, weak Moro reflex, developmental delay, flattened facies, upward-slanted palpebral issues, small dysplastic, low-set ears, congenital heart disease, joint hyperflexibility, short neck with redundant skin, single transverse palmar creases, pelvic dysplasia, gastrointestinal malformations	Most common genetic cause of intellectual disability; life expectancy of 60 years
Klinefelter syndrome	Two X, one Y sex chromosome (male only)	Tall stature with long arms and legs, enlarged breasts, small testes with lack of sperm production, sparse facial/body hair, higher pitched voice	Normal life expectancy
Turner syndrome	One X sex chromosome (female only)	Short stature, congenital lymphedema, patella and hip dislocation, scoliosis, widespread nipples on shield chest, redundant nuchal skin, low posterior hairline, congenital heart disease, hypothyroidism, strabismus, ovarian dysfunction	Life expectancy of 50 years; learning disabilities, but usually normal intelligence
Patau syndrome (trisomy 13)	Three copies of chromosome 13	Cutis aplasia, microphthalmia, microcephaly, sloping forehead, holoprosencephaly, capillary hemangiomas, deafness, congenital heart disorders, missing ribs, clinodactyly, polydactyly, hyperplastic/hyperconvex nails, severe developmental delay, severe growth retardation, renal abnormalities	90%–95% die within first year of life
Edwards syndrome (trisomy 18)	Three copies of chromosome 18	Small appearance, tight palpebral fissures, hypoplastic nose, narrow forehead, prominent occiput micrognathia, cleft lip or palate, microcephaly, congenital heart disease, short sternum, limited hip abduction, clinodactyly, rocker-bottom feet, hypoplastic nails, inguinal or abdominal hernia	95% die within first year of life

Source: Data from Bacino CA, Lee B. Cytogenetics. In: Kliegman RM, St Geme JW, Blum NJ, et al., eds. *Nelson Textbook of Pediatrics.* 21st ed. Philadelphia, PA: Elsevier; 2020:652–676.

abnormalities; developmental delay; and a host of other presentations are likely to receive genetic testing. Such testing may range from karyotyping to more extensive chromosome studies including fluorescence in situ hybridization (FISH) and chromosomal microarray analysis.[25] A research study in a neonatal ICU evaluated the use of clinical exome sequencing in critically ill infants. This analysis uses next-generation sequencing that focuses on only the exons within the genome, saving time and money and identifying the important coding regions of the chromosomes. Of the 278 infants enrolled, 102 received a molecular diagnosis, and that diagnosis affected the management decisions for 53 infants. This study underlines the relative magnitude of genetic disorders, often single gene disorders, presenting as critical illness in early life.[26]

KEY POINTS

- DNA is the molecule of genetic inheritance. Germ cells (egg and sperm) each contain 23 chromosomes: 22 autosomes and one sex chromosome. Upon fertilization, the resulting zygote has the normal human chromosome content consisting of pairs of homologous autosomes, 1 to 22, and two sex chromosomes, XX or XY, for a total of 46 chromosomes.

- DNA is found in the cell nucleus and is made up of long polymers of nucleotides. Each polymer strand is connected to a complementary strand through hydrogen bonds formed between opposite bases.

- There are four DNA bases: adenine (A), cytosine (C), guanine (G), and thymine (T). Complementary base pairing joins A–T pairs with two hydrogen bonds and G–C pairs with three hydrogen bonds.

- The cell cycle enables one cell to give rise to two identical daughter cells. During the cell cycle, all DNA of the parent cell is replicated, doubling the number of chromosomes. At mitosis, the chromosomes are divided equally between daughter cells so that each receives its own copy of the original DNA.

- Germ cells contain only half of the original DNA of a parent cell and are produced through the process of meiosis. In meiosis, after originally duplicating the DNA from a germ cell precursor, the cell goes through two divisions, resulting in germ cells with a single copy of each autosome and one sex chromosome, for a total of 23 chromosomes.

- DNA replication involves a complex of several enzymes working at replication origin sites along the chromosomes. Construction of new complementary strands proceeds from the 5′ to the 3′ direction, reading off a template strand oriented in the 3′ to 5′ direction. Because proofreading capacity is built into the replication machinery, many incorrectly inserted nucleotides are removed before they can create a permanent change in the DNA template.

- Genes, the segments of DNA that code for protein synthesis, are distributed along the chromosomes separated by long stretches of noncoding DNA. Noncoding DNA is not inert; it contributes to the regulation of transcription factor binding and influences gene expression rate.

- Gene expression refers to the process of DNA coding for the synthesis of a new protein. Transcription factors bind and influence the separation of DNA strands and binding of RNA polymerase near the gene promoter region, with subsequent RNA strand elongation until a termination signal is reached. This produces a pre-mRNA.

- Pre-mRNA is modified with the removal of unexpressed introns by spliceosomes, and reconnecting exons that will influence the shape and folding of the protein product. After further modification, the mature mRNA leaves the nucleus to enter the cytoplasm.

- Once in the cytoplasm, ribosomes attach to the mRNA to begin the process of translation. tRNAs bring amino acids to the ribosome for initiation and elongation of a growing polypeptide chain of amino acids held together by peptide bonds.

- Protein folding and other post-translational modifications proceed, with eventual emergence of a fully functional protein.

- Although more than 99.4% of human DNA is identical, when considered base by base there is substantial variability. SNPs (sites where a single nucleotide differs between people) are very common, and these variations can lead to altered function if they occur in or near a gene. DNA mutations are preserved in descendants if they are not lethal mutations and if they have positive or modest negative benefit to the organism, or produce no change in structure or function.

- Even single point mutations can, however, disrupt normal synthesis of the protein coded by a gene; many of these mutations caused by a single base change, termed a *missense mutation*, change an amino acid in the protein product of the gene.

- Nonsense mutations result in a premature stop codon and produce a truncated, nonfunctional protein.

- Many deletion and insertion mutations alter the mRNA's reading frame, resulting in a frameshift mutation that can greatly alter the amino acid sequence of the resulting protein.

- The exact DNA sequence of a person constitutes his or her genotype, whereas the person's physical characteristics and presentation of genetic diseases constitutes his or her phenotype.

- Genes are often represented by two alleles—one on each homologous chromosome. The term *homozygous* indicates that a person has identical alleles at both gene loci, whereas having two different alleles is referred to as being heterozygous.

- Inheritance of traits or genetic disorders depends on the number and strength of the alleles that confer disease susceptibility.

- Autosomal dominant inheritance indicates that the presence of a single mutant allele can confer the phenotype of the disorder—the allele's influence on cell function is sufficient to cause disease.
- With autosomal recessive inheritance, both alleles of a gene must have mutations in order to have the phenotype of the disorder. Having one normal allele is sufficient to suppress the disorder's manifestations.
- Other patterns of inheritance include sex-linked (involving the sex chromosomes X or Y); trinucleotide repeat (involving expansion of a short segment of a repeated 3-base sequence); and mitochondrial inheritance.
- Additional differences in presentation of genetic disorders arise due to variable ability of a mutation to manifest as the disorder 100% of the time, that is, the penetrance of the disorder. Similarly, disease severity can vary in many genetic disorders, a characteristic referred to as expressivity.
- The genotype/phenotype correlation and pathophysiology of single gene disorders such as Marfan syndrome are much clearer in linking etiology to patient presentation. On the other hand, disorders in which a family history (indicating heritability) is present but no single gene is responsible (multifactorial diseases) still need to be elucidated. Complex interactions of genotype, SNPs, environment, experience, and other factors influence the epidemiology and presentation of these disorders.
- Clinical tools in genetics include family history and pedigree development, recognition of genetic "red flags," direct chromosome visualization (karyotyping), hybridization assays and SNP identification, and WGS.
- At the population level, GWAS can identify plausible candidate SNPs involved in genetic risks.
- Epigenetics is the field studying nonmutational influences on gene expression and disease mutations.
- Genetic disorders are often detected in fetuses and neonates by prenatal and newborn screening. In other pediatric cases, abnormalities of physical features (dysmorphisms) or abnormal function detected at birth and during childhood development prompt genetic testing.
- For disorders such as inborn errors of metabolism, early detection through screening and confirmation through advanced genetic testing can be lifesaving or life extending when treatments can be initiated early.

REFERENCES

1. Hegde MR, Crowley MR. Genome and gene structure. In: Pyeritz RE, Korf BR, Grody W, eds. *Emery and Rimoin's Principles and Practice of Medical Genetics and Genomics.* 7th ed. Philadelphia, PA: Elsevier; 2019:53–77.
2. Epstein RS, Moyer TP, Aubert RE, et al. Warfarin genotyping reduces hospitalization rates. Results from the MM-WES (Medco-Mayo Warfarin Effectiveness Study). *J Am Coll Cardiol.* 2010;55:2804–2812.
3. Antonarakis SE, Cooper DE. Human genomic variants and inherited disease: molecular mechanisms and clinical consequences. In: Pyeritz RE, Korf BR, Grody WW, eds. *Emery and Rimoin's Principles and Practice of Medical Genetics and Genomics.* 7th ed. Philadelphia, PA: Elsevier; 2019:125–200.
4. Myerowitz R. Tay-Sachs disease-causing mutations and neutral polymorphisms in the Hex A gene. *Hum Mutat.* 1997;9:195–208. doi:10.1002/(SICI)1098-1004(1997)9:3<195::AID-HUMU1>3.0.CO;2–7.
5. Ogura Y, Bonen DK, Inohara N, et al. A frameshift mutation in NOD2 associated with susceptibility to Crohn's disease. *Nature.* 2001;411:603–606. doi:10.1038/35079114.
6. Hampe J, Cuthbert A, Croucher PJP, et al. Association between insertion mutation in NOD2 gene and Crohn's disease in German and British populations. *Lancet.* 2001;357:1925–1928. doi:10.1016/S0140-6736(00)05063-7.
7. He S, Liang C. Frameshift mutation of UVRAG: switching a tumor suppressor to an oncogene in colorectal cancer. *Autophagy.* 2015;11:1939–1940. doi:10.1080/15548627.2015.1086523.
8. Lee JH, Choi YJ, Je EM, et al. Frameshift mutation of WISP3 gene and its regional heterogeneity in gastric and colorectal cancers. *Hum Pathol.* 2016;50:146–152. doi:10.1016/j.humpath.2015.12.009.
9. Velazquez C, Esteban-Cardenosa EM, Lastra E, et al. A PALB2 truncating mutation: implication in cancer prevention and therapy of hereditary breast and ovarian cancer. *Breast.* 2018;43:91–96. doi:10.1016/j.breast.2018.11.010.
10. Whelan AJ, Ball S, Best L, et al. Genetic red flags: clues to thinking genetically in primary care practice. *Prim Care.* 2004;31:497–508. doi:10.1016/j.pop.2004.04.010.
11. Dupont C, Armant DR, Brenner CA. Epigenetics: definition, mechanisms and clinical perspective. *Semin Reprod Med.* 2009;27:351–357. doi:10.1055/s-0029-1237423.
12. Egger G, Liang G, Aparicio A, Jones PA. Epigenetics in human disease and prospects for epigenetic therapy. *Nature.* 2004;429:457–463. doi:10.1038/nature02625.
13. Bishop KS, Ferguson LR. The interaction between epigenetics, nutrition and the development of cancer. *Nutrients.* 2015;7:922–947. doi:10.3390/nu7020922.
14. Chen SH, Lv QL, Hu L, et al. DNA methylation alterations in the pathogenesis of lupus. *Clin Exp Immunol.* 2017;187;185–192. doi:10.1111/cei.12877.
15. Sekigawa I, Okada M, Ogasawara H, et al. DNA methylation in systemic lupus erythematosus. *Lupus.* 2003;12:79–85. doi:10.1191/0961203303lu321oa.
16. Abdolmaleky HM, Cheng KH, Faraone SV, et al. Hypomethylation of MB-COMT promoter is a major risk factor for schizophrenia and bipolar disorder. *Hum Mol Genet.* 2006;15:3132–3145. doi:10.1093/hmg/ddl253.
17. Nohesara S, Ghadirivasti M, Mostafavi S, et al. DNA hypomethylation of MB-COMT promoter in the DNA

derived from saliva in schizophrenia and bipolar disorder. *J Psychiatr Res.* 2011;45;1432–1438. doi:10.1016/j.jpsychires.2011.06.013.

18. Burzynski SR. Aging: gene silencing or gene activation? *Med Hypotheses.* 2005;64:201–208. doi:10.1016/j.mehy.2004.06.010.

19. Hur K, Cejas P, Feliu J, et al. Hypomethylation of long interspersed nuclear element-1 (LINE-1) leads to activation of proto-oncogenes in human colorectal metastasis. *Gut.* 2014;63:635–646. doi:10.1136/gutjnl-2012-304219.

20. Baxter SK, King M-K. A time to sequence (editorial). *JAMA Pediatr.* 2017;171:e173435. doi:10.1001/jamapediatrics.2017.3435.

21. Latendresse G, Deneris A. An update on current prenatal testing options: first trimester and noninvasive prenatal testing. *J Midwifery Womens Health.* 2015;60:24–36. doi:10.1111/jmwh.12228.

22. Bacino CA, Lee B. Cytogenetics. In: Kliegman RM, St Geme JW, Blum NJ, et al, eds. *Nelson Textbook of Pediatrics.* 21st ed. Philadelphia, PA: Elsevier; 2020:652–676.

23. Scott DA, Lee B. Patterns of genetic transmission. In: Kliegman RM, St Geme JW, Blum NJ, et al, eds. *Nelson Textbook of Pediatrics.* 21st ed. Philadelphia, PA: Elsevier; 2020:640–652.

24. Danecka MK, Woidy M, Zschocke J, et al. Mapping the functional landscape of frequent phenylalanine hydroxylase (PAH) genotypes promotes personalized medicine in phenylketonuria. *J Med Genet.* 2015;52:175–185. doi:10.1136/jmedgenet-2014-102621.

25. Lalani SR. Current genetic testing tools in neonatal medicine. *Pediatr Neonatol.* 2017;58:111–121.

26. Meng L, Pammi M, Saronwala A, et al. Use of exome sequencing for infants in intensive care units: ascertainment of severe single-gene disorders and effect on medical management. *JAMA Pediatr.* 2017;171(12):e173438. doi:10.1001/jamapediatrics_2017.3438.

SUGGESTED RESOURCES

Gunder-McClary LM. *Essentials of Medical Genetics for Nursing and Health Professionals.* Burlington, MA: Jones & Bartlett; 2018.

Jameson JL, Kopp P. Principles of human genetics. In: Jameson JL, Fauci AS, Kasper DL, et al., eds. *Harrison's Principles of Internal Medicine.* 20th ed. New York, NY: McGraw-Hill; 2018:chap 456.

Kasper CE, Schneidereith TA, Lashley FR. *Lashley's Essentials of Clinical Genetics in Nursing Practice.* 2nd ed. New York, NY: Springer Publishing Company; 2016.

Pyeritz RE, Korf BR, Grody W, eds. *Emery and Rimoin's Principles and Practice of Medical Genetics and Genomics.* 7th ed. Philadelphia, PA: Elsevier; 2019.

4

CELL PHYSIOLOGY AND PATHOPHYSIOLOGY

Nancy C. Tkacs, Fruzsina K. Johnson, Robert A. Johnson, and Spencer A. Rhodes

THE CLINICAL CONTEXT

This chapter continues a theme of providing the building block concepts underlying physiology, pathophysiology, and pharmacology. Disorders of membrane transport, cell signaling, and cell death include conditions such as cystic fibrosis (altered ion channel), familial hypercholesterolemia (receptor-mediated endocytosis), receptor-targeting autoimmune disorders (myasthenia gravis and Graves disease), and cancer (failure of apoptosis), among many others. Of at least equal significance for students preparing for independent practice is the fact that many commonly prescribed and over-the-counter drugs target the proteins and mechanisms described in this chapter. For example, common medications to reduce heartburn block histamine receptors or active transport of hydrogen ions (proton pumps), some cardiovascular disorders are treated with calcium channel blockers (ion channels), and selective serotonin reuptake inhibitors used to manage depression and anxiety block a secondary active transport protein. This foundational content on cell biology thus provides the context in which many disease processes can be understood and appropriately managed.

OVERVIEW

As you read this book, what are some of the cells of your body doing?

- Photoreceptor cells in your retinas are detecting patterns on the page or screen.
- Additional neurons are relaying the information to neurons of the cortex that interpret the information as words that add up to concepts and (we hope!) new learning.
- Muscle cells, bones, and joints create movements of holding the book or e-reader, occasionally turning a page.
- Neurons in your brainstem are initiating rhythmic contractions of your diaphragm for regular breathing.
- Red blood cells are carrying oxygen throughout your body.
- White blood cells are producing immune mediators to protect you from infections.
- Cells in the sinoatrial node of the heart are initiating regular heartbeats.
- Gastrointestinal and liver cells are processing the contents of your last meal.
- Kidney cells are processing filtered plasma and producing urine.
- Myriad endocrine cells are synthesizing and secreting hormones that regulate body functions.
- And you are not consciously aware of all of this cellular activity that is keeping you alive and maintaining homeostasis!

The basic unit of life is the cell, and the vast majority of physiological processes are carried out within cells. Pathophysiological alterations at the cellular level underlie many diseases, and medications to treat those diseases often target specific cell proteins and functions. Unique functions of the organs and systems of the body are based on the differentiated structures and functions of the cells making up those organs and systems. This brief review of cell biology builds on the earlier reviews of chemistry, biochemistry, and molecular biology in Chapters 2, Chemical and Biochemical Foundations, and 3, Molecular Biology, Genetics, and

Genetic Diseases, to provide the foundation for the remainder of the book. The organelles and proteins described here make up the "cast of characters" acting out physiology at the cellular level. You will encounter membrane transporters, receptors, contractile mechanisms, and cell death pathways linked to pathophysiology and pharmacology in many different chapters, so this chapter provides a general introduction to prepare you for their roles in specific organs.

CELL COMPONENTS

CELL MEMBRANE

The boundary between intracellular and extracellular fluids is the cell membrane, often referred to as the plasma membrane. The cell membrane is a phospholipid bilayer in which the outer leaflet phospholipids are oriented with their polar head groups facing outward toward the extracellular fluid, and the inner leaflet phospholipids are oriented with their polar head groups facing the intracellular fluid. The nonpolar fatty acid tails of both leaflets make up the hydrophobic core of the membrane, providing the critical barrier that separates intracellular from extracellular fluid.

Molecules of cholesterol are interspersed with the phospholipids, controlling membrane fluidity. One can picture the cell membrane as being like a grilled cheese sandwich, with the outermost bread layers able to mix with water and polar solutes and the melted inner core acting like a barrier, impenetrable to water and to polar and charged solutes.

Integral proteins cross the membrane; some of these function as receptors, others as transporters or channels. Peripheral proteins are often attached to the inner leaflet and work with integral proteins to alter cell function. The outer leaflet is rich in glycoproteins and glycolipids, with complex branching carbohydrates attached. The layer of sugars projecting outward from the cell is referred to as its *glycocalyx*, and it functions in cell–cell recognition. The inner leaflet of the membrane is attached to proteins of the cytoskeleton. The cell membrane functions as a barrier between intracellular and extracellular fluids, as an electrical insulator that allows separation of electrical charges so that a potential difference or membrane voltage can exist between intracellular and extracellular compartments, and as an interface between extracellular messengers and intracellular changes. Within the cell, similar phospholipid membranes form the outer coats of many of the organelles that carry out the work of the cells (**Box 4.1** and **Figure 4.1**).

BOX 4.1
Characteristics of the Cell Membrane

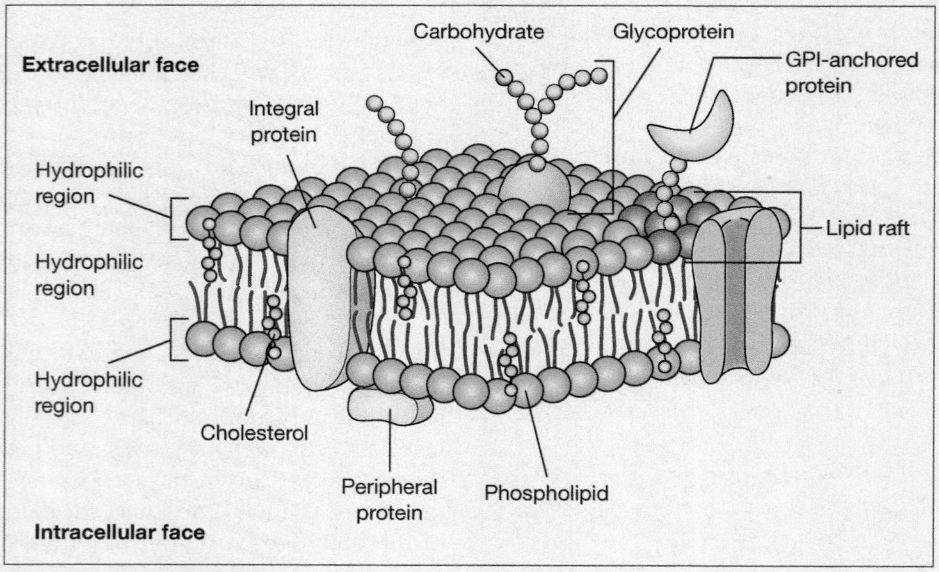

FIGURE 4.1 The cell membrane.

(*continued*)

BOX 4.1 (*continued*)
Characteristics of the Cell Membrane

- The cell membrane (also called the plasma membrane) is a complex phospholipid/cholesterol bilayer with hydrophilic/polar regions of phospholipids and cholesterol facing the extra cellular and intracellular fluids, and a central fatty acid and cholesterol ring core that is hydrophobic and restricts passage of polar/hydrophilic solutes.

- The membrane is studded with proteins—both integral proteins that span the membrane and proteins attached to the inner or outer membrane.

- The membrane is dynamic, moving with motile cells such as white blood cells, conducting exocytosis and endocytosis, and enlarging with cell hypertrophy. Membrane proteins can be internalized and recycled, and new membrane proteins can be inserted from vesicles.

- The clustered lipids shown in red in the figure represent a lipid raft—a region of tighter lipid and cholesterol packing that tends to move as a cohesive unit. A protein is linked to the lipid raft by a GPI anchor, allowing the protein to be associated with the plasma membrane without actual insertion through the membrane.

GPI, glycosylphosphatidylinositol.

CYTOPLASM

The *cytoplasm* refers to the entire contents of a cell. It is made up of cytosol (intracellular fluid), organelles, and other structural components of the cell (**Figure 4.2**). The aqueous intracellular fluid contains dissolved electrolytes, small biomolecules and metabolites, high-energy phosphate compounds, and key intracellular proteins. In muscle cells, the cytoplasm also contains the movement proteins myosin and actin. Protein synthesis and many biochemical processes

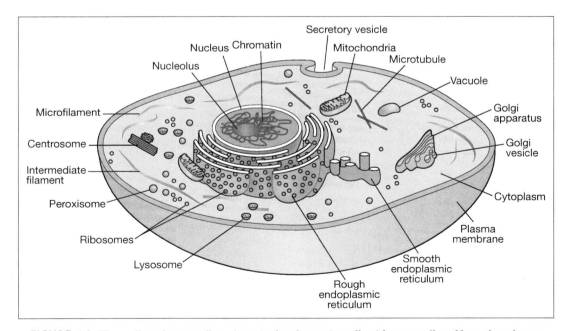

FIGURE 4.2 The cell and organelles. A typical eukaryotic cell with organelles. Note the plasma membrane boundary separating intracellular fluid (cytoplasm) from extracellular fluid. Membrane-bounded organelles include the nucleus and mitochondria (each with two outer membranes), rough and smooth endoplasmic reticulum, Golgi apparatus and vesicle budding from Golgi, lysosomes, peroxisomes, and vacuoles. Ribosomes, centrosome, and protein filaments do not have membranes.

occur in the cytoplasm, while some biochemical reactions occur in specific organelles like the mitochondria or smooth endoplasmic reticulum (SER).

NUCLEUS

The nucleus holds most of a cell's DNA, with the remainder found in the mitochondria. The nucleus also contains a nucleolus that functions in synthesis of ribosomes. Unless a cell is preparing to divide by mitosis, the nucleus contains DNA organized in chromosomes that are wound around histone proteins. The DNA is dispersed throughout the nucleus with regions that are tightly compacted and others that are more loosely arranged. Regions of DNA upstream of genes have binding sites for transcription factors that regulate gene expression. Patterns of gene expression are determined by cell type and differentiation, giving each cell type a unique set of proteins that relate to the functions of that cell within its tissue and organ niche. For example, liver cells produce many proteins for metabolism of glucose and lipids, as the liver is the major organ of energy homeostasis. On the other hand, neurons produce ion channels appropriate to generating action potentials and enzymes to synthesize neurotransmitters, needed for neuronal signaling.

The nuclear membrane has two layers with relatively low permeability; however, nuclear pores allow movement of proteins, signaling molecules, and messenger RNA (mRNA) molecules between nucleus and cytoplasm. Red blood cells do not contain nuclei, and skeletal muscle cells contain multiple nuclei. With these exceptions, each of the body's cells contains one nucleus.

RIBOSOMES AND ROUGH ENDOPLASMIC RETICULUM

Ribosomes are manufactured in the nucleus from RNA and proteins, and then migrate to the cytoplasm. A ribosome is made of large and small subunits that attach to mRNA for the purpose of protein synthesis, as noted in Chapter 3, Molecular Biology, Genetics, and Genetic Diseases. Ribosomes can be found free within the cytoplasm; others are attached to endoplasmic reticulum, forming the rough endoplasmic reticulum, so named for its bumpy appearance. Endoplasmic reticulum is contiguous with the nucleus and is the site of synthesis of proteins that will ultimately be secreted from the cell or moved to a specific cellular location. Within the rough endoplasmic reticulum, proteins fold to assume their secondary, tertiary, and (if applicable) quaternary structures. Rough endoplasmic reticulum is the site of chaperone proteins that detect the progress of protein folding and that mark misfolded proteins for destruction, through the unfolded protein response.

SMOOTH ENDOPLASMIC RETICULUM

SER is an intracellular membrane system connected to rough endoplasmic reticulum and containing enzymes for metabolic processes. It is particularly abundant in liver cells, which do a great deal of metabolic processing of lipid molecules as well as conducting biotransformation of drugs and toxins. SER is the location of some steps in steroid hormone synthesis in certain endocrine gland cells. It is also the site of synthesis of new membranes that can refresh the cell membrane or organelle membranes. SER is a major site of cellular calcium homeostasis, sequestering calcium to keep cytoplasmic free calcium levels low most of the time, and releasing calcium in response to membrane receptor signaling, described later in this chapter. In muscle cells, the specialized SER, called the *sarcoplasmic reticulum*, functions to release calcium ions that initiate muscle cell contraction, subsequently taking up calcium ions and causing muscle cell relaxation.

GOLGI APPARATUS

The Golgi apparatus is a stack of membranes organized in flattened sacks. It functions to sort, modify, and package proteins and lipids that are delivered in vesicles from the nearby endoplasmic reticulum. After proceeding through the Golgi stacks, these substances may leave the cell by exocytosis or be delivered to different intracellular locations. The Golgi apparatus also forms other organelles that are vesicle-type organelles, including lysosomes and other secretory vesicles, as well as being a source of plasma membrane.

MITOCHONDRIA

The mitochondria are the energy powerhouses of the cell, producing much of the cell's adenosine triphosphate (ATP). ATP is the energy source for cellular chemical reactions and ion transport, as well as being the source of phosphate for phosphorylation reactions. Energy-producing reactions of the Krebs cycle and oxidative phosphorylation take place in the mitochondria; thus, they are the site of cellular respiration, consuming oxygen and generating carbon dioxide. Cells with the highest energy requirements have a correspondingly higher number of mitochondria. Other significant aspects of mitochondrial function include the following:

- Mitochondria have two membranes—an outer membrane and a highly folded inner membrane. Some mitochondrial functions and proteins occur within the mitochondrial matrix, while others are localized to the inner membrane.
- Mitochondria contain their own DNA that codes for several mitochondrial proteins.
- Some steps of steroid hormone synthesis and of fatty acid catabolism take place in mitochondria.
- Mitochondria are able to sequester calcium and also play a role in initiating apoptosis (programmed cell death).

LYSOSOMES

Lysosomes contain degradative enzymes that break down aging cell organelles and molecules. The degradative enzymes are in the class called *acid hydrolases*, which depend on low pH for their function. Examples include proteases, which degrade proteins, and phospholipases, which degrade phospholipids and membranes. In phagocytic cells, such as neutrophils, phagocytosis of bacteria is followed by fusion with lysosomes, forming a phagolysosome. The lysosomal degradative enzymes then contribute to bacterial killing. Lysosomes can also contribute to cell death pathways.

PEROXISOMES

Peroxisomes are enriched in enzymes that use oxygen for their reactions. An example is β-oxidation of fatty acids, a pathway of energy generation that is conducted in both peroxisomes and mitochondria. The chemical reactions within peroxisomes often generate hydrogen peroxide (H_2O_2) as a byproduct, and these organelles contain the enzyme catalase to detoxify the H_2O_2.

CYTOSKELETON

The cytoskeleton is made up of protein filaments that extend through the cytoplasm, many of which are anchored to membrane proteins giving the cell its shape. These filaments can be organized by size from small to large: microfilaments (made of actin), intermediate filaments (composed of several proteins), and microtubules (made of tubulin). Organelles and vesicles can move along these filaments, and in mobile cells (such as white blood cells), they are responsible for cell movement. Microtubules contribute to chromosome alignment and movement during mitosis, and drugs that interfere with microtubule functions are used to treat cancer and other diseases. In muscle cells, contractile proteins are anchored to the cytoskeleton and membrane so that the whole cell shortens when actin and myosin cross-links are formed.

MECHANISMS OF MEMBRANE TRANSPORT

As previously noted, the cell membrane provides a lipid barrier between two aqueous solutions of differing composition: the intracellular fluid and the extracellular fluid. Oxygen, carbon dioxide, and steroid hormones and other lipid-soluble substances are able to freely diffuse across the membrane, whereas ions and biomolecules such as glucose and amino acids require specific membrane proteins and mechanisms to cross it. The type of membrane transport mechanism depends on:

- The chemical nature of the substance—primarily whether it is hydrophobic or hydrophilic
- The molecular size of the substance
- The concentration gradient of the substance across the membrane
- The direction of movement: Is the substance moving down its concentration gradient or *uphill* from the side with lower concentration to the side with higher concentration? In the latter case, energy input is required for transport to occur (**Figure 4.3**).

The extracellular and intracellular concentrations of several solutes of interest are listed in **Table 4.1**, along with corresponding pH differences. Note the striking difference in sodium and potassium concentrations—sodium is high extracellularly and potassium is high intracellularly. The concentration gradients for sodium and potassium drive many transport processes and also shape the membrane electrical activity of excitable cells. There is a striking concentration gradient for calcium as well, with extracellular calcium approximately 10,000 times greater than calcium in the intracellular fluid. We will return to the physiological importance of calcium movements several times in the book. Also note the concentration gradient for glucose. Many cells use glucose as their main energy source, keeping intracellular glucose concentration low and favoring glucose movement into the cell. The major classes of membrane transport mechanisms for these and other solutes are described next, with examples.

DIFFUSION

Sometimes called *simple diffusion*, this term describes movement across a barrier without a specific transport protein. Diffusion occurs down a concentration gradient; that is, from an area of high concentration to an area of low concentration (**Figure 4.4**). To diffuse through the cell membrane's lipid core requires a substance that is relatively small, with a hydrophobic, nonpolar chemical structure.

Net diffusion from one side to another is in the downhill direction, in response to the concentration gradient. Oxygen and carbon dioxide are examples, with oxygen entering tissues from capillaries, diffusing into cells and being continually used for cell metabolic processes, lowering its intracellular concentration, and favoring continual diffusion into the cell. Carbon dioxide is produced in many of these metabolic processes, increasing its intracellular concentration and favoring diffusion out of the cell and into capillary blood. In the lungs, thin alveolar walls and a minimal diffusion barrier to pulmonary capillary blood facilitate movement of oxygen and carbon dioxide by diffusion. In alveolar air, partial pressure of oxygen is high and partial pressure of carbon dioxide is low, favoring diffusion of oxygen into pulmonary capillary blood and diffusion of carbon dioxide from pulmonary capillary blood to the alveolus for removal

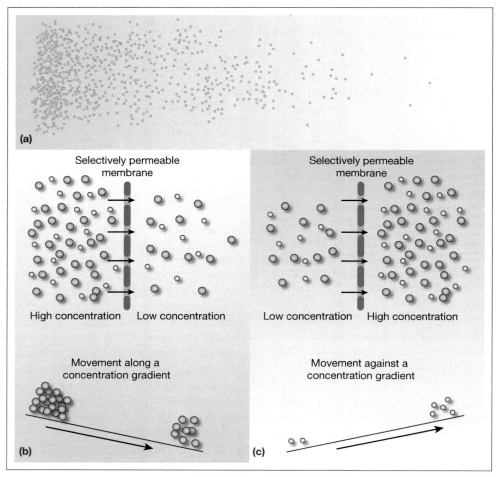

FIGURE 4.3 Concentration gradients. **(a)** Concentration gradient in a solution—no barrier. **(b)** Concentration gradient across a barrier permitting movement from high to low concentration (downhill movement). **(c)** Concentration gradient across a barrier—solute needs energy to be moved from region of low to high concentration (uphill movement, requires energy source).

by respiration. Rate of diffusion for a substance follows Fick's first law of diffusion:

$$J = -DA \frac{\Delta c}{\Delta x}$$

where

  J = flux, the amount of substance that moves across the barrier from a region of higher concentration to a region of lower concentration
  D = the diffusion constant for the substance
  A = the surface area for diffusion
  Δc = concentration gradient for the substance across a barrier
  Δx = thickness of the diffusion barrier

Pathophysiologically, some lung diseases thicken the barrier between alveolar air and capillary blood, reducing the rate of oxygen and carbon dioxide diffusion. In these cases, low levels of oxygen supplementation can increase the partial pressure difference (analogous to the concentration difference, Δc) to compensate for the increased barrier thickness (Δx).

Steroid hormones are relatively hydrophobic and diffuse across cell membranes, binding to intracellular receptors to exert their biological effects. Fatty acids enter cells and can be used as an energy source through oxidation in mitochondria and peroxisomes. Many drugs are hydrophobic and diffuse into cells to produce their biological effects. In summary, substances that are small, uncharged, and nonpolar, and substances that are larger, uncharged, hydrophobic, and nonpolar are all able to cross cell membranes by diffusing through the lipid bilayer. All other substances require other means of transport across this barrier, whether moving from extracellular to intracellular fluid or in the reverse direction.

TABLE 4.1 pH and Concentration Gradients for Physiological Solutes in a Typical Cell

Solutes and pH	Extracellular Concentration	Intracellular Concentration
pH	7.4	7.2
Solutes		
Sodium	135–147 mEq/L	10–15 mEq/L
Potassium	3.5–5.0 mEq/L	120–150 mEq/L
Calcium	2.1–2.8 mmol/L (total) 1.1–1.4 mmol/L (free, ionized)	~10^{-7} mmol/L (ionized)
Chloride	95–105 mEq/L	20–30 mEq/L
Phosphate	1.0–1.4 mmol/L (total) 0.5–0.7 mmol/L (ionized)	0.5–0.7 mmol/L (ionized)
Bicarbonate	22–28 mEq/L	12–16 mEq/L
Magnesium	0.6 mmol/L (ionized)	1 mmol/L (ionized) 18 mmol/L (total)
Glucose	5.5 mmol/L	Very low

Sources: Data from Aronson et al. (2017); Koeppen BM, Stanton BA, eds. *Berne & Levy Physiology.* 7th ed. Philadelphia, PA: Elsevier; 2018.

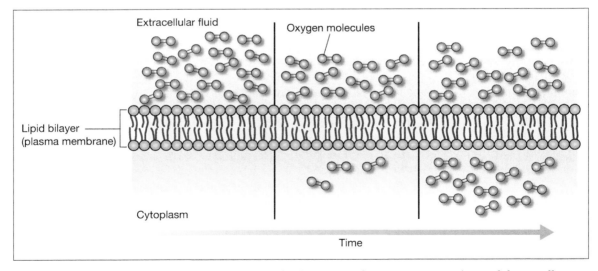

FIGURE 4.4 Simple diffusion. This method of transmembrane movement is used by small, nonpolar molecules, such as oxygen and carbon dioxide, and by lipids such as fatty acids and steroid hormones.

ENDOCYTOSIS AND EXOCYTOSIS

Large molecules such as proteins can be brought into cells or secreted by cells by endocytosis and exocytosis, respectively.

Endocytosis

In endocytosis, a portion of extracellular fluid is engulfed by the cell membrane into a vesicle that pinches off and enters the cell (**Figure 4.5**). Cells are able to conduct surveillance of molecules in their environment through this process. Endocytosis of small amounts of extracellular fluid is referred to as *pinocytosis*. Professional phagocytic cells, such as macrophages and neutrophils, use a similar mechanism to engulf large particles, such as bacteria, internalizing them and destroying them as part of their role in host defense. This process is

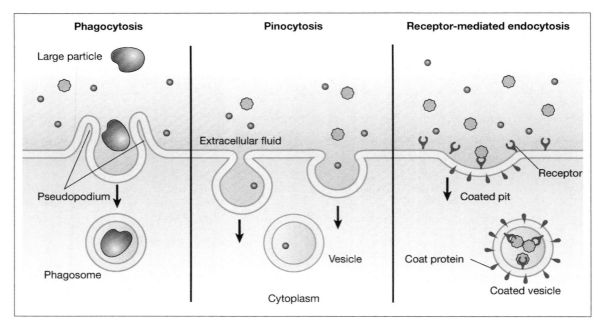

FIGURE 4.5 Endocytosis. Extracellular fluid and particulate matter are pinched off into a vesicle that invaginates into the cell. Phagocytosis is used for larger particles, even cells, while pinocytosis is the internalization of small amounts of fluid and solutes. Receptor-mediated endocytosis is initiated by a specific extracellular particle (such as a low-density lipoprotein) binding to its receptor in the region of a coated pit and signaling for membrane internalization.

referred to as *phagocytosis* to differentiate it as a process most common to phagocytes.

Cells can take up specific extracellular particles such as low-density lipoproteins (LDLs) through interactions between membrane receptors and membrane regions where the cytoskeletal protein clathrin is attached. In this process, termed *receptor-mediated endocytosis*, binding of LDLs, for example, to their receptors signals the underlying membrane and clathrin protein to form an endocytic vesicle. The clathrin protein then folds to enclose the endocytic vesicle, which enters the cell to deliver its contents. This is a selective process enhanced by the presence on a given cell membrane of receptors for a given solute that cell needs to function. The most common form of familial hypercholesterolemia is due to malfunction of LDL receptors that do not trigger endocytosis—this disorder manifests with extremely high cholesterol levels, tissue cholesterol accumulation, and early-onset atherosclerosis.

Exocytosis

The process of exocytosis is essentially the reverse of endocytosis. A membrane-coated vesicle moves to the cell membrane and fuses with it, releasing its contents to the extracellular fluid (**Figure 4.6**). As with endocytosis, there are two prominent modes of exocytosis: general (also referred to as constitutive) and signal-generated (also referred to as *regulated*). General exocytosis is an ongoing process of cells that primarily

function to synthesize secreted proteins—often proteins that will be carried in the blood plasma. Examples include many of the proteins synthesized by the liver (albumin, coagulation proteins, and carrier proteins) or by immune *plasma cells* (immunoglobulins). In these types of cells, protein synthesis may be upregulated or downregulated, but proteins are generally secreted soon after they are synthesized (**Figure 4.6a**).

Regulated exocytosis (see **Figure 4.6b**) is a process in which a molecule or protein destined for secretion is held in intracellular vesicles until a specific event triggers exocytotic release. For neurons, this would involve an action potential reaching an axon terminal, opening of voltage-dependent calcium channels, and release of neurotransmitter vesicles into a synaptic cleft. For β cells of the pancreatic islets, depolarization can occur in response to increased cellular glucose metabolism similarly opening voltage-gated calcium channels, stimulating regulated exocytosis of vesicles containing the hormone insulin. Thus, endocytosis and exocytosis are mechanisms for bulk movement of large numbers of solutes or large solutes such as proteins across the cell membrane by means of membrane-bounded vesicles.

FACILITATED DIFFUSION

Many of the substances that move across cell membranes are polar and hydrophilic, and are thus unable to move by simple diffusion across the membrane's

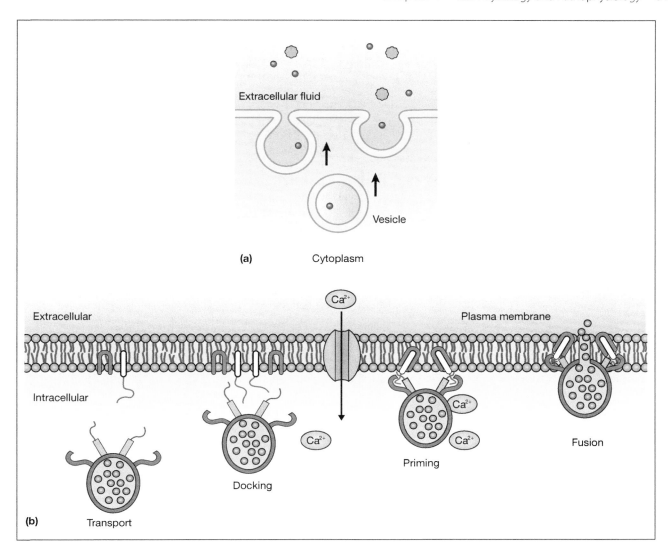

FIGURE 4.6 Exocytosis. **(a)** Constitutive exocytosis. This process basically reverses endocytosis—a substance made in the cell is packaged in a vesicle by the Golgi apparatus, moves to the membrane, and is released to the extracellular fluid. Exocytosis can occur continuously; an example is seen in proteins that must be constantly renewed, as in liver production of albumin and many clotting proteins. **(b)** Regulated exocytosis. Secretion of hormones and neurotransmitters does not occur constantly; rather, a signal is required before they can be released. This is a calcium-dependent process in which vesicles of hormone or transmitter are located near membrane release sites. When intracellular calcium increases, vesicles can dock and fuse with the membrane, followed by exocytosis of vesicle contents.

hydrophobic lipid core. Movement of these substances down their concentration gradient is facilitated by membrane protein transporters, which bind a molecule of the substance on the side of higher concentration and release it on the side of lower concentration. Because the direction of net movement is from higher to lower concentration, this process is referred to as diffusion, and because the movement requires a protein carrier, it is referred to as facilitated (**Figure 4.7**).

Glucose is an example of a biomolecule that commonly enters cells through facilitated diffusion proteins, because it is highly hydrophilic and polar. Many cell types use glucose as their primary fuel, and the continual consumption of glucose keeps intracellular glucose concentration lower than extracellular glucose concentration. Glucose transporters have the generic name GLUT, with the various subtypes identified by number (e.g., GLUT1 through GLUT5).

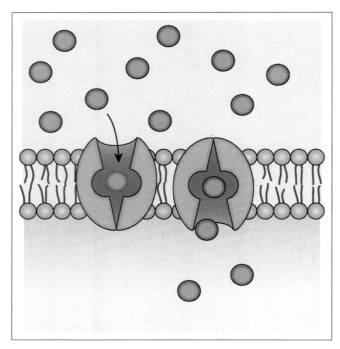

FIGURE 4.7 Facilitated diffusion is used to move polar or charged solutes down a concentration gradient. Thus, the direction is the same as that of simple diffusion, from a region of higher concentration to a region of lower concentration. A protein carrier is needed because the plasma membrane's hydrophobic core blocks passage of the solute and its shell of water. This is the most common way for glucose and amino acids to enter cells.

The GLUT2 protein is particularly associated with moving glucose at high rates in specific sites. Of these, GLUT2 will be highlighted again in Chapters 14, Liver, and 17, Endocrine System, describing the metabolic role of the liver and control of circulating glucose. Glucose can enter liver cells via GLUT2 after a meal, when glucose and insulin levels are high and the liver is metabolizing glucose and also storing it in the form of glycogen. Then, during fasting, liver cells produce glucose through glycogen breakdown and new glucose synthesis (glycogenolysis and gluconeogenesis, respectively). In that state, glucose leaves the liver cells, also via GLUT2, maintaining fasting blood glucose levels in the normal range. GLUT4, on the other hand, is found in vesicles inside muscle and fat cells. When insulin is present, GLUT4 transporters move to the cell membrane and facilitate glucose entry into these cells. This process is discussed further in Chapter 17, Endocrine System, in the context of insulin actions in the body. In summary, facilitated diffusion is a mechanism by which hydrophilic polar and charged substances can move across cell membranes down their concentration gradients.

ACTIVE TRANSPORT

Active transport is a mechanism for moving a solute against its concentration gradient, which requires the input of energy. There are two types of active transport: primary and secondary.

Primary Active Transport

The most abundant primary active transporter of the body is the sodium–potassium pump (Na$^+$/K$^+$ pump), also referred to as the *sodium–potassium ATPase* (adenosine triphosphatase). This protein, found on all cells of the body, splits ATP and, with the energy provided, transports sodium out of the cell and transports potassium into the cell (**Figure 4.8**). Both of these ions are moving against their concentration gradients, and the ability to maintain normal intracellular and extracellular fluid homeostasis is dependent on these transport activities. The concentration gradient for sodium created by the Na$^+$/K$^+$ pump is a source of potential energy in that other solutes can be transported against their concentration gradients by transporters that link their movement to sodium influx into cells. (This process is *secondary active transport*, described later.)

The Na$^+$/K$^+$ pump is active continuously. Beginning with the step of sodium binding, three cytoplasmic sodium ions bind to sites facing the intracellular fluid. ATP then binds to the transport protein and is split, donating a high-energy phosphate group and changing the pump's configuration. The protein shifts its orientation and releases the sodium ions to the extracellular fluid, subsequently binding two potassium ions. This is followed by release of potassium to the intracellular fluid and release of the bound phosphate. The cycle is repeated with the next round of sodium binding and ATP hydrolysis.

Two additional ATP-requiring active transporters are referred to throughout the book (**Figure 4.9**). The first of these is the calcium ATPase, or calcium pump. Another name for this protein is the sarcoendoplasmic reticulum calcium ATPase (SERCA). This pump is found on cell membranes and also on the membrane of the endoplasmic reticulum (or sarcoplasmic reticulum in muscle cells; **Figure 4.9a**). The large calcium gradient between extracellular fluid and intracellular fluid is maintained by these pumps that move calcium across the cell membrane or into the endoplasmic reticulum. Certain cell signaling pathways involved in muscle contraction or receptor activation can release endoplasmic/sarcoplasmic reticulum calcium in brief bursts that cause a cascade of physiological responses. Calcium ATPase activity then restores the low intracellular calcium level and terminates the signal. Finally, the proton pump, or potassium–hydrogen ATPase, is involved in secretion of hydrochloric acid

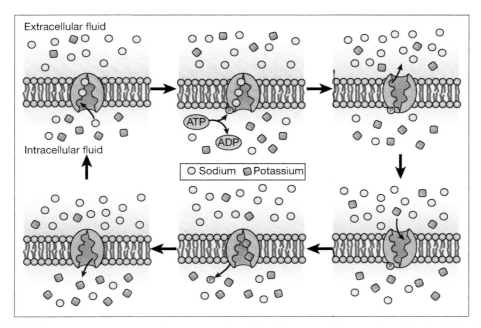

FIGURE 4.8 Active transport: sodium–potassium (Na$^+$/K$^+$) pump. Every cell of the body has Na$^+$/K$^+$ pumps that maintain the proper ionic gradients of high intracellular K$^+$ and low intracellular Na$^+$. These conditions allow the electrophysiological operation of electrically active cells like the cardiac myocytes and the neurons of the brain, and drive transport processes in all tissues. Much of the body's oxygen consumption at rest and during physical activity provides the ATP needed for this continual movement of Na$^+$ and K$^+$ ions against their concentration gradients. When tissues become hypoxic, cells swell and eventually die because of inability to maintain ionic homeostasis. ADP, adenosine diphosphate; ATP, adenosine triphosphate; P, phosphate; Pi, inorganic phosphate.

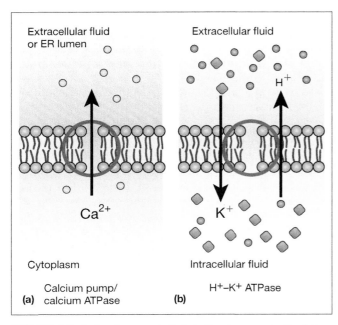

FIGURE 4.9 Active transport. **(a)** Active transport of calcium (Ca^{2+}) and **(b)** hydrogen (H$^+$) and potassium (K$^+$) ions. Uphill movement of the ions is accomplished, in part, by these ATPases that maintain cell ionic and acid–base homeostasis.
ATPase, adenosine triphosphatase; ER, endoplasmic reticulum.

in the stomach and in renal acid–base regulation. The proton pump is the target of drugs that inhibit gastric acid secretion (**Figure 4.9b**).

Secondary Active Transport

Based on the sodium gradient established by the sodium–potassium pump, cells have many transporters that link downhill sodium movement into the cell to drive the uphill movement of other substances against their concentration gradient. This process is called secondary active transport because it does not use ATP, but it does use the favorable energy of allowing sodium to sneak back into the cell after it is actively removed by the Na$^+$/K$^+$ pump. There are numerous examples of secondary active transporters contributing to solute movements in specialized tissues.

Cells of the renal tubules and gastrointestinal tract function to completely remove glucose molecules from one side of an epithelial barrier to the other, against its concentration gradient. The secondary active transport proteins called SGLT1 and SGLT2 (sodium–glucose transporter) accomplish this function in the gastrointestinal tract and renal tubule, respectively. This is an example of cotransport (also referred to as *symport*), in that the sodium and glucose are both moving in the same direction (**Figure 4.10**). SGLT2 is a target of a class of drugs (SGLT2 inhibitors) used in management of type 2 diabetes.

Other secondary active transporters move sodium in the opposite direction of the paired solute. For example, in muscle cells, some of the calcium that enters the cell to cause muscle contraction is removed by a transporter that links entry of three sodium ions to exit of one calcium ion. This opposite movement of ions is referred to as *counter* transport (also known as *antiport*, for example, Na^+/Ca^{2+} exchange [NCX]). Other secondary active transporters described in this book are the sodium, potassium, and chloride cotransporters found in the tubular cells in the kidney that are the target of *loop* diuretic drugs. In the brain, neurotransmitters are removed from synapses by secondary active transporters selective for given transmitters, such as selective serotonin reuptake transporters. **Table 4.2** lists the transporters that are described elsewhere in this book.

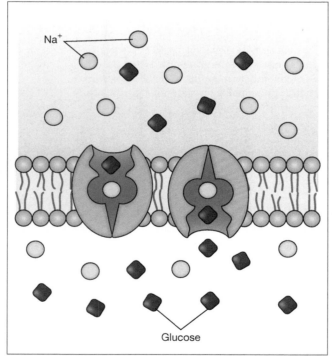

FIGURE 4.10 Secondary active transport. Secondary active transport links the movement of a solute down its concentration gradient (sodium being the most common) to the movement of a second solute against its concentration gradient. This is favorable when cells can benefit from maintaining a concentration gradient of a solute preferentially on one side of the membrane, while sparing ATP. The consumption of ATP by the sodium–potassium pump sustains the sodium concentration gradient so that sodium entry via these transporters is energetically favored. Sodium–glucose transporters are one example of secondary active transport. ATP, adenosine triphosphate.

AQUAPORINS

Although water molecules are polar, it was once thought that they were small enough to be able to freely diffuse across cell membranes. Aquaporins were later identified as channels that serve as the channels that serve as major transport mechanism for water to move into and out of cells, under the influence of osmotic pressure (**Figure 4.11**). Although aquaporin proteins are present in all cells, aquaporin movements are regulated in kidney cells in the distal nephron, where water absorption is controlled by the hormone vasopressin.

ION CHANNELS

Ion channels are transmembrane proteins with a central pore that allow movement of an ion down its concentration gradient. When they are open, ions freely diffuse through until the pores close, or until the ions reach electrochemical equilibrium based on the concentration difference of the ion and the membrane voltage that develops as a consequence of ion movement. Ion channels, by and large, are selective for one ion only. They are named according to the ion that they are selective for, such as sodium channels, potassium channels, and calcium channels (**Figure 4.12**). Ion channels are found in all body cells, but they have a particularly prominent role in electrically excitable cells such as neurons and muscle cells.

The presence of ion channels in the cell membrane contributes to the ability of cells to develop a *resting membrane potential*—a voltage difference across the cell membrane. Most cells have this potential difference as the inside of the cell is electrically negative with respect to the extracellular fluid, with the cell membrane able to separate the charges, maintaining the voltage difference.

The resting membrane potential develops, in part, based on the differential distribution of ions across the plasma membrane (sodium high outside, potassium high inside), as described earlier. In addition, the cell membrane has limited permeability to ions under resting conditions, but is more permeable to potassium than to any other ion. Finally a portion of the resting membrane potential is determined by the Na^+/K^+ pump activity that moves three sodium ions out of the cell for every two potassium ions that enter. How do these factors combine to create the resting membrane potential?

The role of membrane ion channels in producing a resting membrane potential is illustrated in **Figure 4.13**. Study **Figure 4.13a**—a diagram of a barrier separating two fluids of differing composition. As with extracellular fluid, the compartment on the left is high in sodium and low in potassium. As with intracellular fluid, the compartment on the right is high in potassium and low in sodium. Not shown in this figure

TABLE 4.2 Transport Mechanisms Described in This Book

Mode of Transport	Examples	Transporter Names and Locations
Facilitated diffusion	Glucose	GLUT1—red blood cells, blood–brain barrier, many other cells
		GLUT2—liver, pancreatic β cells, renal tubules
		GLUT3—neurons
		GLUT4—muscle and adipose cells (insulin-sensitive)
	Fructose	GLUT5—gastrointestinal tract
	Amino acids	Several transporter types found on most cells, enriched in small intestine and kidney tubules
Active transport (primary active transport)	Sodium–potassium (Na$^+$/K$^+$) pump	Membranes of all cells
	Calcium pump	Cell and endoplasmic reticulum membranes
	Potassium–hydrogen pump	Renal tubules, stomach parietal cells
Secondary active transport	Sodium–glucose cotransport	SGLT1 (gastrointestinal)
		SGLT2 (renal)
	Sodium–calcium exchange	NCX
	Sodium–potassium–2 chloride cotransport	NKCC
	Sodium–chloride cotransport	NCC
	Sodium–hydrogen exchange	NHE
	Sodium–serotonin cotransport	SERT
	Sodium–norepinephrine cotransport	NET
	Sodium–dopamine cotransport	DAT
Ion channels	Potassium leak channels	Many cells—set resting membrane potential
	Delayed potassium channels	Electrically excitable cells—action potential repolarization
	Fast sodium channels	Electrically excitable cells—action potential initiation and propagation
	Slow calcium channels	Muscle cells—some action potential initiation, provide calcium for contraction

are the accompanying anions that give electrical neutrality to each of these solutions. Given an impermeable membrane, none of these ions can move, and no potential difference can develop across the membrane.

Now refer to **Figure 4.13b**. All conditions are the same as in panel (a), but potassium channels are now inserted in the membrane. Now that the potassium ions have a pathway to leave the cell, they flow through the potassium channels, down their concentration gradient, as shown. However, without accompanying anion channels, negative charges are left behind, and

are attracted to the membrane and the greater number of positive charges now on the other side of the membrane. At this point, there is a potential difference across the membrane, with the right side compartment negative with respect to the left side compartment. The negative charge will build up until it attracts potassium ions back through their channels at a rate equal to their movement away. This electrical charge can be calculated based on the concentrations of potassium on each side of the membrane and is known as the *Nernst* potential. Most cells of the body have a resting membrane potential that is negative, owing to these factors:

- *Potassium leak channels* outnumber other open ion channels at rest, so potassium movements are the greatest factor setting the electrical equilibrium.

- The composition of the extracellular fluid and intracellular fluid differs regarding distribution of sodium, potassium, chloride, and calcium, so that each of these has different gradients for movement when ion channels open.
- Constant activity of the Na^+/K^+ pump maintains the proper ion composition of extracellular and intracellular fluids.

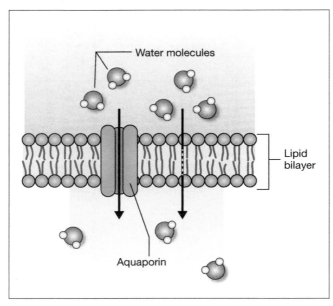

FIGURE 4.11 Aquaporins (water channels). Although some water molecules are able to move across plasma membranes by simple diffusion, the rate of water movement is greatly enhanced by the presence of aquaporin proteins in membranes of most cells. The movement is from a region of lesser osmotic strength to a region of greater osmotic strength, and the water movement is termed *osmosis*.

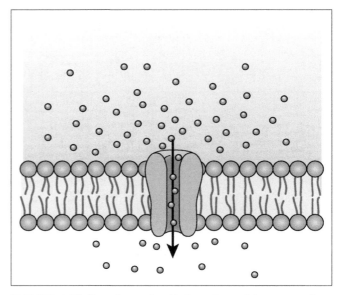

FIGURE 4.12 Ion channels. An ion channel is a pore that, when open, permits a flow of ions in a stream, down its concentration gradient. Most ion channels are selective for one ion, from which they derive their name.

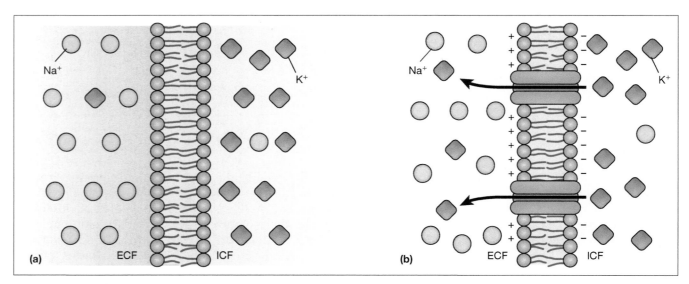

FIGURE 4.13 Potassium leak channels contribute to a resting membrane potential. Potassium (K^+) is high in the ICF and low in the ECF. (**a**) If fluids with this composition are separated by a solid membrane, no ion movement will occur. (**b**) If potassium channels are inserted in the membrane, K^+ will move from ICF to ECF, down its concentration gradient. This will generate a membrane potential difference, with the inside negative with respect to the outside.
ECF, extracellular fluid; ICF, intracellular fluid; Na^+, sodium.

A consequence of having a resting membrane potential is that, for excitable cells, inputs that lead to depolarization (decreased or less negative membrane potential) can open *voltage-gated* channels, some of which produce action potentials—large electrical spikes of depolarization that can be propagated for long distances along axons and ultimately release neurotransmitter molecules into synapses. Action potentials of neurons are the basis of brain activity, and action potentials of muscle cells are the basis of contraction of skeletal and cardiac muscles. Action potentials can also produce contractions of smooth muscle cells, and depolarization can contribute to hormone release from endocrine cells. In summary, ion channels play many roles in cell and organ function and are critical for the function of excitable neurons and muscle cells. Mutations in ion channel genes are the source of many disorders of neuron and muscle function, including epilepsy.

Thought Questions

1. What properties of a solute are relevant in determining the type of transport that moves the solute into and out of cells?

2. Explain the role of the Na+/K+ pump in enabling the function of secondary active transport proteins.

3. What role do potassium leak channels play in creating a negative resting membrane potential?

MECHANISMS OF CELL SIGNALING

OVERVIEW OF SIGNAL TRANSDUCTION

Many rapid homeostatic adjustments are made possible by the autonomic transmitters norepinephrine (sympathetic nervous system) and acetylcholine (parasympathetic nervous system). Adaptations including cardiovascular regulation, airway diameter, gastrointestinal tone and secretions, and kidney functions are modulated by these autonomic mediators. In addition, hormones such as epinephrine, vasopressin, glucagon, and pituitary trophic hormones also have rapid actions to modulate activity of their target cells, glands, and organs. The actions of all of these *ligands* are mediated by binding to membrane G protein–coupled receptors (GPCRs). Growth and development signals, as well as other types of homeostatic adjustments requiring cell division and new protein synthesis, usually involve receptors working through *tyrosine kinase* mechanisms. Finally, steroid and thyroid hormones are able to diffuse through the cell membrane, binding to nuclear receptors and altering cell transcription and translation for long-term effects on cell function. Many of these reactions are reversible once the ligand diffuses away from the receptor, and there are several other mechanisms that stop or reverse the actions of receptor activation, allowing compensatory adjustments to return to normal after a time of altered activity. One can think of these as the *brakes* that slow a system down after a period of applying a *gas pedal*.

AUTONOMIC NERVOUS SYSTEM AND SIGNALING BY G PROTEIN–COUPLED RECEPTORS

The autonomic nervous system is the major rapid regulatory system of the body. Autonomic neurons located within the central nervous system consist of preganglionic neurons that use the neurotransmitter acetylcholine. Parasympathetic preganglionic neurons are located in brainstem cranial nerve nuclei and in the sacral spinal cord, while sympathetic preganglionic neurons are located in thoracic and lumbar spinal segments. These preganglionic neurons have synaptic connections with autonomic postganglionic neurons in peripheral autonomic ganglia, with the parasympathetic ganglia generally located within or close to organs and sympathetic ganglia located lateral to the vertebral column or in front of the vertebral column. Parasympathetic postganglionic neurons are *cholinergic*, releasing the neurotransmitter acetylcholine, and most sympathetic postganglionic neurons are *adrenergic*, releasing the neurotransmitter norepinephrine. Sympathetic postganglionic neurons innervating sweat glands and certain vascular beds are cholinergic.

Much of our knowledge of GPCR mechanisms derives from biochemical, physiological, and pharmacological studies of cholinergic and adrenergic effects on target organs, as these end-organ responses to parasympathetic and sympathetic stimulation are mediated by these receptors. Both autonomic branches have particularly profound effects on cardiovascular control. In addition to autonomic transmitters, many neurotransmitters and hormones act via GPCRs. In this mode of cell signaling, an extracellular hydrophilic ligand binds to a recognition site on its membrane receptor, and this binding initiates a cascade of intracellular reactions in and near the membrane, generating intracellular second messengers that alter target cell activity.

Box 4.2 summarizes characteristics of GPCRs. The GPCRs have certain common structural elements, the chief one being that each is a long protein chain that crosses the plasma membrane seven times (**Figure 4.14**). When the appropriate ligand binds on the extracellular side of the receptor, the receptor's shape changes and it binds to and activates a three-part, guanosine triphosphate (GTP)-binding protein or *G protein* located at the intracellular face of the

BOX 4.2
Characteristics of G Protein–Coupled Receptors

- Found on all cells, GPCRs are the most common mechanism by which hormones and neurotransmitters influence cell and organ function.

- Signaling is amplified as a small group of receptors can activate a larger group of G proteins, ultimately stimulating membrane-bound enzyme production of many molecules of second messengers.

- Second messengers act by turning on protein kinase enzymes that phosphorylate intracellular proteins to change their function to meet the body's changing needs.

- Phosphorylation of some proteins increases their activity, while phosphorylation of other proteins decreases their activity, but in both cases a change in the protein's activity produces the final effect of hormone/receptor signaling.

- The strength and duration of GPCR effects are limited by various inhibitory and off-switches, including inhibitory receptors themselves, an intrinsic timing function of the GTPase activity of G proteins, and protein phosphatase enzymes that remove phosphate groups from proteins.

- Finally, the second messengers can be metabolized, terminating their action. For example, a phosphodiesterase cleaves cAMP and converts it into 5′-AMP, which is inactive.

5′-AMP, 5′-adenosine monophosphate; cAMP, cyclic adenosine monophosphate; GPCR, G protein–coupled receptor; GTPase, guanosine triphosphatase.

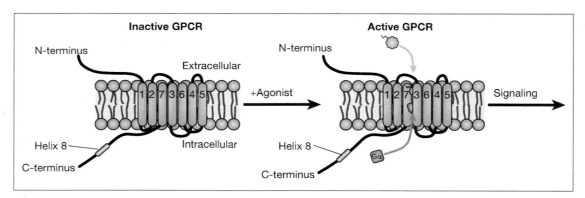

FIGURE 4.14 General features of GPCR structure. These receptors are often described as serpentine, because of the number of bends in the protein as they cross the membrane. Ligand-binding sites for hormones or neurotransmitters face the extracellular fluid, while receptor sites of G protein interactions face the intracellular fluid and inner membrane. GPCR, G protein–coupled receptor.

membrane. The G protein then dissociates, and its active α subunit activates a membrane-bound enzyme that begins to generate intracellular second messenger molecules.

G Protein–Coupled Receptors Linked to Adenylyl Cyclase

The first type of GPCRs discovered were those that stimulate the enzyme adenylyl cyclase and generate the intracellular second messenger cyclic adenosine monophosphate (cAMP). Many hormones and neurotransmitters exert their effects through increasing cAMP levels. The principles of the system are illustrated here by focusing on one of these receptors, the β-adrenergic receptor that responds to the hormone epinephrine and the sympathetic neurotransmitter norepinephrine.

When norepinephrine binds to the β-adrenergic receptor, the receptor undergoes a shape change and increases its affinity for a three-part G_s protein on the inner leaflet of the plasma membrane. The G protein, made up of α_s, β, and γ subunits, dissociates

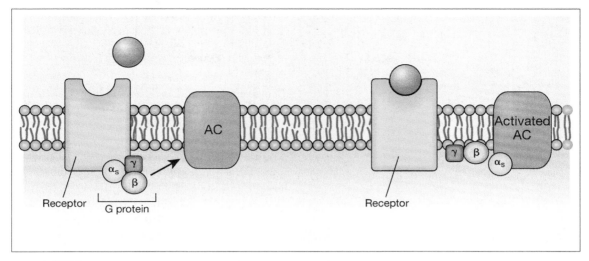

FIGURE 4.15 AC activation by GPCRs. Ligand binding to a stimulatory AC-linked receptor causes the dissociation of the attached G protein, allowing the α_s subunit to move to and activate the enzyme AC. The $\beta\gamma$ subunits remain bound together, but can move within the membrane to modulate the activity of other membrane proteins.
AC, adenylyl cyclase; GPCRs, G protein–coupled receptors.

into α_s, and a $\beta\gamma$ pair (**Figure 4.15**). The α_s moves to the nearby enzyme adenylyl cyclase and increases its activity. Activated adenylyl cyclase converts many molecules of ATP to cAMP, amplifying the signal (**Figure 4.16**). In the next step of the cascade, cAMP molecules diffuse throughout the cytoplasm, activating the enzyme protein kinase A (PKA; **Figure 4.17**). A *protein kinase* is an enzyme that adds a phosphate group onto target proteins. This process of *phosphorylation* occurs on the hydroxyl-containing amino acids serine, threonine, and tyrosine. Many of these protein kinases, including PKA, are serine/threonine kinases, phosphorylating target proteins at sites of the amino acids serine and threonine, thus altering target protein activity level. Each activated PKA can phosphorylate many copies of target protein molecules, further amplifying the signal to quickly change cell function. The end result is that an extracellular signal, in this case norepinephrine, can quickly alter cell and organ function through its GPCRs. β-Adrenergic receptor activation is the mechanism by which the sympathetic nervous system increases heart rate and force of contraction, for example.

The cAMP system is also the target of inhibitory receptors. An example of these is the M_2 subtype of muscarinic acetylcholine receptor. This receptor is found on sinoatrial node cells in the heart and is central to the mechanism used in slowing of heart rate by the parasympathetic transmitter acetylcholine. Activation of M_2 receptors activates a G_i protein that dissociates into α_i and a $\beta\gamma$ pair. The α_i protein inhibits adenylyl cyclase,

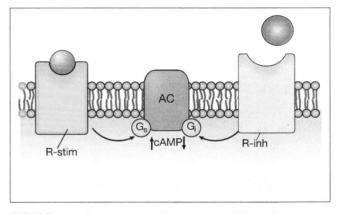

FIGURE 4.16 Stimulatory and inhibitory AC–linked receptors. AC can be stimulated or inhibited, depending on the type of receptor activated. Stimulatory receptors (R-stim) work through G_s to increase AC activity and cyclic adenosine monophosphate (cAMP) production; inhibitory receptors (R-inh) work through G_i to decrease AC activity and cAMP production.
AC, adenylyl cyclase.

decreasing cAMP levels, and the $\beta\gamma$ pair moves within the membrane to increase the activity of inhibitory potassium channels, in this case slowing the heart rate. Again, at each step of this cascade, there is amplification of the signal, so activation of several M_2 receptors can rapidly decrease cell cAMP levels and open many potassium channels, resulting in inhibition. The mechanism of α_i is depicted in **Figure 4.16**. The presence of both stimulatory and inhibitory types of receptors for the adenylyl

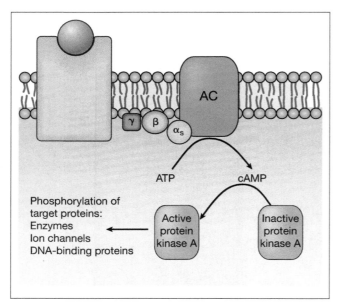

FIGURE 4.17 Downstream effects of cAMP. As an intracellular second messenger, cAMP binds to inactive PKA, releasing the active enzyme. Active PKA, in turn, conducts phosphorylation of intracellular proteins, changing their shape and thus changing their activity. These allosteric modifications depend on addition of phosphate groups to certain serine and threonine amino acids within the target proteins; thus, PKA is called a serine/threonine kinase. Examples of PKA targets are shown. These are specific to the organ and cell sites where receptor stimulation is occurring.

AC, adenylyl cyclase; cAMP, cyclic adenosine monophosphate; ATP, adenosine triphosphate; PKA, protein kinase A.

cyclase system provides for homeostatic adjustments that can upregulate *or* downregulate adaptive changes.

G Protein–Coupled Receptors Linked to Phospholipase C

The second GPCR system has an additional layer of complexity relative to the adenylyl cyclase system. In the phospholipase C–linked signaling cascade, receptors work through the G_q type of G protein, with α_q stimulating the membrane-bound enzyme phospholipase C. Activated phospholipase C splits the membrane phospholipid phosphatidylinositol bisphosphate (PIP_2) into diacylglycerol (DAG) and inositol trisphosphate (IP_3), with DAG remaining in the membrane and IP_3 diffusing into the cytoplasm and serving as an intracellular second messenger (**Figures 4.18** and **4.19**). DAG activates protein kinase C, which then proceeds to phosphorylate target proteins. IP_3 binds to receptors on the endoplasmic reticulum, causing the endoplasmic reticulum to release stored calcium in a burst, transiently increasing cytoplasmic calcium concentrations. The calcium can have several downstream effects, including initiating muscle contraction, binding to calmodulin to regulate many cell activities, and activating other protein kinases. An example of a phospholipase C–linked receptor is the α_1-adrenergic receptor on vascular smooth muscle. When sympathetic nerves innervating blood vessels release norepinephrine, it binds with high affinity to these receptors, increasing intracellular levels of IP_3 and releasing calcium from the endoplasmic reticulum. Calcium elevations lead

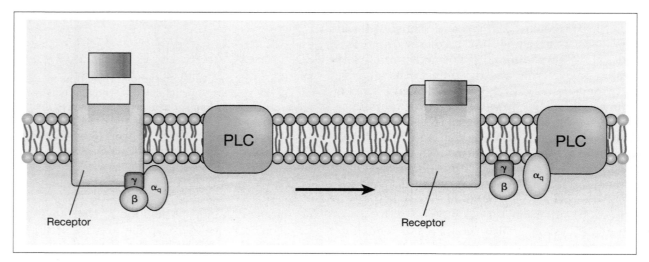

FIGURE 4.18 PLC-activating receptor. In the PLC system, the G_q protein stimulates enzyme activity, and there are no known inhibitory receptors. When a ligand binds to the receptor, the G protein dissociates into an α_q subunit that stimulates PLC and a $\beta\gamma$ pair that may have other physiological actions.

PLC, phospholipase C.

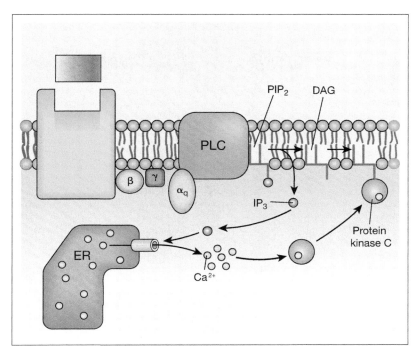

FIGURE 4.19 Consequences of PLC activation. Downstream effects of PLC activation leads to splitting of a membrane lipid phospholipid PIP_2, with the release of DAG, which remains in the membrane and activates protein kinase C, and IP_3, which diffuses to the ER, causing a burst of ER calcium release. Most of the intracellular changes occurring after PLC activation are caused by the increase in intracellular calcium.

DAG, diacylglycerol; ER, endoplasmic reticulum; IP_3, inositol trisphosphate; PIP_2, phosphatidylinositol bisphosphate; PLC, phospholipase C.

to calcium/calmodulin binding and activation of an enzyme that causes cell contraction, ultimately producing vasoconstriction and increasing blood pressure.

An interesting note is that there is also a calcium/calmodulin-activated phosphatase enzyme that reverses phosphorylation, stripping the phosphate away from phosphorylated proteins. This phosphatase, calcineurin, provides a reversal signal, allowing for downregulation of a function once homeostatic adaptation is complete. The major clinical use for calcineurin inhibitors is post-transplantation as these drugs are immunosuppressive.

G Protein GTPase Activity Is a Timing Mechanism

One characteristic held in common by the various G proteins that link to GPCRs is that the α subunits are GTPase enzymes. They are capable of splitting GTP to release guanosine diphosphate (GDP) and a free phosphate group. Before a ligand binds to its GPCR, the associated G protein is initially GDP-bound and inactive. After the ligand binds and activates the receptor, the G protein α subunit GDP is replaced by GTP; the α subunit dissociates from the βγ pair and activates or inhibits the relevant enzyme (adenylyl cyclase or phospholipase C). As the second messenger is generated, the α subunit is also breaking down the bound

GTP, leaving GDP bound to the α protein, returning the βγ proteins to their initial state of binding to α, and turning off second messenger production. If sufficient ligand is present in the extracellular space, it can bind to another receptor and initiate more second messenger production; however, in the absence of additional ligand, the GTPase mechanism will terminate the intracellular signaling cascade (**Figure 4.20**).

CELL SIGNALING BY CYCLIC GUANOSINE MONOPHOSPHATE

On the spectrum of cell signaling from GPCR/second messenger systems and enzyme-linked receptors, signaling by cyclic guanosine monophosphate (cGMP) is something of a hybrid and a novelty, with two major physiologically defined roles. First, cGMP is synthesized in retinal photoreceptor cells and plays a critical role in vision. Second, cGMP acts in vascular smooth muscle as a potent vasodilator. The enzyme that produces cGMP, guanylyl cyclase, occurs in two forms in vascular smooth muscle cells: particulate guanylyl cyclase that is part of membrane-bound receptors for natriuretic hormones, and soluble guanylyl cyclase found in the cytoplasm. Soluble guanylyl cyclase is activated by endothelium-produced nitric oxide that

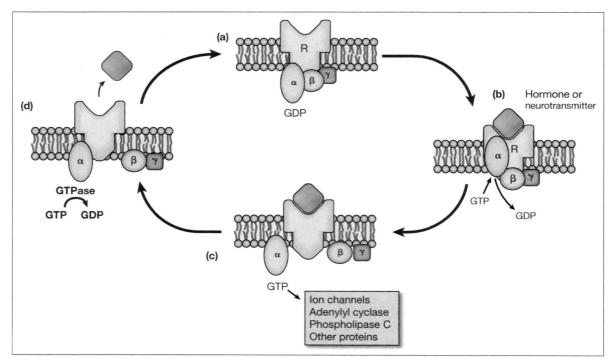

FIGURE 4.20 Hydrolysis of GTP by G proteins limits the duration of hormone-receptor (R) actions. This can be thought of as a timing switch. (**a**) No ligand binds receptor, receptor is inactive and G protein is bound to GDP. (**b**) Hormone binds to the receptor, GDP is replaced by GTP, and the G protein dissociates into α and βγ subunits. (**c**) α subunit activates target enzymes and proteins. (**d**) α subunit intrinsic GTPase activity splits GTP, binding GDP and the βγ subunits, and returning to the inactive state.
GDP, guanosine diphosphate; GTP, guanosine triphosphate; GTPase, guanosine triphosphatase.

diffuses to the blood vessel's smooth muscle layer. The resulting increase in cGMP produces vasodilation and lowers blood pressure.

CELL SIGNALING BY ENZYME-LINKED RECEPTORS

Many of the receptors used for growth, development, and rapid cell proliferation have intrinsic enzyme activity, rather than requiring a G protein to activate an enzyme. In addition, most of these enzyme-containing or enzyme-linked receptors have *tyrosine kinase* activity—they phosphorylate target proteins at tyrosine sites. As a general pattern, ligand binding to these receptors is followed by dimerization, in which two copies of the same receptor (homodimerization) or two different tyrosine kinase receptors (heterodimerization) are drawn together in the membrane. This is followed by autophosphorylation, in which each chain phosphorylates the other. After this self-activation, the tyrosine kinase portions of the receptor begin to phosphorylate additional proteins, some of which attach and build up a complex of proteins along the intracellular portion of the receptor (**Figures 4.21** and **4.22**). Most of these receptors have their greatest activity during

periods of rapid growth and cell proliferation, embryonic and fetal stages, and during childhood. In adulthood, their activity is brief and situation specific, for example, during wound healing or immune responses. Dysregulation of tyrosine kinase signaling pathways is common in cancer, fibrosis, chronic inflammation, and disorders of immune hyper-responses.

The receptors for insulin and insulin-like growth factor (a mediator of growth hormone signaling) do not need to dimerize; they consist of two identical or similar protein subunits bonded together. On the other hand, the epidermal growth factor receptor (EGFR) in its unstimulated form exists as a monomer and requires dimerization for activity. The extracellular portion of both of these receptors is the site of ligand binding, while the intracellular portion contains the tyrosine kinase domain that becomes activated by ligand binding.

One mechanism of dimerization after ligand binding is illustrated in **Figure 4.22**. The ligand has two receptor binding sites, so binding leads to reversible cross-linking of two receptors. This draws the receptors close enough to allow interaction of the intracellular enzyme regions, initiating autophosphorylation.

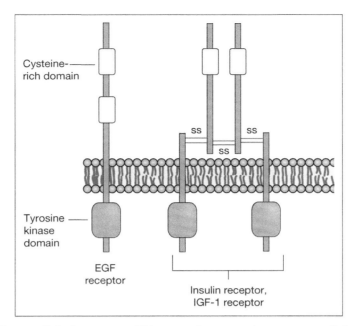

FIGURE 4.21 Enzyme-linked receptors. This type of receptor has an extracellular ligand-binding site, crosses the membrane once, and has an intracellular enzyme site, often consisting of a tyrosine kinase enzyme. The insulin receptor has two identical subunits linked by a disulfide bond, with each subunit consisting of two protein chains also linked together by disulfide bonds (SS). Once two insulin molecules have bound to the insulin receptor, the intracellular portion of the receptor becomes phosphorylated, and its own tyrosine kinase activity begins to phosphorylate nearby proteins. EGF, epidermal growth factor; IGF-1, insulin-like growth factor 1.

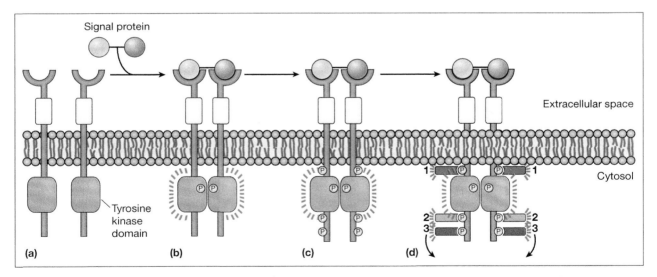

FIGURE 4.22 Intracellular signaling initiated by receptors using tyrosine kinase mechanisms. **(a)** These receptors are present in monomeric form (single, noninteracting chains) and are inactive when no extracellular signal is present. **(b)** Binding of ligands causes the formation of a dimer with two receptor molecules coming to close physical proximity and the tyrosine kinase regions of each phosphorylating the other chain. **(c)** Once phosphorylated, the intracellular portion of each receptor adds more phosphates outside the tyrosine kinase region. **(d)** The newly phosphorylated sites become scaffolds where other signaling proteins (numbered 1–3 in the figure) can bind, be phosphorylated, and exert their own enzyme activities. Some of the tyrosine kinase–type receptors stimulate cell proliferation and are implicated in wound repair and in cancerous transformation of cells. P, phosphate group.

Once phosphorylated, intracellular downstream signaling proteins (many of which are also kinase enzymes) bind and become activated.

The EGFR is particularly well studied, because it is mutated in many cancers, particularly those that involve epithelial tissues, such as colon and breast. In addition, some of the downstream proteins activated by EGFR and other growth-related proteins are also mutated in cancers. The Ras protein was one of the first identified oncoproteins (mutated forms of it are found in many cancers; **Figure 4.23**). EGFR activation turns on several signaling pathways that ultimately alter gene expression, transcription, and translation to increase rates of cell division. While this growth-promoting action of epidermal growth factor is needed during embryonic and fetal development, when it is initiated in an unregulated fashion in adulthood, it promotes cancer formation. A close relative of EGFR encoded by the *HER2/neu* gene is ErbB2—this form of the EGFR is commonly mutated in breast cancer and has been targeted by specific drugs used in treating these cancers.

Cytokines are protein messages of the immune system. Immune responses to foreign proteins include rapid proliferation of clones of immune cells (monocytes and lymphocytes) to fight off invaders. Cytokine receptors do not have intrinsic tyrosine kinase activity; rather, when they are activated by extracellular ligand binding, their intracellular portion changes shape to bind Janus kinase (JAK) proteins—tyrosine kinases that bind to the receptor and begin to phosphorylate target proteins. Many JAK targets are signal transducer and activator of transcription (STAT) proteins (**Figure 4.24**). Although classically associated with cytokine signaling and immune responses, JAK-STAT proteins are also mutated in some cancers and are the target of some antineoplastic drugs.

Transforming growth factor beta (TGF-β) is required for embryonic and fetal development of many tissues. In adulthood, TGF-β can normally inhibit cell proliferation, but its actions reverse to promote proliferation in the context of immune activation, inflammation, and cancer. The TGF-β receptor differs from other receptors in this class in that it has serine/threonine kinase activity rather than tyrosine kinase activity. However, the structure and function of the TGF-β receptor is similar to the tyrosine kinase–type

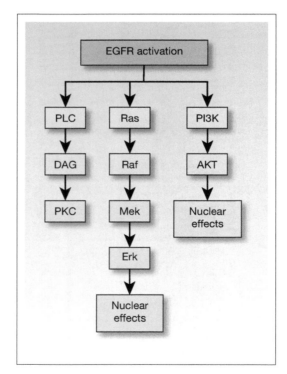

FIGURE 4.23 EGFR intracellular signaling pathways. The nuclear actions of these pathways converge to promote new protein synthesis and to stimulate cell mitosis and proliferation.
AKT, AKR mouse tumor 8 kinase (an oncogene also known as PKB, protein kinase B); DAG, diacylglycerol; EGFR, epidermal growth factor receptor; PI3K, phosphoinositide-3-kinase; PKC, protein kinase C; PLC, phosopholipase C.

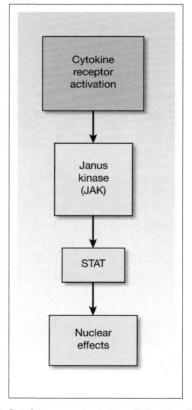

FIGURE 4.24 Cytokine receptor intracellular signaling pathway. The Janus kinase–signal transducer and activator of transcription (JAK-STAT) sequence of activation is strongly associated with cytokine actions in target cells, including leukocyte proliferation and immune cell signaling.

receptors in having a single transmembrane chain with an intracellular kinase domain, and phosphorylating a cascade of intracellular proteins—as shown in **Figure 4.25**, proteins of the Smad family. TGF-β is implicated in pathophysiological induction of fibrosis in a variety of diseases of the lung, liver, blood vessels, and other tissues.

CELL SIGNALING BY CYTOPLASMIC AND NUCLEAR RECEPTORS

Steroid and thyroid hormones are relatively nonpolar and hydrophilic, and are able to move across the cell membrane by simple diffusion. Once inside the cell, one of two pathways is followed: (1) Some steroids bind to receptors in the cytoplasm and are then transported into the nucleus. (2) Other steroid hormones and thyroid hormones diffuse across nuclear membranes to bind to receptors already in the nucleus. In either case, the hormone/receptor complex ultimately binds to regulatory elements on DNA, altering transcription and translation within that cell (**Figure 4.26**). The onset of hormone effects is slower with steroid and thyroid hormones, as they have fewer direct, rapid actions on cells. However,

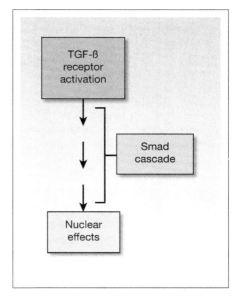

FIGURE 4.25 TGF-β receptor intracellular signaling pathway. The TGF-β receptor is similar to tyrosine kinase–linked receptors in having a single transmembrane protein chain, but it differs in having serine/threonine kinase activity, rather than tyrosine kinase actions.

TGF-β, transforming growth factor beta.

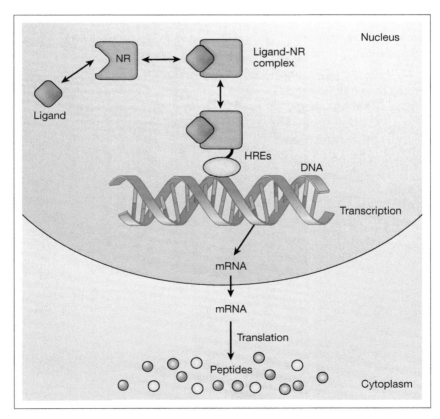

FIGURE 4.26 Signaling by an NR or cytoplasmic receptor. Steroid and thyroid hormone receptors can be found in the nucleus, binding to DNA. Hormone binding activates transcription and translation of target cell proteins. This is a slower and long-lasting mechanism of cell signaling than that associated with G protein–coupled receptors. For some hormones, the receptors are initially located in the cytoplasm, and binding of their ligand first stimulates transport into the nucleus before the DNA binding step occurs.

HRE, hormone response element; mRNA, messenger RNA; NR, nuclear receptor.

by altering cell protein levels, they can induce profound and relatively long-lasting changes in function as well as structure.

SUMMARY OF CELL SIGNALING

Maintaining physiological homeostasis requires the ability to make short- and long-term adaptations to the changing environment within the body and external to the organism. Short-term adaptations mediated by autonomic and endocrine signals often act by way of GPCRs, with rapid onset and several mechanisms of signal termination. Intermediate and longer-term adaptations can be mediated by steroid and thyroid hormone receptors that alter gene expression and protein translation. Finally, some normal and pathophysiological adaptations alter the activity of receptors involved in growth and development, promoting cell proliferation that can be helpful (as in immune responses) or pathophysiological (as in immune hyperreactivity or cancer).

Thought Questions

4. Trace the events involved in signaling by GPCRs that act through the adenylyl cyclase system.

5. List three of the brakes that terminate downstream actions of GPCRs.

6. What are the major points of difference between tyrosine kinase–linked intracellular actions and downstream actions of GPCR signaling?

MECHANISMS OF CONTRACTILE CELLS

OVERVIEW OF CONTRACTILE CELL STRUCTURE AND FUNCTION

There are three types of muscle cells in the body—skeletal muscle, cardiac muscle, and smooth muscle—with further specializations in these types. Historically, muscle cell structures have a unique nomenclature, with the prefix *sarco-*, from the Greek meaning *flesh*. In this fashion, the *sarcolemma* refers to the cell membrane, *sarcoplasm* to the cytoplasm, and *sarcoplasmic reticulum* to the endoplasmic reticulum. There are common elements of force development and cell shortening in each type of muscle, involving crossbridge formation between the proteins myosin and actin, the two strands ratcheting past each other, and a requirement for calcium and ATP. Yet each type of muscle has unique aspects of function and regulation. General mechanisms involved are described here, while other chapters provide additional details regarding certain organ-specific aspects of muscle function and regulation.

THE SARCOMERE OF SKELETAL AND CARDIAC MUSCLE

The microscopic appearance of skeletal and cardiac muscle cells shows a striated appearance, dark bands alternating with light bands (**Figure 4.27**). The repeating unit is the *sarcomere*, the functional

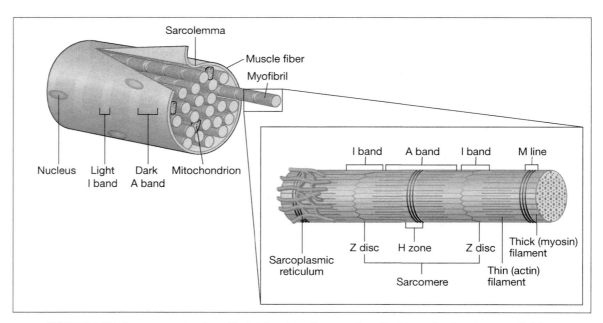

FIGURE 4.27 Sarcomere structure. Skeletal and cardiac muscle cells shorten by forming cross-bridges between actin and myosin filaments highly organized into sarcomeres that shorten as a unit.

unit of muscle contraction. The sarcomeres span from Z disc to Z disc, with darker A bands flanked by lighter I bands, and an M line at the middle of the sarcomere. The fine structure responsible for this appearance includes hundreds of copies each of two linear proteins that reversibly bind together to create muscle contractions. Actin is a protein made up of repeated subunits joined together to form a thin strand, which is further surrounded in a spiral fashion with regulatory proteins troponin and tropomyosin (described later in this section). Myosin is a protein containing two heavy chains and two pairs of light chains. Myosin's heavy chain tail region forms thick interwoven strands with other myosin molecules, while the movable head region contains binding sites for actin, ATP, and regulatory light chains (**Figure 4.28**). Together, these proteins are referred to as *myofibrils.*

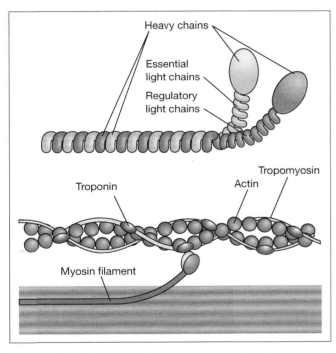

FIGURE 4.28 Proteins of muscle contraction. Each single myosin molecule consists of a heavy chain (divided between a longer tail region and a shorter, angled head region) that binds two light chains near the head region. The tail regions of several myosin molecules twine around each other, forming a thick, straight bundle, with heads projecting off at angles. Within muscle cells, chains of actin molecules line up in parallel, with the accessory proteins tropomyosin (a filamentous protein positioned over actin binding sites) and the tripartite troponin complex holding the tropomyosin molecule in place.

MECHANISM OF MYOFIBRIL CROSSBRIDGE FORMATION AND CONTRACTION

During muscle contraction, myosin heads bind to recognition sites on actin strands and pull the actin strands toward the center of the sarcomere, causing sarcomere shortening and ultimately shortening the whole muscle. Other proteins are involved in holding the actin and myosin strands in alignment and linking sarcomeres together. Actin strands are held in alignment by binding to the Z disks. Myosin strands are held in alignment by binding to a large, elastic protein called titin, which is also anchored to the Z disks. Additional protein complexes connect the sarcomeres to the cell membrane and cytoskeletal proteins so the long muscle fibers shorten as a unit. Genetic mutations of some of these connecting proteins are responsible for some of the hereditary muscular dystrophy syndromes.

At rest, myosin and actin strands are lined up across from each other but are unable to form crossbridges because of the presence of regulatory proteins that block myosin–actin interactions (**Figure 4.29**). Myosin head groups are binding ADP and free phosphate from a previous hydrolysis of ATP. Tropomyosin is a linear protein that physically blocks the sites on actin where myosin binds. A complex of three troponins—troponin I, troponin C, and troponin T—sit at regular intervals along the tropomyosin filament, keeping it in place. Troponin C is the site of calcium binding under conditions of muscle contraction. As sarcoplasmic calcium levels increase, calcium binding shifts the troponin/tropomyosin complex, exposing actin's binding sites and enabling crossbridge formation. As myosin head proteins bind to actin, creating crossbridges, the heads swivel, pulling the actin strands inward, and shortening the sarcomere (**Figure 4.30**). ATP then replaces the ADP, the crossbridges break, and new crossbridges form, ratcheting the actin strands further. This cycle is repeated many times, until the cytoplasmic calcium drops and the troponin/tropomyosin complex returns to its resting state.

As noted earlier, intracellular calcium levels are held very low in comparison to extracellular calcium. One mechanism of calcium entry into muscle cells is by action potentials that depolarize the membrane. Membrane voltage-gated calcium channels allow some calcium entry to initiate contraction. A much bigger source of calcium for contraction comes from the sarcoplasmic reticulum. The structures of the sarcolemma and sarcoplasmic reticulum interact to rapidly increase intracellular calcium concentrations through a structure termed the *triad.* Invaginations of the sarcolemma, the *T-tubules,* propagate the action potential deep into the muscle fiber, near terminal cisterns of

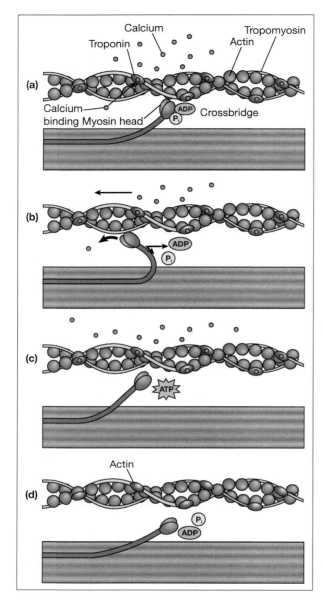

FIGURE 4.29 Myosin–actin crossbridge formation. **(a)** Myosin is bound to ADP and inorganic phosphate (P_i). A spike in cell Ca^{2+} concentration facilitates calcium binding to troponin C, shifting the troponin complex and tropomyosin. This exposes actin binding sites, and the myosin head attaches to myosin. **(b)** The myosin head swivels, pulling myosin and actin in opposite directions in a move called the power stroke. ADP and P_i are released. **(c)** Binding of ATP breaks the crossbridge between myosin and actin. The myosin head returns to its original angle, splits the ATP, and reattaches to an adjacent actin binding site, continuing to pull the actin strand inward toward the center of the sarcomere. **(d)**. When calcium levels drop, tropomyosin shifts back to its original position, myosin–actin crossbridges are released, and the muscle relaxes.

ADP, adenosine diphosphate; ATP, adenosine triphosphate.

the sarcoplasmic reticulum (**Figures 4.31** and **4.32**). As the action potential depolarizes the membrane, a dihydropyridine receptor signals this voltage change to ryanodine receptors on the terminal cisterns, signaling for rapid release of stored calcium. The calcium released from the sarcoplasmic reticulum quickly reaches the troponin proteins and binds to troponin C, initiating muscle fiber contraction.

COMPARISON OF SKELETAL MUSCLE FIBERS AND CARDIAC MUSCLE CELLS

Sarcomere structure and the striated appearance are quite similar between skeletal muscles and cardiac cells. However, there are significant differences in structure, organization, and control. Skeletal muscles carry out involuntary, reflex, and voluntary activity directed by the nervous system, and their contractions are initiated by motor neurons in the spinal cord and brainstem, as described in Chapter 15, Nervous System. The heart contracts autonomously, in response to pacemaker cells of the sinoatrial node, as described in Chapter 10, Heart. Even when denervated, after a heart transplant procedure, for example, the heart will continuously generate rhythmic contractions at a rate of about 60 to 70 beats each minute. Skeletal muscle fibers are elongated and are organized into progressively larger bundles that ultimately transition to tendons that join muscle to bone, allowing purposeful movement. Cardiac cells are short and linked mechanically and electrically to neighboring cells that surround the cardiac chambers. Contraction compresses and squeezes the chambers, ultimately leading to ejection of blood into the vasculature of the body or the lungs. Skeletal muscles are activated in sequence to create a series of movements, whereas the cells in the atria and the ventricles of the heart contract almost simultaneously for efficient ejection.

The strength of contraction of both types of striated muscle fibers is modulated by their length as the contraction starts and by the load the muscle experiences as it contracts. The first property, the length–tension relationship, is demonstrated when a muscle is lengthened prior to contraction. After this initial stretching, the muscle generates greater force when it contracts. Picture a baseball batter or a golfer, stretching his or her arm flexors with a backswing prior to the forward movement of the bat or golf club. A hypothesis for this mechanism is that prior lengthening brings more sarcomeres to an optimal length to conduct crossbridge cycling. The second property, the force–velocity relationship, is demonstrated when the muscle is exposed to a load against which it must work as it is contracting. The greater that load, the slower will be the speed of

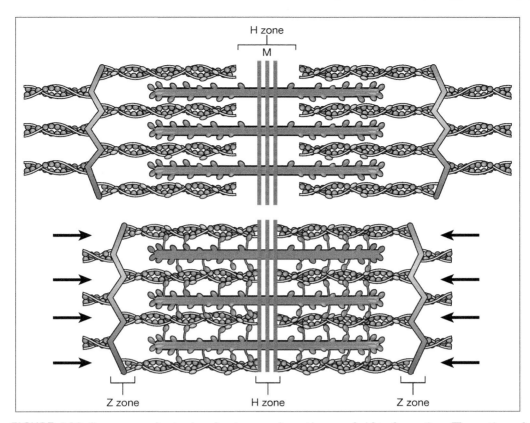

FIGURE 4.30 Sarcomere shortening due to myosin–actin crossbridge formation. The action of many strands of myosin and actin forming crossbridges adds up to the shortening of all sarcomeres in a muscle fiber, producing contractile force and movement.

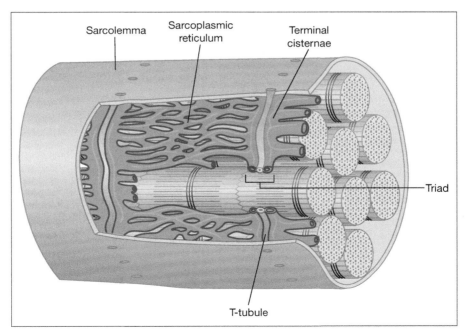

FIGURE 4.31 The triad of structures regulating muscle calcium release. Invaginations of the plasma membrane, T-tubules align next to terminal cisterns of sarcoplasmic reticulum. When the muscle action potential is propagated along the membrane and down the T-tubules, the signal is conveyed to the sarcoplasmic reticulum to release its calcium stores.

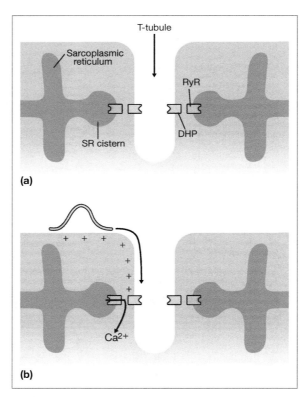

FIGURE 4.32 Close-up view of T-tubule–SR triad at rest and during activation. **(a)** DHP receptors of the T-tubule are adjacent to RyR of the SR cistern. **(b)** Membrane depolarization due to the muscle action potential causes the DHP to activate the RyR, and the SR releases its stored calcium. The wave of calcium quickly diffuses around the actin filaments, binding to troponin, shifting tropomyosin, and allowing myosin–actin crossbridges to form.

DHP, dihydropyridine; RyR, ryanodine receptor; SR, sarcoplasmic reticulum.

contraction. To imagine how this works, picture yourself trying to lift a box of tissues quickly and contrast that with how you would feel lifting a box of weights. These relationships are similar in the heart as well, and are discussed in that context under the topics of *preload* and *afterload*. Characteristics of these two muscle types are compared in **Table 4.3**.

Levels of muscle protein expression are dynamic, with turnover of actin, myosin, and other proteins replacing damaged myofibrils. Increasing the workload on a skeletal or cardiac muscle will increase protein synthesis relative to protein degradation, resulting in hypertrophy. This is a common consequence of strength training for skeletal muscle or hypertension for cardiac muscle. On the other hand, decrease in workload after an acute limb injury (fracture) can result in skeletal muscle atrophy (disuse atrophy), with protein degradation at a greater rate than protein synthesis. A relative increase of muscle protein breakdown over synthesis is

common in aging, resulting in the *sarcopenia* that is a component of frailty in older adults.

MECHANISMS OF SMOOTH MUSCLE CONTRACTION

Smooth muscle cells are found in the walls of hollow organs such as the gastrointestinal tract, bladder, and uterus. They also make up contractile layers of the blood vessels and airways. Contraction and relaxation of vascular and organ smooth muscle layers are primarily regulated by the autonomic nervous system and by local and circulating chemical mediators. Smooth muscles do not have striations or sarcomeres; rather, the actin and myosin filaments are more loosely arranged within the cytoplasm (**Figure 4.33**). Actin and myosin filaments are anchored to dense bodies in the cytoplasm and to the cell membrane, so crossbridge formation and movement of the filaments by crossbridge

TABLE 4.3 Comparison of Skeletal Muscle Fibers and Cardiac Muscle Cells

Characteristic	Skeletal Muscle Fibers	Cardiac Muscle Cells
Cell morphology	Long fibers formed by fusion of precursor cells Contain many nuclei Connect to tendons to generate force across joints	Short cells linked to neighboring cells both mechanically (desmosomes) and electrically (gap junctions) Contain one nucleus
Action potential generation	Acetylcholine released from motor neuron terminals at the neuromuscular junction generates action potentials that propagate along the membrane	Pacemaker cells in the sinoatrial node generate action potentials that propagate along cardiac conduction pathways
Action potential type	Brief twitch in response to one or a few action potentials, *or* Fused contractions (tetany) in response to prolonged firing of motor neurons can sustain muscle contraction for long periods of time, if necessary	Action potentials are discrete; shaped by specialized sodium, calcium, and potassium channels; always ending with repolarization and relaxation Cardiac muscle cannot have tetanic contractions
Mechanism of calcium release from the SR	Depolarization of T-tubules is relayed via the dihydropyridine receptor, activating calcium release via the ryanodine receptor	Calcium entry through the T-tubule dihydropyridine receptor initiates SR calcium release via ryanodine receptor
Metabolism	Anaerobic and aerobic	Primarily aerobic, contain greater numbers of mitochondria
Length–tension relationship	The longer the muscle fiber at the start of contraction, the greater will be the tension it can develop	The greater the filling of the cardiac chamber at the start of contraction, the greater will be the tension it can develop

SR, sarcoplasmic reticulum.

cycling shortens the cell. In most cases, the force generated by smooth muscle cells is weaker than force produced by striated muscles, and ATP requirements of smooth muscle cells are lower. Some smooth muscle cells are able to maintain a state of crossbridge binding without cycling (called a *latch-bridge* mechanism), holding a degree of muscle tone that supports organ or blood vessel function with very low energy cost.

The role of calcium in smooth muscle contraction differs from that in striated muscle (**Figure 4.34**). When intracellular calcium increases in smooth muscle cells, it binds to the protein calmodulin (step 1). This activates calmodulin, and the calcium/calmodulin complex can then bind to the enzyme *myosin light chain kinase*, activating the kinase function (step 2). Myosin light chain kinase then phosphorylates the regulatory light chain of myosin (step 3), causing the head to move closer to the nearby actin filament (step 4), resulting in crossbridge formation and cell contraction (step 5). There are two main mechanisms producing the increase in intracellular calcium in smooth muscle cells (**Figure 4.35**). First, there are voltage-gated calcium channels that can be opened by smooth muscle cell depolarization. Second, many smooth muscle cells have receptors linked to G_q and signaling via the phospholipase C system. As previously noted, a prominent consequence of this pathway is generation of IP_3, which causes the release of calcium from the sarcoplasmic reticulum. For example, in the circulatory system, vasoconstriction by norepinephrine and several other circulating substances (angiotensin II, vasopressin) is due to activation of G_q-linked receptors and IP_3-mediated calcium release.

Relaxation of smooth muscle cells occurs when receptor stimulation or depolarization stops, and the sarcoplasmic reticulum calcium pump reduces intracellular calcium, ultimately reducing myosin light chain kinase activity. Cyclic nucleotides cAMP and cGMP produced by adenylyl or guanylyl cyclase–linked receptors also mediate smooth muscle cell relaxation. An additional mechanism of smooth muscle relaxation is through myosin light chain phosphatase—an enzyme that removes the phosphate from the myosin light chain, restoring myosin to its original position

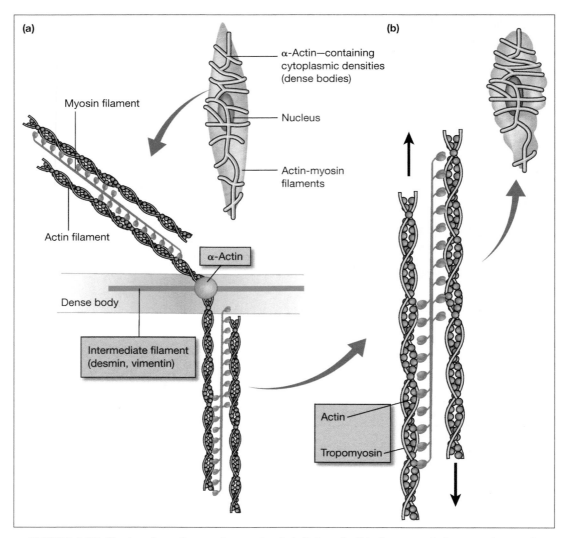

FIGURE 4.33 Contraction of smooth muscle. **(a)** Relaxed. **(b)** Contracted. In smooth muscle cells, actin–myosin strands form a loose meshwork crossing the cell. The strands are anchored by attachments to the plasma membrane and to dense bodies within the cytoplasm. When calcium increases, the cell shortens as shown.

(see **Figure 4.34**, step 6). Certain vasodilating mediators work by increasing myosin light chain phosphatase activity in vascular smooth muscle.

SUMMARY OF MUSCLE CELL FUNCTION

Muscle cells are contractile cells that shorten upon stimulation, providing force for body movements, heart pumping, and contractions of the walls of blood vessels, airways, and internal organs. Actin–myosin crosslinking and crossbridge cycling are responsible for muscle contractions, with crossbridge formation and cycling also requiring calcium ions and ATP. Smooth muscle is regulated differently in the various organs and blood vessels, dependent on the receptors present

on the cell membranes. Throughout this book, specific examples are provided in their organ- or system-specific context.

Thought Questions

7. How do the mechanisms of muscle contraction differ between striated and smooth muscle cells?

8. What are examples of each of these cell types and their function?

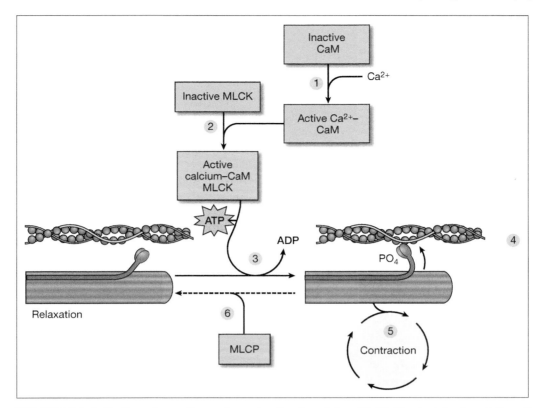

FIGURE 4.34 Activation of smooth muscle contraction by calcium (Ca^{2+}). (See text for description of the numbered steps.)
ADP, adenosine diphosphate; ATP, adenosine triphosphate; CaM, calmodulin; MLCK, myosin light chain kinase; MLCP, myosin light chain phosphatase; PO_4, phosphate.

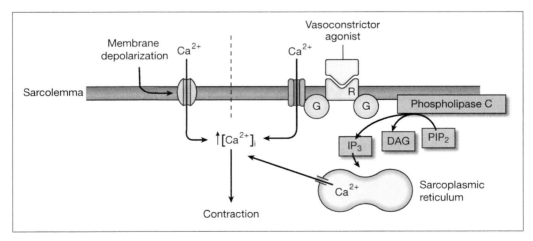

FIGURE 4.35 General mechanisms for activation of the vascular smooth muscle. Electromechanical coupling is shown on the left; a voltage-operated calcium (Ca^{2+}) channel allows calcium entry upon cell depolarization. Pharmacomechanical coupling is shown on the right; a receptor-operated Ca^{2+} channel allows calcium entry upon activation of certain receptors. Other receptors increase $[Ca^{2+}]_i$ through the phospholipase C system and IP_3.
DAG, diacylglycerol; G, GTP-binding protein; IP_3, inositol trisphosphate; PIP_2, phosphatidylinositol bisphosphate; R, agonist-specific receptor; $[Ca^{2+}]_i$, intracellular calcium concentration.

CELL RENEWAL, STRESS, AND CELL DEATH

OVERVIEW OF CELL RENEWAL, MAINTENANCE, AND ADAPTATION

Many cells have finite and short or intermediate life spans, including white and red blood cells, skin cells, and the cells lining the gastrointestinal tract. As these cells die, they must be replaced by stem cells that are self-renewing and give rise to daughter cells that differentiate into the appropriate cell type. In addition to whole cells, individual cells undergo renewal by removal of damaged or malfunctioning proteins and new protein synthesis. Cells that have sustained damage due to injury, infection, or malnutrition can attempt repair pathways, and if not successful they can undergo various patterns of cell death.

Cells exposed to physiological or pathophysiological challenges can also adapt (**Figure 4.36**). Common adaptations include cell enlargement (hypertrophy) by addition of new cell components. As previously described, this is commonly seen in the cells of muscles after strength training. Muscle fibers are nonrenewing cells, so their mode of adaptation is to synthesize additional myosin and actin molecules, increasing fiber

diameter and overall muscle size. For organs containing self-renewing cells, excessive hormone stimulation or workload increases organ mass and volume by *hyperplasia*—production of greater numbers of cells. This is seen in the uterus during pregnancy or in the thyroid gland during Graves disease, in which there is excessive stimulation of the thyroid-stimulating hormone receptor.

Denervation of muscles, disuse, or withdrawal of hormone stimulation results in cell *atrophy*—loss of cell volume or number. These losses are observable on visual inspection of muscle or imaging of organs as an overall decrease in size. Mild organ atrophy is common with aging, for reasons described in the section on Gerontological Considerations. Chronic mechanical or chemical stressors can cause cells to change their tissue-specific characteristics and develop *metaplasia* or an *epithelial–mesenchymal transition*—unstable cell forms with abnormal function and the potential to be transformed to cancer. *Dysplasia* is another form of cell transition in which proper quality control measures of cell division are lost, producing cells that are abnormal in appearance and are also precancerous.

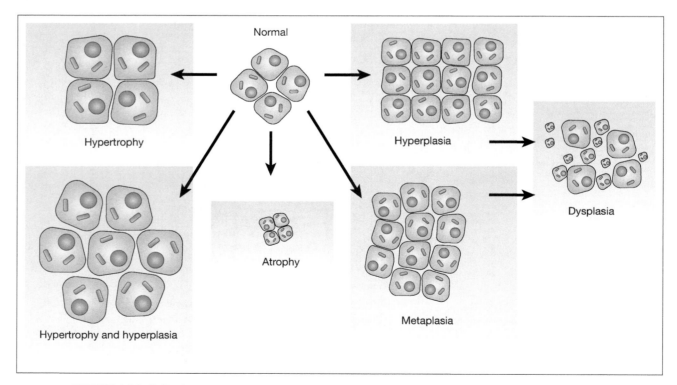

FIGURE 4.36 Cell adaptations to stressors. Adaptations to increased workload can produce cell hypertrophy, hyperplasia, or both. A variety of pathophysiological processes (nutrient deficits, decreased perfusion, neuromuscular disease, growth factor/trophic factor deprivation) can cause cells to atrophy. Chronic injury and inflammation can cause metaplasia and dysplasia, and can proceed to cancerous transformation.

OVERVIEW OF CELL INJURY AND DEATH

The study of pathophysiology and loss of cell function due to disease inevitably connects with the topic of cell injury and death. Cells, tissues, and organs can sustain injury from thromboembolic ischemia, trauma, burns, infections, exaggerated inflammation, chemicals and toxins, neoplastic processes, and radiation. Tissues that lack significant stem cell populations and self-renewing properties, such as brain and heart, may suffer irreversible loss of structure and function. Other tissues that have greater regenerative capacity, such as the liver and the kidney, may rebound from injury and recover close to normal function, depending on the magnitude of the insult. There is ever-increasing knowledge of cell-damaging mediators, cell death pathways, and the overlap between some of these systems with normal healthy aging processes. Specific examples of three cell death pathways are described here.

Tissue Responses to Acute, Severe Ischemia— Necrotic Cell Death

Some of the most devastating health events are those resulting from a blood clot occluding a blood vessel, either in the heart (myocardial infarction) or in the brain (stroke). Although angioplasty to reopen vessels and thrombectomy procedures to remove cerebral clots have successfully limited damage and salvaged function, these events still cause significant organ damage, morbidity, and mortality. In this scenario, many cells will die by the pathway of *necrosis*, creating inflammation and ultimately a scar containing noncontractile tissue (after a myocardial infarction), or a region of reactive gliosis and neuronal loss and atrophy (after a stroke). In stroke, for example, imaging studies aim to identify the region of the core (the center of the area of ischemia that has little or no collateral blood flow) and the region of the penumbra (the outer zone that may be somewhat protected by collateral blood flow).

Cells in the stroke core have the worst hypoxic/ischemic insult, with the following characteristics that lead to cell death by necrosis:

- Rapid loss of ATP production, resulting in diminished membrane potential
- Depressed Na^+/K^+ pump activity
- Intracellular calcium overload
- Cell swelling
- Membrane rupture
- Loss of antioxidant function
- Accumulation of oxygen-derived free radicals (also known as reactive oxygen species [ROS])
- Acidosis
- Activation of degradative enzymes that contribute to membrane rupture and spread of the damage to adjacent cells

Paradoxically, restoring blood flow (reperfusion) may actually worsen cell death by providing oxygen to fuel production of ROS and by recruiting white blood cells that perpetuate the inflammatory response (**Figure 4.37**). Cells in the penumbra vary in their outcomes, with some of the cells proceeding to necrotic cell death, others to apoptotic cell death (a slower pathway with less inflammation), and yet others gradually recovering normal function. Membrane rupture and leakage of cell contents during necrotic cell death can be detected by laboratory evaluation. For example, death of cardiomyocytes as a myocardial infarction evolves is associated with release of the enzyme creatine phosphokinase (MB type) and the cardiac-specific troponin T and I proteins, among others. Acute liver injury resulting from toxic doses of the drug acetaminophen causes hepatocyte death and elevates blood levels of the enzymes alanine aminotransferase (ALT) and aspartate aminotransferase (AST).

Apoptotic Cell Death

Apoptosis is a very common mechanism of cell death that contributes to normal cell turnover, and there are many examples of the utility of apoptotic cell death. During early-life brain development, many more neurons are born than are ultimately retained in the mature brain. The remaining cells die by apoptosis and are removed by macrophages without any pathological remnants. Similarly, development of T lymphocytes in the thymus involves local scrutiny for cells with the potential to become autoreactive and create autoimmune disease. These cells are removed by apoptosis. Cytotoxic T lymphocytes can recognize *self*-cells that are infected with viruses and bacteria, initiating cell death pathways, including death by apoptosis that helps to limit the infection. Cytotoxic T lymphocytes also protect against cancer by recognizing transformed cells (those conducting abnormal cell division and expressing abnormal proteins), and killing them by pathways that include apoptosis. In the context of cell damage due to these various agents, apoptosis is another pathway of cell death, particularly for damage that is limited or lasts a relatively short period of time.

Apoptosis is also known as programmed cell death because the steps follow an orderly sequence (a *death program*) and tissue disruption, organ dysfunction, and inflammation are minimized. Apoptosis can be initiated by extracellular signals (extrinsic pathway) that bind to cell membrane tumor necrosis factor (TNF) receptors, causing assembly of intracellular proteins that can activate the apoptotic enzymes. Apoptosis can also be initiated by intracellular signals (intrinsic pathway) of abnormal cell function that results in release of the enzyme cytochrome C from mitochondria—cytochrome C then triggers a cascade of increases

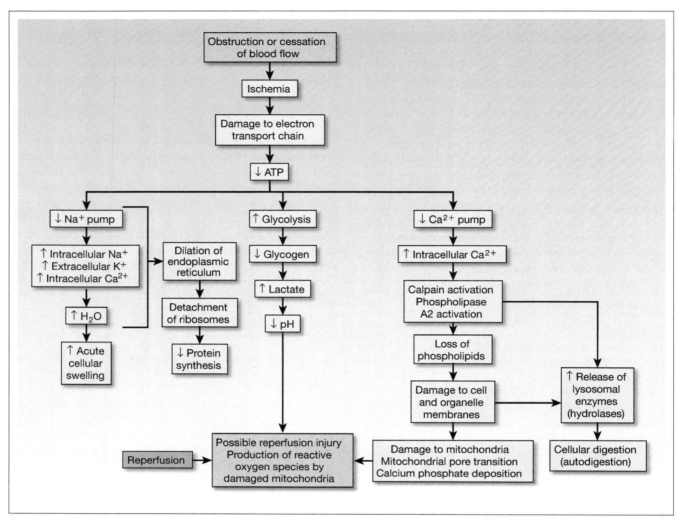

FIGURE 4.37 Cascade of events in ischemic cell injury and death.
Source: From Reisner HM. *Pathology: A Modern Case Study.* McGraw-Hill Education; 2015.

in pro-apoptotic proteins that activate the apoptotic enzymes. The apoptotic enzymes are caspases, and once activated, they begin to degrade cell components. The steps of apoptosis are outlined in **Box 4.3**, and characteristics of necrosis and apoptosis are compared in **Table 4.4**.

Autophagy

Cell adaptation to a nutrient lack, as in malnutrition, starvation, or a local region of poor circulation, can initiate the protective mechanism of *autophagy.* In this pathway, a vacuole forms within the cell and begins to take up some of the cell components—proteins and organelles. That vacuole then fuses with a cell lysosome, and the contents are digested back to small

building blocks—amino acids, sugars, lipids—that can be used to nourish the remaining cells. If deprivation is severe enough, some of the affected cells will also die by autophagy, so this response is on a continuum from mild to severe, with severe cases leading to cell death.

Thought Questions

9. What are the hallmarks of necrotic cell death?

10. Why is it important for cell death programs to exist? How do they contribute to normal physiology and prevention of disease?

BOX 4.3
Steps in Apoptosis

1. Nuclear condensation and clumping of DNA

2. Enzymatic digestion of DNA into segments of uniform length

3. Nuclear membrane fragmentation

4. Cell membrane shrinkage—removal of small pieces of membrane and cytoplasm by blebbing

5. Blebbing—proceeds until the entire cell has been replaced by small fragments termed *apoptotic bodies*

6. Cellular debris and apoptotic bodies are phagocytosed by tissue macrophages

TABLE 4.4 Characteristics of Necrotic and Apoptotic Cell Death Pathways

Characteristic	Necrosis	Apoptosis
Cell size	Cells swell	Cells shrink
Fate of nucleus	Ruptures	Small packages containing fragmented DNA
DNA	Fragment size varies	Fragment size uniform
Cell membrane	Ruptures	Remains intact
Cellular contents	Enzymatic digestion and leakage into surrounding tissue	Enzymatic digestion, then packaged into apoptotic bodies and released
Adjacent inflammation	Frequent	No
Physiological or pathological role	Invariably pathological, resulting from severe tissue injury	Often physiological as a means of eliminating unneeded or diseased cells

Lori St. John

CELLULAR THEORIES OF AGING

Normal healthy aging is associated with decreased numbers and function of cells, in some organ systems more than others. Why do we age? Humankind has tried to answer this question for centuries, and yet the answer remains elusive. Theologists, philosophers, and scientists alike have sought to figure out why we age, how we age, and whether anything can prevent the consequences of aging. Over the years, scientists have put forth theories of what drives aging that range from an evolutionary to a molecular-level focus, although no one theory is sufficient to encompass all aspects of this process.[1] Several of these theories are summarized here.

GLOBAL THEORIES OF AGING

The *programmed* theory states that aging is a genetic program that has developed to direct senescence and death in order to benefit future generations of a species. A variety of genes regulate the aging process, suggesting that aging is innate to our genetic program. Current research, however, has failed to find evidence of any specific gene that has evolved for the sole purpose of aging. Similarly, the *evolutionary* theory argues that the forces of natural selection decline with aging due to accumulation of mutations that are not harmful to fitness early in life and during reproductive years, but are harmful later in life when selection is inefficient to remove them. The *disposable soma* theory postulates that organisms have limited resources that have to be divided for maintenance and reproduction. Because cells cannot use all of their resources for maintenance, protection against insults is not as efficient as it could be, leaving cells vulnerable to accumulating damage and accelerating aging. The *hyperfunction* theory suggests that pathological processes that lead to senescence are a result of gene overactivity rather than damage, breakdown, or failure. Aging can be seen as an increasing mass of pathological events with different causes.[1]

FREE RADICAL THEORY OF AGING

The *free radical* theory of aging was one of the first to focus on the accumulated biochemical effects of constant exposure to these chemically reactive molecules. Free radicals, and more specifically ROS, have been implicated in numerous pathological pathways, so deeper understanding of the pathological nature of these molecules is important to understand this theory and other pathophysiological processes. A free radical is a molecule that has an unpaired electron in its outer orbit that makes it highly chemically reactive. ROS are free radicals that are commonly produced from oxygen as a byproduct of mitochondrial respiration and energy generation. Cells have antioxidant molecules and enzymes that neutralize ROS before they cause molecular damage to membranes, proteins, and DNA. However, if there is a disruption in the removal process or there is an increase in ROS production, cellular damage occurs.

There are three principal cellular targets of ROS-mediated damage. The first target is cell membranes that undergo lipid peroxidation. This process occurs when double bonds in unsaturated fatty acids of the cell membrane lipids are attacked by ROS, leading to the formation of unstable peroxide molecules, causing an autocatalytic chain reaction that can result in extensive cell membrane damage. The next target is proteins that undergo oxidative modification. ROS promote oxidation of amino acid side chains, accelerating protein cross-linking and oxidation of the protein backbone. These molecular changes alter enzyme active sites, disrupt the conformation of structural proteins, and increase degradation of unfolded or misfolded proteins. The third target is DNA. ROS cause single- and double-strand breaks in DNA, DNA strand cross-linking, and adduct formation.[2] This mechanism has been implicated in cell aging and malignant transformation. Whether or not the damage leads to cellular aging or cancer formation is dependent on the amount and location of damage, specific repair, checkpoint, and effector systems involved.[3]

NINE HALLMARKS OF AGING

Aging itself is an abstract concept that is hard to quantify. When does aging start? And how can we tell that something is aging? It is important to identify these concepts as they can guide research to better understand how we age and understand the mechanisms behind age-related pathology. Researchers have posited nine hallmarks that are considered to lead to the aging process and determine the aging phenotype. These processes were chosen because they are all found in normal aging. Also, under experimental conditions, exacerbation or mitigation of these factors could hasten death or increase life span, respectively.[4]

CELLULAR SENESCENCE

Senescence is a phenomenon that only occurs in cells that have the ability to replicate.[5] As cells sustain damage, senescence prevents further propagation of damaged cells and alerts the immune system to degrade and clear them. Senescence is driven by two mechanisms: telomere attrition (discussed later) and activation of tumor suppressor genes. Activation of specific tumor suppressor genes also contributes to replicative senescence. Expression of tumor suppressor protein p16 is most commonly correlated with aging.[4] p16 protects the cells from uncontrolled proliferative signals and pushes cells along the senescence pathway.[2]

Accumulation of senescent cells with aging is potentially a reflection of an increase in the conversion of cells to a senescent state or a decrease in the rate of the death and clearance of these cells. Although preventing the replication of potentially harmful cells is a protection against diseases such as cancer, this mechanism relies on an efficient cell replacement system to clear the senescent cells and signal progenitors to replace the old cells. In older organisms, this system may become inefficient or may exhaust the regenerative capacity of progenitor cells, eventually resulting in the accumulation of senescent cells that may aggravate the damage and contribute to aging.[4]

TELOMERE ATTRITION

Telomere attrition is the mechanism of replicative senescence involving progressive shortening of telomeres, thus resulting in cell cycle arrest. Telomeres are DNA sequences found at the ends of chromosomes and are required for complete replication during the DNA synthesis phase of the cell cycle. With each round of replication, the telomeres grow shorter. As telomeres become shorter, the chromosome ends are less well protected; eventually they are flagged as damaged DNA, signaling cell cycle arrest. Telomere length is extended by telomerase, which is not found in most somatic tissues. Consequently, as somatic cells age, their telomeres become shorter and they eventually cannot produce new cells to replace damaged cells.[2] Since cells are unable to restore telomere length, DNA damage at telomeres is notably persistent and highly efficient in inducing senescence, apoptosis, or both.[4]

GENOMIC INSTABILITY

DNA integrity is threatened by a variety of exogenous challenges (e.g., chemicals or infectious agents), as well as by internal factors such as replication errors and free radicals. DNA alterations can potentially affect important genes and transcriptional pathways, resulting in dysfunctional cells that, if not eliminated, may prevent an organism from carrying out necessary functions of survival. In aging organisms, this is particularly important in stem cells, because damaged progenitor cells can no longer participate in tissue renewal, thus contributing to the overall aging phenotype.

LOSS OF PROTEOSTASIS

Aging is linked to impaired protein homeostasis, or *proteostasis*. Proteostasis has two mechanisms: maintaining proteins in correctly folded configurations (mediated by chaperones) and degrading proteins that have been misfolded.[2] As cells age, the formation of cytosolic and organelle-specific chaperones is significantly impaired, resulting in an increased number of misfolded proteins. Also, the activities of the two main protein degradation systems that assist with protein quality control (the ubiquitin–proteasome system and the autophagy–lysosomal system) decline with aging. This can lead to an accumulation of misfolded proteins, triggering apoptosis and age-associated diseases such as Alzheimer disease.[4]

DEREGULATED NUTRIENT SENSING

Two major pathways that regulate metabolism are the insulin and insulin-like growth factor 1 (IGF-1) signaling pathway and sirtuins. Insulin is secreted from the pancreas, and IGF-1 is produced by the liver in response to growth hormone secreted by the pituitary gland. IGF-1 receptor activation has similar downstream effects as intracellular signaling by insulin, promoting an anabolic state as well as cell growth and replication.

Sirtuins are part of a group of nicotinamide adenine dinucleotide (NAD)–dependent protein deacetylases (enzymes that remove acetyl groups from proteins, including histone proteins that package DNA). They are designed to help the body adapt to environmental stressors, such as nutrient deprivation and DNA damage, and may also promote the expression of genes that increase longevity. These genes have roles in decreasing metabolic activity, reducing apoptosis, stimulating protein folding, and reducing the harmful effects of ROS. They also increase insulin sensitivity and glucose metabolism.[2] Caloric restriction is the only intervention that has been shown to extend a healthy life span in animal models, and it is hypothesized that increased sirtuin levels and reduced insulin signaling are at least somewhat responsible for this extension.

MITOCHONDRIAL DYSFUNCTION

Mitochondrial dysfunction has a major impact on the aging process. As cells age, the efficacy of the respiratory chain tends to decrease, which increases electron leakage and reduces the production of ATP. Mitochondrial deficiencies may affect apoptotic signaling by increasing the mitochondrial permeability changes that precipitate apoptosis. The combination of increased damage and reduced turnover in mitochondria, due to lower biogenesis and reduced clearance, may contribute to the aging process.[4]

STEM CELL EXHAUSTION

As tissues age, their ability to regenerate is significantly reduced due to the inability of stem cells to reproduce. While a decrease in stem cell proliferation clearly impairs the functionality of tissues, excessive proliferation of stem cells can also be dangerous by accelerating the exhaustion of stem cell reserves and leading to premature aging.[4]

EPIGENETIC ALTERATIONS

A variety of epigenetic factors affect cells throughout the life span, including DNA methylation patterns, post-translational modification of histones, and chromatin remodeling. Epigenetic alterations can directly affect regulation of telomere length, one of the other hallmarks of aging discussed earlier. There is also evidence of age-related transcriptional changes in genes that encode key components of inflammatory, mitochondrial, and lysosomal degradation pathways that can contribute to the aging phenotype.[4]

ALTERED CELLULAR COMMUNICATION

Aging does not happen in a vacuum, and there is compelling evidence to suggest that some age-related changes occur with intercellular signaling. Neurohormonal signaling becomes deregulated in the setting of increased inflammatory reactions, decreased immunosurveillance against infectious agents and premalignant cells, and peri- and extracellular environment changes. Evidence also suggests that aging can have a domino effect on other tissues, causing an interorgan aging phenotype. So-called *contagious aging* effects include senescent cells that cause senescence in neighboring cells through gap junction contacts and ROS-mediated processes.[4]

FRAILTY

This book covers the pathological processes of various disease states, but is there a state of disease associated with old age itself? Age is a risk factor in a variety of diseases, such as cancer, cardiovascular disease, and dementia; however, aging can also be pathological in and of itself under the right conditions.

Frailty is a multisystem syndrome that marks a loss of reserve that leaves an individual at an increased risk of death, loss of independence, and decreased mobility.[6] It is a unique state that indicates multisystem physiological changes.[7] Although many older individuals who meet criteria for frailty typically have multiple comorbidities, people can still be classified as frail without having a life-threatening disease process. Frailty is associated with reduced functional reserves and decreased adaptability to both extrinsic and intrinsic stressors.

Clinically, frailty in older adults is often measured by the Fried Phenotype Frailty Index. The five criteria of this index are self-reported exhaustion, reduced physical activity, slow walking speed, reduced grip strength, and unintentional weight loss. A person must meet three or more of the five criteria in order to be classified as frail.[6,7]

INFLAMMATION

An important marker of frailty is inflammation. Chronic levels of inflammation can be a consequence of a variety of different mechanisms. Aging leads to decreased levels of sex steroids, growth hormones, and vitamin D levels, and these declines, in turn, are associated with higher levels of inflammation. Older adults also typically have other comorbid conditions that promote baseline proinflammatory states, such as atherosclerosis or subacute infections. Interleukin 6 (IL-6) is a cytokine that is produced by leukocytes in response to noxious stimuli. High levels of IL-6 are often associated with poor functional status and can predict onset of disability in older adults. Tumor necrosis factor alpha (TNF-α) is a cytokine associated with acute inflammation. TNF-α is strongly associated with death in community-dwelling older adults.[6]

Circulating inflammatory signals such as TNF-α stimulate production of IL-6 and C-reactive protein, which in turn have a catabolic effect on muscles. Muscles store energy in the form of glycogen and proteins that can be used for energy in times of extreme stress or malnutrition. Hormones are produced and catabolized in muscle tissue. Stored amino acids can be used in acute infections to produce antibodies. Loss of muscle can contribute to a reduced response to immunological insults and lower metabolic adaptation.[8]

Despite the many hypotheses of cellular aging, there is much that has not been confirmed by preclinical or clinical research. Active research continues in this field, particularly in individuals and groups who have extraordinary longevity. The intersection of genetic influences with environmental influences on life span is beginning to give clues as to mechanisms of human aging.

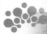

Thought Questions

11. What are the top three classes of cellular biomolecules that are vulnerable to ROS-mediated damage?

12. Explain the role of telomeres in maintaining chromosomal integrity over repeated cycles of mitosis.

KEY POINTS

- Human cells are bounded by a cell membrane consisting of a phospholipid bilayer with polar components facing the outside, and a lipid core made up of fatty acids and cholesterol. The membrane is a hydrophobic barrier between intracellular fluid and extracellular fluid.
- The organelles—nucleus, endoplasmic reticulum, Golgi apparatus, ribosomes, mitochondria, lysosomes, and peroxisomes—carry out the work of the cell, with many reactions being compartmentalized within one or more compartments.
- The membrane's lipid barrier allows movement of small nonpolar substances such as oxygen and carbon dioxide between extracellular and intracellular fluid, but most other molecules require transporters.
- The main factors involved in predicting the mechanism by which a solute will cross the membrane include the degree to which it is polar and hydrophilic (as opposed to nonpolar and hydrophobic); the concentration gradient for the solute across the cell membrane; and the direction of movement relative to that gradient—either downhill (moving from a region of high concentration to a region of low concentration) or uphill (moving from low to high concentration).
- Modes of transport across the cell membrane are diffusion, exocytosis and endocytosis, facilitated diffusion, active transport, secondary active transport, aquaporins, and ion channels.
- Active transport by the sodium–potassium (Na^+/K^+) pump generates and maintains the characteristic ionic composition of extracellular fluid (low potassium, high sodium) and intracellular fluid (high potassium, low sodium).
- In secondary active transport, the movement of one solute down its concentration gradient (often sodium) is coupled to the movement of another solute against its concentration gradient. This mechanism requires ongoing activity of the Na^+/K^+ pump to generate the sodium concentration gradient.
- Ion channels allow ions to move down their concentration gradients. Potassium leak channels are common components of cell membranes and set up a resting membrane potential that is particularly significant in electrically excitable cells such as muscle and nerve cells.

- Cells respond to neurotransmitters and hormones by receptors found in the cell membrane or intracellularly.
- The sympathetic and parasympathetic branches of the autonomic nervous system are the major rapidly acting regulators of organ system adaptations to environmental and internal challenges to homeostasis.
- Receptors for the autonomic neurotransmitters norepinephrine and acetylcholine are examples of GPCRs. Many hormones and other neurotransmitters work by way of GPCRs.
- Cell signaling by GPCRs initiates an amplifying cascade of activated proteins. Following ligand binding to its receptor, a three-part G protein is activated and splits into α and $\beta\gamma$ subunits. The α subunit activates an enzyme within the membrane, and the $\beta\gamma$ subunit may have additional effects. The activated enzyme produces second messengers that diffuse throughout the cytoplasm to initiate changes in intracellular activity.
- Adenylyl cyclase is stimulated by receptors linking to G_s proteins; their activation increases intracellular concentrations of cAMP. The result of increasing cAMP is the activation of PKA, an enzyme that phosphorylates intracellular target proteins to alter their activity, either upregulating or downregulating activity to adapt to homeostatic challenges. PKA is a serine/threonine kinase, adding phosphate groups to proteins specifically at sites of the amino acids serine or threonine.
- Adenylyl cyclase is inhibited by receptors linking to G_i proteins; this inhibition reverses the actions of stimulatory receptors and reduces cAMP levels and PKA activity.
- Receptors linked to G_q activate phospholipase C. This enzyme splits a membrane lipid, PIP_2, producing two second messengers—membrane-bound DAG and intracellular IP_3. IP_3 diffuses to the endoplasmic reticulum and releases calcium from its storage, producing a brief increase of intracellular calcium with a variety of downstream consequences for cell function.
- Several mechanisms terminate the actions of GPCRs: diffusion of neurotransmitter or hormone away from the receptor ends G protein stimulation; the intrinsic GTPase activity of G proteins leads to their inactivation; and intracellular phosphatase enzymes can reverse the actions of protein kinases.

- Certain receptors have an extracellular ligand-binding site and an intracellular enzyme site or binding sites for enzymes. Many of these types of receptors are tyrosine kinases, phosphorylating target proteins on tyrosine sites.
- Tyrosine kinase downstream activities often include activation of cell proliferation, and ligands for tyrosine kinase–linked receptors promote body growth and development and proliferation of immune cells. When dysregulated, many of the receptors and signaling cascade proteins of this class are also oncoproteins—having cancer-promoting activity.
- Steroid and thyroid hormones cross cell membranes and ultimately bind to receptors on DNA, altering transcription and translation for their biological effects.
- Muscle cells produce skeletal movement or organ contractions by interactions between the contractile proteins actin and myosin. Skeletal and cardiac muscle cells are striated muscle, having highly organized bundles of actin and myosin within the functional unit of the sarcomere. Smooth muscle cells found in blood vessels and organs have more loosely arranged bundles of actin and myosin.

- Regulation of striated muscle contraction by calcium depends on troponins and tropomyosin. Regulation of smooth muscle contraction depends on calmodulin and myosin light chain kinase.
- Cells can adapt to a variety of homeostatic challenges by hypertrophy, atrophy, proliferation, dysplasia, or death.
- Necrotic cell death is caused by severe traumatic or ischemic injury, whereas apoptotic cell death is sometimes physiological rather than pathological. Autophagic cell death is slower, and autophagy itself may be a protective mechanism that maintains the cell and prevents cell death.
- The biological cause of aging has not been definitively determined, but humans and other organisms experience gradual losses of cell and organ function that end in death, even in the absence of a specific disease process. Different pathways can contribute to aging, including lifelong exposure to injurious chemicals such as ROS and inflammatory cytokines, and gradual diminishment of cellular quality control systems for integrity of DNA, proteins, and mitochondria.
- Nutrient signaling cascades appear to play a role in aging, and caloric restriction extends life in many animal models.

REFERENCES

1. Gladyshev V. Aging: progressive decline in fitness due to the rising deleteriome adjusted by genetic, environmental, and stochastic processes. *Aging Cell.* 2016;15:594–602. doi:10.1111/acel.12480.
2. Kumar V, Abbas AK, Aster JC, eds. *Robbins and Cotran Pathologic Basis of Disease.* 9th ed. Philadelphia, PA: Elsevier; 2015.
3. Hoeijmakers JHJ. DNA damage, aging, and cancer. *N Engl J Med.* 2009;361:1475–1485. doi:10.1056/NEJM1ra0804615.
4. López-Otín C, Blasco MA, Partridge L, et al. The hallmarks of aging. *Cell.* 2013;153:1194–1217. doi:10.1016/j.cell.2013.05.039.
5. Vicencio JM, Galluzzi L, Tajeddine N, et al. Senescence, apoptosis, or autophagy? *Gerontology.* 2008;58:92–99. doi:10.1159/00129697.
6. Hubbard RE, Woodhouse KW. Frailty, inflammation and the elderly. *Biogerontology.* 2010;11:635–641. doi:10.1007/s10522-010-9292-5.
7. Fulop T, Larbi A, Witkowski JM, et al. Aging, frailty, and age-related diseases. *Biogerontology.* 2010;11:547–563. doi:10.1007/s10522-010-9287-2.
8. Evans WJ, Paolisso G, Abbatecola AM, et al. Frailty and muscle metabolism dysregulation in the elderly. *Biogerontology.* 2010;11:527–536. doi:10.1007/s10522-010-9297-0.

SUGGESTED RESOURCES

Alberts B, Johnson A, Lewis J, et al. Cell signaling. In: Alberts B, Johnson AD, Lewis J, et al., eds. *Molecular Biology of the Cell.* 6th ed. New York, NY: Garland Science; 2015:813–888.

Baynes JW. Aging. In: Baynes JW, Dominiczak MH, eds. *Medical Biochemistry.* 5th ed. Philadelphia, PA: Elsevier; 2019:chap 29.

Boron WF, Boulpaep EL, eds. *Medical Physiology.* 3rd ed. Philadelphia, PA: Elsevier, 2017.

Cantley L. Signal transduction. In: Boron WF, Boulpaep EL, eds. *Medical Physiology.* 3rd ed. Philadelphia, PA: Elsevier; 2017:47–72.

Koeppen BM, Stanton BA, eds. *Berne & Levy Physiology.* 7th ed. Philadelphia, PA: Elsevier; 2018.

Moczydlowski EG. Cellular physiology of skeletal, cardiac, and smooth muscle. In: Boron WF, Boulpaep EL, eds. *Medical Physiology.* 3rd ed. Philadelphia, PA: Elsevier; 2017:228–252.

Reisner HM. *Pathology: A Modern Case Study.* New York, NY: McGraw-Hill; 2015.

5

INFECTIOUS DISEASE

Ross S. Johnson, Jennifer Bailey, and Roseann Velez

THE CLINICAL CONTEXT

Mortality and morbidity rates for infectious diseases vary greatly by geographical location. World Health Organization (WHO) statistics provide striking documentation that deaths due to infectious diseases are much higher in poor countries than in the countries with the highest income levels (Tables 5.1 and 5.2).[1] It is particularly striking that malaria and tuberculosis are significant causes of death in low-resource countries, whereas these diseases are rarely fatal in wealthy countries. Other infectious diseases that are a significant cause of death in low-resource countries are pneumonia, diarrhea, and HIV infection. In lower and middle-resource countries, the top ten causes of death also include lower respiratory infections, tuberculosis, and diarrheal diseases. Although clean water and widespread availability of vaccines and antibiotic medications have reduced the burden of certain communicable diseases, there is always the threat of emerging diseases, antimicrobial-resistant pathogens, international transmission, and local outbreaks that can infect large numbers of people quickly.

In the United States, in 2015, there were about 15.5 million office visits (National Ambulatory Medical Care Survey),[2] as well as 3.7 million ED visits (National Hospital Ambulatory Medical Care Survey),[3] for infectious and parasitic diseases. The Centers for Disease Control and Prevention (CDC) also reported U.S. influenza and pneumonia mortality rate at 14.3% in 2017.[4] It is likely that many acute mild infections do not trigger an office visit, including the common cold, infectious gastroenteritis, cutaneous fungal infections, and genital yeast infections.

OVERVIEW OF INFECTIOUS DISEASE PATHOPHYSIOLOGY

HUMAN–MICROBE INTERACTIONS

Prenatal development occurs in an environment that is generally sterile, with few studies showing bacterial growth from amniotic fluid. During vaginal delivery, neonates experience their first exposure to microbes, the mother's normal vaginal flora. From that point on, for the duration of life, we live in an environment filled with microbes, most of which are not human pathogens. On both skin and mucosal surfaces, colonization with normal flora is common (Box 5.1). Some of the normal flora are neutral, having no harmful effects on the host; some are beneficial, providing protection against pathogens and facilitating normal immune system development; and some are potential pathogens, held in check by surrounding microbiota and immune mechanisms. Although these colonizing organisms may be detected by laboratory pathogen identification, they are not causing disease and do not warrant antimicrobial treatments.

Some body locations are colonized with organisms that are potentially pathogenic, but not in that location. For example, *Streptococcus pneumoniae* bacteria normally colonize the pharynx and would usually be cultured from a throat swab. However, *S. pneumoniae* in the lungs is the most common cause of pneumonia, a serious infection. *Staphylococcus aureus* normally colonizes the skin, but will cause infection if it gains access through the skin from a cut that is not thoroughly cleaned. *Escherichia coli* is part of the normal large intestinal flora, but can cause a urinary tract infection if it enters the urethra or bladder and reproduces there. Table 5.3 contrasts characteristics of colonization and infection.

Some microbes are always pathogenic, and exposure is followed by demonstrable signs and symptoms

TABLE 5.1 Top Ten Causes of Death in 2016—Low-Income Countries

Disease	Number of Deaths	Percent of All Deaths
Lower respiratory infection	**499,839**	**9.33**
Diarrheal disease	**383,400**	**7.16**
Ischemic heart disease	349,076	6.52
HIV/AIDS	**292,097**	**5.45**
Stroke	278,310	5.19
Malaria	**247,602**	**4.62**
Tuberculosis	**225,928**	**4.22**
Preterm birth complications	212,100	3.96
Birth asphyxia and birth trauma	201,395	3.76
Road injury	193,577	3.61

Note: Total deaths and percent of deaths due to infectious disease (bolded): 1,648,866; 30.78%. HIV, human immunodeficiency virus infection; AIDS, acquired immunodeficiency syndrome
Source: Adapted from World Health Organization. The top 10 causes of death. 2019. https://www.who.int/news-room/fact-sheets/detail/the-top-10-causes-of-death.

TABLE 5.2 Top Ten Causes of Death in 2016—High-Income Countries

Disease	Number of Deaths	Percent of All Deaths
Ischemic heart disease	1,724,964	16.78
Stroke	741,425	7.21
Alzheimer disease + other dementias	718,641	6.99
Trachea/bronchus/lung cancer	580,003	5.64
Chronic obstructive pulmonary disease	554,555	5.40
Lower respiratory infection	**438,608**	**4.27**
Colon/rectum cancer	327,925	3.19
Diabetes	271,947	2.65
Kidney disease	220,813	2.15
Breast cancer	187,500	1.82

Note: Total deaths and percent of deaths due to infectious disease (bolded): 438,608; 4.27%.
Source: Adapted from World Health Organization. The top 10 causes of death. 2019. https://www.who.int/news-room/fact-sheets/detail/the-top-10-causes-of-death.

BOX 5.1
Common Body Sites of Colonization

- Eyes
- Nose
- Mouth
- Pharynx
- Skin
- Gastrointestinal tract
- Lower urinary tract
- Vagina

TABLE 5.3 Comparison of Colonization and Infection

Colonization	Infection
Organism documented by culture or other means	Organism documented by culture or other means
No evidence of inflammation	Infection progresses with pathogen numbers increasing, invading tissues
Limited bacterial growth, no progression to infection	Local inflammation: redness, heat, swelling, pain
No signs and symptoms	If upper respiratory infection: cough, airway irritation, mucus production
Sometimes known as "carrier state"	May become systemic: bacteremia, sepsis

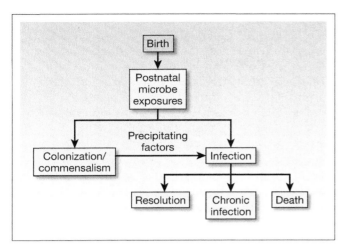

FIGURE 5.1 Human–microbe interactions. Colonization with normal microbial flora begins at birth. Some of the microbes are commensals that help maintain homeostasis, while providing for their own needs for survival and growth. Exposure to pathogens results in infection—during which the body mounts an inflammatory response that clears the pathogen while producing classic signs and symptoms of infection. Many infections resolve, but others may lead to chronic infection or even death. Colonizing organisms of the normal flora, some of which have the capacity to produce infections, are normally held in check and do not cause disease. A variety of host factors can precipitate the transition to microbial disease: Suppressed immunity due to disease or drug treatments, traumatic injuries and burns, and being very young or very old can all lead to infection with a colonizing organism.

of infection such as fever, malaise, anorexia, pain, swelling, exudates, and other manifestations. The course of infections ranges from resolution (with or without pharmacological management, depending on host factors and the nature of the pathogen), to chronic infection, to death (**Figure 5.1**) Host factors vary with age, with comorbidities, and particularly with immune system status. The immunocompromised host is vulnerable to infections and is particularly likely to develop infections from microbes that are common members of normal flora and colonization.

MECHANISMS OF PROTECTION FROM PATHOGENS

As noted, shortly after birth our bodies are colonized with microorganisms, primarily bacteria and a few fungi. These normal flora contribute to the development of the immune system (as described in Chapter 6, The Immune System and Leukocyte Function), help with gastrointestinal immune development and digestive function (as described in Chapter 13, Gastrointestinal Tract), and reduce infections by inhibiting growth of pathogenic microorganisms. Skin and mucosal surfaces are protected by their intact barrier structure and by

secretions such as sweat and tears that contain antimicrobial compounds such as dermcidin and lysozyme. Body regions that have direct contact with the environment—skin, eyes, ears, nose, gastrointestinal tract, respiratory tract, and genitalia—each have their own immune and secretory protective mechanisms. The innate and adaptive immune systems provide powerful mechanisms to kill invading pathogens and to develop specific immunity against many organisms, either following an initial infection or by immunization. Through these mechanisms, many infections are acute and self-limited, cleared by the body's own defenses and not requiring medical interventions. However, these protections are reduced or lacking in populations such as the very young and the very old, individuals with extensive tissue damage due to trauma or burns, and those with chronic debilitating diseases or immunodeficiency states. In these vulnerable hosts, infections can be associated with much greater morbidity and mortality.

PORTALS OF PATHOGEN ENTRY AND TARGETS OF COLONIZATION

A pathogen requires a portal of entry into the host in order to initiate an infection. Entry may be gained by inhalation; oral ingestion; genital, urethral, or anal exposure; contact with membranes of eyes, nose, or ears; a bite from an insect or animal vector; a penetrating wound; or a surgical incision. Retention and movement of the pathogenic organism within the body depend on the structure of the pathogen itself, and its capacity for binding to human cells and tissues. Sites of attachment (e.g., pili projecting from the bacterial cell wall, viral coat glycoproteins) permit adhesion to particular cell and tissue targets, facilitating a stable spot for pathogen growth and multiplication. For example, hemagglutinin, a spike-shaped protein on the surface of the influenza virus, attaches to host cell sialic acid molecules on the membranes of respiratory tract epithelial cells, targeting those cells for invasion and viral replication. In some cases, foreign surfaces, such as artificial heart valves or joints, provide an optimal environment for bacteria to form a biofilm that is highly resistant to immune attack.

PATHOGEN VIRULENCE FACTORS

Organisms vary in the severity and duration of disease they cause. The factors influencing pathogen virulence have been best delineated in the context of bacterial infections and include the following:

- The ability to evade immune phagocytosis, often by formation of a protective capsule or by entry into cells
- Once inside a cell, the ability to resist breakdown by lysosomal enzymes

- Secretion of exotoxins that enter the bloodstream to disrupt function of nearby and remote tissues
- Release of endotoxin that stimulates intense immune system activation
- Expression of superantigens that stimulate intense immune system activation

HOST RESPONSE FACTORS

The severity of infectious disease is also determined by the host. As previously noted, in infants, the relative weakness of immune activity tends to predispose to greater case numbers and more severe presentations of infectious diseases. Older adults are similarly vulnerable, and may also have diminished immune responses that make the onset of infection more subtle and diagnosis more difficult. Patients with chronic diseases, receiving immunosuppressive treatments for immune hyperactivity states or cancer, or with more severe bacterial exposure (e.g., due to massive trauma) have the highest risk. Paradoxically, the magnitude of the host immune response can also amplify the severity of disease presentation. The Spanish flu epidemic in 1918 had high mortality rates in healthy young adults between the ages of 20 and 40 years in addition to young children and older adults. The apparent mechanism for this pattern was the robust inflammatory response in the young adults—their host response to the influenza virus was so intense that the massive cytokine release resulted in septic shock. In a similar fashion, the inflammatory response to viral or bacterial pneumonia can be very robust in an adolescent or young adult, predisposing to alveolar flooding and greatly compromised oxygen exchange.

Thought Questions

1. Define infection and identify the differences between colonization and infection, giving specific examples of each.

2. How does infection start, and what is the usual course?

3. What factors influence the course of an infection? Give specific examples of different trajectories of infection.

MICROBIAL PATHOGENICITY

OVERVIEW

Most microorganisms on this planet are not pathogens—microorganisms with the capacity to transmit a disease to humans. It is estimated that there are about 1,400 pathogenic microorganisms, a miniscule fraction of the estimated 1 trillion microbial species on earth.[5] Similarly, most of the microorganisms that live and thrive on humans (the normal flora, also known as *commensals*) normally do not cause disease without some initiating factor. Different body habitats contiguous with the body surface (skin, mouth, gut, genitalia) contain resident microbial communities that differ by microbial composition and function, whereas other body regions are sterile. (Samples of internal tissues and nongastrointestinal organs, blood, cerebrospinal fluid, and synovial fluid should not grow microorganisms when cultured.)

Pathogenic microbes include prokaryotic cells such as bacteria, eukaryotic cells such as fungi and protozoa, and multicellular helminths (parasitic worms), in addition to nonliving virus and prion particles. Many of these organisms are present in the environment outside the human host or in animal hosts. Infectious microbes can be spread by being passed directly from one person to another, indirectly from contaminated surfaces, or by exposure to an infected member of a different species with transfer by bites, scratches, or inhalation. A few microscopic pathogens have humans as their exclusive hosts; these organisms can be transferred only from human to human. Other human pathogenic microbes are present in environments ranging from soil and water to nonhuman reservoirs, animals, and insects, or are introduced by contamination during food production or harvesting and distribution.

CHARACTERISTICS OF PATHOGEN CLASSES

Bacteria

Bacteria are prokaryotes—single-celled organisms much smaller than human cells that reproduce by binary fission. Different species of bacteria have varying shapes and sizes, from simple spheres and rods to spiral shapes and other configurations (**Figure 5.2**). The bacterial cell structure consists generally of (a) an outer cell wall that varies in numbers of layers and thickness, and (b) cytoplasm that includes a nucleoid (a single coiled circle of DNA, not contained within a nuclear membrane) and ribosomes to conduct protein translation (**Figure 5.3**). Bacterial ribosomes are sufficiently different from eukaryotic ribosomes as to provide a target of antibacterial drugs.

Many of the bacteria that are part of normal human flora can become disease causing if they increase in number or move from their usual body location to a different site. For example, *E. coli* are normal flora of the colon but can be a source of urinary tract infections upon entering the urethra and multiplying there. The broad classes of bacteria that are part of the normal

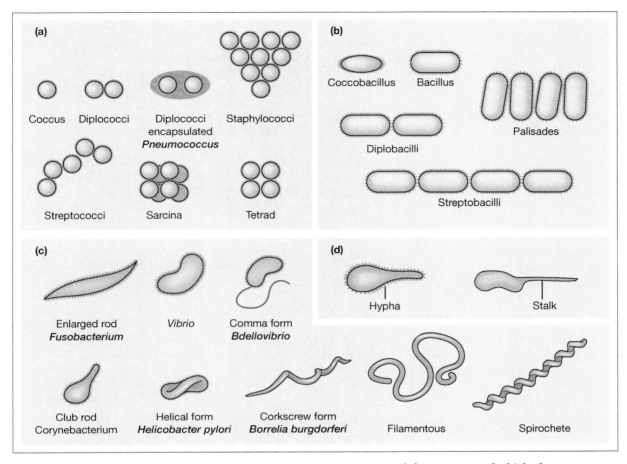

FIGURE 5.2 Bacterial morphology. Bacteria come in a variety of shapes, some of which cluster together, as in diplococci and streptococci (linear clusters) and staphylococci (grouped clusters). **(a)** Cocci appear circular and **(b)** bacilli have a rod-like appearance on microscopic examination. **(c)** More complex shapes such as spiral (spirochetes, *Borrelia burgdorferi*) also occur. **(d)** Some bacteria demonstrate budding and appendages.

flora and sometimes also cause disease are classified as gram positive, gram negative, aerobes, and anaerobes. The Gram stain, developed in 1882 and published in 1884 by the Danish scientist Hans Christian Gram, is the primary method of initial bacterial classification, which is then followed up with cultures and other methods.[6] Gram-positive bacteria have thick cell walls rich in peptidoglycan that retain stain when subjected to the Gram procedure. Gram-negative bacteria have thinner cell walls that do not retain sufficient stain to be seen after the Gram procedure; a different-colored counterstain is used to make these visible on microscopy. Aerobic organisms require oxygen in the environment to grow, whereas anaerobes thrive in low-oxygen environments such as the gut.

Bacterial structural features such as flagella, fimbriae, surface proteins, and capsule proteins can facilitate bacterial adhesion or movement in the human body. For example, *Neisseria gonorrhoeae* membranes are studded with projecting pili that allow adherence to the genital mucosa and movement along the epithelial cells to spread genital infections. The severity of infection is influenced by virulence factors that can include structural elements of the bacterium, its ability to enter cells, and the capacity to produce damaging secretions such as degradative enzymes and exotoxins.

The ability to evade host defenses depends on the specific avoidance factor(s) of the pathogen. After being engulfed by host macrophages, *Mycobacterium tuberculosis* (MTB) avoids further destruction by means of its thick, lipid-rich cell wall and its ability to block lysosomal degradation. Certain bacteria are capable of forming spores—dormant structures with impermeable capsules—that can exist without nutrition and evade destruction for extended periods of time, only to be reactivated to their original form when conditions permit.

Bacterial proliferation and activation lead to infection, in which the host inflammatory and immune

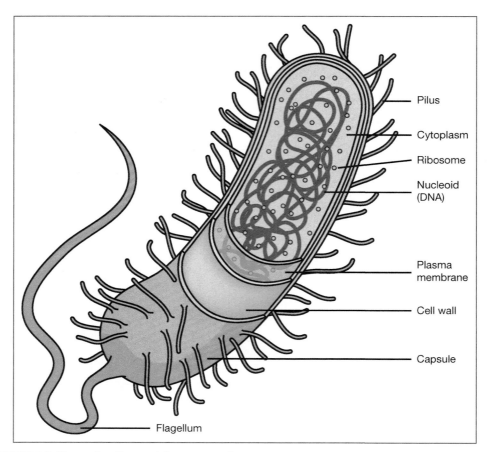

FIGURE 5.3 Example of bacterial structure. A gram-positive bacterium has three coating layers: an inner plasma membrane, an intermediate cell wall that is relatively thick and enriched in peptidoglycan molecules, and a protective capsule. A flagellum allows movement within a host, and pili facilitate attachment to host membranes. DNA is found in a large circular chromosome, the nucleoid, which is located within the cytoplasm, rather than bounded by a nuclear membrane as in eukaryotic cells. Additional DNA may be found in small circular plasmids (not shown). When bacteria reproduce by binary fission, DNA in the nucleoid and plasmids is replicated and divided among daughter cells. This method of reproduction is faster than mitosis of eukaryotic cells. Ribosomes are used for protein translation, as in eukaryotic cells.

responses produce characteristic systemic or local signs and symptoms such as fever, malaise, redness, swelling, and pain. Contributing factors include the following:

- *Bacterial exotoxin secretion:* These exotoxins may have pathophysiological effects on target cells, such as cholera toxin, which promotes massive watery diarrhea, or botulinum toxin, which causes neuromuscular dysfunction and paralysis.
- *Endotoxin release:* Antibiotic treatments or the host complement system may rupture the bacterial cell wall, releasing toxic fragments. This is true for gram-negative bacteria containing membrane-bound molecules of lipopolysaccharide, also known as endotoxin. As host defenses such as complement

break down the cell walls, lipopolysaccharide is released and can provoke a systemic inflammatory response, inducing septic shock.

The differences between prokaryotic and eukaryotic cells provide the foundation for drugs used to treat bacterial infections. Antibiotics that target the cell wall, nucleic acid, and protein synthesis must be able to reach the bacteria in sufficient concentration to be effective (**Figure 5.4**). These drugs may not be as effective against intracellular pathogens such as MTB. In addition, many vaccines have been developed to provide protection against bacterial pathogens, including those causing diphtheria, tetanus, pertussis, pneumococcal pneumonia, and meningitis.

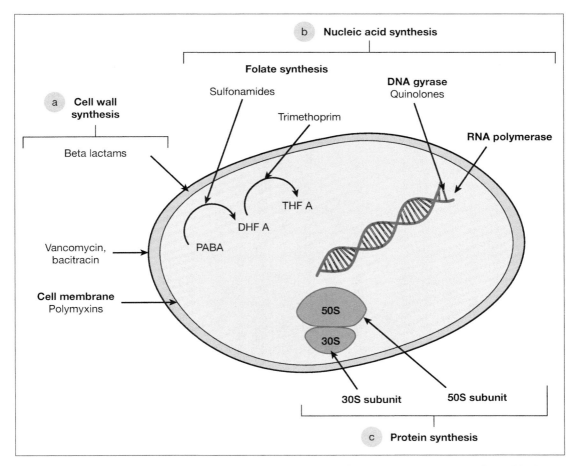

FIGURE 5.4 Cellular targets of antibacterial drugs. **(a)** The earliest widely used antibiotics targeted the synthesis of cell wall components, and new drugs of this class (penicillins, cephalosporins, carbapenems, monobactams) continue to be developed. Early drugs were most effective at eliminating gram-positive bacteria, due to their thick peptidoglycan layer, whereas later generations of drugs gained gram-negative bacteria coverage. **(b)** Nucleic acid synthesis was found to be disrupted by another early antibiotic class, the sulfonamides. The sulfonamides and trimethoprim block sequential steps in the conversion of the precursor para-aminobenzoic acid (PABA) to dihydrofolic acid (DHF A) and to tetrahydrofolic acid (THF A), which is required for purine synthesis needed for DNA replication. Quinolones block bacterial DNA synthesis by inhibiting DNA gyrase. **(c)** Drugs that block bacterial protein synthesis (macrolides, clindamycin, linezolid, chloramphenicol, streptogramins, tetracyclines, aminoglycosides) specifically target bacterial ribosomes while having no effect on eukaryotic ribosomes.
DHF A, dihydrofolic acid; PABA, para-aminobenzoic acid; THF A, tetrahydrofolic acid.

Viruses

Viruses are pathogenic acellular particles much smaller than a host cell (virus diameter ~20–300 nm versus human cell size >~7 μm). They must enter a host cell and use the host cell's enzymes and ribosomes to conduct nucleic acid replication, transcription, and translation to reproduce, using energy provided by the host cell. All virions have similar components: a nucleocapsid composed of a nucleic acid core (DNA or RNA) surrounded by a protein capsid. Viral nucleic acids can be either RNA or DNA (but only one will be present, unlike prokaryotic and eukaryotic cells) and may be either single stranded or double stranded. There are several different forms of capsid: helical, icosahedral, and complex. Icosahedral and helical forms are shown in **Figure 5.5**. Enveloped viruses have an additional outer membranous envelope surrounding the nucleocapsid that is usually derived from the host cell plasma membrane during budding. Capsid proteins (for nonenveloped viruses) and spike proteins projecting from the membranes of enveloped viruses are the antigenic determinants that provoke the host immune response to form neutralizing antibodies

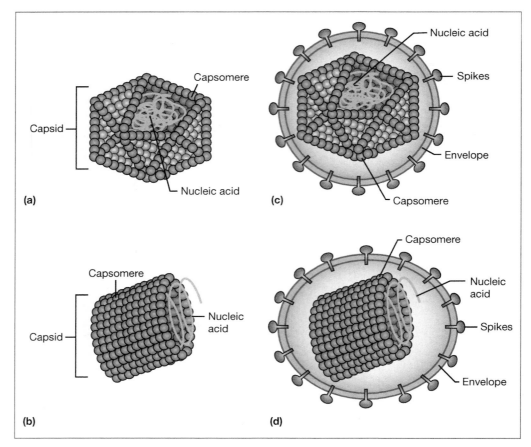

FIGURE 5.5 Viral shapes. A virus consists of a nucleic acid core surrounded by a protein capsule (capsid) made up of capsomere subunits. Enveloped viruses acquire a membrane coat, usually obtained while budding from the host cell. (**a**) Icosohedral structure, naked. (**b**) Helical structure, naked. (**c**) Icosohedral structure, enveloped. (**d**) Helical structure, enveloped.

and to activate cytotoxic T cells to kill host virus-infected cells displaying those proteins.

The basic viral life cycle shown in **Figure 5.6** and described in **Box 5.2** begins with attachment to a host cell, followed by entry into the cell. After removal of the capsid coat, the viral nucleic acid is exposed and viral polymerase as well as host cell polymerases and ribosomes are used for the following functions:

- Replicating many copies of the viral nucleic acid
- Transcribing the viral genome
- Translating viral proteins
- Assembling new virions (hundreds can be produced at this stage)
- Release of the virions locally or systemically

Viruses have characteristic portals of entry, including aerosols inhaled into the respiratory system (rhinovirus and adenovirus, which cause the common cold; influenza virus; measles and mumps viruses); oral ingestion (hepatitis A and E viruses; norovirus; rotavirus, which causes diarrhea); sexual contact (herpesviruses, HIV, hepatitis B virus); blood/injection (HIV, hepatitis B and C viruses); and vertical transmission, from mother to neonate (HIV, hepatitis B virus). In some cases, viral replication primarily involves the entry site, as with viruses that cause acute upper respiratory infection. In other cases, the viruses move from the entry site to their cellular targets, as with hepatitis and HIV infections. The localized response produces cell death that can be observed histologically on biopsy samples as the *cytopathologic effect*. Local stimulation of immune responses causes characteristic signs and symptoms evaluated during a history and physical examination (e.g., coughing, sneezing, and runny nose produced during a common cold).

The time course of a viral infection varies with the virus. Many acute infections resolve within a few days

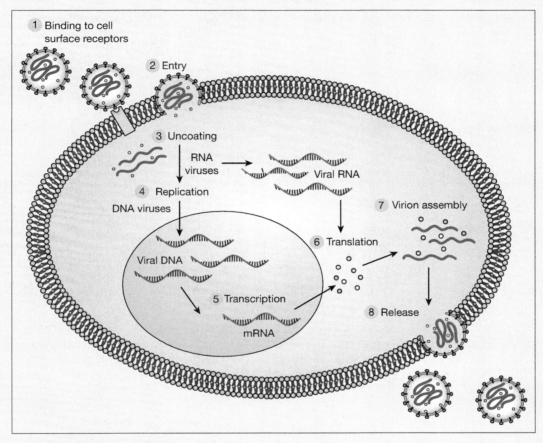

FIGURE 5.6 Life cycle of a virus.

1. Attachment to target cells, often due to highly specific recognition sites on the outer surface of the viral particle that bind specific target cell types.

2. Entering the host cell by endocytosis.

3. Removal of capsid coat to expose nucleic acid.

4. Replication of viral DNA in the nucleus of the host cell, or replication of viral RNA in the cytoplasm of the host cell.

5 and 6. Transcription and translation of viral proteins.

7. Virion assembly: Capsomere subunits often self-assemble surrounding the nucleic acid core.

8. Release may be by cell lysis, killing the host cell. For enveloped viruses, the virions acquire a membrane coat by budding off from the host cell.

to weeks. A very virulent acute virus such as some influenza subtypes may cause intense immune activation and require hospitalization and supportive care. Other viruses may not be completely cleared and enter a *latent* phase during which no viral replication and release take place. At a later time, exposure to stress or altered immunity allows resumption of the viral life cycle and disease expression. This is characteristic of cytomegalovirus, Epstein–Barr virus, and several herpesviruses responsible for cold sores (herpes simplex virus [HSV]-1) and genital herpes (HSV-2). Another well-known example of viral latency is that of the varicella-zoster virus, which causes chickenpox on initial exposure and can be

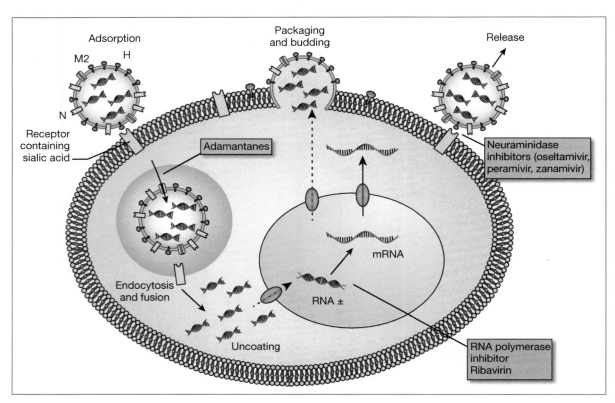

FIGURE 5.7 Targets of drugs to treat influenza infection. Antiviral drugs can target the uncoating phase after virus entry (adamantanes; e.g., amantadine), RNA production (ribavirin), and virion release (neuraminidase inhibitors; e.g., oseltamivir). In addition, viral DNA polymerase is inhibited by acyclovir, vidarabine, foscarnet, and ganciclovir (not shown in this figure).
H, hemagglutinin; N, neuraminidase; M2, a membrane ion channel; mRNA, messenger RNA.

reactivated later in life in the form of shingles (also known as herpes zoster).

In chronic (persistent) viral infections, after an initial acute infection, viral replication drops to very low levels. Rather than being completely inactive, virus is continually produced at low levels, with the capacity to cause gradually accumulating cell and tissue damage. A person may be a carrier, able to infect others, without clinically evident signs of infection, as with hepatitis C and HIV.

Vaccines have been developed to prevent or reduce the risk of many viral infections, including measles, mumps, rubella, varicella, polio, hepatitis A and B, rotavirus infections, influenza, and human papillomavirus infections. This strategy is particularly useful when there is just one serotype of a virus (as is true of the measles virus), but it has limitations when a virus has many serotypes (as with influenza virus) or has a high mutation rate (as with HIV, for which there is currently no vaccination). The steps of viral infection have been the target of antiviral drugs, as shown in **Figure 5.7**, which focuses on influenza drug targets.

Fungi and Yeasts

Of the more than 200,000 known species of fungi, it is estimated that fewer than 400 are pathogenic to humans.[7] Fungi and yeasts are eukaryotic cells with defined nuclei and organelles. Fungi can be multicellular organisms that reproduce sexually or asexually by branching hyphae, whereas yeasts are unicellular organisms. Fungal toxins may cause disease in humans, and airborne fungi are a frequent cause of allergies and diseases. Fungal infections in humans tend to be either superficial or systemic. The most common fungal infections of humans are those that affect skin, skin appendages, and subcutaneous tissue. Superficial fungal infections that do not result in deeply invasive infections include tinea pedis (athlete's foot), tinea capitis (scalp), and tinea corporis (ringworm). Another term for this group of fungi is *dermatophytes*, so called because of their association with the skin and their ability to derive nutrition from the keratin of skin and nails.

Candida albicans is a yeast—a unicellular fungus— often responsible for oral infections (thrush), and a common cause of vaginal infections. Individuals who are immunocompromised, have artificial implants (prosthetic valves, indwelling catheters), or have chronic disease may be at risk for far more serious and life-threatening systemic fungal infections (invasive candidiasis). *Candida glabrata*, *Candida parapsilosis*, and *C. albicans* are the most common organisms associated with invasive candidiasis.[8]

Fungal cells and human cells have shared metabolic and physiological pathways as eukaryotic cells. Most antifungal treatments exploit the differences between human and fungal plasma membrane composition and the composition of the fungal cell wall. In particular, the azoles (e.g., fluconazole, itraconazole) and the allylamines (e.g., terbinafine) block the production of *ergosterol*, a lipid component of fungal cell membranes that is not found in human cells.

Protozoa

Protozoa are single-celled eukaryotic organisms that are abundant in soil and water, and a small number of these are pathogenic. Estimates of global protozoal disease prevalence are extremely high: Amebiasis affects more than 700 million people worldwide; malaria, 300 million people; giardiasis, trichomoniasis, and schistosomiasis, more than 200 million people each; and trypanosomiasis (including Chagas disease), more than 60 million.[9] Major morphological distinctions exist among protozoa, including the flagellates, ameboid organisms, sporozoans, and microsporidia. These characteristics relate to the mode of movement employed by the protozoa, as well as the aspects of their often complex life cycles. Some protozoa reproduce by binary fission, whereas others have a form of sexual reproduction used in a portion of the life cycle. Other classification schemes are organized by site of infection, including intestinal protozoa, urogenital protozoa, and blood and tissue protozoa (including *Plasmodium* species that cause malaria). Some antibacterial agents are also effective in treating certain protozoal infections. An example is the use of metronidazole to treat intestinal *Giardia* infections or vaginal *Trichomonas* infections. Other protozoal infections do not currently have effective or widely available treatments, particularly in under-resourced countries.

Thought Questions

4. Describe the ways in which characteristics of bacteria make them vulnerable to attack by antibacterial drugs.

5. Identify the steps in the viral life cycle and how viral infections spread in the body.

CLINICAL CONCEPTS IN INFECTIOUS DISEASE

METHODS OF PATHOGEN IDENTIFICATION

Direct Observation

It is often possible to take a swab or sample from a region of suspected infection, smear it on a microscope slide, and observe organisms directly, particularly with the assistance of chemical treatments. Gram staining can be done on such a slide for direct visualization of the bacterial cell wall properties and bacterial morphology. Suspected vaginal yeast infections or bacterial vaginosis can be tested in this manner for a rapid evaluation. Red blood cells containing *Plasmodium falciparum* can be visualized in this manner, leading to a diagnosis of malaria. Additional methods are often used to follow up and confirm the initial testing.

Culture-Based Methods

The historical observation of discolored spots on spoiled food gave rise to the invention of growing microorganisms in culture, starting in the 1800s with the work of Louis Pasteur and Robert Koch. This approach worked well for many common bacteria, and the appropriate culture media and environmental requirements have been determined for many human pathogens. Culture media and conditions have been refined over the years, as certain organisms require special conditions in order to grow in culture. Culturing microorganisms is a key method to identify the specific causative pathogen. These techniques involve a multistep process of inoculation, incubation, isolation, inspection, and identification. The process concludes with pathogen identification using metabolic assays, antibody binding, and genetic analysis. In most cases, culture for pathogen identification is combined with testing for antibiotic sensitivity that directs appropriate therapy. Culture techniques are much more difficult for intracellular pathogens such as viruses, but they are commonly used for many bacterial pathogens.

Antigen Identification

Tests for a specific pathogen or a toxin of a specific pathogen are often carried out with immune-based methods (enzyme immunoassays) based on commercial development of antibodies to that particular target. Point-of-care testing, such as a rapid antigen detection test for suspected strep throat or heterophile antibody test for infectious mononucleosis/Epstein–Barr virus (monospot), is useful because results are available quickly, but follow-up testing is often required to confirm a diagnosis. A related indirect identification technique for infectious disease diagnosis measures the levels (titers) of antibodies to a particular pathogen in a patient's blood. A positive result indicates prior exposure to the pathogen.

If the sample is primarily immunoglobulin (Ig) M, it indicates recent infection, whereas the presence of IgG specific to a particular pathogen indicates a prolonged time since initial pathogen exposure.

Molecular Methods

Molecular methods of pathogen identification continue to expand and are often the most accurate and sensitive methods for the pathogen identification. *Nucleic acid amplification testing* (NAAT), involving the polymerase chain reaction (PCR) and nucleic acid hybridization techniques, is now the standard for diagnosis of certain infections, particularly intracellular infections such as those caused by *Chlamydia* spp. and *N. gonorrhoeae*, tuberculosis (TB), and many viral infections. As sequencing of pathogen genomes expands, an increasing number of organisms can be detected by NAAT, and some commercially available products can detect several different pathogens from one sample (multiplex analysis).[10]

DRUG-RESISTANT PATHOGENS

Since the discovery of penicillin in 1928 by Alexander Fleming and the introduction of penicillin as an agent for treatment for bacterial infections in the 1940s, antibiotics have saved the lives of millions. However, over this time frame, resistance to antibiotics has also continually increased (**Figure 5.8**). Antimicrobial resistance occurs when microbes adapt so that they no longer respond to drug therapy that was once effective. Although antibiotic resistance is a natural and somewhat inevitable phenomenon associated with antibiotic exposure, inappropriate or overuse of antibiotics perpetuates resistance. Antibiotic resistance is now a major global threat to health care, associated with poorer outcomes and exaggerated costs, and is predicted to worsen unless significant action is taken.

Resistance can develop to any antimicrobial agent. Genetically acquired resistance can develop from spontaneous mutations or the acquisition of genetic material through horizontal gene transfer between microbes. Spontaneous mutations are promoted by the rapid cell cycle of bacterial growth, and horizontal gene transfer is promoted by *plasmids*—small, circular DNA elements that are replicated during bacterial binary fission and can move from one dividing cell to nearby cells.

Mechanisms of drug resistance depend on the type of organism and are well documented for a variety of bacterial species. Pathogens can develop or acquire genes encoding enzymes that directly alter an antibiotic. A well-known example is the production of β-lactamases by various gram-negative bacteria. These enzymes hydrolyze β-lactam antibiotics such as penicillins and some cephalosporins, rendering them ineffective. Mutations in antibiotic targets can also occur, such as the modification of penicillin-binding proteins (PBPs)—the cell wall–synthesizing enzymes targeted by β-lactam antibiotics. Antibiotic entry into bacteria can also be blocked, as many antimicrobials have intracellular targets and must penetrate the bacterial wall and membrane to exert their effects. Porins, for example, are protein channels that limit entry into bacterial cells. Changes in the number, type, or function of porins may lead to antibiotic resistance. Efflux pumps, which pump molecules out of bacteria, are another mechanism of antibiotic resistance.[11]

WHO has developed a Global Action Plan to combat antimicrobial resistance that includes a Global Antimicrobial Resistance Surveillance System (GLASS) tracking eight priority bacteria in samples of blood, urine, stool, and genital swabs:

1. *E. coli*
2. *Klebsiella pneumoniae*
3. *Acinetobacter* spp.
4. *S. aureus*
5. *S. pneumoniae*
6. *Salmonella* spp.
7. *Shigella* spp.
8. *N. gonorrhoeae*

An early implementation report indicates that many countries are participating in data collection and that trends will be able to be tracked using this system.[12]

The CDC has also identified antimicrobial resistance as a public health threat, reporting that there are more than 2.8 million antibiotic-resistant infections each year in the United States, and that 35,000 deaths result from these infections.[13] Prioritization of the threat level of 18 pathogens is shown in **Table 5.4**.

Control of antibiotic resistance requires a multifaceted approach and the cooperation of many sectors. Individuals can optimize disease prevention through immunization, handwashing/general hygiene, and following medication directions. Health practitioners must take the responsibility for applying antimicrobial stewardship in prescribing (or not prescribing) antimicrobials, whereas researchers need to work to continually develop new medications and diagnostic tests and monitor epidemiological patterns. The agricultural sector must also maintain sound practices in the farming of plants and livestock. Finally, healthcare institutions and policy stakeholders should vigilantly regulate and monitor outcomes and adapt as needed.

ANTIMICROBIAL STEWARDSHIP

Antibiotic stewardship has been defined in a consensus statement by the Infectious Diseases Society of America (IDSA), the Society for Healthcare Epidemiology of America (SHEA), and the Pediatric Infectious Diseases Society (PIDS) as "coordinated interventions designed to improve and measure the

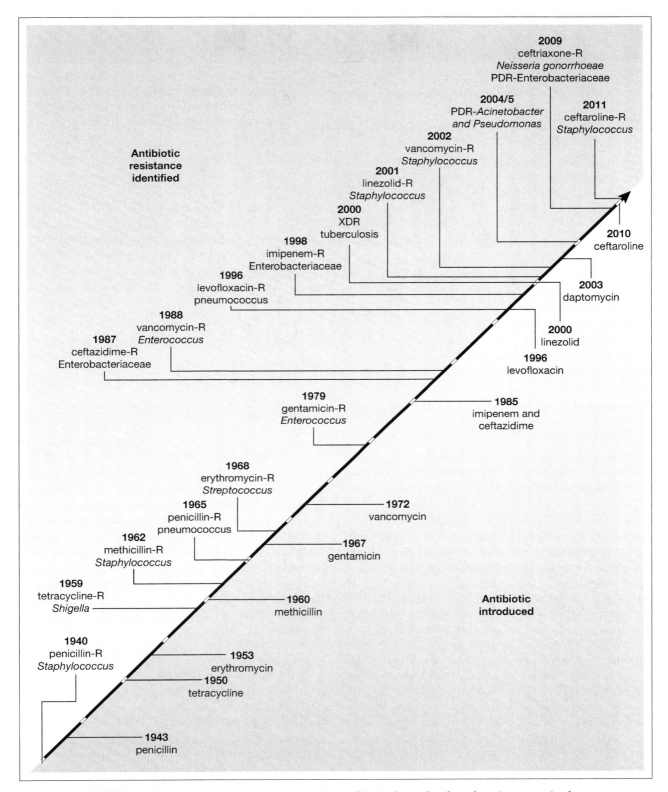

FIGURE 5.8 Timeline of antibiotic resistance. As antibiotics have developed, resistant strains have also been identified, some within just a few years of development.

PDR, pan-drug resistant; R, resistant; XDR, extensively drug resistant.

Note: Authoritative sources state that methicillin was introduced in 1959 and resistance was identified in 1960, within the first year of the drug's use.

Source: From the Centers for Disease Control and Prevention. https://www.cdc.gov/drugresistance/threat-report-2013/pdf/ar-threats-2013-508.pdf

TABLE 5.4 CDC-Identified Threats From Antimicrobial-Resistant Pathogens

Threat Level	Species
Urgent	Carbapenem-resistant *Acinetobacter*
	Candida auris
	Clostridioides difficile (formerly known as *Clostridium difficile*)
	CRE
	Drug-resistant *Neisseria gonorrhoeae*
Serious	Drug-resistant *Campylobacter*
	Drug-resistant *Candida*
	Extended-spectrum, β-lactamase-producing Enterobacteriaceae
	VRE
	Multidrug-resistant *Pseudomonas aeruginosa*
	Drug-resistant non typhoidal *Salmonella*
	Drug-resistant *Salmonella* serotype *typhi*
	Drug-resistant *Shigella*
	MRSA
	Drug-resistant *Streptococcus pneumoniae*
	Drug-resistant *tuberculosis*
Concerning	Erythromycin-resistant group A *Streptococcus*
	Clindamycin-resistant group B *Streptococcus*

CDC, Centers for Disease Control and Prevention; CRE, carbapenem-resistant Enterobacteriaceae; MRSA, methicillin-resistant *Staphylococcus aureus*; VRE, vancomycin-resistant *Enterococcus*; VRSA, vancomycin-resistant *Staphylococcus aureus*.
Source: From Centers for Disease Control and Prevention. 2019 AR Threats Report. Atlanta, GA: U.S. Department of Health and Human Services; 2019.

appropriate use of antimicrobial agents by promoting the selection of the optimal [antibiotic] drug regimen including dosing, duration of therapy, and route of administration."[14] The significant public health threat posed by rising antimicrobial resistance rates led to the development of the National Action Plan for Combating Antibiotic-Resistant Bacteria, driven by the White House and released in March 2015, and intended to serve as a guide to addressing this challenge both domestically and internationally. Part of the National Action Plan called for the establishment of antibiotic stewardship plans in all acute care hospitals and improved stewardship across all healthcare settings.[15] Various strategies in the design and implementation (i.e., policy development, auditing, monitoring/feedback) of these programs should be tailored to the needs, population, structure, and resources of individual institutions. A guideline on the implementation of antibiotic stewardship programs is available from the IDSA and SHEA.[16] The CDC recommends these seven core elements for hospital antibiotic stewardship programs: leadership commitment, accountability, drug expertise, action, tracking, reporting, and education.[17]

Thought Question

6. What options does the clinician have for ordering laboratory pathogen identification in a patient suspected of having an infection? How might these options differ between bacterial and viral infections?

PATHOGENESIS OF SELECTED MICROBES

This section highlights pathogenic mechanisms of selected well-studied disease-causing microbes to illustrate the basic principles of the microbial classes outlined earlier. Clinical textbooks and textbooks of microbiology and infectious diseases are the acknowledged resources for in-depth discussions of major infectious diseases.

Streptococcus pyogenes

S. pyogenes, a gram-positive, group A β-hemolytic streptococcus (GABHS), is the most common cause of **bacterial pharyngitis** and also causes serious skin infections. Although 90% of pharyngitis cases are caused by viruses (including rhinovirus, adenovirus, influenza virus), streptococcal pharyngitis is significant in that it must be treated with antibiotics, whereas **viral pharyngitis** is not responsive to antibiotic treatment. Streptococcal pharyngitis is more common in children than in adults, and children are often asymptomatic carriers of the organism. Those with active infections are most likely to transmit the disorder via aerosolized droplets. If untreated, *S. pyogenes* infections can provoke an autoimmune response against cardiac muscle and valves, resulting in **rheumatic heart disease**. Autoimmune attack against the renal glomeruli can result in **poststreptococcal glomerulonephritis**.[18] Skin infections with *S. pyogenes* can lead to **cellulitis** or **necrotizing fasciitis**.

S. pyogenes can be found in normal flora of the skin and mucous membranes. It has an outer capsule that assists with immune evasion, and it is able to invade epithelial cells, which also provides protection from phagocytosis by neutrophils and macrophages (**Figure 5.9**). Among other virulence factors, the fimbriae of the cell wall contain an M protein that binds fibrinogen and blocks complement fixation to the bacterial surface—another strategy of immune evasion. M protein serotyping is one method of pathogen characterization. *S. pyogenes* also produces exotoxins, among them streptolysin S, which is capable of lysing red blood cells and other tissue cells as the infection spreads through tissues. Group

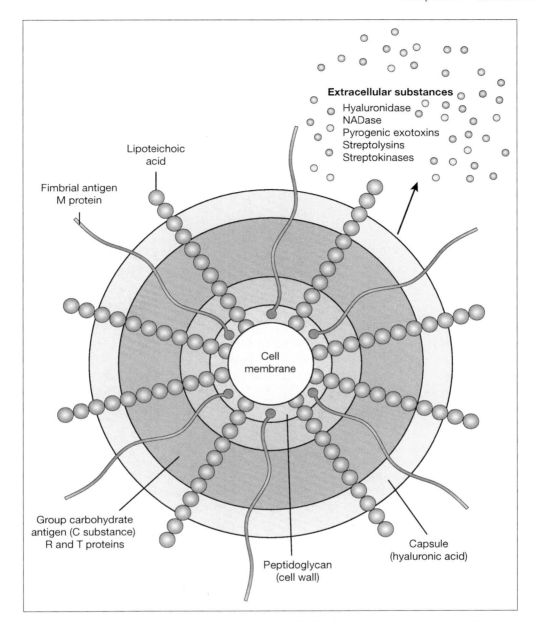

FIGURE 5.9 Schematic of *Streptococcus pyogenes*. The hyaluronic capsule assists with immune evasion, whereas virulence factors include the M protein of fimbriae, lipoteichoic acid, and secreted substances that assist with invasion, cell lysis and tissue damage, and fever.
NADase, nicotinamide adenine dinucleotide nucleosidase.

A streptococcal infections are associated with high fevers due to pyrogenic factors secreted by the bacteria. The organisms can also be transmitted by skin-to-skin contact (skin infections). Pathogen identification is by a rapid antigen detection test and throat culture. The CDC notes that there are no examples of group A streptococci resistant to penicillin, which is the drug of choice for patients who are not allergic to penicillin.[19]

METHICILLIN-RESISTANT *Staphylococcus aureus*

S. aureus is a gram-positive, facultative anaerobic, extracellular pyogenic bacterium that is of intense interest to researchers as the most virulent of the staphylococcal species. *S. aureus* has specific fibronectin-binding proteins that recognize the amino acid sequence arginine–glycine–aspartate in fibronectin, allowing the bacteria to bind closely to cells (**Figure 5.10**).

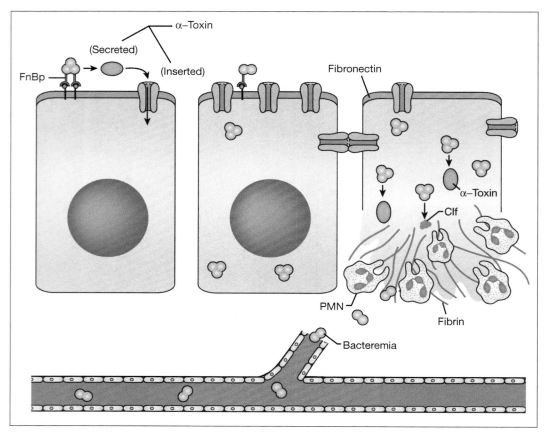

FIGURE 5.10 Cellular mechanisms of *Staphylococcus* pathology. *Staphylococcus* FnBPs mediate cellular attachment, whereas secreted α-toxin forms pores in host cells, ultimately destroying them. Clfs contribute to aggregate formation, and fibrinogen conversion to fibrin is promoted, leading to a walling-off process that can contribute to boil formation.

Clf, clumping factor; FnBP, fibronectin-binding protein; PMN, polymorphonuclear leukocyte.

Infection with *S. aureus* produces inflammation with infiltration of polymorphonuclear leukocytes, macrophages, and fibroblasts, and the infected region can become walled off by fibrin and collagen deposition, sometimes forming a painful boil. *S. aureus* produces a pore-forming α-toxin that destroys host cells, as well as several exotoxins, including a toxic shock syndrome toxin. Some strains produce a Panton–Valentine leukocidin that destroys neutrophils and platelets. The *S. aureus* genome encodes several proteins that neutralize neutrophil lysosomal degradative enzymes and reactive oxygen species and is thus able to evade destruction after being phagocytosed by neutrophils.

In 1952, it was noted that penicillin and other antibiotics were unsuccessful in treating some *S. aureus* infections, and methicillin was introduced in 1959 in the hope that it could treat these resistant strains. Methicillin-resistant *S. aureus* (MRSA) produces an altered PBP, PBP2a, which makes the bacteria unresponsive to penicillin and other β-lactam-containing antibiotics, such as nafcillin, oxacillin, and cefazolin. Resistant strains have

an *mecA* gene, referred to as the staphylococcal cassette chromosome (SCC) gene. The SCC encodes different enzymes capable of excision and insertion of the *mecA* gene into other staphylococcal strains, contributing to the spread of resistance among numerous strains. Resistance to β-lactam antibiotics has increased over the past 20 years, and the incidence of methycillin-resistant *S. aureus* has grown in epidemic proportions globally.

Staphylococcal infections are usually diagnosed by Gram stain, microscopic examination of purulent contents from infected tissue, and NAAT. MRSA infections can be acquired in healthcare facilities, and many healthcare providers are carriers of MRSA, commonly having colonization of the skin and nares. Incidence of community-acquired MRSA is also growing, often in conditions of crowding and athletic facilities in schools. Many cultures are found to be sensitive to trimethoprim/sulfamethoxazole, which is often a first-line treatment in addition to incision and drainage of a boil. Other effective oral options include doxycycline and clindamycin.

Mycobacterium tuberculosis

Historically, **Mycobacterium tuberculosis infection** (TB) has been one of the most feared infectious diseases known to humankind. It is caused by the bacterium MTB. Although most commonly associated with pulmonary infection, MTB may affect virtually every organ and may persist lifelong in its human host. Today, TB infects about one-third of the human population and remains among the leading infectious causes of death worldwide, with substantial geographic variation. The most recent WHO estimates identify MTB as the leading infectious cause of death globally, with 10 million new cases of TB and 1.6 million deaths from TB in 2017.[20]

MTB is one of several species belonging to the MTB complex. Although humans are the only known reservoir of MTB, other mycobacterial species exist that are associated with infections in other animal species. MTB is a nonmotile, non–spore-forming, aerobic bacterium that appears as a thin, straight, or slightly curved rod under microscopy, although variations in appearance may exist. Called tubercle bacilli, the bacteria have complex, waxy cell walls composed of peptidoglycans, polysaccharides, and mycolic acids that protect against host defenses and common antibiotics. The specialized lipid barrier also imparts resistance to decolorization by alcohol. Hence, as with other mycobacteria, MTB is not classified as gram positive or gram negative but is instead characterized by its acid-fastness. Acid-fast bacilli (AFB) smear microscopy is recommended in all patients suspected of having pulmonary TB and may be helpful for other specimens as well. Sputum culture remains the gold standard for diagnosis of pulmonary TB. NAAT may also be used to expedite results in conjunction with other diagnostic tests. Drug susceptibility testing using traditional culture and sensitivity approaches as well as NAAT is necessary to guide the selection of the appropriate therapy.

Differentiation of **TB infection** from **TB disease** is key to understanding its pathogenesis and management. Notably, most humans infected with MTB never actually develop TB disease; rather, the organism is completely cleared through immune responses, or is controlled as a latent infection. Primary TB disease is most likely found in young children, those who are immunosuppressed (there is a significant coinfection rate in people with HIV), and those who developed a later serious health issue, in which case a latent infection may reactivate. Reinfection can also occur in individuals who are repeatedly exposed to MTB and may lead to disease development.

MTB infections are caused by the inhalation of infectious particles, called droplet nuclei, spread via aerosols released when a person with pulmonary TB disease talks, coughs, or sneezes. The infectiousness or bacterial load of the source patient, closeness of physical contact, and frequency and duration of exposure(s) all impact the risk of inoculation of the exposed individual. A person with smear-positive TB disease is more likely to transmit the bacteria. Contacts who are immunosuppressed are also at heightened risk to acquire MTB. Despite these factors, overall, MTB is considered to be only moderately infectious.

Transmission occurs when an uninfected individual inhales the droplet nuclei, which then enter the respiratory tract. Many of the bacilli will be trapped and removed by airway mucociliary clearance, the cough reflex, and other immune protective mediators of the upper airways. However, tubercle bacilli that escape these early defenses may penetrate to the alveoli. This deposition triggers an influx of pulmonary macrophages, which phagocytose and destroy some of the bacilli. Other tubercle bacilli will begin to replicate within the alveolar macrophages. This is the point at which TB infection begins. Infection may subsequently progress to either latent TB infection or, less commonly, active TB disease.

Early spread of the MTB to other lung areas and other tissues is via the lymphatics. In addition to the lungs, the kidneys, long bones, spine, and meninges are sites where TB organisms can multiply. Over the next several weeks, the macrophages induce a cascade of additional immune mediators, such as cytokines and tumor necrosis factor, and then ultimately present TB antigen to T lymphocytes, initiating the adaptive immune response. The bacilli are able to evade complete eradication through several protective mechanisms, including the secretion of enzymes and antioxidants that allow survival despite macrophage ingestion. The accumulation of macrophages and T cells creates a granuloma that surrounds the tubercle bacilli[21] (**Box 5.3** and **Figure 5.11**). Although the granuloma serves to limit bacterial replication and spread, it also allows the bacteria to persist, as latent TB infection, within the host. Within the granuloma, the oxygen becomes depleted, reducing bacterial cell division rates, but not eradicating the bacteria. The granuloma shell may break down over time, allowing the infectious particles to escape, multiply, and lead to TB disease, with the common presentation of fever, night sweats, weakness, anorexia, and weight loss, with later development of cough.

In immunocompetent individuals, there is an average 10% lifetime risk of developing TB. The risk is higher within the first 1 to 2 years following infection. The risk is also higher in young patients (infants to young adults) and in the elderly but may also vary according to bacterial inoculum. Immunocompromised patients face the greatest risk. Individuals with uncontrolled HIV coinfection have an estimated annual risk of up to 10%. Tumor necrosis factor–inhibiting drugs used for autoimmune diseases reduce the effectiveness of innate immune responses and also increase the risk of TB disease progression.

A chest x-ray showing areas of infiltration and cavity formation may be the first indication of TB infection.

BOX 5.3
Steps in Tuberculosis Infection

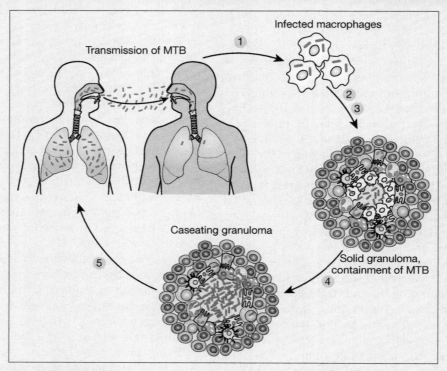

FIGURE 5.11 Stages in *Mycobacterium tuberculosis* infection.

1. Droplets containing MTB bacilli are inhaled and deposit in alveoli, where they are engulfed by alveolar macrophages.

2. Macrophage activation leads to cytokine release, attracting additional immune cells, including T and B lymphocytes, natural killer cells, and neutrophils.

3. A solid granuloma forms around the core of infected macrophages, foam cells, giant cells, epithelioid macrophages, and dendritic cells, surrounded by lymphocytes, neutrophils, and natural killer cells.

4. Macrophage death leads to transition of the solid granuloma to a caseating granuloma with a liquefying center.

5. From this stage, the granuloma may ultimately collapse, releasing the bacilli into the circulation and perpetuating spread of the infection.

MTB, *Mycobacterium tuberculosis.*

In high-resource settings, NAAT is currently used for diagnosing TB and identifying pharmacological susceptibility. In other regions, sputum smear for acid-fast staining and microscopy is commonly used. Culture can be done, but the slow division rate of the bacteria requires at least 2 to 3 weeks of incubation.

Screening for latent TB infection can be done by tuberculin skin testing or the interferon-γ release assay. The establishment of cell-mediated immunity marks the stage by which a tuberculin skin test will become positive. Alternatively, interferon-γ release assays measure the amount of interferon released when white blood cells isolated from the person being screened are exposed to TB antigens. This test has relatively strict requirements for correct performance, but has the advantages of being useful in patients who have previously received treatment with bacille Calmette-Guérin (bCG), as well as not requiring a follow-up appointment to assess the result of the tuberculin skin test.

TB treatment relies on a separate class of antibiotics that are able to penetrate cells and specifically target mycobacteria. Among these, isoniazid, rifampin, ethambutol, and pyrazinamide are often used in combination, and treatment must be prolonged to eradicate the slow-growing mycobacteria. MTB strains readily develop resistance, and early regimens that relied heavily on isoniazid fostered development of strains with resistance to that drug (monoresistance). Multidrug-resistant TB is becoming more common and is characterized by resistance to (at least) isoniazid and rifampin. Extremely drug-resistant TB strains add resistance to fluoroquinolone and at least one second-line drug. Obviously, treatment becomes much more difficult in cases of extreme drug resistance.

Chlamydia trachomatis

C. trachomatis is an obligate intracellular bacterium with a gram-negative–like cell wall that causes the most common sexually transmitted infection in the United States, as well as being a significant cause of blindness in low-resource countries.[22] *C. trachomatis* targets the squamous and columnar epithelial cells of the endocervix and upper genital tract of women and the urethra, rectum, and conjunctivae of men and women. Because of its small genome, the organism has a limited enzyme repertoire and relies on host cells to provide energy and aid in its multiplication. Throughout its life cycle, the bacterium alternates between two forms. Extracellularly, *Chlamydia* exists as infectious *elementary bodies* able to enter host cells. Within several hours of cellular entry, the elementary body converts into a noninfectious *reticulate body* that specializes in nutrient acquisition and replication via binary fission (**Box 5.4** and **Figure 5.12**). The reticulate bodies revert to elementary bodies in an asynchronous manner for release and spread, generally resulting in the death of the host cell.[22]

BOX 5.4
Steps in Chlamydial Infection

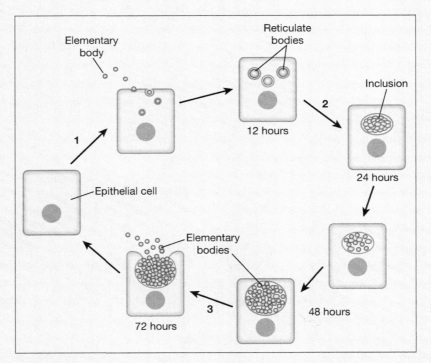

FIGURE 5.12 *Chlamydia trachomatis* life cycle.

1. Exposure to the *Chlamydia* elementary body can occur by sexual transmission or vertical transfer (mother to neonate).

2. Upon entering genitourinary epithelial cells, the bacterium enlarges and transforms to a reticulate body capable of binary fission and rapid enlargement.

3. Within a few days, the reticulate bodies revert to elementary body form and burst out, lysing the cell and spreading infection.

Damage to the epithelial cells induces the secretion of numerous proinflammatory chemokines and cytokines. This results in vasodilation, increased endothelial permeability, and activation of lymphocytes. Antibodies against the chlamydial major outer membrane protein (MOMP) are a component of the protective host immune response. However, antibodies to other proteins, such as the chlamydial 60-kDa heat shock proteins 60 and 10 (cHSP60 and cHSP10), exert both a protective effect and a pathological effect. When released extracellularly, cHSP60 induces a local proinflammatory immune response in fallopian tube epithelial cells. In as many as 70% of primary genital tract infections due to *C. trachomatis*, the immune response is sufficient to clear the pathogen.

In men, **chlamydial infection** initially causes urethritis, but if untreated, it can lead to epididymitis and proctitis. In women, an initial infection can cause cervicitis, urethritis, or endometritis. If infection progresses to the female upper genital tract, pelvic inflammatory disease can develop, causing chronic pain, tubal occlusion, and infertility. Chlamydial infection also has an associated risk of cervical carcinoma. NAAT of urine samples is currently the test of choice for pathogen identification. CDC guidelines recommend treatment with azithromycin and doxycycline. For complicated infections involving the female upper genital tract and pelvic inflammatory disease, hospitalization for prolonged parenteral antibiotic treatment (2 weeks) may be required.[23]

Neisseria gonorrhoeae

Gonorrhea is caused by the bacteria *N. gonorrhoeae*, for which humans are the only natural host. *Neisseria* organisms are gram-negative, nonmotile, non–spore-forming bacteria that often are paired as diplococci with a "dumbbell-like" shape (see **Figure 5.13**). They may grow in aerobic or anaerobic conditions. *N. gonorrhoeae* is well known for its ability to rapidly change its surface structures, such as pili, lipooligosaccharides, and various membrane proteins, to avoid host defenses. *N. gonorrhoeae* coinfection with *Chlamydia* is common.

N. gonorrhoeae organisms most commonly infect the mucosal membranes of the genitourinary tract, but may also infect the eye, throat, and rectum. More specifically, the urethra and cervix are the most common initial infection sites in men and women, respectively. Transmission primarily occurs through sexual contact with an infected individual. There is a greater risk with vaginal intercourse than with anal or oral intercourse. The risk of male-to-female transmission is higher than for transmission from female to male, possibly secondary to host anatomical differences. Vertical transmission can also occur from mother to child during delivery. Dissemination of the pathogen can also lead to arthritis, endocarditis, and meningitis.

The host–pathogen interaction at the epithelial surface is key to the pathogenesis of *N. gonorrhoeae*. Several structural components specifically contribute to its virulence. On the surface of the organism, pili (see **Figure 5.13**) serve to facilitate motility and attachment to host epithelial cells. Opacity-associated bacterial surface adhesion proteins promote adherence between bacterial cells and entry into the host cells. After crossing the epithelial barrier, neutrophils are intensely attracted to the area and phagocytose numerous bacteria. Once inside the neutrophil phagolysosome, *N. gonorrhoeae* bacteria evade killing by enzymes that neutralize neutrophil-reactive oxygen species. Thus, like *Chlamydia*, *N. gonorrhoeae* organisms are primarily intracellular pathogens. A membrane endotoxin-like molecule, lipooligosaccharide, contributes to inhibition of neutrophils, cytokine activation, and host inflammatory response.[24]

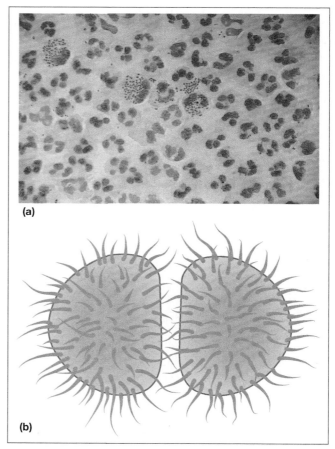

(a)

(b)

FIGURE 5.13 (a) *Neisseria gonorrhoeae* urethritis. Neutrophils in the affected region have phagocytosed many bacteria, others are seen in the extracellular fluid. *N. gonorrhoeae* evade destruction by producing enzymes which neutralize neutrophil reactive oxygen species. **(b)** *N. gonorrhoeae* is a diplococcus with long pili projecting from the cell wall. The pili facilitate initial attachment to mucosal surfaces and movement along and within tissue layers.
Source: (a) Courtesy of Joe Millar/Centers for Disease Control and Prevention Public Health Image Library (PHIL).

In men, *N. gonorrhoeae* infection typically presents as an acute urethritis with symptoms beginning 2 to 7 days after infection.[25] Purulent urethral discharge is common, owing to the combination of the neutrophil response and epithelial cell shedding. An incubation period likely precedes the onset of symptoms. Gonococci have been located within both neutrophils and urethral epithelial cells. It has been proposed that the urethral epithelial cells house and protect the bacteria during early infection. The subsequent release of chemokines, cytokines, and tumor necrosis factor-α from the epithelial cells may then initiate an inflammatory response by triggering the neutrophil influx. The bacteria are released as the epithelial cells are shed from the mucosal surface into the urethral lumen. The cascade would thereby cause the clinical urethritis symptoms, which continues in a cyclical fashion as the infection extends until adequately treated.[25] Gonococcal interaction with the neutrophils may serve to further modulate the efficacy of the host immune response.

In women, the initial exposure occurs at the cervix. However, in contrast to the significant inflammatory response that usually accompanies infection of the male urethra, up to 80% of women with lower genital tract infections are asymptomatic. This finding is further supported by studies that demonstrate a lack of antibody immune response to *N. gonorrhoeae* in cervical secretions. Gonococcal invasion can subsequently ascend to the female upper genital tract through a combination of mechanisms, including twitching motility, additional virulence factors, and the organism's ability to take advantage of hormonal changes of the genital tract.[26] Adhesion to the ciliated cells of the fallopian tubes induces cellular shedding due to various cytotoxic effects. If left untreated, infection that advances to the upper genital tract can cause **pelvic inflammatory disease**, a leading cause of infertility and ectopic pregnancy. The CDC recommends urine testing with NAAT for both *Chlamydia* and *N. gonorrhoeae*, as the rate of coinfection is high.

Clostridioides difficile

C. difficile (formerly known as *Clostridium difficile*) is a gram-positive, rod-shaped, anaerobic bacterium. Its ability to form spores allows the pathogen to survive in unfavorable environmental conditions and facilitates human-to-human transmission. Although many *C. difficile* strains exist, only toxin-producing strains cause disease. **C. difficile infection** (CDI) may encompass varying degrees of severity, from mild diarrhea to pseudomembranous colitis and death. It remains both a significant community-acquired and nosocomial threat. Specifically, it is the leading cause of infectious diarrhea in healthcare settings and the most common hospital-acquired infection.[27]

The formal definition of CDI is based on both clinical and laboratory findings, including the presence of diarrhea (defined as three or more unformed stools in 24 consecutive hours) and a stool test positive for the presence of toxigenic *C. difficile*, its toxins, or colonoscopic or histopathologic findings consistent with pseudomembranous colitis.[28] Diarrhea is typically watery, though it may be associated with mucus or occult blood. Associated symptoms may include fever, cramping, and abdominal pain. Leukocytosis may be present, and it is recommended that CDI be considered in the differential diagnosis of hospitalized patients with unexplained leukocytosis. The most severe complications of CDI may include hypotension, shock, toxic megacolon, intestinal perforation, and acute peritonitis.

It is useful in this context to review the host response mechanisms to pathogenic intestinal bacteria in a person with normal gut function and microbiota (**Figure 5.14**). Factors that resist pathogen infection include the following:

- The normal colon colony of microorganisms, which obtain nutrients and secrete inhibiting factors that reduce the growth of newly arrived bacteria
- Commensal bacteria that produce bacteriocins—microbially produced toxins to other bacterial species
- Certain bile acids that promote *C. difficile* spore formation
- Host IgG and IgA against toxin A, which reduces its toxicity

On the other hand, the following factors promote pathogen infection:

- Antibiotic treatment, particularly with broad-spectrum antibiotics that deplete the normal microbiota
- Proton pump inhibitors, as gastric acid secretion may suppress CDI
- Hospitalization or nursing home environments
- Older age—older adults are more likely to be colonized by *C. difficile*, and CDI is generally more severe in this population
- *C. difficile* ingestion from contaminated food

The pathogenesis of *C. difficile* diarrhea can be differentiated into three phases. The first process, a hallmark of antibiotic-associated diarrhea in general, is the disruption of the normal, protective intestinal flora, or microbiota, in a given individual. This function has been termed *colonization resistance*, and it is lost as a direct consequence of antibiotic use. Although almost all antibiotics have been implicated in CDI, the association is greatest among the third- and fourth-generation cephalosporins, fluoroquinolones, carbapenems, and clindamycin.

Host acquisition of *C. difficile* is likely to occur through the ingestion of spores spread through the fecal–oral route or direct exposure to a contaminated source. During environmental stress, the anaerobe transitions

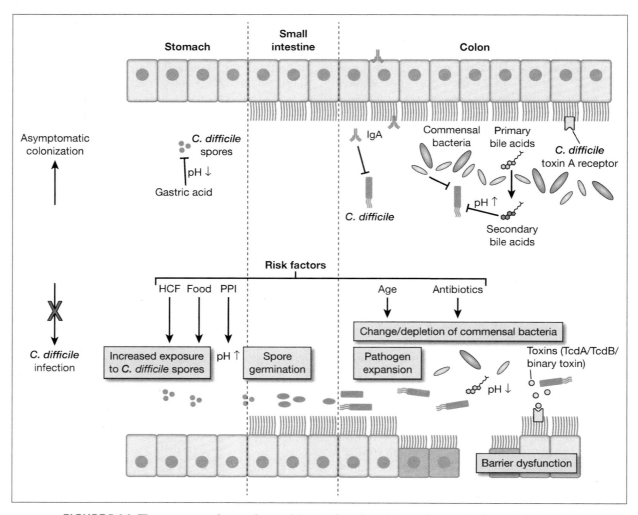

FIGURE 5.14 The presence of normal microbiota and gut function tends to resist the transformation of *Clostridioides difficile* colonization to infection and diarrhea (*top*), by mechanisms described in the text. Inhibition or loss of these mechanisms, by proton pump inhibitors that reduce gastric acid secretion, or changes in microbiota due to aging or antibiotic use, can initiate the transition from the spore colonization state to the active expansion state of the *C. difficile* bacteria. This results in infection and diarrhea production.

HCF, healthcare facility; IgA, immunoglobulin A; PPI, proton pump inhibitor; TcdA, TcdB, *C. difficile* toxin A and B.

to its spore form. In preparation, the cell divides into a smaller component, the forespore, which develops the spore, and a larger component, the mother cell, which prepares for dormancy. The spore is encased in three protective and specialized layers for which mutations in specific proteins have been shown to affect virulence.[29] This robust form is stable to oxygen stress and resists traditional killing methods, such as heat and alcohol-based sanitizers, allowing survival in the environment for extended periods of time. Spores that have been spread to food, objects, or surfaces, often because of incomplete disinfection, may then be ingested by the host.

Upon ingestion by a host with disrupted flora, *C. difficile* can successfully colonize the large intestine,

where it thrives owing to the gut conditions (**Figure 5.14**). Intestinal acids promote germination, and the anoxic environment supports growth and replication of the organism. This complex process is thought to involve more than 500 genes. Once the pathogen is established, it begins to produce the toxins TcdA and TcdB, which wreak havoc on the mucosal epithelial cells. The toxins, characterized as the greatest virulence factors of the pathogen, are taken up by the cells through receptor-mediated endocytosis. Following cleavage, the active subunit is transferred to the host cell cytosol, where it glycosylates cytoskeletal regulatory proteins called guanosine triphosphatases. This action effectively disrupts the cytoskeleton, causing dissociation of the tight junctions between cells and increased cell permeability, ultimately leading to apoptosis and cell death.[30]

The final phase of *C. difficile* pathogenesis involves the host response to infection. Damage to the host mucosal epithelium, as well as the subsequent translocation of gut bacteria into deeper tissues, initiates a rapid and profound host immune response. The release of cytokines and chemokines recruits innate and adaptive immune cells. Neutrophils are of importance in the early host defense and bacterial killing. Although this response is necessary for infection control, the inflammatory process further adds to the epithelial damage.[29] In fact, the diarrhea burden of CDI has been correlated with the degree of intestinal inflammation and not pathogen burden.[31]

Unfortunately, recurrence is common in patients with CDI and is usually seen within 1 to 3 weeks after completion of therapy. Recurrence occurs in up to 25% of patients after the initial episode and rises dramatically with subsequent episodes. The mechanisms of recurrent disease are thought to be unique to the initial pathology, although they are not fully established. The diversity of the host microbiota, the specific infecting *C. difficile* strain(s), the initial host immune response, and CDI treatment itself are some of the proposed factors that influence the risk of disease recurrence.[30] Specifically, the North American pulsed-field type 1, ribotype 027 (NAP1/BI/027) strain has been identified as a hypervirulent strain linked with fluoroquinolone resistance and associated with increased incidence, symptom severity, and mortality.[32]

Pathogen identification involves testing for the organism itself or for toxin production, utilizing NAAT, glutamate dehydrogenase immunoassays, toxigenic culture, cytotoxicity neutralization assay, or enzyme immunoassays for toxins. If a single test is performed, use of NAAT is preferred because of its sensitivity.[30]

Borrelia burgdorferi

B. burgdorferi, the organism that causes **Lyme disease**, is a gram-negative spirochete bacterium with a unique cellular membrane that differentiates it from most other gram-negative organisms. It is a motile parasite whose transmission relies on the complex 2-year life cycle of the *Ixodes* tick, as well as the ability to move between tissues of the host (**Box 5.5** and **Figure 5.15**). The bacterial DNA is composed of both linear chromosomes and many plasmids that are important for adaptation to various host species. Expression of surface proteins varies depending on tick life cycle stage and host species.

The eggs of the *Ixodes* tick (*Ixodes scapularis* in much of the United States) hatch in the spring, resulting in uninfected larvae. Initial transmission of *B. burgdorferi* occurs during the larval feeding, when a tick engorges on an infected animal (usually a white-footed mouse).

The bacteria enter the gut of the tick and remain there until the next blood meal. A fraction of the spirochetes will exit the tick gut, migrate to the salivary glands, and await transfer to the new host. Once the ticks molt into their nymph stage, they feed on additional animal hosts, including mice, deer, and humans, who thereby become new infectious reservoirs. An additional blood feeding that can transmit the disease usually occurs in the life cycle of an adult female tick, which then deposits eggs, beginning the cycle anew. Because of their smaller size, the nymphs are difficult to detect and may have a greater likelihood of completing the blood meal, which must last a few days to complete transmission of the slowly growing spirochetes. For this reason, it is important that potential exposures (hiking in the woods) be followed up immediately by inspection for ticks—if the tick is removed rapidly, it is unlikely that disease will occur.

Lyme disease may be diagnosed based on symptoms, physical examination, and possible tick exposure history. The classic cutaneous sign of erythema migrans, a gradually enlarging "bull's-eye" rash, may or may not be present, so documentation of potential exposures and symptom development is important. Migration of the spirochete to the heart, joints, and nervous system leads to clinical complaints of malaise, headache, musculoskeletal pain, fever, and lymphadenopathy. Severe but rare neurological complications include meningitis and cranial and peripheral neuropathies.[33] Lyme disease can also cause **Lyme carditis**, which often presents with atrioventricular block and may have other cardiac findings such as myocarditis and left ventricular dysfunction.[34] The CDC recommends a two-step lab testing process.[35] In the first step, an enzyme immunoassay (or rarely an immunofluorescence assay) is performed. If it is positive, no further testing is required. If it is negative or the result is inconclusive, a Western blot is performed. Repeat testing may be needed due to slow development of immunoreactivity. Prompt antibiotic treatment usually is successful in treating the infection, although some patients have prolonged symptoms and may require additional treatment. Individuals may spontaneously clear the bacterial infection, but in some cases late manifestations, including arthritis, appear months after the initial infection.[36]

INFLUENZA VIRUS

Influenza (flu) is a contagious respiratory illness that has an impact at the global level each year. The responsible pathogens—differing strains of influenza virus—are enveloped, negative-strand RNA viruses that belong to the family Orthomyxoviridae (**Figure 5.16**). Influenza A, B, and C viruses are all capable of infecting humans; however, influenza A viruses are the best characterized and are the most common cause of epidemics and pandemics. Influenza A envelopes contain prominent spike hemagglutinin (HA) and neuraminidase (NA) proteins used to characterize the strains by the

BOX 5.5
Life Cycle of the *Ixodes* Tick

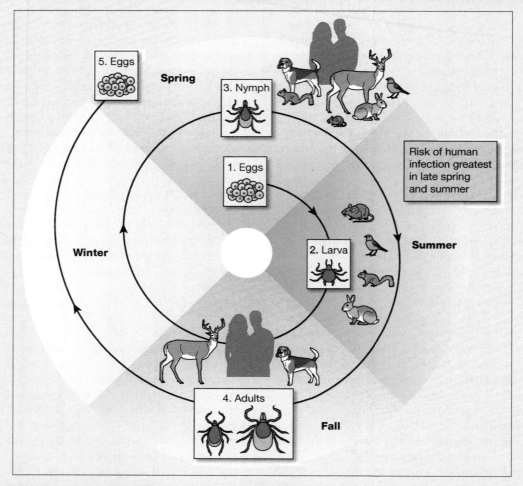

FIGURE 5.15 *Borrelia burgdorferi* transmission via the *Ixodes* tick.

1. Eggs of the female *Ixodes* tick are deposited in the spring, hatch, and become larvae.

2. Larvae obtain their first blood meal—the first exposure that may result in *Borrelia* ingestion.

3. Developing to the nymph phase, the spirochetes move to the *Ixodes* salivary glands and can be transmitted to a mouse, deer, or human host when the tick attaches and begins to feed.

4. Adult female ticks consume an additional blood meal through which they can infect an additional large animal host (e.g., deer, dog, or human).

5. Following the blood meal, the female tick deposits eggs and dies.

Thus, *Ixodes* ticks rely on three critical episodes of blood feeding, during which transmission of *Borrelia* to the host can occur, resulting in creation of new infectious reservoirs.

H/N system (**Figure 5.16a**). Development of an annual vaccine requires selection of strains to be inoculated against, with varying degrees of efficacy in each flu season. Prior infection with one strain does not confer protection against infection with other strains.

As with all viruses, after entering the body (via the respiratory tract and inhalation of aerosolized particles from someone with the infection, or by contact with contaminated surfaces) the influenza virus begins its life cycle with attachment to host cells. HA is the

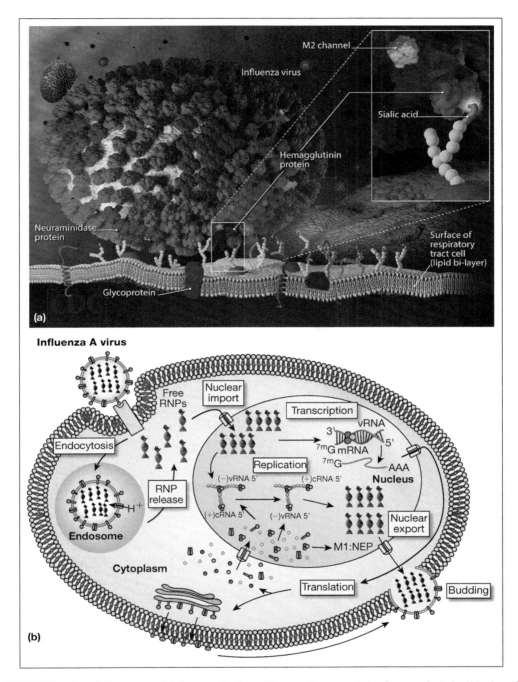

FIGURE 5.16 **(a)** Features of influenza A virus. The envelope proteins hemagglutinin (*blue*) and neuraminidase (*red*), and the M2 ion channel, play functional roles in the viral life cycle of host cell infection. **(b)** Influenza virus life cycle. As with other viruses, influenza A virus attaches to the host cell, in this case, via the hemagglutinin protein attachment to host cell sialic acid. Entry into the cell by endocytosis is followed by uncoating and movement of viral RNA strands to the nucleus for copying into the plus strand RNA that codes for viral protein production and also provides the template for minus strand RNA production to contribute to new virion assembly.

cRNA, complementary RNA; mRNA, messenger RNA; NEP, nuclear export protein; RNP, ribonucleoprotein; vRNA, viral RNA.

Source: (a) From Centers for Disease Control and Prevention. Influenza (flu). https://www.cdc.gov/flu/resource-center/freeresources/graphics/images.htm.

surface protein that binds to sialic residues on host airway epithelial cells (**Figure 5.16b**). Binding is followed by endocytosis and entry of the virus into an endosome. Once in the endosome, the viral membrane M2 channel allows ion entry into the virion, favoring fusion of the viral membrane with the endosome membrane and viral uncoating. Viral RNA moves to the nucleus for transcription, producing mRNA for cytoplasmic viral protein synthesis and also for reproducing the viral genome. Viral nucleic acids and proteins are then packaged into new virions and acquire a membrane envelope by budding from the host cell.[37] NA assists with the membrane fusion and viral exit process. Infection with influenza virus leads to immune system activation and the death of many host cells, contributing to the signs and symptoms of flu infection. Coughing, chills, fever, malaise, headache, myalgias, and arthralgias are all the result of local immune activation and systemic responses to cytokine elevations, as well as the death of infected epithelial cells lining the airways.

Influenza A virus undergoes frequent genetic changes termed *antigenic drift* and *antigenic shift*, in part due to sharing of genes for the different HA proteins (1–18) and NA proteins (1–11). This variability is a contributing factor in the difficulty of flu vaccine production. Major epidemics have been associated with the H1N1 virus (1918 Spanish flu pandemic, 2009 flu pandemic). Other aggressive strains include H5N1 and H7N9.[38] The severity of the disease influenza depends, in part, on the particular strain responsible for the infection and also the strength of the host response—in some cases the host's immune response and cytokine storm precipitate critical illness and septic shock.

Clinical laboratory testing for influenza virus is not necessarily indicated, given the presentation of classic symptoms and knowledge of local prevalence patterns during flu season. If illness severity is sufficient to warrant hospital admission, testing may be useful. Both NAAT and immunoassay tests for influenza are available, including a rapid influenza diagnostic test. Clinical guidelines inform the choice of diagnostic tests for either outpatient or inpatient settings.

HUMAN IMMUNODEFICIENCY VIRUS

HIV, the pathogen that can cause **AIDS**, is a member of the Retroviridae group, lentivirus subdivision. Two forms exist, HIV-1 and HIV-2, of which HIV-1 is the most common in the United States and globally. The classification "retrovirus" refers to the property of an RNA virus having the enzyme *reverse transcriptase* that carries out transcription of DNA from an RNA template, the opposite function of the normal biological process of RNA transcription from a DNA template. The profound implication of retroviral transmission is the ability of these viruses to synthesize double-stranded DNA that can be integrated into the genome of the host cell, residing there permanently. As such, HIV causes a chronic/persistent type of viral infection that can be managed but not cured. To add to this complexity, HIV-infected cells can reside in a quiescent mode sequestered in immune tissues, particularly those of the gut-associated lymphoid tissue, in a state of resistance to antiviral therapies. Activation of viral replication is required for the antiviral medications to be effective.

BOX 5.6
Steps of the HIV Life Cycle

1. Virus attachment occurs when GP120 binds to target cells, primarily macrophages and CD4⁺ T-helper lymphocytes. The host cell membrane protein CD4 is the initial docking site for GP120, and this binding is complemented by binding to a co-receptor, either CCR5 or CXCR4.

2. The first stage of binding allows the transmembrane protein GP41 to bind to the host cell and draw the virion close to the target cell, initiating fusion and entry of the nucleocapsid into the host cell.

3. Uncoating releases the single-stranded viral RNA and enzyme reverse transcriptase.

4. The proviral nucleic acid is synthesized— double-stranded DNA coding for HIV proteins.

5. Proviral DNA is integrated into the host's chromosomal DNA by the viral *integrase* protein. Transcription of messenger RNA (mRNA) for viral proteins begins; additional transcription reproduces the viral RNA needed to produce daughter virions

6. Translation produces the viral pro-protein—a single transcript containing all of the required viral proteins as one long polypeptide strand.

7. Limited proteolysis by viral *protease* produces the proteins that will be packaged inside the virion, including reverse transcriptase, integrase, and protease. Additional translation produces GP120 and GP41 for insertion into the host cell membrane.

8. Budding gives the nucleocapsid a membrane coat that contains the appropriate glycoproteins.

BOX 5.6 (*continued*)
Steps of the HIV Life Cycle

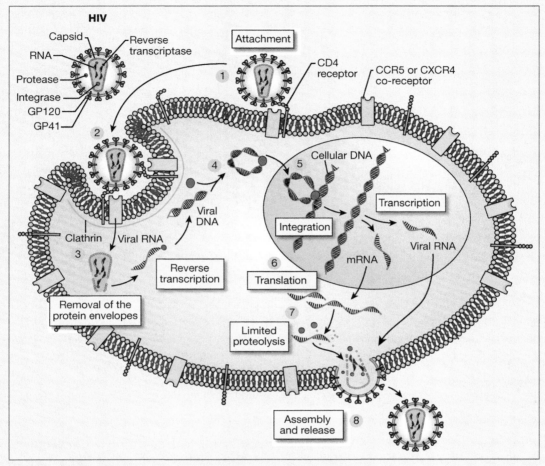

FIGURE 5.17 HIV life cycle.
mRNA, messenger RNA.

The functional anatomy of the HIV virion is that it is an enveloped virus with a nucleic acid core of RNA linked to the enzyme reverse transcriptase and surrounded by the protein capsid. The envelope membrane has many copies of the peripheral glycoprotein GP120, and the integral protein GP41. Mature HIV virions also contain the key proteins integrase and protease. **Box 5.6** and **Figure 5.17** depict the life cycle of the virus.

HIV transmission is by male–female or male–male sexual contact. Penile to vaginal or penile to anal transmission routes are both capable of transmission. In addition, transmission can occur from contaminated percutaneous equipment for drug injection, from needlesticks and other medical devices in healthcare settings, and from mother to child during vaginal delivery and breastfeeding. Overall, HIV transmission risk is very low to nonexistent from other routes such as inhaled aerosols, skin-to-skin

contact, and oral exposure. Transmission risk is heightened by the presence of mucosa breaks of involved genital and anal surfaces, and by coinfection with other diseases, including sexually transmitted diseases such as gonorrhea and chlamydia infection.

The time course of the infection is prolonged after an initial acute phase (**Figure 5.18**). After a 2- to 3-week incubation period, many individuals develop an acute flu-like illness lasting about 2 weeks. During this period, the virus is replicating rapidly and the number of CD4$^+$ T cells rapidly declines. As the host immune response begins, viral load (the measured number of circulating viral particles) decreases and the CD4 T-cell count recovers. During the subsequent chronic phase of the infection, CD4 T-cell numbers slowly decline at a rate that depends on individual factors and presence of coinfections.

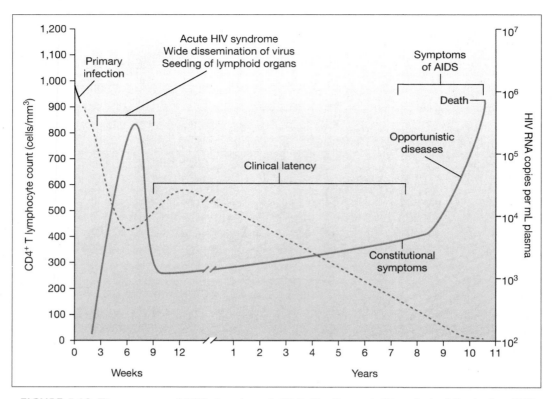

FIGURE 5.18 Time course of HIV viremia and CD4⁺ T-cell count (blue dashed line) after HIV infection. Within weeks of primary infection there is a dramatic rise in viral load (red line) and substantial drop in CD4⁺ T lymphocyte numbers. This is followed by recovery in T lymphocyte population and drop in viral copies that may last for years. In the absence of treatment, viral load gradually increases and lymphocyte numbers gradually drop until a critical level is achieved in which symptoms and opportunistic diseases occur, resulting in death due to AIDS.

As the CD4⁺ T-helper cells are the primary stimulators of both humoral and cell-mediated immunity, their loss represents a serious compromise to the host defense system. Ultimately, the CD4 T-lymphocyte numbers are sufficiently depleted and the host immune response is sufficiently suppressed to begin to allow characteristic opportunistic infections that are used to define AIDS (**Box 5.7**).[39] The duration of latency after HIV infection has been greatly prolonged in resource-rich countries by greater availability of antiretroviral therapy, and efforts have been made to make this therapy more widely available to people in moderate- and low-resource countries.[40]

The primary laboratory-based screening test for HIV is an immune-based test able to detect the HIV p24 antigen and antibodies to HIV-1/2. Follow-up assays may be recommended using NAAT, or assays that differentiate antibodies to HIV-1 and HIV-2. Testing algorithms and standards are provided and updated by the CDC.[41] HIV infection in the United States has become a manageable chronic disease owing to improved understanding of protective lifestyle changes and administration of antiretroviral drugs that target key players in the HIV life cycle, including these drug classes:

- Non-nucleoside reverse transcriptase inhibitors (NNRTIs)
- Nucleoside reverse transcriptase inhibitors (NRTIs)
- Protease inhibitors
- Integrase inhibitors
- Fusion inhibitors
- CCR5 antagonists

PLASMODIUM SPECIES

The *Plasmodium* genus contains over 100 species of which five are capable of infecting humans and causing the disease malaria. **Malaria** is a major global disease; over 200 million people are infected with more than 400,000 deaths each year.[42] The *Plasmodium* species are unicellular parasitic protozoans with a complex life cycle. Transmission to humans is via the female *Anopheles* mosquito.

Malaria infection can be characterized as mild, severe, or relapsing. *P. falciparum* infection, representing 99.7% of cases in Africa, may be mild but more often progresses to severe disease if not treated. It is a major cause of death in children younger than 5 years of age in Africa. *P. vivax* infection, second

BOX 5.7
CDC Listing of AIDS-Defining Conditions

- Bacterial infections, multiple or recurrent[*]
- Candidiasis of bronchi, trachea, or lungs
- Candidiasis of esophagus[†]
- Cervical cancer, invasive[‡]
- Coccidioidomycosis, disseminated or extrapulmonary
- Cryptococcosis, extrapulmonary
- Cryptosporidiosis, chronic intestinal (>1 month duration)
- Cytomegalovirus disease (other than liver, spleen, or nodes), onset at age >1 month
- Cytomegalovirus retinitis (with loss of vision)[†]
- Encephalopathy, HIV related
- Herpes simplex: chronic ulcers (>1 month duration) or bronchitis, pneumonitis, or esophagitis (onset at age >1 month)
- Histoplasmosis, disseminated or extrapulmonary
- Isosporiasis, chronic intestinal (>1 month duration)
- Kaposi sarcoma[†]

- Lymphoid interstitial pneumonia or pulmonary lymphoid hyperplasia complex[*†]
- Lymphoma, Burkitt (or equivalent term)
- Lymphoma, immunoblastic (or equivalent term)
- Lymphoma, primary, of brain
- *Mycobacterium avium* complex or *Mycobacterium kansasii*, disseminated or extrapulmonary[†]
- *Mycobacterium tuberculosis* of any site, pulmonary,[†‡] disseminated,[†] or extrapulmonary[†]
- *Mycobacterium*, other species or unidentified species, disseminated[†] or extrapulmonary[†]
- *Pneumocystis jiroveci* pneumonia[†]
- Pneumonia, recurrent[†‡]
- Progressive multifocal leukoencephalopathy
- *Salmonella* septicemia, recurrent
- Toxoplasmosis of brain, onset at age >1 month[†]
- Wasting syndrome attributed to HIV

[*]Only among children aged <13 years. From Centers for Disease Control and Prevention. 1994 revised classification system for human immunodeficiency virus infection in children less than 13 years of age. *MMWR Morb Mortal Wkly Rep*. 1994;43(RR-12):1–10.
[†]Condition that might be diagnosed presumptively.
[‡]Only among adults and adolescents aged >13 years. From Centers for Disease Control and Prevention. 1993 revised classification system for HIV infection and expanded surveillance case definition for AIDS among adolescents and adults. *MMWR Recomm Rep*. 1992;41(RR-17):1–19.
Source: Centers for Disease Control and Prevention. Appendix A: AIDS-defining conditions. *MMWR Morb Mortal Wkly Rep*. 2008;57(RR10);9. https://www.cdc.gov/mmwr/preview/mmwrhtml/rr5710a2.htm.

in prevalence to *P. falciparum* infection, is generally a milder disorder with lower parasite levels due to preferential infection of reticulocytes. *P. vivax* is uncommon in Africa, as the Duffy antigen, a red blood cell protein it uses for docking is not generally present in those of African ancestral descent. Several genetic blood disorders that are common in individuals of African descent appear to have been evolutionarily favored owing to conferring resistance to malaria infection—these include sickle cell trait, thalassemia, and glucose-6-phosphate dehydrogenase deficiency.

The *Plasmodium* life cycle is characterized by episodes of both asexual and sexual reproduction, depending on site (Figure 5.19). The primary sites of parasite colonization are the intestine of the insect host, and the liver and red blood cells of the human host. The steps of malaria infection are shown in Box 5.8.

Global populations in areas of high transmission of malaria are at risk, but often individuals will develop sufficient immunity to prevent disease following infection. This immunity is short lived once the individual leaves the endemic area. Malaria is a serious and deadly disease for young children. WHO has reported 70% of all malaria deaths occur in children younger than 5 years of age. Other high-risk groups include infants, pregnant women, and people with HIV/AIDS.[42]

Laboratory testing for malaria includes light microscopy of thin and thick blood smears for the characteristic inclusions indicating the different developmental stages of the parasite within red blood cells (Figure 5.20). Additional tests include PCR amplification of parasite DNA, an immune-based rapid diagnostic test (RDT) for parasite antigens, and measures of host antibody response to parasite antigens by immunofluorescene assay (IFA).

Clinical diagnosis is based on the patient's symptoms and on physical findings at examination.[43] Malaria symptoms wax and wane in association with the levels of the asexual erythrocytic or blood stage parasites. There may be a significant lag time between exposure and symptom development. Malaria can be suspected based on the patient's travel history, symptoms, and the physical findings at examination, with the confirming tests as noted previously.

Pharmacological treatment can include provision of prophylactic medication to an individual planning

BOX 5.8
Steps in Malaria Infection

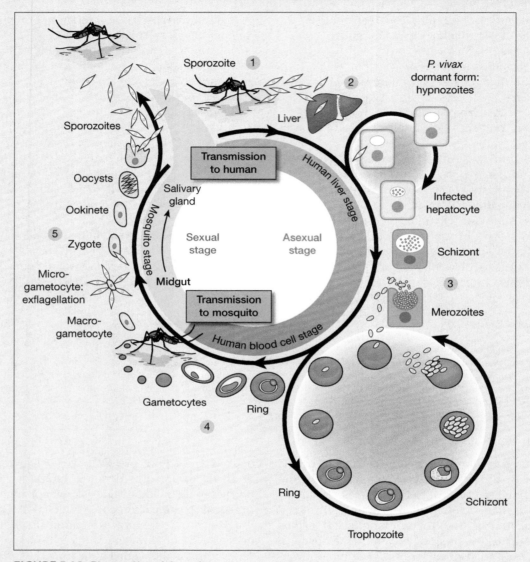

FIGURE 5.19 *Plasmodium* life cycle.

1. A mosquito bites a human, obtaining a blood meal and delivering malarial sporozoites.

2. Sporozoites travel through the bloodstream to the liver, where they enter the hepatocyte and begin to reproduce asexually, forming schizonts (asymptomatic phase).

3. Parasites in the form of merozoites exit hepatocytes and infect red blood cells, visible on light microscopy as ring forms and more advanced forms. After multiplication, more merozoites are released into the circulation as the red blood cell ruptures and dies. (Symptoms may occur.)

4. Some parasites differentiate into gametocytes that circulate freely in the blood. A second mosquito bite and blood meal transmits the gametocytes back to a mosquito.

5. Within the mosquito gut, male and female gametocytes fuse and form a zygote, which progresses through the ookinete stage and produces oocysts that become sporozoites. Upon release of the sporozoites they can then be transmitted to a new human host via a mosquito bite.

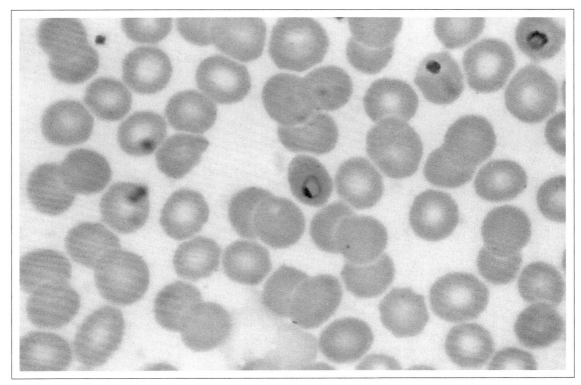

FIGURE 5.20 *Plasmodium*-infected red blood cells. A Giemsa-stained thin blood smear shows ring-form *Plasmodium malariae* parasites.
Source: Courtesy of Mae Melvin. Centers for Disease Control and Prevention, Public Health Image Library (PHIL).

travel to a region of epidemic malaria. Insect repellents and insecticide-treated bed netting are critical preventive measures. Treatment of current infection depends on knowledge of the geographic source and species of *Plasmodium* involved, as well as the detection of resistance. Chloroquine resistance has been recognized since the late 1950s and has spread widely. *P. falciparum* has also demonstrated resistance to several other antimalarial drugs. Combination therapy consisting of artemisinin with other drugs was initially very effective and is still used, but some artemisinin resistance has now been identified. Chloroquine resistance has also been confirmed in *P. vivax* in areas of that species' distribution.[44] Drug development against malaria is ongoing and is informed by new findings in

the details of the parasite life cycle in both mosquito and human hosts.[45] Because no antimalarial drug is completely effective against malaria, personal protective measures should be strongly emphasized, including wearing long sleeves, long pants, and insect repellent, and if possible sleeping in mosquito-free settings.

 Thought Question

7. What resources are available to enable the clinician to get updated clinical information about the infectious diseases most common to their geographical location and practice?

Laura Roettger

Neonates and infants have protection from pathogens in the form of passive immunity: Maternal antibodies circulate to the fetus via the placenta, and breast milk contains secretory IgA. However, after birth, this protection gradually declines and the infant is exposed to an ever-greater number of pathogens. These environmental exposures stimulate immune system development, but are still potentially the source of dangerous infections from which the infant is not yet protected.

Routine immunizations provide the first line of protection against infectious diseases that in earlier centuries caused significant pediatric morbidity and mortality.[46] Prior to immunization, it is important to evaluate whether all adults and older children coming into contact with the infant are up to date on their immunizations. A particular emphasis has been placed on pertussis, as there have been case reports of infants contracting pertussis from adults who were unaware their immunity had lapsed. Many communicable diseases have a more severe course and higher mortality rate in infants and young children than in older children and adults. Among these are influenza, malaria, and forms of gastroenteritis.

Beginning during pregnancy, at birth, and during lactation, there is the potential for transmission of maternal-associated pathogens to the neonate—so-called *vertical transmission*. Prenatal care includes screening tests for these pathogens, including group B streptococcus, *Treponema pallidum* (syphilis), rubella virus, hepatitis B virus, HIV, *C. trachomatis*, and *N. gonorrhoeae*. Depending on maternal geographical, travel, and sexual history, screening for Zika virus may also be appropriate.[47] Other infections that can be transmitted across the placenta include toxoplasmosis, cytomegalovirus infection, and herpes simplex. Treatment of the mother before and during birth or the neonate at birth is often effective at reducing or eliminating vertical transmission of many pathogens.

Beyond the neonatal period, many infants and young children in Western countries are cared for in group daycare settings, which are common sites for transmission of upper respiratory infections, conjunctivitis, dermatophytoses, and viral gastroenteritis. Although in the past, rotavirus was the most common pathogen in pediatric viral gastroenteritis, this infection is now declining owing to widespread vaccination. Norovirus is now a more common cause of pediatric gastroenteritis.

NOROVIRUS

Norovirus and sapovirus are the two viruses in the family Caliciviridae. Both cause viral **gastroenteritis**, but norovirus is the most common pathogen. Both are nonenveloped single-strand RNA viruses, although many different strains have been identified. Groups GI, GII, and GIV infect humans, with the subtype GII.4 isolated in most recent infections. The GII.4 strains also have substantial genetic variability, and prior infection with one form may not confer immune resistance to reinfection because of pathogen mutation rates. The likelihood of infection also varies greatly among hosts, partly depending on the host genotype for human blood group antigen carbohydrates expressed on gastrointestinal epithelial cells (the host cell binding site for norovirus).[48]

Norovirus is the leading cause of acute gastroenteritis in all population groups in the United States.[49] It is highly contagious, requiring as few as 10 to 20 virus particles to induce infection, so norovirus infections spread rapidly, particularly in crowded conditions and daycare centers. Norovirus transmission is via the fecal–oral route, and food contamination is one source of transmission. Aerosols may form during vomiting in a person with norovirus, providing an additional means of transmission. Norovirus is shed primarily in the stool of infected individuals but is also found in the vomitus. The virus can be detected in stool for approximately 4 weeks following infection, and peak viral shedding takes place 2 to 5 days after infection. Up to 30% of assay-verified norovirus infections are asymptomatic, yet these asymptomatic individuals shed virus, which can cause symptomatic infections in other healthy individuals.

Norovirus characteristically presents with rapid onset of severe vomiting, then diarrhea. Abdominal cramping, fever, headache, and myalgias may also occur. Greater severity is common in young children and older adults, and in long-term care settings, with a significant mortality rate of over 200,000 deaths annually, primarily in under-resourced countries.[50] Real-time reverse transcriptase quantitative polymerase chain reaction (RT-qPCR) is used in research settings to detect norovirus, and multiplex nucleic acid assays or enzyme immunoassays may be used clinically. Treatment focuses on supportive care and managing dehydration, as there are no antiviral treatments specifically directed against the norovirus.[51]

MEASLES, MUMPS, AND RUBELLA

In primary and secondary schools and colleges, there has been a resurgence of diseases covered by standard vaccine schedules, so it is useful for clinicians to be familiar with some of these infectious agents.[52]

Measles was eliminated in the United States in 2000, in that there was no documented measles transmission for 12 months. Since that milestone was achieved, however, there have been sporadic outbreaks, and the number of cases reported annually has been rising, with 372 cases reported in 2018.[53] Measles virus is an RNA virus with one serotype, from the genus *Morbillivirus* in the Paramyxoviridae family, and humans are the only hosts. The most highly communicable of all infectious diseases, measles is transmitted by exposure to respiratory droplets, secretions, and aerosols containing the virus. Measles causes necrosis of the infected respiratory epithelium with predominately lymphocytic inflammatory infiltrate. Fever, malaise, cough, and a maculopapular rash are common. Severe complications can occur, and the disease can be fatal. Deaths due to measles are highest in those who are immunosuppressed and in under-resourced settings. Pathogen identification can be done using RT-PCR for viral RNA and also host antibody detection (IgM or IgG).

Cases of **mumps** in the United States surged in 2016 and 2017 to over 6,000 cases per year.[54] Mumps is an RNA virus in the genus *Rubulavirus* of the Paramyxoviridae family. The disease is transmitted through respiratory droplets or direct contact with respiratory secretions or saliva from infected individuals. The virus targets several organs and tissues, including the respiratory tract, nervous system, pancreas, testes, and salivary glands. Salivary gland infiltration produces a characteristic swelling in about two-thirds of cases. In countries with high childhood immunization rates, mumps often occurs in the college years, as the vaccine is not 100% effective. Diagnosis is by RT-PCR or host antibody measurements.

Rubella was eliminated from the United States in 2004, and recent cases have been reported in visitors to the United States, rather than being caused by local outbreaks.[55] Rubella virus is an RNA virus in the Togaviridae family. The disease manifests differently depending on whether it presents congenitally or postnatally. Postnatal rubella is transmitted through inhalation of respiratory droplets or direct contact with an infected person's respiratory secretions. Maternal rubella during pregnancy may result in miscarriage, fetal demise, or a constellation of congenital anomalies. Common anomalies of congenital rubella syndrome include cataracts, pigmentary retinopathy, microphthalmos, congenital glaucoma, patent ductus arteriosus, peripheral pulmonary artery stenosis, sensorineural hearing impairment, behavioral disorders, meningoencephalitis, microcephaly, and intellectual disability.

Measles, mumps, rubella, and other childhood infections have had a resurgence due in large part to parental vaccine refusal or requests for vaccine exemptions in certain geographical locations. The lower the percentage of children who receive vaccinations, the greater the compromise to *herd immunity*—the phenomenon that limits spread of highly contagious infectious diseases due to lack of sufficient unimmunized hosts.

Elizabeth Walsh, Candace Kastner, and Alyssa Bondy

Many infections have more severe manifestations in older adults. This increased severity has been attributed to comorbid conditions, waning immunity, suboptimal nutritional status, and social and environmental factors. Residence in long-term care facilities may be a strong factor in exposure to normal and drug-resistant pathogens.[56] Pneumonia is a common and sometimes fatal infection, whether acquired in the community or in healthcare facilities. With the reduction in adaptive immunity associated with aging, there is sometimes reemergence of latent viruses. Finally, HIV can be acquired and has a somewhat different presentation in adults older than 50 years of age. These examples are described further in this section.

COMMUNITY-ACQUIRED PNEUMONIA

Pneumonia can be classified as either community-acquired pneumonia (CAP) or healthcare-acquired pneumonia (HCAP). HCAP is defined as infection in an individual whose symptoms began after more than 2 days of a hospital stay or 10 to 14 days after being discharged.[57] Distinguishing between the two is key to proper treatment, as the microorganisms accountable for the two types are vastly different.

Recent data show that CAP is the third most common hospitalization diagnosis in adults 65 years of age or older and the leading cause of septic shock. Current guidelines recommend that adults aged 65 years and older receive both the pneumococcal (one dose of the 23-valent vaccine) and the influenza (annual) vaccines.[58] In comparison with the younger population, CAP in the elderly patient carries an increased risk of morbidity and mortality. Because an impaired immune response and other physiological changes that occur with aging create increased vulnerability in this population, fast diagnosis and treatment, and hemodynamic stability, are important when dealing with these patients. Exogenous factors such as frailty, comorbidities, mechanical swallowing disorders, and sedentary lifestyle all contribute to the increased risk of mortality and need for ICU admissions.

Clinical manifestations of CAP in elderly patients differ from findings in younger adults. A subtler presentation may occur; therefore, the absence of typical symptoms such as cough, fever, or elevated white cell count cannot rule out a diagnosis. Additionally, atypical presentations such as altered mental status, frequent falls, anorexia, incontinence, or an overall decline in function may be the only presenting manifestations of the diagnosis in the elder adult.

Diagnosis depends on chest x-ray evidence of opacities. There is much debate over the usefulness of laboratory testing as biomarkers for the diagnosis of CAP in the geriatric patient. Tests such as white blood cell count, C-reactive protein, and procalcitonin are widely used in today's medical practice, but insufficient data over the years have yet to truly prove their sensitivities.[57,58] Age-related alterations in the immune system can create false laboratory results, especially in tests involving inflammatory responses. Other tests that can be useful in supporting a diagnosis are blood cultures, Gram stains, respiratory sputum cultures, and checking the patient's urine for the presence of pneumococcal and *Legionella* antigens. However, in over half of patients, the causative organism cannot be identified.

The most common cause of CAP in older adults is *S. pneumoniae*, followed by *Haemophilus influenzae*. Compared with younger adults, the frequency of atypical strains of pneumonia caused by *Legionella*, *Mycoplasma*, and *Chlamydophila* organisms is lower in the elderly patient.[58] *S. pneumoniae* is part of the normal oral and upper respiratory flora and can enter the lower respiratory passages by inhalation and by aspiration, with the latter being the most common route in older adults. Pneumococcal capsular antigens protect the bacteria from phagocytosis and define serotypes, and several of the antigens are the targets of pneumococcal vaccines. Additional pneumococcal virulence elements include pneumolysin, a pore-forming toxin that promotes host cell damage and death and exacerbates inflammation. Bacterial proteases are able to cleave and inactivate host IgA as well as the mucus protective barrier, disabling mucociliary clearance. Other surface and secreted proteins block complement binding and degrade complement proteins. Respiratory compromise in pneumonia is due to the inflammatory response that promotes fluid entry into alveoli, limiting gas exchange. This is exacerbated when viral and bacterial coinfection occur, synergizing to enhance inflammatory responses.[59]

In addition to acute inflammation and risk of sepsis, pneumonia in older adults is associated with cardiovascular morbidity and mortality. Rates of myocardial infarction and ischemic stroke increase during and after an episode of pneumonia, and this is attributed to hypercoagulability associated with the inflammatory state and bacteremia.[60] In addition, older adults with other comorbidities, including heart failure, atrial fibrillation, and chronic obstructive pulmonary disease, have higher morbidity and mortality rates secondary to pneumonia.[61]

Two important prognostic scales widely used to predict 30-day mortality risk for a patient with CAP are the Pneumonia Severity Index (PSI) and CURB-65. The PSI assigns points for various categories, including both laboratory results and clinical symptoms. Once the points have been tallied, patients are placed into one of five risk categories, increasing in severity, to determine who should be hospitalized. CURB-65 uses a formula based on five markers: (a) confusion, (b) urea level >7 mmol/L, (c) respiratory rate of 30 breaths/min or more, (d) systolic blood pressure <90 mm Hg or diastolic blood pressure ≤60 mm Hg, and (e) patient age of 65 years or older. Studies have shown that one of the biggest flaws in the CURB-65 model is that it does not take into account oxygen saturation or the functional status of the patient. These formulas are intended to supplement the practitioner's diagnosis and help in risk stratification to achieve better long-term outcomes.[57,58]

VARICELLA-ZOSTER VIRUS

Varicella-zoster virus (VZV) is a member of the Herpesviridae family consisting of enveloped, double-stranded DNA-type viruses. As such, the viral DNA is able to reside in the host cell nucleus, forming a latent infection that can be reactivated months and years after the initial exposure. VZV in children causes chickenpox, a highly contagious disease with respiratory transmission and cutaneous lesions that may also spread the infection. Latent infection affects sensory neurons in dorsal root ganglia and cranial nerve ganglia. With aging, as immune protection against VZV wanes, reactivation causes **shingles**—the unilateral painful sensory neuropathy and skin blistering associated with a particular facial or spinal segment (dermatomal distribution). Severe cases may be followed by **postherpetic neuralgia**, a chronic pain syndrome that may last from months to years. Vaccination for VZV is strongly recommended for individuals aged 60 years and older, as the risk of shingles increases with age.[62,63]

HIV

In 2017, 17% of HIV diagnoses were made in people 50 years of age and older. In 2016, Americans aged 55 and older accounted for almost 30% of the population living with HIV infection.[64] Although risk factors for contracting HIV infection remain the same for adults of all ages, the elderly are often less aware of these factors. For this reason, and because of the effects of immunosenescence, diagnosis of HIV in the elderly may occur later in the disease course, often with higher rates of morbidity and mortality and comorbid disease complications. The persistence of immune activation and continued inflammation associated with HIV, combined with the natural effects of aging on the immune system, result in profound havoc; thus, age may be considered to be an independent predictor of clinical progression of HIV.[65,66]

The stages of HIV infection in older adults do not differ from those outlined earlier in the chapter, but as a result of advanced age, these patients may have greater loss of CD4 cells, as well as lower counts of total and functioning CD8 cells, which are crucial for limiting the replication of the HIV. Furthermore, the progression of HIV may be more pronounced in the elderly because the infection itself can inhibit the generation of naive T cells. The net result is greater severity of HIV infection and the potential of more rapid transition to AIDS in older adults, as has been noted for several infections in this population.

CASE STUDY 5.1: A Patient With Acute HIV Infection

Sampath Wijesinghe

Patient Compliant: *"I just got back from a mission trip to Haiti and have been having fevers, sore throat, body aches, and headache for the past 5 days. I thought I'd be feeling better by now, but I don't think I'm improving. I'm wondering if I could have malaria. I didn't have a chance to get this year's flu shot or malaria prophylaxis before my trip."*

History of Present Illness/Review of Systems: A 19-year-old Hispanic man presents to his primary care provider at the university health center during the winter quarter with a 5-day history of fever, sore throat, body aches, and headache. About 4 weeks ago, he went on a mission trip to Haiti. While in Haiti, he had unprotected sex with a female student who was also participating in the trip as well as a male Haitian student. He is concerned about his symptoms as they are not resolving and is requesting an evaluation of his condition. He has been resting and drinking plenty of fluids for the last 5 days, and has also been taking acetaminophen, 500 mg, every 4 hours, as needed for his fever. The fever has decreased slightly and he thinks the acetaminophen has helped with the body ache, sore throat, and headache. The review of systems is positive for fever, fatigue, and anxiousness. The patient reports having headache, sore throat, and myalgia. The review of systems is negative for cough, nausea, vomiting, diarrhea, constipation, abdominal pain, rash, ear pain, dysuria, urinary urgency, back pain, chest pain, and shortness of breath.

Past Medical/Social/Family History: The patient's past medical history is significant for appendectomy (at age 9) and chlamydial infection (at age 17). An HIV test performed at the time of the chlamydia diagnosis was negative. Social history includes drinking a six pack of beer each weekend (Friday and Saturday nights) since age 18 and having three different girlfriends over the last year. He has been living in one of the residence halls on campus. His family history is unremarkable.

Physical Examination: Findings are as follows: temperature of 103°F, blood pressure of 138/89 mm Hg, heart rate of 90 beats/min, and respirations of 19 breaths/min. Body mass index (BMI) is 24 kg/m². His constitutional symptoms include fever and tiredness. He appears anxious. The ear/nose/throat (ENT) and mouth exam is within normal limits, with the exception of mild rhinorrhea. Several cervical lymph nodes are palpable on his anterior neck. His heart rate and rhythm are regular, without murmur or gallop. His lungs are clear, with good air movement throughout.

Laboratory and Diagnostic Findings: A rapid molecular assay result for influenza was negative. Parasite-based diagnostic tools are not readily available at the university health center to rule out *Plasmodium falciparum* infection. His complete blood count (CBC) and complete metabolic panel (CMP) are within normal limits. Results of an HIV fourth-generation test are positive.

CASE STUDY 5.1 QUESTIONS
- *What lab tests should be considered in a first patient visit for possible new HIV infection? If the patient does indeed have a new HIV infection, what are likely to be the lab findings?*
- *Describe the differences between viral infections due to influenza virus and those due to HIV. How would you describe HIV pathophysiology and the appropriate treatment regimen to a new patient?*

CASE STUDY 5.2: A Child With Hand, Foot, and Mouth Disease

Stephanie L. Carper

Patient Complaint: *"My baby was sent home from daycare yesterday because she developed a fever. They told me her temperature was 101, and that she had a rash in her diaper area and behind her knees. She was crying last night, so I gave her some ibuprofen to see if it would bring her fever down."*

History of Present Illness/Review of Systems: A mother has brought her 18-month-old girl to the clinic today. The child was sent home from daycare yesterday because of illness and was still feverish this morning, with a temperature of 102°F, despite being given ibuprofen the night before. The child has not had any vomiting but woke up crying during the night. Mom is concerned because the child refused water and milk this morning, although she had a wet diaper upon waking. She also notes that the girl seems to be drooling more than usual and had a runny nose this morning.

Past Medical/Social History: The patient was a full-term infant, with a birth weight of 7 lb 10 oz, delivered vaginally, with a normal newborn screen. She has been seen at the clinic for routine well-baby care since birth and has no chronic illnesses and no past surgical history. She lives with her mother, father, and older sister (aged 4 years) in a single-family home and attends daycare full time.

Physical Examination: Findings are as follows: temperature of 99.6°F; heart rate of 118 beats/min; and respiratory rate of 26 breaths/min, with peripheral oxygen saturation of 99%. General: The patient is an alert infant and appears mildly ill but in no apparent distress. Her skin is warm and dry, with coalesced erythematous papules noted bilaterally on the popliteal fossa and across the buttocks, and

small, scattered, and annular macular erythematous lesions bilaterally on the palms and soles. Head is normocephalic and atraumatic. Examination of the eyes shows clear sclerae and conjunctivae, with no active discharge; pupils are equal, round, and reactive to light and accommodation (PERRLA); and intact extraocular movements. A moderate amount of clear rhinorrhea is noted, along with moist mucous membranes, pharynx with moderate injection, no tonsillar hypertrophy or exudative tonsils, and a few scattered vesicles on posterior pharynx. There is full range of neck motion, with no cervical lymphadenopathy. Upper extremities have full range of motion, with no gross deformity. Lungs are clear to auscultation bilaterally, with no signs of accessory muscle use or labored breathing. Heart rate and rhythm are regular, with S_1 and S_2 heart sounds present and no murmurs. Abdomen is soft, nontender, and nondistended, with no hepatosplenomegaly. Genitalia are not examined. Lower extremities show full range of motion. Neurological exam reveals an infant who is alert and oriented appropriately for age and development, intact cranial nerves II to XII, normal tone for developmental age, and normal gait for development.

Laboratory and Diagnostic Findings: No tests are warranted for this condition.

CASE STUDY 5.2 QUESTIONS
- *What is the usual course for a mild to moderate acute viral illness, from the prodrome to the resolution?*
- *Hand, foot, and mouth disease can be caused by one of several strains of coxsackievirus. Will a child who has had one episode of this syndrome be protected against future episodes?*

BRIDGE TO CLINICAL PRACTICE

Ben Cocchiaro

PRINCIPLES OF ASSESSMENT

History and Physical Examination

- *Exposure history:* acute illness in family and community contacts, healthcare exposure (especially in older adults), daycare exposures in children, diet, animal contacts (including bites and stings), social history (including travel, substance use, occupational exposure, sexual history, and outdoor activity)
- *Systemic signs and symptoms of infection:* fever, chills, malaise, myalgias, arthralgias, anorexia, vomiting, diarrhea, night sweats, and weight loss
- *Physical examination:* focusing on vital signs (fever, tachycardia, increased respiratory rate) and routes of exposure (eyes, ears, nose, throat, skin, lungs, abdomen, genitalia, lymph nodes)
- *Localized or generalized signs and symptoms of infection:* pain, swelling, redness, heat, rash, rhinorrhea, swollen tonsils (with or without exudate), red pharynx, cough (productive or nonproductive); lung assessment (auscultation for crackles, diminished breath sounds, egophony; palpation for fremitus, percussion for dullness)
- *Vaccination history*

Diagnostic Tools

- Radiography
- CT
- MRI

Laboratory Evaluation

- Complete blood count with differential
- C-reactive protein
- Erythrocyte sedimentation rate
- *Pathogen identification*
  - Microscopy (smears, biopsies)
  - Culture and sensitivity
  - Immune detection (EIA, ELISA, rapid antigen detection, toxin identification)
  - Molecular detection (NAAT)

MAJOR DRUG CLASSES

- *Antibacterials*
  - Cell wall active: penicillins, cephalosporins, carbapenems, monobactams, vancomycin
  - Protein synthesis inhibition: macrolides, clindamycin, linezolid, aminoglycosides, tetracyclines
  - Nucleic acid synthesis and function inhibition: quinolones, trimethoprim/sulfamethoxazole, metronidazole, nitrofurantoin
- *Antivirals:* amantadine, rimantadine, acyclovir, ganciclovir, vidarabine
- *Antiretrovirals:* zidovudine, didanosine, lamivudine, ritonavir, indinavir
- *Antifungals:* azoles, echinocandins, polyenes, flucytosine
- *Antimalarials:* chloroquine, amodiaquine, piperaquine, primaquine, quinine, mefloquine, artemether, artesunate, dihydroartemisinin, pyrimethamine/sulfadoxine, doxycycline, clindamycin

EIA, enzyme immunoassay; ELISA, enzyme-linked immunosorbent assay; NAAT, nucleic acid amplification testing.

KEY POINTS

- Microbes are found on human body surfaces and at sites of interface between humans and the environment. Colonization by the normal microbiota and even by certain pathogens is not associated with disease; rather, the human reaction to pathogens produces the clinically detectable signs and symptoms of infection.
- Immune defenses usually limit the severity and duration of infection, with pathogen elimination commonly occurring after an acute phase. Pathogens have evolved a variety of properties that enable them to evade destruction by the immune system.
- Pathogen virulence features and host susceptibility characteristics contribute to the severity and clinical course of many infections.
- Bacteria are prokaryotic cells that make up the abundant component of the normal microbiota. Bacterial contributions to homeostasis include promoting host immune development as well as inhibition of growth of competing pathogenic bacteria, among other functions.
- Antibacterial drugs target key differences between human cells and bacterial cells to eradicate infection-causing pathogens.
- Viruses are acellular, nonliving particles that are unable to replicate without host cell machinery. They are obligate intracellular pathogens that often kill host cells as part of their life cycle and proliferation. Immune protection against viral infections occurs after an initial exposure, often through immunization.
- The eukaryotic cells of fungi and yeasts are, in some cases, part of the normal human flora, although they are far less common than bacteria. Fungi and yeasts are characterized as eukaryotic cells and are responsible for several common superficial infections.
- Although systemic fungal infections are less common, they can be very severe and even fatal. The major distinction between fungal and human cells is the fungal cell wall containing ergosterol (rather than cholesterol), and unique carbohydrates that can be the target of antifungal drugs.
- Protozoa are single-celled eukaryotes that may have complex life cycles that include colonizations between both vector and host.
- Several laboratory methods have been developed for pathogen identification. Bacteria have long been studied by culture and Gram staining, while culture has been more challenging for viruses.

- Immune-based methods of pathogen identification are often able to determine the presence of antibodies to a virus (indicating prior exposure) or the presence of a viral marker protein, such as a toxin.
- Molecular approaches continue to expand and greatly aid in pathogen identification, screening for antimicrobial resistance, and defining subtypes that vary by pathogenicity.
- Microbes reproduce rapidly and have relatively high mutation rates. Among the beneficial (to the microbe) mutations are those that produce antimicrobial resistance. Widespread use of antimicrobial treatments has led to a dangerous level of resistance of many species to a broad swath of these drugs.
- Antibiotic stewardship calls for judicious prescribing of antimicrobials on an as-needed basis to reduce the development and spread of antimicrobial resistance.
- *S. pyogenes* is the most common bacteria causing pharyngitis, although most pharyngitis is viral. The M protein of *S. pyogenes* fimbriae and several exotoxins are major virulence factors in these infections. Poststreptococcal complications can include damage to heart valves and glomerulonephritis. *S. pyogenes* can also cause serious skin infections.
- MRSA is often a colonizer of human skin and nares. MRSA produces several exotoxins that contribute to infection severity, even to the point of septic shock. Superficial MRSA lesions often present as painful boils. MRSA infection can be community acquired or healthcare acquired.
- MTB has a unique cell wall enriched in long-chain, complex lipids. It is thus protected from host immune attack, and its pathogenic properties include the ability to enter macrophages and resist degradation. Although MTB infection can affect several tissues, the most prominent target is the lungs, as it is spread by respiratory aerosols. Drug-resistant MTB strains have been increasing and provide a global challenge to containment.
- *C. trachomatis* is another intracellular pathogen, and is one of the most common sexually transmitted organisms. *C. trachomatis* infection of the female lower genital tract may be cleared by host immune responses, but spread of the infection to the fallopian tubes may lead to pelvic inflammatory disease. *C. trachomatis* and *N. gonorrhoeae* infections often coexist.

- *N. gonorrhoeae* is a small diplococcus that connects to the epithelial cells lining the male or female genital tract, produces an inflammatory response with robust recruitment of neutrophils, and is phagocytosed by neutrophils where it evades leukocyte destruction. Infected males are generally symptomatic with purulent urethritis, whereas infected females are often asymptomatic. Ascent of the bacteria to the fallopian tubes can lead to pelvic inflammatory disease, tubule scarring, and infertility.
- *C. difficile* is a gram-positive spore-forming rod. People may be colonized and have no infection. However, if normal flora are disrupted by broad-spectrum antibiotics, *C. difficile* can be activated to proliferate and to secrete toxins that create severe diarrhea and colitis. Once acquired, *C. difficile* tends to recur and may require fecal transplants to resolve.
- *B. burgdorferi* is a gram-negative spirochete that infects humans through bites of a tick vector to cause Lyme disease. The disease can affect many tissues and organs with varying degrees of severity.
- Influenza virus has three subtypes—A, B, and C—with A being the most common. It is transmitted via aerosols, with outer hemagglutinin proteins that attach to sialic acid residues on airway epithelial cells. Multiple subtypes of influenza hemagglutinin and neuraminidase can mix and match, making it difficult to tailor the annual vaccine.
- HIV is a retrovirus, with an RNA genome and reverse transcriptase enzyme that synthesizes double-stranded DNA able to integrate with the host genome and remain in a latent state. Viral envelope proteins permit attachment to CD4 T cells, allowing viral entry and the beginning of the viral life cycle. Testing is based on immune-based detection of viral antigen, as well as host antibodies to the infection. Management of HIV is with combination drug approaches that target different steps of the viral life cycle.
- *Plasmodium* species are protozoal parasites with a two-part life cycle in humans. Small sporozoites enter the host from an *Anopheles* mosquito bite, reproduce in the liver, and then infect red blood cells. After several developmental transitions, gametocytes form and circulate freely, are transmitted back to a mosquito, and reproduce to form new sporozoites. Resistance has developed to many early antimalarial drugs, and drug development is ongoing.
- Neonates can acquire maternal infections during pregnancy and delivery. After birth, infants are exposed to many bacteria, rapidly developing their own normal flora. Early exposure to viruses leads to development of many childhood illnesses such as infectious diarrheas and fungal infections of the skin and scalp. Classic childhood viral diseases such as measles, mumps, and rubella are less common now because of widespread immunization, although sporadic outbreaks occur in areas of high vaccine refusal.
- Older adults are more vulnerable to community-acquired pneumonia than those who are younger, and may have a more serious course. Pneumococcal vaccine should be given to those over 65 years of age. Reactivation of dormant VZV can cause shingles, and vaccine immunization is recommended.

REFERENCES

1. World Health Organization. The top 10 causes of death. https://www.who.int/news-room/fact-sheets/detail/the-top-10-causes-of-death. Published May 24, 2018. Accessed July 17, 2019.
2. National Center for Health Statistics. *National Ambulatory Medical Care Survey: 2016 National Summary Tables.* https://www.cdc.gov/nchs/data/ahcd/namcs_summary/2016_namcs_web_tables.pdf. Accessed July 17, 2019.
3. National Center for Health Statistics. *National Hospital Ambulatory Medical Care Survey: 2016 Emergency Department Summary Tables.* https://www.cdc.gov/nchs/data/nhamcs/web_tables/2016_ed_web_tables.pdf. Accessed July 17, 2019.
4. Centers for Disease Control and Prevention, National Center for Health Statistics. Influenza/pneumonia mortality by state. https://www.cdc.gov/nchs/pressroom/sosmap/flu_pneumonia_mortality/flu_pneu-monia.htm. Accessed July 17, 2019.
5. Ballou F, van Dorp L. Q&A: what are pathogens, and what have they done to and for us? *BMC Biol.* 2017;15:91. doi:10.1186/s12915-017-0433-z.
6. University of Pennsylvania Health System. Gram stain. http://www.uphs.upenn.edu/bugdrug/antibiotic_manual/gram1.htm. Accessed July 17, 2019.
7. Rogers PD, Krysan DJ. Antifungal agents. In: Brunton LL, Hilal-Dandan R, Knollmann BC, eds. *Goodman & Gilman's The Pharmacological Basis of Therapeutics.* 13th ed. New York, NY: McGraw-Hill; 2018:1087–1104.
8. Bassetti M, Peghin M, Timsit J-F. The current treatment landscape: candidiasis. *J Antimicrob Chemother.* 2016;71(suppl 2):ii13–ii22. doi:10.1093/jac/dkw392.
9. Pottinger P, Sterling CR. Parasites—basic concepts. In: Ryan KJ, ed. *Sherris Medical Microbiology.* 7th ed. New York, NY: McGraw-Hill; 2018:805–814.
10. Spitzer ED. Infectious diseases. In: Laposata M, ed. *Laposata's Laboratory Medicine: Diagnosis of Disease in the Clinical Laboratory.* 3rd ed. New York, NY: McGraw-Hill; 2019:105–176.

11. Munita JM, Arias CA. Mechanisms of antibiotic resistance. *Microbiol Spectr*. 2016;4(2). doi:10.1128/microbiolspec.VMBF-0016-2015.

12. World Health Organization. *Global Antimicrobial Resistance Surveillance System (GLASS) report: Early Implementation 2017–2018*. Geneva, Switzerland: World Health Organization; 2018. https://www.who.int/glass/resources/publications/early-implementation-report/en. Accessed May 30, 2019.

13. Centers for Disease Control. Antibiotic resistance threats in the United States, 2019. https://www.cdc.gov/drugresistance/biggest-threats.html. Accessed December 19, 2019.

14. Fishman N, Patterson J, Saiman L, et al. Policy statement on antimicrobial stewardship by the Society for Healthcare Epidemiology of America (SHEA), the Infectious Diseases Society of America (IDSA), and the Pediatric Infectious Diseases Society (PIDS). *Infect Control Hosp Epidemiol*. 2012;33:322–327. doi:10.1086/665010.

15. Interagency Task Force for Combating Antibiotic-Resistant Bacteria. *National Action Plan for Combating Antimicrobial Resistant-Bacteria*. https://obamawhitehouse.archives.gov/sites/default/files/docs/national_action_plan_for_combating_antibotic-resistant_bacteria.pdf. Published March 2015. Accessed July 22, 2019.

16. Barlam TF, Cosgrove SE, Abbo LM, et al. Implementing an antibiotic stewardship program: guidelines by the Infectious Diseases Society of America and the Society for Healthcare Epidemiology of America. *Clin Infect Dis*. 2016;62:e51–e77. doi:10.1093/cid/ciw118.

17. Centers for Disease Control and Prevention. *Antibiotic Use in the United States, 2018 Update: Progress and Opportunities*. Atlanta, GA: U.S. Department of Health and Human Services, CDC; 2019. https://www.cdc.gov/antibiotic-use/stewardship-report/pdf/stewardship-report.pdf.

18. Carapetis JR, Beaton A, Cunningham MW, et al. Acute rheumatic fever and rheumatic heart disease. *Nat Rev Dis Primers*. 2016;2:15084. doi:10.1038/nrdp.2015.84.

19. Centers for Disease Control and Prevention. Group A streptococcal (GAS) disease, for clinicians. https://www.cdc.gov/groupastrep/diseases-hcp/strep-throat.html. Accessed July 22, 2019.

20. World Health Organization. *Global Tuberculosis Report 2018*. Geneva, Switzerland: World Health Organization; 2017. https://www.who.int/tb/publications/global_report/en.

21. Ndlovu H, Marakalala MJ. Granulomas and inflammation: host-directed therapies for tuberculosis. *Front Immunol*. 2016;7:434. doi:10.3389/fimmu.2016.00434.

22. Elwell C, Mirrashidi K, Engel J. Chlamydia cell biology and pathogenesis. *Nat Rev Microbiol*. 2016;14:385–400. doi:10.1038/nrmicro.2016.30.

23. Centers for Disease Control and Prevention. *STD Curriculum for Clinical Educators: Chlamydia Module*. Atlanta, GA: CDC; April 2015. https://www.std.uw.edu/custom/self-study/chlamydia

24. Stevens JS, Criss AK. Pathogenesis of Neisseria gonorrhoeae in the female reproductive tract: neutrophilic host response, sustained infection, and clinical sequelae. *Curr Opin Hematol*. 2018;25:13–21. doi:10.1097/MOH.0000000000000394.

25. Pottinger P, Reller LB, Ryan KJ, Weissman S. Neisseria. In: Ryan KJ, ed. *Sherris Medical Microbiology*. 7th ed. New York, NY: McGraw-Hill; 2018:567–582.

26. Edwards JL, Apicella MA. The molecular mechanisms used by Neisseria gonorrhoeae to initiate infection differ between men and women. *Clin Microbiol Rev*. 2004;17:965–981. doi:10.1128/CMR.17.4.965–981.2004.

27. McDonald LC, Gerding DN, Johnson S, et al. Clinical practice guidelines for *Clostridium difficile* infection in adults and children: 2017 update by the Infectious Diseases Society of America (IDSA) and Society for Healthcare Epidemiology of America (SHEA). *Clin Infect Dis*. 2018;66(7):e1–e48. 987–994. doi:10.1093/cid/cix1085.

28. Schäffler H, Breitrück A. Clostridium difficile—from colonization to infection. *Front Microbiol*. 2018;9:646. doi:10.3389/fmicb.2018.00646.

29. Abt MC, McKenney PT, Pamer EG. Clostridium difficile colitis: pathogenesis and host defense. *Nat Rev Microbiol*. 2016;14:609–620. doi:10.1038/nrmicro.2016.108.

30. Gerding DN, Young VB. Clostridium difficile infection. In: Bennett JE, Dolin R, Blaser MJ, eds. *Mandell, Douglas, and Bennett's Principles and Practice of Infectious Diseases*. 8th ed. Philadelphia, PA: Elsevier; 2015:2744–2767.

31. El Feghaly RE, Stauber JL, Deych E, et al. Markers of intestinal inflammation, not bacterial burden, correlate with clinical outcomes in Clostridium difficile infection. *Clin Infect Dis*. 2013;56:1713–1721. doi:10.1093/cid/cit147.

32. Yakob L, Riley TV, Paterson DL, et al. Mechanisms of hypervirulent Clostridium difficile ribotype 027 displacement of endemic strains: an epidemiological model. *Sci Rep*. 2015;5:12666. doi:10.1038/srep12666.

33. Marques AR. Lyme neuroborreliosis. *Continuum (Minneap Minn)*. 2015;21:1729–1744. doi:10.1212/CON.0000000000000252.

34. Fish AE, Pride YB, Pinto DS. Lyme carditis. *Infect Dis Clin North Am*. 2008;22:275–288. doi:10.1016/j.idc.2007.12.008.

35. Centers for Disease Control and Prevention. *Lyme disease: two-step laboratory testing process*. https://www.cdc.gov/lyme/diagnosistesting/labtest/twostep/index.html. Accessed July 23, 2019.

36. Steere AC, Strle F, Wormser GP, et al. Lyme borreliosis. *Nat Rev Dis Primers*. 2016;2:16090. doi:10.1038/nrdp.2016.90.

37. Zheng W, Tao YJ. Structure and assembly of the influenza a virus ribonucleoprotein complex. *FEBS Lett*. 2013;587:1206–1214. doi:10.1016/j.febslet.2013.02.048.

38. Wu X, Wu X, Sun Q, et al. Progress of small molecular inhibitors in the development of anti-influenza virus agents. *Theranostics*. 2017;7:826–845. doi:10.7150/thno.17071.

39. Centers for Disease Control and Prevention. Appendix A: AIDS-defining conditions. *MMWR Morb Mortal Wkly Rep*. 2008;57(RR10):9. https://www.cdc.gov/mmwr/preview/mmwrhtml/rr5710a2.htm.

40. Bennett NJ. HIV infection and AIDS. In: Bronze MS, ed. *Medscape*. https://emedicine.medscape.com/article/211316. Published April 12, 2019. Updated December 2, 2019. Accessed July 23, 2019.

41. Centers for Disease Control and Prevention. *HIV testing, laboratory tests: FDA approved HIV tests, 2018 and 2019 updates*. https://www.cdc.gov/hiv/testing/laboratorytests.html. Updated February 22, 2019. Accessed July 23, 2019.

42. World Health Organization. *World Malaria Report 2018*. Geneva, Switzerland: WHO; November 19, 2018. https://www.who.int/malaria/publications/world-malaria-report-2018/en/. Accessed July 23, 2019.

43. Centers for Disease Control and Prevention. *About malaria*. https://www.cdc.gov/malaria/about/disease.html.

44. Centers for Disease Control and Prevention. Drug resistance in the malaria-endemic world. https://www.cdc.gov/malaria/malaria_worldwide/reduction/drug_resistance.html. Accessed July 23, 2019.

45. Miller LH, Ackerman HC, Su X-Z, Wellems TE. Malaria biology and disease pathogenesis: insights for new treatments. *Nat Med*. 2013;19:156–167. doi:10.1038/nm.3073.

46. Centers for Disease Control and Prevention. Immunization schedules. https://www.cdc.gov/vaccines/schedules/hcp/imz/child-adolescent.html. Accessed July 23, 2019.

47. Snow TM, Coble M. Maternal prenatal screening and serologies. *Adv Neonatal Care*. 2018;18:431–437. doi:10.1097/ANC.0000000000000568.

48. de Graaf M, van Beek J, Koopmans MPG. Human norovirus transmission and evolution in a changing world. *Nat Rev Microbiol*. 2016;14:421–433. doi:10.1038/nrmicro.2016.48.

49. Payne DC, Vinjé J, Szilagyi PG, et al. Norovirus and medically attended gastroenteritis in US children. *N Engl J Med*. 2013;368:1121–1130. doi:10.1056/NEJMsa1206589.

50. Lopman BA, Steele D, Kirkwood CD, Parashar UD. The vast and varied global burden of norovirus: prospects for prevention and control. *PLoS Med*. 2016;13:e1001999. doi:10.1371/journal.pmed.1001999.

51. Shah MP, Hall AJ. Norovirus illnesses in children and adolescents. *Infect Dis Clin North Am*. 2018;32:103–118. doi:10.1016/j.idc.2017.11.004.

52. Baker CJ. *Red Book Atlas of Pediatric Infectious Diseases*. 2nd ed. Elk Grove Village, IL: American Academy of Pediatrics; 2013.

53. Centers for Disease Control and Prevention. Measles cases and outbreaks, 2019. https://www.cdc.gov/measles/cases-outbreaks.html. Accessed July 23, 2019.

54. Centers for Disease Control and Prevention. Mumps cases and outbreaks, 2019. https://www.cdc.gov/mumps/outbreaks.html. Accessed July 23, 2019.

55. Centers for Disease Control and Prevention. Rubella in the U.S. https://www.cdc.gov/rubella/about/in-the-us.html. Accessed July 23, 2019.

56. High K. Infection: general principles. In: Halter JB, Ouslander JG, Studenski S, et al., eds. *Hazzard's Geriatric Medicine and Gerontology*. 7th ed. New York, NY: McGraw-Hill; 2017:1943–1956.

57. González Del Castillo J, Martín-Sánchez FJ. Pneumonia. In: Halter JB, Ouslander JG, Studenski S, et al., eds. *Hazzard's Geriatric Medicine and Gerontology*. 7th ed. New York, NY: McGraw-Hill; 2017:1957–1970.

58. Simonetti A, Viasus D, Garcia-Vidal C, Carratala J. Management of community-acquired pneumonia in older adults. *Ther Adv Infect Dis*. 2014;2:3–16. doi:10.1177/2049936113518041.

59. Weiser JN, Ferreira DM, Paton JC. *Streptococcus pneumoniae*: transmission, colonization, and invasion. *Nat Rev Microbiol*. 2018;16:355–367. doi:10.1038/s41579-018-0001-8.

60. Violi F, Cangemi R, Calvieri C. Pneumonia, thrombosis, and vascular disease. *J Thromb Haemost*. 2014;12:1391–1400. doi:10.1111/jth.12646.

61. Miravitlles M, Anzueto A. Role of infection in exacerbations of chronic obstructive pulmonary disease. *Curr Opin Pulm Med*. 2015;21:278–283. doi:10.1097/MCP.0000000000000154.

62. John AR, Canaday DH. Herpes zoster in the older adult. *Infect Dis Clin North Am*. 2017;31:811–826. doi:10.1016/j.idc.2017.07.016.

63. Mallick-Searle T, Snodgrass B, Brant JM. Postherpetic neuralgia: epidemiology, pathophysiology, and pain management pharmacology. *J Multidiscip Healthc*. 2016;9:447–454. doi:10.2147/JMDH.S106340.

64. Centers for Disease Control and Prevention. *HIV and older Americans*. https://www.cdc.gov/hiv/pdf/group/age/olderamericans/cdc-hiv-older-americans.pdf. Published September 2019. Accessed December 5, 2019.

65. Nguyen N, Holodniy M. HIV infection in the elderly. *Clin Interv Aging*. 2008;3:453–472. doi:10.2147/cia.s2086.

66. Nasi M, Pinti M, De Biasi S, et al. Aging with HIV infection: a journey to the center of inflammAIDS, immunosenescence and neuroHIV. *Immunol Lett*. 2014;162:329–333. doi:10.1016/j.imlet.2014.06.012.

SUGGESTED RESOURCES

Websites

Centers for Disease Control and Prevention websites on infectious disease. https://www.cdc.gov/ncezid/index.html.

National Center for Emerging and Zoonotic Diseases. https://www.cdc.gov/ncezid/index.html.

National Center for HIV/AIDS, Viral Hepatitis, STD, and TB Prevention. https://www.cdc.gov/nchhstp/

National Center for Immunization and Respiratory Diseases. https://www.cdc.gov/ncird/

World Health Organization websites on infectious disease. https://www.who.int/topics/infectious_diseases/en/

U.S. Department of Health and Human Services. *Secretary's Minority AIDS Initiative Fund*. https://www.hiv.gov.

Print Resources

Bennett JE, Dolin R, Blaser MJ, eds. *Mandell, Douglas, and Bennett's Principles and Practice of Infectious Diseases*. 8th ed. Philadelphia, PA: Elsevier/Saunders; 2015.

Levinson W, Chin-Hong P, Joyce EA, et al., eds. *Review of Medical Microbiology and Immunology. A Guide to Clinical Infectious Diseases*. 15th ed. New York, NY: McGraw-Hill; 2018.

Ryan KJ, Ray GC, Ahmad N, et al., eds. *Sherris Medical Microbiology*. 7th ed. New York, NY: McGraw-Hill; 2018.

Wright WF, ed. *Essentials of Clinical Infectious Diseases*. 2nd ed. New York, NY: Springer/Demos Medical; 2018.

THE IMMUNE SYSTEM AND LEUKOCYTE FUNCTION

Jo Kirman and Raffaela Ghittoni

THE CLINICAL CONTEXT

The immune system is exceedingly complex in its constituent cells, molecules, and signaling pathways. Each major component of the immune system is critical for survival; immune activity protects against infections that would quickly be lethal without immune defenses and eliminates cells in the stages of cancerous transformation.

The most common and major disorders of the immune system are related to immune activity that exceeds physiological needs. Hypersensitivity in the form of allergies occurs in 10% to 20% of the population. The prevalence of allergies increased in the developed world from the 1960s through the early 2000s, after which it began to plateau. Allergies were less common in the developing world but are now increasing in prevalence. Autoimmune disorders affect 2% to 5% of people, with a similar pattern of greater prevalence in developed countries but a trend of increasing numbers of cases in the developing world.[1]

Although less common than immune hyperactivity, disorders in which immune activity is below normal leave an individual susceptible to dangerous infections. In some individuals, immune activity is compromised to an extent that those affected are at risk for major illness or even death. Primary immunodeficiency disorders, which generally present in childhood as a result of genetic mutations, are rare but very severe. In 2012, the U.S. prevalence of primary immunodeficiency disorders was 126.8 per 100,000.[2] The most common immunodeficiency disorder occurs secondary to HIV infection. In the United States, an estimated 1.1 million people were living with HIV infection at the end of 2015, about 0.3% of the population.[3] Globally, in 2017, it was estimated that 36.9 million people were living with HIV, almost 0.5% of the population.[4]

ROLE OF THE IMMUNE SYSTEM

The human body is warm, moist, and full of nutrients, with a stable pH—all optimal living conditions for many microorganisms. There are at least as many bacterial cells as human cells in the human body, as well as countless viruses, protozoa, and fungi. Collectively, these organisms are known as the *human microbiota*, and for the most part they consist of commensal organisms that coexist with humans without causing overt disease—even providing physiological benefits such as protection against pathogens and aiding digestion and nutrient absorption. However, the human body constantly faces attack by disease-causing microorganisms known as pathogens. Pathogens express virulence factors that allow them to outcompete their commensal counterparts and, in doing so, cause damage and disease.

To defend ourselves against pathogenic microbial attack, and to maintain homeostasis with commensal organisms, humans have evolved a complex and highly orchestrated system of cells, tissues, and organs that are collectively referred to as the *immune system*. Cytokines are circulating protein molecules produced and secreted by immune cells to promote proliferation and activation of other immune cells. Among the cytokines, there are dozens of interleukins (ILs), so-named because they were originally identified as secreted products of leukocytes (white blood cells). Cells of the immune system are equipped with cell-surface receptors and secreted molecules that act as environmental sensors to detect and respond to foreign or *non-self* molecules and to molecules that are commonly associated with pathogens. The potent immune response systems are held in check by many inhibitory signals and mechanisms, which prevent undue hyperresponsiveness.

In addition to external threats, the immune system is capable of responding to abnormal *self* molecules, such as mutated self-proteins expressed by tumor cells, or organs received from a donor in the case of transplantation. Therefore, the immune system is a multifaceted defense force that serves to protect the human body from infection, toxins, cancer, and any tissue that is detected as an invader or non-self. The cells of the immune system circulate in the bloodstream to the body tissues and via the lymphatic system back to the bloodstream, conducting constant surveillance and attacking invaders.

Like other body systems, in some individuals, the immune system fails to function normally. This can occur from inherited or spontaneous mutations in critical genes encoding molecules of the immune system, or it can be acquired from infectious or environmental exposures. Failure of the immune system to function appropriately can result in aberrant immune responses to harmless molecules in the environments (such as food or pollen, causing *allergy* or *hypersensitivity*) or to self-molecules (leading to *autoimmune disease*). Alternatively, the impaired immune system might fail to respond to pathogens or fail to maintain homeostasis with harmless microbes or commensal organisms, which can lead to severe disease (*immunodeficiency*).

This chapter summarizes the basic concepts of immunology, which is the biomedical science that studies all aspects of the immune system: its cells, molecules, and functions in health and disease. Unlike the other organ systems covered in this text, tools to study the intricacies of immune cell function took many years to develop, and many aspects of immune function are still being elucidated. The complexity and rapid pace of discovery in immunology are exciting and clinically promising, even as they present challenges in staying current in this fast-moving field.

INTRODUCTION TO HOST DEFENSES

Similar to an army that defends its host country by establishing multiple specialized branches, each with highly trained soldiers and equipment, the immune system has three different layers of defense, each with its own specialized cells and molecules. These layers of defense are (a) the physical and chemical barriers, (b) the innate immune system, and (c) the adaptive immune system (**Figure 6.1**). General mechanisms of each of these layers are described in this section,

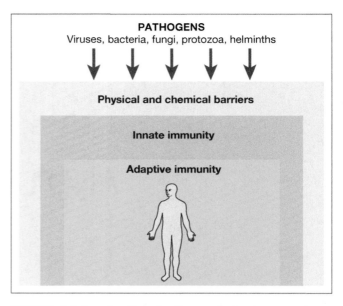

FIGURE 6.1 Levels of protection against microorganisms. There are three levels of protection against pathogens: physical and chemical barriers include surface protections intrinsic to skin and mucous membranes, innate immunity that is nonspecific and results in acute inflammation while also initiating the next step of protection, and adaptive immunity that is specific and long-lasting.

followed by more detailed descriptions of innate and adaptive immune cells and functions.

OVERVIEW OF PHYSICAL AND CHEMICAL BARRIERS

The first layer of immune defense encountered by a pathogen comprises the physical and chemical barriers of the skin and mucosal surfaces (**Figure 6.2**).

- Skin covers the outside of the human body, with an outer layer of dead cells and underlying layers of densely packed living cells (the epidermis and dermis) that provide a strong physical barrier against penetration by pathogenic microorganisms. Regular shedding of the outer, dead cells of the epidermal layer further contributes to the physical removal of microbes.
- Skin also produces chemical defenses against invasion and colonization through the secretion of sebum (a low-pH, oily, waxy substance) and sweat (high in salt, with antimicrobial enzymes) by sebaceous glands and sweat glands in the dermal layer. Antimicrobial peptides secreted by the skin, such as cathelicidins, can be directly antimicrobial and also can activate production of other effector immune molecules. The acidic, salty environment, as well as the production of antimicrobial peptides and enzymes, function together to limit or prevent microbial growth on the skin.

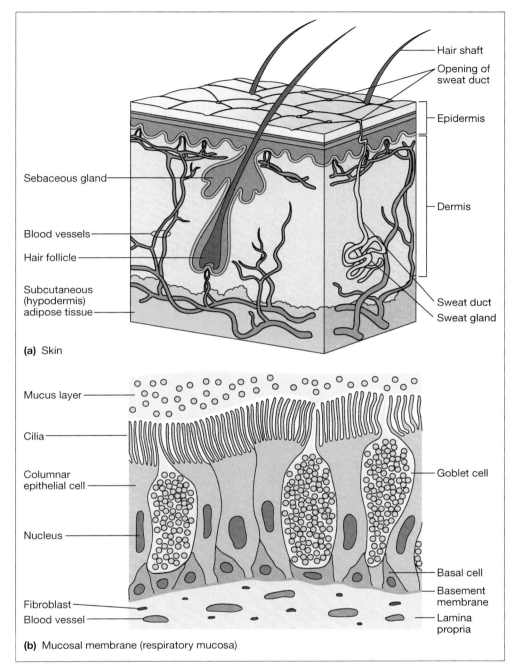

(a) Skin

(b) Mucosal membrane (respiratory mucosa)

FIGURE 6.2 Physical barriers of skin and mucosa. These regions physically interact with substances and microorganisms in the environment and commensals.

- Mucosal surfaces line the cavities of the body that are exposed to air and ingested substances. In contrast to the skin, the outer layer of the mucosa is alive and contains specialized cells that produce mucus, a thick, viscous fluid that coats the outer layer of cells and functions to trap and expel microbes.
- Cells that line the respiratory tract have short hair-like projections on their surface called *cilia*. In healthy individuals, the cilia beat in tandem to expel particles trapped in the mucus up and out of the upper and lower respiratory tract. Failure of the mucociliary transport system can lead to lung disease, such as chronic obstructive pulmonary disease, pneumonia, and increased risk of infection. Cigarette smoking impairs the structure and function of cilia, contributing to the development of smoking-induced respiratory disease.

- The antimicrobial enzyme lysozyme is abundant in mucus and tears, acting as a chemical barrier for mucosal surfaces. Lysozyme functions by disrupting the cell walls of certain bacteria, causing the bacterial cells to rupture and die.

The gastrointestinal tract has its own extensive immune system, summarized briefly here and described in more detail in Chapter 13, Gastrointestinal Tract.

The initial defenses of the immune system effectively parry a vast array of microbial assaults. Nonetheless, at times pathogenic microbes are able to bypass or avoid these physical and chemical barriers, taking advantage of damage or abrasions to enter through the physical barriers or by producing substances that allow them to resist chemical defenses.

OVERVIEW OF THE INNATE IMMUNE RESPONSE

The second layer of immune defense is the innate arm of the immune system. The innate immune system comprises fast-acting cells and molecules that recognize common features of pathogens, rather than specific types of pathogens.

- This broad response is orchestrated by circulating white blood cells and tissue-resident scavenger cells, which act quickly to recruit additional immune cells to sites of infection and trauma using chemical gradients and signals from molecules known as cytokines and chemokines. The innate immune cells become activated to ingest and destroy any invading microorganisms.
- Cells of the innate immune response are generated continuously from multipotent bone marrow stem cells and can rapidly proliferate in response to appropriate signals of infection and pathogen invasion.
- Molecules of innate immunity include proteins of the complement cascade, a system that directly attacks and lyses bacteria, while promoting other aspects of innate and adaptive immunity. The timing of the cell and molecular innate responses is crucial to contain the replication of pathogens and to prevent the spread of the disease in the host.

Innate immunity is generally very efficient, and is not specific to a particular pathogen. Importantly, the cells of the innate arm of the immune response are able to interact and communicate with cells of the third layer of immune defense—the adaptive immune response (**Figure 6.3**).

OVERVIEW OF THE ADAPTIVE IMMUNE RESPONSE

Although slower to respond than the innate arm of the immune system, the adaptive immune response is highly specific for a particular pathogen and qualitatively and quantitatively improves during the course of the response. Upon resolution of the immune response,

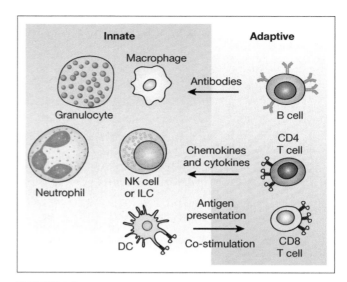

FIGURE 6.3 Cellular and molecular communication between innate and adaptive immune cells. Both arms of the immune system have signals that modulate the responses of the other. DC, dendritic cell; ILC, innate lymphoid cell; NK, natural killer (cell).

a small number of these highly specialized cells are retained in the body and can persist for decades. Some of these cells, such as T-helper lymphocytes, are modulatory and function to promote the activity of other cells. Other adaptive immune cells, such as B lymphocytes and cytotoxic T lymphocytes (CTLs), are *effector* cells that are directly involved in targeting and destroying antigens and foreign cells. Upon any future encounters, these memory cells are able to efficiently promote pathogen neutralization or elimination so quickly that there may not be clinical signs of infection. This remarkable feature of the adaptive response is known as *immunological memory*. Immunological memory by adaptive immune cells is the mechanism upon which vaccination is based.

- B and T lymphocytes mediate adaptive immune responses. Both B and T cells recognize highly specific parts of pathogens, called *antigens*. B cells recognize free antigen located in extracellular compartments of the body, whereas T cells can recognize both intracellular and extracellular peptide antigen but require other cells to *present* the peptides to them on cell-surface molecules called the *major histocompatibility complex* (MHC). A given B or T cell always only recognizes one type of antigen; therefore, each B or T cell has a single specificity.
- When activated, B cells synthesize and secrete highly specific Y-shaped molecules called *antibodies* that can inactivate, neutralize, or label pathogens or toxins. B cells express the same antibody on their cell surface, which forms the antigen-recognition component of the B-cell receptor (BCR). Signaling a naive or antigen-inexperienced B cell through the BCR enables that B cell to become activated and produce

antibodies. Activated B-cell clones start to divide, leading to *clonal expansion*. This expansion can result in many, many thousands of B cells, which all recognize and produce antibody for the same antigen. The antibody-mediated immune response is sometimes referred to as the *humoral immune response*.

- T cells recognize antigen through highly specific receptors, known as T-cell receptors (TCRs), expressed on their cell surface. Although many copies of the TCR are present on the surface of an individual T cell, the TCRs of that cell are all of the same specificity. However, owing to the genetic variation introduced through somatic gene recombination events in the thymus, there are millions of different T cells present in the body, each with their own TCR specificity and the capacity to proliferate upon recognition of their specific antigen.
- There are two types of T cells: the *CD4 T cell*, which is sometimes referred to as a *T-helper cell* (*Th cell*), and the *CD8 T cell*, sometimes referred to as a CTL. CD4 T cells primarily function to produce cytokines, which can activate innate cells and support B-cell and CD8 T-cell responses. CD8 T cells function to lyse cells infected by intracellular bacteria,

virus-infected cells, or tumor cells. CD refers to cluster of differentiation, and signifies specific membrane proteins found on the surface of lymphocytes and many immune cells.

Although the innate and adaptive immune responses have distinct characteristics (summarized in **Table 6.1**), their functions overlap and are interconnected. The innate and adaptive immune cells cooperate through a mutual exchange of signals and mediators to provide efficient protection from pathogens, toxins, and cancer (see **Figure 6.3**). These processes are described in more detail in the next sections.

Thought Questions

1. What is the "big picture" of the role of the immune system in maintaining homeostasis?

2. What are the general principles involved in protection provided by the innate and adaptive immune systems?

TABLE 6.1 Characteristics of Innate and Adaptive Immunity

Feature	Innate	Adaptive

Pathogen recognition	Broad—pathogen recognition receptors for:
	• PAMPs
	  › Pathogen surface markers: lipopolysaccharide, flagellin, di- and tri-acyl-lipopeptides, peptidoglycan, zymosan, mannose
	  › Intracellular pathogen markers—dsRNA, ssRNA, unmethylated CpG, DNA
	• DAMPs—tissue injury signals (sterile inflammation)
		Highly specific—epitopes of microorganisms, foreign proteins, modified self-proteins, modified self-cells

Initiation time	Fast; minutes to hours	Slow; days to weeks
Memory	Absent or broad enhancement *"trained immunity"*	Specific enhanced (faster and better quality) responses to subsequent exposure
Diversity of response	Low	Extremely high; increases during the course of the response
Major molecules and mechanisms	Physical and chemical barriers; antimicrobial molecules; phagocytosis; complement; cytokines; chemokines	Antigen-specific receptors: BCR and TCR, antibodies, cytokines, cytolysis
Major cell types	Phagocytes (macrophages, dendritic cells); granulocytes (neutrophils, eosinophils, mast cells, basophils); innate lymphoid cells (NK cells and ILCs)	B and T lymphocytes

BCR, B-cell receptor; unmethylated CpG, dinucleotide cytosine-guanine sequences common to microbes; DAMP, danger-associated molecular pattern; dsDNA, double-stranded DNA; ILC, innate lymphoid cell; NK, natural killer; PAMP, pathogen-associated molecular pattern; ssRNA, single-stranded RNA; TCR, T-cell receptor.

FUNCTIONAL ANATOMY OF THE IMMUNE SYSTEM

The specialized organs and tissues of the immune system are termed *lymphoid organs* and *lymphoid tissues*. They are separated into primary and secondary lymphoid organs and tissues based on their function (**Figure 6.4**). Primary lymphoid organs and tissues are the site of immune cell development and include the thymus, where T cells develop, and the bone marrow, where B cells develop. Both T and B cells, as well as cells of the innate immune system, develop from multipotent precursor stem cells that reside in the bone marrow. The secondary lymphoid organs and tissues are the sites of adaptive immune cell activation and include the lymph nodes and lymphatic vessels, in which cells respond to damage and infection of the tissues, and the spleen, where immune responses to blood-borne pathogens are initiated. The lymphatic network provides T and B cells with the ability to recirculate through the tissues, lymph, and blood, allowing them to constantly patrol and survey the body for signs of infection.

HEMATOPOIESIS

In humans, hematopoiesis occurs in the bone marrow, where multipotent precursor stem cells, known as hematopoietic stem cells (HSCs), are supported to survive, proliferate, and differentiate by mesenchymal stem cells. HSCs are self-renewing, meaning that they can divide to make more precursor cells. The HSCs can develop into the major cellular constituents of blood: red blood cells, platelets, and white blood cells of the innate and adaptive immune system (**Table 6.2**).

The three blood lineages that develop from HSCs are the *erythroid lineage*, which develops into red blood cells (also referred to as erythrocytes) and platelet-producing megakaryocytes, and the *myeloid* and *lymphoid lineages*, which both can develop into white blood cells (also referred to as leukocytes). The myeloid lineage

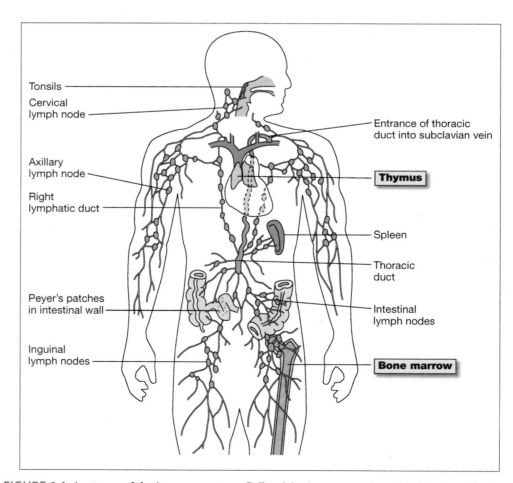

FIGURE 6.4 Anatomy of the immune system. Cells of the immune system circulate from the bone marrow to primary and secondary lymphoid tissues, moving through blood and lymph vessels, and sometimes stationary in primary and secondary lymphoid tissues.

TABLE 6.2 Concentration and Frequency of Cells in Human Blood

Cell Type	Cells/mm³	Total Leukocytes (%)
Red blood cells	5.0×10^6	
Platelets	2.5×10^5	
Leukocytes	7.3×10^3	
Neutrophil	$3.7–5.1 \times 10^3$	50–70
Lymphocyte	$1.5–3.0 \times 10^3$	20–40
Monocyte	$1–4.4 \times 10^2$	1–6
Eosinophil	$1–2.2 \times 10^2$	1–3
Basophil	$<1.3 \times 10^2$	<1

Source: From Owen JA, Punt J, Stranford SA. Kuby Immunology. 7th ed. W.H. Freeman Company; 2013, Table 2-1.

originates from a specialized progenitor cell derived from the HSC, known as the common myeloid progenitor, which can differentiate into granulocytes (neutrophils, eosinophils, basophils, and mast cells) as well as mononuclear cells, including monocytes, macrophages, and certain dendritic cells. The lymphoid lineage develops from the common lymphoid progenitor and gives rise to T and B lymphocytes, natural killer (NK) cells, innate lymphoid cells (ILCs), and some types of dendritic cell (**Figure 6.5**).

CELLS AND TISSUES OF THE IMMUNE SYSTEM

B Cells Develop in the Bone Marrow

To recognize the vast array of different carbohydrates and proteins expressed by different pathogens with a high degree of specificity, an equally vast range of B cells, each with its own unique antigen specificity, must exist. As previously noted, B cells recognize antigen through their BCR. The BCR has the same structure and specificity as the antibody it goes on to secrete during an immune response. Each B cell expresses $\sim 10^5$ BCRs on its cell surface, all with the same antigen specificity. Therefore, billions of different B cells exist in the body, each able to respond to a unique specific antigen.

To encode such a vast range of different BCRs, the human genome, which encodes only ~20,000 proteins, would need to be orders of magnitude larger. To circumvent this, the genes that encode the antigen-binding (variable) region of the BCR are expressed in segments (**Box 6.1** and **Figure 6.6**). Dozens of different options for each gene segment combine together in a kind of mix-and-match fashion to create the great BCR diversity required with very few genes. This process, called

somatic gene rearrangement, occurs in B-cell precursors in the bone marrow. Because the BCR has two chains, heavy and light, and each rearranges its genes encoding the variable region independently, this process increases the possibility of generating different unique antigen-binding sites on the receptor.

Gene rearrangement does not depend on antigen, so an antigen-specific B cell can develop well before exposure to a given pathogen. As the gene rearrangement process occurs, the new BCRs are tested. During development, B cells with nonproductive BCRs or self-reactive BCRs are deleted or made nonresponsive so that the B cells that survive are functional and unlikely to lead to autoimmune disease. Each day billions of new B cells enter the circulation from bone marrow. Naive B cells survive for only a few weeks if they do not encounter antigen. Therefore, the process of developing new B cells continues in the bone marrow throughout life.

T Cells Develop in the Thymus

The thymus is a primary lymphoid organ critical for T-cell development early in life. At birth, the human thymus is fully developed; however, after 1 year of age, the thymus begins to involute (shrink) and its function reduces. Naive (antigen-inexperienced) T cells generated by the thymus are long-lived or self-renewing in the periphery, meaning that loss of thymic function with age does not impair T-cell driven immunity over a lifetime.

Progenitor cells from the bone marrow enter the thymus, becoming *thymocytes*—cells that are committed to the T-cell lineage. In a manner similar to the way B-cell precursors in the bone marrow rearrange the antibody variable genes, thymocytes in the thymus undergo a process of somatic gene rearrangement that leads to the development of an antigen-specific TCR.

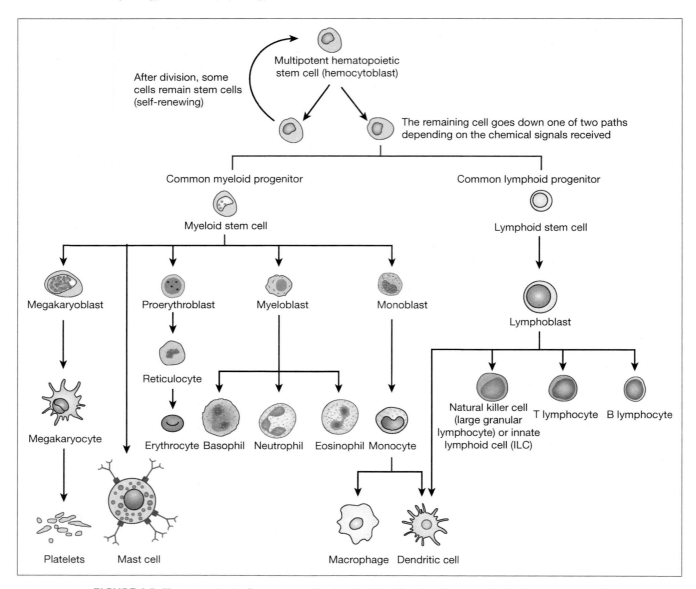

FIGURE 6.5 Hematopoiesis. Generation of red and white blood cells occurs in the bone marrow. A multipotent stem cell can follow a myeloid or lymphoid path before further differentiating to final forms of the cells shown.

The TCR is made up of two polypeptide chains: most commonly, the TCR α chain and the TCR β chain (**Box 6.2** and **Figure 6.7**). Each chain has a variable region and a constant region. The variable domain includes the region that recognizes peptide antigens that are bound to MHC molecules. Similar to the gene segments that encode the antigen-binding regions of BCRs, the TCR variable region is also encoded by gene segments, and for each segment of the TCR there are multiple distinct alternatives encoded in the germline genome. In a developing T cell, one option for each gene segment is selected to recombine with the other selected segments to create a unique TCR. In this way,

enormous diversity in the TCRs expressed in the human body is achieved with a limited number of genes.

Each developing T cell will express multiple TCRs of a single specificity on its cell surface. Therefore, each T cell will recognize only one type of antigenic peptide. Most T cells will express an αβ TCR, which is made up of the α and β chains. However, a small number of T cells express a different type of receptor made up of γ and δ chains; these cells are referred to as γδ T cells. The γδ TCR is encoded by a different set of gene segments, and this different type of TCR leads to different cellular functions.

Developing T cells commit to becoming a CD4 T cell or a CD8 T cell in the thymus, by expressing

- B-cell receptors and antibodies are composed of two heavy (H) chains and two light (L) chains forming the shape of the letter Y (**Figure 6.6**). The stem is the Fc (constant fragment) region, consisting only of heavy chain components and having consistent amino acid composition determined by an antibody's class. The two antigen-binding regions (Fab) are made up of the terminal ends of heavy and light chains.

- The genes coding for these regions have multiple diverse segments (shown as different blocks within the gene's diversity and variable regions) that are shuffled during B-cell development. Unused portions of the genes are discarded, and the remaining portions are rejoined in a relatively random fashion, producing the *rearranged DNA*. Because of this gene rearrangement, proteins translated from the final light and heavy chain genes are extraordinarily diverse.

- Each B cell recognizes its specific antigen out of millions of possible antigens, and the millions of B cells constitute a repertoire able to respond to most if not all possible antigens encountered throughout a lifetime.

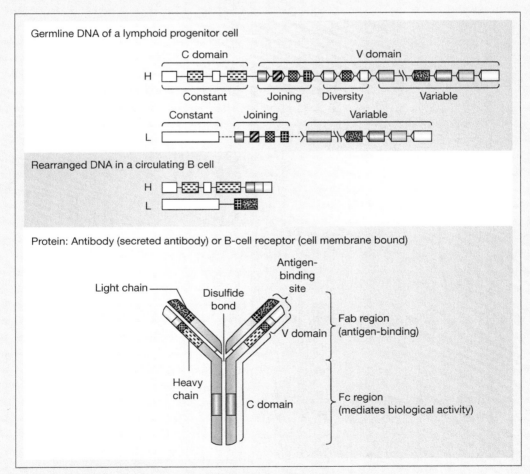

FIGURE 6.6 B-cell receptor gene arrangement and antibody structure.

either the CD4 or the CD8 *co-receptor* along with the TCR on their cell surface. Although these co-receptors do not directly bind antigen, they do bind to the MHC molecules that present the antigen to the TCR. Because CD4 T cells recognize only MHC class II and CD8 T cells recognize only MHC class I, the type of peptide antigens recognized by CD4 T cells and CD8 T cells is different. Once mature, CD4 and CD8 T cells go on to play distinct roles in the immune response, described later in this chapter.

BOX 6.2
T-Cell Receptor Gene Rearrangement

- The process of gene rearrangement with variable and constant regions is similar between B cells and T cells. Most T-cell receptors (TCRs) are of the $\alpha\beta$ type, where the gene coding for α chains has several possible variable (V) and joining (J) regions and a constant (C) region, and the gene coding for the β chains has V and J regions as well as diversity (D) regions (**Figure 6.7**).

- As with B cells, rearrangement of coding sequences for both α and β chains confers tremendous diversity of antigen-recognition sites of TCRs, and a broad repertoire of recognition sites for antigens encountered throughout the life span.

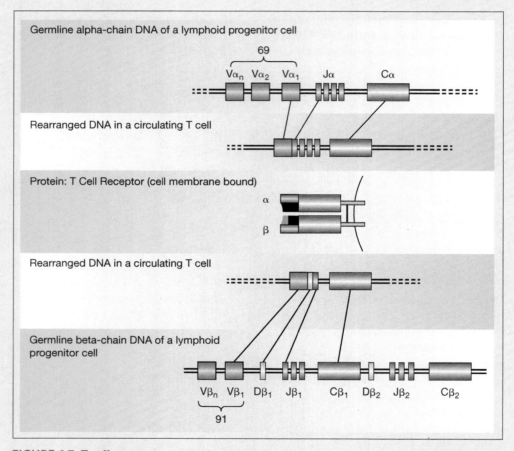

FIGURE 6.7 T-cell receptor gene rearrangement.

The gene rearrangement process enables the development of highly diverse TCRs to create a broad and rich repertoire of antigen-specific T cells throughout the body. This is important so that T cells are able to recognize the great diversity of antigens expressed by pathogens to which the human body is routinely exposed. A cost of the gene rearrangement process is that some of the TCRs either will not be functional or will recognize and respond to self-antigen. Because recognition of self-antigen can lead to autoimmunity, the newly expressed TCRs are tested in the thymus to ensure they are functional (a process termed *positive selection*), and they are tested for self-reactivity and deleted if they are activated by self-antigen (a process termed *negative selection*). Negative selection prevents the release of lymphocytes that could potentially damage body tissues and trigger an autoimmune response. Alternatively, some developing self-reactive T lymphocytes survive but become unresponsive (*anergic*) or differentiate into suppressive cells known as *regulatory T cells* (Tregs).

B Cells and T Cells Circulate Through the Lymphatic System

Lymphatic vessels drain interstitial fluid and allow movement of white blood cells from the tissues. After entering these vessels, the fluid is known as lymph. The fluid moves through the network of lymph nodes that are located at the junction of lymphatic vessels, eventually returning to the blood via the thoracic duct (see **Figure 6.4**). Lymph flow is powered by muscle contractions during body movement, and backflow is prevented by one-way valves in the lymphatic vessels. Lack of movement or damage to the lymphatic vessels or valves can lead to accumulation of lymph in the tissues, known as **edema**. This type of swelling in the arms and hands is a common complication following radiation therapy or cancer surgery and is due to damage to the local lymphatic network.

The lymph node has a highly structured architecture that aids immune surveillance (**Figure 6.8**). Cells and fluid from the tissues enter the lymph node via *afferent lymphatic vessels*. Then, responding to chemical gradients, newly arriving T and B cells move into separate parts of the lymph node. Lymphoid follicles are predominantly populated with B cells, and as B cells respond and proliferate in response to antigen they form circular structures known as germinal centers within the B-cell follicle. The germinal center is highly dynamic, increasing in size as the immune response progresses and decreasing in size as the response resolves. This can lead to enlarged lymph nodes, which are common during infection, particularly under the chin (submandibular) or in the neck (cervical), armpits (axillary), and groin (femoral and inguinal lymph nodes). Discrete T-cell areas are adjacent to the lymphoid follicles, allowing T and B cells to interact. Cells leave the lymph node to return to the blood via the *efferent lymphatic vessel*.

The Spleen

The spleen is composed of red pulp, where damaged or senescent red blood cells are removed, and scattered nodules of white pulp, in which T and B cells respond to blood-borne antigen (**Figure 6.9**). Like the lymph node, the white pulp of the spleen is organized into clear T- and B-cell areas, with T cells mainly located near the arteriole in the periarteriolar lymphoid sheath and B cells within the lymphoid follicle, adjacent to the T cells. A unique feature of the spleen is the presence of the marginal zone, which surrounds the white pulp and is bordered by the perifollicular zone. Resident within the marginal zone are specialized macrophages as well as innate-like B cells, known as marginal zone B cells, which are clonally distinct from conventional adaptive B cells. In humans, marginal zone B cells can circulate throughout the body, and they are associated with protection from bacterial and viral infections, including HIV.

Following injury or rupture, the spleen may be removed to stem internal bleeding. Individuals whose spleen is removed, as well as those with the rare condition of congenital asplenia, are predisposed to the development of several bacterial infections. This susceptibility highlights the critical function of the spleen in controlling blood-borne pathogens.

Gut-Associated Lymphoid Tissue

The mucosal immune system, separate from the immune system surveying the blood, protects the surfaces where

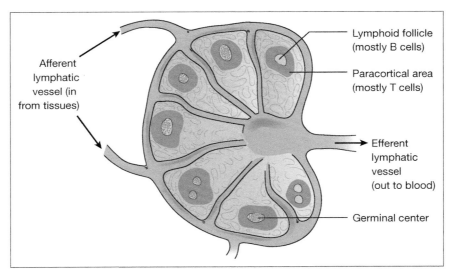

FIGURE 6.8 The lymph node. Lymph nodes are located along lymphatic vessel pathways from the tissues to the thoracic and right lymphatic ducts that empty into the systemic venous circulation. Within lymphoid follicles, T cells and B cells that are specific to the same antigen can be drawn together and provide co-stimulation that promotes development of mature lymphocytes, antibody production, and ultimately memory cells.

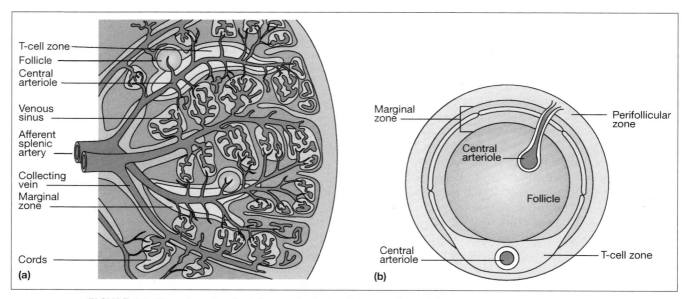

FIGURE 6.9 The spleen has both hematological and immunological functions. **(a)** The splenic artery enters the organ and branches into central arterioles. White-pulp areas represent lymphoid zones, containing a T-cell zone, B-cell follicles, and arterioles. The red pulp consists of cords transitioning into venous sinuses that drain to the splenic vein. **(b)** The white pulp.

pathogens often invade: body orifices and surfaces that come in contact with the environment (eyes, nose, mouth, throat, gut, lungs, vagina, uterus). Here we highlight the highly developed gut-associated lymphoid tissue (GALT). GALT comprises three secondary lymphoid tissue types: the Peyer patches, the isolated lymphoid follicles, and the mesenteric lymph nodes. The GALT is the largest lymphoid organ in the human body, functioning to support tolerance to highly diverse commensal gut microorganisms, while maintaining the ability to respond to food-borne pathogens. As with the spleen and peripheral lymph nodes, GALT tissues have a highly organized structure with distinct T- and B-cell zones. Outside the secondary lymphoid tissue, effector lymphocytes are scattered throughout the gut epithelium and lamina propria. In addition to their presence in the blood and lymphoid tissues, noted previously, cells of the immune system can be found throughout the body. Innate and adaptive immune cells are strategically positioned within the peripheral tissues, fat, and organs, as well as in skin and mucosal tissue, poised to combat invading pathogens, neutralize toxins, and kill cancerous cells.

Thought Questions

3. **What are the major tissues and organs of the immune system, and what is the role of each?**

4. **How does gene rearrangement endow B and T cells with the ability to recognize a wide variety of potential antigens?**

INNATE IMMUNITY

Innate immunity immediately leaps into action when protective barriers such as skin and mucous membranes are breached. There are many different cells of the innate immune system, each with its own specialized function. A major function of the innate immune response is to *vacuum up* debris and pathogens in a process known as phagocytosis. The term *phagocyte* comes from the Greek words *phagos* meaning *eat* and *cyte* meaning *cell*; therefore, in phagocytosis the cell ingests solid particles, such as microorganisms or cellular debris. Neutrophils, macrophages, and dendritic cells are all highly phagocytic cells that help engulf and then destroy pathogens.

Various molecules—including those derived from arachidonic acid, cytokines, reactive nitrogen and oxygen species, proteases, and enzymes of the complement system—contribute to escalate the innate immune response and destroy invading pathogens to restore healthy tissue structure and function.

ACUTE INFLAMMATION

Acute inflammation develops as a consequence of innate immune activation. Mast cells, macrophages, and related sentinel cells detect tissue damage and invasion, rapidly initiating the inflammatory cascade. Pathogen-specific signals activate tissue-resident innate cells and trigger components of the complement system, leading to the production of chemotactic signals that stimulate the movement of leukocytes (mainly neutrophils and monocytes) from the circulation into the tissue at the site of injury or infection. Activated mast cells and macrophages at the site of injury or infection release chemical mediators, such as histamine, that increase blood vessel permeability and cause local blood vessels to dilate, increasing blood flow to the area. Endothelial cells lining the blood vessels upregulate membrane proteins that bind to leukocytes to assist their movement from blood to tissue. Once in the tissue, neutrophils and monocytes differentiate into a highly active state, with increased ability to phagocytose pathogens and generate additional inflammatory mediators. Activated phagocytes kill microbes and contribute to escalating vasodilation, leukocyte recruitment, and inflammation. **Box 6.3** and **Figure 6.10** visually summarize these steps in the acute inflammatory response.

INNATE IMMUNE CELLS

Innate immunity depends on circulating leukocytes and on sentinel cells within tissues that conduct ongoing surveillance for chemical signals of tissue damage and pathogen invasion. White blood cells include the granulocytes (containing cytoplasmic granules) and agranulocytes (see **Table 6.2**). Neutrophils, eosinophils, and basophils are the granulocytes, in descending order of abundance in the blood. Mast cells are similar to basophils in containing histamine granules, but they reside in tissues, rather than in the circulation. Agranulocytes have smaller granules, not visible by light microscope. Monocytes and lymphocytes are the circulating agranulocytes. Monocytes continuously leave the circulation and enter the tissues, where they enlarge and differentiate, becoming macrophages. Lymphocytes circulate between the blood, lymph vessels, and lymph nodes. The principal leukocytes that mediate acute inflammation are neutrophils and monocytes/macrophages.

Neutrophils

Neutrophils, also known as polymorphonuclear leukocytes (PMNs) for the multilobed shape of their nucleus, are highly motile and phagocytic and become activated quickly in response to tissue injury and infection.[5] They are by far the most abundant white blood cells circulating in the blood, representing 50% to 70% of all leukocytes.

A complete blood count with differential white cell count (*CBC with differential*) is the laboratory evaluation of absolute and relative numbers of leukocytes (see **Table 6.2**). In cases of acute infection, it is common to observe leukocytosis, an increase in white cell count, generally associated with an increase in neutrophil count. The neutrophil production rate can increase up to ten times in response to infection and the associated increase in colony-stimulating factors secreted by macrophages.

In severe acute infection, the blood smear composition can reveal significantly increased numbers and proportions of immature neutrophils. The relative increase in immature cells detected in the blood sample is the result of rapid movement of mature neutrophils into tissues,

and increased bone marrow production and release of immature neutrophils. The immature cells, called *band* or *stab* cells, are easily recognizable by the characteristic shape of their nucleus. Compared with mature neutrophils, in which chromatin appears in three to five clumps, the nucleus of immature neutrophils is less segmented, appearing as a single *band* across the cell.

The neutrophil life span averages 24 hours. After entering the circulation from the bone marrow, neutrophils circulate in the vascular system for up to 12 hours before being recruited into tissues to respond to injury or invasion. Once in the tissue, the neutrophils conduct their job of phagocytosis of invaders before dying. Macrophages remove the cellular debris of dead neutrophils and other remnants of the inflammatory response from tissues.

Neutrophils are highly phagocytic cells, able to ingest and kill thousands of bacteria before dying. They have two mechanisms of bactericidal activity: exposure of bacteria to toxic oxygen compounds known as reactive oxygen species (ROS), and degradation of bacteria by protease and other enzymes. Specialized neutrophil organelles and enzymes generate ROS as oxygen-derived free radicals via a burst of oxidative chemical activity. Together with ROS, phagocyte lysosomes contain many proteases that are able to break down bacterial proteins. These chemicals are very efficient in eliminating pathogens but are also highly toxic, potentially causing secondary tissue damage to the host. Consequently, the oxidative burst is limited to states of strong neutrophil activation resulting from the presence of bacteria or other alert signals. Moreover, the body has endogenous processes protecting against the ROS and the proteases released from neutrophils and macrophages. One example of these protective compounds is the enzyme α_1-antitrypsin, which counteracts the action of particular proteases.

An additional defense mechanism restricted to neutrophils has been recently identified. When faced with overwhelming numbers of bacteria, neutrophils can combine and organize themselves into a *neutrophil extracellular trap* (NET). Activated neutrophils in the process of dying release their DNA into the extracellular space (**Figure 6.11**). At this point, chromatin from many neutrophils starts to aggregate, generating a sticky trap for bacteria. Antimicrobial enzymes and ROS contained in neutrophil granules are also released in the extracellular compartment, targeting the entrapped bacteria for destruction. NETs are implicated in the pathophysiology of cystic fibrosis complications, preeclampsia, and some autoimmune diseases.[6]

Basophils, Mast Cells, and Eosinophils

Among the granulocytes, three other cell types are present in the blood or tissue: basophils, mast cells, and eosinophils. Basophils and mast cells are related nonphagocytic granulocytes. Although rare, basophils

Steps in the Acute Inflammatory Response

TISSUE DAMAGE ACTIVATES RESIDENT CELLS (FIGURE 6.10a)

- Trauma damages tissue and allows pathogen invasion, signaled by danger- and pathogen-associated molecular patterns.

- Mast cells and macrophages release histamine and cytokines, respectively.

- Vasodilation and increased vascular permeability begin, increasing blood flow and delivery of cells and proteins to the injured region.

WHITE BLOOD CELLS MOVE TO THE INJURED REGION BY CHEMOTAXIS (FIGURE 6.10b)

- Cytokines, chemokines, and complement protein fragments promote chemotaxis of neutrophils and monocytes to the injured region.

- Antibodies and complement proteins coat bacteria to aid phagocytosis.

- Increased capillary filtration promotes local swelling and edema formation.

- Neutrophils phagocytose bacteria, killing them via an oxidative burst that generates reactive oxygen species and via fusion with lysosomes containing degradative enzymes, particularly proteases.

INFLAMMATION CESSATION AND REPAIR INITIATION (FIGURE 6.10c)

- Macrophages engulf apoptotic neutrophils, cleaning up the injury debris, while releasing antiinflammatory mediators and cytokines to recruit fibroblasts and cells capable of rebuilding the tissue.

RESOLUTION AND RECOVERY (FIGURE 6.10d)

- Macrophage signals stimulate fibroblasts and endothelial cells to support regrowth of tissue and its vascular supply, restoring tissue integrity.

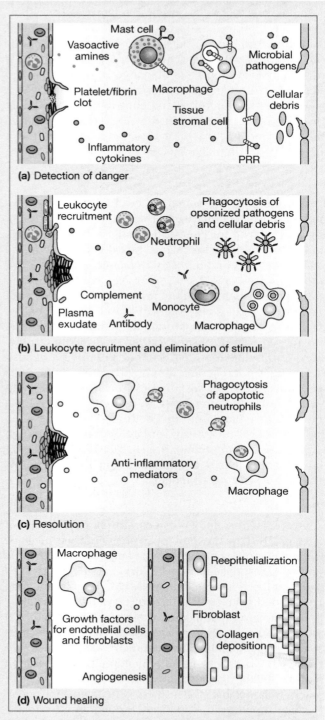

FIGURE 6.10 Steps of acute inflammation: **(a)** detection of danger; **(b)** leukocyte recruitment and elimination of stimuli; **(c)** resolution; **(d)** wound healing. PRR, pattern recognition receptor.

Source: From Raynes JG. *Inflammation: Acute.* Wiley Online Library: eLS (Encyclopedia of Life Sciences). https://doi.org/10.1002/9780470015902.a0000943.pub3

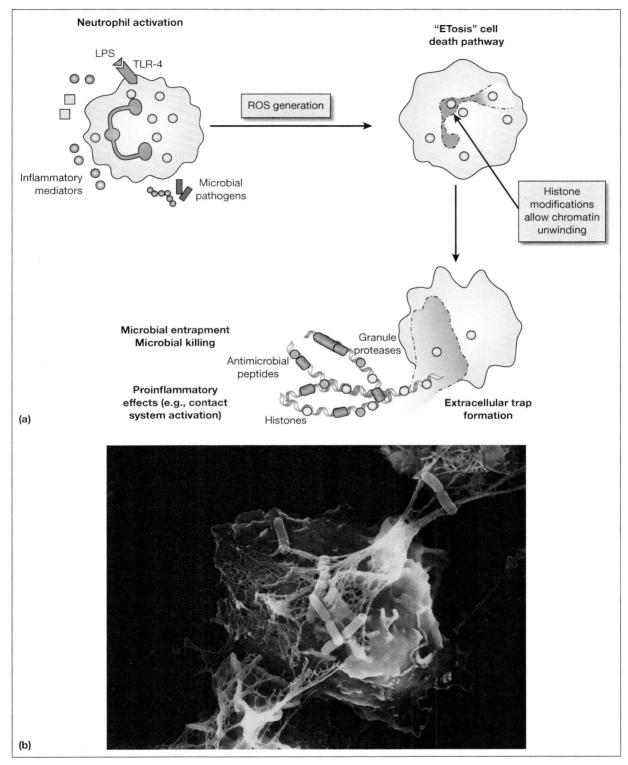

FIGURE 6.11 Neutrophil extracellular traps. (**a**) When neutrophils encounter large numbers of pathogens, they can respond by extruding their DNA and granules as a sticky net that traps and rapidly kills many bacteria at one time. (**b**) Electron micrograph of bacteria (orange) caught in neutrophil extracellular trap (yellow). Although effective at microbe removal, because this is an extracellular reaction, it has the potential to create secondary tissue injury.

ET, extracellular trap; LPS, lipopolysaccharide; ROS, reactive oxygen species; TLR, toll-like receptor.
Source: (b) From Max Planck Institute for Infection Biology.

circulate in the bloodstream, while mast cells reside in tissues, particularly in the connective tissue of skin, on mucosal surfaces, and adjacent to blood vessels. Basophils and mast cells contain granules of proinflammatory chemicals such as histamine. Immediately after tissue injury or during the early phase of an allergic response, these cells degranulate, releasing histamine, a potent mediator of vasodilation. In an allergic response, prompt antihistamine administration can counteract the action of basophils and mast cells and reduce the systemic allergic reaction.

Eosinophils, like neutrophils, are phagocytic granulocytes. Their cytoplasm is filled with granules containing toxic enzymes that are released by exocytosis onto specific targets. Eosinophil granules are capable of killing large targets, such as parasites (helminths), which are too big for phagocytosis. However, eosinophils have a critical role in allergy and hypersensitivity reactions because they tend to participate in the late phase of allergic responses. In asthma, eosinophils in the lung contribute to airway hyperresponsiveness, mucus production, tissue damage, and airway remodeling, as described in Chapter 11, Lungs.

Monocytes and Macrophages

Monocytes, macrophages, and dendritic cells represent other groups of highly phagocytic cells among the agranulocytes. Monocytes generated in the bone marrow enter the bloodstream where they circulate as an immature form of a macrophage. Monocytes migrate into tissues before differentiating into macrophages. In the tissue, monocytes increase their size and phagocytic capacity. There are two types of macrophages. The first type operates beneath epithelial tissue and in several organs, patrolling as sentinels ready to ingest any microorganism able to get through the tissue. The second type circulates between lymph and bloodstream, conducting surveillance for any foreign material. Some cells of the macrophage lineage reside in specific tissue locations to exert their function and are identified by unique names (**Table 6.3**). For example,

TABLE 6.3 Specialized Cells of the Macrophage Lineage

Location	Cell Type
Lung	Alveolar macrophage
Bone	Osteoclast
Connective tissue	Histiocyte
Liver	Kupffer cell
Brain	Microglia
Intestine	Intestinal macrophage
Joint	Synovial macrophage

macrophages found in the liver are known as Kupffer cells. In the central nervous system, microglia display macrophage functions. Synovial macrophages share similar activity in the joints, and alveolar macrophages are found in the lung airways. Macrophages are also located throughout the primary and secondary lymphoid tissues, where they exhibit a range of different phenotypes and functions, depending on their specific location and local signaling mediators.

When infection or injury occurs, sentinel macrophages detect cell damage and migrate to that area by *chemotaxis*, the movement of a cell toward or away from a chemical stimulus (see **Figure 6.10**). Phagocytes use pseudopods to move toward microorganisms or damaged cells to arrive promptly at the site of infection. Pseudopods are temporary cytoplasmic extensions, reaching out from the cell to allow movement. The term *pseudopod* is derived from the Greek words *pseudes* and *podos*, meaning *false feet*. Chemotactic substances that attract monocytes and macrophages include microbial products, components of damaged cells, chemicals released by other white blood cells, and peptides derived from the complement system. Upon activation, macrophages begin to secrete cytokines, particularly IL-1 and tumor necrosis factor (TNF), that contribute to chemotaxis, activate other leukocytes, and signal bone marrow to produce more leukocytes.

Dendritic Cells

The dendritic cell is the most critical cell type for communication between the innate and adaptive arms of the immune response. Derived from either myeloid or lymphoid precursors, dendritic cells are a diverse subset of immune cells located throughout the body, including the skin (Langerhans cells and dermal dendritic cells), primary lymphoid tissues (e.g., follicular dendritic cells in the thymus), secondary lymphoid tissues (e.g., splenic or lymph node dendritic cells), and blood (**Figure 6.12**). Immature dendritic cells are highly phagocytic.

Upon maturation, which occurs following recognition of broad features of pathogens or damage through receptors on their surface, dendritic cells lose their phagocytic abilities and instead focus on a process termed *antigen presentation*. Maturation triggers dendritic cells in the tissues to move to secondary lymphoid tissues, where they activate cells of the adaptive immune response through antigen presentation and co-stimulation.

Opsonization and Phagocytosis

Neutrophils, macrophages, and dendritic cells are able to conduct phagocytosis of pathogens as one of their functions within immune protection. The first step in the process of phagocytosis is adherence of the plasma membrane of phagocytes to glycoproteins on the surface of the microorganism (**Figure 6.13**). To promote this first step, antibodies or complement proteins from the host coat the microbe surface, a

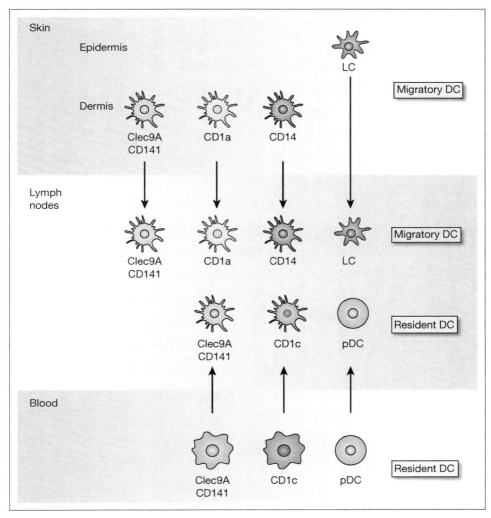

FIGURE 6.12 DCs are professional antigen-presenting cells (they express MHC class II proteins and can activate T cells) and are found in locations throughout the body. Resident DCs tend to remain in lymph nodes, while migratory DCs are able to circulate between tissues, blood, and lymph nodes. DCs, including LCs of the skin, are perfectly positioned to encounter antigens arriving by the cutaneous route. After engulfing the antigen or microbe, the DCs move to lymph nodes where they can interact with resident cells and lymphocytes newly arrived from the blood to activate the next steps of the immune response.

DC, dendritic cell; LC, Langerhans cell; MHC, major histocompatibility complex; pDC, plasmacytoid dendritic cell; CD, cluster of differentiation; Clec, C-type lectin receptor.

process termed *opsonization*. These proteins can then bind to receptors on the phagocyte cell, facilitating adherence to the cell. The proteins that coat the microbe and thereby enhance phagocytosis are called *opsonins*.

The next steps include the formation of a pseudopod, which extends out from the cell, surrounding the particle, and engulfing it. The cell membrane fuses together, forming the *phagosome*, a circular membrane-bound body filled with extracellular fluid and the engulfed particles that is situated in the cytoplasm of the phagocytic cell. The phagosome then merges with *lysosomes*, small fluid-filled vesicles that contain digestive enzymes, ROS, and other

antimicrobial substances. The resulting structure is called a *phagolysosome*. Digestion of most bacteria is complete within 10 to 30 minutes. After phagocytosis, the remaining debris is eliminated from the cell by *exocytosis*, in which the phagolysosome fuses with the plasma membrane and expels its contents.

INNATE LYMPHOID CELLS

A group of innate cells that derive from the lymphoid lineage were only recently identified. Like CD4 T cells, their main function is cytokine production; however, unlike T cells, these cells do not express a genetically recombined antigen receptor. Known as ILCs, these

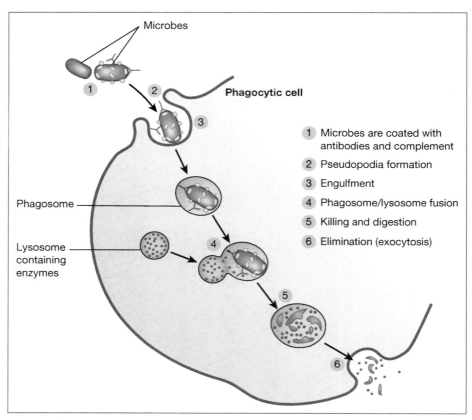

FIGURE 6.13 Phagocytosis. The steps in phagocytosis depend on the ability of professional phagocytes like macrophages to deform their plasma membrane to move toward a microbe by pseudopod formation, attach to the microbe (a process facilitated by opsonization), ingest the microbe, fuse the phagosome with an intracellular lysosome, and kill off the microbe.

cells do not express the lineage markers of other immune cells but instead respond to their local environment by recognizing cytokines, chemokines, and other chemical signals through receptors on their cell surface. In this way, they function to augment the nonspecific reactions of innate immunity, providing broad protection against a variety of pathogens.

ILCs can be categorized according to their functions and cytokine expression (**Figure 6.14**). These include ILC1s, a group that includes cytotoxic NK cells; ILC2s, which are found in fat, liver, lung, and skin, are thought to be important for fighting helminth infection, and may mediate asthma and wound repair; and ILC3s, which are found in the gut and lung and may be important for maintaining homeostasis in mucosal tissues. The ILC3 group also includes lymphoid tissue inducer cells, which are critical for establishing secondary lymphoid structures during development.[7]

NK cells were identified decades before the other ILCs, and are therefore much better characterized. NKs can recognize and directly kill cells that appear abnormal, such as virus-infected or tumor cells. Armed by a series of surface receptors and cytoplasmic granules containing toxic substances, NK cells scan for the presence of unusual ligands on cell plasma membranes. Ligand and receptor interactions can modulate NK cell effector properties. For example, the absence of normal MHC class I expression on the surface of a target cell, which can occur in virus-infected cells or certain tumors, can induce the activation program in NK cells.

Once activated, NK cells orientate and release their granules in the extracellular space toward the target cells. Granules contain mainly two substances: perforin and granzyme B. Perforin creates a channel in the plasma membrane, altering the membrane integrity and inducing cytolysis of the target cell. Moreover, membrane pores allow the entrance of the second compound, granzyme B, a protease able to engage the apoptosis pathway leading to cell destruction.

ACTIVATION OF THE INNATE INFLAMMATORY RESPONSE

Recognition of Pathogens and Tissue Damage

Unlike T cells and B cells, which recognize pathogens with great specificity, innate immune cells respond to pathogen invasion by recognizing molecules that are common to entire classes of pathogens. They are also able to sense tissue damage by recognizing molecules

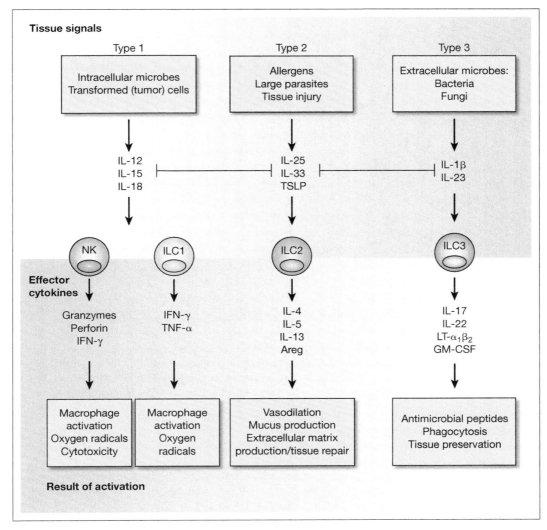

FIGURE 6.14 Innate lymphoid cells. The role of NK cells in innate immunity has long been recognized, particularly their ability to recognize and kill virus-infected cells. Recently, additional lymphoid cell types were found to contribute to innate immunity, reinforcing the work of the myeloid cells, which are the workhorses of acute inflammation.

Areg, amphiregulin; GM-CSF, granulocyte/macrophage colony-stimulating factor; IFN-γ, interferon gamma; IL, interleukin; ILC, innate lymphoid cell; LT-α₁β₂, lymphotoxins alpha-1, beta-2; NK, natural killer; TNF-α, tumor necrosis factor alpha; TSLP, thymic stromal lymphopoietin.

produced by damaged or stressed tissue. The innate cells sense these molecules through cell surface and cytoplasmic protein receptors called *pattern recognition receptors* (PRRs).

Among the PRRs are several types of toll-like receptors (TLRs) that recognize common bacterial cell wall components such as lipopolysaccharide from gram-negative bacteria, viral or bacterial nucleic acids, and fungal carbohydrates (**Figure 6.15**). The generic term for such ligands is *pathogen-associated molecular patterns* (PAMPs). PRRs are found within and on the surface of macrophages and dendritic cells as well as epithelial cells. Local engagement of these receptors promptly stimulates phagocytosis and triggers the

secretion of other signaling agents, including chemokines and cytokines that mediate acute inflammation and enhance antigen processing and presentation.

The cells of innate immunity can also recognize and become activated by signals of tissue damage, cellular stress, and cell death. These triggers can occur in the presence or absence of infection, and are referred to collectively as *danger-associated molecular patterns* (DAMPs). When tissue damage occurs without pathogen invasion and infection (think of a bad ankle sprain that occurs without a break in the skin, or a myocardial infarction), the innate immune response is referred to as **sterile inflammation**, and the DAMPs are the originating signals. DAMPs are also recognized by PRRs,

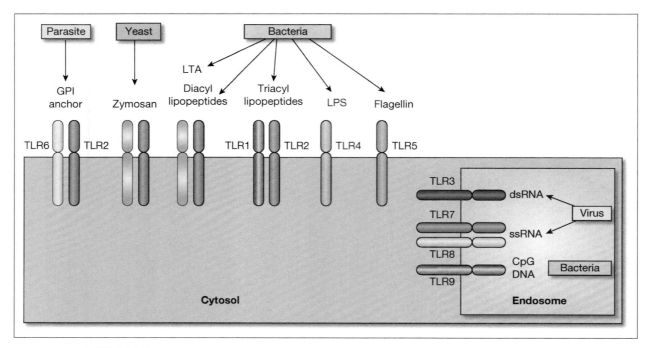

FIGURE 6.15 TLRs are a subset of pattern recognition receptors that mediate pathogen recognition in the innate immune system. There are many types and combinations of TLRs, as shown here. Many TLRs recognize components of bacterial, yeast, or parasite cell membranes; other TLRs are found on endosomes and recognize components of invading bacteria and viruses. This is a nonselective way of distinguishing between self and non-self that characterizes innate immunity. CpG, pathogen DNA sequence of unmethylated CG dinucleotides recognized by TLR9; dsRNA, double-stranded RNA; GPI, glycosylphosphatidylinositol of protozoal membranes; LPS, lipopolysaccharide; LTA, lipoteichoic acid of gram-positive bacteria cell wall; ssRNA, single-stranded RNA; TLR, toll-like receptor.
Source: From Zaru R, European Bioinformatics Institute EMBL-EBI, UK. Pattern recognition receptors (PRRs): toll-like receptors. © British Society for Immunology. https://www.immunology .org/public-information/bitesized-immunology/receptors-and-molecules/pattern-recognition -receptors-prrs.

including TLRs and an intracellular multiprotein complex called the *inflammasome.*

The inflammasome is able to recognize PAMPs as well as DAMPs. The inflammasome is an essential mediator of innate immunity and inflammation by activating caspase-1 and the cytokines IL-1 and IL-18. Secretion of these cytokines can lead to activation and cytokine secretion by other innate cells, including ILCs and NK cells, as well as cell death of infected cells.

SEQUENCE OF INFLAMMATION AND INFLAMMATORY MEDIATORS

Initiation of the innate immune response triggers inflammation. The inflammatory response can be local and confined, or systemic, involving the entire body (e.g., fever, leukocytosis). The cardinal signs of inflammation are redness in the area, swelling, pain, and heat—and in some cases, loss of function.

Acute inflammation occurs in order to destroy any injurious agent causing the tissue damage, while simultaneously preventing spread of the infectious agent,

limiting its effects on the body, and later leading to tissue repair (see **Figure 6.10**). During the first stages of inflammation, PAMPs and DAMPs activate endothelial cells, ILCs, and tissue-resident sentinel macrophages to release early phase, local proinflammatory chemicals. Histamines, prostaglandins, kinins, and leukotrienes cause local vasodilation, increase capillary permeability, and stimulate pain fibers. Macrophages release cytokines such as IL-1 and TNF locally and to the circulation, stimulating the bone marrow to produce more leukocytes and the liver to secrete another class of proinflammatory substances, known as acute phase proteins. These acute phase proteins include C-reactive protein (CRP) and serum amyloid A protein. Concentrations of both proteins increase in the blood by several hundredfold during inflammation or tissue damage, and therefore can be used diagnostically as an indicator of infection or inflammation. Another important acute phase protein is mannan binding lectin (MBL), which can bind to mannose sugars, found in abundance on some microbial pathogens, particularly yeasts.

These proinflammatory chemical mediators induce systemic responses, including fever, anorexia, hypotension, increased heart rate, and the release of the stress hormone cortisol. Histamine and other proinflammatory molecules cause local vasodilation and increased vascular permeability, facilitating migration of cells and molecules out of the bloodstream and into the inflamed area. This increased blood flow and local swelling results in redness, heat, and pain associated with inflammation. At the same time, if there is damage to blood vessels, other components of the blood lead to activation of the coagulation system, which drives the formation of blood clots. The blood clots act to seal off the area, preventing the infection from spreading.

Chemotactic inflammatory mediators attract circulating neutrophils and monocytes. In response, these leukocytes adhere to blood vessel walls through a process called margination (**Figure 6.16**). IL-1 and TNF released by macrophages cause the endothelial cells to upregulate cell membrane proteins called selectins. Selectins have affinity for selectin ligand proteins on the surface of neutrophils. Neutrophils become attracted and loosely attach to the vessel wall, rolling along the surface of the blood vessel. Neutrophils upregulate a membrane protein called integrin, which can bind to integrin receptors also upregulated on the endothelial cells. This interaction provides a tight connection, so the neutrophil stops rolling and becomes firmly attached to the side of the blood vessel. The adhered neutrophils squeeze through the epithelial cells in a process called diapedesis to reach the site of inflammation.

After leaving the vessel, neutrophils and monocytes, which mature into macrophages or inflammatory dendritic cells, rapidly engulf microbes by phagocytosis and destroy them through intracellular killing mechanisms, such as ROS production and

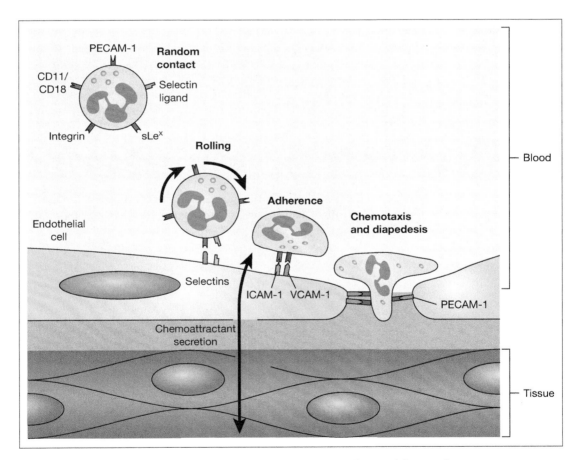

FIGURE 6.16 Margination and diapedesis of neutrophils. Neutrophils are the most numerous and active cells responding to a penetrating injury with bacterial invasion. Chemotactic signals generated in injured tissue upregulate selectins on vascular endothelial cells, promoting binding of selectin ligands on neutrophils. The neutrophils begin to roll along the blood vessel wall, responding to the chemotaxic compounds by upregulating additional adhesion molecules that allow firm sticking to endothelial cell adhesion molecules ICAM–1 and VCAM-1. Finally, neutrophils activate their membrane adhesion molecule, PECAM-1, and begin to move out of the blood into the tissue by squeezing between endothelial cells (diapedesis).
ICAM-1, intercellular adhesion molecule 1; PECAM-1, platelet-endothelial cell adhesion molecule 1; sLe^x, sialyl Lewis X motif; VCAM-1, vascular cell adhesion molecule 1.

release of lysosomal enzymes. Antigen-presenting cells (APCs), such as dendritic cells, traffic to the local draining lymph nodes, where they initiate the adaptive immune response through antigen presentation. Other leukocytes begin to arrive at the inflammatory site and start producing their mediators, including arachidonic acid metabolites (prostaglandins) and cytokines, which amplify the inflammatory response in a cascade effect. After engulfing large numbers of microorganisms and damaged tissue, the phagocytes die. In some cases, dying phagocytes form pus; in other cases, significant numbers of phagocytes (particularly neutrophils) die and release their content of killing mediators, including ROS and proteases. This can cause a second wave of tissue injury, as seen in reperfusion injury after myocardial infarction. The principal cell types and mediators of inflammation are summarized in **Table 6.4**.

Resolving an Inflammatory Response

The final stage of inflammation is tissue repair. After an inflammatory event or tissue injury, innate and adaptive immune cells as well as nonhematopoietic cells, including fibroblasts, epithelial cells, and endothelial cells, work together to resolve inflammation and initiate and regulate the wound-healing response. Ideally, this leads to restoration of normal tissue architecture; however, aberrant wound-healing responses can yield fibrotic and scarred tissue that interferes with normal function or leads to development of chronic wounds. Macrophages can be subdivided into two types, one of which is acutely activated and proinflammatory, secreting proinflammatory cytokines such as IL-1 and TNF-α; the other type is antiinflammatory, secretes IL-10 and transforming growth factor-β (TGF-β), and participates in wound healing.

As inflammation resolves and progresses to the stage of wound healing, activity of antiinflammatory macrophages increases, resulting in increased levels of platelet-derived growth factor (PDGF), vascular endothelial growth factor alpha (VEGF-α), and TGF-β1. The cytokine IL-13, produced by other types of innate cells and certain T cells, also can promote TGF-β production. Together, these growth factors promote cell proliferation and development of blood vessels. Macrophages also produce chemokines to recruit fibroblasts and myofibroblasts to mediate wound closure, and additionally regulate the balance of matrix metalloproteinases (enzymes that control extracellular matrix turnover and fibrosis). Wounds characterized by persistence of proinflammatory macrophages producing IL-1 and TNF are associated with impaired or delayed

TABLE 6.4 Inflammatory Mediators

Class of Mediators	Principal Sources	Major Functions
Vasoactive amines (histamine, serotonin)	Mast cells, basophils, platelets	Histamine: vasodilation, increased capillary permeability Serotonin: vasoconstriction
Kinins (bradykinin, kallikrein)	Liver	Vasodilation, increased capillary permeability, pain, coagulation
Complement	Liver	Microbe opsonization, chemotaxis, bacterial killing via membrane attack complex
Arachidonic acid metabolites (prostaglandins, leukotrienes, lipoxins)	Leukocytes, endothelial cells	Proinflammatory—vasodilation, increased capillary permeability, pain Anti-inflammatory (lipoxins)
Reactive oxygen species (superoxide, hydrogen peroxide, hypochlorous acid)	Neutrophils and macrophages	Bacterial killing, release into tissues perpetuates injury
Lysosomal degradative enzymes (proteases, lysozyme)	Neutrophils and macrophages	Bacterial killing, release into tissues perpetuates injury
Acute phase proteins (C-reactive protein, serum amyloid A)	Liver	Markers of inflammatory response, inhibit pathogen growth, proinflammatory
Cytokines and chemokines	Leukocytes	*Proinflammatory:* IL-1, IL-6, TNF, IL-18, others *Antiinflammatory:* IL-10, TGF-β *Chemokines:* CCL and CXL families—chemotaxis and co-stimulators

CCL, CC-motif chemokine ligand; CXL, CX-motif chemokine ligand; IL, interleukins; TGF-β, transforming growth factor-beta; TNF, tumor necrosis factor.

BOX 6.4
Overview of the Complement Pathway

- Complement proteins are designated with an uppercase C and are numbered from 1 to 9, based on order of discovery rather than the order in which they act. Complement proteins that are activated by cleavage produce two subunits that are indicated with lowercase letters *a* or *b*.

- There are three different ways in which the complement system can be activated: the classical, alternative, or lectin pathways. All three pathways directly or indirectly lead to death of the invading pathogen (see **Figure 6.17**).

- Although they are initiated in different ways, all three pathways converge at the cleavage of C3 into C3a and C3b (see **Figure 6.18**). From this point, the complement pathways lead to the outcomes of (a) recruiting inflammatory cells to the site of infection; (b) labeling or *opsonization* of pathogens for enhanced uptake and destruction by phagocytic cells; or (c) formation of the *membrane attack complex (MAC)*, which forms pores in pathogen membranes.

---

tissue repair after injury, infection, or sterile inflammation, leading to chronic inflammation.

THE COMPLEMENT PATHWAY

The complement pathway is a series of proteins that are produced by the liver, and can be found throughout the body in extracellular fluids, lymph, and blood (**Box 6.4**). Many of the complement proteins are proteolytic enzymes that exist in an inactive state, similar to proteins of the coagulation cascade (see Chapter 8, Blood and Clotting). When activated by signals of pathogen invasion, complement proteins initiate a cascade of activation whereby one enzyme cleaves and activates the next in the series.

There are three initiating pathways for the complement cascade. In the classical pathway, either antibody (produced by B cells or plasma cells) or the acute phase protein CRP binds to a pathogen. The antibody- or CRP-bound bacterium then interacts with the C1 protein complex triggering its activation and releasing an active protease. The active protease cleaves C2 and C4, generating C2a and C4b (**Figure 6.17**). C2a and C4b combine to form *C4bC2a*, also known as a *C3 convertase*. This is the point in the cascade at which C3 is cleaved to produce C3a and C3b.

The main pathway triggering the complement cascade early in infection is the alternative pathway. This pathway is initiated as a result of the ability of C3 and protein B to bind to the surface of the invading microbe, leading to cleavage of C3 and protein B, with formation of an active and potent C3 convertase known as *C3bBb*. Thus, activation on the bacterial surface of a small amount of C3 and factor B to C3bBb can trigger the activation of greater numbers of C3 molecules.

The most recently discovered pathway of initiation of the complement cascade is the lectin pathway.

Mannan-binding lectin (MBL) is an acute phase protein produced by the liver during an inflammatory response. MBLs circulating in plasma bind to mannose sugars on the surface of the pathogen. This binding triggers the MBL polyprotein to become enzymatically active and able to cleave C4 and C2 to form the C4bC2a C3 convertase as seen in the classical pathway. It is here that the pathway converges with the alternative and classical pathways, and complement effector functions are elicited by the C3 cleavage products: C3a and C3b. The complement cascade interacts with both innate and adaptive immunity, with three main outcomes (**Figure 6.18**):

1. Cleaving larger precursor proteins C3 and C5 generates smaller proteins, C3a and C5a, that are potent inflammatory signals. They are also known as anaphylatoxins because they promote mast cell degranulation with histamine release. C5a is particularly effective at promoting leukocyte chemotaxis.

2. C3b is an opsonin that binds to bacterial cell walls to promote efficient phagocytosis by neutrophils and macrophages. C3b also promotes B-cell antibody production.

3. The final steps of the complement cascade on bacterial surfaces involve sequential activation of complement proteins 5, 6, 7, and 8, leading up to insertion of several copies of C9 into bacterial membranes, forming the membrane attack complex (MAC). MACs form cylinder-shaped large pores in the cell wall or membrane of the invading pathogen, which allows water to move into the pathogen, causing swelling and resulting in cell death by cytolysis. Gram-negative bacteria have two membrane layers separated by only a thin peptidoglycan layer and are more susceptible to cytolysis than are gram-positive bacteria.

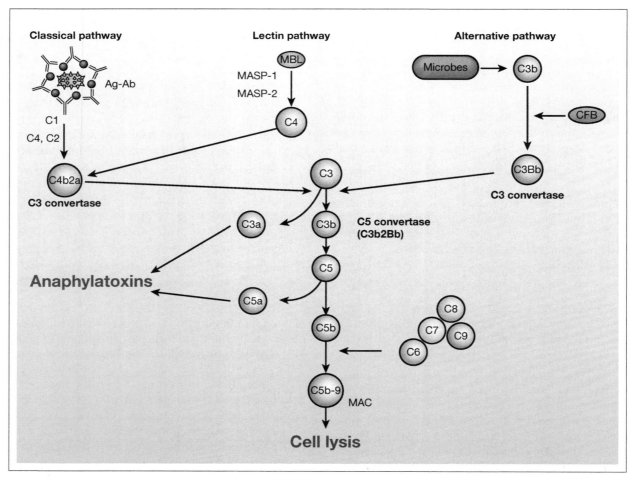

FIGURE 6.17 Pathways of complement activation. In the classical pathway, bacteria are coated by antibodies that attract and activate the complement cascade. In the alternative pathway, complement binds to the bacterial wall itself, initiating its own cascade. The lectin pathway depends on MBL (a circulating protein synthesized by the liver) to attach to the bacteria before activating the complement cascade.

Ag-Ab, antigen-antibody; CFB, complement factor B; MAC, membrane attack complex; MASP, mannan-binding lectin-associated serine protease; MBL, mannan-binding lectin.

The complement cascade is the target of regulatory proteins that suppress activation in the absence of pathogen invasion. In addition, activated complement proteins are quickly degraded to prevent excess tissue damage. Mutations in complement genes may predispose to greater incidence of infection. Notably, deficiencies in C5 to C9 result in exquisite susceptibility to *Neisseria* spp., some of which cause life-threatening invasive meningococcal meningitis.

INNATE RESPONSES TO VIRAL INFECTION

Viruses are exclusively intracellular pathogens. After gaining access to the body via respiratory, gastrointestinal, and other routes, viruses use the host cell machinery to conduct replication, transcription, and translation of viral DNA and RNA. During viral infection, viral nucleic acid can be detected in the cytoplasm by cytosolic PRRs. Binding to intracellular PRRs—RIG-I-like receptors (RLRs), nucleotide-binding domain-leucine-rich repeat-containing molecules (NLRs), or cytosolic DNA sensors such as cyclic guanosine monophosphate–adenosine monophosphate synthase (cGAS)—leads to the production of type I interferons (IFNs) and other proinflammatory cytokines. Type I IFNs are a group of structurally related cytokines that induce antiviral responses within infected cells and alert neighboring cells to upregulate molecules that antagonize virus replication. Produced early during viral infection, type I IFNs are also essential for activating NK cell effector functions.

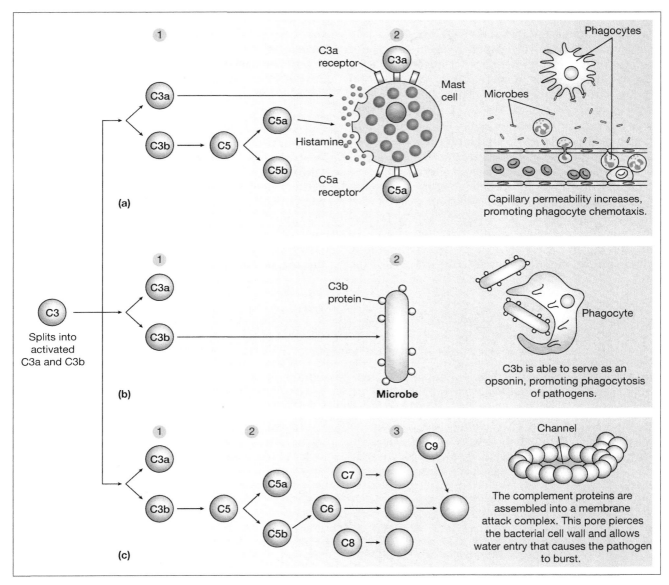

FIGURE 6.18 Mechanisms of complement effector functions diverge after C3 splits (step 1). **(a)** C3a and C5a are small fragments (anaphylatoxins) that promote histamine release and phagocyte chemotaxis (step 2). **(b)** C3b fragments opsonize (coat) microbes (step 2). **(c)** C3b initiates the full complement cascade (steps 2 and 3), resulting in MAC formation and pathogen lysis.

Upon binding their cell-surface receptors, type I IFNs stimulate expression of more than 300 genes (known as IFN-stimulated genes), which leads to inhibition of viral replication, assembly, and release, as well as promoting adaptive immune responses.

CHRONIC INFLAMMATION

Cancer, autoimmunity, allergy, obesity and metabolic dysfunction, infection, genetic diseases, aberrant responses to the microflora, and aging can all lead to **chronic inflammation**. While acute inflammation is short lived, chronic inflammation occurs when an inflammatory response fails to resolve, leading to sustained inflammation that lasts months or even years. Chronic inflammation heightens the risk of developing many harmful diseases, including cardiovascular disease, chronic kidney disease, cancer, and even depression.

Inflammatory responses typically resolve when neutrophil recruitment to the tissue stops, and those neutrophils present in the tissue die and are engulfed by phagocytic macrophages. The local macrophages then adopt a wound-healing, antiinflammatory phenotype. Other cells, including regulatory or IL-13–producing T cells, also contribute to the resolution of inflammation.

Multiple mechanisms can lead to failure of the antiinflammatory response, resulting in chronic inflammation.

Genetic susceptibility can contribute to chronic inflammation; for example, certain variants of the *IL-1β gene* are associated with lower or higher serum concentrations of proinflammatory cytokines. Noncoding microRNAs (miRNAs) that can regulate inflammation decrease with aging and may contribute to the inflammatory phenotype observed in older people. Other causes of chronic inflammation include production of proinflammatory mediators by adipocytes in obesity; increased gut permeability leading to translocation of gut organisms into the bloodstream; alterations in the gut microflora leading to proinflammatory responses; the inflammatory tumor microenvironment in cancer; type 2 diabetes, which leads to a heightened risk for cardiovascular disease, chronic inflammation, and infections; and chronic infectious processes such as lung granuloma formation in tuberculosis, cirrhosis of the liver in hepatitis B, or recurrent severe lower respiratory tract infections that lead to fibrosis and permanent structural airway damage in cystic fibrosis and bronchiectasis. In some individuals, chronic inflammation persists after an infection or injury has resolved. In other cases, it occurs when there have been no obvious initiating factors.

Early modulation of chronic inflammation is important to prevent health decline. Broad-acting pharmaceuticals already in clinical use, such as aspirin, metformin, and rapamycin, are known to have antiinflammatory activity and can improve the overall health and life span in animal models. Other tissue- and disease-specific biologically targeted therapeutics are available, such as the TNF inhibitors used in rheumatoid arthritis (**Box 6.5** and **Figure 6.19**) and inflammatory bowel disease, and many more are in development.

BOX 6.5
Rheumatoid Arthritis Exemplifies Chronic Inflammation

Rheumatoid arthritis (RA) is an autoimmune disease found in 0.5% to 1% of persons globally. RA is two to three times more common in women than in men, and generally develops at a younger age in women. Clinical hallmarks include joint swelling, pain, and stiffness; fevers; anemia; increased erythrocyte sedimentation rate; and increased acute phase protein levels, as well as antibodies to citrulline-modified proteins (anti citrullinated protein antibodies, or ACPAs) and the autoantibody *rheumatoid factor*. Although the precipitating event has not been identified, genetic risk contributes to RA development, with 15% concordance in monozygotic twins and 5% concordance in dizygotic twins.

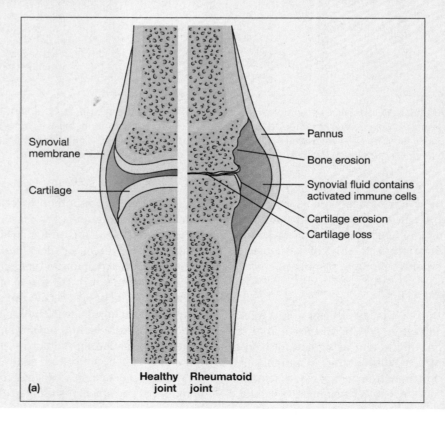

Synovial membrane
Cartilage
Pannus
Bone erosion
Synovial fluid contains activated immune cells
Cartilage erosion
Cartilage loss

(a) Healthy joint Rheumatoid joint

(continued)

The focus of tissue damage in RA is the synovial joints, with the accumulation of Th1 and Th17 cells, macrophages, B cells, fibroblasts, and synovial cells (**Figure 6.19b**). The joints in individuals affected by RA are characterized by chronic, nonresolving inflammation. The persistence of T cells chronically activates macrophages to secrete IL-1, TNF, and IL-6, promoting osteoclast activity and bone resorption, and causing progressive bone deformity, joint degeneration, swelling, fluid accumulation, and pain (**Figure 6.19a**). Targeted therapy with *disease-modifying antirheumatic drugs* (DMARDs) usually involves monoclonal antibodies that inactivate one of these cytokines or their receptors.[8]

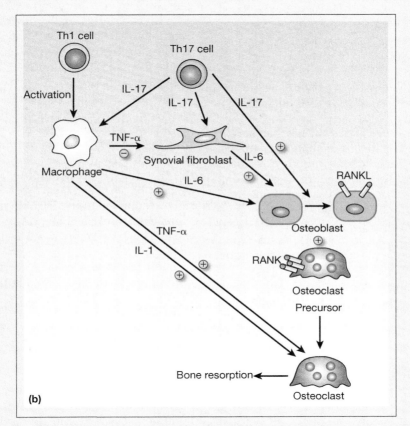

FIGURE 6.19 (a) The joint damage from chronic inflammation in RA includes loss of cartilage cushioning the joint, loss of bone contributing to deformity, excess synovial fluid containing inflammatory cells and mediators, and thickening of the synovial membrane with pannus formation. **(b)** Cells and mediators of the chronic inflammatory process in RA. Although synovial fluid normally has very few cells, RA is associated with infiltration of inflammatory cells, including macrophages, dendritic cells, B cells, and T-helper cells (Th1 and Th17). Fibroblasts and osteoclasts can also accumulate in the joint. Inflammatory fluid and cells cause proliferation of the synovial membrane, which enlarges, forming a pannus. The chronic inflammatory cells produce proinflammatory cytokines, particularly TNF, IL-6, and IL-17. These cytokines promote activation of synovial fibroblasts, which proliferate and also begin to secrete IL-6. The cytokine milieu alters the activity of nearby osteoblasts and osteoclasts with subsequent degradation of bone at the margins of the joint and adjacent cartilage, creating the joint deformities associated with RA.
IL, interleukin; RA, rheumatoid arthritis; RANK, receptor activator of nuclear factor kappa B; RANKL, RANK ligand; TNF, tumor necrosis factor.

TRAINED INNATE IMMUNITY

The ability to react more effectively and efficiently against specific pathogens is a mechanism restricted to the adaptive immune system. The innate immune system, however, possesses a type of immunological memory, known as *trained immunity*, which lacks specificity but still offers enhanced protection against pathogenic organisms.

Evidence from epidemiological and preclinical studies has hinted at this mechanism for some time, but the science of trained immunity of the innate system has only recently gained attention. It has been known for many years that vaccines can have beneficial off-target effects. For example, even as far back as its first use in the 1920s, the tuberculosis vaccine, bacille Calmette-Guérin (BCG), was suggested to prevent death in neonates that extended far beyond its ability to prevent tuberculosis. This was subsequently confirmed by epidemiological and preclinical studies, and other vaccines have been shown to act in a similar way.

It was only in the last decade that the mechanism for this curious feature of the innate immune system was elucidated. It was discovered that monocytes could undergo epigenetic and metabolic reprogramming after exposure to certain organisms or molecules from pathogens. This reprogramming results in a heightened functional state that enables the monocyte to respond more effectively against a subsequent infectious insult, whether it be by the same pathogen or another, unrelated pathogen.

Trained immunity may play an important role in chronic inflammation. Trained monocytes have been proposed to drive atherosclerotic lesion development, leading to cardiovascular disease, and they may also play a role in the development and maintenance of autoimmune and autoinflammatory diseases. This area of research is still very much in its infancy, but offers great potential for providing new therapeutic targets.

TRANSITION FROM INNATE TO ADAPTIVE IMMUNITY: ANTIGEN PRESENTATION AND THE MAJOR HISTOCOMPATIBILITY COMPLEX

In certain phagocytic cells, some of the proteins from the pathogen are broken down further in the phagolysosome into small peptides. These peptides (typically 13 to 25 amino acids long) associate with a transmembrane protein called MHC class II or human leukocyte antigen (HLA)-DM, -DO, -DR, -DQ, or -DP. MHC molecules present the peptide antigen in a cleft of their tridimensional protein structure (**Figure 6.20**). Antigen processing and presentation on MHC II is a critical process that involves dendritic cells, B cells, and macrophages—collectively referred to as APCs—but not neutrophils. Unlike B cells, which can recognize free antigen, T cells can only recognize antigen that is displayed to them on MHC by APCs. Antigen presentation is thus a critical step linking innate immunity with adaptive immunity.

There are two main classes of MHC proteins: MHC I and MHC II. MHC II is expressed only by APCs; however, MHC I is expressed by nearly all nucleated cells. While MHC II presents peptides from phagocytized material of extracellular organisms, the peptides presented on MHC I are processed in a different way and are predominantly sourced from intracellular pathogens such as viruses or intracellular bacteria. Because viruses can infect many different cell types, it is important that T cells can be alerted to which cells are infected through antigen presentation on MHC I. CD4 T cells recognize antigen on MHC II; CD8 T cells recognize antigen on MHC I.

Smaller peptides (typically eight to ten amino acids long) are presented on MHC I. These cytosolic peptides are produced from within the cell using the *immunoproteasome*, which produces peptides able to bind to MHC I. These peptides are transported to the endoplasmic reticulum by a special *transporter associated with antigen processing* (TAP). The peptides are loaded onto MHC I in the endoplasmic reticulum, then the MHC I–peptide complex is exported to the cell surface, ready for presentation to CD8 T cells (**Figure 6.21**).

Each individual expresses a genetically distinct combination of MHC molecules of both classes. There are six MHC I isotypes: HLA-A, HLA-B, HLA-C, HLA-E, HLA-F, and HLA-G. There are multiple different alleles of each isotype, with HLA-A, HLA-B, and HLA-C being the most polymorphic. For MHC II, HLA-DP, HLA-DQ, and HLA-DR are also highly polymorphic.

Besides their role in antigen presentation, highly polymorphic MHC I molecules, which are expressed by almost every cell in the body, play an important role in rejection of transplanted tissue. The antigenic differences between host MHC and donor MHC can lead to an immune response initiated against the graft, leading to transplant rejection. Conversely, HSCs used in bone marrow transplantation can develop into T cells that recognize the host MHC as a foreign antigen, leading to a potentially serious condition known as **graft-versus-host disease**. Tissue typing prior to transplantation evaluates the degree of similarity of donor and recipient HLA proteins—the closer these proteins are, the less likely that transplant rejection will occur. Therefore, correct matching of HLA of the donor and recipient is necessary for successful tissue transplantation.

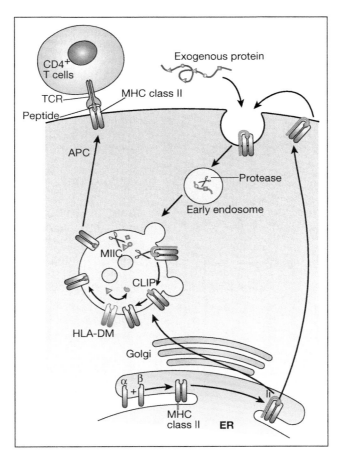

FIGURE 6.20 Presentation of exogenous, extracellular antigens on MHC II proteins is conducted by professional antigen-presenting cells. MHC II presentation is a multistep process, initiated by synthesis of MHC II. The antigen-binding site of MHC II is protected by an invariant peptide (Ii). MHC II can move to the membrane or to an intracellular compartment, the MIIC. Foreign proteins are brought into the APC by endocytosis, forming the early endosome, where they are broken down by proteases into small fragments. Fusion of the endosome with the MIIC allows cleavage of the invariant protein and replacement of the resulting CLIP with the antigen fragment. The final complex of antigen fragment and MHC II protein are displayed on the membrane of the APC for presentation to CD4+ T cells.
APC, antigen-presenting cell; CLIP, class II-associated Ii peptide; ER, endoplasmic reticulum; HLA, human leukocyte antigen; MHC, major histocompatibility complex; MIIC, MHC class II compartment; TCR, T-cell receptor.

 Thought Questions

5. **What is the role of the endothelium in acute inflammation?**

6. **What is the role of neutrophils in acute inflammation?**

7. **What is the role of complement in acute inflammation?**

8. **How do macrophages contribute to tissue surveillance, acute inflammation, and chronic inflammation?**

9. **How do dendritic cells aid the transition from innate to adaptive immunity?**

ADAPTIVE IMMUNITY

The adaptive immune response contrasts with the broad innate immune response by being highly specific. Its precision is such that adaptive immune cells can recognize a particular strain of a pathogen while failing to recognize a different strain of the same pathogen. An example of the problems posed by such specificity relates to the large number of different viral strains that cause influenza. Immunizations to reduce infection with and transmission of the influenza virus attempt to cover viral strains that are predicted to be in circulation over the coming year, because it is not practical to immunize against all possible strains. If the predictions are incorrect, the

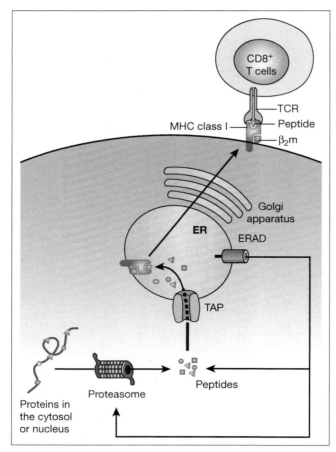

FIGURE 6.21 Intracellular antigenic peptides are presented on MHC class I molecules to CD8 T cells following antigen degradation by the proteasome. The peptides generated are translocated via TAP into the lumen of the ER, then loaded onto MHC I molecules. Peptide–MHC I complexes are transported to the plasma membrane via the Golgi apparatus for presentation to CD8 T cells.

β_2m, β_2-microglobulin; ER, endoplasmic reticulum; ERAD, ER-associated protein degradation; MHC, major histocompatibility complex; TAP, transporter associated with antigen processing; TCR, T-cell receptor.

flu vaccine may be relatively ineffective in any given year. Fortunately, other viruses that are targeted by vaccines, such as measles, chickenpox, and hepatitis A, have stable structures and routine immunizations are very effective at preventing infections.

A remarkable feature of the adaptive immune response is its ability to specifically recognize and respond more quickly and more effectively to a second exposure with the same pathogen. This is the underlying principle of vaccination. B and T cells are the main cellular mediators of adaptive immunity; however, they are heterogeneous groups of cells and vary greatly in the types of responses they produce (**Figure 6.22**). The cells, mediators, and mechanisms of adaptive immunity are detailed in this section.

B CELLS ARE RESPONSIBLE FOR HUMORAL IMMUNITY

The main effector mechanism of the B-cell response is the secretion of antibodies, a specialized class of circulating glycoproteins that are a soluble version of the BCR, as described earlier (**Figure 6.22a**). Circulating antibodies are effector proteins that bind antigen on pathogens or toxins with high specificity. This binding provides protection through three general mechanisms, as follows:

1. Antibody binding may neutralize target proteins. For example, a patient with tetanus can be treated with antitoxin—antibodies that bind to tetanus toxin molecules throughout the circulation and tissues and prevent their effects on the body.
2. Coating a microbe with antibodies is a form of opsonization that facilitates phagocytosis and destruction by neutrophils and macrophages.
3. Antibodies can also lead to bacterial killing by triggering activation of the classical complement pathway (discussed earlier; **Figure 6.23**).

Antibody Structure

As noted earlier, all antibodies generally share common molecular and structural characteristics, as illustrated in **Figure 6.24**. They are made up of four protein chains: two heavy chains and two light chains. These are held together by disulfide bonds, forming a Y-shaped molecule. Each arm of the immunoglobulin consists of a light chain held to the upper portion of the heavy chain. Then the two heavy chains, or *stalk*, are also held together by disulfide bonds. Functionally, antibodies have two regions: one end (with two arms) to bind antigen and one end that is constant across their class and is able to bind to receptors and recognition sites. When cleaved by an enzyme, papain, the antibody generates two fragments. The portion with variable amino acid sequence based on B-cell gene rearrangement is within the *fragment antigen-binding* (Fab) region. Although the Fab regions are extremely variable and differ between immunoglobulins of different B-cell clones, the remaining *constant fragment*, or Fc, region is the same in all immunoglobulin molecules of a given class.

The Fc region of an antibody interacts with different immune effector cells, such as neutrophils, mast cells, NK cells, and macrophages, by binding to immunoglobulin class-specific Fc receptors expressed on the cell membrane. The specificity of the Fc receptors for the different immunoglobulin isotypes and the type of cells expressing the Fc receptor determines the different effector outcomes.

Antibody Classes

The five immunoglobulin classes or antibody isotypes are IgM, IgD, IgG, IgA, IgE; their functions are

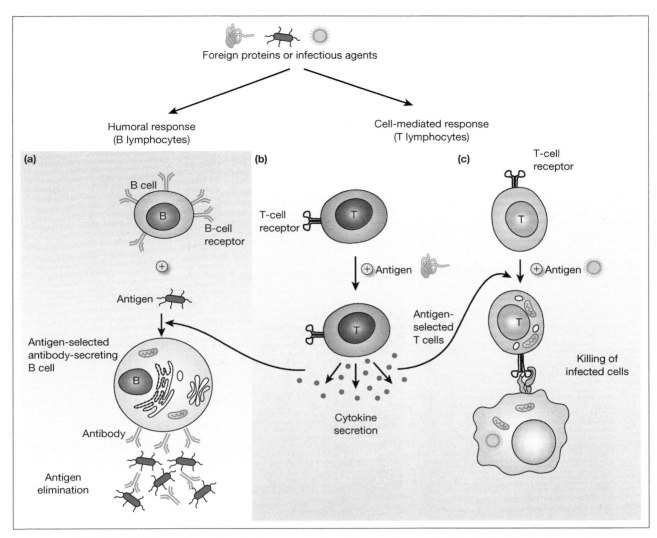

FIGURE 6.22 Overview of adaptive immunity. Adaptive immunity is divided into humoral responses mediated by B cells and antibody secretion (**a**), and cell-mediated responses (**b and c**). Cell-mediated immunity is carried out by cytotoxic T lymphocytes (**c**) that can kill virus-infected or abnormal (cancerous) self-cells. Both humoral and cell-mediated immunity require stimulatory factors produced by related antigen-specific T-helper lymphocytes (**b**).

summarized in **Table 6.5**. Each heavy chain gene is given a Greek letter that corresponds to the class of antibody it encodes. For example, the IgM heavy chain is encoded by μ, IgD is encoded by δ, and so on. Monomeric IgM and IgD are the first immunoglobulin types expressed on the surface of a mature naive B cell. These cell-surface antibodies function as the BCR.

IgM is the first secreted antibody of the immune response and is secreted as a pentamer. IgM can be expressed by some B cells even in the absence of prior immunization and antigen exposure, contributing to *natural* humoral immunity. Although the antigen-binding sites of IgM are, in general, low affinity, their multivalent structure helps them to create very effective antigen–antibody complexes. Compared with the effector functions of other immunoglobulin

classes, IgM has the highest ability to activate complement to help destroy the invading pathogen. Secretion of IgD is rarely observed; however, IgD is used as a marker for B-cell maturation because its surface expression changes according to different B-cell maturation stages. The functions of IgD are still largely unknown, despite its being a highly conserved immunoglobulin across many species. There are indications that IgD on B-cell membranes promotes responses to foreign proteins while reducing responses to self-antigens. Secreted IgD, although present in relatively low concentrations, may contribute to mucosal immunity.

Three quarters of circulating immunoglobulin is monomeric IgG, the most abundant immunoglobulin isotype. IgG is good at activating the complement

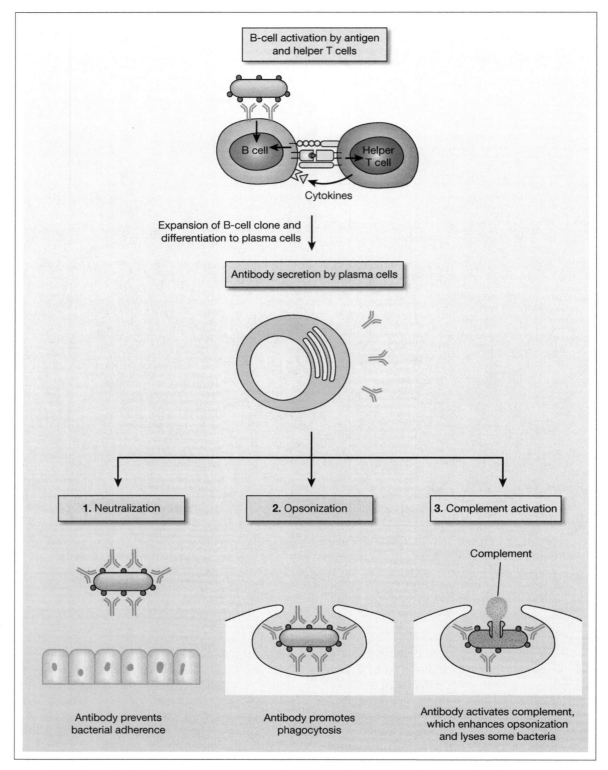

FIGURE 6.23 The effector actions of antibodies. Antibodies provide protection from toxins and pathogens by three major mechanisms: **(1)** In neutralization, antitoxin antibodies bind toxin molecules into antigen–antibody complexes that can be removed by macrophages. **(2)** In opsonization, antibodies bind to pathogens as opsonins, facilitating macrophage phagocytosis. **(3)** Antibodies binding to pathogens initiate complement via the classical pathway of complement activation, leading to MAC formation and cytolysis.

MAC, membrane attack complex.

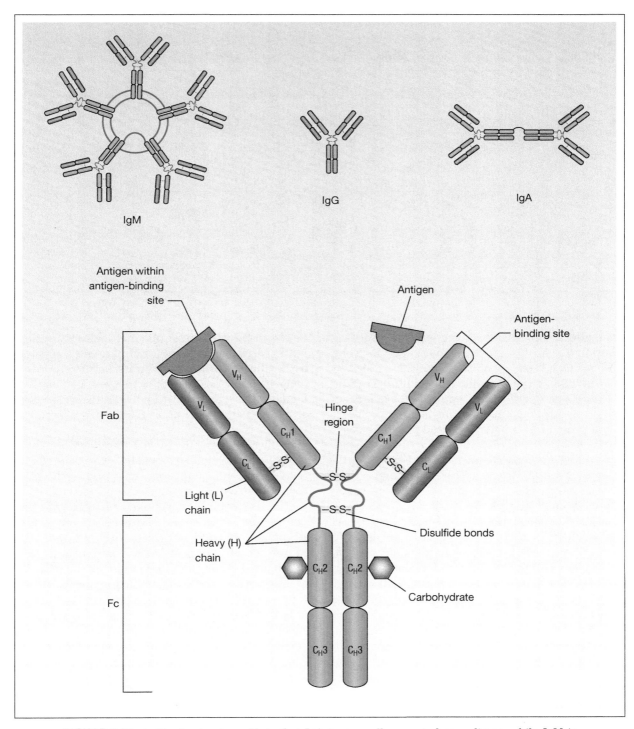

FIGURE 6.24 Antibody structure. Note that IgA is generally secreted as a dimer, while IgM is usually a pentamer.

C_H, constant domain heavy chain; C_L, constant domain light chain; Fab, fragment, antigen-binding; Fc, fragment, crystallizable (or constant); IgA, immunoglobulin A; IgG, immunoglobulin G; IgM, Immunoglobulin M; V_H, variable domain heavy chain; V_L, variable domain light chain.

TABLE 6.5 Characteristics of the Major Antibody Classes

Feature	IgM	IgD	IgG	IgA	IgE
Heavy chains	μ	δ	γ	α	ε
Number of units	5	1	1	1 or 2	1
% of total immunoglobulin (Ig)	10	<1	75	15	<1
Complement activation	++++	−	++	−	−
Crosses placenta	−	−	+	−	−
Binds to macrophages and neutrophils	−	−	+	−	−
Binds to mast cells and basophils	−	−	−	−	+
Crosses epithelial membranes	−	−	−	+	−

cascade and eliminating pathogens, promoting opsonization and MAC complex formation on microbe surfaces. With a half-life of approximately 3 weeks, IgG is a long-lasting immunoglobulin. Fc receptors specific for IgG antibodies are highly expressed on macrophages and neutrophils, making this isotype the most efficient at promoting opsonization and phagocytosis.

Notably, IgG is the only isotype able to cross the placenta, providing protection to the fetus during pregnancy and the neonate in the weeks after birth. While greatly beneficial in most cases, the ability of IgG to cross the placenta can cause fetal loss or death of the newborn if the mother produces IgG antibodies against the blood type (rhesus factor) of the fetus. This can occur if the mother and fetus have incompatible blood types. This condition is now easily detectable and treatable.

IgA is secreted as either a monomer or dimer. Monomeric IgA represents about 15% of the total immunoglobulin circulating in the bloodstream. One of its exclusive characteristics is the ability to cross epithelial membranes and to be expressed abundantly in body secretions that protect mucosal tissues and body openings. Mucus in the airways and in the urogenital and gastrointestinal tracts, as well as tears, sweat, and saliva, contain dimeric IgA. In these locations, it is strategically positioned to bind and inactivate invading pathogens, preventing their entrance into the body. IgA is also abundant in breast milk and provides protection for neonates and infants whose immune systems are still developing.

In the healthy individual, IgE is the least abundant immunoglobulin class, making up less than 1% of total immunoglobulin in the bloodstream. IgE binds to mast cells and basophils interacting with its specific Fc receptor that is present on these innate cells. Binding to the Fc receptors triggers the release of preformed granules containing histamines and inflammatory molecules. IgE is particularly useful for eliminating parasites such as helminth worms. Despite its extremely low blood concentration, IgE is very potent and can cause tissue damage; it is associated with hypersensitivity type 1 diseases, also known as atopic diseases or allergies.

Steps in B-Cell Activation and Maturation

B cells are activated when the BCRs on their cell surface bind to free antigen. In some cases, when the antigen is repetitive in nature (e.g., flagellin on flagellated bacteria), the BCRs become cross-linked or aggregate together on the cell surface, and the B cell receives a strong enough signal to be activated without any T-cell help. In most cases, though, B cells require help from T cells in order to be fully activated (**Figures 6.22b** and **6.25**). B cells can internalize their BCR and process the antigen for presentation to CD4 T cells on the MHC II molecules. CD4 T cells that recognize the antigen can then support B-cell activation through the upregulation of cell-surface co-stimulatory receptors or through cytokine production. The activated B-cell clone, while proliferating, starts simultaneously to increase the production of IgM, and differentiates into effector cells (antibody-secreting plasma cells). This process constitutes the first phase of the adaptive humoral immune response.

Follicular helper T (T_{fh}) cells are specialized CD4 T cells that are located within B-cell follicles in secondary lymphoid tissues. T_{fh} cells are critical for the formation and maintenance of germinal centers, the site of intense B-cell proliferation, because they support B-cell survival and differentiation. Following the first stage of activation, and with the support of T_{fh} cells, B cells form the germinal center. There, they begin to proliferate and some cells differentiate into plasma cells. Plasma cells have prominent secretory organelles and

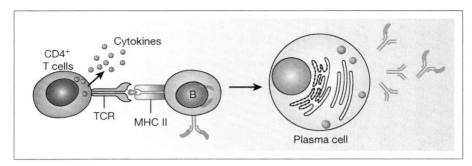

FIGURE 6.25 CD4 T-cell help for B-cell activation. B cells can interact with the T_{fh} cells specific for the same antigen by way of antigen presentation. Like macrophages and dendritic cells, B cells express MHC class II receptors for antigen presentation to T_{fh} cells and other helper T cells. Within lymphoid follicles, B and T_{fh} cells programmed to respond to the same antigen encounter each other and bind through their complementary TCRs and MHC protein. The T_{fh} cell then secretes cytokines that expands the clone of B cells and promotes maturation to plasma cells that act as prolific antibody factories.

MHC, major histocompatibility complex; TCRs, T-cell receptors; T_{fh} cell, follicular helper T cell.

serve as *antibody factories*, secreting large amounts of specific antibody that circulates through the blood, lymph, and extracellular fluids.

The daughter B cells and plasma cells usually bear the same BCR on their surface and produce the same type of secreted antibody as the parent B cell. However, as the germinal center reaction progresses, the B cells undergo a process called *isotype class-switching*. During isotype class-switching, the B cells, which initially produce pentameric IgM, are able to class switch and swap the gene segment used to encode the constant region of the heavy chain. This process is governed by the local cytokine environment induced by the T_{fh} cells. Thus, in the first days of a B-cell immune response, membrane-bound and secreted IgM antibodies are produced by the B cell; however, at later stages different isotypes of antibody are expressed, with IgG being the most common.

Another fascinating feature of B cells, touched on earlier, is their propensity to undergo point mutations in antigen-binding regions of their heavy and light chain variable domains during the germinal center reaction. This process is called *somatic hypermutation* and can affect the strength of binding between the antibody and antigen. The tighter the bond, the more effective the antibody. Some mutations, of course, are deleterious or have no effect; however, this is a small price to pay for the chance to produce a better antibody. B cells that produce a more tightly binding antibody undergo a process known as *affinity maturation*. In this process, B cells that produce higher affinity (or more tightly binding) antibody preferentially survive and outcompete their lesser counterparts. Therefore, as the germinal center progresses, the affinity of the antibody for the antigen improves. The B cells and their daughter cells and plasma cells are now able to produce high-affinity antibody of the most appropriate class to fight the infection or toxin.

B-Cell Memory

A further remarkable feature of B cells is their ability to remember (**Figure 6.26**). During the B-cell response, high-affinity, class-switched B cells are able to differentiate into long-lived memory B cells, which can survive for many years. These memory cells, now present in high numbers, are at the ready to produce high levels of high-affinity, class-switched antibody upon reexposure to the same pathogen. The impressive ability of memory B cells to recall over long periods of time was illustrated by the resistance of the elderly population in the remote Faroe Islands of the North Atlantic to the measles virus. An epidemic of measles had occurred in the islands 65 years earlier, with no further measles cases until an outbreak many decades later.[9] That immunity to the virus had persisted for 65 years is nothing short of amazing!

B cells can also differentiate into long-lived plasma cells able to secrete antibody for months after infection. These cells exist in the bone marrow, and their survival is supported by bone marrow stromal cells. Long-lived plasma cells help prevent reinfection with the same organism, particularly if it remains circulating in the population during an epidemic.

Antibody Production

Compared with the immediacy of the innate immune response, the B-cell response process takes at least 3 to 4 days before being detectable (latent or lag phase; see **Figure 6.26**). IgM levels peak in the serum between 5 and 10 days after infection and then decrease, becoming undetectable in about 20 days, although the kinetics of the antibody response may differ according to the type of pathogen or toxin, exposure route, dose of antigen, and intensity of the initial innate response.

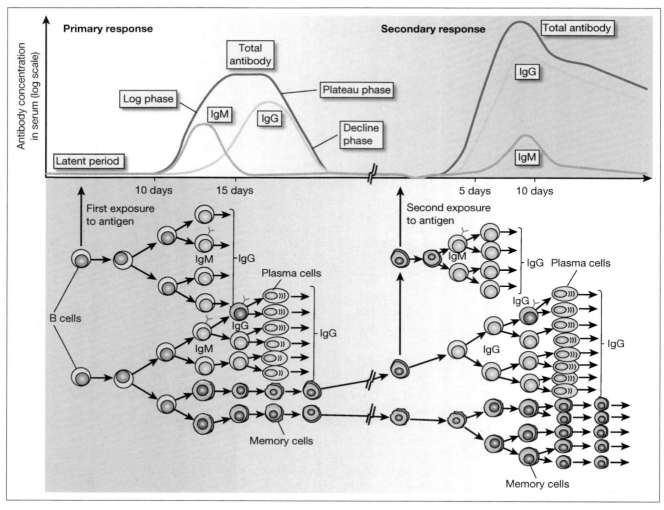

FIGURE 6.26 Primary and secondary (memory) B-cell responses. First presentation of antigen, either due to infection or vaccination, produces a delayed and relatively weak response, with IgM produced first, transitioning to IgG. This stage results in B cells diverging to become either plasma cells or memory cells. Upon a second exposure (or booster shot), antibodies are rapidly produced, the total amount of antibody released increases, and there is very little IgM response. The clone of memory cells expands further. Any further exposures to the antigen will elicit a robust response, providing protection that can last a lifetime.

IgM, immunoglobulin M; IgG, immunoglobulin G.

Source: From Willey J, Sherwood L, Woolverton CJ. *Prescott's Microbiology.* 10th ed. McGraw-Hill; 2016, Figure 34.16.

During the first exposure to a pathogen, IgG production is delayed compared with IgM, and peak levels of IgG are lower than peak levels of IgM. On the other hand, IgG antibodies are long lasting, and during the late stages of the response long-lived plasma cells are able to maintain an active serum level of IgG, which provides protection for weeks and months after the infection has resolved.

Clinical Applications of Antibodies

Antibodies or immunoglobulins constitute about 20% of human plasma proteins. Concentrations of immunoglobulins (titers) specific for antigens on pathogens such as rubella, hepatitis B, and measles viruses can be measured in the blood. Analysis of antibodies for a pathogen-specific antigen can reveal whether an individual has been previously exposed to or vaccinated against that pathogen, and can determine whether the infection is recent (IgM-dominated) or had occurred in the past (IgG-dominated).

As previously mentioned, neutralizing antibodies are often administered as a treatment against specific toxins. Purified preparations of antibodies are used in the ED to neutralize foreign toxins. Snake antivenom is a preparation of purified antibodies specific against snake toxins. Prompt injection of antivenom helps to neutralize snake toxin and allows its clearance from the body before it causes long-term effects and irreversible tissue damage.

Large amounts of pure antibody can be produced for clinical use. Fusing a B-cell clone to an immortal tumor cell creates a B-cell hybridoma. Each B-cell hybridoma can divide seemingly endlessly in culture while producing antibodies that bind to the same antigenic epitope, meaning that all of the antibodies produced have exactly the same specificity. The antibody can be designed to specifically target certain molecules, receptors, or cytokines that modify the response in vivo to reduce or eliminate disease. Over the past 10 years, the use of monoclonal antibodies as therapeutic agents has escalated dramatically. Monoclonal antibodies belong to a class of drug known as *biologics* that have propelled us into an exciting new era of highly targeted drug development. The earliest cytokine-directed antibodies for autoimmune diseases targeted IL-1 and TNF; the targets have now expanded to include IL-17A, IL-22, IL-23, and many others. In addition, monoclonal antibodies are used to treat conditions as varied as cancer, hypercholesterolemia, postpercutaneous coronary intervention, and recurrent *Clostridioides difficile* diarrhea. For a brief list of monoclonal antibodies approved by the Food and Drug Administration (FDA), their targets, and indications, see **Table 6.6**.

Thought Questions

10. How do B cells recognize their antigen and the T$_{fh}$ cells that facilitate their activation?

11. What are the general structural characteristics of antibodies, and what are the features and characteristics of the different antibody types?

T-CELL FUNCTIONS

The T-cell response, sometimes referred to as the *cell-mediated immune response*, involves activation of T cells through the highly specific TCRs, which recognize antigen presented to them in the context of MHC, as previously described. T cells respond to activation by proliferating and producing effector molecules, which include cytokines and cytotoxic molecules. Cytokines are able to act on other cells, including B cells and many cells of innate immunity, sending signals through cytokine receptors that trigger effector mechanisms of immune protection.

Although the functions of CD4 and CD8 T cells overlap, broadly speaking, CD4 T cells function to produce cytokine and are sometimes termed *T-helper* (*Th*) cells whereas CD8 T cells have cytolytic functions in addition to their cytokine-producing abilities. Therefore,

CD8 T cells are often referred to as CTLs. CTLs play a critical role in combating intracellular bacterial and viral infections, as well as cancer cells. Many infections lead to CD4 and CD8 T-cell responses, as well as B-cell responses. The balancing of the different types of response depends on the context of exposure to the antigen and the type of antigen. Cooperation between CD4 and CD8 T cells, B cells, and cells of the innate immune system is responsible for the incredible effectiveness of the adaptive immune system. Humans depend on this system to neutralize and kill pathogens before they cause disease and to limit the duration of a disease once it is established. For this reason, many infectious diseases are acute and limited in duration, and for some diseases, just one infection with the pathogen may protect against having the same disease again.

Major Histocompatibility Complex Restriction

As T cells develop and mature in the thymus, they become committed to expressing either the CD4 co-receptor or the CD8 co-receptor. These receptors dictate the type of antigen that the T cell will recognize. As noted earlier, CD4 T cells only recognize antigen presented by MHC II found on specialized APCs; CD8 T cells only recognize antigen presented by MHC I found on most nucleated cells. This is referred to as *MHC restriction*. Because T cells respond only to antigen that is presented on an MHC molecule, the ability of MHC proteins to associate with different antigen epitopes is critical for determining whether an adaptive immune response will develop against a specific antigen. To optimize and enhance antigen presentation to T cells, the HLA gene locus for MHC class I and MHC class II each encodes for three different co-dominantly expressed proteins. Both sets of inherited alleles are normally expressed. Each MHC gene is highly polymorphic, so thousands of different gene variants (alleles) exist in the human population. This varability in MHC genes and their resulting proteins contributes to phenomena such as transplant rejection. Improving diversity in antigen presentation is an evolutionary strategy to ensure development of efficient adaptive immune responses. However, this diversity may also create different vulnerabilities such that people may have varying levels of susceptibility to a given pathogen or to developing autoimmune diseases.

CD4 T-Cell Responses

CD4 T cells have a key role of coordinating the activation of both arms of the adaptive immune response as well as the effector function of innate cells; most CD4 T-helper cells work to promote and sustain other immune cells to expand, differentiate, or elicit their effector functions (**Figure 6.22b**). Conversely, some CD4 T cells—the Tregs—do exactly the opposite and prevent other immune cells from expanding,

TABLE 6.6 Monoclonal Antibodies Approved for Clinical Use

Antibody	Target	Indication
Abciximab	Platelet glycoproteins	Percutaneous coronary intervention
Adalimumab	TNF	Rheumatoid arthritis
Alirocumab	PCSK9	Hypercholesterolemia
Belimumab	B-lymphocyte stimulator	Systemic lupus erythematosus
Bezlotoxumab	*Clostridioides difficile* toxin B	Recurrent *C. difficile* diarrhea
Certolizumab	TNF	Crohn disease
Daclizumab	IL-2R	Multiple sclerosis
Denosumab	RANKL	Postmenopausal osteoporosis
Golimumab	TNF	Rheumatoid arthritis, ankylosing spondylitis
Infliximab	TNF	Crohn disease, other autoimmune diseases
Ipilimumab	CTLA-4	Metastatic melanoma
Natalizumab	α4 integrin	Multiple sclerosis
Nivolumab	PD-1, immune checkpoint	Metastatic melanoma
Omalizumab	IgE	Asthma
Pembrolizumab	PD-1	Metastatic melanoma
Rituximab	CD20	B-cell non-Hodgkin lymphoma
Secukinumab	IL-17A	Plaque psoriasis
Tocilizumab	IL-6R	Autoimmune arthritis (several)
Trastuzumab	*HER2*	Metastatic breast cancer
Ustekinumab	IL-12 IL-23	Plaque psoriasis

CTLA-4, cytotoxic T lymphocyte–associated protein 4; IgE, immunoglobulin E; HER2, human epidermal growth factor receptor 2; IL, interleukin; PCSK9, proprotein convertase subtilisin/kexin type 9; PD-1, programmed cell death protein 1; RANKL, receptor activator of nuclear factor kappa-B ligand; TNF, tumor necrosis factor.

differentiating, or exerting their effector functions. CD4 T cells recognize antigen in the context of MHC class II, which is expressed only on *professional* APCs.

Antigen on MHC class II molecules mostly originates from extracellular sources. Antigen displayed on MHC class II molecules is detected by the TCR at an *immunological synapse* along with T-helper cell CD3 and CD4 proteins. An additional set of membrane proteins provide co-stimulation signals, the APC CD80 or CD86 proteins bind to T-helper cell CD28. Activation of both the TCR complex and the co-stimulation complex are required for full T-helper cell activation (**Figure 6.27**). Once this dual activation occurs, T-helper cells upregulate expression of genes that encode cytokines and

molecules that can stimulate and support other T cells, B cells, and innate cells. Simultaneously, activated CD4 T cells start to replicate and can generate antigen-specific memory T cells as well. CD4 T cells differentiate into different types of helper cells that are classified based on their cytokine secretion profile and their expression of certain transcription factors that are associated with their effector function.

T-Helper Subsets

The context of antigen presentation to naive CD4 T cells is an important factor for determining the type of T-helper response that will develop. Important factors affecting the context of presentation include (a) type of antigen, (b) amount of antigen, (c) type

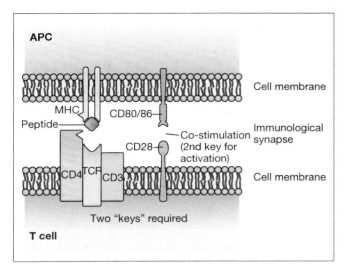

FIGURE 6.27 Antigen presentation to activate T cells. In addition to the TCR–MHC interaction (the first key for T cell activation), effective antigen presentation requires additional co-stimulatory signals and changes in gene expression mediated by the transcription factor CREB in the T cell nucleus. APC, antigen-presenting cell; CREB, cyclic adenosine monophosphate response element-binding protein MHC, major histocompatibility complex; TCR, T cell receptor.

of APC, and (d) local cytokine environment at the time of activation. APCs produce different cytokines depending on the PRR signals they receive and the different receptors they express, so early innate events can lead to different local cytokine environments, which dictate the type of adaptive T-helper response that develops.

The cytokines produced by APCs can reprogram the patterns of gene expression within the T-helper cell, enabling the cell to produce the most effective immune response for a given pathogen. Naive T-helper cells have been characterized as developing into one of five broad T-helper subsets currently described: Th1, Th2, Th17, T$_{fh}$, and Tregs (**Figure 6.28**).

- Th1 cells are characterized by their expression of the transcription factor Tbet, and their secretion of the cytokine interferon gamma (IFN-γ). Th1 cells promote mechanisms of innate cells, such as phagocytosis and antigen presentation, and on the adaptive side, support development of CTLs against intracellular pathogens.
- Th2 cells express the transcription factor GATA3 and secrete the cytokines IL-4, IL-5, IL-9, and IL-13. This subset supports B-cell responses and drives isotype class-switching to IgE, which is important for degranulation of mast cells and basophils to fight helminth infections. On the one hand, the Th2 response has an important role in tissue repair following injury; on the other hand,

it can contribute to the acute allergic responses, progressive fibrosis, and chronic inflammation that occur in asthma, atopic dermatitis, and other allergic disorders.

- T$_{fh}$ cells, discussed earlier in this chapter, are found in secondary lymphoid tissues, where they support maturation and proliferation of B cells.
- IL-17–producing Th17 cells express the transcription factor retinoic-acid receptor-related orphan nuclear receptor gamma (RORγt) and are important for immune responses against extracellular bacteria as well as fungal infections. Like Th2 cells, Th17 cells have a dichotomous nature. Th17 cells can drive inflammatory disorders, such as the autoimmune disease multiple sclerosis; yet Th17 cells are also critical for maintaining homeostasis and barrier protection in the gut. It may be that Th17 cells differ from one another depending on how they are induced; however, this area requires more study.
- Lastly, Tregs function to damp down immune responses, and are essential for preventing autoimmune responses, providing tolerance to the gut microbiota and quenching inflammation once a pathogen has been eliminated. There are two types of Tregs. The first type develops in the thymus; the second type develops when a naive T cell is stimulated in a particular cytokine environment that encourages the expression of FoxP3, the transcription factor associated with Treg function. Tregs exert their effect through immune-suppressive cytokines, such as IL-10, or through cell-to-cell contact and expression of inhibitory molecules, such as cytotoxic T lymphocyte–associated protein 4 (CTLA-4). Blocking inhibitory receptors such as CTLA-4 has revolutionized cancer therapy and led to the development of a new class of medicines known as checkpoint inhibitors.

CD8 T-Cell Responses

Activated through their TCR complex following recognition of antigen on MHC I in conjunction with co-stimulatory signals, CD8 T cells divide and differentiate into effector CTLs. These effector cells are able to identify virus-infected cells or cancer cells through their expression of antigen on MHC I and eliminate them directly by inducing cell lysis or burst (**Figures 6.22c** and **6.29**). Cytolysis protects nearby cells from virus infection and limits tumor cell proliferation. Cytotoxic T cells also produce cytokines such as IFN-γ that can lead to macrophage activation to destroy engulfed pathogens.

In the case of infected or cancerous cells, peptides within the cytosol (from the virus) or abnormal self-proteins (found within tumor cells) are presented on top of MHC class I. These complexes are recognized

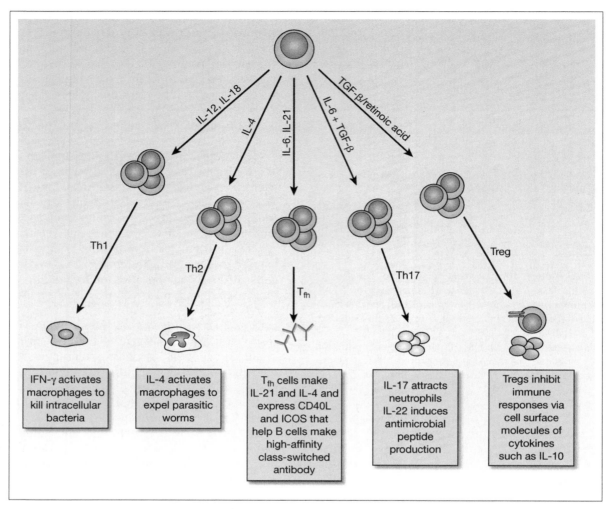

FIGURE 6.28 T-helper (Th) cell subsets and functions.
ICOS, inducible T-cell co-stimulator; IFN, interferon; IL, interleukin; T_{fh} cell, follicular helper T cell; TGF-β, transforming growth factor beta; Treg, regulatory T cell.

by CTLs, which in turn release proteolytic granules to kill the infected or cancerous cell, activating apoptosis. Alternatively, expression of Fas ligand on the membrane of the cytotoxic T cell can initiate apoptosis in the target cell by engaging the apoptotic receptor, Fas.

Unconventional T Cells: γδ T Cells, Mucosal-Associated Invariant T, and Invariant Natural Killer T Cells

The T cells discussed previously are known as conventional T cells and express a TCR known as the αβ TCR. However, a minor subset of T cells that also develop in thymus are termed γδ T cells; these cells express a TCR known as the γδ TCR. They make up only 1% to 5% of circulating T cells but are much more common in epithelial tissues, such as the skin and intestine. γδ T cells are important for tissue homeostasis, thermogenesis in adipose tissue, and epithelial repair. They also

contribute to immune responses against infection and cancer.

Mucosal-associated invariant T (MAIT) cells, as their name suggests, are found in mucosal sites, as well as the skin, liver, and blood. They express an αβ TCR but have an invariant α chain, meaning that they recognize a reduced set of small molecules. These are predominantly vitamin B metabolites from bacteria and fungi, and are not presented on MHC, but rather a related molecule called MR1. MAIT cells can also be activated independently of MR1, through cytokines such as IL-12 and IL-18. MAIT cells are important for controlling bacterial and fungal infections at mucosal sites through secretion of cytokines. They also produce cytolytic granules like conventional CD8 T cells. Owing to their reduced antigen specificity and ability to be activated without antigen, these cells straddle the innate and adaptive arms of the immune response.

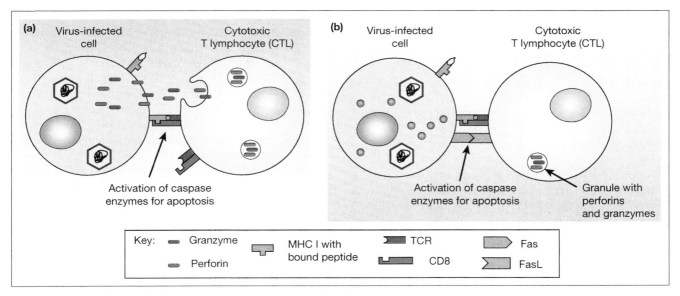

FIGURE 6.29 Mechanisms of cytolysis by CD8 T cells. (**a**) Upon recognizing a virus-infected self-cell, the T cell releases perforin, which penetrates the membrane of the infected cell, and granzyme, an enzyme that enters the cell and initiates apoptosis. (**b**) In addition, the T cell FasL engages the target cell Fas protein, initiating apoptosis of the infected cell.

FasL, Fas ligand; MHC, major histocompatibility complex; TCR, T-cell receptor.

A further unconventional, innate-like T-cell subset comprises the invariant NK T (iNKT) cells. These cells have a semi-invariant TCR that recognizes self and microbial lipid-based antigen presented by MHC I–like CD1d molecules. iNKT cells rapidly produce cytokines after stimulation through their TCR and also have cytotoxic activity. iNKT cells have roles in autoimmunity, infectious diseases, and cancer.

T-Cell Memory

As an adaptive immune response resolves, most responding T cells that have clonally expanded in response to the antigen die. However, a small pool of T cells remains, and these cells survive long term to act as memory T cells that can respond more quickly and more effectively upon subsequent exposures to the same antigen.

Because of the higher numbers of antigen-specific T cells that exist in the memory T-cell pool compared with the naive T-cell pool, when antigen is reencountered, the T cells can expand to higher numbers than in the first, naive T-cell response. Moreover, epigenetic changes that have occurred during the first exposure to antigen endow the remaining memory T cells with the ability to produce effector molecules more quickly than naive T cells. The T cells retain their functional polarization that was established during the initial antigen exposure. For example, if a CD4 T cell had been polarized to a Th1 phenotype and developed into a memory cell, when it reencounters its cognate antigen, it would continue to express the transcription factor Tbet and produce IFN-γ.

Memory T cells are very heterogeneous. Both CD4 and CD8 T cells form distinct subsets of memory T cells that can be identified based on their anatomical location, recirculation patterns, and the types of cell-surface receptors that they express. Resident memory T cells establish in the tissue in which the immune response first occurred; for example, the skin or the lung. These cells do not recirculate but are strategically located to respond to a second infection, which is most likely to occur in a similar location. Effector memory T cells circulate among the tissues, blood, and lymphatics, and central memory T cells, which have a more *resting* phenotype, are typically located in the bone marrow and secondary lymphoid tissues.

As humans age, the ratio of naive T cells to memory T cells changes, with naive T cells predominating at first, during the years in which thymic output is at its greatest. Memory T cells accumulate following infectious exposures, exposure to the commensal microbiota, and vaccination during childhood and adolescence. By adulthood, memory T cells outnumber naive T cells. Interestingly, cytomegalovirus (CMV), which infects the majority of the human population but is usually asymptomatic in immune-competent individuals, leads to a very strong T-cell response. In the elderly, the memory CD8 T-cell pool is often dominated by CMV-specific CD8 T cells in a process known as *memory inflation*.

PATHOGEN–HOST IMMUNE EVASION MECHANISMS

Despite their amazing and intricate immune system, humans still succumb to infectious disease. As the immune system has evolved, so too have pathogens. Viruses, bacteria, fungi, protozoa, and helminths have all devised ways to escape the immune assault that they encounter in the human body.

Many viruses evade immune responses by continually changing their antigens; they do so by introducing mutations in the genes that encode the immunogenic proteins. High antigenic variation can lead to evasion of the adaptive immune response, enabling the virus to infect its host unchecked. Influenza is an example of such a virus, with different variants predominating each year, each encoding antigenically distinct hemagglutinin and neuraminidase viral glycoproteins.

Even though viruses have very small genomes, most pathogenic viruses include genes that encode immune-subverting molecules. Some viruses encode proteins that bind to their nucleic acid, precluding its sensing by host PRRs. Other viruses encode molecules, such as proteases, that degrade components of the inflammasome, preventing its activation. Yet others encode molecules that interfere with antigen presentation, cytokine production, or cytokine signaling. These virally encoded molecules can cleave host proteins or act as cytokines or as decoy cytokine receptors that bind host cytokines, preventing normal immune activation.

Similar to viruses, bacteria also encode proteins to evade host immune responses. Group B streptococcus, which causes severe disease in the very young and very old, blocks the type I IFN response. Group A streptococcus (*Streptococcus pyogenes*), which causes a range of diseases including pharyngitis, scarlet fever, and skin infections, expresses a range of different proteins that inactivate or inhibit components of the complement cascade. Another major cause of human skin infections and more severe systemic disease, *Staphylococcus aureus*, can inhibit complement. *S. aureus* also possesses mechanisms enabling it to modulate and evade neutrophil bactericidal actions, such as producing leukocidins that form pores in the neutrophil membranes and cause them to lyse. Some bacteria, including *S. aureus*, escape phagocytosis by secreting extracellular material that forms a capsule or slime layer. *Mycobacterium tuberculosis*, the cause of the potentially deadly lung disease tuberculosis, also interferes with phagocytosis by preventing formation of the phagolysosome, enabling its survival intracellularly.

More complex organisms, such as the *Plasmodium* species that cause malaria, possess multiple immune evasion strategies. Different stages of the *Plasmodium* life cycle expose the immune system to different antigens, and the organisms are located in different tissues at each stage of the life cycle. This means an adaptive immune response against one stage of the life cycle may not affect the next stage. Notably, during the blood stage *Plasmodium* organisms live intracellularly within erythrocytes, one of the few cell types that does not express MHC I on its surface. This enables the organisms to evade the CD8 T-cell response.

Many other evasion mechanisms exist among pathogens. The complexity and intricacy of the immune system can be appreciated and understood, given the ongoing battle that exists between the human host and the invading microorganisms that constantly develop new mechanisms to escape immune attack.

VACCINATION

Vaccination is the medical procedure by which immunological memory is induced in an individual without requiring an active infection. This prevents the individual from developing severe disease when he or she is subsequently exposed to a given pathogen. If sufficient individuals in a community are immunized against a pathogen, it causes *herd immunity* and prevents disease transmission within the population (**Figure 6.30**).

Vaccines generally contain noninfectious material from a pathogen that still includes the pathogen-specific antigens necessary to stimulate the adaptive immune response. This material can be in many forms, such as proteins, live weakened (attenuated) viruses or bacteria, inactivated viruses, virus-like particles, and inactivated toxins (toxoids). Live vaccines typically elicit a more robust immune response and greater protection than other types of vaccines. Live vaccines are able to replicate in the immunized individual and therefore amplify the antigen available. They also contain PAMPs that can elicit strong innate responses.

Nonlive vaccines require the use of adjuvants, which potentiate the immune response by activating PRRs to drive an innate immune response alongside the adaptive response. Moreover, nonlive vaccines often require more boosts than live vaccines. Boosting occurs when an individual is revaccinated to create a larger antigen-specific memory B- and T-cell pool. Most vaccines require at least one boost to induce a protective memory immune response.

Vaccination has led to major strides in human health. The devastating lethal disease caused by infection with smallpox virus was eradicated through vaccination. Poliovirus, which causes a potentially deadly paralytic disease in some infected individuals, has been eradicated in many countries through vaccination.

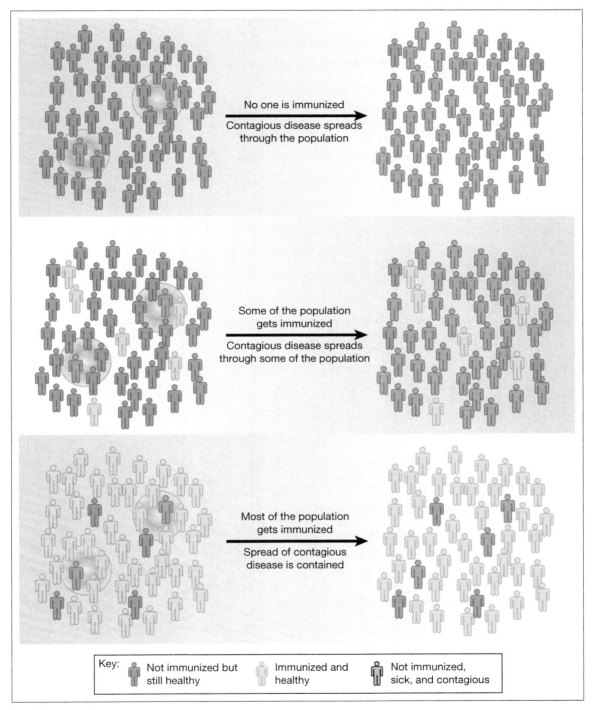

FIGURE 6.30 Herd immunity. In general, the greater the percentage of the population that receives recommended vaccinations, the broader the protection for all.

In countries with strong immunization programs, diseases that were once commonplace, such as measles, diphtheria, mumps, rubella, and tetanus, are now very infrequent.

Vaccines are under development and in clinical trials for the global *big three* infectious disease killers: tuberculosis, HIV, and malaria. Although the BCG vaccine already exists for tuberculosis and is used to protect neonates and young children in countries where the disease is endemic, it does not reliably protect adults against the disease. As new infectious diseases emerge, or old threats reemerge, developing new and better vaccines remains a global health priority.

Although vaccines are subject to rigorous clinical testing for safety, very rarely they can have serious adverse effects. Some people may have a serious allergic response to a vaccine component, so careful monitoring immediately after vaccination is necessary. Immune-compromised individuals are cautioned to avoid vaccination with live vaccines, as there is a risk they can develop disease. Maintaining high levels of vaccination in healthy individuals is, therefore, very important to protect vulnerable individuals in the community through herd immunity. Among the very common mild adverse effects after vaccination are short-lived pain at the vaccination site, fever, and malaise.

Despite the great improvements in human health that vaccination has achieved, there is a small but very vocal resistance against it. This antivaccination movement gained attention in the past few decades through a study published in a reputable medical journal that falsely linked the early childhood vaccine for measles–mumps–rubella (MMR) with autism. Even though some of the data in the study were fabricated, the study design was faulty, and the publication was eventually retracted, the hype that the original publication generated led to some intense public mistrust of vaccination. Evidence for a link between the MMR vaccine and autism has not been supported by large population studies.[10] Furthermore, studies of safety of all vaccines include continuous and ongoing monitoring of adverse events to ensure that the benefits of vaccine use far outweigh any risks.[11]

Despite these and other sources supporting vaccine safety and the greater danger of vaccine avoidance to the individual and population health, false information about the dangers of vaccination is widely available on the Internet, and social media enables the fast spread of this type of misinformation. It is therefore vital that healthcare professionals appreciate the real fears that parents may have around vaccination, and take the time to explain the importance of vaccination for their own children and why vaccination is critical for preventing disease transmission to vulnerable members of society.

HYPERSENSITIVITY

In a large and increasing proportion of individuals in developed countries, the immune system mistakenly generates an immune response to a harmless molecule from the environment, such as food or pollen. Reexposure to that molecule can lead to a strong inflammatory response that causes varying degrees of discomfort and, in very severe cases, death. This type of reaction is known as **hypersensitivity**, **atopy**, or **allergy**. There are four types of hypersensitivity reaction (**Figure 6.31**).

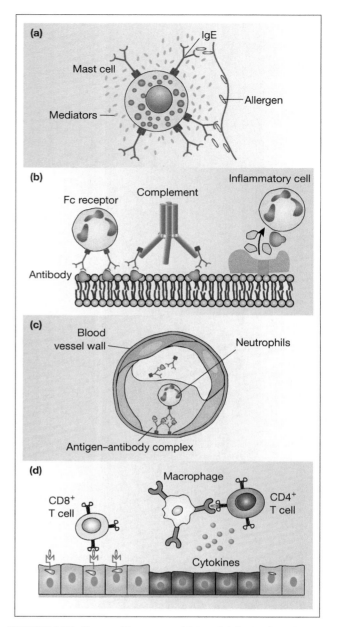

FIGURE 6.31 Types of hypersensitivity. (**a**) Immediate hypersensitivity (type 1). Mast cell degranulation releases histamine, prostaglandins, and cytokines. Cytokines recruit eosinophils and other granulocytes; leukotrienes and eosinophil mediators perpetuate tissue damage. (**b**) Antibody-mediated (type 2). \Specific antibodies alter function of receptors and other membrane proteins. Antibodies bound to tissues attract and activate complement and granulocyte attack mechanisms. (**c**) Immune complex–mediated (type 3). Antigen–antibody complexes deposit in subendothelial tissues, particularly in the kidneys and joints. Complement activation worsens tissue damage. (**d**) T cell–mediated (Type 4). Helper T cells and their cytokines provoke local cell recruitment and inflammation. Cytotoxic T cells kill altered self-cells.

Fc, constant fragment; IgE, immunoglobulin E.

Type 1: Immediate Hypersensitivity

Type 1 reactions are known as immediate hypersensitivity (**Figures 6.31a** and **6.32**). This response is mediated by the production of IgE that recognizes an environmental antigen (in this case, referred to as an *allergen*). Once synthesized and secreted by B cells, IgE circulates throughout the body and binds to high-affinity IgE receptors on the membranes of mast cells and basophils. Upon later exposures, the allergen binds to IgE, causing mast cell and basophil degranulation with immediate release of histamine and development of allergic inflammation. The conditions that develop from type 1 reactions include **hives, eczema, allergic rhinoconjunctivitis** (hayfever, allergic rhinitis), **allergic asthma, food allergy,** and **anaphylaxis**. Although the initial allergic reaction occurs immediately, late-stage reactions occur several hours after allergen exposure as newly synthesized effector molecules take effect. Sustained allergic inflammation can occur, for example, in chronic asthma and eczema.

The pathogenesis of type 1 hypersensitivity is not completely understood. It is thought to involve an interaction between genetic predisposition and environmental exposures. There is a strong familial risk, with identical twins having 50% concordance for allergic disorders.[1] The major step leading to the development of allergies occurs when the body reacts to an allergen with activation of Th2 cells and a subset of T_{fh} cells that direct a stimulated B cell to switch from IgM or IgG production to IgE production. The cytokines released (**Figure 6.32**) direct this class-switching within the lymphoid follicle tissue, after which the B cell produces IgE specific to the allergen. Allergen exposures may come via the skin, causing atopic dermatitis (eczema); through the airways, producing asthma; or through the gastrointestinal tract, producing food allergies. As these disorders commonly present in childhood, additional information is provided in the later section on Pediatric Considerations.

Type 2: Antibody-Mediated Hypersensitivity

Type 2 hypersensitivity reactions can occur when a host cell surface molecule becomes modified by exposure to a chemically reactive molecule, leading the immune system to perceive the host molecule as non-self (**Figure 6.31b**). B cells produce IgM or IgG against the modified host molecule, and IgG binding to host tissue leads to inflammation and cell death mediated by complement and cell-mediated cytotoxicity. An example of this is hypersensitivity caused by the antibiotic penicillin. In other situations, type 2 hypersensitivity can be a mechanism in autoimmune disease (see later discussion).

Type 3: Immune Complex–Mediated Hypersensitivity

In type 3 hypersensitivity responses, IgM or IgG is produced against soluble foreign protein, leading to immune complex formation. Immune complexes are complexes of antigen, usually with IgG, that circulate in the blood and can also form deposits in tissues and activate the complement cascade, leading to inflammation within that tissue and tissue damage. Examples include **poststreptococcal glomerulonephritis**, in which immune complexes deposit in the kidneys, and rheumatoid arthritis, in which immune complexes to endogenous antigens are deposited in the joints (**Figure 6.31c**).

Type 4 (Delayed): T-Cell–Mediated Hypersensitivity

Type 4 hypersensitivity is known as delayed-type hypersensitivity because it occurs several days after exposure to the antigen (**Figure 6.31d**). This response is mediated by CD4 Th1 cells or CD8 T cells and most commonly manifests as a blistering skin rash. The delayed-type hypersensitivity response can be elicited by metals in jewelry such as nickel. Nickel ions that enter the skin can be chelated by histidine residues in host proteins, which are processed and presented to CD4 T cells as non-self. Other examples include the reaction that occurs to the oils on the leaves of poison ivy, and the reaction to proteins from tuberculosis that have been applied to the skin of an infected individual (formerly used as a diagnostic test for tuberculosis [the Mantoux test]).

AUTOIMMUNITY

Autoimmune diseases occur as an aberrant and destructive immune response against self. These responses can occur when immunological tolerance mechanisms break down. In primary lymphoid tissues (bone marrow and thymus), only B and T cells that do not respond to self-proteins, and therefore are tolerant to self, are able to survive and mature. This is known as central immunological tolerance.

Secondary mechanisms of inducing tolerance also exist, because primary immunological tolerance is not perfect, and some self-reactive cells do escape negative selection in the primary lymphoid tissues and go on to mature. These peripheral mechanisms of tolerance include inducing unresponsiveness (anergy) or death in self-reactive cells when they encounter antigen without any additional activating signals, and inducing self-reactive cells to become Tregs or to be suppressed by Tregs.

When both central and peripheral tolerance fail, autoimmunity can occur. The diseases caused by autoimmunity are wide and varied in terms of the tissues and organs affected and the severity of disease. Some autoimmune disorders target one particular cell and tissue type (e.g., pancreatic β cells in **type 1 diabetes mellitus**, acetylcholine receptors in **myasthenia gravis**), while others have evidence of a variety of targets (e.g., rheumatoid arthritis [see **Box 6.5**, earlier], **systemic lupus erythematosus, Sjögren syndrome**). In many cases, assessment of antibody titers is part of the diagnosis, indicating inappropriate activity of both B cells and T cells. Despite the rarity of individual autoimmune diseases, considered together, they are a major cause of disease in developed countries.

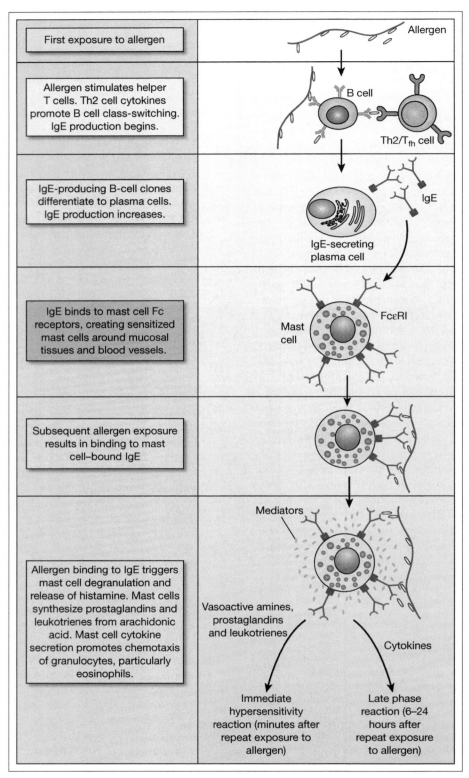

FIGURE 6.32 Pathogenesis of type 1 hypersensitivity. Note that a critical step in the production of allergies is class-switching, which stimulates B cells to change from IgM or IgG to IgE production. Because mast cell membranes have IgE receptors, the IgE molecules can bind onto mast cells and sensitize them to degranulate (release granules of histamine) upon the next antigen exposure. Fc, constant fragment; FcεRI, high-affinity IgE receptor; IgE, immunoglobulin E; IgG, immunoglobulin G; IgM, immunoglobulin M; T_{fh} cell, follicular helper T cell; Th2, T-helper type 2 cell.

Factors that contribute to autoimmunity risk include female sex, older age, environmental exposures (cigarette smoking, obesity), and genetic factors (e.g., HLA genes, loss of function mutations in transcription factors required for negative selection in the thymus or for Treg development). Notably, primary immunodeficiency is a strong risk factor for developing autoimmunity, with over a quarter of patients with primary immunodeficiency reporting one or more autoimmune or inflammatory symptoms. One further relatively new risk for developing autoimmunity is through the use of checkpoint inhibitors in cancer immunotherapy.

Although many of the risks associated with the development of autoimmunity are known, aside from the few loss of function genetic mutations that have been identified, the specific mechanisms involved in this process are largely unknown and are an area of intense research. The earliest stages of autoimmunity evade clinical detection until proposed environmental triggers, acting on someone with a genetic susceptibility, result in the production of autoantibodies at detectable levels. As the condition progresses, tissues come under direct attack by antibodies and complement, as well as by immune complex deposition in tissues resulting in disease signs and symptoms. Ongoing stimulation of T and B cells increases cytokine levels, perpetuating the immune response, and producing tissue destruction and fibrosis (Figure 6.33).

Increasingly, biologic agents, such as monoclonal antibodies, are being used to provide a more targeted approach for treating autoimmune disease than the older, broadly immunosuppressive drugs, thus reducing the risk of infection. It is important to acknowledge that all current therapies are disease modifying rather than curative.

IMMUNODEFICIENCY

There are two main categories of **immunodeficiency**: (a) primary, which are inherited or genetic immune deficiencies, and (b) secondary, which are acquired during life as a result of infection, other diseases, medical intervention, or environmental factors such as stress and poor nutrition.

Primary immune deficiencies affect over 10 million people worldwide. More than 150 different types, affecting both innate and adaptive arms of the immune response, have been defined. Primary immune deficiencies typically present early in life, as soon as protection against infection mediated by maternal antibody in the newborn has waned.[12]

Primary immune deficiencies can result from loss of function mutations in immune cell receptors, cytokines, chemokines, transcription factors, or complement components. These can lead to failure of a particular cytokine pathway or the complement cascade, or to broader

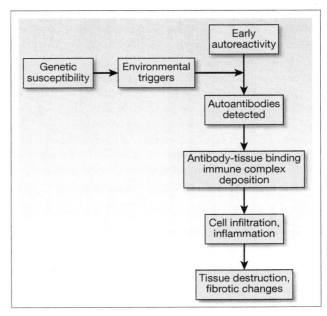

FIGURE 6.33 General mechanisms in autoimmunity. The mechanisms underlying predisposition to autoimmune disease are not known, but family history is usually positive for members with one or more types of autoimmune disease. Against this background, it is thought that environmental exposures or prior infections can trigger autoreactivity. Autoantibodies are often present before any overt disease symptoms. Over time, the autoimmune response increases, with tissue damage resulting from immune and complement activation.

deficiencies involving loss of whole immune cell subsets (e.g., severe combined immunodeficiency [SCID]). Many primary immune deficiencies are X-linked; thus, males are fully affected whereas females are chimeric and retain normal function in some cells.

Defects in specific pathways lead to susceptibility to certain pathogens but not others. For example, individuals with deficiencies in the MAC proteins of the complement cascade are exquisitely susceptible to infection with *Neisseria* species, but are able to defend against many other bacterial infections and have normal responses against viral infection.

Loss of function mutations in the enzymes or cytokine receptors that orchestrate BCR and TCR gene rearrangement and B- and T-cell development, respectively, can lead to SCID as B and T cells fail to develop in the primary lymphoid organs. Affected individuals are devoid of conventional B and T cells and therefore are highly susceptible to a broad range of infections.

For severe primary immunodeficiency, the best outcomes occur with hematopoietic stem cell transplantation. For specific immune deficiencies, regular intravenous immunoglobulin, careful monitoring, prophylactic antimicrobial use, and increased hygiene can help prevent severe infection.

The most prevalent cause of secondary immunodeficiency is **HIV** infection. HIV infects CD4 T cells and some macrophages, and if untreated, leads to significant loss of immune cells throughout the body. This results in broad immune suppression, known as **AIDS**, in which infected individuals become susceptible to *opportunistic infection* with organisms that typically do not cause disease in immune-competent individuals. Until recently, HIV/AIDS was the leading cause of death by a single infectious agent. Robust public health measures to reduce transmission through sexual contact and needle sharing, together with the development and implementation of antiretroviral therapy (ART) that can eliminate the risk of transmission, have contributed to the impressive global reduction in deaths due to HIV/AIDS.

Thought Questions

12. **What are the similarities and differences in development, antigen recognition, and function between CD4- and CD8-bearing T cells?**

13. **What are major differences in cytokine secretion and function between the T-cell subtypes: Th1, Th2, Th17, T$_{fh}$, and Tregs?**

14. **How would a tissue biopsy sample from a region of allergic inflammation compare with one from a region of acute injury–induced (nonallergic) inflammation, in terms of cell types and mediators?**

IMMUNE RESPONSES ACROSS THE LIFE SPAN

The immune system is significantly weaker in infancy and older adulthood than during the rest of the life span (**Figure 6.34**). During prenatal development, the fetus is protected by maternal antibodies that cross the placenta and confer passive immunity. The fetus can tolerate exposure to maternal antigens due to the higher activity of Tregs and Th2 cells, combined with low activity of Th1 and B cells. Similarly, the pregnant woman is tolerant of fetal antigens, due in part to increases in Treg and Th2 activity with lower Th1 activity. At birth, a neonate immediately begins to experience colonization with commensal bacteria: from the vagina during a vaginal delivery, from the skin in a cesarean delivery, and via skin, gastrointestinal, and respiratory routes thereafter. In infancy, maternal passive immunity continues in the form of IgA that is secreted into milk during lactation.

Throughout early childhood development, natural and vaccine exposures increase the immunological repertoire, helped by progressive maturation of lymphocyte function and lymphoid tissue development and function. Exposure to pathogens trains helper and effector cells that reach full functioning between the ages of 10 and 20 years. In older adults, Th2 responses are preserved, while activity of Th1 and B cells declines. In older adults, infections such as influenza have higher morbidity, mortality, and risk of developing secondary bacterial pneumonia.[13,14] Specific concerns in pediatric and gerontological populations follow.

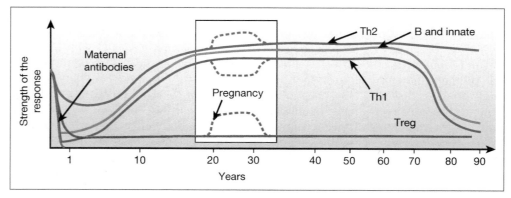

FIGURE 6.34 Immune responses across the life span.
Th, T-helper cell; Treg, regulatory T cell.

Jane Tobias

As noted earlier, most or all of a child's exposure to bacteria starts at birth, beginning the development of immune responsiveness. These exposures can vary with mode of birth (vaginal versus cesarean delivery), antibiotic exposure of the mother or infant, and adoption of breastfeeding. Bacterial colonization of the gut is thought to have primary importance in shaping immune responses throughout the childhood[15] (Figures 6.35 and 6.36). Tolerance of commensal bacteria requires a balance of immunosuppressive activity during early development, with greater activity of Treg and Th2 cells and cytokines IL-10, IL-6, and IL-23. Adaptive immune responses are weak in infants, and immunoglobulin class-switching and affinity maturation do not occur. Thus, infants are susceptible to infections, and vaccines must be boosted to achieve protection.[15]

Later in childhood, environmental exposures to greater numbers of people and animals (siblings and extended family, pets, daycare) and locations (urban versus rural) continue to contribute challenges that mature the immune system (see Figure 6.35). This leads to greater activity of the innate immune system and greater lymphocyte diversity. The *hygiene hypothesis* posits that increased prevalence of type 1 hypersensitivity disorders in the developed world is due to decreased diversity of microbial exposures in early life. Trends in allergy prevalence are consistent with this hypothesis, with allergies increasing and then plateauing in resource-rich countries over the past 40 years, while allergies are now increasing in developing countries that are acquiring more resources for clean air, water, and vaccinations.[16]

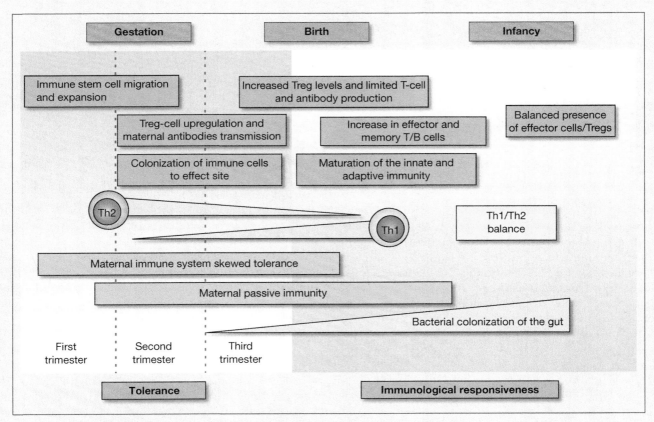

FIGURE 6.35 Stages of immune development from gestation through infancy. Before birth, the fetal immune system is suppressed and does not respond to maternal antigens. Passive immunity is derived from the maternal antibodies that cross the placenta (before birth) and maternal IgA in breast milk (after birth). After birth, normal flora begins to colonize the gut and skin. The gradual increase in microbial diversity occurs against a background of increasing immune competence of the infant such that immune protection increases dramatically in the first year of life.

Th, T-helper cell; Treg, regulatory T cell.

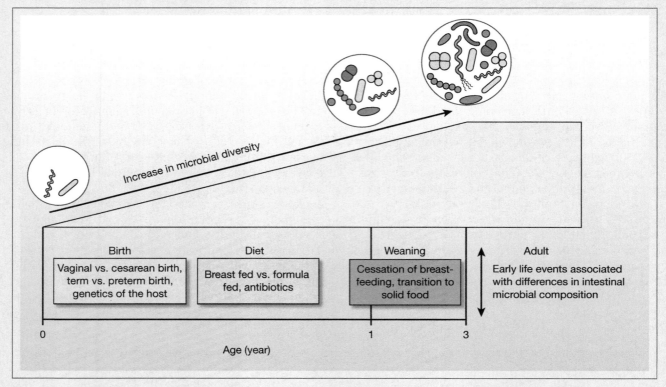

FIGURE 6.36 Postnatal development of diversity of commensal bacteria. The trajectory of colonization with normal flora and infant microbial diversity is influenced by mode of birth (vaginal versus cesarean delivery), breastfeeding versus bottle-feeding, antibiotic exposure, and introduction of solid foods, as well as environmental exposures. Microbial diversity influences immune development and may influence later risk of autoimmune and hypersensitivity disorders.

TYPE 1 HYPERSENSITIVITY IN CHILDREN AND ADOLESCENTS

The global prevalence of allergy-related disorders in adolescents is reported to be greater than 40% (for any disorder), with allergic rhinoconjunctivitis (12.9%) and atopic dermatitis (8.1%) having the highest prevalence. There is a high rate of comorbidity for allergic rhinitis, atopic dermatitis, and asthma.[17] Allergies often begin in childhood, with atopic dermatitis a common disorder in early childhood, and they may wane in intensity through adulthood.[18] Family history generally is positive for siblings or parents with a history of allergy, although a specific gene has not yet been identified for all allergies.

MEDIATORS IN TYPE 1 HYPERSENSITIVITY

The central pathways of type 1 hypersensitivity have been identified (see **Figure 6.31** and earlier discussion). Allergen exposure and release of IL-4 and IL-13 stimulate the Th2 phenotype, promoting B-cell class-switching from IgG production to IgE production. IgE production is critical to allergic responses as it is a step that sensitizes mast cells. Upon repeat exposure

to allergen, the mast cell coated with IgE degranulates, immediately releasing histamine, proteases, and cytokines, and begins to synthesize additional mediators.

Histamine rapidly produces vasodilation and increased vascular permeability, in addition to producing the sensation of itch (in atopic dermatitis) or mucosal irritation (in allergic rhinitis and asthma). Proteases produce local tissue damage and perpetuate inflammation. Cytokines induce chemotaxis in granulocytes (particularly eosinophils), and continue to perpetuate the immune response.

Of the arachidonic acid metabolites formed during an allergic response, prostaglandin D2 and leukotriene C4 have end-organ effects that contribute to the state of allergic inflammation. Prostaglandin D2 promotes vasodilation, facilitating granulocyte chemotaxis. Leukotrienes promote irritation and inflammation. In asthma, leukotrienes are implicated in bronchoconstriction and epithelial damage. Hours after an initial provocation, the late phase of an allergic response may result from the release of major basic protein, a toxic eosinophil mediator[1,19] (**Figure 6.37**). Allergies are similar to disorders of chronic inflammation in that the affected tissue has persistent changes with the presence of long-lived immune cells: T cells, B cells,

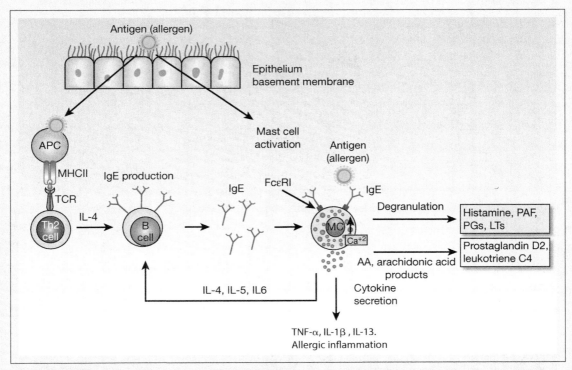

FIGURE 6.37 Cells and mediators of type 1 hypersensitivity. Th2 cytokines IL-4 and IL-13 contribute to B-cell class-switching. Primed MCs reinforce the cytokine milieu with secretion of IL-4, IL-5, and IL-6. Allergen exposure causes mast cell degranulation and production of inflammatory PGs, LTs, and PAF, while also recruiting eosinophils and neutrophils to the allergic inflammatory site. Hours after the acute episode, tissue damage can result from eosinophils releasing major basic protein, a toxic protein.

AA, arachidonic acid; APC, antigen-presenting cell; FcεRI, high-affinity IgE receptor; IgE, immunoglobulin E; IL, interleukin; LTs, leukotrienes; MCs, mast cells; MHC II, major histocompatibility complex class II; PAF, platelet-activating factor; PGs, prostaglandins; TCR, T-cell receptor; Th2, T-helper 2; TNF-α, tumor necrosis factor alpha.

and macrophages. Differences between these chronic states include the predominance of IL-4 and IL-13 in allergic inflammation, along with systemic titers of IgE, and local persistence of eosinophils in an allergic focus. Both states may produce local scar tissue and fibrotic changes that lead to permanent structural alterations.

ATOPIC DERMATITIS

The natural history of **atopic dermatitis** is given here as an example of the pathogenesis of allergic disorders. An early insult that disrupts the epithelial layer initiates the cascade of events shown in **Figure 6.38**. The potential role of epithelial damage is highlighted by the fact that some individuals with atopic dermatitis and other immunological skin disorders have mutations in the filaggrin gene that encodes the epidermal cell protein filaggrin. Abnormal function of this protein is one pathway to epidermal disruption leading to antigen entry. Langerhans cells are APCs of the skin and are the

first responders to antigens that come through the damaged skin barrier. They interact with dermal dendritic cells and migrate to the draining lymph node, where activation of Th2 cells occurs. Th2 cells secrete IL-4, promoting B-cell class-switching to IgE production for the invading antigen. IgE binds to mast cells, which are now primed to degranulate upon further encounters with antigen, releasing histamine, which causes vasodilation, redness, and intense itching.[20] A vicious cycle ensues, with additional skin disruption, antigen invasion, and immune cell proliferation that ramps up the inflammatory response.

Th2 cytokines, IL-4, IL-13, and IL-31, are particularly involved in perpetuation of the inflammatory response, but several categories of T cells contribute. As with other atopic disorders, eotaxin is secreted and recruits eosinophils to the region. Eosinophil secretion of major basic protein contributes to tissue injury and inflammation. A child or adolescent with atopic dermatitis is more prone to begin to react to other skin-associated antigens, resulting in allergic contact dermatitis. These children will have a positive skin

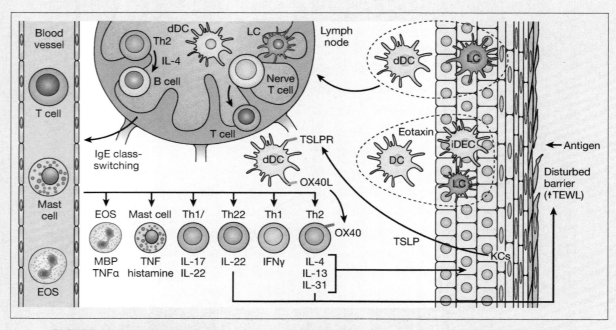

FIGURE 6.38 Cells and mediators in atopic dermatitis. Atopic dermatitis is another form of type 1 hypersensitivity. The cell types involved begin their interaction in the lymph node, but long-term alterations in cytokine levels predispose to ongoing lesion production in affected skin.
DC, dendritic cell; dDC, dermal DC; EOS, eosinophil; iDEC, inflammatory dendritic epidermal cell; IFN-γ, interferon gamma; IgE, immunoglobulin E; IL, interleukin; KCs, keratinocytes; LC, Langerhans cell; MBP, (eosinophil) major basic protein; OX40, stimulatory receptor on Th2 cell; OX40L, OX40 ligand; TEWL, transepidermal water loss; TNF, tumor necrosis factor; TSLP, thymic stromal lymphopoietin; TSLPR, TSLP receptor.

prick response to allergy testing, as well as positive tests for circulating IgE.[20]

FOOD ALLERGIES

In the pediatric patient, almost any food can produce an immune response triggering a reaction. Reactions to foods can occur at any age; however, **food intolerance** usually manifests in early childhood. Although gastrointestinal exposure to most foreign proteins is usually tolerance inducing, up to 6% of children experience food allergic reactions in the first 3 years of life, including approximately 2.5% with cow's milk allergy, 1.5% with egg allergy, and 1% with peanut allergy. Peanut allergy prevalence has tripled over the past decade. Most children *outgrow* milk and egg allergies, but approximately 80% to 90% of children with peanut, nut, or seafood allergy retain their allergy for life.[21]

Food intolerances result from a variety of mechanisms, whereas the pathophysiology of food allergy is predominantly IgE and cell mediated.[22] Similar to other atopic disorders, exposure to the particular food in a susceptible pediatric patient results in the formation of specific IgE antibodies that bind to receptors on the mast cells, basophils, macrophages, and dendritic cells. Air-borne exposure to vegetable antigens may also result in allergies to the ingested food. It is through the release of histamine and other mediators that the pediatric patient demonstrates both local and systemic reactions.

Symptoms manifested during IgE-mediated food reactions are not restricted to the gastrointestinal tract. Skin reactions include urticaria, angioedema, and flushing. Respiratory symptoms include nasal congestion, rhinorrhea, nasal pruritus, sneezing, laryngeal edema, dyspnea, and wheezing. Gastrointestinal symptoms include oral pruritus, nausea, abdominal pain, vomiting, and diarrhea. Severe reactions may proceed to shock and anaphylaxis. Food reactions are the single most common cause of anaphylaxis seen in hospital EDs in the United States.

Until recently, families were encouraged to avoid the exposure of infants to allergenic foods. This management actually tended to increase rates of food allergy. Current recommended practice is exclusive breastfeeding for 4 to 6 months, followed by gradual introduction of all foods. Slow introduction should include common food allergens including cow's milk, other dairy products, eggs, wheat, peanut, and soy.

Nancy Tkacs

Immune system activity decreases with age, with adaptive immunity impaired more than innate immunity (**Table 6.7**). This phenomenon has been referred to as *immunosenescence*.[23] Age-related immune system alterations lead to an increased number of infections, as well as greater infection-associated morbidity and mortality rates; diminished wound healing; decreased effectiveness of adaptive immunity, including responses to vaccines; and decreased immune surveillance, contributing to increased cancer incidence. At the same time, there are two opposing changes in innate immunity: (a) Decreased function of neutrophils, monocytes/macrophages, dendritic cells, and NK cells increases vulnerability to infections, while (b) there is a general increase in inflammatory mediators, particularly IL-1β and IL-6, and TNF-α. The process of immunosenescence explains, in part, why older adults often have multiple comorbid conditions and conditions with an inflammatory component.

IMMUNE CELLULAR SENESCENCE AND DISEASE

Throughout the life, the adaptive immune system builds up an armament against pathogens through T-cell–directed cellular and humoral activity. Both T cells and B cells acquire memory of pathogens following exposures to their antigens and are able to launch fast and effective responses following subsequent exposures. These cells and related cell receptors of the adaptive immune system are maintained into the sixth decade, and then gradually decline with age. Multipotent stem cells in the bone marrow generally reduce replication rates, potentially due to shortening of telomeres. The bone marrow's lymphocyte production rate specifically decreases, with a shift to greater numbers of cells progressing to the myeloid lineage. Specific to T cells, throughout adulthood, the thymus gland undergoes involution, leading to a decline of naive T cells. Thymic involution accelerates after age 70. With slow but progressive losses in naive and memory T and B cells, susceptibility to pathogens increases.[13,14]

The progressive weakening of adaptive immunity with aging is manifested in a number of ways:

- Vaccinations are less effective and may need additional boosters, adjuvants, or higher doses.
- Latent infections may reemerge—the most common of these is the reactivation of varicella zoster virus, producing shingles.
- Cancer occurrence increases owing to inadequate immune surveillance.
- An additional consequence is that the recently developed immune-based cancer therapies may not be as effective in older adults as in younger adults.

TABLE 6.7 Immune Changes With Aging

Type of Tissue	Changes
Primary lymphoid tissue: bone marrow	↓ lymphoid progenitors ↓ progenitor self-renewal ↑ DNA damage
Primary lymphoid tissue: thymus	↓ thymus tissue mass (involution) ↓ T-cell seeding from bone marrow ↓ thymus cellular output ↑ adipose deposition in thymus
Secondary lymphoid tissue: spleen and lymph nodes	↓ naïve T-cell numbers ↓ follicular cell developmental network ↓ dendritic cell antigen presentation ↑ inflammatory cytokines ↑ TGF-β ↑ pool of memory T cells
Tissues and organ systems	↓ specific immune protection ↓ proliferation of naïve and memory T cells ↓ effector molecule production and secretion ↑ nonspecific inflammation

TGF-β, transforming growth factor beta.

INFLAMMAGING

The concept of **inflammaging** is based on observations that the levels of inflammatory mediators generally increase with aging. Accelerated stimulation by pathogens (PAMPs of bacteria and viruses) and altered self-proteins and cells (DAMPs released from damaged and dying cells) are detected by PRRs, stimulating the pathways of innate inflammation, including cytokine release. At the cellular level, cell senescence is a state reached as cells stop replicating because of injury or aging and telomere shortening. These cells can transition to the senescence-associated secretory phenotype (SASP) in which they release damage signals and proinflammatory mediators. Proinflammatory conditions such as atherosclerosis, insulin resistance and type 2 diabetes mellitus, increased adiposity, cancer, and alterations in gut microbiota all contribute to this heightened inflammatory state in a vicious cycle that also worsens those conditions (**Figure 6.39**).[24-28]

With the increased inflammatory state, the damaging effects of innate immune activation are perpetuated, including oxidative stress; nucleic acid and protein damage; and cell, tissue, and organ dysfunction. Heightened inflammation may contribute to frailty, loss of function, and earlier death. Rates of age-related progression into this state are very variable and are influenced by genetics, environment, diet, activity level, stress, social determinants of health, and numerous psychosocial factors. The biological pathways and mechanisms connecting aging to the heightened inflammatory state and its associated effects on morbidity and mortality remain to be elucidated.

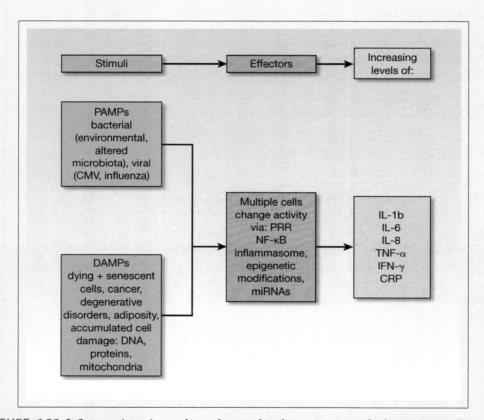

FIGURE 6.39 Inflammaging. A number of age-related exposures and changes contribute to increased levels of chronic inflammatory cytokines and other mediators in some older adults. This inflammatory milieu may then accelerate age-related dysfunction.

CMV, cytomegalovirus; CRP, C-reactive protein; DAMP, danger-associated molecular pattern; IFN-γ, interferon gamma; IL, interleukin; miRNA, microRNA; NF-κB, nuclear factor kappa B; PAMP, pathogen-associated molecular pattern; PRR, pattern recognition receptor; TNF, tumor necrosis factor.

CASE STUDY 6.1: A Patient With Allergic Rhinitis

Linda W. Good

Chief Complaint: *"I'm here for my sinuses. I know what I have, and I always need a Z-pak to get over this," the patient states as he enters the examination room. This healthy-appearing 27-year-old Caucasian man then describes 10 days of alternately stuffy and runny nose, postnasal drip, sneezing, and "that deep itch that I can't get to scratch." He explains, "This happens every year at this time and I take Sudafed, which keeps me from sleeping and leaves me tired and less able to work, so now I've started Afrin instead, because I can't breathe without it."*

History of Present Illness/Review of Systems: You elicit the following additional facts: The patient has had no fevers and no pain or pressure in the ears or face, but has had mild sore throat that is worse in the mornings. Upon closer questioning, you suspect that the patient's inability to breathe is related to nasal obstruction and not the lungs. He denies wheezing, shortness of breath, coughing, or sputum production, but admits to tearing and burning of his eyes. Review of systems is negative for any cardiovascular, gastrointestinal, musculoskeletal, or neurosensory concerns. His sleep has been somewhat disrupted, and appetite and energy a little low, which he attributes to the decongestant medication.

Past Medical/Family History: The patient's past medical history is significant for childhood asthma and eczema. He had otitis media frequently growing up and his mother told him he was on repetitive courses of antibiotics as a child. Both parents were smokers, but he never smoked. He grew up with cats and thought that they might have caused his asthma, so he has only had dogs as pets since he left home. He works as an inspector for the water company, which requires going into basements of homes.

Physical Examination: Findings are as follows: temperature of 97°F, blood pressure of 116/70 mm Hg, heart rate of 60 beats/min, and respirations of 12 breaths/min. BMI is 22 kg/m². You note good landmarks and normal color of the tympanic membranes; no palpable facial tenderness or cervical adenopathy, but mildly erythematous oropharynx with cobblestoning of the posterior pharyngeal wall. Nasal turbinates are swollen bilaterally, with clear rhinorrhea visible anteriorly. Lungs are clear and abdominal examination is benign. Routine CBC and CMP results are normal.

CASE STUDY 6.1 QUESTIONS
- *What factors in the patient's history indicate sources of upper airway irritation?*
- *What mediator released during a type 1 hypersensitivity reaction can contribute to mucosal edema and swelling, nasal stuffiness, and itchy nose and eyes?*

BMI, body mass index; CBC, complete blood count; CMP, comprehensive metabolic panel.

BRIDGE TO CLINICAL PRACTICE

Ben Cocchiaro

PRINCIPLES OF ASSESSMENT

History

Evaluate:

- *Constitutional symptoms:* fevers, pain (joint pain and other), weight loss, anorexia, fatigue
- *Potential exposures in suspected allergies:* pets, work environment, associations with food and drink
- *System-specific symptoms related to:*
  - Allergic rhinitis: ENT—stuffy nose, runny nose, sneezing, itchy eyes, postnasal drip, and cough
  - Asthma—chest tightness, dyspnea, cough, wheezing, worsening with exposures
  - Atopic dermatitis—intense itching, inflammatory papules
  - Rheumatoid arthritis—joint pain, swelling, and stiffness, difficulties with activities of daily living, constitutional symptoms
- *Suggestive findings in immune disorders:* patients may have more than one autoimmune or hypersensitivity disorder; family history is common; note history of exacerbations and remissions
- *History of drug allergies must focus on specific reactions:* nonspecific rash, nausea, and vomiting (less likely to be true allergy); hives, difficulty breathing (more likely to be true allergy)
- Recurrent infections may be a sign of immunodeficiencies

Physical Examination

Findings may be specific to organ system:

- *ENT:* boggy nasal mucosa, red and watery eyes, erythema and *cobblestoning* of pharynx
- *Asthma:* wheezing, use of accessory muscles of respiration, cyanosis if airflow severely limited
- *Arthritis:* swollen, deformed joints with redness and warmth
- *Atopic dermatitis:* redness, popular rash, scaly, thickened skin

Diagnostic Tools

- Radiography for joint-related disorders
- MRI—can be used in multiple sclerosis
- Tissue biopsy

Laboratory Evaluation

- Complete blood count with differential
- C-reactive protein (acute phase protein): nonspecific indicator of inflammation
- *ESR:* nonspecific indicator of inflammation
- *Immunoassays of IgG, IgM (autoantibodies, vaccine titers):* specific antibodies are diagnostic for certain autoimmune disorders
  - Systemic lupus erythematosus—ANA
  - Rheumatoid arthritis—rheumatoid factor and anticyclic citrullinated peptide antibodies
  - Type 1 diabetes—antiislet antibodies, antiglutamic acid decarboxylase (GAD) antibodies
- Allergy skin testing

MAJOR DRUG CLASSES

- *Glucocorticoid steroids:* generally immunosuppressive, may be directly applied to target tissues (inhaled corticosteroids for asthma, topical corticosteroids for atopic dermatitis, intraarticular injection for joint disorders). Localized or short-term systemic use is preferable to avoid adverse effects of long-term administration
- *Antihistamines:* often used to reduce allergic responses
- *Nonsteroidal antiinflammatory drugs:* inhibit production of arachidonic acid metabolites prostaglandins and leukotrienes. Adverse effects can occur, particularly in older adults.
- *Disease-modifying antirheumatic drugs* (DMARDs)
- *Synthetic immunosuppressants:* methotrexate, azathioprine, chloroquine, cyclophosphamide, cyclosporine, leflunomide, sulfasalazine, tofacitinib
- Biologics *(monoclonal antibodies):* adalimumab, etanercept, infliximab, rituximab, golimumab (see also **Table 6.6**)

ANA, antinuclear antibodies; ENT, eyes/nose/throat; ESR, erythrocyte sedimentation rate; GAD, glutamic acid decarboxylase; IgG, immunoglobulin G; IgM, immunoglobulinM.

KEY POINTS

- The immune system comprises body mechanisms that protect from microbial invaders and cancerous cells at the levels of physical barriers (skin and mucous membranes); a rapidly activated, nonselective, innate immune system; and a slowly developing but highly specific adaptive immune system.
- The innate immune response recognizes general molecular patterns of pathogens and rapidly recruits many phagocytic cells to engulf and destroy the pathogens.
- The adaptive immune response recognizes specific patterns of pathogens called antigens and stimulates limited numbers of B and T lymphocytes responsive to those antigens to proliferate and generate immune defenses.
- The primary lymphoid organs are the bone marrow, site of lymphocyte production and B-cell development, and the thymus gland, where T cells develop.
- Lymph nodes are secondary lymphoid organs and are the sites of communication between antigen-presenting cells, T cells, and B cells during the developing immune response to antigen.
- B lymphocytes express B-cell receptors with antigen-recognizing characteristics similar to the antibodies they will eventually secrete. Gene rearrangement is the method by which a small number of B-cell receptor genes can code for a huge number of potential antibodies.
- T lymphocytes express T-cell receptors from genes that have undergone gene rearrangement, creating a great diversity of antigen-recognition possibilities. T cells, however, can only recognize antigens presented on membrane proteins termed major histocompatibility class (MHC) proteins.
- The lymph nodes, spleen, and gut-associated lymphoid tissues are the major sites of antigen presentation and interactions of T cells and B cells.
- The innate immune response is initiated when tissue injury and invasion stimulates sentinel cells such as macrophages and mast cells.
- Acute inflammation ensues, with release of chemotactic factors that rapidly recruit additional neutrophils and monocytes into the region of injury.
- Leukocyte chemotaxis is added by the release of histamine and prostaglandins that produce vasodilation and increased capillary permeability.

- Neutrophils and macrophages phagocytose invading organisms and release cytokines that stimulate further chemotaxis, as well as promoting bone marrow leukocyte proliferation.
- Complement proteins are synthesized by the liver and circulate as pro-proteins that need cleavage for activation (similar to the clotting cascade). Complement is activated by bacterial exposure, antibody binding, and mannose-binding lectin. The cascade generates proteins that directly opsonize and kill bacteria, and promote chemotaxis.
- NK cells are *innate lymphoid* cells in that they have lymphoid origins but function like cells of the innate immune system. They are particularly active at killing virus-infected and cancerous cells. The roles of recently identified innate lymphoid cells are still being defined.
- Chronic inflammation is a pathological state in which a localized immune response does not proceed to normal wound healing. Instead, long-lived macrophages, T cells, and B cells perpetuate a response to one or more tissue antigens, creating pain, swelling, and impaired function.
- Adaptive immunity allows for specific targeting of one antigen or invading organism and neutralizing it by a combination of antibodies that mark circulating extracellular antigens for destruction and cell-mediated immunity: lysis of self-cells infected with intracellular pathogens.
- B cells recognize circulating antigens through their B-cell receptors, migrate to lymph nodes and tissues, and are stimulated to maturation and activation by T-helper cells selective for the same antigen.
- Once mature, B cells proliferate and secrete antibodies, beginning with IgM and maturing to IgG secretion. Continued presence of the antigen stimulates affinity maturation of B cells to produce antibodies with increasing affinity for antigen.
- B cells ultimately differentiate into (a) plasma cells—large cells with greatly enhanced capacity for antibody secretion, and (b) memory cells—long-lived cells that can rapidly activate in response to a later encounter with their antigen. Memory B cells can provide protection for many years to decades.
- Antibodies can bind to and neutralize toxins, opsonize bacteria to promote phagocytosis, and bind to bacteria to activate complement-mediated killing. When a pathogen is encountered for the second time, the rapid production

of antibodies clears the pathogen, often before any illness is experienced.

- IgG is the most abundant antibody, whereas IgA predominates at mucosal surfaces. IgE is present at very low levels but is elevated in individuals with allergies.

- T cells can be subdivided based on their membrane proteins. The marker CD4 is associated with T-helper cells, whereas the marker CD8 is associated with cytotoxic T cells.

- CD4 T cells recognize antigen presented by specialized APCs on the APC cell MHC II molecules. Once activated, many CD4 cells stimulate B-cell responses and other responses of adaptive immunity. These cells are further subdivided into Th1, Th2, Th17, T_{fh}, and Tregs, each with a unique spectrum of activity.

- All nucleated cells express MHC I proteins on their membranes. Intracellular protein turnover is linked to the presentation of protein fragments on MHC I. When a virus-infected or cancerous cell begins to display abnormal protein antigens on MHC I, CD8 cells bind via their T-cell receptors.

- CD8 cells release perforin and granzyme enzymes to lyse infected/abnormal cells, and can also trigger apoptosis via the Fas pathway.

- Additional lymphocyte classes provide protection of epithelia, secrete cytokines, and have NK cell attributes.

- Memory T cells of both the CD4 and CD8 types are produced throughout the life span. They may reside in the tissue where their antigen was first encountered, or circulate through the blood, tissues, and lymph tissues.

- Through vaccination, people are exposed to antigenic determinants or whole (weakened) injections of major infectious pathogens, provoking a primary immune response and memory cell formation. A booster dose leads to a secondary immune response and long-lasting protection. Empirical evidence determines the need for additional booster shots at certain intervals.

- Hypersensitivity reactions are excessive immune responses to normally innocuous stimuli. The most common form, type 1 hypersensitivity, is also known as atopy or allergy. In allergy, individuals respond to allergen exposure with Th2-promoted class-switching of B cells to produce IgE instead of IgG. Mast cells become sensitized through IgE binding to mast cell membrane receptors for the IgE constant region. Subsequent exposures lead to mast cell degranulation and generation of an allergic inflammatory response in the exposed tissue.

- Hypersensitivity can also overlap with autoimmunity when antibodies are produced to self-proteins. This is termed type 2 hypersensitivity.

- Autoimmunity is the pathological immune response to one's own cells and tissues. The genetics of autoimmunity involves, in part, certain classes of HLA genes that code for the MHC proteins. Vulnerable individuals often have more than one autoimmune disorder.

- Immunodeficiency disorders are less common than hypersensitivity and autoimmunity. The most common immunodeficiency is secondary, occurring in patients with HIV infection who have loss of CD4 cells to viral attack.

- Fetal development includes development of the main features of the immune system, but the cells and tissues are in a latent stage until birth. At birth, neonates have circulating IgG that crossed the placenta from the mother's blood. In the early postnatal period, vulnerability to infections is high, as this passive protection wanes.

- Colonization with commensal bacteria begins at birth, and the spectrum of bacteria varies with method of delivery (vaginal versus cesarean). In the first several months of life, the infant is exposed to many environmental microorganisms, and often has many immunizations. Thus, within the first year of life, the immune system has gained experience and strength in responding to pathogens.

- Early in life, treatment with antibiotics or failure to experience certain exposures may lead to later life immune vulnerabilities, particularly allergies.

- In older adults, the thymus gland involutes, with decreased immune function and accumulation of fatty, nonfunctional tissue. Few naive T cells are produced, and the diversity of the T-cell repertoire decreases. Infections induce greater morbidity and mortality, and vaccines are less effective.

- The cells of innate immunity are less active in older adults, but other cells can develop an inflammatory phenotype. Cytokine levels tend to be higher in older adults, and contribute to age-related decline in function, in the phenomenon of inflammaging.

REFERENCES

1. Abbas AK, Lichtman AH, Pillai S. *Basic Immunology: Functions and Disorders of the Immune System*. 5th ed. Philadelphia, PA: Elsevier; 2016.

2. Rubin Z, Pappalardo A, Schwartz A, et al. Prevalence and outcomes of primary immunodeficiency in hospitalized children in the United States. *J Allergy Clin Immunol Pract*. 2018;6:1705–1710. doi:10.1016/j.jaip.2017.12.002.

3. Centers for Disease Control and Prevention. Statistics overview: HIV surveillance report. https://www.cdc.gov/hiv/statistics/overview/index.html. Accessed February 12, 2019.

4. UNAIDS. Global HIV & AIDS statistics—2018 fact sheet. http://www.unaids.org/en/resources/fact-sheet. Accessed February 12, 2019.

5. Kolaczkowska E, Kubes P. Neutrophil recruitment and function in health and inflammation. *Nat Rev Immunol*. 2013;13:159–175. doi:10.1038/nri3399.

6. Papayannapoulos V. Neutrophil extracellular traps in immunity and disease. *Nat Rev Immunol*. 2018;18:134–147. doi:10.1038/nri.2017.105.

7. Ebbo M, Crinier A, Vély F, et al. Innate lymphoid cells: major players in inflammatory diseases. *Nat Rev Immunol*. 2017;17:665–678. doi:10.1038/nri.2017.86.

8. Smolen JS, Aletaha D, Barton A, et al. Rheumatoid arthritis. *Nat Rev Dis Primers*. 2018;4:18001. doi:10.1038/nrdp.2018.1.

9. Panum PL. *Observations Made During the Epidemic of Measles on the Faroe Islands in the Year 1846* (A translation from the Danish). Originally published in the Bibiliothek for Laeger, Copenhagen, 3R, 1847;1:270–344. http://www.med.mcgill.ca/epidemiology/courses/EPIB591/Fall%2010/midterm%20presentations/Paper9.pdf.

10. Hviid A, Hansen JV, Frisch M, Melbye M. Measles, mumps, rubella vaccination and autism: a nationwide cohort study. *Ann Intern Med*. 2019;170(8):513–520. doi:10.7326/M18-2101.

11. DiPasquale A, Bonanni P, Garçon N, et al. Vaccine safety evaluation: practical aspects in assessing benefits. *Vaccine*. 2016;34:6672–6680. doi:10.1016/j.vaccine.2016.10.039.

12. Rubin Z, Pappalardo A, Schwartz A, et al. Prevalence and outcomes of primary immunodeficiency in hospitalized children in the United States. *J Allergy Clin Immunol Pract*. 2018;6:1705–1710. doi:10.1016/j.jaip.2017.12.002.

13. Simon AK, Hollander GA, McMichael A. Evolution of the immune system in humans from infancy to old age. *Proc R Soc B*. 2015;282:20143085. doi:10.1098/rspb.2014.3085.

14. Goronzy JJ, Gustafson CE, Weyand CM. Immune deficiencies at the extremes of age. In: Rich RR, Fleisher TA, Shearer WT, et al., eds. *Clinical Immunology: Principles and Practice*. 5th ed. Philadelphia, PA: Elsevier; 2019:chap 38, 535–543.

15. Dzidik M, Boix-Amorós A, Selma-Royo M, et al. Gut microbiota and mucosal immunity in the neonate. *Med Sci*. 2018;6:56. doi:10.3390/medsci6030056.

16. Gensollen T, Blumberg RS. Correlation between early-life regulation of the immune system by microbiota and allergy development. *J Allergy Clin Immunol*. 2017;139:1084–1091. doi:10.1016/j.jaci.2017.02.011.

17. Christiansen ES, Kjaer HF, Eller E, et al. The prevalence of atopic diseases and the patterns of sensitization in adolescence. *Pediatr Allergy Immunol*. 2018;27:847–853. doi:10.1111/pai.12650.

18. Thomsen SF. Epidemiology and natural history of atopic diseases. *Eur Clin Respir J*. 2015;2:24642. doi:10.3402/ecrj.v2.24642.

19. Amin K The role of mast cells in allergic inflammation. *Respir Med*. 2012;106:9–14. doi:10.1016/j.rmed.2011.09.007.

20. Gittler JK, Krueger JG, Guttman-Yassky E. Atopic dermatitis results in intrinsic barrier and immune abnormalities: implications for contact dermatitis. *J Allergy Clin Immunol*. 2013;131(2):300–313. doi:10.1016/j.jaci.2012.06.048.

21. Nowak-Wegrzyn A, Sampson HA, Sicherer SH. Food allergy and adverse reactions to foods. In: Kliegman RM, Stanton BF, St Geme JW, et al., eds. *Nelson Textbook of Pediatrics*. 20th ed. Philadelphia, PA: Elsevier; 2015:chap 151, 1137–1143.

22. Sampson HA, O'Mahony L, Burks AW, et al. Mechanisms of food allergy. *J Allergy Clin Immunol*. 2018;141:11–19. doi:10.1016/j.jaci.2017.11.005.

23. Nikolich-Zugich J, Davies JS. Homeostatic migration and distribution of innate immune cells in primary and secondary lymphoid organs with ageing. *Clin Exp Immunol*. 2017;187:337–344. doi:10.1111/cei.12920.

24. Fougere B, Boulanger E, Nourhashémi F, et al. Chronic inflammation: accelerator of biological aging. *J Gerontol A Med Sci*. 2017;72:1218–1225. doi:10.1093/gerona/glw240.

25. Stout MB, Justice JN, Nicklas BJ, et al. Physiological aging: links among adipose tissue dysfunction, diabetes, and frailty. *Physiology*. 2017;32:9–19. doi:10.1152/physiol.00012.2016.

26. Wagner K-H, Cameron-Smith D, Wessner B, et al. Biomarkers of aging: from function to molecular biology. *Nutrients*. 2016;8:338. doi:10.3390/nu8060338.

27. Weyand CM, Goronzy JJ. Aging of the immune system: mechanisms and therapeutic targets. *Ann Am Thorac Soc*. 2016;13:S422–S428. doi:10.1513/AnnalsATS.201602-095AW.

28. Franceschi C, Garagnani P, Parini P, et al. Inflammaging: a new immune-metabolic viewpoint for age-related diseases. *Nat Rev Endocrinol*. 2018;14:576–590. doi:10.1038/s41574-018-0059-4.

SUGGESTED RESOURCES

Boehm T, Takahama Y, eds. *Thymic Development and Selection of T Lymphocytes*. Vol. 373. Berlin, Germany: Springer-Verlag Berlin Heidelberg; 2014.

Brubaker SW, Bonham KS, Zanoni I, et al. Innate immune pattern recognition: a cell biological perspective. *Ann Rev Immunol*. 2015;33:257–290. doi:10.1146/annurev-immunol-032414-112240.

Buckner JH. Mechanisms of impaired regulation by CD4+/CD25+/FOXP3+ regulatory T cells in human autoimmune diseases. *Nat Rev Immunol*. 2010;10:849–859. doi:10.1038/nri2889.

Dendrou CA, Fugger L, Friese MA. Immunopathology of multiple sclerosis. *Nat Rev Immunol.* 2015;15:545–558. doi:10.1038/nri3871.

Galli SJ, Borregaard N, Wynn TA. Phenotypic and functional plasticity of cells of innate immunity: macrophages, mast cells, and neutrophils. *Nat Immunol.* 2011;12:1035–1044. doi:10.1038/ni.2109.

Galli SJ, Grimbaldeston M, Tsai M. Immunomodulatory mast cells: negative, as well as positive, regulators of immunity. *Nat Rev Immunol.* 2008;8:478–486. doi:10.1038/nri2327.

Girard J-P, Moussion C, Förster R. HEVs, lymphatics and homeostatic immune cell trafficking in lymph nodes. *Nat Rev Immunol.* 2012;12:762–773. doi:10.1038/nri3298.

Goldberg AC, Rizzo LV. MHC structure and function—antigen presentation, part 1. *Einstein (Sao Paulo).* 2015;13:153–156. doi:10.1590/S1679-45082015RB3122.

Goldberg AC, Rizzo LV. MHC structure and function—antigen presentation, part 2. *Einstein (Sao Paulo).* 2015;13:157–162. doi:10.1590/S1679-45082015RB3123.

Hussain A, Ali S, Hussain S. The anti-vaccination movement: a regression in modern medicine. *Cureus.* 2018;10:e2919. doi:10.7759/cureus.2919.

Iwasaki A, Foxman EF, Molony RD. Early local immune defenses in the respiratory tract. *Nat Rev Immunol.* 2017;17:7–20. doi:10.1038/nri.2016.117.

Kabashima K, Honda T, Ginhoux F, et al. The immunological anatomy of the skin. *Nat Rev Immunol.* 2019;19:19–30. doi:10.1038/s41577-018-0084-5.

Kaplan DH, Igyártó BZ, Gaspari AA. Early immune events in the induction of allergic contact dermatitis. *Nat Rev Immunol.* 2012;12:114–124. doi:10.1038/nri3150.

Kirman JR, Henao-Tamayo MI, Agger EM. The memory immune response to tuberculosis. *Microbiol Spectr.* 2016;4(6). doi:10.1128/microbiolspec.TBTB2-0009-2016.

Kondo M. Lymphoid and myeloid lineage commitment in multipotent hematopoietic progenitors. *Immunol Rev.* 2010;238:37–46. doi:10.1111/j.1600-065X.2010.00963.x.

Kumar V, Abbas AK, Aster JC. Inflammation and repair. In: Kumar V, Abbas AK, Aster JC, eds. *Robbins Basic Pathology.* 10th ed. Philadelphia, PA: Elsevier; 2018: chap 3.

Kumar V, Abbas AK, Aster JC. Diseases of the immune system. In: Kumar V, Abbas AK, Aster JC, eds. *Robbins Basic Pathology.* 10th ed. Philadelphia, PA: Elsevier; 2018: chap 5.

Kurashima Y, Kiyono H. Mucosal ecological network of epithelium and immune cells for gut homeostasis and tissue healing. *Ann Rev Immunol.* 2017;35:119–147. doi:10.1146/annurev-immunol-051116-052424.

Lenette LL, Suscovich TJ, Fortune SM, et al. Beyond binding: antibody effector functions in infectious diseases. *Nat Rev Immunol.* 2018;18:46–61. doi:10.1038/nri.2017.106.

McCusker C, Upton J, Warrington R. Primary immunodeficiency. *Allergy Asthma Clin Immunol.* 2018;14(suppl 2):61. doi:10.1186/s13223-018-0290-5.

Mebius RE, Kraal G. Structure and function of the spleen. *Nat Rev Immunol.* 2005;5:606–616. doi:10.1038/nri1669.

Melchers F. Checkpoints that control B cell development. *J Clin Invest.* 2015;125:2203–2210. doi:10.1172/JCI78083.

Mori L, Lepore M, De Libero G. The immunology of CD1- and MR1-restricted T cells. *Ann Rev Immunol.* 2016;34:479–510. doi:10.1146/annurev-immunol-032414-112008.

Netea MG, Joosten LA, Latz E, et al. Trained immunity: a program of innate immune memory in health and disease. *Science.* 2016;352(6284):aaf1098. doi:10.1126/science.aaf1098.

Punt J, Stranford S, Jones P, et al. *Kuby Immunology.* 8th ed. San Francisco, CA: WH Freeman; 2018.

Randolph GJ, Ivanov S, Zinselmeyer BH, et al. The lymphatic system: integral roles in immunity. *Ann Rev Immunol.* 2017;35:31–52. doi:10.1146/annurev-immunol-041015-055354.

Rappuoli R, Mandl CW, Black S, et al. Vaccines for twenty-first century society. *Nat Rev Immunol.* 2011;11:865–872. doi:10.1038/nri3085.

Sallusto F. Heterogeneity of human CD4+ T cells against microbes. *Ann Rev Immunol.* 2016;34:317–334. doi:10.1146/annurev-immunol-032414-112056.

Schmidt ME, Varga SM. The CD8 T cell response to respiratory virus infections. *Front Immunol.* 2018;9:678. doi:10.3389/fimmu.2018.00678.

Shim JM, Kim J, Tenson T, et al. Influenza virus infection, interferon response, viral counter-response, and apoptosis. *Viruses.* 2017;9:223. doi:10.3390/v9080223.

Solano-Gálvez SG, Tovar-Torres SM, Tron-Gómez MS, et al. Human dendritic cells: ontogeny and their subsets in health and disease. *Med Sci (Basel).* 2018;6(4):E88. doi:10.3390/medsci6040088.

Taniguchi K, Karin M. NF-κB, inflammation, immunity and cancer: coming of age. *Nat Rev Immunol.* 2018;18:309–324. doi:10.1038/nri.2017.142.

Tokuhara D, Kurashima Y, Kamioka M, et al. A comprehensive understanding of the gut mucosal immune system in allergic inflammation. *Allergol Int.* 2019;68:17–25. doi:10.1016/j.alit.2018.09.004.

Urry LA, Cain ML, Wasserman SA, et al. *Campbell Biology.* 11th ed. Englewood Cliffs, NJ: Pearson; 2016:chap 43.

Varol C, Mildner A, Jung S. Macrophages: development and tissue specialization. *Ann Rev Immunol.* 2015;33:643–675. doi:10.1146/annurev-immunol-032414-112220.

Vignesh P, Rawat A, Sharma M, et al. Complement in autoimmune diseases. *Clin Chim Acta.* 2017;465:123–130. doi:10.1016/j.cca.2016.12.017.

Vinuesa CG, Linterman MA, Yu D, et al. Follicular helper T cells. *Ann Rev Immunol.* 2016;34:335–368. doi:10.1146/annurev-immunol-041015-055605.

Weisel F, Shlomchik M. Memory B cells of mice and humans. *Ann Rev Immunol.* 2017;35:255–284. doi:10.1146/annurev-immunol-041015-055531.

Wiley J, Sherwood L, Woolverton CJ. *Prescott's Microbiology.* New York, NY: McGraw-Hill: 2016.

Wynn TA, Vannella KM. Macrophages in tissue repair, regeneration, and fibrosis. *Immunity.* 2016;44:450–462. doi:10.1016/j.immuni.2016.02.015.

Yu W, Hussey Freeland DM, Nadeau KC. Food allergy: immune mechanisms, diagnosis, and immunotherapy. *Nat Rev Immunol.* 2016;16:751–765. doi:10.1038/nri.2016.111.

7

NEOLASIA

Kolbrun (Kolla) Kristjansdottir, Thomas M. Bodenstine, and Sandhya Noronha

THE CLINICAL CONTEXT

The annual incidence of **cancer** in the United States is estimated at 439.2 per 100,000 persons, with an annual rate of deaths due to cancer of 163.5 per 100,000 persons. As a cause of death in the United States, cancer ranks second, just behind heart disease.[1] Data from 2013 to 2015 indicate that about 38% of men and women in the United States will be diagnosed with cancer sometime in their lifetime.[2] Worldwide estimates of cancer cases are 18.1 million new cancer cases and 9.6 million cancer deaths annually.[3]

Over the past 25 years, death rates have dropped in the United States for cancers of the lung and bronchus, prostate, colon and rectum, and stomach, while liver cancer death rates have increased. At least 42% of cancer cases in the United States may be preventable with lifestyle changes such as smoking cessation, weight loss, physical activity, alcohol use reduction or avoidance, improved nutrition, use of sunblock, and avoidance of tanning devices. Vaccination or antibiotic use can reduce incidence of cancer-causing infections such as those due to hepatitis B and C viruses, human papillomavirus, and *Helicobacter pylori*. Clinicians should educate their patients about these cancer-reduction strategies as well as promoting evidence-based screening tests to reduce cancer morbidity and mortality.[4]

OVERVIEW OF CANCER PATHOPHYSIOLOGY

In the United States, cancer remains a leading cause of death, with nearly one in four deaths resulting from this disease.[5] Unique to cancer cells is the acquisition of traits that impart a proliferative capacity that bypasses many of the inherent safety features designed to prevent abnormal growth. This uninhibited cell division, even in a single tissue or organ, harbors the potential to cause demise of the entire body. In line with this, the ability of cancer cells to spread to additional organs and form new tumors remains the most clinically relevant aspect of the disease. As discussed in this chapter, a diverse array of molecular alterations leads to key changes in cellular function, survival, and proliferation.

Although cancer remains heterogeneous in its development, experimental molecular evidence, animal model characterization, and analysis from clinical studies have elucidated key features common to cancer cells. Most cases of cancer arise sporadically from the accumulation of changes in DNA that may be influenced by environmental interactions. This feature is highlighted by the fact that overall cancer incidence increases with age. Characterization of heritable forms of cancer in individuals with a strong family history has further increased our understanding of the genetic basis of cancer. Importantly, our knowledge in this area has been supplemented by genomic-based approaches that continue to delineate the complex and interrelated changes underlying cancer initiation and progression. Taken together, these studies have propelled the development of novel therapies aimed at disrupting the signaling mechanisms responsible for promoting various aspects of cancer cell function.

As uncontrolled cellular growth is the central flaw in a cancer cell, we begin this chapter with a brief overview of the cell cycle to highlight important aspects of growth initiation and control. We then expand our discussion to encompass tumor terminology and phenotypic changes that drive the aggressive qualities of a cancer cell and distinguish it from its normal counterparts. Finally, we examine specific examples of mutations that initiate and promote the progression of cancer from a clinical perspective, and discuss genotyping in cancer diagnosis and treatment.

THE CELL CYCLE

The steps of cell division, collectively referred to as the cell cycle, encompass a complex system of interacting molecules. In multicellular organisms, coordinated cell division gives rise to tissues and organs during embryogenesis that are subsequently maintained by a balance between cell growth and cell death. Rates of cell division vary widely among mammalian cells. For example, mature cardiac cells and neurons exhibit low rates of division, whereas cells lining the gastrointestinal tract and blood cell precursors of the bone marrow divide rapidly. The steps of the cell cycle must proceed in a careful, regulated manner to ensure proper production of new cells. Consequently, the cell cycle exhibits distinct phases, each with its own molecular signatures and specific functions to accomplish the generation of viable new cells. To achieve this feat, cells not only manage their internal machinery, but integrate cues from the extracellular environment, including the influence of growth factors, availability of nutrients, and physical interactions with neighboring cells. During this process, tight regulation of cellular proliferation must exist to avoid pathological consequence. As discussed later in this chapter, an inability to control cell division remains the fundamental defect in cancer.

Although researchers have learned much about the regulation of cell division from experimental models such as the fruit fly, nematode, and amphibian, our discussion focuses on the division of human somatic cells, which account for the majority of cells present within the body. (Stem and reproductive cells exhibit specialized forms of division.) In its simplest categorization, the cell cycle is divided into two broad stages (**Figure 7.1**). *Interphase* describes the period in which the cell grows, replicates its DNA, and activates factors necessary for cell division. *M phase*, or the *mitotic phase*, entails separation of chromosomes and cytoplasm. Thus, cells prepare for division in interphase and carry out this division in M phase. Although the molecular complexities of the cell cycle and its regulation are extensive, brief descriptions of its basic components are provided here.

INTERPHASE

Cells spend the majority of their time in interphase. It is during this period that they evaluate whether conditions are appropriate for cell division, irreversibly commit to the process, and complete the necessary preparations required for successful duplication. Interphase is characterized by three subphases referred to as G_1 (first gap phase), S (synthesis), and G_2 (second gap phase), as illustrated in **Figure 7.1a**.

G_1 is the most variable portion of interphase in regard to duration, and the amount of time cells spend in this period depends on cell type. Cells with high rates of division spend less time in G_1 than cells with less frequent division. Throughout G_1, high RNA and protein synthesis rates support cell growth. Organelles such as mitochondria and lysosomes begin their own process of biogenesis in preparation for providing each new cell with the necessary repertoire of organelles that will support cell function. It is also during this time that cells make a commitment to completing the remaining steps of cell division.

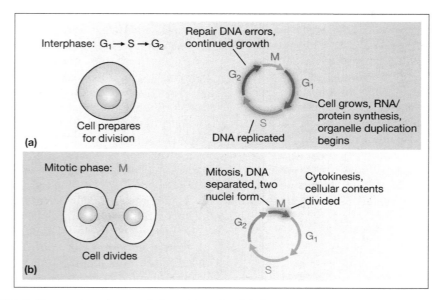

FIGURE 7.1 Two major phases of the cell cycle. **(a)** During interphase, the cell prepares for division. In G_1, the cell grows, organelles begin duplication, and RNA and protein synthesis are increased to complete replication of DNA in S phase. Integrity of DNA is assessed and repaired if necessary during G_2. **(b)** The mitotic phase (M phase) details the process by which replicated DNA is separated, forming two nuclei. During cytokinesis, the contents of the cell are separated as two new cells form.

S phase is so named because the primary function involves DNA synthesis within the nucleus. During this phase, DNA from all 46 chromosomes is replicated, with each new copy remaining linked to the original by cohesive proteins. These connected chromosomes are referred to as *sister chromatids*. Production of histone proteins increases during S phase, and DNA becomes tightly coiled around these proteins. This creates a DNA–histone complex known as *chromatin*, which helps organize, condense, and package DNA in later stages of the cell cycle.

Following DNA duplication, the cell enters G_2, in which integrity of the DNA is checked for errors and corrected if necessary by DNA repair pathways. This ensures that new cells inherit DNA that is free from mistakes that would compromise its ability to carry out the vital tasks of the cell, tissue, or organ. Following completion of G_2, the cell has reached a critical size, doubled its internal contents, replicated and checked its DNA, and is now ready to divide.

M PHASE (MITOTIC PHASE)

Upon completing interphase, the cell must separate its DNA and cellular contents to properly form two new cells in the intricate process known as M phase (**Figure 7.2**).

This phase can be described in two stages: (a) Mitosis, with its own set of subphases, encompasses the process of breaking down the nuclear membrane and dividing the now duplicated chromosomes, while (b) cytokinesis entails equal splitting of the cell membrane and all of the components contained within it (**Figure 7.1b**).

Mitosis involves five distinct subphases: prophase, prometaphase, metaphase, anaphase, and telophase. These processes are shown in **Figure 7.2a** and described in **Box 7.1**. Interpreting the steps of mitosis allows us to understand the process by which cells perform the critical task of dividing their genomic content.

Cytokinesis completes the final phase of the cell cycle by separating the cellular contents and finalizing the formation of the new cells, each with their own nuclei. By this time, a ring composed of actin and myosin has formed and been positioned toward the center of the cell. Known as the cleavage furrow, the ring begins to separate the cytoplasm as it contracts, ultimately sealing off the plasma membrane on each side (**Figure 7.2b**). At the end of cytokinesis, the cell cycle is now complete, resulting in the production of two daughter cells, each with its own set of DNA and cytoplasm to support function and survival.

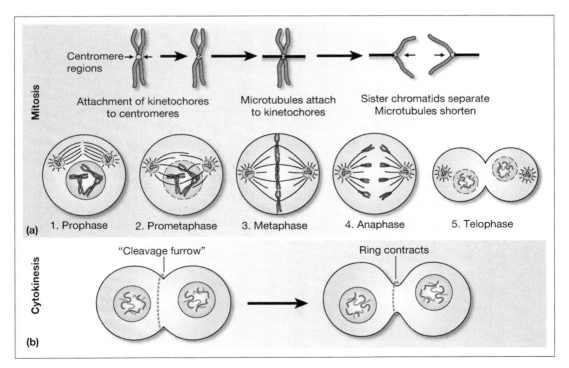

FIGURE 7.2 Details of M phase. (**a**) The process of mitosis involves condensation of DNA into chromosomes during prophase while centromeres move toward opposite ends of the nucleus. Kinetochore complexes attach to centromere regions of chromosomes in prophase, while the nuclear membrane begins to break down, allowing binding of microtubules to kinetochores. Chromosomes are lined up during metaphase and separated by shortening microtubules in anaphase. Nuclear membranes form around newly separated chromosomes, which begin to decondense during telophase. (**b**) During cytokinesis, an actin and myosin ring aligned at the center of the dividing cell begins to contract. This serves to separate the cellular components and seal off the membranes of each new cell.

BOX 7.1
Subphases of Mitosis

PROPHASE

- During the initial step of mitosis, *prophase*, the chromatin condenses into chromosomes, a process that involves regulated compaction of DNA while the nuclear membrane remains intact.

- A protein complex known as the kinetochore assembles on each sister chromatid at specialized regions known as centromeres. These structures will be important for separation of the sister chromatids by microtubules, dynamic protein structures that constitute part of the cytoskeleton.

- In each cell, microtubules are organized in a structure known as the centrosome. Centrosomes duplicate during cell division and move toward opposing sides of the nucleus during prophase, awaiting dissolution of the nucleus.

PROMETAPHASE

- In *prometaphase*, the nuclear membrane breaks down and exposes the sister chromatids to the microtubules of the centrosome.

- Microtubules from opposite centrosomes bind to the bound kinetochore protein complexes of each sister chromatid, forming a tight connection and creating tension on the proteins holding them together.

METAPHASE

- During *metaphase*, the microtubules align sister chromatids toward the center of the cell. This creates an appearance sometimes referred to as the metaphase plate or equatorial plane due to the alignment of the sister chromatids along the center. The next phase of mitosis will not occur until all kinetochores are attached to microtubules and properly aligned.

ANAPHASE

- With sister chromatids aligned at the center of the cell and microtubules attached to kinetochores, the proteins linking the chromatids are released and bound microtubules begin to shorten during *anaphase*. As this occurs, the chromatids are effectively separated and pulled to opposite ends of the cell by the shortening microtubules.

TELOPHASE

- Following this separation, in *telophase*, kinetochores and their attached microtubules disassemble while two nuclear membranes begin to form around the now separated and decondensing chromosomes. At this stage, the replicated DNA has been split and moved to opposite ends, but the cell must still effectively divide the cytoplasm.

EXIT AND REENTRY OF THE CELL CYCLE

While replicating cells continue to move through additional rounds of the cell cycle, a cell may leave this progression and enter a state known as G_0. In G_0, cells remain both viable and functional, but do not actively proliferate. A cell may permanently leave the cycle and enter G_0 once it has matured and performs a specific function. This is true for cells such as cardiac myocytes and neurons. These cells are said to be *terminally differentiated*, indicating that they carry out their function but no longer divide. This is a primary reason that ischemic damage of heart and brain often results in long-term and potentially permanent consequences. In addition to differentiation, most cells have a finite number of division cycles that they can complete as the ends of their chromosomes (telomeres) become progressively shorter with each division, a process known as *replicative senescence*. Once a critical length is reached, DNA cannot be appropriately replicated and the cells enter a permanent state of G_0. Collectively, terminally differentiated and senescent cells are thus thought to be in a state of irreversible G_0.

Compared to heart and brain, liver cells maintain a much higher capability of compensatory growth, and portions of liver can regrow following injury. These liver cells have the capacity to exit G_0 and reenter the cell cycle. Cells possessing this ability are said to be quiescent, in that they can enter G_0 but later resume the cell cycle if necessary by returning to G_1. In an additional example, memory T cells of the immune system follow patterns of quiescence. During exposure to a pathogen, activated T cells increase in number as part of the immune response. Following resolution of the infection, a portion of these cells remains in the body in a quiescent state of G_0. Should the body again encounter the same pathogen, these cells will rapidly reenter the cell cycle and proliferate.

CONTROL OF THE CELL CYCLE

While the cell cycle itself has been well characterized experimentally and its phases documented in detail through microscopy, the underpinnings of these functional events lie at the molecular level in an enormously complex network of signaling interactions. Any discussion of these mechanisms must include a basic understanding of cyclins, cyclin-dependent kinases (CDKs), and CDK inhibitors (CKIs). Although these molecules are not the only contributors to control of the cell cycle, our understanding of the regulation of cell division stems largely from what has been discovered about them.

CDKs are a family of kinase proteins that, when active, phosphorylate a specific set of protein substrates. These phosphorylation events set in motion various stages and transition points in the cell cycle by activating or inhibiting a multitude of proteins at key times. The activity of CDKs is regulated by their own phosphorylation signatures, and as the name implies, depends on the binding of proteins known as cyclins, which increase CDK function. As such, active CDKs exist as a heterodimer with cyclins and have both a cyclin-binding domain and a kinase domain that increases in activity following cyclin binding. Various CDKs have roles in the cell cycle (e.g., CDK1, CDK2, CDK4, CDK6), and different combinations of CDKs and their cyclins are important for regulation (e.g., cyclin D/CDK4, cyclin E/CDK2, cyclin B/CDK1). A key feature of these interactions is that while cellular levels of CDKs remain relatively constant, the levels of cyclins rise and fall as the cell cycle progresses (**Figure 7.3**). Thus, cell cycle regulation is controlled in part by fluctuations in the amount and type of cyclins present. This allows the process to occur in a sequential order, and activity of some CDK/cyclin complexes will upregulate levels of the cyclin required for the next phase. For example, cyclin D/CDK6, which guides the cell through G_1, upregulates the levels of cyclin E, which is important for the transition from G_1 to S phase through its association with CDK2.

Of equal importance to cell cycle progression is the ability to halt the cycle when necessary. If a cell experiences alterations to its DNA through damage or mutations, the cell must be prevented from proceeding through cellular division so as not to produce daughter cells with the same genetic alterations. Additionally, cells must ensure that the necessary nutrients and building blocks are present before proceeding through the steps of division. One regulatory protein of cell division, the retinoblastoma protein (pRb), inhibits the cell cycle from progressing through G_1 by binding and inhibiting the activity of necessary transcription factors. As levels of cyclin D rise in response to growth factor—and nutrient-induced signaling—the cyclin D–activated CDKs phosphorylate pRb, leading to a change in its structure. This structural shift causes the release of the bound transcription factors and allows the cell to continue through G_1.

CKIs represent additional modes of cell cycle control and include the <u>in</u>hibitors of <u>k</u>inase <u>4</u> (INK4) family (p15, p16, p18, p19) and <u>C</u>DK-interacting <u>p</u>rotein/<u>k</u>inase <u>i</u>nhibitory <u>p</u>rotein (CIP/KIP) inhibitors (p21, p27, p57). These molecules have potent inhibitory activities on numerous cyclin/CDK complexes and interactions. Of these inhibitors, p21 is of particular note in that it is capable of disrupting numerous cyclin/CDK combinations and, as a result, possesses the ability to halt the cell cycle at multiple stages.[6,7]

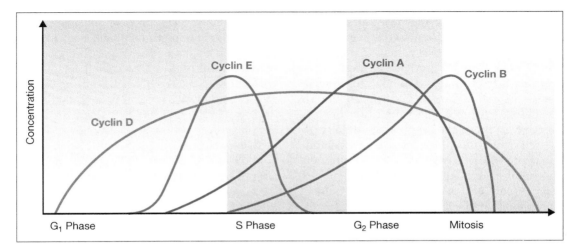

FIGURE 7.3 Levels of cyclins vary through the cell cycle. While cellular levels of cyclin-dependent kinases stay relatively constant throughout the cell cycle, levels of their activating proteins, the cyclins, fluctuate with the cell cycle phases. Along with additional activating mechanisms, these fluctuations determine the timing of transitions between phases, controlling the rate of cell division.

Equally important as the inhibitors are the molecules that control inhibitor expression and activity. The *TP53* gene encodes the protein p53, which is critical to halting the cell cycle when DNA is damaged or the cell has suffered injury—two scenarios in which progression through the cell cycle would be detrimental. Several proteins and complexes survey the genome for damage and, when present, initiate signaling pathways that lead to activation of p53. The p53 protein enters the nucleus and functions as a transcription factor, inducing the expression of numerous genes capable of halting the cell cycle, activating DNA repair pathways, or inducing cell death if defects cannot be reversed. In the case of its inhibitory cell cycle effects, p53 mediates this in part, by increasing the expression of p21. The link between p53 and the suppression of neoplastic growth was first proposed following experiments utilizing colorectal carcinoma cells in which loss of p53 function was consistently observed.[8] This finding was later supported by additional evidence in other types of cancer, solidifying the idea that loss of the p53 *brakes* of the cell opened the door to unregulated cell proliferation.[9,10]

CHECKPOINTS

Multiple *checkpoints* are present within the cell cycle machinery to ensure the cell undergoes division appropriately. Progression through a G_1 checkpoint, also known as the restriction point, ensures the presence of necessary growth conditions and commits the cell to the remainder of the division process. Up to this point, the cell is influenced by the presence of external growth factors, which increase the activation of signaling pathways that promote cell division by increasing cyclin D, as previously discussed. Thus, this checkpoint ensures that nutrients and growth factors are present and the extracellular environment is favorable for cell division. Once the cell has reached necessary levels of this activation, it moves through this checkpoint and proceeds through the remainder of the cell cycle without the need for extracellular factors. Additional checkpoints exist within the cell; for example, a DNA damage checkpoint ensures that DNA has been correctly replicated and is free of alterations prior to mitosis, while an M-phase checkpoint assesses that all kinetochores are bound to microtubules before chromosome separation begins. Failure to pass any of these checkpoints results in cessation of the cell cycle until the issues are corrected. Each of these checkpoints is regulated by an elaborate system of coordinated molecular interactions.

Collectively, cell division is characterized by numerous phases and an abundance of coordinated intracellular activity. This setup ensures that these complex functions occur in a regulated manner. Nonetheless, control mechanisms are often circumvented in cancer cells, leading to unregulated growth that threatens the body.

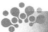

Thought Questions

1. What is the fundamental feature of all cancer cells?

2. How does regulation of the cell cycle relate to cancer development?

PROPERTIES OF NEOPLASMS

TUMOR TERMINOLOGY

A *tumor* is defined as "[a]n abnormal mass of tissue that results when cells divide more than they should or do not *die* when they should."[11] Similarly, a *neoplasm* refers to a new and uncontrolled proliferation of cells that can be benign (noncancerous) or malignant (cancerous). It is important to note that not all malignant cellular proliferations form a tumor. Hematological malignancies are the most common examples of those that do not form discrete tumors. For example, acute lymphoblastic leukemia (ALL) is a malignant proliferation of lymphoblasts in the bone marrow and the peripheral blood without overt formation of a tumor. Histopathological examination of a tissue biopsy sample, or observation of a blood smear, together with knowledge of the salient clinical features (derived from the history, physical examination, and imaging results), helps to make a diagnosis of a malignancy.

A *benign* tumor is typically slow growing and on macroscopic examination appears to be well circumscribed. On microscopic examination, the tumor cells do not infiltrate into the adjacent tissue. The term *dysplasia* is used to describe a change or an alteration in a cell. Dysplastic cells, when viewed on a stained tissue section, show variation in the size and shape of their nuclei (nuclear pleomorphism), and the nuclei may appear darkly stained (hyperchromatic). An increased number of mitoses may be seen in tissue sections along with mitotic figures that are atypical. For example, infection of human ectocervical epithelial cells with the human papillomavirus (HPV) can result in dysplasia. Dysplasia may be low grade or high grade. In low-grade dysplasia, the cells in the lower third of the ectocervical epithelium are altered, and in high-grade dysplasia, the altered cells extend into the middle and upper thirds of the cervical epithelium (**Figure 7.4**).

The term **carcinoma in situ** has been used to describe aggregates of abnormal cells that have not extended beyond the basement membrane. For example, **ductal carcinoma in situ of the breast** refers to a condition in which neoplastic cells fill some of the

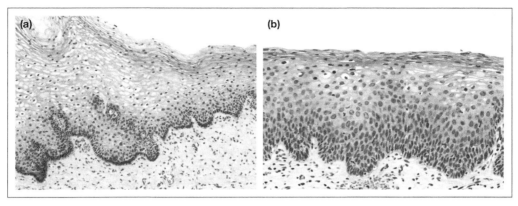

FIGURE 7.4 Micrographs of normal cervical epithelium **(a)** and level II cervical intraepithelial neoplasia **(b)**. Abnormal cells **(b)** have larger and darker nuclei and are found in the lower third of the epithelial layer but do not breach the basal lamina.

ducts in breast tissue. The neoplastic cells are contained within the ducts and do not breach the basement membrane, which is a specialized matrix to which the cells are attached. An invasive cancer occurs when the neoplastic cells break through this basement membrane and extend into the underlying stroma.

A *malignant* tumor is composed of cells that are able to infiltrate into the adjacent stroma or connective tissue. Macroscopic examination of the tumor reveals the tumor margins to be poorly circumscribed. Microscopic examination reveals infiltration of the tumor cells into the surrounding connective tissue, which may allow the malignant cells to extend into lymphatics or blood vessels and to disseminate to distant organs where the tumor cells can form new tumors—a process known as *metastasis*. Malignant tumors (cancers) are named based on the tissue from which they develop. A **carcinoma**, for instance, is a malignant tumor derived from cells of epithelial origin; examples are squamous cell carcinoma, adenocarcinoma, and small cell carcinoma.

- A **squamous cell carcinoma** is a malignant tumor arising from squamous epithelial cells. For example, a squamous cell carcinoma of the skin is derived from squamous cells in the epidermis of the skin.
- **Adenocarcinomas** are malignant tumors arising from glandular epithelial cells. For example, an adenocarcinoma of the lung is derived from glandular epithelial cells lining the tracheobronchial tree in the lungs.
- A **small cell carcinoma** arises from neuroendocrine cells that occur normally in various tissues in the body. For example, a small cell carcinoma of the lung arises from neuroendocrine cells in lung tissue.

Sarcomas are malignant tumors arising from mesenchymal tissue (e.g., blood vessels, cartilage, bone,

muscle) and are rare in comparison to carcinomas. The prefix of a sarcoma designates its origin; for example, an osteosarcoma arises from bone tissue, whereas a liposarcoma indicates a sarcoma arising from adipose tissue. Additional examples are chondrosarcoma (cartilage), leiomyosarcoma (smooth muscle), rhabdomyosarcoma (skeletal muscle), and angiosarcoma (blood vessels).

In **hematopoietic neoplasms**, there is an abnormal proliferation of cells in the bone marrow, peripheral blood, or other hematopoietic tissues such as the lymph nodes, spleen, or liver. A **lymphoma** refers to a malignant tumor that results from a monoclonal proliferation of lymphoid cells such as B lymphocytes or T lymphocytes. **Leukemia** occurs secondary to a monoclonal proliferation of early hematopoietic cells (blast cells) in the bone marrow, accompanied by an arrest in the normal maturation of the cells.

Other malignant tumors likely to be encountered in clinical practice include melanoma, brain tumors, and teratoma. **Melanoma** arises from melanocytes such as those seen within the skin. **Tumors of the brain** may arise from a multitude of cells in the nervous system, including neurons, glial cells, choroid plexus, and meninges. Brain tumors commonly seen in clinical practice include glial tumors, meningioma, and secondary tumors that have metastasized to the brain from other sites in the body. A **teratoma** is a tumor that arises from germ cells and is composed of tissues derived from one or more of the embryological germ cell layers. For example, a mature cystic teratoma, also known as a dermoid cyst, may occur in organs such as the testes or ovaries, and may be composed of an aggregate of mature tissues representing various organs in the body; for example, skin and hair (ectoderm), lungs and intestines (endoderm), and bone and cartilage (mesoderm).

Thought Questions

3. What features help to differentiate a benign tumor from a malignant tumor?

4. What tissues give rise to a carcinoma, a sarcoma, and a lymphoma?

CHARACTERISTICS OF A CANCER CELL

The development of a malignant neoplasm, or cancer, is a stepwise process that includes a series of genetic changes in a normally functioning cell that gradually transform the cell into a cancer cell. These genetic changes result in the inability of the body to restrain cell division and can lead to the spread of the cancer cells around the body. Collectively, the characteristics that a cell acquires when it becomes cancerous are referred to as the *hallmarks of cancer*.[12,13] Some of these characteristics include uncontrolled proliferative signaling, evading growth suppressors, genomic instability, enabling cell immortality, resisting cell death, hijacking or generating blood supply sources for nourishment, and acquiring invasive and metastatic abilities.

Proto-Oncogenes, Oncogenes, and Tumor Suppressor Genes

As a general principle, the genetic changes that promote the stepwise progression from normal cell function to malignancy alter the amount, activity, or regulation of two types of genes.

First, some genes possess the ability to promote cellular proliferation and survival, but are subject to careful regulation to limit these functions to appropriate circumstances. Genes with these characteristics are known as *proto-oncogenes*, and the majority of these proto-oncogenes are involved in regulation of the cell cycle and responses to growth factor activation. Proto-oncogene mutations may lead to loss of proper regulation and result in disease due to overactivity of their inherent properties. This conversion from proto-oncogene to *oncogene* leads to sustained activity of their encoded proteins, resulting in unchecked growth that may progress to neoplasia. Such mutations are referred to as *gain-of-function* mutations because the resulting protein has an increase in activity.

Second, many protective genes encode proteins that inhibit uncontrolled cell division and conduct surveillance of DNA. Signals of DNA damage or deranged cell function result in DNA repair (if possible) or initiation of apoptosis if the cell is beyond repair. These genes can collectively be referred to as *tumor suppressor genes*. As described next, the loss of normal function of a single tumor suppressor gene allele is not sufficient to induce loss of normal protein function; both copies of

the gene must be mutated in order for decreased tumor suppressor activity and promotion of cancer. These mutations are referred to as *loss-of-function* mutations because absence of the normal protein function is integral to cancer promotion (**Figure 7.5**).

Uncontrolled Proliferative Signaling

An oncogene may be formed as a result of mutations within the proto-oncogene or as a consequence of larger alterations such as chromosomal translocations that disrupt normal controls on oncogene expression. One of the most commonly observed oncogenes is mutated *Ras*, found in about 20% of all human cancers. Ras is an important intracellular signaling protein that, when properly stimulated, transmits signals that activate cell growth for a brief time before being turned off. Mutated Ras results in continuous stimulation that fuels tumor growth. Another proto-oncogene codes for the membrane epidermal growth factor receptor (EGFR) a member of the ErbB family of growth-promoting tyrosine kinases. Increased levels of EGFR or mutated forms of EGFR are frequently present in cancers, resulting in unregulated cell division due to the continual activation of its signaling properties. Inhibitors that bind to EGFR and decrease cellular growth are used in the treatment of some breast, pancreatic, and colon cancers.

Evading Growth Suppressors

Cells have many mechanisms to regulate cell proliferation in response to activation of oncogenes or cell stress, including halting cell division, inducing DNA repair, and initiating cell death. The tumor suppressor genes controlling these processes include many cell cycle inhibitors and regulators. When a tumor suppressor is inactivated or *turned off*, the likelihood of cancer development is increased. As such, the actions of a normally functioning tumor suppressor will inhibit proliferation, but upon loss of its function unregulated growth can occur. Over half of all human cancers have mutations in the *TP53* tumor suppressor gene, illustrating its vital importance in maintaining genome integrity and eliminating irreversibly altered cells. When the p53 protein is not functional, DNA damage goes unrepaired and mutations accumulate in cells, leading to acquisition of other cancer cell characteristics. *RB1* represents an additional tumor suppressor gene and its product, pRb, has the capacity to stop the cell cycle in G_1. The consequence of losing this function is underscored by the common findings of *RB1* mutations in retinoblastoma, osteosarcoma, and carcinomas of breast, lung, and colon.

Genomic Instability

Defects in *DNA repair pathways* are not directly oncogenic; however, because the DNA cannot be effectively repaired, DNA mutations accumulate. The genome becomes unstable, significantly increasing the risk of mutations occurring in processes that regulate cell

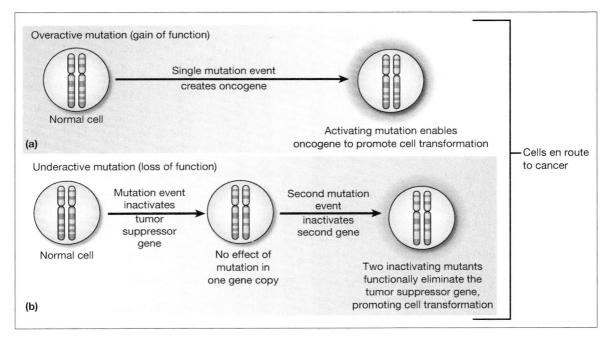

FIGURE 7.5 Two major groups of genetic mutations favor progression of cells to malignancy. **(a)** A proto-oncogene within a normal cell is mutated, becoming an oncogene. The oncogene product stimulates excessive and unregulated cell division. **(b)** A tumor suppressor gene is inactivated by a mutation. The remaining normal allele sustains cell protection from proliferation; however, if the second allele develops an inactivating mutation, tumor suppressor function and this pathway of protection from malignancy are lost.

growth, such as tumor suppressors, proto-oncogenes, and cell death pathways. For example, patients with the disease **xeroderma pigmentosum** have germ-line mutations in nucleotide excision repair pathways, decreasing their ability to correct DNA damage caused by ultraviolet (UV) light. As a result, these patients are extremely susceptible to UV-induced burns and skin damage. Without protection from sun or other UV sources, about half of these patients will develop their first skin cancer by age 10 years.[14]

Enabling Replicative Immortality

The human body must maintain equilibrium between the replacement of old cells and generation of new ones. The cell cycle continuously produces new cells, but each cell has a limited number of cell divisions before it undergoes a process called cellular aging, or *senescence*. Senescent cells function but are no longer able to enter the cell cycle and divide. A hallmark of cancer cells is the ability to bypass senescence and continue cell division. This occurs, in part, because of increased levels of *telomerase*, an enzyme that maintains chromosome length, making cancer cells in essence immortal. This property is supported by the fact that many cancer cell lines derived from cancer patients can survive indefinitely in the laboratory if maintained under appropriate growth conditions. Telomerase inhibitors are promising

anticancer agents because telomerase is expressed in the majority of cancer cells and is not present, or is present in very low amounts, in normal cells.

Resisting Cell Death

Cell death can occur through two primary routes. *Necrosis* represents an uncontrolled form of cell death that often occurs in response to an acute cellular injury. The plasma membrane is ruptured and intracellular contents spill into the surrounding tissues, promoting inflammation and tissue damage. *Apoptosis* is a regulated and programmed form of cell death. Under normal conditions, cells that sustain extensive or unrepairable damage to their DNA undergo apoptosis due to intracellular surveillance mechanisms. Abnormal or pathogen-infected cells will also be targeted for apoptosis or outright lysis by immune cells. Thus, apoptotic mechanisms serve a protective function in the body and represent a challenge to the development of cancer. Cancer cells, however, have found ways to evade apoptosis by upregulating anti-apoptotic factors such as inhibitors of apoptosis (IAPs) or decreasing production of proapoptotic factors such as Fas. This enables cancer cells to resist induction of apoptosis. Avoiding this built-in mechanism of cell death allows a cell with mutated DNA to continue to grow and divide, gaining mutations that make the cell more tumorigenic and ultimately malignant.

Promotion of Angiogenesis

Blood vessels provide oxygen and nutrients to tissues and are crucial for cell function and survival. Tumors that are not in close proximity to blood vessels are limited in growth to several millimeters diameter before cells in the hypoxic core become quiescent or die. In order for tumors to continue to grow, they must develop an *angiogenic* ability to generate new blood vessels or expand the existing vascular tree. The resulting vasculature feeds growing tumors with the newly developed blood supply, allowing tumors to enlarge and the cancer cells to invade adjacent tissues, promoting metastasis. To accomplish this, many cancer cells have increased local levels of proangiogenic factors such as vascular endothelial growth factor (VEGF). Molecules such as these normally induce blood vessel formation during development or in response to vascular injury but are repurposed by cancer cells to provide themselves with a blood supply. Scientists have developed angiogenesis inhibitors with the goal of starving the cancer of its needed blood supply. Bevacizumab is an example of a VEGF inhibitor used in the treatment of cancers that have metastasized or recurred, including glioblastoma multiforme, renal cell cancer, and ovarian cancer.

Invasive and Metastatic Ability

Cancer cells have the ability to spread from the original tumor site to distant areas of the body, through the process of *metastasis*. In order to metastasize, cells must separate from the original tumor; invade the surrounding tissues; enter and survive in the circulation, lymphatics, or peritoneal space; and settle in a distant target organ where they adapt, survive, and proliferate. To do this, metastatic cancer cells typically develop alterations in their shape and in their attachment to other cells and to the extracellular matrix. The *epithelial–mesenchymal transition (EMT)* is an important process that allows transformed epithelial cells to invade tissues, resist apoptosis, and spread. Increased expression of EMT transcriptional regulators results in a loss of adherence, an associated conversion from an epithelial to a fibroblastic, or spindle-like morphology, expression of matrix-degrading enzymes, and increased cell motility. E-cadherin, a key adhesion molecule, is lost in many cancer cells, allowing tumor cells to detach from surrounding cells, and increasing the risk of invasion and metastasis. The cancer hallmarks and examples of proteins and processes altered are summarized in **Table 7.1**.

RECENTLY IDENTIFIED CANCER CELL CHARACTERISTICS

The concept of cancer hallmarks was further elaborated in 2011, with the inclusion of *evasion of immune destruction* and *altered metabolism* as additional emerging hallmarks.[13]

TABLE 7.1 Cancer Characteristics and Exemplar Causative Factors

Cancer Cell Characteristics or Hallmarks	Associated Protein or Key Process
Uncontrolled proliferative signaling	Ras, EGFR
Evading growth suppressors	p53, pRb
Genomic instability	DNA repair
Enabling replicative immortality	Telomerase
Restricting cell death	Apoptosis
Promotion of angiogenesis	VEGF
Invasive and metastatic ability	EMT, E-cadherin

EGFR, epidermal growth factor receptor; EMT, epithelial–mesenchymal transition; VEGF, vascular endothelial growth factor.

Evasion of Immune Destruction

Classical immunology proposes that cytotoxic T lymphocytes, among other effector cells, are capable of killing not only virus-infected self-cells, but also self-cells that have undergone cancer-causing mutations and unregulated proliferation. Interestingly, having cancer promotes a state of increased generalized inflammation, with elevated cytokine levels both within a tumor and systemically that may promote cancer cell proliferation. In addition, lymphocytes are found within tumor tissue, but they are not always cytotoxic lymphocytes. Rather, regulatory T cells (Tregs) may be present in tumors and downregulate the ability of the immune system to clear the tumor cells. Cancer cells may develop characteristics that activate immune system inhibitory signaling, particularly through the activation of cytotoxic T lymphocyte-associated protein 4 (CTLA-4), which downregulates immune responsiveness. Similarly, cancer cells produce a ligand that activates programmed cell death 1 (PD-1) receptors found on T cells, B cells, and natural killer cells, and suppresses immune activity, hindering clearance of the cancer cells.[15]

Immune-based cancer treatments continue to evolve.[16] Chimeric antigen receptor–T cell (CAR-T cell) is a method of altering T-cell receptors to attack antigens associated with a tumor. Monoclonal antibodies are also successfully used, and several types have been developed that specifically target proteins unique to a given cancer type. Monoclonal antibodies can opsonize tumor cells, marking them for phagocytic destruction. At the same time, destruction of the cells increases the reactions of antigen-presenting cells that can drive T-helper– and cytotoxic T-lymphocyte–mediated tumor destruction. Finally, some tumors have signals that inhibit lymphocyte proliferation by activating checkpoints that block their entry into the cell cycle needed for clonal proliferation. Checkpoint inhibitor drugs block those cell membrane signals, allowing the lymphocytes to respond with proliferation and immune-mediated eradication of tumor cells.

Cancer Cell Metabolic Alterations

As previously noted, a growing tumor will have varying degrees of oxygen supply, depending on proximity to existing or newly formed blood vessels. The collection of cells will consist of tumor cells in varying states of genetic alteration, each having somewhat different characteristics and energy requirements, plus surrounding tissue cells, called the stroma. Cell types making up the tumor include the cancer stem cells that propagate their own growth, immune cells (lymphocytes, macrophages, dendritic cells) stimulated by inflammatory signals of the tumor, fibroblasts, and cells undergoing the EMT. The microenvironment of the tumor depends on interactions between these cell types and determines the type of metabolism needed by cells in different stages of tumor progression. One model proposes that hypoxia-stressed cells in the center of a tumor adopt the properties of increased survival, treatment resistance, and immune evasion, ultimately becoming more likely to develop mutations favoring invasion and metastasis[17] (**Figure 7.6**).

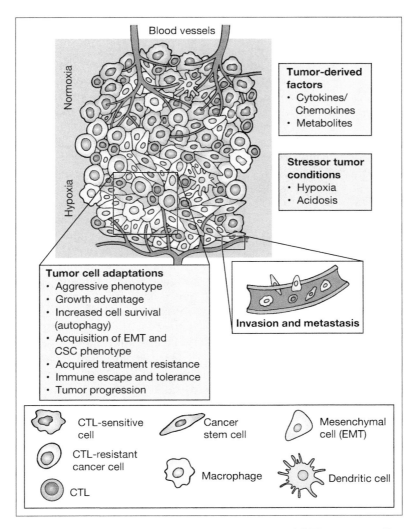

FIGURE 7.6 Events in tumor progression. A tumor is made up of CSCs, cancer cells, stroma cells (of the original tissue), lymphocytes, macrophages, dendritic cells, and cells in some phase of the EMT. The tumor region closest to a blood vessel has normal oxygen supply and has cells that may maintain normal sensitivity to killing by CTLs. The tumor region at a distance from the blood vessel has a hypoxic and acidotic environment that induces cell stress. This may promote acquisition of cancer cell immune resistance and development of immune tolerance, as well as favoring mutations that enable invasion and metastasis.

CTL, cytotoxic T lymphocyte; CSC, cancer stem cell; EMT, epithelial–mesenchymal transition.

Early studies of tumor cell metabolism indicated a high rate of glucose uptake due to increased levels of glucose transporter 1 (GLUT1). This alteration is clinically useful, as the accelerated glucose uptake forms the basis of PET scanning for fluorodeoxyglucose uptake to localize tumors and metastases. Rapidly dividing and aggressive tumor cells often rely on glycolysis for energy production. The glycolytic pathway does not produce as much adenosine triphosphate (ATP) as the usual metabolic pathways of glycolysis, Krebs cycle, and oxidative phosphorylation, but it is rapid and produces lactate, which can be used to synthesize new cell components to support further cell division.[18]

In summary, accumulation of sporadic mutations can result in the acquisition of cancer cell characteristics. A mutated cell acquires more mutations over time, resulting in a heterogeneous tumor composed of cells with a range of cancer cell characteristics. Genomic instability accelerates mutation rates, and some of those mutations further promote the rate of cellular growth and division. A benign neoplasm can, over time, become malignant, highlighting the importance of early identification and treatment. Even established malignant tumors continue to accumulate mutations, adapting to their surroundings and acquiring more cancer characteristics. Each hallmark of cancer presents a pathway of targeted therapy development to improve clinical outcomes.

Thought Questions

5. What is an oncogene?

6. How do cancer cells obtain sufficient oxygen and nutrients in a large tumor?

7. Why does genomic instability increase cancer risk?

CLINICAL ASPECTS OF NEOPLASIA

PATHOPHYSIOLOGY OF CANCER MANIFESTATIONS AND TREATMENT SEQUELAE

Cancer and cancer treatments are associated with a number of pathophysiological alterations at the systemic level, in addition to localized manifestations resulting from solid tumors. Chief among these are inflammation, with elevated cytokine production that may cause fevers and suppress appetite while also promoting clotting. Hypercoagulability also commonly accompanies cancer, particularly in early stages. Some patients originally diagnosed with deep vein thrombosis

and pulmonary embolism are subsequently found to have cancer. In addition, fatigue that is disproportional to effort is common, particularly in more advanced cancer. Poor appetite and wasting can also occur in advanced cancer, as well as resulting from chemotherapy-induced nausea and vomiting. Endocrine-related syndromes can result from tumors that are ectopic sources of hormones and hormone-like substances. An example is parathyroid hormone–related protein, which can cause hypercalcemia and bone loss, and tumor-produced vasopressin, which can cause the syndrome of inappropriate antidiuretic hormone secretion (SIADH).

Tumor lysis syndrome is an acute generalized reaction to massive cell death caused by cancer treatment. Although tumor lysis syndrome can be a spontaneous event, it is generally precipitated after initiating a round of treatment that results in robust and rapid killing of malignant cells. The cells then release their contents, causing hyperuricemia, hyperkalemia, hyperphosphatemia, and hypocalcemia. The ensuing electrolyte imbalance can cause instability of excitable tissues, resulting in cardiac arrhythmias and neurological seizures. Acute renal failure is also a potential outcome. Risk stratification to reduce tumor lysis syndrome is aided by estimating tumor volume, cell lysis potential of the treatment, and patient factors such as fluid and electrolyte status and renal function. Careful monitoring is required to manage the onset of this complication with fluid supplementation and measures that reduce uric acid, phosphate, and potassium.[19]

Other cancer- and therapy-associated complications and symptoms include pain, anemia, neutropenia, thrombocytopenia, nausea and vomiting, stomatitis, fatigue, radiation-induced tissue injury, sleep disturbance, and dysphoria. Providers in oncology centers continue to refine evidence-based strategies to care for patients with cancer with the aim of optimizing quality of life and function. This is a critical step with the striking evolution of novel, highly effective gene- and immune-based therapies that have a high risk of unpredictable adverse reactions.

BIOLOGICAL ASPECTS OF GENE MUTATIONS AND CANCER RISK FACTORS

Cancers may occur as a result of hereditary or sporadic gene mutations in somatic or germline cells. *Germline mutations* are mutations that occur in the DNA of germ cells such as ova and spermatozoa. Inheritance of a germline mutation results in every cell in the body having the mutation. *Somatic mutations* are mutations that occur in the cells spontaneously or as a result of mutagen exposures. For example, skin cells that have been repeatedly exposed to UV rays may develop a somatic mutation. A somatic mutation is inherited by the progeny of the cell with the mutation but does not occur in all cells in the body and cannot be inherited by offspring.

Sporadic gene mutations occur more commonly than inherited gene mutations. It has been estimated that only about 5% to 10% of cancers are inherited.[20] Typically, sporadic gene mutations accumulate in the tissues over time prior to the development of a tumor. For example, benign adenomatous polyps of the colon accumulate gene mutations over time before developing into a malignant tumor. Screening procedures such as colonoscopy are extremely important to detect and remove benign polyps of the colon before they become malignant. Some risk factors thought to play a role in the development of cancer include age, race and ethnicity, smoking, alcohol consumption, excessive exposure to UV light, exposure to environmental toxins, lack of exercise, and obesity. For example,

- Smoking has been identified as the leading cause of lung cancer and is linked to many other cancers.
- Excessive exposure to UV light has been linked to the development of skin cancer.
- Age is a risk factor for the development of prostate cancer, which typically occurs in older men, and men of African descent appear to have a higher risk of prostate cancer.
- A diet low in fruits and vegetables and rich in red meats is a risk factor for the development of colon cancer.
- Excessive consumption of alcohol is a risk factor for liver and other cancers.
- Exposure to asbestos has been linked to the development of mesothelioma, a tumor arising from the pleura of the lung.
- Obesity and a lack of physical activity have also been implicated as increasing development of many cancers.

Hereditary gene mutations also play a role in the development of neoplasia, and typically occur in patients at an earlier age than neoplasia due to sporadic mutations. For example, the inheritance of germline mutations in DNA mismatch repair genes such as *hMSH2*, *hMLH1*, *hMSH6*, and *hPMS2* has been implicated in the development of **Lynch syndrome**, also known as hereditary nonpolyposis colorectal cancer (HNPCC). Mismatch repair genes are genes that play a role in ensuring the accurate pairing of DNA base pairs. Microsatellites are short DNA sequences that may be altered due to mutations in the mismatch repair genes, which may then result in a genomic instability called microsatellite instability. Patients with mismatch repair gene mutations are at an increased risk for the development of tumors, especially colorectal and endometrial cancers, as well as cancers in organs such as the duodenum, kidneys, liver, stomach, and ovaries.[21]

Mutations in tumor suppressor genes may be inherited. Affected individuals are heterozygous, being born with two alleles, of which one has normal function and the other lacks that function. In **Li-Fraumeni syndrome**, a germline mutation of the tumor suppressor gene *TP53* is inherited. Patients with Li-Fraumeni syndrome are at an increased risk for the development of tumors at an early age. Tumors include sarcoma of the bone and soft tissue, breast cancer, brain tumors, and tumors of the adrenal cortex.[22] The breast cancer genes 1 and 2 (*BRCA1* and *BRCA2*) are tumor suppressor genes that are often germline mutations, and inheritance of a copy of the mutated gene significantly increases the risk for the development of early breast and ovarian cancer. The inheritance of mutated *BRCA1* and *BRCA2* has also been associated with the development of cancers in other organs such as the fallopian tube, peritoneum, prostate, and the male breast.[23]

Chromosomal alterations due to deletions or translocations may also result in oncogene activation and the development of neoplasia. For example, a follicular lymphoma may develop following the overexpression of the oncoprotein (resulting protein produced from an oncogene) BCL-2 in B lymphocytes. In the vast majority of patients, BCL-2 overexpression occurs secondary to a t(14;18) chromosomal translocation. The overexpression of BCL-2 prevents normal cell death or apoptosis of B lymphocytes, resulting in the development of a B-cell lymphoma. Acute promyelocytic leukemia (APL; or acute myeloid leukemia–M3) is a condition in which a t(15;17)(q24.1;q21.2) chromosomal translocation leads to the production of an oncoprotein that prevents the normal maturation of promyelocytes to neutrophils in the bone marrow.

The chromosomal translocation t(9;22), a balanced translocation between the breakpoint cluster region gene *BCR* on chromosome 22 and the *ABL* gene on chromosome 9, results in the generation of the Philadelphia chromosome, first identified at two research laboratories in Philadelphia. The translocation is visible upon karyotyping and labeling, and the chromosomal rearrangement forms an abnormal *BCR-ABL* fusion gene (**Figure 7.7**). This abnormal gene produces oncoproteins that have proliferation-promoting tyrosine kinase activity that can no longer be *switched off*. Uncontrolled proliferation of granulocytic cells ensues and is associated with the development of a chronic myeloid leukemia (CML).

VIRAL CAUSES OF CANCER

Adding to the potential mechanisms of cancer initiation, several viruses have been implicated in the development of human cancers. The Epstein–Barr

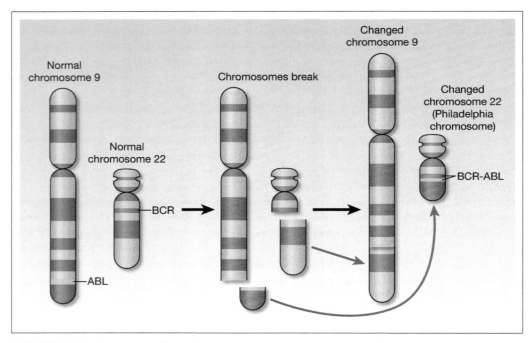

FIGURE 7.7 A chromosomal translocation activates an oncogene. Chromosomal translocation between chromosomes 9 and 22 produces a mutant Philadelphia chromosome that positions a *BCR* (breakpoint cluster region) gene next to the *ABL* proto-oncogene. The protein encoded by the fusion gene *BCR-ABL* is a continually activated protein tyrosine kinase that stimulates cells to continually divide, bypassing normal controls of the cell cycle. Presence of this gene is common in leukemias, particularly in chronic myelogenous leukemia.

virus is a herpesvirus that can infect B lymphocytes. The virus has been associated with a t(8;14) chromosomal translocation and the development of a B-cell lymphoma called **Burkitt lymphoma**. The hepatitis B virus is a DNA virus that has been associated with the development of **hepatocellular carcinoma**. The mechanism by which hepatitis B viruses may induce the development of a tumor is complex but is likely related to changes that occur secondary to the integration of the hepatitis B viral DNA into the genome of patients with chronic hepatitis B. Hepatitis C is caused by an RNA virus that also increases risk of hepatocellular carcinoma.[24]

HPV is a small, sexually transmitted DNA virus. There are more than 200 genotypes of HPV. Subtypes 6 and 11 are associated with the development of lesions such as cutaneous and anogenital warts in adults and laryngeal papillomas in children, and HPV subtypes 16 and 18 have been implicated in the development of **head and neck** and **anogenital cancers**. The mechanism by which HPV induces neoplasia has been studied extensively. The virus produces six early (E) proteins and two late (L) proteins. The E6 and E7 proteins are involved in degradation of the pRb tumor suppressor, which allows viral replication in the cell infected with HPV. The E6 protein

also interacts with the p53 protein, resulting in the degradation of p53 and a decrease in apoptosis or cell death. In addition to p53 and pRb, many other cellular proteins are also targeted, which leads to an uncontrolled proliferation of cells and an increased risk for neoplasia.[25] Vaccines are available against viruses such as hepatitis B and HPV. Immunization with these vaccines is important to decrease the risk of infection with the viruses and, therefore, decrease the risk of developing a cancer. Newer therapies for hepatitis C have played a significant role in clearing the virus from the body and reducing the risk of cancer development.

Thought Questions

8. What is the molecular basis for the development of the Lynch syndrome and the Li-Fraumeni syndrome?

9. What is the Philadelphia chromosome?

10. What viruses are associated with the development of neoplasia?

GENOTYPING IN CANCER DIAGNOSIS AND TREATMENT

Approaches to the treatment of cancer depend on the type, location, and progression of the tumor at the time of diagnosis. Included in these options are traditional strategies such as surgery, radiation, and chemotherapy. Surgery is commonly used to excise solid tumors and has the greatest success when tumors have not spread and remain accessible. A subset of cancers responds to radiation treatment, and the technology and accuracy of this approach has dramatically improved over the past several decades.

Given that cancer cells often have fast growth rates, chemotherapy can be used to nonspecifically target any rapidly growing cells by damaging DNA or inhibiting its replication. Because chemotherapy is distributed systemically, it can be used to treat advanced cancers that have spread from their primary site of origin. However, because normal cells are also affected by the chemotherapeutic agents, side effects of chemotherapy are frequent and often severe. The discovery of common cancer cell characteristics, the mechanism behind cancer development, and technological advancements have resulted in the identification of numerous targeted cancer drugs that have revolutionized diagnosis and treatment.

Cancers can now be genotyped, identifying cancer-associated genetic abnormalities using a wide variety of techniques, including whole genome sequencing, targeted polymerase chain reaction (PCR), and immunological methods. These genetic abnormalities can affect patient outcomes and can be used for diagnosis, prognosis, and, in some cases, to determine therapeutic approach. For example, the detection of the *BCR-ABL* fusion gene, described earlier, confirms the diagnosis of CML. Treatment with a specific tyrosine kinase inhibitor such as imatinib will *switch off* the growth-promoting activity of the BCR-ABL fusion protein and has resulted in a dramatic improvement in the prognosis for patients with CML. Patients with APL can be diagnosed by the translocation causing the disease, and then treated with all-*trans* retinoic acid, which induces the promyelocytes to differentiate to neutrophils. The addition of all-*trans* retinoic acid to the treatment regimen of patients with APL has significantly reduced the mortality and morbidity rates of patients with this disease.

Amplification of the *HER2* gene occurs in about 30% of breast cancers and causes the cancer cells to grow and divide rapidly.[26] Patients with breast cancer are routinely tested for *HER2* amplification to determine whether they are candidates for treatment with drugs such as trastuzumab or lapatinib that can *turn off HER2* activity. Interestingly, diverse cancers can have the same genetic abnormalities. For example, some metastatic stomach or gastroesophageal junction cancers also have an amplification of the *HER2* gene and can thus be treated with the same *HER2*-targeting drugs as those used in breast cancer. Thus, genetic mutations shared by tumors, irrespective of their tissue of origin, make it possible to treat vastly different cancers with the same targeted drugs. These newer drug therapies are sometimes combined with radiation therapy and chemotherapy.

Thought Questions

11. What is the benefit of testing for genetic abnormalities in cancers?

12. Why is it sometimes possible to treat different types of cancer with the same targeted drug?

OVERVIEW OF PEDIATRIC CANCER

Cancer in children differs from that in adults in that it is not often of epithelial origin, as it is in adults, and cannot be explained by environmental exposure. The most commonly occurring broad categories of cancer in children are of hematopoietic origin, followed by nervous system tumors and those of embryonic origin.[26] Just as the origin of cancer in children differs from that in adults, the presenting signs and symptoms may differ[27,28] (Box 7.2).

LEUKEMIAS

Leukemia is classified as either lymphocytic or myelogenous; each type may occur as either an acute or chronic form of malignancy. The leukemias account for at least a third of all childhood cancer, and ALL accounts for 75% of cases of childhood leukemia.[29] Chronic leukemias occur less frequently in children. A primary malignancy of the bone marrow, leukemia, results in the normal bone marrow components being supplanted by abnormal white blood cells. The abnormal cells demonstrate a growth advantage over normal cells. Rampant overgrowth of the abnormal cells causes displacement of other blood cells, which can result in pancytopenia leading to anemia and bleeding. The exact cause of leukemia remains unknown, although numerous chromosomal and genetic abnormalities have been identified in leukemic cells.[30]

ACUTE LYMPHOBLASTIC LEUKEMIA

Risk factors for the development of acute lymphoblastic leukemia (ALL) include numerous genetic conditions, with Down syndrome being the most frequent. Ionizing radiation exposure is a known environmental risk factor.[30] The presentation of ALL is usually nonspecific and may include intermittent low-grade fever, anorexia, malaise, fatigue, and irritability. Lower extremity bone pain may also occur. ALL may metastasize to the central nervous system, resulting in signs of increased intracranial pressure such as headache, vomiting, or vision changes. Genetic studies indicate that aneuploidy (having more or less than two copies of each chromosome), particularly trisomy of chromosomes 4, 10, and 17, predicts likelihood of treatment success. On the other hand, children born with trisomy 21 (Down syndrome) are ten to 20 times more likely to develop ALL.[31]

ACUTE MYELOGENOUS LEUKEMIA

Risk factors for the development of acute myelogenous leukemia (AML) are similar to those for ALL. Signs and symptoms are also similar, although in AML subcutaneous hemolytic purpuric nodules (often termed *blueberry muffin lesions*) may occur.[30]

BOX 7.2
Signs and Symptoms of Cancer in Children

Continued, unexplained weight loss

Headaches, often with early-morning vomiting

Increased swelling or persistent pain in bones, joints, back, or legs

Lump or mass, especially in the abdomen, neck, chest, pelvis, or armpits

Development of excessive bruising, bleeding, or rash

Constant infections

A whitish color behind the pupil

Nausea that persists or vomiting without nausea

Constant tiredness or noticeable paleness

Eye or vision changes that occur suddenly and persist

Recurrent or persistent fevers of unknown origin

Source: From Feist P. Signs of childhood cancer. *Pediatric Oncology Resource Center.* http://www.ped-onc.org/diseases/SOCC.html#anchor75392.

BONE TUMORS

In children and adolescents, **bone tumors** result in localized pain, which may be worse at night or with activity; tender soft tissue mass; and limp or movement limitations.[29,32] **Osteosarcoma** is an aggressive bone tumor affecting the long bones near the metaphyseal plate. It accounts for less than 2% of childhood cancer and is most frequently diagnosed in teenagers.[28] **Ewing sarcoma** is a small, round cell undifferentiated tumor that is believed to be of neural crest origin. Children with a small nonmetastatic Ewing sarcoma have a good prognosis, but if metastasis is present at diagnosis, the long-term survival rate is much poorer.[32]

NERVOUS SYSTEM TUMORS

The second most frequently occurring type of cancer in children and adolescents is malignant **brain and spinal cord tumors**.[27,29] Exposure to ionizing radiation or certain inherited disorders may be risk factors for brain tumor development. Presenting symptoms of nervous system tumors are most often consistent with signs and symptoms of increased intracranial pressure resulting simply from tumor presence or blockage of cerebrospinal flow, or both.

There are more than 100 histological categories of brain tumors. In children, **medulloblastoma** (primitive neuroectodermal tumor) and pilocytic **astrocytoma** are the most common, although several other central nervous system tumors may also occur. Medulloblastoma is an embryonic cerebellar tumor, diagnosed most often by the ages of 5 to 7 years, which can spread via cerebrospinal fluid and can cause fourth ventricle obstruction. Cerebellar dysfunction is often present with this tumor. Astrocytoma also occurs most often in the cerebellar area. Histologically, in the compact area of the tumor, Rosenthal fibers (condensed glial filament masses) are present.[33]

NEUROBLASTOMA

Neuroblastoma occurs only in children, usually younger than 10 years of age, with an average age at diagnosis of 18 months. The tumor arises from primordial neural crest cells (neuroblasts) of the sympathetic nervous system. The tumors can develop in the adrenal medulla and sympathetic ganglia, and commonly have metastasized by the time of diagnosis. Neuroblastoma cells have gene and chromosomal alterations, in most cases involving the *MYCN* and *ALK* genes. Approximately half of all children who develop neuroblastoma before age 12 months will experience complete spontaneous regression, whereas children diagnosed later are more likely to require treatment. The most disabling complications of neuroblastoma are spinal cord compression in up to 10% of patients, and a rare condition termed *opsoclonus myoclonus syndrome*.[34]

RETINOBLASTOMA

Retinoblastoma is a rare cancer that occurs only in children. It develops either as a hereditary disease, due to an abnormality of the *RB1* gene, or sporadically (70% of cases).[29,35] Located on chromosome 13q14, the *RB1* gene is responsible for encoding pRb, which is a tumor suppressor protein. In the heritable form, the *RB1* gene mutation is inherited through germinal cells, with a second mutation occurring in somatic retinal cells. The noninherited type of retinoblastoma occurs as a result of two mutations in the somatic retinal cells. The tumor arises from the inner surface of the retina and then spreads into the retina, resulting in leukocoria—a white appearance to the red reflex, commonly called cat-eye reflex—which is most often first identified by the child's parents.[35]

WILMS TUMOR

Wilms tumor usually presents in young children as a unilateral, painless abdominal mass that is most often initially observed by parents.[29,36] An embryonal malignancy of the kidney, it is thought to be due to a genetic predisposition to nephrogenic rests (fragments of embryonic tissue retained in the developed kidney). Rests that persist are thought to develop into Wilms tumor after undergoing further genetic mutation. Genes for Wilms tumor continue to be identified. In addition to abdominal mass presence, some children may exhibit hematuria or hypertension.[36]

Rita M. Jakubowski and Janet H. Van Cleave

Between 2015 and 2050, the segment of the U.S. population aged 65 years and older is projected to undergo rapid growth from nearly 48 million people to 88 million.[37] As older adults carry a disproportionate share of the cancer burden in the United States, this increase has implications for cancer care. Adults aged 65 years and older currently make up 15% of the U.S. population, yet account for 53% of cancer diagnoses.[37,38] As a result, the incidence of cancer in the United States has been projected to increase by approximately 45% between 2010 and 2030.[39]

To deliver appropriate care for older adults with cancer, clinicians must have a fundamental understanding of the association between aging and cancer. This section describes the physiological processes of aging that may promote cancer development and implications for practice.

PHYSIOLOGICAL PROCESSES OF AGING THAT MAY PROMOTE CANCER DEVELOPMENT

Four processes of aging that may promote cancer development are (a) a favorable environment for cancer, (b) an accumulation of cellular mutations, (c) a decline in immune function, and (d) alterations in hematopoietic stem cells.

FAVORABLE ENVIRONMENT FOR CANCER

Research supports the observation that cancer increases with aging,[39–41] and in fact, its incidence increases exponentially beginning at approximately the midpoint of the life span.[42] The mechanisms underlying this association have not been fully determined. A number of explanations for increased cancer incidence with increased age are summarized in **Figure 7.8** and include the following:

- Longer time of exposure to environmental and endogenous sources of DNA mutations, leading to accumulating mutations
- Decline in DNA repair mechanisms
- Inevitable telomere shortening that may destabilize DNA structure
- Decreased immune surveillance
- Increase in senescent cell number and progression to the senescence-associated secretory phenotype that promotes chronic inflammation[43]

ACCUMULATION OF CELLULAR MUTATIONS

As outlined earlier in this chapter, cancer originates from the mutation of DNA sequences in cells that reroute pathways regulating tissue homeostasis, cell survival, or cell death.[44] These mutations may result in the activation of oncogenes or the loss of tumor-suppressing proteins. Often multiple mutations must occur over many years before the cell actually becomes a cancer stem cell, thus explaining the increased incidence of cancer with aging. As we age, our cells are more likely to accumulate mutations and to develop one that triggers the development of cancer.[45] When such mutations disrupt genes that regulate cell division and growth, the cells begin to grow uncontrollably. A few cells quickly multiply and then increase rates of cell division, eventually becoming a tumor. These abnormal cells acquire phenotypes that increase their ability to proliferate, migrate, and colonize at abnormal sites within the body, to survive hostile tissue environments, and to escape immune system surveillance.

DECLINE IN IMMUNE FUNCTION (IMMUNE SENESCENCE)

The immune system is a major defense mechanism against the development of cancer, monitoring tissue homeostasis to protect against invading pathogens and eliminate damaged cells.[44] It performs these functions by:

- Eliminating or suppressing viral infections to protect the host from virus-induced tumors
- Eliminating pathogens and promptly resolving inflammation to prevent an environment conducive to the development and growth of tumors
- Identifying and eliminating tumor cells by the recognition of specific antigens[45]

The thymus is the major site of T-cell development and maturation. A gradual decline in thymic output of T cells has been proposed as another aspect of the aging process that can aid the development of cancer through a decline in immune function (immunosenescence).[46] The decline in functional immunity is not only more permissive to tumor formation but may also promote it by contributing to chronic low-level inflammation. Age-related declines in T-cell numbers and responsiveness (described in Chapter 6 , The Immune System and Leukocyte Function) contribute to reduced immune surveillance. They help to explain the decreased

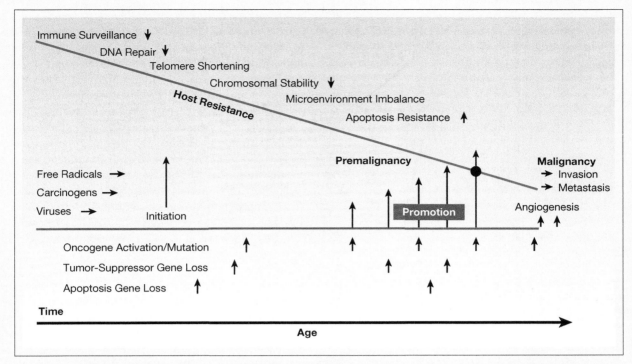

FIGURE 7.8 Increased cancer incidence with aging can be related to a number of changes across the life span. There are potentially multiple sporadic DNA-damaging exposures (free radicals, carcinogens, viruses), leading to altered expression of oncogenes, tumor suppressor genes, apoptosis genes; *initiation* of altered phenotype with increased cell proliferation; accumulation of additional gene alterations; *promotion* of the transition to malignancy with gradual acquisition of invasive and metastatic capacity; and tumor expansion later supported by angiogenesis—all of which are occurring against the natural backdrop of declining host resistance. When factors favoring malignancy outweigh factors inhibiting malignancy, cancer develops.
Source: From Halter JB, et al. *Hazzard's Geriatric Medicine and Gerontology.* 7th ed. McGraw-Hill Education. www.accessmedicine.com. All rights reserved.

ability of the elderly to resist infections to which they were not previously exposed, or to respond to the appearance of tumor antigens, as well as to respond adequately to reinfection or to retain memory for antigens expressed by relapsing tumors.

ALTERATIONS IN HEMATOPOIETIC STEM CELLS

The unique ability of stem cells to proliferate, differentiate, and self-renew allows them to play a major role in homeostasis, replacing cells that are weakened or destroyed by aging.[47] This activity occurs through precise coordination of signaling processes throughout the body. Aging brings a cascade of changes in homeostasis, including a decline in organ function that affects the hematopoietic system, primarily stem cells. To replace blood cells that are constantly being lost due to splenic destruction or tissue utilization, hematopoietic stem cells continuously regenerate circulating cells of the blood and immune system throughout life. Hematopoietic reserves, however, are depleted during

aging, and their ability to renew deteriorates. The ability of stem cells to differentiate into different cell types is also altered, with maintenance of myeloid cell production better than lymphoid cell production.

With aging, there is a decline in stem cell functioning but not numbers.[48] Because of their long life span and ability to replicate, stem cells are subject to damage from both intracellular and extracellular sources. Intracellular sources include the oxidative chemical reactions occurring within the cell. Stem cells undergo repetitive DNA replications during their lifetime, and such repetitive replications can cause random errors. As a result, genetic damage occurs and may accumulate. Instability of stem cells exists to a greater degree in bone marrow of older adults, which suggests a progressive decrease in DNA repair process.[49] Such a decrease or defect in this process may contribute to the increased incidence of leukemia and **myelodysplastic syndrome** (MDS) in older individuals.

Cancers of the hematopoietic system (leukemias) are thought to originate within the normal stem cell through the acquisition of mutations, genetic alterations, and chromosomal translocations.[50] Over time, these changes transform cells from normal to malignant. As previously discussed, the altered cells are able to escape apoptosis and have an endless ability to replicate. AML has an increased incidence among older adults and is an example of a cancer that is thought to originate from an accumulation of genetic mutations occurring over the lifetime of an individual.

AGING AND CANCER: PRACTICE IMPLICATIONS

Screening and treatment recommendations for cancer in older adults take into consideration the functional status of the individual, indications of frailty, and personal preference. Frequency of mammography, cervical cancer screening, and colonoscopy may be reduced after the age of 75, depending on an individual's risk factors and desire for testing. Similarly, frail older adults with reduced functional reserve may be at higher risk for delayed recovery or severe adverse effects after cancer surgeries and conventional chemotherapies. Altered liver and renal drug clearance must be assessed prior to chemotherapy initiation. For these reasons, careful evaluation and consultation with the patient and family are imperative in designing treatment strategies for older adults with a new cancer diagnosis.

Remarkable scientific advances over the past 30 years have generated new therapies that are changing the landscape of cancer treatment. First, the growing number of people with AML or MDS, in conjunction with improvements in transplantation science, has increased the use of allogeneic hematopoietic cell transplantation as a treatment in older adults. Allogeneic hematopoietic cell transplantation is a process whereby stem cells from either a related or an unrelated donor are infused into a patient with the goal of replacing the patient's immune and hematopoietic systems. Data from 103 transplant centers between 2000 and 2013 show that the percentage of allogeneic hematopoietic

cell transplantations in adults aged 70 years and older increased from 0.1% of transplants in 2000 to 3.85% in 2013. Nearly 40% of this population was alive 2 years after transplantation.[51] These findings suggest that, in the context of a growing older adult population, the use of hematopoietic cell transplantation in older adults will continue to increase. Furthermore, advances in hematopoietic stem cell transplantation have allowed the development of reduced-intensity conditioning as a preparative regimen prior to transplantation for some populations of patients. These regimens use less chemotherapy or radiation therapy, or both, than standard myeloablative conditioning regimens, thereby decreasing the potential for organ toxicity. This option has afforded older patients the opportunity for potentially curative therapy.

Second, myriad novel, targeted biological therapies to kill cancer cells are either being used in clinical practice or are under development. One example of a novel targeted therapy is ipilimumab, an immune checkpoint inhibitor, which has demonstrated improvement in survival rates in patients who have undergone surgical resection for stage III melanoma. This therapy blocks CTLA-4 to augment antitumor immune responses.[52] However, while proven to be beneficial, such drugs can induce varying degrees of adverse reactions ranging from rashes to pneumonitis.[53]

One of the major issues in the care of older adults with cancer is the ability of older adults to tolerate these novel therapies. Some evidence supports the contention that older adults tolerate these novel therapies as well as their younger counterparts.[54] However, older adults are underrepresented in cancer clinical trials; thus, the data on the toxicities of targeted therapies experienced by this special population are limited.[55] Because of this limited knowledge regarding the toxicities of novel therapies in older adults, it is important that practitioners who care for older adults with cancer understand the physiological basis of these novel targeted therapies to enable early detection and intervention of treatment toxicities.

CASE STUDY 7.1: A Patient With Breast Cancer

Beth Boyer

Patient Complaint: *"About 2 months ago the skin on my chest felt itchy for several days. It started gradually, but after several days seemed persistent and wouldn't go away. I performed a self-exam and noticed a new lump in the upper outer corner of my right breast that hadn't been there before. I'm very concerned because of my family history of breast cancer."*

History of Present Illness/Review of Systems: Your patient is a 55-year-old postmenopausal African American woman who first noticed itching of both breasts that began in the inframammary ridge area but extended to both breasts. The itching was not relieved with use of oral antihistamine and hot and cold packs. She does not have a visible rash or hives, and has noticed no change to the skin. She performed a breast self-examination and noted a lump in the superior right breast. She has not been on any hormone replacement and experienced menopause at age 50.

The review of systems is negative for fever and infections, vision or hearing changes, headaches, and memory loss. The patient reports no abdominal pain and no nausea, vomiting, diarrhea, or constipation. There are no enlarged lymph nodes and no new problems with bleeding or bruising, no back pain or bone pain, and no peripheral neuropathy. She continues to experience mild itching over her right breast without any rash or hives; however, she noted that this is much better than when she first noticed the itching sensation. She reports no itching or skin changes anywhere else. She has no chest pain, palpitations, or dyspnea, and remainder of her review of systems is negative.

Past Medical/Social/Family History: The patient's past medical history is notable for hypertension and hyperlipidemia. Obstetrical history includes gravida 2, para 2, and pregnancy number 1 at age 29 years; she breastfed both her son and her daughter. Her surgical history includes left knee surgery in 2008 and left axilla lipoma excision in 1992. Social history includes exercise one to two times per week (running) and alcohol intake of one glass of wine daily. She is a former smoker of one pack per month for 10 years; she quit 17 years ago. Oncological family history is negative for ovarian cancer but positive for breast cancer in her sister at age 44, her maternal aunt at age 61, and her maternal grandmother in her 60s. There is no other contributory family history.

Physical Examination: Findings are as follows: temperature of 98.4°F, blood pressure of 110/76 mm Hg, heart rate of 84 beats/min, respirations of 14 breaths/min. Body mass index (BMI) is 30 kg/m². In general, the patient appears well and in no apparent distress. Her heart rate is regular, lungs are clear, and abdomen is soft. Breast examination is performed with the patient sitting and supine. Examination of the left breast demonstrates no evidence of dominant mass, skin change, nipple discharge, or changes within the nipple–areolar complex on the left side. Examination of the right breast reveals a 2- to 3-cm dominant firm mass at the 12 o'clock position, with no overlying skin change, nipple discharge, or change the nipple–areolar complex. There is no supraclavicular or infraclavicular axillary adenopathy on either side.

Laboratory and Diagnostic Findings: Both the CBC with differential and the chemistry panel are normal. Bilateral digital diagnostic mammogram and static ultrasound images are obtained, as follows:

- *Mammogram* indicates that breast tissue is heterogeneously dense. In the left breast, there are no significant findings or changes. In the right breast at 12 o'clock, there is a suspicious mass, correlating with an area of palpable concern as indicated by a metallic marker. Spot compression views show a few punctate calcifications associated with the mass. There are no other suspicious findings in the right breast; specifically, there is no mammographic abnormality in an additional area of palpable concern in the inferior right breast as indicated by a metallic marker.
- *Static ultrasound images* labeled *right breast 12:30*, 5 to 6 cm from the nipple, demonstrate a suspicious solid mass with calipers demarcating measurements of 12 × 18 × 14 mm. This correlates with both the palpable area in the superior breast and mammographic finding. There is no sonographic abnormality in the other area of palpable concern in the right breast 4 to 5 o'clock position.

(continued)

(continued)

- *Pathology ultrasound-guided needle core biopsy:* Right breast, 12:30, 5 to 6 cm from nipple: Invasive ductal carcinoma, Nottingham grade 3 of 3; 1 cm in greatest dimension. Lymphovascular invasion is identified.
- *Immunohistochemical stains* performed at an outside institution demonstrate that the neoplastic cells are immunoreactive for ERs and PRs (75% to 100% strong). The

HER2 (sometimes referred to as HER2/neu) immunohistochemical stain performed at the outside institution is negative (1+).

CASE STUDY 7.1 QUESTIONS
- *What consequences does this patient's case have for the daughter of the patient? Is there a rationale for genetic testing in this case?*
- *Research tamoxifen and describe the rationale for treating the patient with tamoxifen.*

CBC, complete blood count; ERs, estrogen receptors; HER2, human epidermal growth factor receptor 2; PRs, progesterone receptors.

BRIDGE TO CLINICAL PRACTICE

Ben Cocchiaro

PRINCIPLES OF ASSESSMENT

History and Physical Examination
- *Constitutional symptoms:* weight loss, night sweats, anorexia, fever, and fatigue
- *Organ-specific signs and symptoms:*
  - Lung: chronic cough, hemoptysis, chest pain, dyspnea, hoarseness
  - Colon: change in bowel habits, hematochezia, change in stool caliber, bowel obstruction
  - Pancreas: jaundice, abdominal pain, nausea, dark urine, hepatomegaly
  - Breast: breast mass, nipple discharge (especially unilateral)
  - Prostate: urinary retention, nodular, lumpy prostate on examination
  - Skin: lesions with high potential for malignancy often feature asymmetry, uneven borders, multiple colors, diameter greater than ¼″, and change over time
- *Vaccination history:* The HPV and hepatitis B vaccines prevent cancers of the cervix and liver, respectively

Screening Tests
- *Age- and risk-appropriate cancer screenings:* As many neoplasms have long asymptomatic periods in which they are more easily treatable, screening programs have been developed for many of the most common cancers. These include cancers of the breast, colon, cervix, and lung. See recommendations from the USPSTF for more information.

Diagnostic Tools
- *Imaging studies:* The diagnostic evaluation of isolated masses frequently begins with ultrasonography. In contrast, patients with suspected neoplasia of unknown origin often undergo CT scanning of the chest and abdomen. PET imaging is a useful tool for identifying metastases as it highlights areas with high metabolic activity.
- *Biopsy:* Once a suspicious mass has been identified, tissue must be obtained from the mass and sometimes from nearby lymph nodes in order to guide treatment. Genotyping and special histological stains for tumor cell surface proteins can identify the tissue of origin of a mass as well as guide therapy.
- *TNM staging:* To help in prognosis and treatment of most cancers, a standardized staging classification has been developed based on characteristics of the primary tumor (T), lymph node (N) biopsies, and the identification of metastases (M).

Laboratory Evaluation
- *Complete blood count and peripheral smear:* useful in the diagnosis of hematological malignancies
- *Specific tumor markers:* Several dozen biomarkers have been associated with various cancers, but lack of sensitivity and specificity limits their utility to measuring therapeutic response or recurrence in previously diagnosed patients. PSA is a notable example in that while it is still used for prostate cancer screening, providers are encouraged to

have in-depth discussions with patients regarding the risks of false-positive test results.

MAJOR THERAPEUTIC MODALITIES AND DRUG CLASSES
Surgery:
- Surgical removal of affected and adjacent tissue
  - Surgery may be augmented by immediate analysis (frozen section) of the primary lesion and surrounding tissue to evaluate completion of removal of malignancy.
  - PET scanning can also identify patterns of lymph node drainage to target lymph nodes to biopsy for signs of metastasis.
- Chemotherapeutic or radioactive (brachytherapy) beads are sometimes implanted within cancerous tissue.

Radiotherapy:
- Taking advantage of cancer cells' limited ability to repair DNA damage compared with healthy cells, ionizing radiation is frequently used in cancer treatment to target tumors.

Chemotherapy drug classes:
- Nucleic acid synthesis (DNA or RNA) inhibitors
- Protein synthesis inhibitors
- Microtubule inhibitors
- Enzyme inhibitors (intracellular signaling cascades)
- Immune checkpoint inhibitors (promote endogenous immune attack)
- Hormone receptor antagonists
- Tumor-targeting T lymphocytes (CAR-T cells).

CAR-T cells, chimeric antigen receptor–T cells; HPV, human papillomavirus; PSA, prostate-specific antigen; USPSTF, United States Preventive Services Task Force.

KEY POINTS

- The cell cycle is a series of events in the life of a cell in which cell components are grown and DNA is completely replicated, followed by mitosis: division into two daughter cells, each containing the identical genetic information as the parent cell.
- Cells spend varying amounts of time in G_1 (or in the dormant state of G_0) before cell signals, particularly levels of cyclin proteins, initiate entry into the cell cycle. After a number of divisions, cells may enter replicative senescence after which they will not reenter the cell cycle.
- Control of the cell cycle is dependent on tissue needs, but also on signals internal to the cell indicating that sufficient supplies are available for DNA duplication and, later, that DNA replication has produced a normal result. Cell cycle checkpoints assure cell readiness and healthy status prior to cycle progression.
- The protein p53 is a critical signal for blocking cell cycle progression when DNA damage has occurred.
- Cancer is a state in which cell proliferation proceeds uninhibited by the usual control mechanisms, producing tumors made up of progressively more abnormal cells.
- Malignant tumors are named by their tissue of origin and share the properties of invasion

(cell growth beyond usual tissue boundaries) and metastasis (ability of tumor cells to break off from the original site and travel through blood or lymph to distant organs).
- Cancer is a genetic disorder in which a single cell with a few gene mutations produces generations of cells that have progressive mutations favoring the development of uncontrolled cell division and, ultimately, invasion and metastasis.
- Proto-oncogenes may be activated into oncogenes (a gain-of-function mutation), stimulating unregulated cell proliferation.
- Tumor suppressor genes may be turned off (loss-of-function mutation), reducing protective reactions such as DNA repair and cell cycle arrest when DNA damage has occurred.
- The hallmarks of cancer include uncontrolled proliferative signaling, evasion of growth suppressors, genomic instability, telomerase activity, apoptosis evasion, angiogenesis promotion, epithelial–mesenchymal transition that contributes to invasion and metastasis, evasion of immune destruction, and metabolic alterations that promote cell survival.
- Cancer may be localized to a specific organ or may affect bone marrow blood cell precursors, producing leukemias and lymphomas. Whether localized or generalized, cancer can produce systemic changes and symptoms, including inflammation, hypercoagulability, changes in

blood count, mucosal lesions, fatigue, fevers, pain, anorexia, changes in mood, and sleep disturbance. Treatment with chemotherapy or radiation therapy often has similar effects, while sometimes resulting in the critical state of tumor lysis syndrome.

- Approximately 90% to 95% of cancers result from sporadic DNA mutations, including those that activate proto-oncogenes to oncogenes. Some of these sporadic mutations are chromosomal translocations that turn on oncogenes. Cancer genetics also include hereditary cancers in which a germline mutation in a tumor suppressor gene confers risk of cancer development in later life. Cancer-causing viruses can directly alter oncogene or tumor suppressor gene expression in the affected cell.

- Genotyping tumor cells at various stages of disease progression enables targeted therapies that can be very effective across a wide variety of cancer types.

- Cancers in children often have hematopoietic origin, or target brain or bone. Signs and symptoms may be somewhat different than in adults with cancer. Within the hematological cancers, those affecting lymphoid cells are more common in children and adolescents than in adults.

- Cancer incidence increases with age, and age also influences management choices for patients with cancer. Possible explanations for age as a risk factor for cancer include the greater number of years of exposures to DNA-damaging environments, chronic inflammation (inflammaging), increased numbers of sporadic DNA mutations, and diminished adaptive immunity (immunosenescence).

- Age-associated alterations in hematopoietic stem cells predispose greater activity of myeloid precursors, relative to lymphoid, plus a tendency to develop myelodysplasia, a potential cancer precursor.

REFERENCES

1. Heron M. Deaths: leading causes for 2016. *National Vital Statistic Reports*, 67(6). Hyattsville, MD: National Center for Health Statistics; 2018. https://stacks.cdc.gov/view/cdc/57988.
2. National Cancer Institute. Cancer statistics. https://www.cancer.gov/about-cancer/understanding/statistics. Updated April 27, 2018. Accessed January 16, 2019.
3. Bray F, Ferlay J, Soerjomataram I, et al. Cancer statistics 2018: GLOBOCAN estimates of incidence and mortality worldwide for 36 cancers in 185 countries. *CA Cancer J Clin*. 2018;68:394–424. doi:10.3322/caac.21492.
4. American Cancer Society. *Cancer Facts & Figures 2018*. Atlanta, GA: American Cancer Society; 2018. https://www.cancer.org/content/dam/cancer-org/research/cancer-facts-and-statistics/annual-cancer-facts-and-figures/2018/cancer-facts-and-figures-2018.pdf.
5. Siegel RL, Miller KD, Jemal A. Cancer statistics. *CA Cancer J Clin*. 2018;68:7–30. doi:10.3322/caac.21442.
6. Serrano M, Hannon GJ, Beach D. A new regulatory motif in cell-cycle control causing specific inhibition of cyclin D/CDK4. *Nature*. 1993;366:704–707. doi:10.1038/366704a0.
7. Zhang H, Xiong Y, Beach D. Proliferating cell nuclear antigen and p21 are components of multiple cell cycle kinase complexes. *Mol Biol Cell*. 1993;4:897–906. doi:10.1091/mbc.4.9.897.
8. Baker SJ, Markowitz S, Fearon ER, et al. Suppression of human colorectal carcinoma cell growth by wild-type p53. *Science*. 1990;249:912–915. doi:10.1126/science.2144057.
9. Baker SJ, Fearon ER, Nigro JM, et al. Chromosome 17 deletions and p53 gene mutations in colorectal carcinomas. *Science*. 1989;244:217–221. doi:10.1126/science.2649981.
10. Nigro JM, Baker SJ, Preisinger AC, et al. Mutations in the p53 gene occur in diverse human tumour types. *Nature*. 1989;342:705–708. doi:10.1038/342705a0.
11. National Cancer Institute. NCI dictionary of cancer terms. https://www.cancer.gov/publications/dictionaries/cancer-terms/def/tumor. Accessed April 26, 2019.
12. Hanahan D, Weinberg RA. The hallmarks of cancer. *Cell*. 2000;100:57–70. doi:10.1016/s0092-8674(00)81683-9.
13. Hanahan D, Weinberg RA. Hallmarks of cancer: the next generation. *Cell*. 2011;144:646. doi:10.1016/j.cell.2011.02.013.
14. Kraemer KH, Lee MM, Andrews AD, Lambert WC. The role of sunlight and DNA repair in melanoma and nonmelanoma skin cancer. The xeroderma pigmentosum paradigm. *Arch Dermatol*. 1994;130:1018–1021. doi:10.1001/archderm.1994.01690080084012.
15. Chen DS, Mellman I. Oncology meets immunology: the cancer-immunity cycle. *Immunity*. 2013;39:1–10. doi:10.1016/j.immuni.2013.07.012.
16. Sukari A, Nagasaka M, Al-Hadidid A, et al. Cancer immunology and immunotherapy. *Anticancer Res*. 2016;36:5593–5606. doi:10.21873/anticanres.11144.
17. Chouaib S, Janji B, Tittarelli A, et al. Tumor plasticity interferes with anti-tumor immunity. *Crit Rev Immunol*. 2014;34:91–102. doi:10.1615/critrevimmunol.2014010183.
18. Lehuédé C, Dupuy F, Rabinovitch R, et al. Metabolic plasticity as a determinant of tumor growth and metastasis. *Cancer Res*. 2016;76:5201–5208. doi:10.1158/0008-5472.CAN-16-0266.
19. McBride A, Trifilio S, Baxter N, et al. Managing tumor lysis syndrome in the era of novel cancer therapies. *J Adv Pract Oncol*. 2017;8:705–720. doi:10.6004/jadpro.2017.8.7.4.

20. National Cancer Institute. The genetics of cancer. https://www.cancer.gov/about-cancer/causes-prevention/genetics. Accessed November 26, 2018.

21. Vasen HF, Boland CR. Progress in genetic testing, classification, and identification of Lynch syndrome. *JAMA*. 2005;293:2028–2030. doi:10.1001/jama.293.16.2028.

22. Malkin D. Li-Fraumeni syndrome. *Genes and Cancer*. 2011;2:475–484. DOI: 10.1177/1947601911413466.

23. Grignol VP, Agnese DM. Breast cancer genetics for the surgeon: an update on causes and testing options. *J Am Coll Surg*. 2016;222:906–914. doi:10.1016/j.jamcollsurg.2016.01.005.

24. Tsai WL, Chung RT. Viral hepatocarcinogenesis. *Oncogene*. 2010;29:2309–2324. doi:10.1038/onc.2010.36.

25. Yeo-Teh NSL, Ito Y, Jha S. High-risk human papillomaviral oncogenes E6 and E7 target key cellular pathways to achieve oncogenesis. *Int J Mol Sci*. 2018;19(6): E1706. doi:10.3390/ijms19061706.

26. Slamon DJ, Clark GM, Wong SJ, et al. Human breast cancer: correlation of relapse and survival with amplification of the HER-2/neu oncogene. *Science*. 1987;235:177–182. doi:10.1126/science.3798106.

27. Asselin A. Epidemiology of childhood and adolescent cancers. In: Kliegman RM, Stanton BF, St. Geme JW, Schor NF, eds. *Nelson Textbook of Pediatrics*. Vol 2. 20th ed. Philadelphia, PA: Elsevier; 2016:2416–2419.

28. Feist P. Signs of childhood cancer. Pediatric Oncology Resource Center. http://www.pedonc.org/diseases/SOCC.html#anchor75392. Updated January 11, 2018. Accessed March 10, 2019.

29. Barbel P, Peterson K. Recognizing subtle signs and symptoms of pediatric cancer. *Nursing*. 2015;45:30–37. doi:10.1097/01.NURSE.0000461852.18315.b5.

30. Tubergen DG, Bleyer A, Ritchey AK, Friehling E. The leukemias. In: Kliegman RM, Stanton BF, St. Geme JW, Schor NF, eds. *Nelson Textbook of Pediatrics*. Vol 2. 20th ed. Philadelphia, PA: Elsevier; 2016:2437–2452.

31. Kato M, Mahabe A. Treatment and biology of pediatric acute lymphoblastic leukemia. *Pediatr Int*. 2018;60:4–12. doi:10.1111/ped.13457.

32. Arndt CAS. Malignant tumors of bone. In: Kliegman RM, Stanton BF, St. Geme JW, Schor NF, eds. *Nelson Textbook of Pediatrics*. Vol 2. 20th ed. Philadelphia, PA: Elsevier; 2016:2471–2474.

33. Ater JL, Kuttesch JF. Brain tumors in childhood. In: Kliegman RM, Stanton BF, St. Geme JW, Schor NF, eds. *Nelson Textbook of Pediatrics*. Vol 2. 20th ed. Philadelphia, PA: Elsevier; 2016:2453–2461.

34. Matthay KK, Maris JM, Schleiermacher G, et al. Neuroblastoma. *Nat Rev Dis Primers*. 2016; 2:16078. doi:10.1038/nrdp.2016.78.

35. Terek N, Herzog CE. Retinoblastoma. In: Kliegman RM, Stanton BF, St. Geme JW, Schor NF, eds. *Nelson Textbook of Pediatrics*. Vol 2. 20th ed. Philadelphia, PA: Elsevier; 2016:2476.

36. Daw NC, Huff V, Anderson PM. Wilms tumor. In: Kliegman RM, Stanton BF, St. Geme JW, Schor NF, eds. *Nelson Textbook of Pediatrics*. Vol 2. 20th ed. Philadelphia, PA: Elsevier; 2016:2464–2467.

37. United States Census Bureau. 2014 national population projections tables. https://www.census.gov/data/tables/2014/demo/popproj/2014-summary-tables.html. Updated May 9, 2017. Accessed March 10, 2019.

38. National Cancer Institute. Cancer statistics at a glance, 2017. http://seer.cancer.gov/statfacts/html/all.html. Accessed March 10, 2019.

39. Smith BD, Smith GL, Hurria A, et al. Future of cancer incidence in the United States: burdens upon an aging, changing nation. *J Clin Oncol*. 2009;27:2758–2765. doi:10.1200/JCO.2008.20.8983.

40. Hakim FT, Gress RE. Immunosenescence: immune deficits in the elderly and therapeutic strategies to enhance immune competence. *Expert Rev Clin Immunol*. 2005;1:443–458. doi:10.1586/1744666X.1.3.443.

41. White MC, Holman DM, Boehm JE, et al. Age and cancer risk: a potentially modifiable relationship. *Am J Prev Med*. 2014;46:S7–S15. doi:10.1016/j.amepre.2013.10.029.

42. Berger NA, Savvides P, Koroukian SM, et al. Cancer in the elderly. *Trans Am Clin Climatol Assoc*. 2006;117:147–156.

43. Rao AV, Cohen HJ. Oncology and aging: general principles. In: Halter JB, Ouslander JG, Studenski S, et al., eds. *Hazzard's Geriatric Medicine and Gerontology*. 7th ed. New York, NY: McGraw Hill; 2017:1423–1440.

44. de Visser KE, Eichten A, Coussens LM. Paradoxical roles of the immune system during cancer development. *Nat Rev Cancer*. 2006;6:24–37. doi:10.1038/nrc1782.

45. Falandry C, Bonnefoy M, Freyer G, et al. Biology of cancer and aging: a complex association with cellular senescence. *J Clin Oncol*. 2014;32:2604–2610. doi:10.1200/JCO.2014.55.1432.

46. Foster AD, Sivarapatna A, Gress RE. The aging immune system and its relationship with cancer. *Aging Health*. 2011;7:707–718. doi:10.2217/ahe.11.56.

47. Bell DR, Van Zant G. Stem cells, aging, and cancer: inevitabilities and outcomes. *Oncogene*. 2004;23:7290–7296. doi:10.1038/sj.onc.1207949.

48. Liu L, Rando TA. Manifestations and mechanisms of stem cell aging. *J Cell Biol*. 2011;193:257–266. doi:10.1083/jcb.201010131.

49. Kenyon C. The plasticity of aging: insights from long-lived mutants. *Cell*. 2005;120:449–460. doi:10.1016/j.cell.2005.02.002.

50. Reya T, Morrison SJ, Clarke MF, et al. Stem cells, cancer, and cancer stem cells. *Nature*. 2001;414:105–111. doi:10.1038/35102167.

51. Muffly L, Pasquini MC, Martens M, et al. Increasing use of allogeneic hematopoietic cell transplantation in patients age 70 years and older in the United States. *Blood*. 2017;130:1156–1164. doi:10.1182/blood-2017-03-772368.

52. Eggermont AMM, Chiarion-Sileni V, Grob JJ, et al. Prolonged survival in stage III melanoma with ipilimumab adjuvant therapy. *N Engl J Med*. 2016;375:1845–1855. doi:10.1056/NEJMoa1611299.

53. Rubin KM. Understanding immune checkpoint inhibitors for effective patient care. *Clin J Oncol Nurs*. 2015;19:707–717. doi:10.1188/15.CJON.709-717.

54. Townsley CA, Pond GR, Oza AM, et al. Evaluation of adverse events experienced by older patients participating in studies of molecularly targeted agents alone or

in combination. *Clin Cancer Res.* 2006;12(7 Pt 1):2141–2149. doi:10.1158/1078-0432.CCR-05-1798.

55. Kelly CM, Power DG, Lichtman SM. Targeted therapy in older patients with solid tumors. *J Clin Oncol.* 2014;32:2635–2646. doi:10.1200/JCO.2014.55.4246.

SUGGESTED RESOURCES

Alberts B, Johnson A, Lewis J, et al. Cancer. In: Alberts B, Johnson A, Lewis J, et al., eds. *Molecular Biology of the Cell.* 6th ed. New York, NY: Garland Science; 2015:1091–1144.

Anderson G, Francis J, Cornell C. The genetic basis of cancer. In: Kasper CE, Schneidereith TA, Lashley FR, eds. *Lashley's Essentials of Clinical Genetics in Nursing Practice.* 2nd ed. New York, NY: Springer Publishing Company; 2016:389–428.

Bunz F, Vogelstein B. Cancer genetics. In: Jameson JL, Fauci AS, Kasper DL, et al., eds. *Harrison's Principles of Internal Medicine.* 20th ed. New York, NY: McGraw-Hill; 2018:chap 7.

Clark JW, Longo DL. Cancer cell biology. In: Jameson JL, Fauci AS, Kasper DL, et al., eds. *Harrison's Principles of Internal Medicine.* 20th ed. New York, NY: McGraw-Hill; 2018:chap 68.

Kumar V, Abbas AK, Aster JC. Neoplasia. In: Kumar V, Abbas AK, Aster JC, eds. *Robbins and Cotran Pathologic Basis of Disease.* 9th ed. Philadelphia, PA: Elsevier; 2015:265–340.

8

BLOOD AND CLOTTING

Allison Rusgo, Megan E. Schneider, Daniela Livingston, and Patrick C. Auth

THE CLINICAL CONTEXT

Blood disorders vary from the very common (iron-deficiency anemia) to the rare (hereditary spherocytosis) and encompass disorders of red blood cell production and function, platelet disorders, and disorders of bleeding and clotting. Anemia has been identified as one of the greatest global health challenges, ranking fourth among the top five causes of disability globally.[1] In the United States, the National Health and Nutrition Examination Survey (NHANES) data show anemia prevalence to be 5.6%, with the highest rates in women (7.6% versus 3.5% of men) and older adults (12.4% and 19.4% for age groups 70 to 79 and 80 to 85, respectively). There is a striking racial disparity in the prevalence of anemia, with rates of 4.0% in non-Hispanic Whites and 14.9% in non-Hispanic Blacks, compared with 5.1% in Hispanics and 6.1% in all others.[2]

Atherosclerosis and atrial fibrillation are very prevalent in the United States. The most common cause of death is myocardial infarction, often caused by blood clot formation secondary to coronary atherosclerosis; and atrial fibrillation promotes clot formation, which significantly increases risk of stroke. Among the top 200 prescribed drugs in the United States are several that affect blood clotting and are used to reduce morbidity and mortality from coronary artery disease and stroke. Risk reduction in patients diagnosed with acute coronary syndrome includes treatment with the antiplatelet agents aspirin (no. 39 on the top 200 list) and clopidogrel (no. 40). Patients at risk for embolism due to atrial fibrillation or venous

thrombosis are managed with anticoagulants such as warfarin (no. 42), rivaroxaban (no. 131), and apixaban (no. 185).[3] Management of both anemia and anticoagulant therapy is common in primary care settings, which are also the sites of initial identification of many other disorders of red blood cells, platelets, and clotting.

OVERVIEW OF BLOOD AND CLOTTING

Blood circulates throughout the cardiovascular system in order to supply oxygen and nutrients to the body's tissues and organs. Without adequate blood supply, tissues become ischemic and can die. The essential functions of the blood are carried out by the many and various components of the blood. Red blood cells (RBCs) deliver oxygen to the tissues and remove byproducts of cellular metabolism, such as carbon dioxide. Blood also transports white blood cells, platelets, and proteins of the coagulation, complement, and kinin systems to sites of injury and pathogen invasion. Additional functions of blood include regulating body temperature, maintaining acid–base balance, transporting nutrients to tissues and discarding wastes, and carrying hormones to target tissues.

Blood is composed of plasma and formed elements. Plasma makes up approximately 55% of the whole blood volume. Ninety percent of plasma is water; the remaining volume is composed of electrolytes (sodium [Na^+] and chloride [Cl^-] being the most abundant), plasma proteins (such as albumin, globulins, fibrinogen, and prothrombin), nutrients (glucose, amino acids, and lipids), wastes (creatinine, bilirubin, and urea), and dissolved gases (oxygen and carbon dioxide). The remaining 45% of the whole blood volume is composed of formed elements. More than 99% of the cells in the formed elements are RBCs, with white blood cells and platelets making up the remaining cells. White blood cells and their disorders are discussed in Chapters 6, The Immune System and Leukocyte Function, and 7, Neoplasia.

RED BLOOD CELLS

RBCs (also known as red cells or erythrocytes) are the most abundant blood cells. Each milliliter of blood contains approximately 5 billion RBCs. The primary purpose of the RBC is to travel between the lungs and the tissues carrying oxygen to the tissues (site of oxygen utilization), where it picks up carbon dioxide for removal by the lungs. RBCs lack nuclei, organelles, and ribosomes in order to accommodate a large amount of hemoglobin, which maximizes oxygen-carrying capacity. Without nuclei and other organelles, RBCs are unable to undergo mitotic division or conduct cell repair, resulting in their limited life span (100 to 120 days). Continual production of new RBCs through erythropoiesis is required to maintain an adequate red cell count. RBCs constitute approximately 34% to 47% of the blood volume in adult women and 39% to 54% in adult men; this value is termed the *hematocrit*. Total hemoglobin is measured by lysing the cells in a blood sample to measure the total protein. Hemoglobin in adult women averages 11 to 16 g/dL; in adult men it averages 14 to 18 g/dL. Lower values for hematocrit or hemoglobin are diagnosed as anemia.

In order to carry oxygen to the tissues of the body, RBCs must have a size and shape that allow them to travel through very small capillaries. The biconcave disk of the RBC is 7 to 8 μm in diameter and 2 μm thick, which allows for optimal diffusion of gases across the membrane. RBCs also have the capacity to be reversibly deformed, which allows the cells to become more compact to squeeze through smaller capillaries, which can be only 5 μm in diameter, and then return to their original shape. Specific characteristics of the cells are quantified using several key indices:

- RBC size is estimated as the *mean cell volume (MCV)*, calculated by the laboratory as the hematocrit divided by the red cell count. Differential diagnosis of many RBC disorders includes identification of macrocytosis (increased MCV, >100 fL), microcytosis (decreased MCV, <80 fL), or normal cell volume (80–100 fL).
- Conditions such as sickle cell disease (SCD), hemolysis, and thalassemia are associated with greater than normal variability of RBC size. The index of RBC size variability is the *red cell distribution width (RDW)*. Abnormally high RDW is also termed *anisocytosis*, indicating greatly varying RBC sizes observed in a blood smear.
- Additional RBC characteristics calculated by the clinical laboratory are the *mean cell hemoglobin* (MCH; defined as the total hemoglobin value divided by the red cell count) and *mean cell hemoglobin concentration* (MCHC; defined as the hemoglobin value divided by the hematocrit).
- RBC *color* is evaluated qualitatively from the blood smear and can be characterized as normal (normochromic) or pale (hypochromic).

ERYTHROPOIESIS

In adults, the only sources of RBC formation are multipotent stem cells in the bone marrow. There are two types of bone marrow: red and yellow. Red bone marrow is capable of cell production, whereas yellow bone marrow is not. Yellow marrow is high in fat content and gradually replaces red marrow during childhood; however, red marrow persists in a few locations throughout the body into adulthood (sternum, ribs, and proximal long bones). Red bone marrow is the source of RBCs, white blood cells, and platelets (**Figure 8.1**). The rapid production rate of both red and white blood cells mandates a high rate of DNA synthesis to support quick cell cycling of precursors. Vitamin B12 and folate are required for DNA synthesis and must be adequate to support bone marrow production of red and white blood cells.

All of the formed elements in the blood are produced from a single cell type, the multipotent stem cell. In erythropoiesis, the multipotent stem cell produces a colony-forming unit (CFU) progenitor of the myeloid blood cell line, referred to as the colony-forming unit–granulocyte-erythrocyte-monocyte-megakaryocyte (CFU-GEMM). The CFU-GEMM cell differentiates into burst-forming units–erythrocytes (BFU-Es), which are precursors committed to the erythroid lineage. Stimulated by erythropoietin, stem cell factor, granulocyte-macrophage colony-stimulating factor (GM-CSF), and interleukin 3 (IL-3), BFU-Es proliferate into about 1,000 daughter cells that mature into colony-forming units–erythrocytes (CFU-Es). CFU-Es proliferate into 50 to 70 daughter cells (proerythroblasts). BFUs and CFUs cannot be distinguished from other bone marrow precursors by microscopy, although these erythroid precursors do have unique membrane proteins, such as the receptor for erythropoietin. The rapidly repeated cycles of BFU-E and CFU-E cell division require high rates of DNA synthesis. Under the influence of the proper cytokines, and pending availability of folate and vitamin B12, the CFU-Es mature into large, nucleated proerythroblasts. Cell division continues until the midpoint of the polychromatic erythroblast stage (**Figure 8.2**).

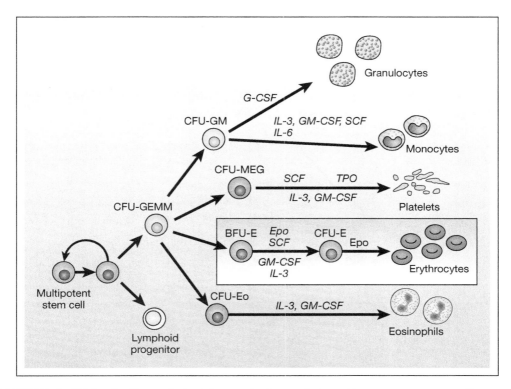

FIGURE 8.1 All blood cells are derived from a single population of bone marrow stem cells. BFU-E, burst-forming unit–erythrocytes; CFU-E, colony-forming unit–erythrocytes; CFU-Eo, colony-forming unit–eosinophils; CFU-GEMM, colony-forming unit–granulocyte-erythrocyte-monocyte-megakaryocyte; CFU-GM, colony-forming unit–granulocyte-macrophage; CFU-MEG, megakaryocytic colony forming unit; Epo, erythropoietin; G-CSF, granulocyte colony-stimulating factor; GM-CSF, granulocyte-macrophage colony-stimulating factor; IL, interleukin; M-CSF, monocyte colony-stimulating factor; SCF, stem cell factor; TPO, thrombopoietin.

Maturation from basophilic (bluish color), through polychromatic (many color) and orthochromatic (uniform color) phases of erythroblast development coincides with the production of hemoglobin, which relies on the availability of iron. The maturing erythroblast begins eliminating intracellular structures while accommodating a growing number of hemoglobin molecules. The final organelle to be eliminated is the nucleus, which contracts and is expelled from the erythroblast, marking the stage at which no further transcription is possible. The cell is now a reticulocyte that leaves the bone marrow to enter the circulating blood. A reticulocyte lacks a nucleus, but contains a network of ribosomal RNA, ribosomes, and possibly a few mitochondria.

Once in the blood, reticulocytes lose the remaining organelles (and thus the ability to synthesize protein), becoming mature RBCs. The mature cells are smaller than reticulocytes and assume the biconcave disk shape. With the loss of the mitochondria and ribosomes, the RBC is no longer able to synthesize hemoglobin or DNA. Approximately 2 to 2.5 million RBCs

are produced per second, or about 200 billion per day, which equals the daily rate of splenic removal of aging RBCs. Reticulocytes normally make up approximately 1% of the red cell count, and the reticulocyte count (expressed as a percentage of RBCs) is a useful measure of RBC production.

Erythropoiesis is stimulated by erythropoietin. Erythropoietin is a glycoprotein synthesized and secreted by the kidneys into the bloodstream that circulates to the bone marrow. Erythropoietin increases RBC progenitor proliferation and differentiation, especially of CFUs. Tissue hypoxia, as in the case of anemia, hemorrhage, chronic lung disease, or high-altitude environments, stimulates increased erythropoietin production. Severe tissue hypoxia may increase RBC production up to six times the normal level. Patients with chronic kidney disease have reduced erythropoietin production, which can lead to anemia, while patients with chronic lung disease and hypoxemia may develop compensatory polycythemia. Secondary polycythemia can develop in individuals who are heavy smokers or who take exogenous testosterone.

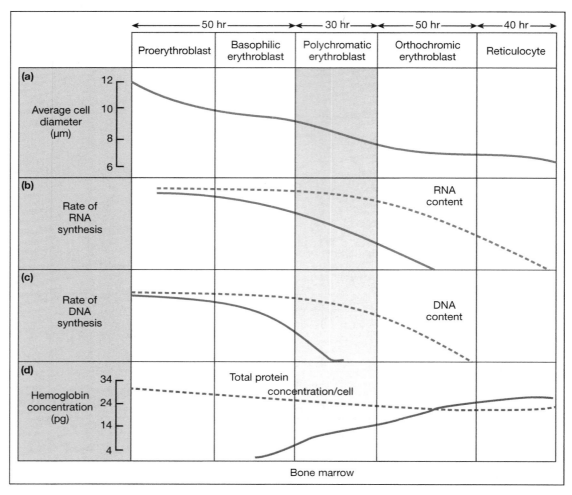

FIGURE 8.2 Stages of bone marrow red blood cell development end at the reticulocyte, at which point the cell leaves the bone marrow and enters the circulation. Shading of the polychromatic erythroblast stage indicates that cell division stops at this stage.
Source: Adapted from Keohane E, Smith L, Walenga J. *Rodak's Hematology: Clinical Principles and Applications.* Elsevier; 2015.

 Thought Questions

1. **What organelles are present in a mature red blood cell?**

2. **What proteins does a mature red blood cell synthesize?**

HEMOGLOBIN

RBCs are essentially packages built to contain high concentrations of the body's oxygen-carrying protein hemoglobin. Hemoglobin production begins during the basophilic erythroblast stage, and continues through the reticulocyte phase, as long as hemoglobin RNA is present. Each hemoglobin molecule is composed of two pairs of polypeptide chains (the globins) and four heme/iron complexes (**Figure 8.3**). The structure of the polypeptide chains varies and influences the hemoglobin

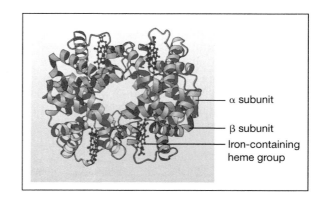

FIGURE 8.3 Model of a hemoglobin molecule. The α chains are blue, β chains are red, and heme groups are shown in gray.

molecule's oxygen affinity. During most of fetal development, RBCs contain hemoglobin F (HbF), with two alpha and two gamma chains ($\alpha_2\gamma_2$). Beginning at about 38 weeks of gestational age, there is a transition to hemoglobin A (HbA), containing two alpha and two beta chains ($\alpha_2\beta_2$). The heme groups are bound to the polypeptide chains and are able to reversibly bind oxygen molecules at their iron ion.

⚕ *Genetic Hemoglobinopathies*

Mutations in the genes coding for the α or β chains can produce hemoglobinopathies. **Sickle cell disease (SCD)** and **sickle cell trait** are due to a single base (missense) mutation in the β-globin gene, resulting in substitution of the hydrophobic amino acid valine for the charged, hydrophilic amino acid glutamate at position 6. Hemoglobin S (HbS) is the primary hemoglobin produced in homozygotes; these individuals are referred to as having SCD. Heterozygotes are referred to as having the sickle cell trait and have fewer clinical manifestations than homozygotes. HbS has a surface hydrophobic region due to the prominent position of the valine at position 6 of the β chain. Transition of hemoglobin to the deoxy form changes the protein conformation to expose a complementary hydrophobic site on the α chains, potentially precipitating a nucleation event in which two HbS molecules are held together by hydrophobic interactions. Nucleation is followed by chain elongation, with the addition of more HbS molecules lengthening the polymer (**Figure 8.4**). Finally, elongated HbS polymers can align and deform the RBC into the sickle shape. This reaction is facilitated under

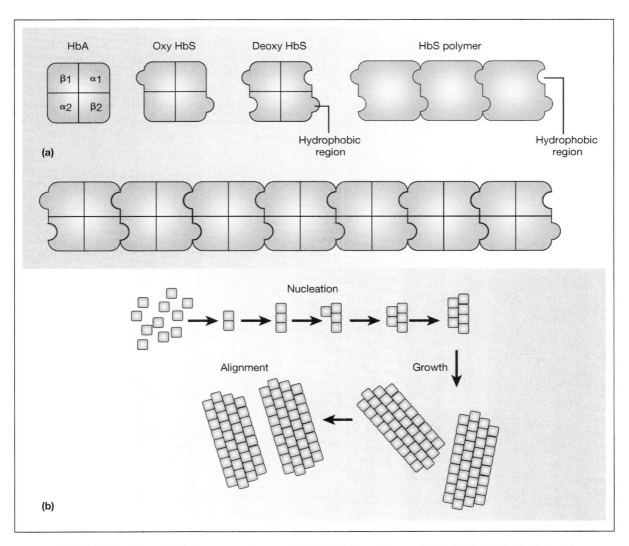

FIGURE 8.4 **(a)** and **(b)** Diagram of hemoglobin A (HbA) and hemoglobin S (HbS). The β chain of hemoglobin S has valine substituted for glutamate at position 6. This forms a hydrophobic *sticky* spot on the outside of the molecule. Deoxygenation exposes a complementary hydrophobic site on the α chain, where two hemoglobin molecules can stick together by hydrophobic attraction (nucleation). This process repeats until long polymers of hemoglobin S molecules are produced and deform the red blood cell into the elongated *sickle* shape.
Deoxy, deoxygenated; Oxy, oxygenated.

conditions of dehydration, which concentrates the hemoglobin within the RBC cytoplasm. Hypoxia and acidosis further favor sickling. The misshaped RBCs block small blood vessels and produce severe pain secondary to tissue ischemia. The abnormally shaped cells are removed at higher than usual rates by macrophages in the spleen (extravascular hemolysis), so splenectomy is sometimes performed to reduce this source of blood cell loss. Most of the severe consequences of SCD begin in childhood and are described in the Pediatric Considerations section.

Thalassemia is the term for a group of genetic disorders that result in abnormal production of either α- or β-hemoglobin chains. β-Thalassemias are associated with hypochromic, microcytic anemia due to the reduction in RBC hemoglobin concentration. α-Thalassemias vary in prevalence and severity, depending on the number of α genes that are abnormal (of the four genes coding for α-globin chains). Thalassemia can alter RBC function both through the reduced production of the specific globin chains and the buildup of abnormal levels of the unaffected globin chains, some of which form cellular precipitates that lead to hemolysis.

IRON

Iron is required for hemoglobin production. Total body iron is approximately 3 to 4 g, with at least half of that contained in hemoglobin molecules. Iron is poorly soluble in plasma, so it is transported in the blood by the binding protein transferrin. The transferrin–iron complex carries iron to the bone marrow, where it binds to transferrin receptors on erythroblasts. After the complex has moved into the erythroblast, iron is dissociated from transferrin, and transferrin is returned to the plasma for reuse. Transferrin bound to iron is referred to as saturated transferrin, and the percentage of transferrin saturation varies from 20% to 50% in healthy individuals. Iron used for hemoglobin synthesis comes from two sources: 5% is obtained from gastrointestinal (GI) absorption of dietary iron, which takes place in the duodenum, and 95% is recycled from breakdown of aging RBCs in the spleen (**Figure 8.5**). Body iron losses occur daily with sloughing of GI epithelial cells, totaling approximately 1 mg/day, and dietary iron absorption adds 1 mg of new iron to the body daily. Iron absorption is very inefficient: Dietary intake is about 10 to 15 mg/day, so absorption by the duodenum represents only 5% to 10% of ingested iron.

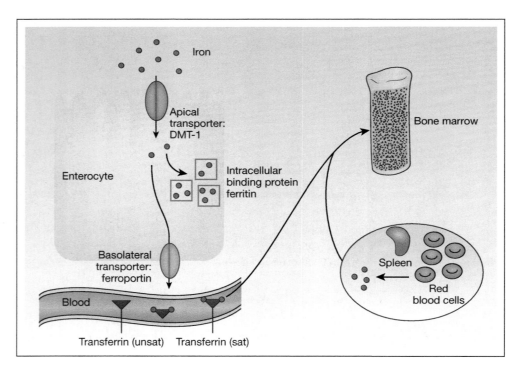

FIGURE 8.5 Splenic macrophages break down aging red blood cells, releasing 95% of the iron needed for red blood cell synthesis. The iron is released from the spleen and then binds to the plasma carrier protein transferrin for transport to the bone marrow. GI absorption of dietary iron involves a DMT-1 on the apical side of the epithelial cell. Some iron is stored in ferritin in gut epithelial cells (enterocytes), and the remainder leaves the cell by the basolateral ferroportin transporter. Iron then binds to circulating transferrin for transport to the bone marrow.
DMT-1, divalent ion membrane transporter; GI, gastrointestinal; sat, saturated; unsat, unsaturated.

Iron is also stored intracellularly, with the greatest storage in the liver and in macrophages of the reticuloendothelial system. The intracellular storage protein apoferritin is synthesized in these and other cells. Iron ions accumulate in apoferritin; the resulting iron-laden molecule is then referred to as ferritin. Iron can move from ferritin-bound to free inside cells. Some ferritin is present in plasma, and the blood ferritin level is measured in the differential diagnosis of anemia.

Iron balance is disrupted by inadequate intake or absorption or by excessive demands. States of high iron requirements include infant and childhood development, adolescence, pregnancy, and normal or excessive menstruation. In older adults, GI losses associated with malignancy can cause excessive iron demand. GI malabsorptive disorders such as Crohn disease, celiac disease, or those secondary to weight loss surgeries compromise iron absorption and require supplementation (usually parenteral) to maintain erythropoiesis. In all cases, if dietary supply and body stores in the liver and other tissues are inadequate, iron-deficiency anemia will result.

VITAMIN B12 AND FOLATE

Rapid proliferation of bone marrow RBC precursors requires a sufficient supply of vitamin B12 and folate, both of which are needed for nucleotide production to support DNA synthesis. Deficiency states of folate are relatively uncommon in the United States, as many foods have supplemental folate added. The dietary source of vitamin B12 is animal products, including meat, eggs, and milk, and deficiency may be seen in people on vegetarian or vegan diets. Dietary absorption of vitamin B12 occurs in a multistep process. Gastric parietal cells secrete the protein intrinsic factor into the stomach lumen; the intrinsic factor then binds to vitamin B12, either in the stomach or in the small intestine. The B12–intrinsic factor complex travels through the remaining small intestine until docking to receptor sites on ileal epithelial cells. Once inside the cells, the complex dissociates and vitamin B12 is absorbed into the circulation. The binding protein transcobalamin transports vitamin B12 through the portal vein to the general circulation, with a first-pass removal, allowing some vitamin B12 to be stored in the liver.

Thought Questions

3. What are the dietary sources of iron, vitamin B12, and folate?

4. Who may be at risk for inadequate dietary intake of these nutrients, predisposing them to anemia?

GENERAL CONCEPTS IN ANEMIA

Anemia is defined as decreased RBC mass or hemoglobin content of the blood. The blood smear in anemia allows characterization based on normal, decreased, or increased RBC size (normocytic, microcytic, or macrocytic) and on normal or pale color (normochromic or hypochromic). Homeostatic compensation for anemia depends on the rate and duration of blood loss. **Hemorrhage** induces rapid loss of RBCs and plasma, with an abrupt decrease in hemoglobin, hematocrit, and blood volume. These changes elicit dramatic hypotension with compensatory tachycardia and tachypnea. Blood pressure decreases, sometimes to the point of circulatory hypovolemic shock. Slow, chronic blood loss, as in menorrhagia, or GI losses associated with cancer or other source of GI bleeding are compensated by renal sodium and fluid retention, and relative maintenance of blood volume and pressure accompanied by low hematocrit. Severe **chronic anemia** with volume compensation still results in tachycardia and tachypnea, as the remaining RBCs are circulated more rapidly to compensate for decreased blood oxygen-carrying capacity. Patients present with pallor of skin and mucous membranes, fatigue, exercise intolerance, and, in severe cases, syncope. A general overview of the most common forms of anemia is presented here. Additional discussion of iron-deficiency anemia appears later in this chapter, under the section Pediatric Considerations, and anemia in older adults can be found under the section Gerontological Considerations.

IRON-DEFICIENCY ANEMIA (MICROCYTIC ANEMIA)

As noted previously, iron deficiency is the most common cause of anemia in adults and children in the United States and globally. The clinical features of **iron-deficiency anemia (microcytic anemia)** depend on the degree of anemia. Some individuals may be asymptomatic or may have mild to severe signs and symptoms, including fatigue, generalized weakness, dyspnea on exertion, orthostatic lightheadedness, restless legs syndrome, and tachycardia. Signs of GI bleeding may be present, ranging from melena to stools containing bright red blood. Anemia of long duration can be associated with pica and the appearance of a smooth tongue and brittle nails. In middle-aged women, iron-deficiency anemia may present with dysphagia due to esophageal webbing, also known as Plummer–Vinson syndrome.

Laboratory studies in iron-deficiency anemia reveal decreased red cell count, hemoglobin, and hematocrit; decreased serum iron and ferritin; increased total iron-binding capacity and transferrin levels; low transferrin saturation; and microcytic, hypochromic RBCs. MCV will be below the normal range (<80 fL). The bone marrow biopsy is the gold standard to confirm the diagnosis but is not commonly ordered owing to the invasive nature of the procedure. Gastroenterology evaluation is appropriate if occult blood loss or malabsorption is suspected. The management of iron-deficiency anemia consists of treatment of the underlying disorder. Oral iron replacements should be given to a menstruating woman. Parenteral iron replacement may be used in patients with poor absorption and for individuals who require more iron than oral therapy can provide or individuals who cannot tolerate oral ferrous sulfate.

VITAMIN B12 DEFICIENCY ANEMIA (MACROCYTIC ANEMIA)

The most common cause of **vitamin B12 deficiency anemia (macrocytic anemia)** is an inability to absorb vitamin B12. **Pernicious anemia** is an autoimmune disorder with destruction of gastric parietal cells. The resulting lack of intrinsic factor prevents vitamin B12 absorption. Individuals with chronic gastritis due to *Helicobacter pylori* infection are also vulnerable to vitamin B12 deficiency. Malabsorptive conditions such as Crohn disease reduce ileal surface area, with the resulting loss of vitamin B12 absorption. Bariatric surgery that dramatically reduces the size of the stomach also reduces the number of parietal cells available to synthesize intrinsic factor, resulting in poor vitamin B12 absorption. Parasitic infections of the small intestine, as well as certain medications (including metformin and cholestyramine), can block vitamin B12 absorption.

The laboratory manifestations of vitamin B12 deficiency anemia include decreased vitamin B12, increased serum methylmalonic acid and homocysteine, anisocytosis with a predominance of large (macrocytic) RBCs, reduced white cell and platelet counts, and abnormal neutrophils with hypersegmented nuclei. A bone marrow biopsy may show megaloblasts and erythroid hyperplasia. Vitamin B12 is required for myelin formation, and demyelination can accompany vitamin B12 deficiency anemia. In severe and prolonged cases, demyelination of the posterior columns, lateral corticospinal tracts, and spinocerebellar tracts may occur. This leads to a loss of position and vibratory sensation (particularly in the lower extremities), ataxia, and upper motor neuron signs, such as increased deep tendon reflexes, spasticity, weakness, and an extensor Babinski sign. Sensory paresthesias may also be present. The management of megaloblastic anemia due to vitamin B12 deficiency generally involves oral or parenteral administration of vitamin B12. Treatment completely reverses the anemia and white blood cell findings, but neurological damage may not be completely reversible with treatment.

ANEMIA OF CHRONIC INFLAMMATION

Anemia of chronic inflammation (ACI) is an umbrella term for a subset of anemias that occur secondary to infections, malignancies, or connective tissue diseases lasting at least 1 month. Infections resulting in ACI include subacute bacterial endocarditis, osteomyelitis, pyelonephritis, or late stage HIV. In oncology care, there are several mechanisms whereby tumors function as catalysts for inflammatory responses that cause ACI. Some tumors, either because of normal function or abnormal gene expression, secrete cytokines that cause an inflammatory response, while other tumors invade healthy cells and tissues for a similar result. Additionally, certain tumors undergo necrosis due to decreased oxygen and nutrient supply; this process also leads to the secretion of inflammatory mediators and subsequent ACI. Lastly, autoimmune connective tissue disorders represent a significant portion of diseases that cause ACI. The most common culprits are rheumatoid arthritis, systemic lupus erythematosus (SLE), and polymyalgia rheumatica. It should also be noted that with SLE, there is increased RBC destruction from autoantibodies and associated renal insufficiency, which also cause anemia. Therefore, patients with SLE are at an increased risk of several types of concurrent anemias and should be monitored accordingly.

Pathophysiologically, ACI is associated with low levels of circulating iron. Normally, in the process of removing aging RBCs from the circulation, iron storage occurs in the macrophages of the spleen. Additional stores can be found in macrophages in bone marrow and liver. In the setting of chronic inflammatory disorders with elevated cytokine levels, liver production of the circulating iron-regulatory protein hepcidin and the intracellular storage protein apoferritin increase. Hepcidin suppresses the membrane transporter ferroportin, which normally releases iron from cells. Thus, when hepcidin levels increase, less iron moves into the circulation from gut absorptive cells and splenic macrophages.

Despite adequate body intracellular iron stores in the form of ferritin, circulating iron decreases, erythropoiesis is reduced, and RBC production slows, and there is a low reticulocyte index. This process explains the somewhat paradoxical findings of increased intracellular iron stores and decreased circulating iron in patients with ACI. Clinically, this decrease in iron availability rarely causes hemoglobin levels to decrease below 8 g/dL, which is often the threshold used to determine the necessity of interventions such as blood transfusions. From a treatment perspective, patients with ACI benefit from continued management of their primary disease process, and in some instances, recombinant erythropoietin therapy can also be used.

ANEMIA IN CHRONIC KIDNEY DISEASE

Anemia of chronic kidney disease is extremely common in patients in renal failure. The pathophysiological mechanisms are multifactorial. The primary mechanism is the loss of erythropoietin production by the failing kidneys. In clinical practice, this has been managed with exogenous erythropoietin and its analogues. However, iron deficiency may contribute to anemia in these patients, so iron status should be evaluated. In addition, chronic kidney disease is associated with chronic inflammation and increased hepcidin production, so there is an overlap between ACI and chronic kidney disease. Finally, dialysis itself is associated with a modest blood loss, contributing to the overall factors causing anemia in patients with chronic kidney disease.

HEMOLYTIC ANEMIA

Hemolytic anemia results when RBCs are destroyed before their normal life span of 100 to 120 days. Assuming adequate nutritional status and normal bone marrow, the homeostatic response is to increase erythropoiesis, leading to an elevated reticulocyte count. If erythropoiesis cannot keep up with the destruction of RBCs, anemia results. Hemolytic anemia resulting from factors external to RBC defects occurs in immune hemolysis, in mechanical hemolysis (e.g., prosthetic heart valves), in some clotting disorders, and as an adverse effect of certain medications. Hemolysis resulting from intrinsic RBC defects is often genetic and occurs in patients with hemoglobin abnormality (e.g., SCD, thalassemia), membrane defects (i.e., hereditary spherocytosis, paroxysmal nocturnal hemoglobinuria), and enzyme defects (e.g., glucose-6-phosphate dehydrogenase [G6PD] deficiency).

Hemolytic anemia is classified based on the predominant site of hemolysis. Intravascular hemolysis occurs within the blood vessels, and extravascular hemolysis occurs within the reticuloendothelial system, primarily the spleen. Intravascular hemolysis can occur secondary to clotting disorders that block small blood vessels, termed **microangiopathic hemolytic anemia**, as seen in thrombotic thrombocytopenia purpura, hemolytic uremic syndrome, or HELLP (hemolysis, elevated liver enzymes, low platelets) syndrome of pregnancy.

The increased rate of RBC breakdown, particularly when it occurs intravascularly, releases the iron and heme components of hemoglobin into the blood at a rapid rate. The fate of heme groups is conversion to biliverdin, which is then metabolized to bilirubin (**Figure 8.6**). As bilirubin production precipitously increases, bilirubin levels may overwhelm the ability of the liver to conjugate and secrete bilirubin into bile (described in Chapter 14, Liver), producing jaundice and dark urine. In hemolytic anemia, blood levels of unconjugated (indirect) bilirubin rise more than conjugated bilirubin. Other laboratory manifestations of

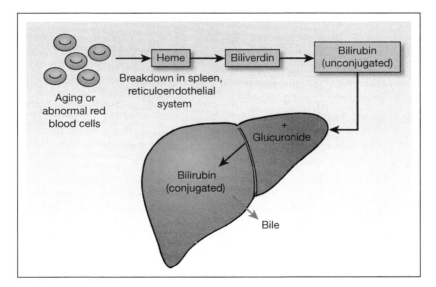

FIGURE 8.6 Breakdown of red blood cells releases hemoglobin. The protein chains of hemoglobin are broken down to their constituent amino acids, and the iron atoms travel in the circulation, bound to transferrin, to return to the bone marrow for synthesis of new hemoglobin. The heme component of hemoglobin is metabolized first to biliverdin, then bilirubin. Unconjugated bilirubin is hydrophobic, and it binds to plasma albumin for transport to the liver. Liver cells take up the bilirubin and conjugate it, increasing its water solubility, and excreting much of this conjugated bilirubin into bile.

acute hemolysis include low red cell count, hemoglobin, and hematocrit; anisocytosis with the appearance of schistocytes (RBC fragments); increased reticulocyte count; and elevated serum iron and lactate dehydrogenase. Other manifestations of hemolytic anemia include splenomegaly, hepatomegaly, and gallstones.

Glucose-6-Phosphate Dehydrogenase Deficiency

Glucose-6-phosphate dehydrogenase (G6PD) is a metabolic enzyme that catalyzes the first reaction in the pentose phosphate pathway, a route of glucose metabolism that generates reduced nicotinamide adenine dinucleotide phosphate (NADPH). NADPH is required to generate reduced glutathione, a critical cellular antioxidant that protects cells from oxidative stress. The G6PD gene is located on the X chromosome, so **G6PD deficiency** has an X-linked inheritance pattern. Males are hemizygotes (they have only one X chromosome) and are more severely affected. There are several variants that differ in severity, with some variants producing little or no evidence of hemolysis.

As noted earlier, RBCs lack the DNA, RNA, and ribosomes needed for transcription and translation, so patients with G6PD deficiency are unable to compensate for the decreased half-life of the mutant G6PD enzyme by synthesizing new protein. Stimuli that increase oxidative stress, therefore, can exhaust the RBC supply of reduced glutathione, precipitating oxidative damage to the globin chains of hemoglobin and accelerating RBC removal by splenic macrophages. Oxidizing medications are the most common sources of oxidative stress that precipitate hemolytic reactions in individuals with G6PD deficiency. These drugs include several antimalarial drugs, sulfonamides, and the antibiotic nitrofurantoin. Dietary oxidants can also precipitate hemolysis, in particular, ingestion of fava beans. An acute hemolytic episode precipitated by such exposures resolves after removal of the cause.[4] Management of a person with G6PD is relatively straightforward: avoidance of certain medications and foods (particularly fava beans) is sufficient to prevent hemolytic episodes.

Autoimmune Hemolytic Anemia

Autoimmune hemolytic anemia (AIHA) is an uncommon condition characterized by the body's production of anti–RBC autoantibodies. The anemia is secondary to rupture of RBCs caused by binding of antibodies, complement, or both to the RBCs, or by uptake and destruction of antibody-coated cells by macrophages. AIHA may have a primary cause or may be secondary to other events, including SLE and other autoimmune diseases, infections, and certain medications. In 50% of cases, AIHA is idiopathic.

Laboratory tests classify AIHA by the optimal temperature at which the anti–RBC autoantibodies bind to a patient's RBCs and cause lysis, with warm or cold subtypes. Warm AIHA accounts for about 80% of all AIHA cases, and is immunoglobulin G (IgG) mediated. Cold agglutinin disease results from binding of IgM or complement, or both, and is often idiopathic. Complement binding and formation of the membrane attack complex in cold agglutinin disease results in intravascular hemolysis, whereas binding of IgG and opsonization of RBCs in warm AIHA often result in extravascular hemolysis in the spleen or the liver. As with other hemolytic anemias, AIHA is accompanied by compensatory reticulocytosis and elevated bilirubin and, often, urine urobilinogen or hemoglobinuria following intravascular hemolysis.

Thought Questions

5. How does the physical appearance of blood cells differ among the various types of anemia: iron deficiency, vitamin B12 or folate deficiency, hemolytic anemia, and SCD?

6. What is the main source of bilirubin in the blood? Why does the blood concentration of unconjugated bilirubin increase in hemolytic anemia?

HEMOSTASIS

Hemostasis (blood clotting) is a vital defense system contributing to homeostasis by preventing hemorrhage or reducing blood loss when there is a break or injury in the vasculature. Hemostasis is a tightly regulated cascade of responses to injury, involving endothelial cells, extracellular matrix (ECM), platelets, and plasma proteins. This cascade leads to platelet plug formation, followed by the production of a stable clot. Hemostasis is a very rapid and localized process. Platelets and protein components of the hemostatic system circulate in inactive forms but are rapidly activated upon tissue injury. Clot formation needs to be initiated quickly, but must be limited to the site of injury to prevent excessive blood vessel occlusion. After tissue healing and regrowth of blood vessels, the clot must be removed. Thus, from the beginning of the hemostatic process, the opposite reactions of anticoagulation and fibrinolysis are initiated, particularly in normal regions adjacent to areas of injury and blood vessel breakage.

The hemostatic system may be divided into two stages:

1. In *primary hemostasis*, vessel constriction (due to endothelin released by endothelial cells and serotonin from platelets) is rapidly followed by platelet adhesion and aggregation to form a platelet plug.
2. In *secondary hemostasis*, zymogens (protease enzymes in their precursor and active forms) and cofactors undergo a series of activations leading to a stable clot made out of fibrin deposited on and within the platelet plug.

PLATELET STRUCTURE AND FUNCTION

Platelets are nonnucleated fragments of bone marrow megakaryocytes. Platelets have a life span of 7 to 10 days and high turnover rate, with daily losses and replacement averaging 1×10^{11} platelets. Platelets circulate between the vasculature (for potential clot production) and the spleen (for storage and eventual destruction). Patients who undergo splenectomy commonly develop thrombocytosis; patients who have immune-mediated alteration of platelet membranes often develop splenomegaly and thrombocytopenia. Production of platelets is stimulated by thrombopoietin, a protein synthesized by liver and kidneys, and chemokine CXCL12, which is produced by the bone marrow stroma. Platelet production is also stimulated by cytokines such as IL-3, IL-6, and GM-CSF, thus explaining the thrombocytosis associated with many inflammatory states.

Circulating quiescent platelets are small and oval shaped, and contain several types of granules, the enzyme cyclooxygenase, and a microtubule network that supports rapid shape change upon activation. The resting platelet membrane contains receptors (in an inactive state) and glycoproteins (GPs) that contribute to their rapid activation and clotting function. Activation of platelets occurs after injury to the blood vessel wall strips away the endothelial lining and exposes subendothelial ECM and collagen. Circulating von Willebrand factor (vWF) adheres to the ECM and attracts platelets, which adhere to the vWF via a membrane glycoprotein, GP Ib.[5] This initial binding event rapidly triggers additional platelet changes that promote clot formation, as illustrated in **Box 8.1** and **Figures 8.7, 8.8,** and **8.9.**

MODULATION OF CLOTTING AND ANTICLOTTING BY PRODUCTS OF ARACHIDONIC ACID METABOLISM

The injury-induced flip from production of *healthy endothelial cell* prostacyclin to the production of *activated platelet* thromboxane A_2 (TXA$_2$) is a key event in clot initiation. Focusing strictly on these two cell types, the pathway from arachidonic acid is shown in **Figure 8.10**. Platelet cyclooxygenase-1 (COX-1) is stimulated by platelet

---

BOX 8.1

Clot Formation: A Stepwise Process of Activation and Expansion

1. As a first step in clot formation, the platelet changes shape from oval to spiked, with cell extensions and membrane GPIb-IX-V that can strongly adhere to vWF/ECM and to other platelets, contributing to plug formation (**Figure 8.7**).

2. Platelets degranulate, releasing the contents of their α granules (including ADP, serotonin, and thrombin). These agents attract and activate additional platelets arriving in the region.

3. Platelet cyclooxygenase is activated, synthesizing TXA$_2$, a potent stimulator of vasoconstriction and platelet aggregation.

4. ADP, thrombin, and TXA$_2$ bind to platelet membrane G protein–coupled receptors, perpetuating and enhancing platelet activation.

5. A membrane integrin (also known as GP IIb/IIIa) changes to an active conformation and begins to bind to the damaged vessel wall and to other platelets through vWF and fibrinogen. This has a cross-linking effect that builds up the platelet plug.

6. Large granules containing factor V, platelet factor 4, vWF, and fibrinogen release their contents, supporting the initiation of the coagulation cascade.

7. Once platelet activation and aggregation have produced an initial plug, the platelet surface is used as the site of binding of coagulation cofactors and activation of coagulation cascade proteases. Strands of fibrin are generated and bind, further stabilizing the clot (**Figures 8.8** and **8.9**).

ADP, adenosine diphosphate; ECM, extracellular matrix; GP, glycoprotein; TXA$_2$, thromboxane A$_2$; vWF, von Willebrand factor.

(continued)

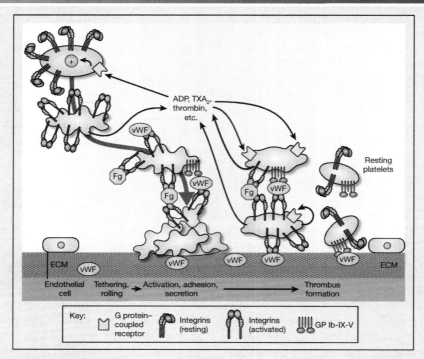

FIGURE 8.7 Clots form at sites of vascular damage, in particular when the endothelial cell layer is disrupted and the ECM is exposed. Formation of the primary clot depends on platelet adherence to ECM, mediated by glycoprotein Ib-IX-V (GP Ib-IX-V) and vWF; platelet activation and shape change, mediated by ADP, TXA_2, and thrombin binding to G protein–coupled receptors; and platelets binding to fibrinogen (Fg) and to each other by activated integrin $\alpha_{IIb}\beta_3$ (also known as glycoprotein IIb/IIIa). ADP, adenosine diphosphate; ECM, extracellular matrix; TXA_2, thromboxane A_2; vWF, von Willebrand factor.

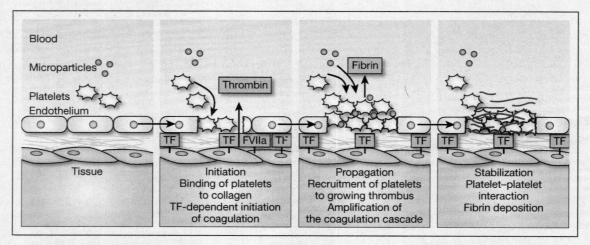

FIGURE 8.8 Summary of steps in clot formation. As platelets are undergoing activation and adhesion to the region of vascular damage, TF and factor VIIa begin to cleave factor X, which converts prothrombin to thrombin (factor IIa). Thrombin contributes to platelet activation as well as activating other clotting factors and breaking down fibrinogen into fibrin strands that begin cross-linking among the aggregated platelets. The platelet surfaces are the site of deposition and activity of clotting cascade proteins of the intrinsic and common pathways, providing local positive feedback to accelerate fibrin deposition and clot formation.
TF, tissue factor.

BOX 8.1 (*continued*)

Clot Formation: A Stepwise Process of Activation and Expansion

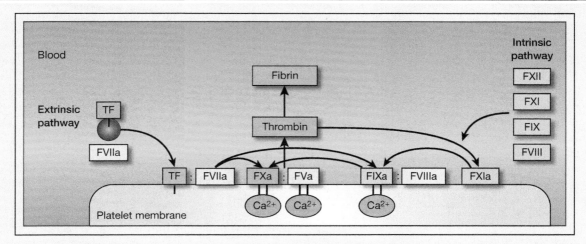

FIGURE 8.9 The coagulation cascade takes place on the membrane of activated platelets, where zymogens and cofactors are stabilized on the phospholipid surface by calcium ion binding. Proteases VIIa, IXa, and Xa are stabilized by TF, cofactor VIII, and cofactor V, respectively. Tissue damage initiates clotting by the extrinsic pathway, as shown on the left. Factor VIIa initiates the common pathway, generating factor Xa, which, stabilized by factor Va, functions as *prothrombin convertase*, cleaving prothrombin to release active thrombin. Factor VIIa also activates factor IX, adding intrinsic pathway reinforcement of the early extrinsic pathway activity. TF, tissue factor.

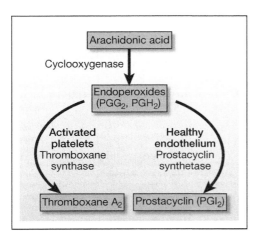

FIGURE 8.10 Two products of arachidonic acid metabolism, prostacyclin and thromboxane A_2, are particularly significant in the balance of anticoagulant and procoagulant forces in healthy and damaged vessels, respectively. Normal, healthy endothelial cells continuously produce and secrete prostacyclin. Prostacyclin reduces platelet adherence to endothelium and also promotes vasodilation. On the other hand, in regions of vascular damage and disrupted endothelium, prostacyclin production is inhibited. In these regions of injury, platelets adhere and become activated, producing thromboxane A_2, which promotes platelet activation, aggregation, and vasoconstriction. PGG_2, prostaglandin G_2; PGH_2, prostaglandin H_2; PGI_2, prostaglandin I_2 (also known as prostacyclin).

activation, and begins to produce TXA_2, which further stimulates platelet function and vasoconstriction. Aspirin is an irreversible inhibitor of COX-1, inhibiting clot formation for the remaining life span of the platelet exposed to it. For this reason, discontinuing aspirin use is often recommended before surgery. Other nonsteroidal anti inflammatory drugs (NSAIDs) reversibly inhibit COX-1 and do not have long-lasting effects on blood clotting.

 Thought Questions

7. What changes occur in a platelet as it transitions from the resting state to the fully activated state of participation in the platelet plug?

8. At what stage in platelet development does it acquire the enzyme cyclooxygenase?

COAGULATION CASCADE

The coagulation cascade occurs on the surface of platelets as a coordinated step-by-step activation of multiple circulating plasma protein factors leading to the deposition of insoluble fibrin on the platelet plug and transforming it into a stable clot. The two major categories of clotting proteins are the *zymogens* and the *cofactors*, and virtually all of these proteins are synthesized by the liver. The cofactors, tissue factor (TF) and factors V and VIII, provide a stable scaffold for zymogen activity, often on the surface of activated platelets (see **Figure 8.9**). The zymogens are protein precursors of proteolytic (protease) enzymes. At each step in the coagulation cascade, an activated protease cleaves an inactive zymogen, releasing the next activated protease. This sequence continues until the conversion of zymogen prothrombin to protease thrombin (factor IIa). Thrombin cleaves the large, soluble plasma protein fibrinogen, releasing small, sticky fibrin monomers that attach to the platelet surface and are cross-linked, forming a tightening web of fibrin strands in and around the platelet plug. A platelet/fibrin clot can be formed by activation of either the intrinsic or extrinsic pathway; however, clotting secondary to tissue damage with blood vessel breakage is initiated by the extrinsic pathway (**Figure 8.11**; see also **Figures 8.8** and **8.9**).

Tissue damage exposes TF, a transmembrane protein found in many cells in the blood vessel walls. Local damage signals also stimulate movement of TF to the membrane of activated platelets, and may recruit TF-bearing microparticles from the circulation. The initiating step in hemostasis occurs when TF (also known as thromboplastin) binds to activated factor VII on the surface of activated platelets, achieving the extrinsic pathway of coagulation (see **Figure 8.9**). In this first step, the TF/factor VIIa complex cleaves factor X. Simultaneously, the TF/factor VIIa complex cleaves factor IX. Factor IXa works with activated cofactor VIIIa to cleave and activate more factor X, strongly reinforcing the actions of factor VII. Factor Xa forms a complex with factor Va, held by calcium ions on the phospholipid surface of the platelets, making up the prothrombinase complex. This complex cleaves prothrombin, releasing thrombin (factor IIa), as seen in **Figures 8.9** and **8.11**.[6]

The small amount of thrombin activated during the initial activation event has many procoagulant activities.

- Thrombin binds to receptors on platelets, contributing to rapid platelet activation.
- Thrombin cleavage of fibrinogen begins to generate fibrin monomers in and around the platelet plug.
- Thrombin cleaves and activates cofactors V and VIII, increasing the local concentration of activated cofactors (see **Figure 8.9**).
- Thrombin cleaves and activates factor XI, leading to accelerated activation of factor IX. Factors IXa and VIIIa bind to the platelet surface to increase the rate of factor X activation. As a result, much of factor X activation during a prolonged injury-induced clotting event results from the factor IX pathway. This important contribution of the factor IX/factor VIII complex explains the severe bleeding events that occur in patients with hemophilia A (factor VIII deficiency) or hemophilia B (factor IX deficiency), as discussed later under Pediatric Considerations.
- Finally, thrombin's procoagulant activity includes activation of factor XIII, the agent that cross-links fibrin strands to tighten the clot. Thrombin also has anticoagulant activity, including binding to thrombomodulin, an endothelial cell membrane protein, to activate protein C, an anticoagulant protein.

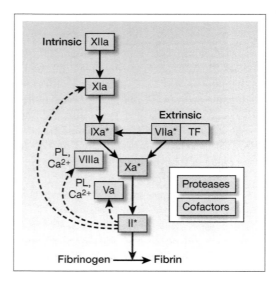

FIGURE 8.11 As the coagulation cascade accelerates, thrombin (factor IIa) provides positive feedback by activating cofactors V and VIII, and factor XI of the intrinsic pathway, further accelerating fibrin deposition. Asterisks indicate clotting factors II, VII, IX, and X that are subjected to carboxylation during synthesis in the liver. This posttranslational modification is blocked by the drug warfarin, which reduces the effectiveness of the clotting cascade.
Ca^{2+}, calcium ion; PL, phospholipid; TF, tissue factor.

The intrinsic pathway is a cascade initiated by factor XII, also known as contact factor and Hageman factor. Factor XII is a protease activated by contact with clot-promoting surfaces, and its properties have been studied in vitro to a much greater extent than in vivo. Once activated by contact with negative charges (clay or glass beads in vitro), factor XII cleaves and activates factor XI and high-molecular-weight kininogen. In this way, contact activation stimulates both clotting and inflammatory responses through the kinin pathway of inflammation. Interestingly, individuals born with factor XII deficiency do not develop excessive bleeding, so it seems that this pathway contributes to clotting more through its later proteases, principally factor IX. However, the intrinsic pathway is very likely to contribute to pathological clotting in the context of blood stasis and endothelial injury, as described later.

LABORATORY ASSESSMENT OF CLOTTING

Laboratory evaluation of the clotting process takes anticoagulated blood, isolates the plasma, and separates it into two aliquots. The first aliquot is exposed to TF and calcium, and the time to clot formation is reported as the prothrombin time (PT). This method tests the extrinsic and common coagulation pathways (**Figure 8.12**). Standardization of the PT is usually reported as the international normalized ratio [INR], which expresses the patient's PT as a ratio of a laboratory standard sample. Thus, a normal PT should have an INR of 1.0. This allows cross-lab comparisons and also guides dosing for the anticoagulant drug warfarin. The second aliquot is exposed to phospholipid, an activator, and calcium, and the time to clot formation is reported as the (activated) partial thromboplastin time (aPTT). This method tests the intrinsic and common coagulation pathways (**Figure 8.13**).

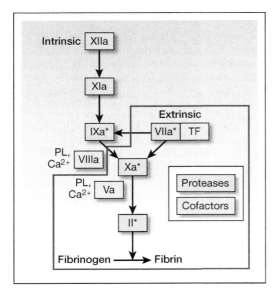

FIGURE 8.12 In the PT laboratory test, tissue factor is added to a blood sample and time to clot formation is measured. This test primarily evaluates the extrinsic pathway and normally takes 10 to 14 seconds. In addition to assessing the extrinsic pathway, the PT and the related INR are used to assess degree of anticoagulation in people taking the drug warfarin. Asterisks indicate clotting factors II, VII, IX, and X that are subjected to carboxylation during synthesis in the liver. This posttranslational modification is blocked by the drug warfarin, which reduces the effectiveness of the clotting cascade.
Ca^{2+}, calcium ion; INR, international normalized ratio; PL, phospholipid; PT, prothrombin time; TF, tissue factor.

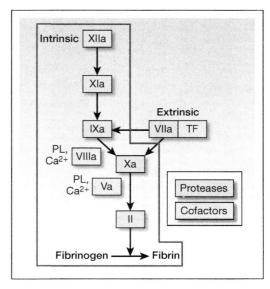

FIGURE 8.13 In the PTT laboratory test, a source of negative charges is added to a blood sample and time to clot formation is measured. This test primarily evaluates the intrinsic and common pathways and normally takes 32 to 45 seconds. The protease clotting factors, XII, XI, IX, VII, X, and II are inactivated by antithrombin in a reaction that is accelerated by exogenous heparin. The PTT can be prolonged in disease states like hemophilia, disseminated intravascular coagulation, and liver failure, and in people taking the drug heparin.
Ca^{2+}, calcium ion; PL, phospholipid; PTT, partial thromboplastin time; TF, tissue factor.

CONTROL OF THE CLOTTING PROCESS

Clot formation must be tightly regulated and restricted to regions of tissue injury with vessel breakage. The consequences of excessive clotting or clotting in the absence of tissue injury are severe, such as local tissue ischemia and infarction. Clots that dislodge from their formation sites are called emboli and travel through the circulation to other organs, where they lodge and cause ischemia and infarction. Endogenous anticoagulation mechanisms limit these risks. These mechanisms are similar to the procoagulant forces in having some factors fixed in tissue (generally associated with endothelial cells) and some factors that circulate in plasma, often in an inactive form.

Endothelial Influences on Clotting

All blood vessels are lined with a layer of endothelial cells. As such, subendothelial collagen is shielded and unable to bind vWF and to attract platelets to initiate clot formation. Under normal, healthy conditions, endothelial cells have the following properties that inhibit platelet adhesion and activation (**Figure 8.14**).

- Endothelial cells constitutively express nitric oxide synthase (NOS) and release nitric oxide (NO), a potent inhibitor of platelet activation and aggregation.

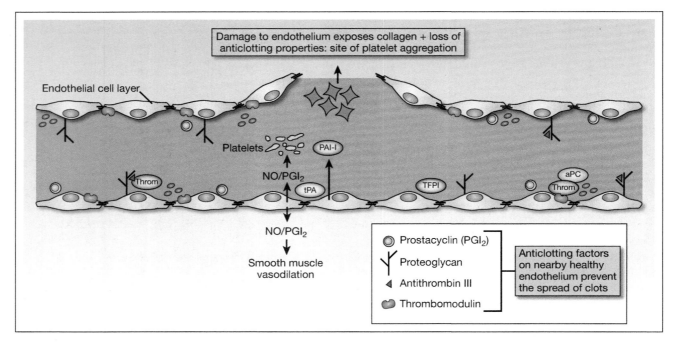

FIGURE 8.14 Healthy endothelial cells in an intact blood vessel have several anticoagulant properties. They secrete prostacyclin and nitric oxide (NO) into the blood vessel and to the underlying smooth muscle layer. Both agents inhibit platelet activation and promote vasodilation, maintaining a steady stream of blood flow that reduces blood pooling and intrinsic pathway activation. Intact endothelial cells display the membrane proteins proteoglycans—heparin-like molecules that bind antithrombin, and thrombomodulin, which binds thrombin (Throm). Antithrombin inactivates thrombin and many other coagulation proteases in the vicinity. The thrombin/thrombomodulin complex activates protein C to cleave cofactors V and VIII. They secrete TFPI and tPA, inhibiting clot formation and promoting clot lysis. They express adenine diphosphatase (ADPase), which splits and inactivates ADP.

ADP, adenosine diphosphate; aPC, activated protein C; PAI-1, plasminogen activator inhibitor-1; TFPI, tissue factor pathway inhibitor; tPA; tissue plasminogen activator.

- Endothelial cells also tonically metabolize arachidonic acid to prostacyclin, a potent local inhibitor of platelet activation and aggregation.
- Endothelial cell membranes express the enzyme adenosine diphosphatase (ADPase), which breaks down adenosine diphosphate (ADP) released from granules of activated platelets.

Endothelial cells also contribute to inhibition of coagulation cascade proteases and cofactors.

- Heparin-like molecules (heparin proteoglycans) projecting from endothelial cell membranes can bind and activate circulating antithrombin III (AT-III), which in turn inhibits thrombin and factors IXa, Xa, XIa, and XIIa.
- Endothelial cell membranes display thrombomodulin, a cofactor that binds thrombin and activates protein C. Activated protein C (aPC) binds to protein S and inactivates the coagulation cascade cofactors VIII and V.
- Endothelial cells synthesize and bind TF pathway inhibitor that binds to factor Xa and inhibits the TF/factor VII complex.

Plasmin and the Fibrinolytic Process

From the very beginning of the activation of the coagulation cascade, preparations are in place for the counteracting system of fibrinolysis. The fibrinolytic pathway promotes dissolution of a clot after injuries heal and also prevents extension of clotting in regions adjacent to an injury (see **Figure 8.15**). Fibrinolysis is triggered by tissue plasminogen activator (tPA) and urokinase-type plasminogen activator (uPA), enzymes that convert the precursor plasminogen into plasmin. Plasmin degrades fibrin clots and releases fibrin degeneration products that are unable to polymerize. The

D-dimer is a laboratory test used as a marker of thrombotic states; it measures levels of one of the fibrin degradation products that result from plasmin action on cross-linked fibrin. Active plasmin in the circulation is inhibited by binding to α_2-antiplasmin. During the early response to tissue injury, plasminogen activator inhibitor-1 (PAI-1) is released by endothelial cells, suppressing plasminogen activation. As vessel healing occurs, tPA is released, cleaving the plasminogen trapped in the clot, and accelerating the fibrinolytic process (**Figures 8.15** and **8.16**).

Cessation of Clotting Activity

To limit excessive spread of clot formation, several mechanisms inactivate the clotting proteases and cofactors (**Figure 8.17**). First, circulating activated

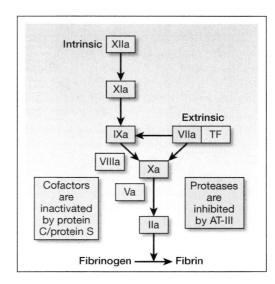

FIGURE 8.17 Inhibition of clotting is critical once a clot has formed, to prevent extension of this process to adjacent healthy regions of vasculature. Two main systems are in place to inhibit either the coagulation proteases (in yellow) or the cofactors (in blue). The circulating mediator AT-III binds to endothelial cell proteoglycans and inactivates proteases. Protein C and protein S work together to cleave and inactivate proteins VIII and V, the required cofactors for factors IX and X.
AT-III, antithrombin III; TF, tissue factor.

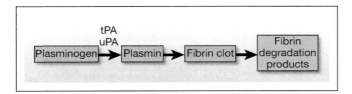

FIGURE 8.15 The plasmin system is responsible for breaking down clots when healing has occurred. tPA and uPA cleave the protein plasminogen in the circulation and bound in the clot to release plasmin. Plasmin is an enzyme that breaks down cross-linked fibrin within the clot, dissolving the clot and releasing fibrin breakdown products such as D-dimer.
tPA, tissue plasminogen activator; uPA, urokinase-type plasminogen activator.

clotting factors are taken up by the liver and are degraded. Second, antithrombin (AT, also known as AT-III) inactivates the major (activated) coagulation proteases: XII, XI, IX, VII, X, and II. AT activity is potentiated by binding to endothelial cell membrane heparin proteoglycans, and is further potentiated by binding to exogenous heparin given to manage patients with pathological thrombus formation. Third, the protein C/protein S system cleaves and inactivates cofactors VIII and V. Cleavage of protein C is greatly accelerated by thrombin binding to endothelial thrombomodulin. This is one way in which the spread of a clot is limited to regions of damaged endothelium—spread to adjacent healthy endothelium is limited by the presence of thrombomodulin to bind thrombin and activate protein C.

Modulation of Clotting Activity by Anticoagulant Drugs

Factors II, VII, IX, and X require calcium ion (Ca^{2+}) binding to exert their protease activity. At the molecular level, this requirement is due to a post-translational modification during hepatic synthesis of these factors, as well as proteins C and S. Near the amino terminal of the protein chains of these factors, there are nine to 13 glutamate residues. The

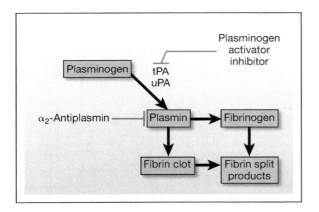

FIGURE 8.16 The plasmin system is regulated by the plasma protein α_2-antiplasmin, which blocks the action of circulating plasmin, and plasminogen activator inhibitor-1 (PAI-1), produced by endothelial cells and other cell types. PAI-1 increases in response to inflammatory mediators, including cytokines, providing one link between inflammation and hypercoagulable states. Red bars indicate inhibition, while black arrows indicate sequential reactions.
tPA, tissue plasminogen activator; uPA, urokinase-type plasminogen activator.

enzyme carboxylase adds a second carboxyl group to each of the glutamates, resulting in a Gla region (carboxylated glutamate) with two anionic prongs for each glutamate (**Figure 8.18**). The double negative charges provide the binding site for extracellular calcium to bind to the clotting factor and to the negatively charged membrane phospholipids on the surface of activated platelets. Thus, calcium functions as a *glue*, securing the proteases to the platelet membrane during their successive cleavage and activation reactions (see **Figure 8.9**).

Vitamin K is a required cofactor that is oxidized in this carboxylation reaction. Reduction of oxidized vitamin K is catalyzed by the enzyme vitamin K epoxide reductase complex (VKORC1) in a reaction that is inhibited by warfarin. There is substantial genetic heterogeneity in the *VKORC1* gene, as well as in the gene for CYP2C9, responsible for hepatic metabolism of warfarin, such that effective drug dosing can be very variable. For this reason, as well as the dietary restrictions that limit warfarin treatment, newer anticoagulants have been developed that are more narrowly focused on one clotting factor.

Thrombin (factor II) activation is central to clotting, and inhibiting thrombin activity greatly slows clotting.

Factor X, in conjunction with factor V, phospholipids, and calcium, makes up prothrombinase—the common pathway step that releases active thrombin. Factors X and II are targeted by the direct oral anticoagulants. Drugs such as rivaroxaban and related compounds directly inhibit active factor X, while dabigatran directly inhibits thrombin. As mentioned earlier, aspirin inhibits COX-1, reducing platelet thromboxane production and suppressing platelet activation. Drugs such as clopidogrel and prasugrel inhibit platelet activation by blocking the receptor responsive to ADP released from platelet granules during activation and aggregation.

Thought Questions

9. Which interactions of the clotting cascade mediators provide positive feedback to accelerate clotting?

10. Which interactions of the clotting cascade mediators provide negative feedback to limit clotting?

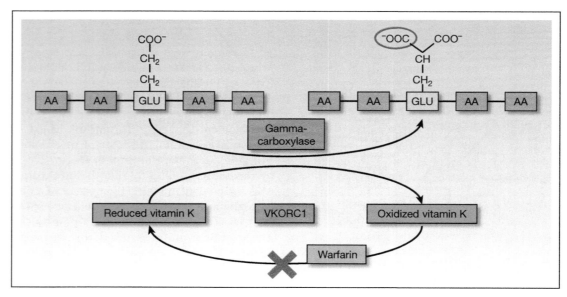

FIGURE 8.18 The AA sequences of factors II, VII, IX, and X include an N-terminal region enriched in glutamate (GLU) residues. The glutamate carboxyl group is normally deprotonated and therefore negatively charged at physiological pH. The liver enzyme gamma-carboxylase adds one more carboxyl group (red oval) to these glutamates in a post-translational reaction. This reaction adds a negatively charged extension to the protein, facilitating binding to platelet surfaces by calcium once the precursor zymogen has been activated. Vitamin K serves as a cofactor in this reaction, transitioning from the reduced to the oxidized state. The enzyme VKORC1 regenerates reduced vitamin K and is inhibited by the anticoagulant drug warfarin.

AA, amino acid; VKORC1, vitamin K epoxide reductase complex.

THROMBOEMBOLIC STATES

Three major factors contribute to abnormal blood clotting in the absence of frank vascular breaks: endothelial injury, venous stasis, and hypercoagulability. Together, these variables comprise the *Virchow triad*, postulated by Dr. Rudolf Virchow in the mid-19th century. Excessive clotting contributes strongly to the global burden of disease. The World Health Organization (WHO) calculates that the top causes of death worldwide are ischemic heart disease and strokes. These disorders account for 15 million deaths annually, representing more than one fourth of all deaths internationally.[7] Understanding patient risk factors and identifying optimal management strategies is a clinical imperative to reduce these numbers.

Endothelial injury can be a catalyst for intravascular clot formation, particularly in the arterial circulation (**Figure 8.19**). The most common context for thrombus formation is fissuring or rupture of an atherosclerotic plaque. Within regions of atherosclerosis, endothelial cells lose their normal antithrombotic properties and, instead, develop prothrombotic characteristics. In addition, the fibrous cap of an atherosclerotic plaque is prone to fissure or rupture, exposing the inflammatory plaque core and its procoagulant components, including TF. These mechanisms may lead to acute myocardial infarction.

Venous stasis and other states of low blood flow promote pooling of the blood, prolonged contact with endothelium that may reduce some of its anticlotting properties, and activation of the intrinsic clotting pathway (see **Figure 8.17**). Clinically, this phenomenon can occur acutely or chronically. For example, people who are immobile during a long trip (e.g., long airplane flight) or patients with reduced mobility secondary to an orthopedic procedure or prolonged illness are at risk for venous stasis and blood clots, such as **deep vein thrombosis** (DVT) or an associated **venous thromboembolism** (VTE). VTEs can break off from their formation site and travel through the right side of the heart into the pulmonary vasculature to cause a **pulmonary embolism** (PE) or multiple pulmonary emboli. In the setting of chronic illness, patients with atrial fibrillation lack effective atrial contractions, so blood pools in the atria. This promotes clot formation, most commonly in the left atrial appendage, producing clots that can travel to the cerebrovascular system, causing transient ischemic attack or stroke/cerebrovascular attack. To summarize, endothelial injury is most characteristic of thrombi that form in arteries, while blood stasis is most characteristic of thrombi that form in veins, particularly those draining the legs, and in the atria of patients with atrial fibrillation.

The final component of the Virchow triad is hypercoagulability. Many genetic (e.g., factor V Leiden [FVL]) and autoimmune (e.g., antiphospholipid syndrome [APS]) conditions predispose to hypercoagulability,

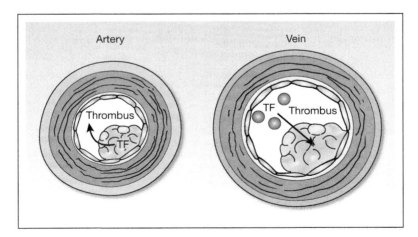

FIGURE 8.19 Arterial thrombi often form at the sites of atherosclerotic plaque. Endothelial cells are diseased in the vicinity of the plaque, losing their normal antithrombotic properties and becoming sites of platelet aggregation and clot formation. In a catastrophic plaque rupture situation, the cap of the plaque fissures, exposing large amounts of TF and other procoagulant substances. This can quickly lead to a massive thrombus that completely occludes the vessel and causes a myocardial infarction or stroke. Venous thrombi are often formed in areas of blood stasis, such as the deep veins of the legs. Circulating TF may accumulate here, along with surface activation of intrinsic pathway proteins, to produce clots. These clots may break off and travel through the right side of the heart to the lungs, forming pulmonary emboli.
TF, tissue factor.

but it is likely that the most common population-wide cause is chronic inflammation. Hypercoagulability is associated with metabolic syndrome, an obesity-related pathological state comprising hypertension, truncal obesity, dyslipidemia, and insulin resistance. The syndrome is highly prevalent, particularly in the United States, and is associated with increased levels of proinflammatory markers.[8] Individuals with chronic inflammatory conditions such as metabolic syndrome and rheumatoid arthritis, or acute inflammatory conditions such as influenza or pneumonia, are prone to myocardial infarctions. In these states, any underlying endothelial dysfunction is heightened by inflammatory mediators, and clots may form more easily owing to elevated levels of procoagulant factors, including PAI-1.

Other examples of hypercoagulable states include pregnancy and use of oral contraceptives or hormone replacement therapy. Estrogens increase liver synthesis of clotting proteins and decrease synthesis of protein S and AT-III, thus promoting clot formation. Patients with malignancies are also hypercoagulable and at risk for blood clots, most often VTEs and PEs, apparently because tumor cells have an innately increased ability to activate the coagulation cascade.

SPECIFIC DISORDERS OF HYPERCOAGULATION

Factor V Leiden and Other Genetic Disorders

Factor V Leiden (FVL) results from an autosomal dominant mutation of the human *F5* gene with incomplete penetrance. FVL most commonly affects ethnic Caucasian Europeans with an estimated 3.2% to 6% prevalence in the United States.[9] FVL is produced by a single base missense mutation in which guanine (G) is replaced by adenine (A), resulting in an amino

acid substitution of glutamine for arginine at position 506 (**Figure 8.20**). This position is the natural site at which aPC cleaves and inactivates factor V, and the mutation greatly slows the action of aPC, creating aPC resistance. The resulting prolongation of the active form of factor V increases the duration of prothrombinase activity, causing hypercoagulability.[9] Between 2% and 15% of Caucasians are heterozygotes for this trait, which carries a ten-fold increased risk of thromboembolic events, while homozygous individuals have a 30- to 140-fold increased risk of a hypercoagulable-related diagnosis. Healthy young patients with an unexplained DVT or PE should be screened for FVL.

Additional genetic disorders associated with hypercoagulability and increased risk of venous thromboses include a prothrombin G20210A mutation and congenital deficiencies of AT, protein C, or protein S. Any of these states may present with DVT or PE, particularly after known procoagulant exposures such as immobility, pregnancy, or use of oral contraceptives.

Antiphospholipid Syndrome

Antiphospholipid syndrome (APS) is an autoimmune condition that results in increased clotting. APS can occur secondary to another autoimmune disease, most commonly SLE; the remaining cases are primary APS, and the patients have no other autoimmune diagnosis. Patients with APS have elevated levels of antibodies against the phospholipid-binding plasma proteins cardiolipin or β_2-glycoprotein I, or both, in addition to lupus anticoagulant antibodies. The exact mechanism by which the antibodies promote clotting is not understood. Clinically, APS is suspected in patients with recurrent thromboembolic events and in women

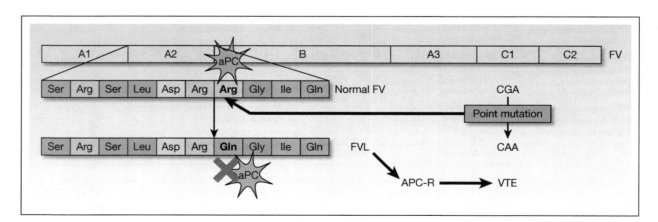

FIGURE 8.20 FVL production results from a missense mutation in the FV gene that results in an arginine (Arg) to glutamine (Gln) substitution at amino acid position 506. This is the site where factor V is cleaved and inactivated by protein C. The mutation makes FVL resistant to protein C's action (conferring aPC-R), promoting a hypercoagulable state and increasing risk of VTE.

aPC, activated protein C; aPC-R, activated protein C resistance; FV, factor V; FVL, factor V Leiden; VTE, venous thromboembolism.

with repeated pregnancy losses or complications, with no other identifiable cause.

Patients with APS can present with thrombi in the coronary arteries, cerebrovascular system, pulmonary system, extremities, or other tissue/organ locations (e.g., kidney, eye, liver). Patients with one or more late-term (>10 weeks of gestation) spontaneous abortions, multiple consecutive spontaneous abortions (<10 weeks of gestation), or premature births (<34 weeks of gestation) secondary to eclampsia/preeclampsia should be tested for APS. As with FVL evaluation, providers should consider laboratory screening for APS in patients (male younger than 55 years; female younger than 65 years) with a myocardial infarction, PE, or stroke without any risk factors or comorbid conditions.

STATES OF EXCESS BLEEDING

Dysfunction of hemostasis can produce signs and symptoms of excess bleeding, ranging from superficial **petechiae** to large **ecchymoses**, deep **hematomas**, and **hemarthroses** (bleeding into the joints). These disorders can be present from birth as a result of genetic mutations, or can be secondary to acquired, often immune-mediated, disorders. Finally, excess bleeding can result from abnormalities of platelets, clotting factors, or both.

THROMBOCYTOPENIA

Thrombocytopenia is classified as a blood platelet level lower than the normal 150,000 to 450,000 cells/µL. As the platelet count decreases, there is increased bleeding after trauma, and at extremely low platelet levels (<5,000 platelets/µL) spontaneous superficial bleeding may be evident in the form of petechiae and mucosal bleeding. Thrombocytopenia arises from three general mechanisms: decreased bone marrow production, increased sequestration, or increased destruction. Decreased bone marrow production is not usually specific to platelets; rather, it occurs in the context of broader bone marrow dysfunction or suppression, such as aplastic anemia, chemotherapy medications, or vitamin B12 deficiency. Increased splenic sequestration of platelets often occurs secondary to liver failure with portal hypertension and splenomegaly.

Increased platelet destruction due to immune mechanisms, although rare, can produce the greatest degree of thrombocytopenia. As in hemolytic anemia, increased platelet destruction stimulates the bone marrow to release young platelets that are larger than normal, with reticular staining and, importantly, greater clot-promoting activity. Acute-onset **immune thrombocytopenic purpura** (ITP) can occur spontaneously or after an infection and is more common in children. The symptoms associated with ITP can range in severity according to the degree of thrombocytopenia, from cutaneous findings of petechiae and purpura to the most serious complication of intracerebral hemorrhage (highest risk if platelets <10 × 10^6/µL). Pediatric postinfectious ITP often resolves without treatment.

Unlike self-limiting acute ITP, chronic ITP is a classic autoimmune illness. There is no associated prodrome in chronic ITP, and patients usually present because of skin manifestations (petechiae/purpura) or excess bleeding (gingival, menorrhagia, or epistaxis). Antibodies are produced against platelet membrane GPs or human leukocyte antigen (HLA) proteins. Antibody binding targets the platelets for destruction by macrophages in the spleen and the liver. In contrast to patients with acute ITP, which rarely requires treatment, those affected with chronic ITP require oral or intravenous corticosteroids (first-line therapy) or intravenous immunoglobulin G (IVIG) infusions.

Many drugs are associated with platelet destruction, and management is straightforward: cessation of the drug effectively ends the episode. **Heparin-induced thrombocytopenia** is the exception to this principle, because it predisposes patients to thrombotic events, as opposed to excess bleeding (**Box 8.2**).

VON WILLEBRAND DISEASE

Von Willebrand disease (vWD) is the most common inherited bleeding disorder, occurring in up to 2% of the population.[10] It is a heterogeneous disease that occurs because of either a dysfunction or a lack of the vWF protein. Its six subtypes (types 1, 2A, 2B, 2M, 2N, and 3) are classified according to quantitative (type 1 and type 3) or qualitative (all type 2) defects in vWF. This section focuses on type 1, which represents >70% of all cases and is an autosomal dominant mutation of the *VWF* gene with incomplete penetrance. Mutations can lead to more rapid clearance of vWF from the circulation or decreased secretion of vWF, or both.

vWF is a large, multimeric glycoprotein that is coded by chromosome 12 and is similar in size to factor VIII. It is made and released from tubular storage compartments within platelets, megakaryocytes, and endothelial cells. Secretion of vWF is stimulated by factors such as thrombin, fibrin, histamine, and various cytokines. vWF circulates bound to factor VIII, and the half-life of factor VIII in the circulation is extended by this transport. Synthetic DDAVP (desmopressin acetate) has been shown to stimulate release of vWF (and factor VIII) into circulation.

vWF has two major roles—facilitating platelet aggregation at sites of vascular injury, and helping to bind factor VIII to the platelet plug, which is an important step in the production of thrombin, fibrin, and eventual clot formation. In type 1 vWD, there is a 20% to

---

BOX 8.2

Heparin-Induced Thrombocytopenia

- HIT results from development of IgG antibodies to platelet membrane complexes of heparin bound to platelet factor 4. It occurs within 5 to 10 days of heparin exposure and can carry life-threatening complications.

- The antibodies bind to the platelet surface, stimulating platelet activation. With this activation, there is an abundant release of procoagulants and consumption of platelets; thus, thrombocytopenia ensues.

- Although it may seem counterintuitive that thrombocytopenia increases thrombosis risk, with HIT there is an increased production of thrombin as well as stimulation of inflammatory mediators. This cascade causes endothelial

injury and increases the risk of large-vessel arterial or venous thromboses.

- Findings in affected individuals include mild to moderate thrombocytopenia (platelets rarely <15 × 10^9/L), but the hallmark test is either an immunoassay for the antibodies to the heparin–platelet factor 4 complex or a functional study looking at platelet aggregation when exposed to heparin.

- Management of patients with HIT includes the discontinuation of all heparin-based products and the use of other anticoagulants for treatment and prophylaxis against thrombotic events. With few exceptions, lifelong avoidance of all heparin-containing products is required.

HIT, heparin-induced thrombocytopenia.

50% decrease in circulating vWF, resulting in failure of platelets to properly agglutinate. This is accompanied by decreased factor VIII levels; thus, bleeding time is increased and clot formation is inadequate.

The most common clinical manifestation of type 1 vWD is mucosal bleeding, and epistaxis occurs in 60% of patients. Additionally, affected individuals report hematomas following mild to moderate trauma, menorrhagia, excessive postpartum bleeding, gingival bleeding, and occasional GI bleeding. Those with type 1 vWD also experience excessive bleeding after procedures such as dental extractions and invasive surgeries.

Type 1 vWD can be difficult to detect with conventional hematology laboratory studies. Routine coagulation studies—including PT and aPTT—are not diagnostic, although some patients have increased aPTT values. Levels of vWF and factor VIII are decreased. Functional activity of vWF is assessed by measuring platelet agglutination in the presence of the patient's serum and the chemical ristocetin, which normally stimulates platelet binding to vWF. This test is referred to as vWF:RCo (ristocetin cofactor) analysis. Because vWD is often diagnosed in childhood, manifestations in pediatric patients are discussed separately (see Pediatric Considerations, later in this chapter).

The treatment of choice for type 1 vWD patients is DDAVP, which is a synthetic antidiuretic hormone that works on type 2 vasopressin receptors to increase secretion of vWF and factor VIII. This medication can be used prophylactically before surgical procedures or dental extractions. Patients on this medication also need to be monitored for side effects, particularly dilutional hyponatremia, because of DDAVP's antidiuretic properties.

COAGULATION CASCADE–ASSOCIATED DISORDERS

Excessive bleeding can be due to lack or dysfunction of the proteases and coagulation cofactors. This section focuses on two disorders that are associated with coagulation cascade abnormalities: hemophilia A and cirrhosis.

Hemophilia A

Hemophilia A, or factor VIII deficiency, is an X-linked recessive genetic disease that occurs in approximately one out of every 5,000 to 7,000 live male births. According to the Centers for Disease Control and Prevention, it is four times more common than hemophilia B (factor IX deficiency) and affects approximately 20,000 individuals in the United States and 400,000 worldwide.[11] Hemophilia A is often considered an inherited disorder; however, 30% of cases arise from a spontaneous mutation of the *F8* gene, and thus are not associated with a family history of the disorder.

In hemophilia A, a mutation in the *F8* gene results in a reduced amount of the active factor VIII protein, either because of an improperly functioning protein or an overall decrease in its production. Factor VIII is produced in the liver and in the reticuloendothelial cells throughout the circulation. Once factor VIII enters the circulation, it binds to vWF via noncovalent bonds, an interaction that stabilizes factor VIII and prevents degradation. The half-life of factor VIII without vWF is 2 hours, but this increases to 12 hours when the two are bound. As previously described, the clotting cascade is usually initiated by the extrinsic pathway in which factor VII binds to TF to activate factors X and IX (see **Figure 8.12**). Soon after this initial event, TF pathway inhibitor blocks additional activation by this pathway. However, the initial step activates thrombin, which proceeds to activate factor XI. Factor XI then activates factor IX, which, in the presence of factor VIII, is able to continue activating factor X. It is clear that this reinforcement of clotting by these final steps of the intrinsic pathway is critical for normal bleeding cessation, since factor VIII deficiency produces extensive deep tissue bleeding.

In families with a history of the disorder, factor VIII deficiency has an X-linked inheritance pattern in which all sons of an affected father are unaffected and all daughters are carriers. The male offspring of female carriers have a 50% chance of inheriting the disease, whereas the daughters in that lineage have a 50% chance of being carriers. Although it is rare, girls can be diagnosed with either type of hemophilia A. For this to occur, the affected daughter would have a hemophiliac father and a mother who is a carrier for the trait. Hemophilia A can also affect girls with other X-chromosome abnormalities, such as Turner syndrome and X chromosomal mosaicism. This information is important because genetic testing (via direct gene sequencing) is used for females with close or remote family histories of hemophilia (which can skip generations) or those who are known trait carriers.

Hemophilia A patients are categorized into three groups according to disease severity. This designation is based on serum levels of factor VIII—severe (<1%), moderate (1% to 5%), and mild (6% to 30%)—and those with severe hemophilia A represent more than half of all cases. Patients with severe hemophilia A have a high risk of joint-related hemarthroses, spontaneous hematuria, mucous membrane bleeding, and hematoma formation that are managed with clotting factor replacement. In addition, these patients can have intracranial bleeding, either spontaneously or as a result of minor trauma, which is the leading cause of death for hemophiliacs. Patients with moderate disease can have hemorrhages after surgery or trauma, but spontaneous bleeding episodes occur only occasionally. Patients with a mild form of the disease usually go undiagnosed unless there is significant bleeding after a trauma or invasive surgical procedures. Hemophilia A patients usually have a prolonged aPTT with normal PT and thrombin clotting time. However, diagnosis and categorization are based on factor VIII assays.

Severe hemophilia A has traditionally been managed with intravenous infusions of virus-inactivated purified factor VIII or recombinant factor VIII. This approach sometimes results in patients developing neutralizing antibodies to the factor. Newer treatments aim to prolong the half-life and reduce antigenicity of factor VIII analogues, to augment procoagulant activity with agents that block TF pathway inhibitor, or to replace the defective gene with gene therapy. Many of these treatments are still being studied for efficacy and safety.

Cirrhosis-Related Coagulation Dysfunction

As the site of synthesis of most of the clotting factors, the liver has an integral role in the body's ability to maintain hemostasis. Hepatocytes constitutively synthesize and secrete not only most of the coagulation factors, but also many proteins associated with anticoagulation, including protein C, protein S, and AT-III; therefore, patients with chronic cirrhotic liver disease are prone to **cirrhosis-related coagulation dysfunction**. More than half of patients with chronic liver failure have thrombocytopenia (platelets <150,000/ µL) due to lack of liver thrombopoietin production. Patients with portal hypertension develop splenomegaly, accelerating platelet destruction by splenic macrophages. Patients with cirrhosis have decreased levels of all clotting factors synthesized by the liver: fibrinogen; factors II, V, VII, VIII, IX, X, XI, XII, and XIII; and proteins C and S. Deficiencies of bile salt production impair gut absorption of fat-soluble vitamins, including vitamin K, further exacerbating the bleeding tendency.

The liver is also responsible for production of most of the fibrinolytic and plasmin-related proteins except tPA and PAI-1; thus, affected individuals have a decrease in all of the pro- and antifibrinolytic-related proteins. tPA, however, is elevated because of an increase in its endothelial cell secretion and a decrease in its clearance by the liver.

Patients with liver failure may manifest a variety of bleeding-related complications. The sequelae of hemostatic derangement range from mucosal bleeding, menorrhagia, and excessive bruising to GI bleeding secondary to peptic ulcer disease; however, spontaneous bleeding episodes are rare. The recommended treatment modalities for hemostatic-related bleeding in cirrhotic patients are based on the cause. For example, minor bruising, purpura, and gingival bleeding are usually self-limiting while fibrinolysis inhibitors, such as tranexamic acid, can be used for significant epistaxis. If cirrhotic patients do present with severe bleeding and thrombocytopenia (platelets <50,000/µL), platelet transfusions should be administered as would be done for any patient regardless of liver function status. In mild to moderate liver disease, PT and INR are prolonged, and as the disease progresses, aPTT may also be prolonged.

 Thought Questions

11. How does the process of pathological clot formation in arteries differ from clot formation in veins?

12. When a child is born with vWD, what precautions may parents need to take to reduce the child's risk of bleeding?

Stephanie L. Carper

Children are more likely than adults to present with certain blood and clotting disorders, and management considerations can vary greatly from those of the adult patient. RBC indices fluctuate throughout childhood and adolescence, reflecting changes in physiological demands as children age. At birth, neutrophil levels are high, declining quickly to normal levels by 1 month. The white blood cell differential count shows a distinctive pattern of relatively high lymphocyte numbers and percentage from the first month through 2 years of life, after which values transition to normal adult levels (see Bridge to Clinical Practice at the end of this chapter). Platelets and clotting indices show smaller differences from birth through childhood.

DEVELOPMENTAL CHANGES IN RED BLOOD CELL MEASURES

The red cell count, hematocrit, and hemoglobin are all highest at birth, decreasing over the first 12 weeks of life. At birth, the neonate transitions from a relatively hypoxic uterine environment, with a Pao_2 of approximately 45 mm Hg, to a relatively oxygen-rich environment, with a Pao_2 of approximately 90 to 100 mm Hg. During prenatal development in hypoxic conditions, erythropoietin is released from the kidneys, resulting in an overall increased state of erythropoiesis in the fetus to ensure adequate oxygen delivery to the tissues while in utero. A term neonate's RBC volume is composed mostly of RBCs containing fetal hemoglobin (HbF). Fetal RBCs have a life span of approximately 45 to 70 days, after which they are degraded. During fetal development, RBC precursors switch from the production of γ chains to β chains, transitioning to HbA synthesis ($\alpha_2\beta_2$). At term birth, HbF represents 70% to 80% of hemoglobin, with HbA representing 25% to 30%. As breakdown of fetal RBCs continues after birth, the hemoglobin level drops to its nadir at about 60 days of life, usually reaching values of approximately 11.5 g/dL.

During this period, from birth to physiological nadir, erythropoiesis is relatively low. There is little stimulation to the bone marrow to increase RBC production, as the surplus of fetal RBCs is able to adequately oxygenate the tissues. However, as these fetal RBCs begin to reach the end of their life span, the neonate's hemoglobin level starts to decline. Once the hemoglobin reaches values of approximately 10 mg/dL, erythropoietin is released from the kidneys, stimulating bone marrow

erythropoiesis. As erythropoiesis starts to increase the red cell count again, the hemoglobin level also increases.

Other factors in addition to reduced erythropoiesis influence the decrease in neonatal red cell counts over the first few months of life. During the first 2 months of life, the neonate is undergoing profound growth at more rapid rates than at any other time in infancy. Rapid growth with accompanying increases in plasma volume, in conjunction with relative bone marrow suppression in the first 2 months, produces a clinical picture of decreasing red cell counts in the neonate. Additionally, the RBCs are macrocytic at birth. The MCV at birth is approximately 110 fL, decreasing to normal adult values of approximately 80 to 100 fL by 3 to 6 months of age. In premature infants, the physiological nadir for hemoglobin occurs sooner, between 6 and 8 weeks of age, and achieves a lower level. Premature infants can reach physiological nadirs of 6.5 to 9.0 mg/dL.[12] These changes are summarized in Figure 8.21.

IRON-DEFICIENCY ANEMIA

Iron-deficiency anemia is the most common RBC disorder of childhood and the most commonly encountered anemia in pediatric populations.[13] Periods of rapid growth increase demand for iron as well as other critical nutrients and elevate the risk of this disorder. Children are most vulnerable to development of iron-deficiency anemia in the years from infancy through early toddlerhood, and again in adolescence.

In utero, the fetus builds up iron stores based on maternal iron consumption; these stores sustain the infant's iron requirements for hemoglobin synthesis during rapid periods of growth and development in early infancy. Higher maternal serum ferritin correlates to higher infant iron stores and lower incidence of iron-deficiency anemia in the newborn and later infancy; conversely, infants born to women with lower serum ferritin are at a higher risk for anemia. Premature infants, born before 37 weeks of gestation, may have decreased iron stores because of truncated time in utero, leading to lower iron stores and increased risk of iron-deficiency anemia during the first year of life.

During early infancy, between 6 and 8 weeks, the change in conditions from the hypoxic uterine environment to the oxygen-rich external environment yields a physiological nadir in hemoglobin production as iron stores are shifted from hemoglobin production to intracellular stores. As erythropoiesis increases to

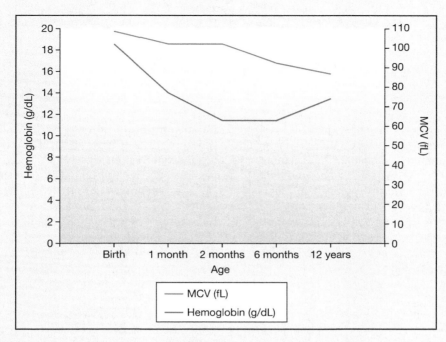

FIGURE 8.21 At birth, both MCV and hemoglobin concentration are higher than normal adult levels. MCV gradually decreases during childhood, while hemoglobin rapidly reaches a nadir within the first 6 months, then recovering by the teen years. MCV, mean cell volume.

accommodate rapidly increasing rates of growth in the infant, iron is released from intracellular stores and relocated to the bone marrow for hemoglobin synthesis.[14]

The exclusively breastfed infant has a higher risk of developing iron-deficiency anemia in the first year of life because of poor transmission of iron through breast milk. Formula-fed infants receive supplemental iron through fortification of commercial infant formulas. As breastfed infants begin to supplement their diet with solid foods, their iron consumption increases, but iron intake from readily bioavailable sources must be constant and sufficient in order to maintain normal hemoglobin levels. These infants may present with significantly decreased hemoglobin by the time they are routinely screened at 9 to 12 months of age. Cow's milk, often introduced at 12 months, is low in iron, increasing the risk for iron-deficiency anemia.

Adolescence is a period of rapid growth, accompanied by pubertal changes and the start of menses in girls. Menses is an obvious source of blood and iron loss, and adolescent girls who experience menorrhagia, or excessive uterine bleeding during menses, are at an even higher risk for developing iron-deficiency anemia. Additionally, vegetarian and vegan diets that may be initiated during adolescence, along with poor dietary habits, may limit the consumption of iron-rich foods and can contribute to iron-deficiency anemia in adolescence.

HYPERBILIRUBINEMIA

Hyperbilirubinemia is a common and potentially life-threatening hematological condition in infancy, predominantly occurring within the neonatal period. There are several types of hyperbilirubinemia of the neonate, including physiological jaundice, breastfeeding jaundice, and pathological jaundice. Regardless of the cause, exceedingly high levels of bilirubin can have severe and potentially life-threatening effects, including hearing loss, intellectual disability, and encephalopathy.

Physiological jaundice is the most commonly encountered type of hyperbilirubinemia in the neonatal period. Contributing factors include the production of bilirubin as fetal RBCs, with a relatively short life span, are removed by the spleen, combined with decreased ability of the neonatal liver to conjugate and excrete bilirubin. In most cases, the hyperbilirubinemia resolves without significant intervention or major sequelae. Physiological jaundice usually appears either within the first 24 to 72 hours of life or on day 4 or 5 of life. It typically persists for 10 to 14 days, usually reaching peak levels between the fifth and seventh days of life. Physiological hyperbilirubinemia usually presents as yellow discoloration of the skin (jaundice), scleral icterus, lethargy, decreased ability to feed, decreased urine and stool output, and dehydration. All of these signs and symptoms exist in varying degrees depending upon the serum concentration of bilirubin. Unconjugated bilirubin, measured through the indirect bilirubin or total bilirubin on serology, typically does not exceed 15 to 20 mg/dL.

Pathological jaundice is a category of hyperbilirubinemia that comprises several types of disease processes. Hemolytic processes of the RBCs that produce neonatal pathological jaundice include ABO incompatibility and Rh factor hemolytic disease. Congenital and neonatal hyperbilirubinemia can also result from liver disorders (see Chapter 14, Liver). Pathological jaundice is characterized by increased bilirubin within the first 24 hours of birth, as well as prolonged hyperbilirubinemia persisting longer than 2 weeks, or exceedingly high serum concentrations of bilirubin.

ABO incompatibility between mother and newborn can cause **antibody-mediated hemolysis**. Maternal immunoglobulins attack fetal or neonatal RBCs, causing hemolysis; this process results in jaundice in a manner similar to adult hemolytic anemia. **Rhesus hemolytic disease of the newborn** (also known as **Rh incompatibility**) can produce severe hemolytic anemia that can be fatal. As with ABO incompatibility, Rh incompatibility and hemolytic disease occur when an Rh-negative mother is carrying an Rh-positive fetus. On exposure to Rh-positive fetal blood, the Rh antigen is recognized as non-self and anti-Rh antibodies develop in the mother. These antibodies cause hemolysis of the fetal Rh-positive RBCs, causing marked hyperbilirubinemia. Hemolysis can be so severe that fetal or neonatal death can occur if not treated promptly and appropriately.

SICKLE CELL DISEASE

The genetic basis of SCD was noted earlier in this chapter. The abnormal hemoglobin HbS is susceptible to polymerization, leading to RBC sickling when exposed to acidosis, hypoxia, and dehydration. Children with SCD begin to manifest the complications of sickling and blood vessel occlusion as the RBCs transition from HbF to HbS production.

Hemoglobin polymerization may result in either reversibly or irreversibly sickled cells. The ability of the RBCs to be irreversibly sickled depends upon how many times the individual cell has undergone conformation changes. Cells that have never undergone sickling tend to be able to revert back to their normal shape once the sickling conditions cease. Pathophysiological consequences of hemoglobin polymerization and sickling are related to shortened RBC survival and the consequences of microvasculature occlusion. Repeated sickling of the RBC causes the life span of the cell to shorten to

approximately 45 days. Increased hemolysis of abnormal RBCs causes anemia, jaundice, and bilirubin gallstones. Hepatosplenomegaly is also readily apparent, due to extramedullary hematopoiesis and vascular congestion of the microvasculature of these organs.

Children with SCD have an enlarged spleen in infancy. During early childhood, episodic enlargement of the spleen during times of acute microvasculature obstruction and splenic infarction causes splenic sequestration—a life-threatening event. RBC sickling causes obstruction and congestion in the sinusoids of the spleen. This prevents adequate outflow of blood, and in extreme cases no outflow, causing engorgement of the spleen. The amount of blood that can become sequestered in the spleen accounts for a significant portion of the child's blood volume and hemoglobin, tantamount to internal hemorrhage. During episodes of splenic sequestration, hemoglobin can drop from baseline to as low as 2 g/dL.

As the child ages and experiences subsequent episodes of RBC sickling and splenic infarction, the spleen undergoes physical changes. School-age children develop a nonpalpable spleen, due to repeated episodes of infarction during sickle cell crises. Repeated infarction of the spleen causes atrophy of the splenic tissue, referred to as autosplenectomy. This should not be mistaken for surgical splenectomy. Surgical splenectomy is indicated for children who have at least two episodes of splenic sequestration.

The child's other organs are also susceptible to the consequences of vaso-occlusive events. Painful episodes (crises) localized to muscle, bone, and abdomen are common clinical presentations of sickling. As these organs become infarcted because of obstruction of the microvasculature, extreme pain results. Additionally, the distal appendages, such as hands and feet, can frequently be subject to these pain crises. Acute chest syndrome, a manifestation of occlusion of the pulmonary microvasculature, is associated with high mortality rate. Sickling in the pulmonary capillary beds results in severe hypoxemia and lung infarction, leading to impairment of respiratory function and gas exchange.

Occlusion of the cerebral microvasculature can lead to long-term sequelae and central nervous system manifestations. Strokes are the most significant of these events, and children younger than 5 years of age are the most susceptible. For children with SCD, routine transcranial Doppler imaging is performed starting at age 2 years, assessing for narrowing of the large cerebral arteries, which determines susceptibility for strokes. In addition to stroke, obstruction of the cerebral microvasculature can contribute to learning disabilities and cognitive impairment.

Micro-occlusive events of the kidneys contribute to renal disease and sickled nephropathy in adulthood. Loss of renal tissue from chronic infarction can lead to significant difficulty in concentrating urine. In states of dehydration, children with SCD are unable to concentrate urine, making them susceptible to further dehydration that promotes sickling. SCD impacts the heart indirectly. The child's anemic state and associated hypoxemia demand increased cardiac output through tachycardia and increased stroke volume, which leads to cardiomegaly.

Pathological changes to the spleen noted previously leave children with SCD more susceptible to infection, and this increased susceptibility can be life threatening. The reticuloendothelial cells of the spleen are responsible for phagocytizing encapsulated bacteria, such as pneumococci, *Haemophilus influenzae* type B (Hib), and meningococci. In SCD, the ability of the splenic macrophages to phagocytize the encapsulated bacteria is impaired, owing to increased phagocytosis of sickled RBCs. Children with SCD are more susceptible to sepsis and meningitis as a result of infection with these organisms. Management includes prophylactic treatment with penicillin. Additionally, the timely administration of immunizations for pneumococcal, meningococcal, and Hib illnesses is imperative in protecting children with SCD.[15]

VON WILLEBRAND DISEASE

vWD, introduced earlier in this chapter, is the most common genetic disorder of excess bleeding. Affected children present similarly to children with hemophilia and other coagulopathies, but vWD differs from the hemophilias in having many subtypes that vary in severity. The more severe the phenotype, the earlier the disease is likely to be diagnosed. In children, vWD typically manifests as an increased propensity for bleeding. Patients complain of gingival bleeding when brushing teeth, frequent and recurrent epistaxis, excessive bleeding with minor abrasions, or severe bruising from injuries involving relatively minor impact. Excessive bruising may raise concerns about

abuse that need to be pursued until the bleeding disorder diagnosis is identified. Adolescent girls with vWD are likely to have menorrhagia. Bleeding is typically mild to moderate in severity for the most common forms of vWD, but may be severe and life threatening in patients with more severe types of vWD. Bleeding tendencies may also be modified by concurrent medication use. For example, NSAID use may exacerbate bleeding, and oral contraceptives may reduce bleeding tendencies. The coagulopathy may also become readily apparent following a surgical procedure, when bleeding is prolonged and exceeds normal variations. Commonly, severe vWD or hemophilia is detected in male neonates following circumcision.

When vWD is suspected in a pediatric patient, a coagulation workup should be completed. This workup should include a complete blood count (CBC) with platelets to discern platelet numbers and morphology, PT, PTT, fibrinogen, vWF assays (vWF:Ag, vWF:Rco), and factor VIII assay. vWF:Ag measures the concentration of the vWF protein in the serum, and vWF:Rco measures the ability of the vWF protein to interact with platelets. If the history and physical examination are not suggestive of a severe bleeding disorder, an initial battery of hemostasis tests—including CBC with platelets, PT, PTT, and fibrinogen—may be sufficient, without the addition of the vWF and factor VIII assays. This evaluation approach might be appropriate in healthcare settings where high cost or limited resources restrict the ability to obtain laboratory tests. If the PTT is prolonged, then the factor assays should also be completed.

In general, management of vWD is aimed at reducing bleeding and providing prophylactic treatment prior to surgical interventions. Patients should be advised to avoid use of aspirin and other NSAIDs which inhibit platelet activity. Children should receive immunizations, especially hepatitis A and B, at recommended ages, according to the Centers for Disease Control and Prevention schedule (found at https://www.cdc.gov/vaccines/schedules/hcp/imz/child-adolescent.html).

Linda L. Herrmann

Age-related changes in blood and clotting include changes in red cell count, hemoglobin, and hematocrit (anemia); changes in bone marrow; hypercoagulability; and effects related to medications commonly used in older adult populations.

ANEMIA

Research has repeatedly shown the association between anemia and various comorbidities and complications in hospitalized and community-dwelling older adults.[16] Three forms of anemia are prevalent in older adults: (a) anemias related to nutritional deficits of iron, vitamin B12, or folic acid; (b) anemia of chronic disease; and (c) anemia of unknown origin.[17] The most common type of nutrient-deficient anemia is iron-deficiency anemia, which is the cause of anemia in one third of anemic older adults.

Anemia of inflammation is generally seen in older adults, particularly in patients with chronic illness, cancer, and rheumatoid disorders. It is thought to be attributed to age-related changes within the GI tract. Many studies since NHANES III have explored hepcidin, the antimicrobial peptide synthesized in the liver that controls iron metabolism. As previously noted, hepcidin downregulates cellular activity of the iron export protein ferroportin. Thus, iron is retained intracellularly and remains inaccessible in the stores, resulting in a state of functional iron deficiency.[18,19] The state of inflammation potentiates hepcidin synthesis, thereby increasing iron trapping, resulting in the low circulating iron that is seen in ACI.[20] Clinically, older adults have low serum iron, low iron-binding capacity, and an elevated serum ferritin level, all of which are typical descriptors of anemia of inflammation. As previously noted, there is an overlap between anemia of inflammation and anemia of chronic kidney disease, which also is more prevalent in older adults.

Unexplained anemia, or, anemia of unknown origin, in older adults is not well understood and is seen in approximatively one third of older adults with anemia.[17] Hematological changes were attributed to *inflammaging*—an age-related chronic inflammatory state with increased levels of proinflammatory cytokines, IL-1, IL-6, tumor necrosis factor, and transforming growth factors that contribute to anemia because they reduce the stem cell sensitivity to erythropoietin.[20] Unexplained anemia may occur secondary to reduced erythropoietin levels, as well as reduced sensitivity of early erythroid precursors (BFU) to erythropoietin.[21]

CHANGES IN BONE MARROW

Bone marrow in older adults changes in composition, containing more adipose tissue (due to decline in growth hormone production) and fewer stem cells, and showing a decline in the percentage of hematopoietic tissue (20% to 40%) compared with younger adults (40% to 60%).[22] This residual area of bone marrow, once occupied by hematopoietic tissue, is then replaced by adipose tissue, which further compromises the regulation of the bone marrow composition. These changes parallel an age-related decrease in thymic mass (Figure 8.22). In otherwise healthy older adults, clinical manifestations of these changes in bone marrow and thymic mass are mild anemia and immune deficiency. Immune deficiency increases the risk of infection (e.g., dormant tuberculosis) and neoplasms.[23] These changes in bone marrow composition have detrimental effects on stem cell function, decreasing overall systemic cellular rebuilding and resilience after injury.[22]

HYPERCOAGULABILITY

Older adults are inclined to have a hypercoagulable state at baseline, thus increasing their risk of DVT, PE, cardiac emboli, and myocardial infarction. Research has shown that increased platelet activity in older adults is related to three distinct but associated alterations: (a) a decrease in the number of prostacyclin receptors, thus reducing inhibition of platelet aggregation; (b) increased phosphoinositide turnover; and (c) increased vWF production.[22]

MEDICATION EFFECTS ON BLOOD AND CLOTTING

Clinicians must also be mindful of the effects that medications (over-the-counter and prescribed) have on blood and clotting function in older adults. Cardiovascular, cerebrovascular, and peripheral vascular diseases are often treated with drugs that affect clotting: aspirin, warfarin, direct oral anticoagulants, or platelet ADP-receptor antagonists

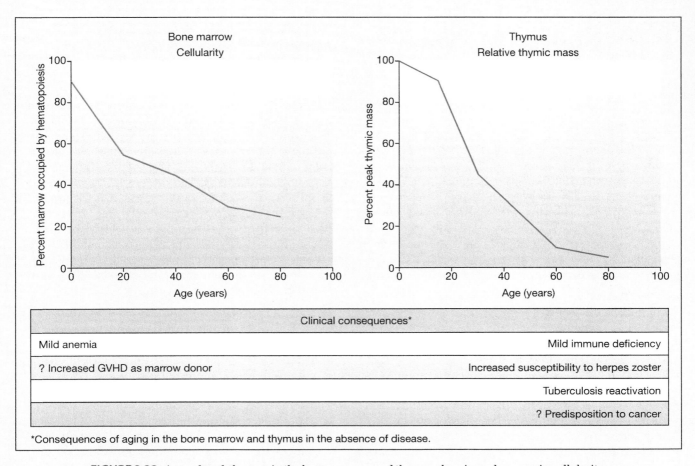

FIGURE 8.22 Age-related changes in the bone marrow and thymus showing a decrease in cellularity that parallels a decrease in thymus mass.
GVHD, graft-versus-host disease.

(prasugrel, clopidogrel). These medications make patients vulnerable to GI bleeding—a scenario that should be ruled out in older adults with unexplained anemia. At the same time, many older adults take proton pump inhibitors or histamine-2 receptor antagonists that reduce gastric acid secretion. This change in gastric acid may make absorption of iron less efficient and contribute to iron-deficiency anemia.[24]

Evaluation of laboratory studies in older adults is comparable to that in younger adults, and should include a CBC and peripheral blood smear. Laboratory values should be reviewed for changes in RBCs (namely, MCV), macrocytosis, leukopenia, leukocytosis, or platelet or white blood cell dysplastic features that may be indicative of myelodysplastic syndrome, which increases with age. Review of the reticulocyte count can clarify a hyper- or hypoproliferative anemia.

CASE STUDY 8.1: A Patient With Pernicious Anemia

Allison Rusgo and Michelle Zappas

Patient Complaint: *"I recently retired from my job as an executive assistant after 35 years and was looking forward to staying active and enjoying my free time, but lately, I'm so tired that all I want to do is rest on the couch. I try to play with my grandchildren, but my legs have been feeling numb, on and off, and I'm afraid that I might lose my balance. Several friends and family members asked if I'm dieting because my clothes seem to be fitting more loosely. I haven't been trying to lose weight, but I haven't had much appetite. I'm quite concerned because I've never experienced anything like this before."*

History of Present Illness/Review of Systems: You observe a fatigued, thin, and somewhat anxious-appearing 67-year-old Hispanic woman sitting on the examination table. The patient explains that her constellation of seemingly unrelated symptoms over the past several months has prompted her to seek medical attention. She reports generalized fatigue despite having 8 hours of consistently uninterrupted sleep per night. She also indicates waxing and waning numbness and paresthesias in her lower extremities that have caused her to almost lose her balance on several occasions. The patient is particularly concerned about this because she babysits her young grandchildren regularly and is afraid that she might fall while holding one of them. Lastly, she notes that her appetite has been poor over the past 2 months, with postprandial epigastric discomfort after most meals. She has tried antacids and avoiding spicy foods while maintaining a well-balanced diet; however, her symptoms have persisted. The patient estimates that she has lost 10 pounds over the past month, and notes that she needed to purchase clothes in a smaller size. The patient denies any other symptoms except those mentioned in the history of present illness, including hematochezia, hematuria, fevers, chills, sweats/night-sweats, and syncope. She also denies any chest pain, palpitations, shortness of breath, or dyspnea on exertion.

Past Medical/Family History: The patient's past medical history is significant for alcohol use

disorder 35 years ago, but she reports abstinence from all substances since receiving treatment at that time. She denies a history of hypertension, coronary artery disease, diabetes mellitus, osteo/rheumatoid arthritis, or any hematological or neurological diseases. The patient has never been hospitalized or undergone any invasive surgical procedures. She does not use any daily over-the-counter or prescription medications except for a multivitamin, and does not report any medication allergies. The patient's family history is significant for an older sister with Hashimoto thyroiditis, and her mother has rheumatoid arthritis.

Physical Examination: Findings are as follows: temperature of 98.6°F (oral), blood pressure of 132/74 mm Hg (left arm, sitting), heart rate of 98 beats/min (regular), respirations of 16 breaths/min (unlabored). Body mass index (BMI) is 17.9 kg/m². There is conjunctival pallor bilaterally. The remainder of the cardiovascular, respiratory, and abdominal examination is within normal limits. The neurological examination is significant for decreased lower extremity muscle strength (3/5) and deep tendon reflexes (1+) bilaterally. Vibratory sense is decreased bilaterally at ankles and wrists, the patient is slow to stand from a sitting position, and her gait also appears slower than expected.

Laboratory Findings: Hemoglobin and hematocrit are decreased; reticulocyte count is decreased; platelets and white blood cells are normal. MCV is increased, with normal MCH and MCHC. Ferritin and serum iron are normal, folic acid mildly decreased, and vitamin B12 decreased. She is anti-IF antibody positive. A blood smear shows hypersegmented polymorphonuclear leukocytes. Liver, kidney, and thyroid function levels are all within normal limits.

CASE STUDY 8.1 QUESTIONS
- *What is the reason for the patient's tachycardia?*
- *What is the most likely diagnosis?*
- *What is the mechanism of the neurological findings?*

IF, intrinsic factor; MCH, mean cell hemoglobin; MCHC, mean cell hemoglobin concentration; MCV, mean cell volume.

CASE STUDY 8.2: A Patient With Deep Venous Thrombosis

Allison Rusgo and Michelle Zappas

Patient Complaint: *"I'm concerned because I noticed some swelling in my left calf that started 4 days ago. I'm 27 weeks' pregnant with my second child, and at first, I thought it was just a normal part of pregnancy, but in the past 24 hours it's become more noticeable. I've been elevating my legs when I have a chance, but I spend most of the day chasing after my 3-year-old and I've also been busy getting the nursery ready. I was afraid to take any medications because I don't want to affect my baby. I called my OB-GYN yesterday when I noticed that my left calf seemed red, too. I'm nervous because I had a blood clot in my lungs before the birth of my first child. My OB-GYN sent me to the emergency department to be evaluated. I hope I don't have another blood clot, because my partner and I were hoping for an uneventful pregnancy this time."*

History of Present Illness/Review of Systems: You observe a well-developed, well-nourished, pregnant 32-year-old White woman who is lying supine on the examination table with her feet elevated. That patient reports that she has been feeling well throughout her pregnancy. She has remained physically active and denies any fatigue or nausea. She notes that her symptoms began gradually 4 days ago when her partner noticed that her left calf appeared mildly swollen. The patient initially ignored that observation, convincing herself that she was retaining some fluid in her feet, as she experienced during her previous pregnancy. Over the past 2 days, she states that the swelling became more pronounced despite elevating her left leg for several hours per day. Yesterday, the patient noticed that the same calf appeared red and felt warm to the touch. She also notes some discomfort at the area when she bends (dorsiflexes) her foot. She has not used any medication for these symptoms and denies any prior similar symptoms. Upon further review of symptoms, the patient confirms only recent leg cramps that are worse at night, without any chest pain, shortness of breath, dyspnea on exertion, palpitations, or syncope. The patient has not had any recent illnesses, prolonged immobility, bed rest, surgery, or trauma, and has not traveled recently.

Past Medical/Family History: The patient's past medial history is significant for a pulmonary embolism during her first pregnancy 3 years ago. Her only daily medication is a prenatal vitamin, and she reports no allergies to medication. She is a nonsmoker, has abstained from alcohol during her pregnancy, and never used any illicit substances. The only notable family history is that her mother was also diagnosed with a pulmonary embolism when pregnant with the patient's older brother 35 years ago.

Physical Examination: Findings are as follows: temperature of 99.2°F (oral), blood pressure of 128/62 mm Hg (left arm, sitting), heart rate of 68 beats/min (regular), respirations of 16 breaths/min (unlabored). The patient is alert, oriented, and in no acute distress. Her cardiovascular, respiratory, and abdominal examinations are within normal limits. Other findings include mild warmth and erythema in conjunction with moderate tenderness and edema to the affected posterior aspect of the left calf. There is no evidence of lesions, rashes, cellulitis, or venous congestion. Lower extremity pulses are 2+ bilaterally, and sensation is intact.

Diagnostic Findings: A venous duplex ultrasound examination of the patient's left lower extremity reveals an area of incompressibility and impaired venous blood flow within a distal segment of the posterior peroneal vein.

CASE STUDY 8.2 QUESTIONS
* *What factors can contribute to increased tendency to form clots in the absence of trauma?*
* *What might lead you to suspect a genetic disorder in this case? What specific genetic disorder could be responsible for these findings?*

BRIDGE TO CLINICAL PRACTICE

Ben Cocchiaro

PRINCIPLES OF ASSESSMENT

History

Evaluate:

- Changes in weight, exercise tolerance, bowel habits, menstrual patterns, skin color (i.e., jaundice, pallor, ecchymosis) or neurological status (i.e., paresthesias or gait abnormalities)
- Mucosal bleeding, prolonged epistaxis (nosebleed), hemarthrosis (bleeding into a joint), or menorrhagia
- Family history of blood disorders
- Dietary patterns, including vegetarianism or veganism

Physical Examination

- Assess skin for pallor, jaundice (or scleral icterus), capillary refill, ecchymoses, petechiae, or purpura.
- Observe for oropharyngeal abnormalities, particularly atrophic glossitis (concerning for nutritional deficiencies), mucosal bleeding, and pallor of the mucous membranes.
- Examine thyroid; auscultate for carotid bruits, and palpate lymph nodes for any signs of infection/inflammation.
- Palpate liver and spleen for enlargement and tenderness.
- *Neurological assessment:* Focus on vibratory sense, position sense, and gait.
- *Rectal examination:* Look for occult blood or obvious bleeding.

Laboratory Evaluation

- *Complete blood count:* Quantitative description of the peripheral blood, including counts (RBCs, WBCs) and sizes (MCV, RDW); useful in diagnosing anemias, infections, and hematological malignancies. The reticulocyte count provides a window into hematopoiesis that can help differentiate anemias caused by RBC loss or destruction from those caused by deficient RBC production. Platelet counts provide important information regarding the body's ability to form clots.
- *Peripheral blood smear:* Qualitative description of the size, shape, and color of RBCs and WBCs; useful in the evaluation of hemolytic anemias, thrombocytopenias, toxic metal exposures, parasites, and hematological malignancies.

- *Iron studies:* Measures of blood iron content; useful in the confirmation of iron-deficiency anemias as well as iron overload. Tests include iron, transferrin saturation (%), and ferritin.
- *Relevant nutritional assessment:* Determine vitamin B12 and folic acid levels.
- *Coagulation studies:* PT and PTT are useful in the evaluation of unexplained bleeding and in the monitoring of patients on certain forms of anticoagulant therapy. The INR is a standardized measure of PT crucial for monitoring patients on warfarin (Coumadin).
- *D-dimer:* This sensitive, though nonspecific, quantitation of fibrin degradation products is used for the evaluation of suspected deep vein thromboses, pulmonary emboli, and disseminated intravascular coagulation.

MAJOR DRUG CLASSES

- *Nutritional supplements:* Ferrous iron salts, cobalamin, or folate may be indicated once the diagnosis of anemia secondary to nutritional deficiencies is confirmed.
- *Recombinant erythropoietin:* Used to treat anemia of chronic kidney disease; can be used to treat anemia resulting from certain drug treatments.
- *Anticoagulants* (parenteral or oral): Warfarin (oral), heparin or enoxaparin (parenteral), or direct oral anticoagulants that inhibit factors II or X (dabigatran, apixaban, rivaroxaban, and edoxaban) can be used to treat thromboembolic disease and to reduce clot formation in conditions such as atrial fibrillation.
- *Antiplatelet agents* (e.g., prasugrel, clopidogrel, and ticagrelor): Block ADP receptors; can be used after percutaneous coronary intervention for acute coronary syndrome. Aspirin irreversibly inhibits platelet TXA_2 synthesis.
- *Fibrinolytics* (e.g., tissue plasminogen activator): Enhance plasmin activity to break up existing clots; may be used for myocardial infarction or stroke.
- *Factor replacements:* Factors VIII and IX are indicated in deficiency states such as hemophilia.
- *DDAVP:* Stimulates factor VIII and von Willebrand factor synthesis; indicated for transient use in hemophilia A and vWD.

ADP, adenosine diphosphate; INR, international normalized ratio; MCV, mean cell volume; PT, prothrombin time; PTT, partial thromboplastin time; RBC, red blood cell; RDW, red cell distribution width; TXA_2, thromboxane A_2; WBC, white blood cell.

KEY POINTS

- All blood cells and platelets are derived from multipotential precursor cells (stem cells) in the bone marrow. Blood cell production rates depend on several growth factors, such as IL-3, erythropoietin, thrombopoietin, and GM-CSF.
- The most numerous blood cells are RBCs (red cells or erythrocytes). Lacking nuclei and other organelles, these are small, highly flexible biconcave disks that function to carry large amounts of hemoglobin throughout the bloodstream for oxygen delivery to tissues.
- Hemoglobin is made up of four protein chains with four iron-containing heme groups. The iron is the site of oxygen binding.
- Anemia is the most common blood disorder. There are several forms of anemia: iron deficiency (the most common), macrocytic, hemolytic, and anemias due to abnormal RBC proteins. Within these large categories, there are further subdivisions that need to be evaluated in the differential diagnosis of anemia. Along with the history and physical examination, the CBC and peripheral blood smear provide critical information in diagnosing anemia.
- Iron-deficiency anemia can result from inadequate iron intake or absorption or from chronic blood loss that accelerates body iron requirements. Owing to lack of hemoglobin production, cells are small and pale. Iron-deficiency anemia is the most common form of anemia across all age groups.
- Macrocytic anemia can result from vitamin B12 or folate deficiency, leading to slowing of DNA synthesis and delayed cell maturation. Cells are large and fragile, exacerbating the anemia because they have a shorter life span. A distinguishing characteristic of vitamin B12 deficiency is that it can have neurological consequences in addition to anemia.
- Anemia due to increased rate of hemolysis can have several causes: (a) Cells can be abnormally shaped because of abnormal hemoglobin (SCD). (b) Cells can be vulnerable to oxidative stress because of enzyme deficiency (G6PD deficiency). (c) Cells can be abnormally fragile because of cytoskeletal mutations (spherocytosis). (d) Cells can be targeted by antibodies for destruction. (e) Cells can be destroyed by intravascular clots in a microangiopathic hemolytic process (HELLP syndrome, thrombotic thrombocytopenia).
- The abnormal hemoglobin of SCD polymerizes in response to oxidative stress or cellular dehydration, leading to sickling of cells, occlusion of blood vessels, and rapid cell destruction. Tissue ischemia due to blood vessel occlusion produces severe pain and organ damage.
- Hemostasis, or the ability to stop bleeding when a blood vessel is damaged, involves a tightly regulated sequence of events. First, the cut blood vessel constricts, reducing blood flow. Second, platelets become activated and aggregate to form a plug. Third, the plasma protein clotting cascade is activated and deposits a mesh of fibrin strands in and around the platelet plug. Finally, the clot retracts, squeezes out excess fluid, and becomes a compact plug.
- Platelets produce several important mediators to assist the clotting cascade. Activated platelets synthesize and release ADP and thromboxane A_2 as well as serotonin (stored in granules). These factors and others recruit more platelets to become activated in a positive feedback system. Platelets also provide phospholipids as cofactors for the clotting cascade, and platelets are activated by thrombin as the clotting cascade occurs around the platelet plug. Platelet membrane GPs are important contributors to the clotting process.
- The clotting cascade is a carefully controlled series of enzymes that, when activated, split target proteins resulting in products that are, themselves, activated protease enzymes. This chain reaction rapidly accelerates and amplifies the clotting signal so that bleeding can be stopped quickly. The process also depends on protein cofactors (proteins VIII and V) and on calcium and phospholipids.
- Liver post-translational carboxylation of clotting factors requires vitamin K, a fat-soluble vitamin produced by gut bacteria and absorbed with the assistance of bile salts.
- Anticoagulant factors work to prevent clotting when it is not appropriate or to reduce the spread of clotting once it has started. Important signals include prostaglandin I_2 (prostacyclin), antithrombin III, thrombomodulin, and proteins C and S—each of which works by a different mechanism of action.
- When no longer needed, clots are broken down by plasmin, a protein split from the precursor plasminogen by the action of tPa and other compounds.
- States of excess bleeding can occur from genetic deficiencies in clotting proteins and

factors. Among these heritable states are vWF, factor VIII, and factor IX deficiencies.

- Even without tissue damage, pathological clots can form via the intrinsic pathway of coagulation in cases of damaged endothelium, states of slow blood flow, or blood stasis.
- A fairly common genetic disorder that promotes abnormal clot formation is a mutation causing production of FVL. This mutation causes factor V to resist cleavage and inactivation by protein C. This condition is also referred to as *aPC resistance*.
- Iron-deficiency anemia is a prominent RBC disorder in infancy and childhood, primarily due to increased iron requirements during growth and development.
- Genetic disorders of RBCs and bleeding also typically manifest early in life with lifelong consequences, including SCD, vWD, and hemophilia.
- Healthy older adults have few changes in blood and clotting. However, given the prevalence of chronic diseases among the elderly, there is an increased incidence of anemia (prominently, nutritional anemia and anemia of inflammation, as well as unexplained anemia) in this population. The prevalence of chronic disease also manifests in hypercoagulability, which is promoted by chronic inflammation. Consequently, risks of myocardial infarction, stroke, and thromboembolic disorders are more common with aging.

REFERENCES

1. Global Burden of Disease 2016 Disease and Injury Incidence and Prevalence Collaborators. Global, regional, and national incidence, prevalence, and years lived with disability for 328 diseases and injuries for 195 countries, 1990–2016: a systematic analysis for the Global Burden of Disease Study 2016. *Lancet.* 2017;390: 1211–1259. doi:10.1016/S0140-6736(17)32154-2.

2. Le CHH. The prevalence of anemia and moderate-severe anemia in the US population (NHANES 2003–2012). *PLOS ONE.* 2016;11:e0166635. doi:10.1371/journal .pone.0166635.

3. Fuentes AV, Pineda MD, Venkata KCN. Comprehension of top 200 prescribed drugs in the US as a resource for pharmacy teaching, training, and practice. *Pharmacy.* 2018;6:43. doi:10.3390/pharmacy6020043.

4. Allister LM, Torres C, Schnall J, et al. Jaundice, anemia, and hypoxemia. *J Emerg Med.* 2017;52:93–97. doi:10.1016/ j.jemermed.2016.07.113.

5. Offermans S. Activation of platelet function through G protein-coupled receptors. *Circ Res.* 2006;99:1293–1304. doi:10.1161/01.RES.0000251742.71301.16.

6. Mackman N, Tilley RE, Key NS. Role of the extrinsic pathway of blood coagulation in hemostasis and thrombosis. *Arterioscler Thromb Vasc Biol.* 2007;27:1687–1693. doi:10.1161/ATVBAHA.107.141911.

7. World Health Organization. Disease burden and mortality estimates. http://www.who.int/healthinfo/global_ burden_disease/estimates/en/index1.html. Accessed September 28, 2018.

8. van Rooy M-J, Pretorius E. Metabolic syndrome, platelet activation and the development of transient ischemic attack or thromboembolic stroke. *Thromb Res.* 2015;135:434–442. doi:10.1016/j.thromres.2014.12.030.

9. Jadaon MM. Epidemiology of activated protein C resistance and factor V Leiden mutation in the Mediterranean region. *Mediterr J Hematol Infect Dis.* 2011;3:e2011037. doi:10.4084/MJHID.2011.037.

10. Roman E, Larson PJ, Manno CS. Transfusion therapy for coagulation factor deficiencies. In: Hoffman R, Benz Jr EJ, Silberstein LF, et al., eds. *Hematology: Basic Principles and Practice.* 7th ed. Philadelphia, PA: Elsevier; 2018: 1769–1780.

11. Centers for Disease Control and Prevention. Hemophilia: data and statistics. https://www.cdc.gov/ncbddd/ hemophilia/data.html. Accessed November 6, 2018.

12. Roberts IAG, Murray NA. Haematology. In: JM Rennie, ed. *Rennie and Roberton's Textbook of Neonatology.* 5th ed. Philadelphia, PA: Elsevier; 2012:755–790.

13. Wang M. Iron deficiency and other types of anemia in infants and children. *Am Fam Physician.* 2016;93:270– 278. Retrieved from https://www.aafp.org/afp/2016/0215/ p270.html.

14. Hernell O, Fewtrell MS, Georgieff MK, et al. Summary of current recommendations on iron provision and monitoring of iron status for breastfed and formula-fed infants in resource-rich and resource-constrained countries. *J Pediatr.* 2015;167:S40–S47. doi:10.1016/j .jpeds.2015.07.020.

15. Azar S, Wong TE. Sickle cell disease: a brief update. *Med Clin North Am.* 2017;101:375–393. doi:10.1016/j .mcna.2016.09.009.

16. Ershler WB, Artz AS, Kanapuru B. Hematology in older persons. In: Kaushansky K, Lichtman MA, Prchal JT, et al., eds. *Williams Hematology.* 9th ed. New York, NY: McGraw-Hill; 2016:129–142.

17. Lanier JB, Park JJ, Callahan RC. Anemia in older adults. *Am Fam Physician.* 2018;98:437–442. Retrieved from https://www.aafp.org/afp/2018/1001/p437.html.

18. Röhrig G, Rucker Y, Becker I, et al. Association of anemia with functional and nutritional status in the German multicenter study "GeriAnaemie2013." *Z Gerontol Geriatr.* 2017;50:532–537. doi:10.1007/s00391-016-1092-3.

19. Vanasse GJ. Anemia. In: Williams BA, Chang A, Ahalt C, et al., eds. *Current Diagnosis & Treatment: Geriatrics.* 2nd ed. New York, NY: McGraw-Hill; 2014: 314–320.

20. Burney S, Ahmad SQ, Masroor R. Aenemia in elderly: a benign condition or an early warning? A hospital based

study. *Pakistan Armed Forces Med J*. 2016;66:400–406. Retrieved from https://pafmj.org/index.php/PAFMJ/article/view/1334.

21. Gowanlock Z, Sriram S, Martin A, et al. Erythropoietin levels in elderly patients with anemia of unknown etiology. *PLOS ONE*. 2016;11:e0157279. doi:10.1371/journal.pone.0157279.

22. Fischer PE, DeLoughery TG, Schreiber MA. Hematologic changes with aging. In: Yelon JA, Luchette FA, eds. *Geriatric Trauma and Critical Care*. New York, NY: Springer; 2014:55–60.

23. Prabhaker M, Ershler WB, Longo DL. Bone marrow, thymus, and blood: changes across the lifespan. *Aging Health*. 2009;5:385–393. doi:10.2217/ahe.09.31.

24. Lam JR, Schneider JL, Quesenberry CP, et al. Proton pump inhibitor and histamine-2 receptor antagonist use and iron deficiency. *Gastroenterology*. 2017;152:821–829. doi:10.1053/j.gastro.2016.11.023.

SUGGESTED RESOURCES

Aster JC, Bunn HF. *Pathophysiology of Blood Disorders*. 2nd ed. New York, NY: McGraw-Hill; 2017.

Goodnough LT, Schrier SL. Evaluation and management of anemia in the elderly. *Am J Hematol*. 2014;89:88–96. doi:10.1002/ajh.23598.

Hoffman R, Benz EJ, Silberstein LE, et al. *Hematology: Basic Principles and Practice*. 7th ed. Philadelphia, PA: Elsevier; 2018.

Kaushansky K, Lichtman MA, Prchal JT, et al., eds. *Williams Hematology*. 9th ed. New York, NY: McGraw-Hill; 2016.

Kumar V, Abbas AK, Aster JC. Hemodynamic disorders, thromboembolism, and shock. In: Kumar V, Abbas AK, Aster JC, eds. *Robbins Basic Pathology*. 10th ed. Philadelphia, PA: Elsevier; 2018:97–119.

Lanzkowsky P, Lipton JM, Fish JD. *Lanzkowsky's Manual of Pediatric Hematology and Oncology*. 6th ed. Philadelphia, PA: Elsevier; 2016.

Lönnerdal B, Georgieff MK, Hernell O. Developmental physiology of iron absorption, homeostasis, and metabolism in the healthy term infant. *J Pediatr*. 2015;167:S8–S14. doi:10.1016/j.jpeds.2015.07.014.

Schaan MD, Schwanke CHA, Bauer M, et al. Hematological and nutritional parameters in apparently healthy elderly individuals. *Hematol Transfus Cell Ther*. 2007;29:136–143. doi:10.1590/S1516-84842007000200011.

9

CIRCULATION

Fruzsina K. Johnson, Robert A. Johnson, and Spencer A. Rhodes

THE CLINICAL CONTEXT

Cardiovascular disease is the most common cause of adult morbidity and mortality, accounting for 31% of deaths worldwide.[1] The most common disorder of the vascular system is hypertension, defined by the American College of Cardiology and the American Heart Association (AHA) as blood pressure >130/80 mm Hg. In the United States, from 2015 to 2016, hypertension prevalence was 29% overall. Blood pressure tends to increase with age, and the prevalence of hypertension was 63.1% in people aged 60 years and older during this period. The same report noted that about half of patients with hypertension achieved blood pressure control, although controlled hypertension was more likely for women than for men.[2]

Complications of hypertension include accelerated atherosclerosis, myocardial infarction, stroke, kidney failure, and aneurysm. There is substantial overlap between hypertension and atherosclerosis, the second most common vascular disorder. Patients with atherosclerosis are at risk for development of ischemic heart disease (including myocardial infarction), stroke, and peripheral arterial disease. Ischemic heart disease caused almost 9 million deaths globally in 2015, and 3 million deaths resulted from ischemic strokes.[3] This chapter focuses on the structure, function, and diseases of the circulation, and Chapter 10, Heart, focuses on the heart.

OVERVIEW OF CIRCULATORY STRUCTURE AND FUNCTION

HOMEOSTATIC FUNCTIONS OF THE CIRCULATORY SYSTEM

Historically, William Harvey (in 1628) was the first to hypothesize that blood traveled through the body by means of a series of blood vessels that led away from and then returned to the heart. The circulatory (or vascular) system provides an essential connection among all organ systems in the body as they work together toward the common goal of maintaining homeostasis. The primary roles of blood as it travels in the circulatory system are to transport:

- Oxygen from the lungs to the tissues and carbon dioxide from the tissues for elimination from the lungs
- Nutrients from the digestive tract to the tissues
- Metabolic waste products from the tissues to their point of elimination
- Hormones from their point of production to the site of action
- Immune system components

Most tissues are in continuous need of oxygen delivery for adenosine triphosphate (ATP) production; only a few minutes of complete interruption of blood flow (termed *no-flow ischemia*) can lead to irreversible tissue damage (*infarction*). Vascular diseases can also cause long-term reductions in blood flow, resulting in inadequate oxygen delivery for the tissue's metabolic demand (*ischemia*), and thus chronically compromising tissue function without overt infarction.

ORGANIZING PRINCIPLES OF THE CIRCULATORY SYSTEM

The circulatory system has three primary components:

1. Blood (the focus of Chapter 8, Blood and Clotting)
2. The heart (the focus of Chapter 10, Heart)
3. Blood vessels (the primary focus of this chapter)

The heart has four chambers and acts as a dual pump, simultaneously pumping blood in both cardiovascular circuits: the systemic and the pulmonary circulation (**Figure 9.1**). The two vascular circuits are coupled in series; thus, total blood flow (cardiac output) is the same in both systems. Movement of blood (flow) requires pressure—blood flows from regions of high pressure (generated by the ventricles pumping into the systemic and pulmonary vessels) to regions of lower pressure (the right and left atria, respectively). The biophysical principles noted in the next section govern this flow and associated pressures and have consequences for vascular structure, function, and vulnerability to disease.

The Pulmonary Circulation

The pulmonary circulation originates from the right ventricle with the pulmonary artery. The primary goal of the pulmonary circulation is to oxygenate blood and remove carbon dioxide; thus, 100% of the cardiac output (volume of blood pumped by the ventricle per minute, normally ~5 L/min) flows through the lungs. Oxygenated blood is returned to the left atrium by means of the pulmonary veins. Despite the same amount of total blood flow, pressure and vascular resistance are about five- to ten-fold lower in the pulmonary circulation compared with that in the systemic circuit.

The Systemic Circulation

The systemic circulation starts with the aorta, which receives output from the left ventricle, and branches into numerous parallel vascular circuits, each receiving a fraction of the cardiac output. Distribution of blood flow through these parallel circuits dynamically adapts to the tissues' metabolic needs—flow increases in active tissues and decreases in inactive tissues.

At rest, the kidneys, the gastrointestinal system, and the skeletal muscle each receive about 20% of the cardiac output, while skin blood flow is only 4% to 5% (**Figure 9.2**). During exercise, cardiac output, skeletal muscle, and skin blood flow increase greatly, while renal and gastrointestinal blood flow decrease. This redistribution of blood flow is an adaptive mechanism that ensures that blood is being directed to areas with greater metabolic need during times of increased activity. Vital organs such as the brain are always active and receive similar blood flow under both conditions.

STRUCTURE AND PROPERTIES OF BLOOD VESSELS

General Structure of Blood Vessels

All blood vessels, except for capillaries, have a three-layer wall structure (**Figure 9.3**).

The inner layer, called the tunica intima (or simply *intima*), consists of a single layer of endothelial cells forming the vessel lining, basement membrane, and a layer of elastic fibers (internal elastic lamina). Endothelial cells play crucial roles in maintaining vascular health in large arteries (highlighted later in this chapter, in the discussion of atherosclerosis) as well as

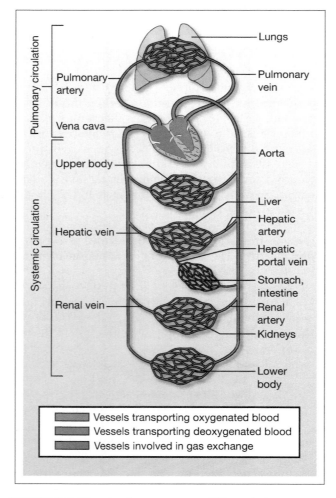

FIGURE 9.1 The circulatory system, differentiating systemic and pulmonary circulation.

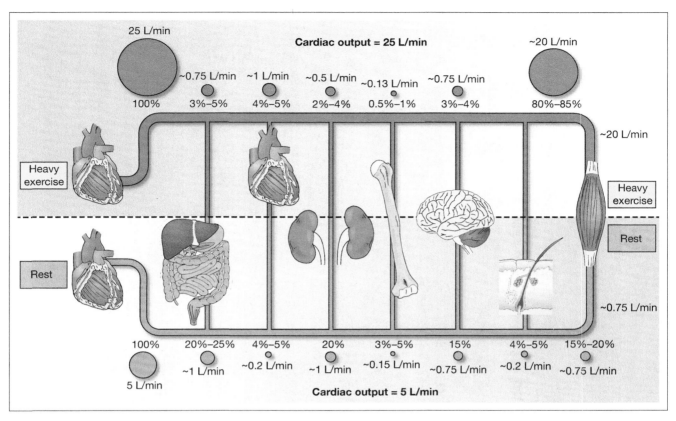

FIGURE 9.2 Blood flow distribution to organs and tissues at rest (bottom) and redistribution during exercise (top). Average absolute rates are shown, as well as the percentage of total cardiac output perfusing each organ.

regulating vascular resistance and function in smaller arterioles. Folds of the intima in limb veins form one-way valves that are essential in facilitating venous return, especially from the lower limbs when a person is standing upright.

The middle layer, the tunica media (or *media*), is mostly composed of concentric layers of vascular smooth muscle (VSM) cells. Changing contractile activity of VSM is the primary mechanism of second-to-second regulation of arteriolar resistance and thus tissue blood flow (described later in this chapter, in the context of VSM contractile properties and regulation). Surrounding the smooth muscle is another layer of elastic fibers (the external elastic lamina).

The outermost layer, the tunica externa (or *adventitia*), is composed of strong connective tissue that helps to keep the blood vessels intact.

Comparative Structure of Blood Vessels

The size and ratio of wall components in blood vessels vary greatly, depending on their primary functions in the circulation (see **Figure 9.3**). Blood flow in the systemic circulation is driven by the pumping action of the left ventricle (as described in Chapter 10, Heart). The pressure is highest in the aorta and falls throughout the circuit as a result of vascular resistance. The aorta branches into successively smaller arteries that distribute blood flow to various organs. Arteries have much thicker walls compared with veins and thus are able to withstand much higher pressures.

Arteries branch into arterioles, which represent the primary site (70% to 80%) of systemic vascular resistance and give rise to microcirculatory networks with an abundance of capillaries. As the ideal site for exchange between the blood and tissues, capillaries have uniquely thin walls composed of only endothelial cells and basement membrane (no elastic fibers or VSM). Blood flow from capillaries is collected into venules and increasingly larger veins that serve an important blood reservoir function and regulate venous return to the heart.

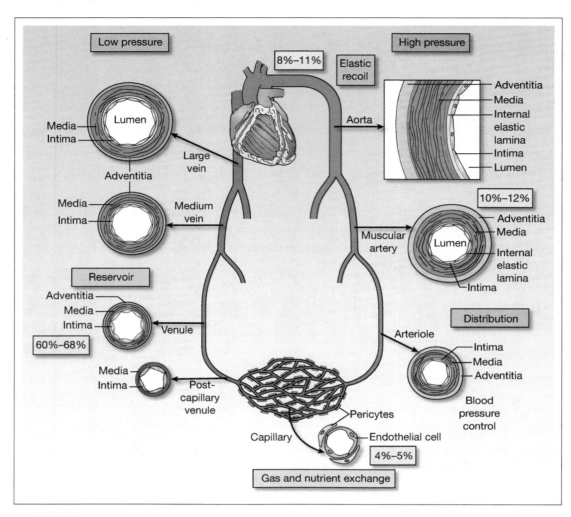

FIGURE 9.3 Structure and function of the different classes of blood vessels. Structurally, the walls of arteries are thicker than veins at each level of organization. Eight percent to 11% of the total blood volume is found in the heart, with 10% to 12% in arteries and arterioles, 4% to 5% in capillaries, and 60% to 68% in veins. Veins have the greatest capacity to store blood at low pressure, but can constrict to mobilize blood to the heart during hypotension and hypovolemia.

PROPERTIES AND DISORDERS OF LARGE ARTERIES

OVERVIEW OF LARGE ARTERY STRUCTURE AND FUNCTION

Large arteries have three primary functions:

1. Deliver blood from the heart to the tissues (conduit vessels)
2. Distribute blood flow to the multiple parallel circuits of the systemic circulation
3. Maintain blood pressure and blood flow during diastole

These functions require large arteries to be able to withstand high blood pressures, branch extensively, and be able to stretch during systole and return to their original size during diastole—but they also leave them vulnerable to injury. Biophysical properties such as wall tension, compliance, and blood flow characteristics determine the structure/function relationships of large arteries in health and disease.

Biophysics of Vascular Wall Tension (Law of Laplace)

Blood pumped into the aorta by the left ventricle generates hydrostatic pressure—a *push* on the vessel wall in the outward direction. This pressure is highest in the aorta and large arteries, and contributes to wall tension. Wall tension is pictured in **Figure 9.4** as the variable *T*—the force that would contribute to rupturing the vessel wall if there were an area of weakness or a tear. The law of Laplace describes determinants of wall tension in blood vessels as follows:

$$T = \frac{(P \times r)}{h}$$

where

T = wall tension
P = pressure in the blood vessel
r = radius of the blood vessel
h = wall thickness of the blood vessel

Wall tension (T) is increased by both pressure (P) and radius (r), but decreased by wall thickness (h). Large arteries have to withstand high pressure at a relatively large radius, which both increase wall tension. To reduce wall tension and avoid rupture, large arteries have much thicker walls compared with walls of veins of similar size.

Vascular Hypertrophy

As previously noted by the law of Laplace, the compensatory mechanism for increased vascular pressure is to increase wall thickness in blood vessels (**vascular hypertrophy**). This increase in wall thickness helps to offset the effect of increased pressure and decrease wall tension. However, if elevated blood pressure is sustained over time (as in poorly controlled hypertension), the thicker vascular walls become fibrotic and can lead to secondary problems, such as kidney failure.

Vascular Aneurysm

Another consequence of the law of Laplace for blood vessels is that high arterial pressure can cause a progressive increase in vascular radius if the arterial wall becomes weakened, often by atherosclerosis. Initial compensation with wall hypertrophy may progress to wall ischemia that ultimately weakens the wall. This sets

up a vicious cycle in which the vessel begins to dilate, further increasing its radius, and therefore wall tension. This forms a **vascular aneurysm** that tends to progressively enlarge over time and may eventually lead to catastrophic rupture of the vessel wall. Men ages 65 and older with a history of hypertension and atherosclerotic cardiovascular disease (ASCVD) have the highest risk of **abdominal aortic aneurysm**. Aneurysm rupture has a very high mortality rate, but if an aneurysm is detected prior to rupture, surgery can be performed to remove the enlarged area and replace it with a vascular graft.

Biophysics of Vascular Compliance

Compliance describes the ability of three-dimensional structures to stretch (increase in volume) in response to an increase in pressure. Real-life experience teaches us that objects with varying structures have varying compliance. It is much easier to blow air to inflate a (more compliant) party balloon than it is to pump air to fill a (less compliant) bicycle tire! This relationship is described in the following equation:

$$C = \frac{\Delta V}{\Delta P}$$

where

C = compliance
ΔV = volume change
ΔP = pressure change

All blood vessels stretch under pressure, but to different degrees (**Figure 9.5**). Arteries are less compliant than veins, but are subjected to greater pressure changes as they receive the stroke volume of the heart during systole. The aorta and large arteries contain an abundance of elastic fibers that stretch during systole and return

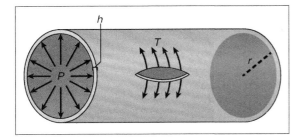

FIGURE 9.4 The determinants of wall tension (the force tending to rupture the vessel wall) include intravascular pressure, radius, and wall thickness. These relationships are quantified in the law of Laplace.

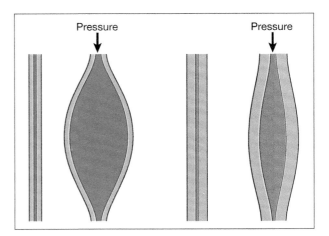

FIGURE 9.5 Compliance (*stretchability*) of arteries (right) versus veins (left). Veins are more compliant than arteries, therefore at an equal amount of input pressure, they stretch to hold a greater volume of blood.

to their original shape and size during diastole. The tendency to return to their original size is referred to as their elastic recoil function. This elastic recoil of the large arteries helps to maintain diastolic blood pressure and thus tissue perfusion between heart beats. With age-related changes and vascular disease (e.g., atherosclerosis), arterial walls become less compliant, leading to an increase in systolic blood pressure and a decrease in diastolic pressure and blood flow. Veins are much more compliant than arteries, which make them ideally suited to function as a blood reservoir, referred to as *capacitance*. In fact, 60% to 68% of the circulating blood volume is typically stored at relatively low pressures in the systemic veins and venules (see **Figure 9.3**).

The elastic properties of large arteries allow them to stretch to accommodate the stroke volume ejected by the left ventricle, and then to maintain pressure on the blood as they return to their original size after ejection ends (**Figure 9.6**). Diastolic pressure is thereby maintained, to continue to drive blood flow into small arteries and arterioles. Arterial compliance receives the blood ejected from the ventricle while yielding to stretch with a moderate elevation of systolic pressure; elastic recoil contributes to diastolic pressure that maintains blood flow during diastole. Vessels that develop stiffness due to vascular damage and aging receive the stroke volume and develop elevated systolic pressure, but have decreased recoil, leading to decreased diastolic pressure and flow.

Biophysics of Blood Flow Velocity and Shear Stress

As large arteries branch into smaller arteries, arterioles, and capillaries, the cross-sectional area at each segment of the circulation becomes greater. The blood flows into many more channels, lowering the velocity of flow in these segments. In other words, blood flow velocity and cross-sectional area are inversely related (**Figure 9.7a**). Thus, blood velocity is highest in the aorta and large arteries and lowest in the capillaries. Blood flow velocity is important, because it is directly related to shear stress (friction of the blood sliding past and pulling on the endothelial cell surface parallel to the direction of flow, as shown in **Figure 9.7b**), as well as the chance of turbulence. Slow blood velocity is also the foundation for capillary function, as these vessels are the regions of exchange of water and blood-borne substances between blood and interstitial fluid (see Properties and Disorders of Capillaries, later in this chapter).

Laminar flow in a large blood vessel refers to layers of blood traveling smoothly parallel to the long axis of the vessel, with the blood in the middle of the vessel having the greatest velocity, and the surrounding layers traveling more slowly (**Figure 9.7b**). This type of

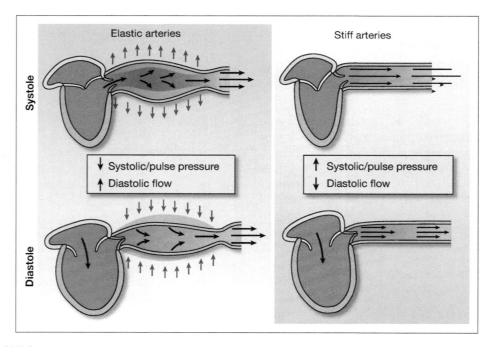

FIGURE 9.6 The elastic recoil of large arteries (left) and changes with arterial stiffening (right). Blood ejected from the left ventricle distends the artery, which stretches with a moderate elevation of systolic pressure. Elastic recoil contributes to diastolic pressure that maintains blood flow during diastole. In vessels that develop stiffness due to vascular damage and aging, ejection from the left ventricle produces higher systolic pressure but with little distention, and pressure rapidly falls during diastole, reducing diastolic flow.

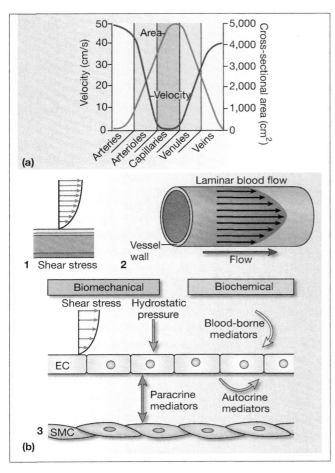

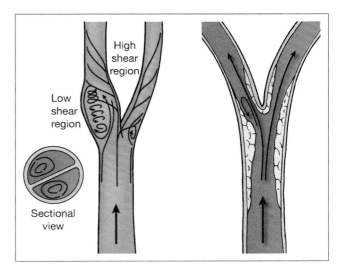

FIGURE 9.8 Laminar versus turbulent flow at the bifurcation of the carotid artery. Flow is laminar and shear stress is uniform in the main vessel. At the bifurcation, the larger internal carotid artery has reduced shear stress, while the external carotid artery is smaller and has higher shear stress. Greater plaque formation occurs on the side of the internal carotid artery, which may also experience reverse blood flow.

FIGURE 9.7 Biophysical and biochemical forces acting on the vascular walls. (**a**) Blood velocity varies with vessel cross-sectional area across the systemic vasculature. (**b**) Mechanical forces acting on the ECs within the vascular wall include (**1**) longitudinal shear stress and (**2**) the presence of smooth laminar flow. (**3**) Biomechanical and biochemical factors influence EC production of paracrine mediators and autocrine mediators of SMC and EC function. EC, endothelial cell; SMC, smooth muscle cell.

blood flow is low vibration and highly efficient. Picture the blood slipping smoothly past the endothelial cells lining the blood vessel wall: with smooth laminar flow, there will be little friction between the formed elements of the blood (cells and platelets) and the vessel lining. Blood flow can become turbulent at narrowed areas and at branch points (**Figure 9.8**). Turbulent flow causes vibration of the vascular wall, resulting in bruits that can be auscultated over narrowed vascular segments.

Normally, laminar flow and high velocity in large arteries cause shear stress, a tugging force on the endothelial layer lining the vessel. Hydrostatic pressure further acts on the vessel wall by maintaining a perpendicular distending force that contributes to wall tension. In response to these forces, the endothelial cell

and smooth muscle layers generate and respond to a variety of biochemical mediators. The most important of these is the production of *nitric oxide* by endothelial cells that diffuses to the underlying smooth muscle layer and promotes vasodilation, maintaining vessel patency and vascular wall health and lowering blood pressure.

Having a relatively constant level of shear stress and normal blood pressure stimulates endothelial nitric oxide production and release. In areas of turbulent flow, such as downstream from an atherosclerotic plaque and in areas of vascular branching, endothelial shear stress is reduced, leading to decreased nitric oxide production. Decreased endothelial nitric oxide production is a hallmark of endothelial dysfunction that contributes to and accompanies atherosclerosis. In contrast, during hypertension, increased blood pressure causes elevated shear stress with the background of endothelial dysfunction and decreased nitric oxide production. In this case, elevated sheer stress cannot increase nitric oxide production, but rather contributes to endothelial damage and exacerbates atherosclerosis.

ATHEROSCLEROSIS: THE MOST COMMON DISEASE OF LARGE ARTERIES

Overview of Large Vessel Diseases

Vascular diseases cause more morbidity and mortality than any other human disease category. Arterial diseases are the most common and have two principal presentations: (a) atherosclerotic narrowing or complete obstruction of the vessel lumen, leading to tissue ischemia; and (b) weakening of the vascular wall, leading to dilation (aneurysm), rupture, and hemorrhage. These two mechanisms can be closely related and may cause one another, such as an abdominal aorta aneurysm forming downstream from a lumen-narrowing atherosclerotic plaque. The most common sites of atherosclerosis, in order of frequency, are the following:

1. Abdominal aorta
2. Coronary arteries
3. Thoracic aorta, femoral and popliteal arteries
4. Carotid arteries
5. Vertebral, basilar, and middle cerebral arteries

Overview of Atherosclerosis

Atherosclerosis is the buildup of plaque within the walls of large conduit arteries and is seen to varying degrees in most humans, beginning in adolescence and early adulthood. Worldwide, 85% of cardiovascular deaths are due to myocardial infarction and stroke.[1] Atherosclerosis underlies the pathogenesis of coronary, cerebral, and peripheral vascular disease. Atherosclerosis is a chronic inflammatory response to the accumulation of lipids (low-density lipoprotein [LDL] cholesterol) and macrophages in the artery wall. It often starts during childhood and is initially characterized by clinically silent arterial intimal plaques that grow and become more complex for years to decades. While atherosclerosis develops in many people, particularly in developed societies, certain risk factors accelerate the process and cause disease and death at an earlier age. Progression to critical vessel narrowing can be due to acute changes in complex plaques that trigger thrombus formation and lead to severe narrowing (stenosis) or complete obstruction of the artery, resulting in target organ ischemia.

Stages of Atherosclerosis Development

The initial atherosclerotic lesion is a *fatty streak*. Endothelial cell injury initiates the process of increased endothelial permeability, soon followed by movement of LDLs into the intima. These events are promoted by elevated levels of LDLs and by systemic inflammation, associated with increased levels of the acute phase protein C-reactive protein (CRP) and the cytokine tumor necrosis factor-α (TNF-α). Upregulation of endothelial adhesion molecules recruits monocytes to the intima, where they differentiate into macrophages and they begin to phagocytose LDLs.

Plaque growth begins with recruitment of additional inflammatory cells. T lymphocytes, dendritic cells, platelets, and mast cells are recruited in response to inflammatory signals such as macrophage- and T-lymphocyte–secreted cytokines. Cholesterol accumulation continues to swell the evolving lesion, giving it a fatty appearance, but without elevation and encroachment on the vessel lumen.

Recruitment of vascular smooth muscle (VSM) cells initiates the next phase of plaque growth. VSM cells invade the intima and become activated to proliferate and produce extracellular matrix, increasing the intima-media thickness (IMT). VSM cells produce fibrous cap over the plaque, beneath which inflammatory interactions and cholesterol deposition continues.

After months and years of growth, many of the foam cells die, leaving behind cholesterol crystals and inflammatory debris. The necrotic plaque core is highly thrombogenic but is initially covered by a fibrous cap and endothelial cells that keep blood from coming in contact with it. This is called the *complex plaque* (or atheroma) stage that causes vascular lumen narrowing. IMT and vascular calcification can be measured clinically as indicators of atherosclerotic progression.

Cells and mediators of atherosclerosis are outlined in **Box 9.1** and the accompanying **Figure 9.9**.

Fate of Atherosclerotic Plaques

Endothelial cells overlying the plaque are highly dysfunctional, with diminished synthesis of nitric oxide and prostacyclin (PGI$_2$). These factors normally cause vasodilation, as well as inhibit platelet aggregation, so their diminished production sets the stage for *thrombus formation*. As the plaque enlarges, the artery's own blood vessels that supply the vascular wall (vasa vasorum) may grow into the plaque (neovascularization). Plaques can develop internal hemorrhages from these blood vessels, causing rapid expansion of the plaque and more severe narrowing of the lumen.

Depending on the size of the inflammatory lipid core and the thickness of the fibrous cap, plaques can be divided into stabilized or vulnerable plaque categories. Vulnerable plaques are more likely to rupture, allowing the thrombogenic lipid core to come in contact with blood. This, in turn, causes the rapid formation of a large thrombus that can completely occlude the artery, resulting in infarction. Ruptured plaques can heal with fibrosis, leading to a very narrow lumen that causes critical stenosis (with clinical symptoms even at rest). If thrombus formation is avoided, plaque rupture can cause cholesterol crystal embolization of smaller downstream arteries.

Stages of Plaque Growth and Vessel Narrowing

The initial stages of plaque growth swelling the intima is accompanied by an increase in vessel outer diameter (**Figure 9.10**). Thus, the size of the vessel lumen is preserved and the patient is asymptomatic. This compensation is most effective at mild to

BOX 9.1
Cells and Mediators of Atherosclerosis

1. *Fatty streak initiation:* Endothelial cell (EC) injury permits low density lipoprotein (LDL) particles to migrate from the blood to the subendothelial layer (intima). This is promoted by increased levels of LDL, acute phase proteins (e.g., CRP), and inflammatory cytokines such as TNF-α.

2. *Local inflammatory mediator generation:* Endothelial cells upregulate adhesion molecules (Adh), promoting recruitment of monocytes (Mon). Monocytes differentiate into macrophages (Mac) and continue production of cytokines and reactive oxygen species (ROS). LDL particles undergo oxidation, leading to modified lipoproteins (MLp).

3. *Inflammatory cells are recruited and activated:*
   - Mac upregulate scavenger receptors and ingest MLp, becoming immobilized foam cells (FC).
   - Platelets (Pl), T lymphocytes (TLy), Dendritic cells (DC) and mast cells are recruited into the growing plaque, producing their own inflammatory mediators and cytokines.

4. *Smooth muscle cells (SMCs) are recruited to the intima:* SMCs produce extracellular matrix (ECM), including proteins like collagen that contribute to plaque growth and stiffness. SMC proliferation swells the bulk of the plaque and forms a fibrous cap.

5. *Growth of complex plaque:* Continuation of the above processes promotes plaque growth. Within the plaque, some cells are dying by apoptosis even as others are proliferating. Death of foam cells leaves cholesterol crystals (cc), apoptotic cells contribute inflammatory debris, and calcification cores (Ca) harden the plaque.

6. *Thrombogenic potential:* Platelets are recruited to the inflammatory lesion, and overlying endothelial cells lose their anti-platelet characteristics. Platelet adherence and activation can promote thrombus formation.

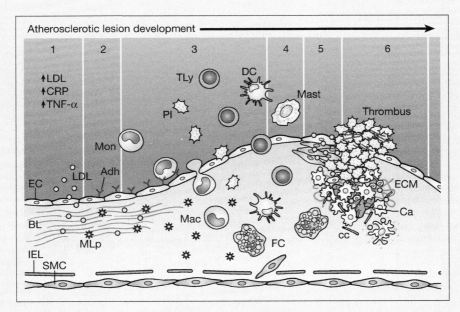

FIGURE 9.9 Cells and mediators implicated in progression of atherosclerosis. BL, basal lamina; cc, cholesterol crystal; CRP, C-reactive protein; DC, dendritic cell; EC, endothelial cell; ECM, extracellular matrix; FC, foam cell; IEL, internal elastic lamina; LDL, low-density lipoprotein; Mac, macrophage; MLp, modified lipoproteins; Mon, monocyte; Pl, platelet; SMC, smooth muscle cell; TLy, T lymphocyte; TNF-α, tumor necrosis factor alpha.

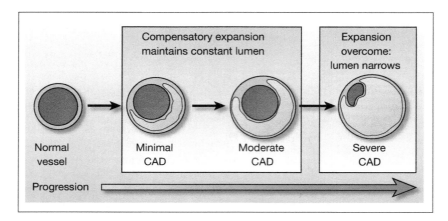

FIGURE 9.10 Progression of vessel enlargement in atherosclerosis. Expansion of the vessel compensates for narrowing of the lumen by plaque.
CAD, coronary artery disease.

moderate stages of coronary artery disease (CAD), but as lesions progress, they occlude ever greater percentages of the lumen.

Plaque Growth and Aneurysm Formation

A vascular aneurysm may develop just downstream from a large atherosclerotic plaque. This is most common in the abdominal aorta where the vascular wall supply is less developed compared with the thoracic aorta. Narrowing due to the atherosclerotic plaque changes hemodynamic factors, causing turbulent flow just behind the plaque. As the vascular wall stretches, it weakens and the aneurysm starts to form, causing increased vascular diameter. This leads to further changes in hemodynamic forces that increase wall tension, which in turn causes the aneurysm to progressively grow and eventually rupture, creating an acute emergency (**Figure 9.11**).

Risk Factors for Atherosclerosis

Population studies have identified several factors associated with ASCVD development.[4] **Table 9.1** lists major known risk factors for atherosclerosis that are often divided into modifiable and nonmodifiable categories. A variety of risk calculators for clinical use allow providers to enter data to calculate a patient's 10-year risk of a cardiovascular event and to guide interventions targeting lifestyle modifications and lipid levels. Family history and genetic risk factors continue to be identified, including diseases that cause elevated blood lipid levels, especially LDL cholesterol. Ongoing research is uncovering the mechanisms by which the clinically identified risk factors contribute to endothelial cell injury and initiation of atherosclerosis.

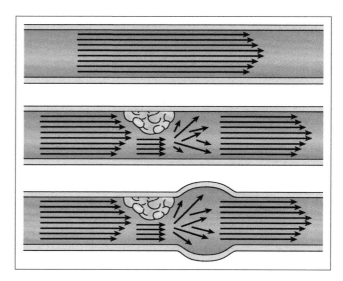

FIGURE 9.11 Aneurysm formation behind an atherosclerotic plaque is promoted by hemodynamic factors (increased velocity, turbulent flow, increased lateral pressure, and increased wall tension).

TABLE 9.1 Major Risk Factors for Atherosclerosis

Nonmodifiable	Modifiable
Older age	Elevated total and LDL cholesterol
Male sex	
Race/ethnicity	Decreased HDL cholesterol
Family history	Hypertension
	Cigarette smoking
	Diabetes

HDL, high-density lipoprotein; LDL, low-density lipoprotein.

Endothelial Vulnerability and Risk Factors Contributing to Atherosclerotic Plaque Development

Endothelial Vulnerability

The endothelium plays a critical role in maintaining vascular health in all blood vessels. The healthy endothelium secretes various substances, most importantly nitric oxide, which is vital in maintaining normal vascular endothelial and smooth muscle cell function and inhibiting platelet adhesion. Healthy endothelial cells are impermeable to large molecules (such as lipoproteins, LDL) and provide an intact lining layer that protects the vascular wall. Normal endothelial cells are also smooth and present a surface that does not support adhesion of leukocytes or thrombus formation. Damaging forces, including altered shear stress, local turbulent flow, hypertension, smoking, inflammation, dyslipidemia, and hyperglycemia, contribute to early stages of endothelial injury and activation.

Once cells are activated, the endothelial barrier is breached, allowing LDL particles to enter and accumulate in the intima. In addition, activated endothelial cells express adhesion molecules that allow leukocytes (monocytes initially) to enter the vascular wall and phagocytose LDL particles, mounting an inflammatory response that plays a fundamental role in the development of complex atherosclerotic plaques (refer to Box 9.1, earlier).

Dyslipidemia: Altered Blood Lipoprotein Levels

LDL normally contributes to homeostasis by serving as the major source of cholesterol for tissues such as steroid hormone–producing cells (see Chapter 2, Chemical and Biochemical Foundations, Table 2.2). However, as endothelial damage occurs, LDL molecules enter the vascular wall and become trapped there by interacting with the extracellular matrix of the intima. This LDL deposition is a critical step in initiating atherosclerosis. Clinically, risk increases progressively with **dyslipidemia**, characterized by high levels of LDL cholesterol, elevated VLDL (triglyceride), low levels of HDL cholesterol or some combination of these findings. Rare genetic disorders that produce extreme LDL levels (such as familial hypercholesterolemia [FH]) greatly accelerate atherogenesis. High-density lipoprotein (HDL) normally picks up cholesterol from tissues and returns it to the liver for disposal. Having lower levels of HDL cholesterol increases the risk for atherosclerosis.

Hypertension

As blood pressure increases, hydrostatic pressure perpendicular to the vascular wall and shear stress parallel to the vascular wall both increase, predisposing to endothelial injury and atherosclerosis.

Smoking

Epidemiological studies link smoking to development of atherosclerosis, and mechanistic studies have provided some links between the two. These include increased oxidative stress, inflammatory reactions to inhaled particulate matter, increased vascular constriction and reactivity, and hypercoagulability.

Diabetes Mellitus

Atherosclerotic macrovascular diseases are among the most common complications of type 1 and type 2 diabetes mellitus. Hyperglycemia is often accompanied by dyslipidemia, due to increased lipid production, with increased triglyceride and cholesterol levels, including LDL cholesterol. Chronically elevated glucose levels contribute to abnormal glycosylation of circulating and tissue proteins. Nonenzymatic addition of glucose to proteins fosters later cross-linking and formation of advanced glycation end products that promote inflammatory responses and abnormal tissue function.

Interactions Among Risk Factors

The **metabolic syndrome** refers to a constellation of findings that tend to have a high rate of comorbidity and association with cardiovascular disease. Guidelines for diagnosis were developed by the National Cholesterol Education Program Adult Treatment Panel III and were updated by the AHA. Metabolic syndrome is diagnosed in people having three or more of the following findings:

- Waist circumference >102 cm (40 in.) in men or >88 cm (35 in.) in women
- Blood triglycerides ≥150 mg/dL
- HDL cholesterol <40 mg/dL in men or 50 mg/dL in women
- Blood pressure ≥130/85 mm Hg or taking medication for hypertension
- Fasting plasma glucose level ≥110 mg/dL or taking medication for diabetes mellitus[5]

The metabolic syndrome combination of central obesity, dyslipidemia, hypertension, and diabetes or insulin resistance is particularly significant for atherosclerosis development.

Inflammation

LDL deposition and monocyte recruitment and activation are early consequences of endothelial injury and activation. As in acute inflammation, monocyte attachment to damaged endothelium is followed by movement, in this case to the intima, and differentiation into macrophages. Macrophages begin to ingest (phagocytose) LDL molecules. ROS are generated, causing LDL oxidation. As macrophages detect oxidized LDL, they begin to express scavenger receptors that increase phagocytosis of LDL. As they accumulate cholesterol, macrophages turn into foam cells and can no longer leave the now growing atherosclerotic plaque. Macrophages secrete cytokines that recruit T lymphocytes (T cells) to the plaque. T cells further perpetuate the inflammatory process (see Figure 9.10). The metabolic syndrome is associated with increased chronic inflammation that likely contributes to atherosclerosis progression. In addition, acute inflammation in older adults with high cardiovascular risk can precipitate myocardial infarction. For example, myocardial infarction incidence increases after influenza and upper respiratory infections.[6]

Genetics of Familial Hypercholesterolemia

Familial hypercholesterolemia is an autosomal dominant disorder that is associated with lifelong elevated levels of LDL cholesterol. Prevalence varies depending on ethnicity and ancestral background, but the heterozygous form (HeFH) may affect as many as one in 200 to 250 persons in the United States. The homozygous form (HoFH) is very rare and affects less than one in 250,000 people.[7] There are a variety of responsible gene mutations, but the most common is a defect in the LDL receptor that reduces its ability to bind circulating LDL particles and to remove them into cells by receptor-mediated endocytosis. The condition is considered to exhibit a *gene dosage* effect, in which the consequences of homozygous mutations are much more severe than those of the heterozygous genotype.

For most people with HeFH, cholesterol levels are elevated the throughout life and need to be managed with statin drugs and other cholesterol-lowering medications. Individuals with HoFH are often recognized early, based on family history and the physical findings of xanthomas (lipid growths) on tendons and fingers, and arcus corneae, a gray ring around the cornea. These individuals have very high LDL cholesterol levels unless they are aggressively treated. Myocardial infarction can occur in their 20s or 30s without treatment.

A related genetic disorder that promotes hypercholesterolemia is a gain-of-function mutation in the gene coding for proprotein convertase subtilisin/kexin 9 (PCSK9), a protein that reduces the number of LDL receptors on cells. Clinical genetic studies indicated that individuals with elevated PCSK9 activity have higher LDL levels, and those with reduced PCSK9 activity have lower LDL levels and greatly reduced rates of atherosclerotic diseases. These findings led to the development of a new class of monoclonal antibody drugs, PCSK9 inhibitors, for use in the management of hypercholesterolemia that is not adequately managed by high-dose statin and other therapies.[7]

Risk Reduction

Acknowledging the role of modifiable lifestyle factors in altering cardiovascular risk, the AHA has identified seven steps for reducing risk (Box 9.2). The AHA encourages all clinicians to use online cardiovascular risk calculators to assess their patients' risk, and to promote these healthy lifestyle changes as the first-line management of atherosclerosis risk, before starting and during drug therapy (usually involving statin drugs).[8]

Atherosclerotic Peripheral Arterial Disease

Peripheral arterial disease (PAD) is a disorder caused by stenosis or occlusion of the aorta or arteries of the limbs. Atherosclerosis is the leading cause of PAD in patients older than 40 years of age, with highest incidence in the sixth and seventh decades of life.[5] PAD is most common in the legs and can result in vascular rupture, dissection, and thromboembolism.

Many patients are asymptomatic or may have slow or impaired gait. The most common presentation is intermittent claudication—pain, ache, cramp, or fatigue of muscles that occurs during exercise and is relieved by rest. Intermittent claudication always presents below the site of stenosis. Physical examination typically finds diminished pulses below the stenosis. The ankle–brachial index (ABI) is based on bilateral

---

BOX 9.2
Reducing Risk: The American Heart Association's Emphasis on Health Promotion[8]

- Managing blood pressure with a goal of systolic <120 mm Hg and diastolic <80 mm Hg

- Controlling cholesterol through lifestyle changes and medications as necessary

- Reducing blood glucose level

- Increasing physical activity

- Eating a healthy diet (reasonable portions; a variety of fruits, vegetables, whole grains, poultry, and fish; and avoiding added salt, sugar, and saturated and trans fats)

- Losing weight

- Stopping smoking

measurements of systolic blood pressure made while the person is in the supine position.

- Brachial systolic pressure is measured using standard techniques from both right and left arms, and using the highest systolic pressure.
- Ankle systolic pressure is measured using a standard cuff and Doppler flow probe to detect systolic blood flow from both posterior tibial (PT) and dorsalis pedis (DP) arteries, and taking the highest value from the right and left sides.

> *Right ABI* = higher of the right ankle pressure (PT or DP)/higher arm pressure
>
> *Left ABI* = higher of the left ankle pressure (PT or DP)/higher arm pressure

The lower of the right or left ABI is then the overall ABI

- ABI >0.9 is normal; ABI <0.9 suggests PAD; and ABI <0.5 suggests severe stenosis.

The risk factors for PAD are the same as those for atherosclerosis, with diabetes mellitus and smoking being particularly important.

Thought Questions

1. What are the structural and functional characteristics of large and medium-sized arteries?

2. How do the biophysics of flow in large arteries contribute to the tendency to develop atherosclerotic plaque and form aneurysms?

3. What is known of the connection between atherosclerosis risk factors and the formation of atherosclerotic plaque?

PROPERTIES AND DISORDERS OF ARTERIOLES

OVERVIEW OF ARTERIOLE STRUCTURE AND FUNCTION

Arterioles provide resistance to support blood pressure, while regulating flow to tissues. The pressure inside each vascular segment serves a physiological purpose and is maintained within a relatively narrow range. Normal arterial pressure is critical for driving blood flow through the series of narrowing vessels and for ensuring normal perfusion pressure to all organs. The upright posture of humans creates a gravitational pull on the columns of blood held within the vascular system such that vascular pressures are higher below the heart, and lower above it. For an adult man of average height, having a systolic pressure of 120 mm Hg at the level of the heart, this means that in the upright position systolic pressure will be about 70 mm Hg at the brain and about 190 mm Hg at the feet. A constant supply of oxygen to the brain is essential for maintaining consciousness, and arterial pressure ensures adequate flow while standing. For this reason, the arteriolar resistance limiting outflow and maintaining arterial pressure is central to upright posture and normal ambulatory function.

After flowing through large, then small arteries, blood arrives at the arterioles. The arterioles have a relatively small diameter and thin walls consisting of intima, media containing smooth muscle layers that are one to two cells thick, and a thin adventitia. The lumen of an arteriole averages 30 μm in diameter. Arterioles are abundantly innervated by the sympathetic nervous system, and their smooth muscle cells display G protein–coupled and other receptors for norepinephrine as well as circulating and locally generated mediators. Mediators that cause smooth muscle contraction produce *vasoconstriction*, and mediators that cause smooth muscle relaxation produce *vasodilation*. Regulation of this VSM by circulating substances can cause whole-body changes in vascular resistance, thus altering blood pressure. In addition, VSM is under local control that regulates tissue perfusion according to need or in response to local tissue damage and inflammation. Disorders of these resistance vessels include *hypertension*, a state of inappropriately high vascular resistance, and *shock*, a state of inappropriately low vascular resistance.

Biophysical Determinants of Blood Pressure

Mean arterial pressure (MAP) is the average driving pressure in the circulatory system. MAP can be estimated from systolic (SBP) and diastolic (DBP) blood pressures as follows:

$$MAP = DBP + \frac{(SBP - DBP)}{3}$$

assuming a typical cardiac cycle (total length = 1/3 systole + 2/3 diastole; **Figure 9.12**).

Ohm's law, originally developed to explain current flow in electrical circuits, has been applied to the circulatory system to state the relationship of flow (*F*)—in this case, cardiac output, driving pressure (*P*), and vascular resistance (*R*):

$$F = \frac{P}{R}$$

Vascular resistance refers to the tendency of the branching and narrowing blood vessels to hinder blood flow (**Figure 9.13**).

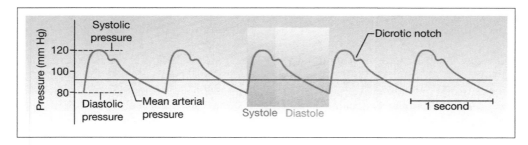

FIGURE 9.12 Arterial blood pressure. Typical arterial pressure waves showing the peak (systolic) and trough (diastolic) pressures. The dicrotic notch indicates a brief increase of pressure when the aortic valve closes and pressure rebounds against the now closed valve. At resting heart rate, about one third of the time is spent in systole, and two third in diastole. Systolic pressure is influenced by cardiac stroke volume and pressure and by properties of the aorta and large arteries. Diastolic pressure is influenced by properties of the aorta and large arteries, as well as by vascular resistance.
Source: From PhysiologyWeb at http://www.physiologyweb.com/calculators/figs/aterial_pressure_fluctuations_jpg_gp5wnM4ioge6G2Rr68jaW0DCmB9bG9QZ.html.

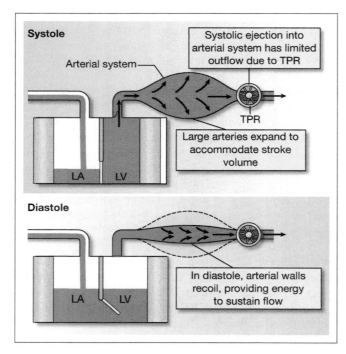

FIGURE 9.13 TPR hinders blood flow from the LV and is a major determinant of blood pressure.
LA, left atrium; LV, left ventricle; TPR, total peripheral resistance.

Technically, the pressure gradient driving flow in the systemic circulation is MAP minus central venous pressure (CVP), but because CVP is normally much lower than MAP it is often not included in calculations. Applying Ohm's law to the entire systemic circulation, the equation then becomes:

$$CO = \frac{MAP}{TPR}$$

or, rearranged to show the determinants of pressure,

$$MAP = CO \times TPR$$

where

CO = cardiac output (total flow in the systemic circulation)
MAP = mean arterial pressure
TPR = total peripheral resistance

To summarize (**Figure 9.14**), arterial blood pressure (MAP) is primarily determined by two factors: cardiac output and peripheral resistance. Although influenced by aortic pressure (afterload), cardiac output is primarily determined by cardiac factors (as described in Chapter 10, Heart) and constitutes the total body blood flow in the systemic vascular circuit. The distribution of cardiac output between the parallel vascular beds is further regulated by local changes in vascular resistance. The sum of these resistances is total peripheral resistance.

Determinants of Vascular Resistance

The Poiseuille–Hagen formula relates flow and pressure to the individual factors that determine vascular resistance:

$$F = \left(P_A - P_B\right) \times \left(\frac{\pi}{8}\right) \times \left(\frac{1}{\eta}\right) \times \left(\frac{r^4}{L}\right)$$

where

F = flow
$P_A - P_B$ = pressure difference between the two ends of the tube
η = viscosity of blood
r = radius of the tube
L = length of the tube

Rearranging the equation, the Poiseuille–Hagen formula shows the determinants of resistance (R) as:

$$R = \frac{8\eta L}{\pi r^4}$$

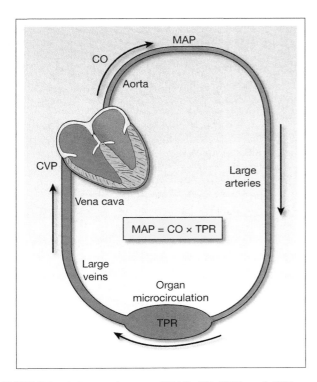

FIGURE 9.14 Determinants of MAP: CO, TPR, and CVP. CO, cardiac output; CVP, central venous pressure; MAP, mean arterial pressure; TPR, total peripheral resistance.

Because 8 and π are constants, the primary determinants of vascular resistance are the following:

- Length of the blood vessel (L): Under normal conditions, this changes very little once a person is fully grown.
- Viscosity of blood (η): Blood viscosity decreases in anemia and increases in polycythemia, but otherwise stays relatively constant and stable under standard ambulatory conditions.
- Radius of the vessel (r): This is the main factor controlling vascular resistance on a minute-to-minute basis. Resistance is directly related to the radius raised to the fourth power, so even small changes in vascular radius translate to large inverse changes in resistance. For example, increasing the radius (vasodilation) by just 19% would cause a 50% drop in resistance. On the other hand, reducing the radius by just 16% doubles the resistance.

Distribution of Vascular Resistance in the Systemic Circulation

The general principle in the systemic circulation is that pressure is highest in the left ventricle during cardiac ejection (systole) and drops throughout the cardiovascular circuit as vascular resistance (**Figure 9.15**) hinders flow of blood. Flow will only

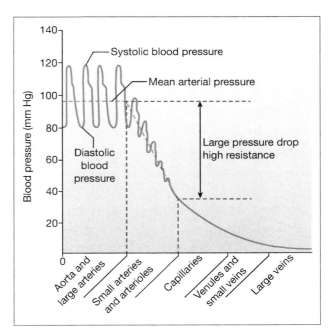

FIGURE 9.15 Vascular pressures in the systemic circulation. Vascular pressures drop throughout the systemic circuit, and the difference between the initial pressure in the aorta and the final pressure in the right atrium is the force driving blood flow through the circuit. The greatest pressure drop is at the level of arterioles, as they are the sites of greatest resistance. Pulsatility also ends at the arterioles. Pressure in the capillaries determines fluid movement across the capillary walls.
Source: From Kibble JD, Halsey CR. *The Big Picture: Medical Physiology.* Fig. 4-28, McGraw-Hill.

occur from an area of higher pressure to an area of lower pressure.

Blood pressure is pulsatile in the left ventricle (120/0 mm Hg) owing to the intermittent nature of the cardiac pump. Pressure remains pulsatile in the aorta (120/70 mm Hg), but the pressure changes are smaller because of the elastic recoil of the aorta and large arteries that help to maintain diastolic pressure and blood flow. Pulse pressure (systolic pressure minus diastolic pressure) increases slightly in the large arteries, then decreases in small arteries. The greatest drop in MAP and pulse pressure occurs at the arterioles, as they represent the greatest amount (~70%) of resistance in the systemic circulation. At the level of the capillaries, pulsations are gone and the pressure continues to drop. Pressure in the largest veins is very low, just above that of the right atrial pressure.

Because most of the vascular resistance is at the level of the arterioles, these vascular segments are in a unique position to regulate blood pressure in both the arteries (systemic blood pressure) and the capillaries downstream from the arterioles. As illustrated in **Figure 9.16**, increasing arteriolar resistance by arteriolar constriction (analogous to stepping on a garden hose) will increase

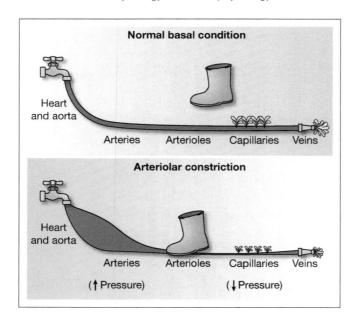

FIGURE 9.16 Dual role of arterioles. The resistance of arterioles regulates blood pressure in the aorta and large arteries, while also regulating tissue blood flow at the level of capillaries. Top panel shows normal basal condition; bottom panel represents arteriolar constriction.

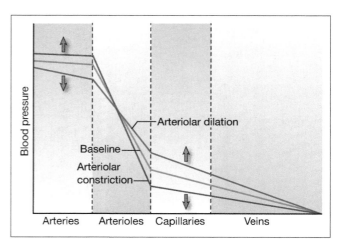

FIGURE 9.17 Effect of changes in arteriolar resistance on vascular pressures. *Green line*, normal baseline condition; *blue line*, decreased arteriolar resistance due to vasodilation; and *purple line*, increased arteriolar resistance due to vasoconstriction. Arrows show the direction of vascular pressure changes.
Source: From Mohrman DE, Heller LJ. *Cardiovascular Physiology*. 8th ed. Fig. 6-7. McGraw Hill Education; 2014.

pressure in the arteries (the hose segment between the faucet and the boot), but decrease pressure in the capillaries following those arterioles (the hose segment after the boot). In this scenario, arterial pressure increases due to the increase in vascular resistance, while capillary pressure decreases, because increased arteriolar resistance causes a greater pressure drop at the level of the arterioles. In contrast, vasodilation reduces the arteriolar resistance. Decreased total peripheral resistance reduces arterial pressure while increasing pressure reaching the capillaries (**Figure 9.17**).

Under normal conditions arteriolar resistance is regulated by local and systemic factors that balance metabolic demands of individual organs with whole-body requirements. Shifts of flow between vascular beds and changes of cardiac output can adapt cardiovascular function to changing need. Global changes in flow come into play during intense exercise, during which cardiac output can increase up to five times normal (see **Figure 9.2**, earlier). Muscle and cardiac flow increases four- or five-fold as a percentage of cardiac output, with absolute flow to brain, gastrointestinal tract, and kidney showing stable values or small increases or decreases. This capacity underlies the extraordinary performance of elite athletes and the improved performance of anyone engaged in regular aerobic physical activity.

Under pathological conditions such as hypertension, arteriolar resistance may be too high, causing an elevation in blood pressure and the potential for reduced tissue perfusion due to decreased capillary pressure and flow. In contrast, decreased arteriolar resistance,

as in shock, can cause a dangerous decrease in arterial blood pressure and the potential for loss of fluid into the tissues due to increased capillary pressure and flow (see **Figure 9.17**).

Thought Questions

4. What is the overall role of peripheral resistance exerted by arterioles in maintaining homeostasis of the circulatory system?

5. Explain the effect of temporary generalized vasoconstriction on mean arterial pressure and on the pressure in capillaries.

REGULATION OF BLOOD PRESSURE

Overview of Blood Pressure Control

Blood pressure is controlled by short-term (minute to minute) and long-term (hours to days) mechanisms (**Figure 9.18**). Short-term mechanisms are primarily neural (baroreceptor reflex by the autonomic nervous system), humoral (circulating mediators such as angiotensin II and vasopressin), and local mediators such as nitric oxide, bradykinin, endothelin, and prostaglandins. These mechanisms alter vascular resistance by changing arteriolar diameter, and cardiac output by changing heart rate, contractility, and preload.

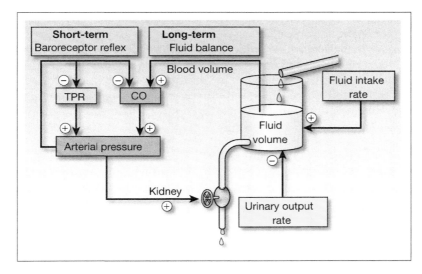

FIGURE 9.18 Long-term versus short-term blood pressure regulation. Short-term control of blood pressure is accomplished by the rapid activity of the baroreflex—a neural mechanism relaying the signal of increased or decreased blood pressure to the brainstem, leading to appropriate adjustments of parasympathetic and sympathetic cardiovascular outflow. Long-term control of blood pressure over hours and days is accomplished by sensors that detect circulating blood volume and blood pressure and adjust fluid intake and renal fluid excretion to alter total body fluid volume.
CO, cardiac output; TPR, total peripheral resistance.
Source: From Raff H, Levitzky M. *Medical Physiology: A Systems Approach*. Fig. 29-5. McGraw-Hill LANGE.

Long-term mechanisms are primarily endocrine and include hormones that affect fluid balance, such as aldosterone (secreted by the adrenal cortex), vasopressin (secreted by the posterior pituitary), and natriuretic peptides (secreted by the heart). These mechanisms alter blood volume by modulating fluid output (renal sodium and water excretion) as well as fluid intake (via the hypothalamic sodium and water appetite).

Blood pressure is regulated at four anatomical sites:

1. *Resistance arterioles:* Arterioles represent the primary site of vascular resistance maintaining normal blood pressure. Their radius is directly regulated by intrinsic mechanisms, including action potential activity that opens voltage-gated calcium channels. Extrinsic regulation is by neural and humoral vasoconstrictor and vasodilator substances. Many antihypertensive drugs work by altering cellular mechanisms of contraction and relaxation of VSM.

2. *Capacitance venules:* Veins and venules can alter cardiac output and blood pressure by regulating venous return (amount of blood returned to the right atrium). Normally, veins and venules store a substantial portion of blood volume (capacitance function). During times of hypotension and hypovolemia, the sympathetic nervous system stimulates venoconstriction, increasing venous return (preload) and restoring cardiac output.

3. *Heart pump output:* Cardiac output = heart rate × stroke volume, so increasing heart rate or stroke volume, or both, will increase cardiac output and thus blood pressure (see Chapter 10, Heart).

4. *Kidneys (regulation of fluid volume):* Blood volume is primarily regulated by the kidneys (see Chapter 12, Kidneys), which conserve sodium (regulated by aldosterone and natriuretic peptides) and water (regulated by vasopressin, also known as antidiuretic hormone).

Maintenance of Vascular Smooth Muscle Tone: Intrinsic, Neural, and Local Mechanisms

VSM is in a constant state of moderate contraction, termed *vascular tone*, due to intrinsic VSM properties. Action potentials open voltage-gated calcium channels, initiating smooth muscle cell contraction. Once contracted, the actin–myosin cross-bridges do not completely relax; rather, they stay in a state of moderate contraction. This state is supported by low levels of tonic firing of sympathetic vasoconstrictor fibers. These mechanisms are important for overall blood pressure maintenance. Picture what would happen if you opened the taps on all of the sinks and showers in a house, while simultaneously running the dishwasher and washing machine—there would be very low water pressure! In a similar way, dilation of all of the resistance vessels throughout the body simultaneously could precipitously drop arterial pressure, as described later in relation to shock. Pathophysiologically, generalized loss of sympathetic vasoconstrictor tone can occur after a high spinal cord injury that disrupts excitatory pathways from the medulla to spinal sympathetic neurons, resulting in neurogenic shock and hypotension.

In summary, there is a basal state of vascular and sympathetically supported vasoconstriction that maintains arterial pressure. Short-term homeostasis of blood pressure involves increases and decreases of sympathetic nervous system vasoconstrictor activity to meet the demands of the body, while long-term blood pressure homeostasis is maintained by renal regulation of body sodium and water balance.

Concurrent with the intrinsic and sympathetic maintenance of vasoconstrictor tone, there is a balancing vasodilator influence of nitric oxide. Normal healthy endothelial cells forming the inner layer of all blood vessels express the enzyme nitric oxide synthase (NOS). As previously noted, arteries are subjected to shear stress by the relatively high pressure and movement of blood along their length. This moderate shear stress promotes production of nitric oxide gas, which diffuses past the intima to reach the media, the smooth muscle layer in the blood vessel wall. Nitric oxide induces vasodilation. Normal homeostasis, then, involves a balance of tonic vasoconstriction mediated by VSM and sympathetic tone, with nitric oxide–mediated vasodilation. The VSM cell integrates these two signals and those of other circulating and local mediators in setting the level of vascular resistance.

The Cellular Basis of Vascular Smooth Muscle Control

Resistance in the vascular system is regulated at the level of VSM cells. As noted in Chapter 4, Cell Physiology and Pathophysiology, factors that increase smooth muscle calcium concentration produce cell contraction and, thus, vasoconstriction. The intracellular pathway is via calcium/calmodulin activation of myosin light-chain kinase (MLCK). Some mechanisms intrinsic to the VSM cells are involved in ongoing vasoconstriction. For example, membrane voltage-gated calcium channels are one source of calcium entry to support contraction. As electrically excitable cells, smooth muscle cells can have action potentials that open these voltage-gated calcium channels and cause contraction. Vascular calcium channels are the target of one class of antihypertensive medications: calcium channel blockers.

Vascular Autoregulation

The mechanism of autoregulation is also important in controlling blood flow to many organs, most notably the brain, kidneys, and heart. Autoregulation is defined as the ability of an organ to maintain constant blood flow over a range of perfusion pressures. For example, an abrupt decrease in blood pressure that would normally decrease organ blood flow elicits compensatory vasodilation, restoring flow toward normal. Conversely, an abrupt increase in blood pressure that would normally increase

organ blood flow elicits compensatory vasoconstriction that restores blood flow to normal (**Figure 9.19**).

Autoregulation has been explained by the *myogenic hypothesis* in which the acute pressure-induced stretch of the arterial and arteriolar walls stimulates immediate constriction, possibly through stretch-activated membrane ion channels, while a rapid pressure drop elicits vasodilation. The *metabolic hypothesis* of autoregulation posits that decreased pressure and flow result in buildup of vasodilator metabolites that produce vasodilation, while increased pressure and flow wash out vasodilator metabolites, producing vasoconstriction. Finally, the organs with the highest degree of autoregulation, the kidneys and the brain, have additional tissue-specific mechanisms maintaining relatively constant flow despite varying perfusion pressures.

Extrinsic Vascular Regulation

A major extrinsic influence on vasoconstriction and vasodilation is the presence of receptors on VSM that allow responses to circulating and local mediators. Receptors that cause vasoconstriction are linked to G_q and phospholipase C activation. This leads to IP_3 generation and release of calcium from intracellular stores. VSM relaxation, and thus vasodilation, occurs through inhibition of MLCK and activation of myosin light-chain phosphatase (MLCP). G_s-coupled receptors increase intracellular cyclic adenosine monophosphate (cAMP), which inhibits MLCK. Mediators that increase cyclic guanosine monophosphate (cGMP) activate MLCP. **Table 9.2** summarizes the major mediators of vasoconstriction and vasodilation and their intracellular mechanisms.

Neural and Endocrine Mediators That Regulate Vascular Smooth Muscle Contraction and Arteriolar Resistance

Five key mediators help to regulate VSM contraction and arteriolar resistance:

1. *Norepinephrine* is the sympathetic neurotransmitter mediating tonic vasoconstriction. This vital mechanism maintains normal blood pressure, especially in an upright position. Drugs that block α_1-adrenergic receptors can cause very low blood pressure and severe postural (orthostatic) hypotension. Hypotension and hypovolemia can increase firing of sympathetic venoconstrictor fibers (also α_1 mediated) that contract VSM cells of the veins, increasing venous return and supporting cardiac output.

2. *The renin-angiotensin-aldosterone system (RAAS)* has multiple effects that support blood volume and blood pressure through its actions in the kidneys and on VSM cells (**Figure 9.20**). Low blood pressure is detected by the juxtaglomerular apparatus of the nephrons of the kidney, and renin is secreted by granular cells in the walls of the afferent arterioles. Renin is an enzyme that cleaves the precursor protein angiotensinogen, releasing the decapeptide angiotensin I. Angiotensin I circulates through the systemic and

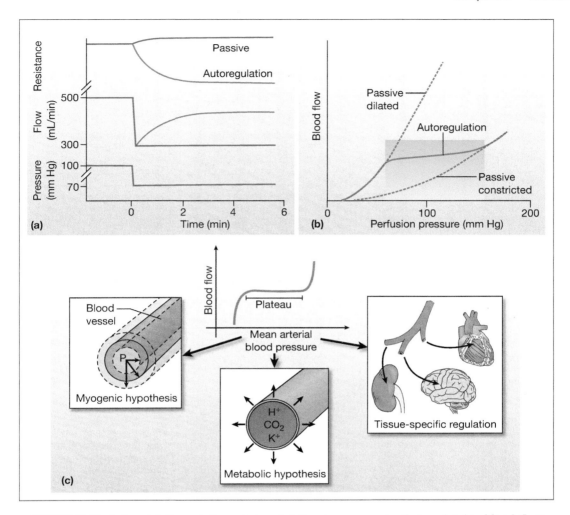

FIGURE 9.19 Autoregulation of flow. Autoregulation is a property that maintains blood flow relatively constant over a wide range of perfusion pressures. **(a)** With autoregulation present, a decrease in pressure is compensated for by a decrease in resistance, restoring flow relative to the condition of passive responses to the pressure change. **(b)** A system with autoregulation can vary between dilated vessels and constricted vessels to maintain a relatively constant flow despite altered perfusion pressures. **(c)** Mechanisms that can account for autoregulation include myogenic responses and control by tissue metabolism.
Source: (a) From Klabunde RE. *Cardiovascular Physiology Concepts.* 2nd ed. Lippincott; 2012. (b) From Rivera-Lara L, et al. Cerebral autoregulation-oriented therapy at the bedside: a comprehensive review. *Anesthesiology.* June 2017;126:1187–1199. http://anesthesiology.pubs. asahq.org/article.aspx?articleid=2618829.

pulmonary circulations and is converted to angiotensin II by angiotensin-converting enzyme (ACE), which is particularly abundant in the lungs. Angiotensin II is a vasoconstrictor at vascular AT_1 receptors and is also the key regulator of adrenal aldosterone secretion. Aldosterone, the final mediator of the RAAS, stimulates sodium conservation through its actions on the distal nephron. Angiotensin II acts within the hypothalamus to stimulate thirst, further promoting fluid acquisition and retention to support blood volume.

3. *Vasopressin (arginine vasopressin [AVP])* is a posterior pituitary hormone that regulates renal water retention and prevents whole-body hypertonicity. AVP is released in response to increased blood osmolality or by hypovolemia and hypotension. Although the vasoconstrictive effects of AVP at V_1 receptors is not always active at the normally low levels of circulating AVP, hypotension-induced increases in AVP levels activate vascular receptors and augment compensatory vasoconstriction.

4. *Epinephrine* released from the adrenal medulla in response to sympathetic nervous system stimulation is also important in blood pressure regulation. Although epinephrine primarily has cardiac effects

TABLE 9.2 Mediators and Mechanisms That Regulate Vascular Resistance

Vascular Effect	Mediator	Receptor	G Protein	Second Messenger	Type of Regulation
Constriction/ increased resistance	NE	α_1	G_q	IP_3—calcium release	Neural
	Epinephrine				Endocrine
	Angiotensin II (ATII)	AT_1			Endocrine
	Vasopressin (AVP)	V_1			
	Endothelin-1 (ET1)	ET_A			Paracrine
	Thromboxane A_2 (TXA_2)	TP			
Dilation/ decreased resistance	Epinephrine	β_2	G_s	cAMP ↑	Endocrine
	Adenosine	A_2			Paracrine
	Prostacyclin (PGI_2)	IP			
	Nitric oxide (NO)	sGC	None	cGMP ↑	Paracrine
	Atrial natriuretic peptide (ANP)	NPR (pGC)	None		Endocrine

cAMP, cyclic adenosine monophosphate; cGMP, cyclic guanosine monophosphate; IP_3, inositol triphosphate; NE, norepinephrine; pGC = particulate guanylyl cyclase; sGC, soluble guanylyl cyclase.

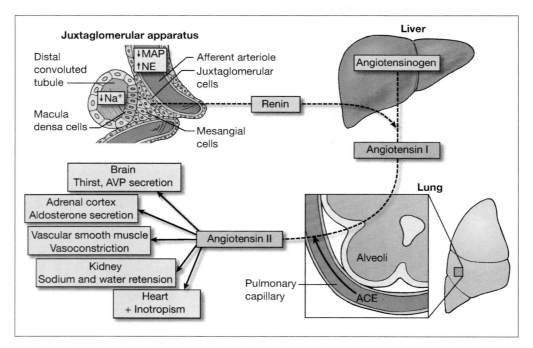

FIGURE 9.20 The renin-angiotensin-aldosterone system (RAAS). Granular cells in the wall of the kidney's afferent arterioles sense sodium (Na^+) and chloride concentration reaching the macula densa at the junction of the ascending limb of the loop of Henle and the distal convoluted tubule, and release renin if sodium and chloride levels fall. Renin circulates in the plasma, cleaving angiotensinogen produced by the liver and releasing angiotensin I. Angiotensin I is cleaved by ACE, releasing angiotensin II. Angiotensin II activates body systems of sodium conservation, water repletion, and vasoconstriction, restoring normal blood pressure and glomerular filtration.
ACE, angiotensin-converting enzyme; AVP, arginine vasopressin; MAP, mean arterial pressure; NE, norepinephrine.

(increased heart rate and contractility via β_1-adrenergic receptors on cardiac muscle cells), it can also play an important role in regulation of vascular resistance. Epinephrine can stimulate α_1-adrenergic receptors, causing vasoconstriction, although it is not as potent as norepinephrine. Epinephrine also can stimulate β_2-adrenergic receptors in skeletal muscle arterioles, causing vasodilation and increased muscle blood flow during exercise.

5. *Natriuretic peptides* are produced in the heart and other tissues, and include atrial natriuretic peptide (ANP), B-type natriuretic peptide (BNP), and a third form, C-type natriuretic peptide (CNP). ANP and BNP are the major effectors in human tissues. ANP and BNP are released from cardiac tissue when it is stretched under conditions of hypervolemia. The natriuretic peptides act on the kidneys to promote glomerular filtration and to reduce sodium reabsorption, thereby promoting excretion of sodium and water and lowering body fluid volume. This hypotensive effect is reinforced by the actions of the natriuretic peptides to promote VSM relaxation and vasodilation through natriuretic peptide receptors linked to guanylyl cyclase. BNP is inactivated by the enzyme neprilysin.

Local Mechanisms of Vascular Smooth Muscle Control
VSM is also controlled by local mechanisms that are typically subdivided by the origin of the mediators, as follows:

1. *VSM cells intrinsically respond to stretch* (due to increased blood pressure or blood volume) *by contraction* (myogenic mechanism). This response, which helps regulate renal blood flow and maintain glomerular filtration rate (GFR), is most likely mediated by stretch-gated ion channels.

2. *Endothelium-derived mediators play a vital role.* The primary endothelium-derived mediators are the vasodilators nitric oxide and prostacyclin and the vasoconstrictor endothelin-1 (ET1).

   a. Endothelium-produced nitric oxide is essential for maintaining normal blood flow during physiological conditions. Nitric oxide is produced in the endothelial cells by endothelial nitric oxide synthase (eNOS) in response to blood flow (shear stress) and receptor stimulation (acetylcholine— M_3 cholinergic receptors; histamine—H_1 receptors; bradykinin—B_2 receptors; **Figure 9.21**). These G_q protein–coupled receptors increase cytosolic calcium concentrations resulting in activation of eNOS, which produces nitric oxide gas from an amino acid precursor, L-arginine. Nitric oxide diffuses out of the endothelial cells to the underlying smooth muscle and causes relaxation by increasing cGMP production. Endothelial dysfunction is common in diabetes, hypertension, and atherosclerosis, causing decreased nitric oxide production and contributing to vascular pathology.

   b. Prostacyclin (PGI_2) is another endothelium-derived vasodilator. In endothelial cells, PGI_2 is produced from arachidonic acid by cyclooxygenase-2 (COX-2) and other enzymes. COX is inhibited by nonsteroidal anti inflammatory drugs (NSAIDs) such as aspirin, ibuprofen,

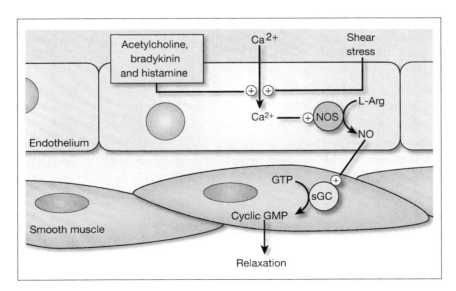

FIGURE 9.21 Endothelium-derived nitric oxide (NO) as a vasodilator. Circulating mediators and shear stress stimulate endothelial cell nitric oxide synthase (NOS) to synthesize NO, which then diffuses through the internal elastic lamina and into VSM cells, where it activates guanylyl cyclase, producing VSM relaxation and vasodilation.
GMP, guanosine monophosphate; GTP, guanosine triphosphate; L-Arg, L-arginine; sGC, soluble guanylyl cyclase; VSM, vascular smooth muscle.

and naproxen. Usually, the vasoconstrictor effect of decreased endothelial PGI_2 production (due to COX-2 blockade in the endothelium) is balanced by the vasodilator effect of decreased thromboxane A_2 (TXA_2) production in platelets (due to COX-1 inhibition). As a side effect, selective COX-2 inhibitor drugs (celecoxib) can cause ischemia, resulting in myocardial infarction or ischemic stroke in patients who are at high risk of atherosclerotic disorders.

c. ET1 is an endothelium-derived vasoconstrictor peptide. ET1 activates ET_A receptors on VSM to cause vasoconstriction. Vascular trauma releases ET1, resulting in rapid vasoconstriction that reduces blood loss from the broken vessel—the first stage in hemostasis. Under healthy physiological conditions, ET1 production is minimal. However, increased ET1 production has been implicated in the pathogenesis of primary pulmonary arterial hypertension, and ET_A receptor antagonists can be used in the management of that condition.

3. *Tissue-derived mediators are usually vasodilators.* These mediators occur or are released from tissue during increased metabolic activity (CO_2, K^+, H^+, adenosine) and are important in matching tissue blood flow to metabolic demand. In certain tissues, such as the heart, metabolic regulation dominates and overrides systemic control mechanisms.

4. *Mediators released in response to tissue inflammation and trauma include both vasodilators and vasoconstrictors.* Histamine, bradykinin, and prostaglandins (also known as eicosanoids) all contribute to the local vasodilation and increased vascular permeability that characterize the redness, swelling, and warmth of inflammation. TXA_2 released from platelets in response to activation and initiation of clotting is a vasoconstrictor, helping to reduce blood loss from a damaged vessel.

To summarize (**Figure 9.22**), arteriolar resistance is determined by the balance of local and systemic vasodilator and vasoconstrictor influences in health and disease. As discussed earlier, arterioles serve a dual role, regulating systemic blood pressure (MAP) by regulating peripheral resistance while also regulating blood flow to individual organs according to organ oxygen demand. Changes in arteriolar resistance elicit opposite changes in arterial pressure (MAP) and capillary pressure. This complex regulatory scheme continuously weighs the whole body's needs (need to maintain blood pressure to ensure blood flow to other organs) against

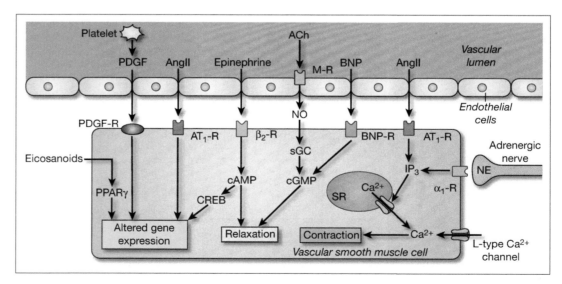

FIGURE 9.22 VSM cells integrate many signals. Calcium entry through L-type calcium channels stimulates VSM contraction, which is also modulated by several types of G protein–coupled receptors. Agents that increase intracellular calcium promote vasoconstriction, while increased cyclic nucleotides cAMP and cGMP promote vasodilation. Long-term changes in VSM gene expression account for the development of hypertrophy in the context of hypertension and vascular disease.

ACh, acetylcholine; AngII, angiotensin II; AT_1-R, angiotensin type 1 receptor; BNP, B-type natriuretic peptide; cAMP, cyclic adenosine monophosphate; cGMP, cyclic guanosine monophosphate; CREB, cyclic AMP response element-binding protein; IP_3, inositol triphosphate; M-R, muscarinic receptor; NE, norepinephrine; NO, nitric oxide; PDGF, platelet-derived growth factor; PPARγ, peroxisome proliferator-activated receptor gamma; R, receptor; SR, sarcoplasmic reticulum; VSM, vascular smooth muscle.

the metabolic demands of individual tissues and organs (need for oxygen delivery). Vasoconstrictor dominance can cause tissue ischemia (decreased capillary pressure and blood flow) and hypertension (elevated MAP due to increased resistance), whereas vasodilation can cause potentially life-threatening hypotension (distributive shock) and tissue edema. Drug classes targeting vasoconstricting and vasodilating mediators and their receptors are used extensively to manage hypertension, heart disease, and hypotensive states.

Integration of Mediators Regulating Peripheral Resistance

With so many mediators that influence VSM contraction, most of which have low but measurable blood levels at all times, how do the smooth muscle cells put all of these signals together to maintain normal blood pressure? **Table 9.3** summarizes the contributions these mediators make to blood pressure under resting conditions and in response to physiological and pathophysiological challenges.

Baroreflexes and Circulatory Control

Rapid adaptation to short-term changes in blood pressure occurs through a negative feedback system—the baroreceptor reflex that regulates autonomic outflow to the blood vessels and heart. This reflex is triggered by changes in blood pressure. Stretch-sensitive sensory endings in the carotid sinus and the aortic arch respond to increases or decreases in vessel distention. Increased pressure stretches the sensory endings, increasing their action potential firing rates. Decreased pressure relaxes the stretch on the sensory endings, decreasing their action potential firing rates. These fibers terminate in the nucleus of the tractus solitarius (NTS) in the medulla (**Figure 9.23**).

Abrupt increases of arterial pressure increase baroreceptor sensory fiber activity to the NTS. This stimulates NTS neurons that project to the parasympathetic nucleus ambiguus, resulting in rapid compensation by increased vagal outflow to the sinoatrial node that slows heart rate. NTS neurons also project to caudal ventrolateral medullary (CVLM) neurons that inhibit the main sympathetic region in the rostral

TABLE 9.3 Mediators and Mechanisms of Vascular Smooth Muscle Contraction		
Mediator	**Source**	**Major Function in Resistance, Regulation in Health or Disease**
NE	Sympathetic vasoconstrictor fibers	Blood levels show circadian rhythm, highest when awake at upright posture Tonic activity at α_1 receptors is the primary factor in normal blood pressure maintenance Prevents orthostatic hypotension
Epinephrine	Adrenal medulla	Blood levels lower than NE, highest when awake at upright posture Some activity at α_1 receptors Levels increase with exercise contributing to β_2-mediated vasodilation supplying skeletal muscles
Angiotensin II (ATII)	Renin, ACE generated	Blood levels low at rest Primary effects are on sodium and blood volume regulation Vasoconstricting activity at AT_1 receptors complements other renal and cardiovascular effects and potentiates NE effects Growth factor for cardiac and vascular smooth muscle, potentially contributing to deleterious cardiac and vascular hypertrophy Major target of antihypertensive drugs, particularly ACE inhibitors and ARBs that lower blood pressure and protect kidneys from hypertensive injury
Vasopressin (AVP)	Posterior pituitary hormone	Major role in water conservation by the kidneys Increased secretion stimulated by hypotension and hypovolemia augments sympathetic vasoconstriction AVP and its analogues can be used pharmacologically to support blood pressure during hypotensive/shock states
Atrial natriuretic peptide/BNP	Released from cardiac atria/ventricles in response to stretch	Normally low circulating levels; BNP increases in heart failure Primary action is on the kidneys, reducing circulating volume by stimulating natriuresis and diuresis Secondary action is vascular smooth muscle relaxation Breakdown by the enzyme neprilysin is targeted by the heart failure drug sacubitril
Prostacyclin (PGI_2)	Normal endothelial cells	Tonically produced; inhibits platelet aggregation and promotes vasodilation

(continued)

TABLE 9.3 Mediators and Mechanisms of Vascular Smooth Muscle Contraction (*continued*)

Mediator	Source	Major Function in Resistance, Regulation in Health or Disease
Nitric oxide (NO)	Normal endothelial cells	Tonically produced; diffuses to smooth muscle layer and promotes vasodilation Mechanism of vasodilation produced by acetylcholine and bradykinin Target of nitrate vasodilator drugs
Endothelin (ET)	Damaged endothelial cells	Potent vasoconstrictor Mediates trauma-induced vasoconstriction, limiting blood loss Endothelin antagonism is effective at reducing pulmonary arterial hypertension
CO_2, H^+, K^+, adenosine	Local tissues with high metabolic activity	Mediators of local flow increase in response to high metabolic demand, producing vasodilation This is proposed as the mechanism of metabolic autoregulation
Bradykinin	Produced locally in areas of tissue inflammation	Contributes to cardinal signs of inflammation: redness, swelling, heat, and pain, through vasodilation
Histamine	Released by mast cells in areas of trauma or allergic responses	Contributes to inflammatory and allergic vasodilation and increased vascular permeability Can cause severe tissue swelling and contribute to anaphylactic shock
PGD_2 and PGE_2	Released by white blood cells in the process of inflammatory responses	Contribute to inflammatory and allergic vasodilation PGE_2 and PGI_2 increase vasodilation and blood flow in the renal medulla
TXA_2	Released by platelets in conditions of vascular and tissue trauma	Contributes to vasoconstriction that reduces blood loss after vascular trauma

ACE, angiotensin-converting enzyme; ARBs, angiotensin receptor blockers; BNP, B-type natriuretic peptide; NE, norepinephrine; PGD_2, prostaglandin D_2; PGE_2, prostaglandin E_2; TXA_2, thromboxane A_2.

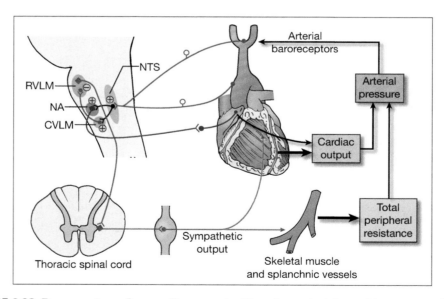

FIGURE 9.23 Baroreceptor reflex arc. Baroreceptor fibers have stretch-sensitive nerve endings in the aortic arch and carotid sinus—their firing rate increases when blood pressure increases, and decreases when blood pressure decreases. Baroreceptors synapse in the NTS, where relay neurons project to vagal preganglionic neurons in the NA and to the rostral and caudal ventrolateral medullas (RVLM and CVLM), centers that stimulate sympathetic neurons in the spinal cord. An acute increase in blood pressure will elicit an acute decrease in heart rate and a decrease in tonic sympathetic vasoconstriction.

CVLM, caudal ventrolateral medulla; NA, nucleus ambiguus; NTS, nucleus of the tractus solitarius; RVLM, rostral ventrolateral medulla.

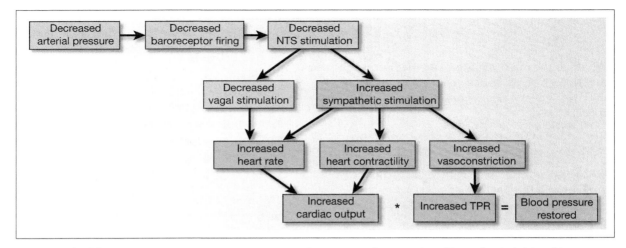

FIGURE 9.24 Response of the baroreceptor reflex to acute hypotension. The reflex is initiated by a decrease in mean arterial pressure. The compensatory responses act to increase arterial pressure back to normal.
NTS, nucleus of the tractus solitarius; TPR, total peripheral resistance.

ventrolateral medulla (RVLM). This circuit decreases firing of spinal cord sympathetic neurons that regulate vasoconstriction. The combination of decreased heart rate (which decreases cardiac output) and decreased sympathetic vasoconstriction (which decreases peripheral resistance) returns blood pressure to normal levels.

Decreased arterial pressures also elicit circulatory adjustments via the baroreceptor reflex (**Figure 9.24**). Sudden decrease in arterial pressure reduces action potential firing rate of baroreceptors. Medullary responses include decreased vagal flow to the heart and increased sympathetic cardiovascular activation. Sympathetic stimulation of the sinoatrial node increases heart rate, and stimulation of the cardiac ventricles stimulates contractility. These adjustments both increase cardiac output. At the same time, sympathetic vasoconstrictor activity increases, resulting in VSM contraction and increased peripheral resistance. The effect of these alterations is to restore normal arterial pressure. This reflex is critical for short-term adaptation to postural changes as well as the integrated responses to major blood loss and other hypotensive episodes. Increased sympathetic tone also includes α_1-mediated venoconstriction, pushing blood from the venous reserves back to the heart to improve cardiac preload. Through this series of events, the baroreceptor reflexes help restore both cardiac output and arteriolar resistance to return arterial pressure toward normal levels.

The baroreceptor reflex is important in beat-to-beat regulation of blood pressure and plays a vital role in preventing postural (orthostatic) hypotension when moving from a supine to an upright position. This homeostatic system is responsible for short-term compensation for altered blood pressure, rather than chronic alterations. However, long-term changes in blood pressure, as in hypertension, lead to accommodation of the baroreceptor fibers and resetting to a new, higher level of blood pressure.

Long-Term Blood Pressure Control by Hormones That Control Blood Volume and Vascular Tone

As previously noted (see **Table 9.3**), angiotensin II and AVP increase blood pressure control by two mechanisms:

1. Direct stimulation of VSM contraction, increasing peripheral resistance
2. Increasing body sodium and water content through actions on the kidneys and other tissues

An increase in sodium and water retention increases blood volume filling the circulatory system, increasing blood pressure. Secretion of these hormones is controlled by both high-pressure arterial baroreceptors in the carotid sinus and aortic arch, and low-pressure and low-volume receptors in the atria, ventricles, and pulmonary arteries. Finally, intrarenal baroreceptors in the juxtaglomerular apparatus of the nephron also regulate renin release.

ANP and BNP decrease blood pressure in the opposite fashion: When the heart is stretched by increases in circulating blood volume, ANP and BNP are secreted. These hormones cause vasodilation and decreased peripheral resistance, lowering blood pressure. They also act on the kidney to promote natriuresis and diuresis, reducing blood volume.

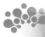

Thought Questions

6. What are the major systems and mediators that function on an essentially continuous basis to maintain normal arterial pressure and tissue blood flow?

7. How many of these systems work directly on VSM, renal sodium and water retention, or both?

8. What are examples of other vasoconstricting and vasodilating mediators, and under what circumstances are they regulating vasoconstriction and dilation?

PATHOPHYSIOLOGY OF ELEVATED VASCULAR RESISTANCE: HYPERTENSION

Definition and Causes of Hypertension

According to the AHA, **hypertension** is defined as a blood pressure of >130 mm Hg systolic or >80 mm Hg diastolic pressure.[9] About 90% of all hypertension cases are primary or essential hypertension in which the cause remains unknown. Prevalence increases with age, greater African ancestral descent, and increased obesity or diabetes. The consequences of untreated or undertreated hypertension are severe and include stroke, coronary heart disease, left ventricular hypertrophy, PAD, heart failure, and chronic kidney disease. Patients with essential hypertension usually present with mild elevations in blood pressure that are persistent and that chronically damage vulnerable organs. The condition develops insidiously, as there are no symptoms, so the earliest changes in cardiovascular function may never be observed. At the time of diagnosis, the patient with essential hypertension generally presents with normal heart rate, urinary sodium excretion, cardiac output, and sympathetic tone.

There are two major hypotheses regarding the origin of primary hypertension. The first hypothesis proposes an initial defect in sodium and water retention that increases vascular volume and cardiac output. This is predicted to result in vasoconstriction by generalized autoregulation. Over time, the cardiovascular system achieves a new steady state, with normal cardiac output but higher vascular resistance maintained by increased tone and hypertrophy of VSM. The second hypothesis of the origin of hypertension is chronically increased sympathetic tone that leads to vasoconstriction and RAAS activity, as shown in **Figure 9.25**. These hypotheses are not mutually exclusive, and data also support a role for increased sodium intake, obesity, and a state of chronic inflammation as contributing factors to the hypertension seen as a component of the metabolic syndrome.

Hypertension is generally asymptomatic, so it is generally detected by random screening or when blood pressure is measured during medical visits for other reasons. Family history is important in screening for hypertension, and the condition is polygenic, with many potential genetic factors contributing and interacting with the environment to produce the disorder. An isolated finding of elevated blood pressure at one visit should be followed up with repeat measurements. Psychological factors can influence blood pressure in the form of *white coat hypertension*—elevated pressure associated with the office visit. Ambulatory blood pressure recording is an option to identify the pattern

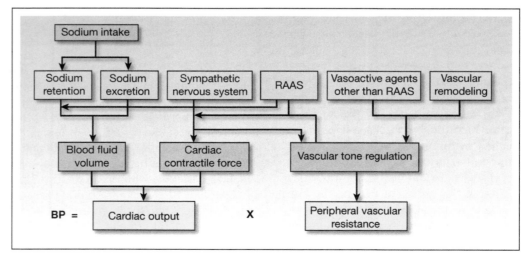

FIGURE 9.25 Systems involved in initiating and maintaining hypertension.
BP, blood pressure; RAAS, renin-angiotensin-aldosterone system.
Source: From Ohishi, M. Hypertension with diabetes mellitus: physiology and pathology. *Hypertens Res.* 2018;41:389–393. doi:10.1038/s41440-018-0034-4

of blood pressure changes in someone who has white coat hypertension or other evidence of variable blood pressure data.

At the time of diagnosis of mild hypertension, the usual presentation includes normal heart rate and cardiac output, urinary sodium and water balances that appear typical, and no evidence of suppression of sympathetic tone or increased parasympathetic outflow that would indicate baroreflex compensation. This profile leaves increased vascular resistance as the likely cause of elevated blood pressure. It appears as if a physiological *set point* for systemic regulatory activities has simply shifted to a higher pressure. Because the basis for the elevated pressures cannot be identified, treatment focuses on reducing blood pressure to normal levels through lifestyle changes and medications. Hypertension cannot be cured, so lifelong treatment is necessary. Maintaining blood pressure as close to normal as possible is key to preventing the many serious complications of hypertension.

In 5% to 10% of hypertension cases, an underlying cause can be identified. This is known as secondary hypertension; in these patients, hypertension is a symptom for some underlying condition, particularly kidney or endocrine disorders. Chronic kidney disease produces hypertension through dysregulation of body salt and water balance. Renovascular hypertension is due to narrowing of the renal arteries (often due to atherosclerosis) that results in chronically elevated RAAS activity. Endocrine disorders that present with hypertension include Cushing disease, hyperthyroidism, and pheochromocytoma. Once identified, these secondary forms of hypertension are usually readily treatable by correcting a causative factor.

Hypertension Damages Several Organs

As previously noted, hypertension is generally asymptomatic, and patients will not generally know whether or not their blood pressure is controlled by medication. Statistics show that in about 50% of patients with hypertension, blood pressure is not controlled, so persistent organ damage contributes to hypertension-associated morbidity and mortality.[2] Elevated blood pressures tend to promote compensatory thickening of the blood vessel wall (by the law of Laplace), as well as endothelial damage and vascular expression of inflammatory cytokines that accelerate atherosclerosis formation. Endothelial dysfunction reduces nitric oxide formation and promotes platelet aggregation and clot formation, increasing the risk of deep vein thrombosis, pulmonary emboli, and cerebral infarctions.

The main concern with chronic untreated or undertreated hypertension is the resulting damage to several organs (Table 9.4). The heart responds to the increased demands of generating ever higher systolic pressures by developing left ventricular hypertrophy. The hypertrophy increases myocardial oxygen demand, increasing the risk of angina and myocardial infarction, particularly in the context of hypertension-accelerated atherosclerosis. Over time, hypertension is a major cause of myocardial infarction or later heart failure. The brain is quite sensitive to blood pressure variation. Hypertension also affects the cerebral circulation, predisposing to ischemic and hemorrhagic stroke and rupture of cerebral aneurysms. Cognitive decline is also accelerated by hypertension.

The kidneys are highly vascular, and hypertension is the second most common cause of chronic kidney disease after diabetes. High pressures in the afferent arterioles increase wall tension, resulting in smooth muscle hypertrophy and nephrosclerosis (thickening of extracellular matrix in the walls of small arteries and arterioles), which then reduces the vessel radius. Proteins are deposited in the media, producing a microscopic feature termed *hyaline arteriosclerosis*.[10] Patient monitoring in hypertension should include periodic

TABLE 9.4 Complications of Hypertension

Complication	Contributing Factors
Atherosclerosis	Shear stress, endothelial injury, inflammation
Coronary heart disease	Atherosclerosis, left ventricular hypertrophy, increased myocardial oxygen demand
Heart failure	Increased afterload, myocardial remodeling
Stroke	Atherosclerosis, inflammation/hypercoagulability, aneurysm rupture
Kidney disease	Vascular wall hypertrophy and hyaline arteriosclerosis of renal vessels
Retinopathy	Endothelial damage, leakiness and rupture, vessel narrowing
Aneurysm formation and rupture	Turbulent flow, high pressure, vascular wall thickening and ischemia
Peripheral arterial disease	Atherosclerosis, endothelial injury, inflammation

measures of renal function as well as urinary albumin excretion. As previously noted, aneurysm formation and rupture are increased by the high vascular pressures and increased atherosclerosis induced by chronic hypertension. Finally, small vessels of the eye are vulnerable to endothelial damage, leakage into the retina, narrowing, or hemorrhage in response to sustained hypertension, comprising hypertensive retinopathy.

Of the estimated 30.3 million people in the United States diagnosed with diabetes in 2015, almost 75% had hypertension or were on medications for hypertension.[11] All of the end-organ complications of hypertension are accelerated by comorbid diabetes. Management of hypertension alone or coexisting hypertension and diabetes with lifestyle modifications and pharmacological treatments reduces the complication-associated morbidity and mortality risks. These responses are graded, so greater clinical benefit is achieved the closer blood pressure and glucose levels are to target levels.

Management of Hypertension

Secondary forms of hypertension are treated by correcting the initiating insult, but essential hypertension is usually managed through lifestyle changes and drug therapies. Lifestyle changes include reduced sodium intake, increased dietary fiber and potassium (e.g., vegetables), heart-healthy dietary approaches to stop hypertension (DASH) diet or Mediterranean diet, weight loss, exercise, and smoking cessation. Pharmacological management most commonly includes drugs that promote sodium excretion (e.g., chlorothiazides) and agents that block the effects of RAAS (ACE inhibitors, angiotensin receptor blockers). The advantage of blocking RAAS is that it promotes both vasodilation and sodium excretion. These agents also reduce the cardiovascular inflammatory and fluid-retaining effects of angiotensin II and aldosterone. Calcium channel blockers that target VSM calcium channels and β-blockers that reduce heart rate and cardiac output are also commonly used. Although none of these agents cures hypertension, they reduce end-organ damage, morbidity, and mortality associated with essential hypertension.

PATHOPHYSIOLOGY OF DECREASED BLOOD PRESSURE AND PERIPHERAL RESISTANCE: SHOCK

Definition of Shock

Shock is a clinical state of severely decreased blood pressure and blood flow that greatly reduces tissue perfusion and oxygenation. If this state is not quickly corrected, irreversible tissue damage occurs and can lead to death. There are many forms of circulatory shock that can be initiated by different events, display dissimilar symptoms, and require specific treatments. Ultimately, however, they all constitute conditions of reduced blood flow to the tissues that can ultimately progress to widespread tissue hypoxia, ischemia, and cell death.

Common Shock Progression

Shock can be initiated by a variety of events, including trauma with hemorrhage, anaphylaxis, sepsis, obstructed blood flow, and myocardial infarction (see **Table 9.5**). In each case, blood volume or blood pressure is insufficient to perfuse tissues, particularly in the upright position. Many of these cases involve complications of hospitalization, but for those initiated in the outpatient population, syncope is usually one of the first indications of inadequate blood flow and pressure. At first, the intensity of the insult may be masked by numerous neural, hormonal, and local mechanisms that customarily contribute to blood pressure regulation through the baroreflex. As perfusion worsens, the system progresses from compensated to decompensated shock, and eventually to circulatory collapse.

Compensated Shock

This initial phase, often referred to as compensated shock, constitutes a period when arterial pressures may not reflect the full magnitude of the insult. Any acute reduction in systemic blood pressure triggers an immediate baroreflex-mediated increase in the heart rate via withdrawal of parasympathetic tone. The fall in blood pressure also activates sympathetic nervous system–mediated increases in heart rate, contractility, and vasoconstriction, and RAAS activation, which can help to restore blood pressure. These adjustments are evident by tachycardia and decreased peripheral perfusion, leaving the extremities cool to palpation.

As blood flow diminishes to the periphery, CO_2 accumulates and lactic acid levels rise, along with other products of tissue hypoxia. The generation of these factors triggers the chemoreceptors of the aortic and carotid bodies to further increase sympathetic discharge to increase the cardiac output and peripheral vasoconstriction. This peripheral response helps divert blood flow from the limbs to the heart, brain, and other vital organs. However, long-term reduction of blood flow to the limbs and organs causes tissue hypoxia and damage that counteracts vasoconstrictor influences and promotes progression from compensated shock toward complete multiorgan system failure.

Decompensated Shock

A transitional phase of decompensated shock signals the development of tissue damage, which reduces the likelihood for recovery. Decreased velocity of blood allows for greater contact between red blood cells and the formation of rouleaux. These *stacks* of red blood cells, commonly detected in blood smears, block capillaries and decrease blood delivery to the tissues. Tissue damage becomes widespread, and severely ischemic tissues release a host of cytokines and other damage signals of disrupted cellular ATP formation. Severe hypoxia promotes anaerobic metabolism, resulting in widespread lactic acidosis. If the systemic pH drops severely, then α_1-adrenergic receptors become unresponsive to sympathetic stimulation, leading to loss of sympathetic tone and rapid circulatory collapse.

Irreversible Shock and Circulatory Collapse

Once severe widespread damage has developed, the body reaches a point at which recovery is no longer possible. A patient in irreversible shock may still be alive but is usually unresponsive. The widespread vascular decay is evident as blood settles and pools into the lowest regions. These broad red and purple patches on the skin indicate that the heart is no longer able to support the circulation, vascular damage is extreme, and death is imminent.

Forms of Shock

Four types of shock are differentiated based on the underlying physiological disturbance: hypovolemic, distributive, cardiogenic, and obstructive[12] (Table 9.5).

Hypovolemic Shock

Any event that causes a decrease in circulating blood volume can cause **hypovolemic shock**. Examples include traumatic or surgical hemorrhage/severe blood loss, dehydration, and severe gastrointestinal fluid loss. Severe blood loss reduces the circulating volume, thus decreasing cardiac preload. This in turn decreases cardiac output and lowers the blood pressure. Baroreflex compensation increases sympathetic activity to increase heart rate and cardiac contractility,

and to promote α_1-adrenergic receptor–mediated vasoconstriction. The RAAS is also activated to further raise the blood pressure through increased vascular resistance. Increased resistance may compensate and maintain blood pressure near normal, but the individual still has low cardiac output and may still progress to decompensation. The likelihood that a patient will progress into circulatory collapse is directly related to the rate and the magnitude of volume loss. The key to treating hypovolemic shock is rapid replacement of the circulating volume. Patients treated in such a manner have an excellent chance for full recovery.

It is critical to maintain blood pressure as close to normal as possible despite hypovolemia, as MAP is the driving force for blood flow in the systemic circulation. As the various vasoconstrictor mechanisms increase peripheral resistance to maintain blood pressure, they also further compromise tissue blood flow and capillary perfusion pressure (see **Figures 9.16** and **9.17**). Clinically, this presents as slowed capillary refill observed on physical examination.

Distributive Shock

Events producing massive vasodilation can produce **distributive shock**. Blood volume is initially normal, but massive vasodilation reduces peripheral resistance, abruptly dropping the blood pressure. Distributive shock includes anaphylactic shock, septic shock, and neurogenic shock, among other forms. Anaphylactic shock is the worst-case response of severe type 1 hypersensitivity (allergy) that causes widespread release of histamine, resulting in profound vasodilation. Blood pools in the dilated vessels, decreasing venous return and therefore cardiac output, while

TABLE 9.5 Different Types of Shock			
Type of Shock	Examples	Primary Problem	Initial Hemodynamic Change
Hypovolemic	Blood loss Dehydration	Low circulating volume	↓ Preload, ↓ CO, ↑ TPR
Distributive	Anaphylactic reaction (type 1 hypersensitivity) Systemic infection (septic shock)	Generalized decrease of peripheral resistance	↓ TPR, blood pooling in periphery, ↓ venous return, ↓ preload, ↓ CO
	Neurogenic shock (spinal cord injury, drug overdose)	Loss of sympathetic tone	↓ TPR, blood pooling in periphery, lack of cardiac compensation, ↓ CO
Cardiogenic	Myocardial infarction Papillary muscle rupture	Impaired cardiac contractility Acute mitral regurgitation	↓ CO, ↑ TPR
Obstructive	Cardiac tamponade, pulmonary embolism, tension pneumothorax	Physical block of vasculature or of cardiac filling	↓ CO, ↑ TPR

↓, decreased; ↑, increased; CO, cardiac output; TPR, total peripheral resistance.

simultaneously arteriolar dilation reduces total peripheral resistance, causing blood pressure to collapse to the level of shock.

Septic shock is the catastrophic response to overwhelming systemic infection. It occurs in both children and adults, with increased risk seen in compromised patients with multiple morbidities, including chronic cardiac, lung, or kidney disease. Infections from any source, if undetected and untreated, may progress to this critical stage, characterized by widespread vasodilation, vascular insensitivity to the actions of vasoconstrictors, and cardiac insensitivity to the actions of cardiostimulatory drugs. Multiple organ dysfunction syndrome (MODS) is the final stage and represents failure of several organs concurrent with death of peripheral tissues. Sepsis morbidity and mortality rates are high and remain among the most challenging of disease syndromes to manage.

Neurogenic shock results when there is complete cessation of firing of vasoconstrictor sympathetic neurons. Spinal cord injuries, drug overdoses, and complications from spinal anesthesia all have the potential to interrupt the spinal sympathetic outflow. With the withdrawal of sympathetic nervous system tone, the vessels dilate and peripheral resistance drops precipitously as does blood pressure. The loss of brainstem stimulation of sympathetic tone also prevents baroreflex stimulation of heart rate and cardiac contractility. After spinal cord injury and the initial stage of spinal shock, over time there is recovery of a certain degree of tonic vasoconstriction that permits blood pressure maintenance in the upright position.

Cardiogenic Shock

Heart attacks can dramatically reduce cardiac output, resulting in **cardiogenic shock**. The sympathetic nervous system and RAAS respond to increase heart rate and promote vasoconstriction. Because reduced cardiac contractility is the initiating event, CVP becomes elevated but cardiac output remains low. Cardiac output cannot be improved by volume expansion, which can promote pulmonary edema. The focus for treating cardiogenic shock is to restore cardiac contractility as quickly as possible.

Obstructive Shock

Disease conditions that reduce cardiac filling or obstruct blood flow can acutely and critically reduce cardiac output and blood pressure, resulting in **obstructive shock**. Examples include severe restrictive pericarditis and pericardial tamponade that restrict cardiac filling. Impairment of lung blood flow can also produce obstructive shock, as caused by pulmonary emboli or tension pneumothorax.

Management of Shock

All forms of shock are managed with urgent, invasive support measures with close monitoring, fluid replacement, and administration of pressor agents. The distinctive aspect across all forms of distributive shock, relative to hypovolemic, cardiogenic, and obstructive shock, is the inability to compensate by vasoconstriction and increased peripheral resistance. Blood pooling restricts cardiac filling, reducing cardiac output; when combined with reduced peripheral resistance, hypotension is severe.

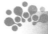
Thought Questions

9. How do antihypertensive medications interact with determinants of cardiac output and peripheral resistance to reduce blood pressure?

10. What are the most common complications of untreated or undertreated hypertension?

11. Based on the equation relating mean arterial pressure, peripheral resistance, and cardiac output, explain the causes of low blood pressure in the different forms of shock.

PROPERTIES AND DISORDERS OF CAPILLARIES

OVERVIEW OF CAPILLARY STRUCTURE AND FUNCTION

Principles Governing Capillary Fluid Exchange

Capillaries are a collection of narrow branching blood vessels that are located between the arterioles and venules. The capillary walls are a single endothelial cell thick with a small amount of basement membrane. This thin-walled and permeable structure makes them specialized sites for gas, nutrient, fluid, and waste exchange between circulating blood and tissues. The rate of exchange is based upon the size, solubility, and charge of the substances. Exchange is also affected by the charge, abundance, and size of pores between the endothelial cells. These features vary substantially among the common types of capillaries (**Figure 9.26**).

Continuous capillaries are the most abundant type and are found throughout all tissues. Their capillary walls have a continuous layer of endothelial cells, but possess small pores (clefts) in between. These pores allow for fluid exchange, including water, electrolytes, and other small water-soluble molecules (glucose, amino acids, etc.). The pores, however, are too small to

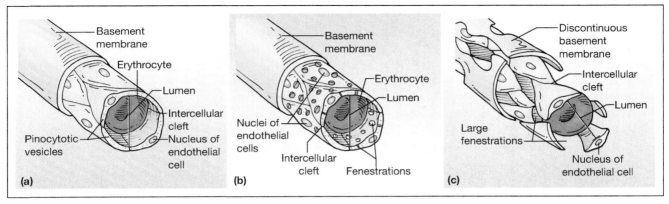

FIGURE 9.26 Capillary types have different permeabilities: (**a**) continuous (least permeable),
(**b**) fenestrated (intermediate permeability), (**c**) sinusoid (most permeable).

permit movement of plasma proteins, which remain in the vessel and exert a force called colloid osmotic pressure that helps retain fluid within the capillary lumen. Capillaries in the intestines, kidneys, and endocrine organs display loose endothelial junctions. These *fenestrated capillaries* allow higher rates of fluid exchange, and often greater exchange of molecules such as small proteins. The functions of the spleen, liver, and bone marrow require the passage of large proteins and even cells across their capillary walls. This purpose is served by *sinusoids*, modified capillaries with large gaps between endothelial cells, and having discontinuous basement membranes.

Net fluid exchange across capillary walls is influenced by a summation of capillary and interstitial pressures. Both sides have *hydrostatic pressures* that *push* water and small dissolved molecules away from the source across the capillary walls. Both regions also have *colloid osmotic pressures* created by proteins that have little ability to move across capillary walls. Colloid osmotic pressure *pulls* water and small dissolved molecules toward the source across the capillary walls. It is the balance of these pressures that establish the net movement of fluid and solutes across capillary walls. The rate of transport is also influenced by a filtration coefficient that is affected by the density and properties of the filtration pores. These elements can be used to estimate net fluid movement through a capillary wall according to the Starling equation, as follows:

$$\text{Net fluid movement} = k[(P_c - P_i) - (\pi_c - \pi_i)]$$

where

k = filtration coefficient
P_c = capillary hydrostatic pressure
P_i = interstitial hydrostatic pressure
π_c = capillary colloid osmotic (also known as oncotic) pressure
π_i = interstitial colloid osmotic pressure

The values for both capillary and interstitial hydrostatic pressures vary widely in different tissues and organs. In some cases, interstitial hydrostatic pressure is negative, favoring filtration. Capillary colloid osmotic pressure is not as variable, although it changes over the long term in the context of liver production of plasma proteins. For continuous capillaries, the average capillary hydrostatic pressure is about 26 to 28 mm Hg, while the interstitial hydrostatic pressure is thought to vary from –1 to +3 mm Hg; thus, the net hydrostatic pressure gradient favors *filtration*—fluid movement outward across the wall. The colloid osmotic pressure in the capillary lumen is normally about 25 to 28 mm Hg, with the most abundant plasma protein being albumin. A lesser interstitial colloid osmotic pressure that is derived from the proteins of the interstitial matrix, and some escaped albumin, is about 0 to 3 mm Hg; thus, the net colloid osmotic pressure gradient favors *reabsorption*—inward movement of fluid across the wall. With this milieu, capillaries are thought to have a small net outflow of fluids into the interstitium, with a net driving force of approximately 1 to 5 mm Hg (**Figure 9.27**).

Capillary hydrostatic pressure is intermediate between the hydrostatic pressure initially reaching the arteriole–capillary junction and pressure within the venule as the capillary joins it. As the capillary hydrostatic pressure gradually drops from the arteriole end to the venous end, the rate of fluid movement across the wall changes accordingly. Consequently, capillary filtration is relatively high in the arteriolar end of the capillary, but a substantial portion is reabsorbed in the venous end of the capillary. This allows plasma fluids to be filtered and cleansed by extravascular processes while also facilitating nutrient delivery and waste removal.

Lymphatics
Interstitial fluid arising from capillary filtration forms lymph that returns to the circulation via an extensive

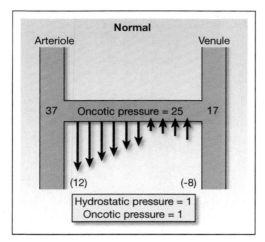

FIGURE 9.27 Normal filtration and reabsorption along a typical capillary in the systemic circulation. Black arrows represent the magnitude and direction of fluid exchange. Pressure values are shown in millimeters of mercury (mm Hg). Hydrostatic pressures at the arteriolar and venular ends of the capillary are shown in their respective locations. The yellow rectangle represents pressures in the interstitium. Parentheses indicate effective (net) filtration pressures at the arteriolar and venular end of the capillary. The value of capillary oncotic (colloid osmotic) pressure is displayed within the capillary.

specialized network of lymphatic capillaries. These capillaries converge and feed into low-pressure lymphatic vessels with one-way valves that facilitate lymph transport. Beyond the feeder capillaries, the lymph vessels become lined with smooth muscle that slowly contracts when filled with lymph (**Figure 9.28**). Lymph vessels eventually converge at lymph nodes that filter fluid proteins and are active in immune responses. The lymph then proceeds back into the circulation, primarily through the subclavian vein. The fact that capillary filtration slightly exceeds reabsorption in most tissues is evident from the daily lymph flow of 2 to 4 L.[13]

Principles Governing Capillary Fluid Movement and Edema Formation

Normal capillary function relies on fluid filtration at a rate that is matched by lymphatic clearance back into the circulation. If lymph is formed at a rate that is faster than it can be cleared, then it can accumulate in the interstitium to produce **edema** (**Box 9.3** and **Figure 9.29**). Conditions favoring this interstitial fluid accumulation include the following:

- *Dilation of arterioles*—The associated decrease in resistance means pressure does not drop as much from arteries to capillaries, elevating capillary hydrostatic pressure.
- *Elevated venous pressure or restriction of venous flow* causes blood to be retained in capillaries and increasing capillary hydrostatic pressure.

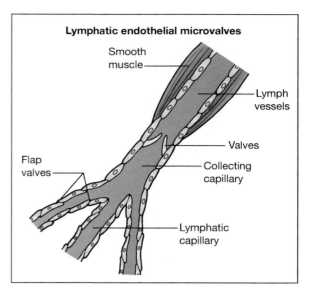

FIGURE 9.28 Lymphatic capillaries and larger lymph vessels with valves.

- *Decreased plasma protein concentration* reduces capillary colloid osmotic pressure.
- *Lymphatic obstruction* blocks removal of interstitial fluid and proteins.

Thought Question

12. All other factors remaining equal, what is the effect on capillary filtration and potential edema formation of the following changes? Give a rationale for your answers.
    a. Decreased arterial pressure
    b. Increased venous pressure
    c. Local inflammation with release of histamine

PROPERTIES AND DISORDERS OF VEINS

OVERVIEW OF VENOUS STRUCTURE AND FUNCTION, AND VULNERABILITY TO PRESSURE ELEVATIONS

Veins have greater radius with proportionally thinner walls and smooth muscle layers than arteries and arterioles. These characteristics confer the compliance needed for their capacity to store up to two thirds of the blood volume. The downside of this structure is that they are prone to dilation and deformation when they are exposed to high intravascular pressure. In the upright position when movement is not occurring, venous pressure in the legs is

BOX 9.3

Conditions Associated With Altered Lymphatic Clearance and Edema Formation

VASODILATION

- Arteriolar vasodilation allows higher hydrostatic pressure to be sustained to the level of the capillaries (**Figure 9.29a**; see also **Figure 9.17**). This, in turn, enhances the rate of lymph formation to an extent that it can exceed the clearance rate of the lymphatics.

- **Vasodilatory edema** is a hallmark of **local inflammation**. When tissue trauma triggers an innate immune response, histamine is released into the region. Histamine promotes vasodilation and increased capillary permeability, both of which favor filtration over reabsorption and produce the cardinal inflammatory sign of swelling.

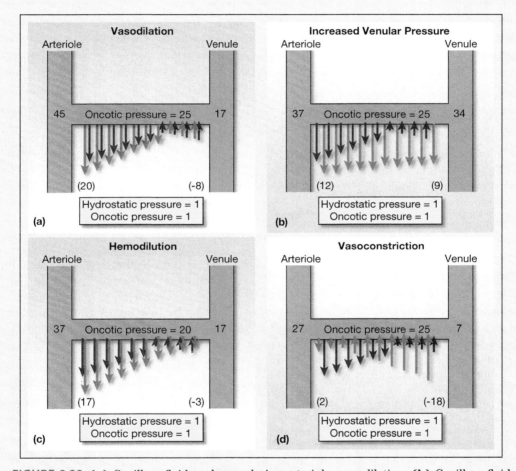

FIGURE 9.29 **(a)** Capillary fluid exchange during arteriolar vasodilation. **(b)** Capillary fluid exchange during increased venous pressure. **(c)** Capillary fluid exchange during decreased plasma oncotic pressure. **(d)** Capillary fluid exchange during arteriolar vasoconstriction. Arrows represent the magnitude and direction of fluid exchange. Gray arrows represent normal fluid exchange as shown in **Figure 9.27**; red arrows show altered fluid exchange due to the precipitating condition. Pressure values are shown in millimeters of mercury (mm Hg). Capillary hydrostatic and oncotic pressures are shown within the capillary and the yellow rectangle shows interstitial hydrostatic and oncotic pressures. Parentheses indicate effective (net) filtration pressures at the arteriolar and venular end of the capillary.

(continued)

BOX 9.3 (*continued*)
Conditions Associated With Altered Lymphatic Clearance and Edema Foundation

INCREASED VENOUS PRESSURE

- **Venous obstruction** in the context of deep venous thromboses increases venous pressures in the affected region (usually the leg). This pressure greatly increases capillary hydrostatic pressure and promotes filtration along the capillary length (**Figure 9.29b**). This is manifested by edema in the affected limb.

- **Right-sided heart failure** is also known to cause fluid retention and increase systemic venous pressures, promoting peripheral edema that is most prominent in the dependent body regions, feet, and ankles. Diuretics are often used to enhance water excretion, reduce capillary hydrostatic pressures, and reduce edema.

- Finally, **venous hypertension** can occur in the legs, particularly in older adults, due to incompetence of venous valves and decreased effectiveness of leg muscle activity to compress the leg veins. One of the main signs of this syndrome of venous insufficiency is ankle edema.

PLASMA PROTEIN DEFICIENCY AND HEMODILUTION

- Liver disease, malnutrition, and some kidney diseases can lead to reductions of circulating albumin and other proteins, reducing the colloid osmotic pressure. This loss of the restoring force favoring reabsorption promotes widespread edema (**Figure 9.29c**).

- Hemodilution that reduces colloid osmotic pressure is also a prevalent scenario in EDs, where patients are volume expanded with intravenous fluids containing glucose and electrolytes, but no proteins, after major hemorrhagic losses.

LYMPHATIC OBSTRUCTION

- Although relatively rare, any condition that impairs the return of lymph to the circulation will also cause lymph to accumulate and edema to form. In patients with cancer, a variety of sites may develop tumors that block lymph flow and produce edema of the affected region.

- Several parasites are also known to impair lymphatic flow. The most commonly recognized is *Wuchereria bancrofti*, which causes **lymphatic filariasis**, often referred to as elephantiasis.

HYPOTENSION AND HYPOVOLEMIA INCREASE CAPILLARY REABSORPTION

- The opposite changes in capillary Starling forces and fluid movements are seen in pathophysiological adaptation to severe hypotension and hypovolemia. Baroreflexes promote intense sympathetic vasoconstriction that maintains arterial pressure but greatly reduces capillary hydrostatic pressure (**Figure 9.29d**; see also **Figures 9.17** and **9.18**). The balance of Starling forces now favor reabsorption of fluid along the length of the capillaries, a phenomenon sometimes termed *autotransfusion*.

- **Loss of skin turgor** is a physical manifestation of this fluid shift, particularly in children and youth who have abundant tissue elasticity. This sign is less prominent in older adults, owing to reduced elasticity of skin and interstitial tissues. Capillary refill is also slowed due to the generalized vasoconstriction.

significantly higher than in other body regions, so leg veins are particularly prone to pathological changes[14] (**Figure 9.30**).

Two types of veins drain the legs: superficial veins and deep veins. The deep veins are surrounded by muscles, and muscle compression assists the flow of blood *uphill*—against the force of gravity to larger collecting veins. Venous pressure in the legs increases while in the standing position, then decreases when walking. Connecting veins bridge between superficial and deep veins and allow the deep veins to accommodate some flow from the superficial veins, reducing pressure within the superficial veins. Veins have bicuspid valves at regular intervals that close behind the blood flowing upward to the vena cava; competent valves prevent reflux toward the feet (**Figure 9.31**).

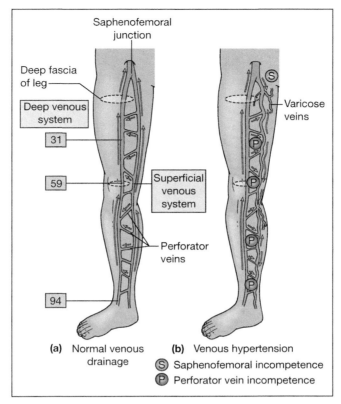

FIGURE 9.30 Anatomy of leg veins under **(a)** normal conditions and **(b)** with venous hypertension. Venous drainage of the leg is through deep and superficial veins that are connected by perforator veins. Gravitational pull on the blood increases venous pressure as shown in the blue boxes, numbers are pressures in mm Hg. The highest venous pressures are at the feet and ankles. Contractions of leg muscles compress the deep veins, facilitating their emptying and reducing venous pressure. Perforator veins allow superficial veins to drain to the deep veins that are emptied by the muscle pump. With aging or primary venous disease, superficial veins fail to empty and become tortuous and dilated. Flow from deep veins can reflux into superficial veins, worsening pressures and dilation that ultimately contributes to valve incompetence.

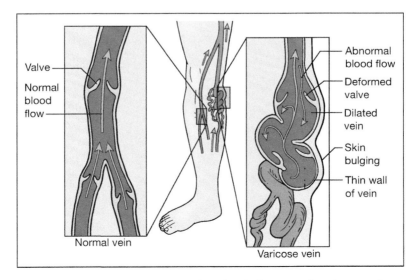

FIGURE 9.31 Varicose veins. Individuals with a family history of varicose veins are prone to these deformations of superficial leg veins. Varicose vein formation is promoted by pregnancy, occupations requiring prolonged standing, and older age.

Venous Disorders

Varicose Veins

Varicose veins have a high prevalence, affecting about 23% of U.S. adults with a female-to-male ratio of 2:1.[15] Risk factors include occupations that involve much time spent standing, family history, multiple pregnancies, obesity, and congenital valve dysfunction. Increased venous pressures lead to increased vessel diameter and length, resulting in tortuous, bulging veins, particularly affecting the superficial veins (see **Figure 9.31**). Increased venous diameter near valves causes valve incompetence with reflux of blood, worsening the venous pressure and vessel dilation. Varicose vein development is also promoted after **deep venous thrombosis** (DVT) of proximal great veins such as the femoral vein.

Some varicose veins are asymptomatic and treatment is performed for cosmetic reasons, while other varicose veins are painful and associated with a host of other symptoms including leg heaviness, itching and burning sensations, paresthesias, night cramps, and changes of the overlying skin. A distinguishing characteristic between venous and arterial malfunction is that pain associated with venous disorders can lessen with physical activity (presumably due to the additional muscle compression), whereas peripheral arterial disorders affecting the legs generally have increased pain with physical activity.

Deep Venous Thrombosis

Factors contributing to abnormal clotting (the Virchow triad) are discussed in Chapter 8, Blood and Clotting. The leg veins are a common site of pathological thrombus formation owing to the relatively slow rate of blood flow combined with the tendency for compression to obstruct blood flow in this region. Superficial veins such as the greater saphenous vein may develop thrombophlebitis due to inflammation, whereas deep veins more commonly develop thrombosis without inflammation. Factors that increase the risk for deep venous thrombosis (DVT) include hypercoagulability (genetic, or related to another disease process such as cancer), immobility due to recent surgery (particularly orthopedic surgery), and family history of DVT. Signs and symptoms include pain, edema, swelling, and localized tenderness of the affected leg. Development of a large DVT is a major risk for embolization to the lungs, causing **pulmonary embolism** and, in some cases, death.

Thought Questions

13. How does gravity contribute to the location and pathogenesis of vein disorders?

14. What is the rationale for prescribing compression stockings for individuals with vein disorders?

Randall L. Johnson

EMBRYOLOGICAL DEVELOPMENT OF THE CIRCULATORY SYSTEM

All structures of the cardiovascular system—heart and blood vessels—are lined with a single layer of endothelial cells. In fact, endothelial cells make up the first tube-like structures that will develop into heart and vessels. Cardiac development is described in Chapter 10, Heart; vessels must develop simultaneously, to deliver oxygen and nutrients to support embryonic and fetal growth. From the earliest stages of endothelial tubes, the vessels destined to become arteries develop distinctive characteristics first, followed by the vessels destined to become veins. The properties of pulmonary vessels and the embryonic circulation that brings oxygenated blood from the placenta prenatally are determined by the unique requirements of fetal circulation. After birth, pulmonary vascular resistance decreases and connecting vessels normally close. The postnatal pattern of blood flow is then established—from the right side of the heart to the lungs, and back to the left side of the heart for pumping to the systemic circulation—as the fetal circulation adjusts to extrauterine existence. There is a brief, though slightly variable, time period as the neonate transitions during which circulation may be reduced or impaired until structures have modified to their final pattern.

BLOOD PRESSURE AND PEDIATRIC HYPERTENSION

Hypertension is the most common disorder of the circulatory system in children, and prevalence is increasing, partly because of sedentary lifestyle, obesity, and type 2 diabetes mellitus. The child's blood pressure should be measured annually during well-child visits in an ambulatory setting. Appropriately sized equipment must be used for accuracy. Bladder cuff length should be 80% to 100% of the circumference of the arm, and the width should be around 40% of the arm length.[16] Although screening with an oscillometric device validated for pediatric use is acceptable, confirmation of elevated blood pressure should be performed with auscultatory measures. Recommendations for the frequency of obtaining blood pressure in children are adjusted for other conditions, such as obesity, diabetes, or kidney disease.

The determination of elevated blood pressure is based on normative tables that were revised in 2017. The tables are different for boys and girls and are adjusted for age and height. Up to the age of 13 years, the identification of elevated blood pressure, stage 1 or stage 2 hypertension, is based on measurements falling between the 90th and 95th percentiles for age, sex, and height; greater than the 95th percentile and less than the 95th percentile plus 12 mm Hg; or greater than the 95th percentile plus 12 mm Hg.[17] After the age of 13, the current ranges for adults apply. Elevated blood pressure should be confirmed with three separate measurements and should be measured by auscultation, as the tables were generated from auscultated measurements. It is estimated that 3.5% of children without diabetes, obesity, or kidney disease have primary hypertension, whereas the rate of hypertension in children with type 2 diabetes is about 9.5%.[18]

The clinical significance of early identification and treatment of pediatric hypertension is high: pediatric hypertension induces early vascular aging. Thus, the types of vascular changes associated with aging—including vascular wall stiffness, inflammation, endothelial damage, and increased left ventricular mass—are promoted in children with hypertension, accelerating their development of cardiovascular disease in later life.[19]

Susan Krekun and Linda L. Herrmann

VASCULAR CHANGES WITH AGING

Blood vessels are dynamic structures that are remodeled by complex pathways throughout the life span. Remodeling of the vascular system with aging influences the structural and functional changes of nearly all other organ systems in the body, especially the heart. In fact, this is an independent significant risk factor for the development of cardiovascular disease as we age.

Two major changes occur in arteries with aging: endothelial dysfunction and increased arterial stiffness (arteriosclerosis), which propagates throughout the vascular beds centrally to peripherally. The role of the endothelium has been well described earlier in this chapter. The endothelium secretes factors that positively and negatively influence VSM tone, inflammation, thrombosis, and oxidative stress. The endothelium's role in maintaining vascular homeostasis is altered in aging; these changes contribute to atherogenesis and thrombosis over time[20] and occur widely throughout the vasculature.

ENDOTHELIAL CHANGES WITH AGING

Endothelial dysfunction as we age is signaled by changes in balance of the vasodilators nitric oxide and PGI_2 and the vasoconstrictors ET1, TXA_2, and angiotensin II, with a net reduced ability of the vessel to dilate and a reduction of antithrombotic properties. Nitric oxide is a very important mediator in this balance; aging results in not just decreased production of nitric oxide, but also increased degradation.

In animal studies, reduced production of nitric oxide is due to reduced function of the synthetic enzyme eNOS and is also related to decreased bioavailability of cofactor BH4 (tetrahydrobiopterin), as well as reduced availability of the nitric oxide precursor L-arginine. When BH4 is in short supply, the ROS superoxide anion, O_2^-, increases. Notably ROS inactivates eNOS, leading to a decrease in nitric oxide production (called eNOS uncoupling). L-arginine is less available because arginase, an enzyme that competes for L-arginine, increases with aging and coopts the available substrate, leaving less for conversion to nitric oxide.

Chronic inflammation and changes in neurohormonal signaling increase the degradation of nitric oxide as well, further limiting its availability. As chronic inflammation increases, more ROS are generated that deplete nitric oxide. Neurohormonal signaling by the

RAAS is thought to also contribute to decreasing nitric oxide concentrations whereby increases in angiotensin II trigger increasing concentrations of ROS. An increase in ROS promotes inflammation, propagating a pathological cycle that promotes vasoconstriction and reduces vasodilation.

Circulating vasoconstrictors contribute to the impaired ability of the vasculature to dilate. Circulating levels of ET1 increase, impairing vasodilation. Other vasoconstrictors, such as prostaglandin H_2, TXA_2, and prostaglandin F_2, also increase with age, with a concomitant fall in the vasodilator PGI_2. All of these changes are accentuated by a decrease in the ability of the endothelium to regenerate as the number of endothelial progenitor cells decreases, curtailing the capacity to replace those lost through senescence.[21]

ARTERIAL STIFFNESS INCREASES WITH AGING

Increased arterial stiffness is the second major change seen with aging. The intimal and medial walls become thicker, the result of migration of VSM cells into the intimal layer that begins with the large central elastic arteries and progresses distally through the vasculature. Matrix and, particularly, collagen production is increased by the activity of the transforming growth factor-β, which induces VSM cells to produce more collagen. The RAAS is also thought to be involved in this process; increased activity of the RAAS system induces collagen production. Not only is there an increase in production of collagen, but its degradation declines because of increased cross-linking of collagen fibers, which makes them more resistant to breakdown.

Elastin is degraded more rapidly as proteases and compounds that break it down, such as matrix metalloproteases, increase due to inflammatory mediators. This process is also affected by RAAS, which not only stimulates collagen synthesis but also induces elastin degradation (**Figure 9.32**).

The stiffening of arteries increases systolic blood pressure. Arterial pressure is determined by central artery stiffness and resistance of small arteries and arterioles, so systolic and diastolic blood pressure will change with concomitant changes of the arterial beds. Systolic pressure increases steadily as it reflects the stiffening central arteries. The diastolic blood pressure, in contrast, increases up until the age of 50, then levels off for a period of time, and decreases after age 60 due to loss of elastic recoil of the aorta and larger arteries.

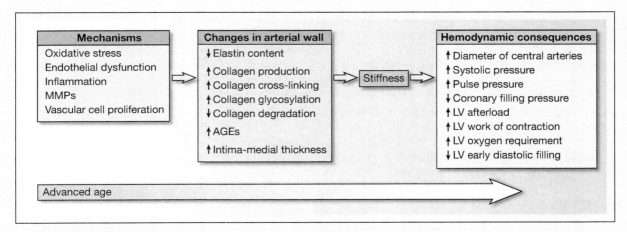

FIGURE 9.32 Molecular mechanisms that increase arterial stiffness with aging and hemodynamic consequences.
AGEs, advanced glycation end products; LV, left ventricle; MMPs, matrix metalloproteinases.
Source: From Dai X, et al. Cardiovascular physiology in older adults. *J Geriatr Cardiol.* 2015; 12:196–201.

This is seen as a widening of the pulse pressure. The process of stiffening is measured by pulse wave velocity (PWV), which simply represents the velocity at which a blood pressure pulse propagates through the circuit of arteries. It can be easily measured by placing two pressure catheters a known distance from one another along an arterial tree (most typically the carotid artery to the femoral artery). With aging, the PWV increases, and this has been shown to be a reliable predictor of cardiovascular disease events independent of blood pressure.[22]

The increased PWV can result in decreased coronary artery perfusion. Normally, when a pulse wave travels down the arterial tree, a reflected wave is pushed back when the forward wave reaches an area of narrowed, branching vessels. In younger individuals, the wave rebounds to the proximal aorta in diastole, aiding in blood flow that increases in coronary arteries during diastole. The changes that stiffen the arteries cause the pulse wave to arrive sooner, and often in late systole; this can compromise coronary filling.[23] Another consequence of decreased arterial compliance and the widened pulse pressure is that small changes in volume can cause a large shift in blood pressure, causing end-organ damage in the cardiac, renal, and central nervous systems.[21]

In the heart, the increased arterial stiffness increases afterload on the left ventricle, resulting in left ventricular hypertrophy and stiffness. These factors contribute to the greater incidence of heart failure, atrial fibrillation, and myocardial ischemia in older adults. Consequences of these vascular changes for the brain are strokes and dementia. In the renal system, chronic kidney disease and renal failure can occur.

AGING-ASSOCIATED VASCULAR DISORDERS

Age-related changes in the vasculature predispose to the development of complications in each vascular bed. The concomitant development of atherosclerosis plays a significant role in the development of these complications; however, there is some evidence that some people experience these changes as result of aging alone. In a large study of 3.6 million self-referred individuals conducted between 2003 and 2008, the overall incidence of any vascular disease (carotid artery stenosis, PAD, or abdominal aortic aneurysm) increased with each decade of life (**Table 9.6**).[24]

TABLE 9.6 Prevalence of Having Any Vascular Disease Diagnosis Stratified by Age per Decade

Age in Years	Prevalence
40–50	2%
51–60	3.5%
61–70	7.1%
71–80	13.0%
81–90	22.3%
91–100	32.5%

Source: Adapted from Savji N, et al. Association between advanced age and vascular disease in different arterial territories. A population database of over 3.6 million subjects. *J Am Coll Cardiol.* 2013; 61:1736–1743. https://doi.org/10.1016/j.jacc.2013.01.054

Age-related changes are an independent risk factor for diseases of the central arteries and peripheral arterial (carotid, upper extremity, mesenteric, aortoiliac, femoropopliteal, and infrapopliteal) segments and corresponding venous segments. There is significant overlap between age and other risk factors in the development of the vascular disease, making it difficult to distinguish what is specifically attributable to aging. That said, common disorders that increase with aging include aneurysms, dissections, intramural hematomas, and ulcerations of arterial vessels.

ANEURYSMS

Arterial aneurysms can occur anywhere along the arterial tree from the proximal, thoracic aorta to the abdominal aorta, and from the iliac, femoral, and popliteal arteries up to the carotid and cerebral arteries. Abdominal aortic aneurysm tends to be the most common type of aneurysm, typically occurring below the level of the renal arteries.[25] It is more common in the elderly and is five times more common in men than women. The prevalence increases with age: rates are 1.3% in men and 0 in women aged 45 to 54 years, but 12.5% in men and 5.2% in women aged 75 to 84.[26] The altered architecture of the arterial walls with aging, combined with the effects of hypertension, atherosclerosis, and the other risk factors, can predispose to the formation of aneurysms. These are defined by abdominal aortic diameter >3 cm. While often asymptomatic, in the elderly they can sometimes present as failure to thrive (secondary to mesenteric ischemia), acute renal insufficiency, or thromboembolic disease. The most significant complication is rupture, which carries a very high mortality rate—up to 90% by some reports. Rupture becomes a significant threat when the aneurysm is >5 cm and when the rate of enlargement accelerates.

Dissections develop when tears occur in the intimal layer, allowing blood entry into the arterial wall and creating a channel or false lumen. The false lumen can extend distally (and proximally to the aortic valve) and can sometimes compress the true lumen of the vessel, causing ischemic complications in the distal distribution of the vessel.[27] It is not entirely clear why or how this occurs in some individuals, but the age-related changes in the vessels and perhaps uncontrolled hypertension are thought to play large roles in the pathogenesis.

Symptomatically, the most common complaint associated with dissection is chest pain, often described as tearing and radiating to the back. Hypertension is fairly common, but patients may also present with hypotension if rupture has occurred. Also noted can be pulse and blood pressure discrepancies between limbs and diastolic heart murmurs, but these are highly variable findings. In the elderly, syncope, stroke, and heart failure symptoms may predominate.[28] Alternative presentations may include focal neurological manifestations such as paraplegia or paraparesis.

AGING VEINS: CHRONIC VENOUS INSUFFICIENCY, VARICOSE VEINS, AND VENOUS ULCERS

As explained earlier in this chapter, nearly two thirds of human blood volume resides on the venous side, a low-pressure system. As such, the venous system plays a significant role in the overall capacity and function of the cardiovascular system. Age-related changes in the venous system include fibrous thickening of the subintimal layer; fibrotic changes within the tunica intima, tunica media, and tunica adventitia; thinning of elastin; and increase in cross-linkage of collagen, thus contributing to venous stiffening and decreased venous compliance.[29,30] These age-related changes in capacity, compliance, and venous constriction create a shift, reallocating venous blood to the arterial system. The totality of these changes, coupled with the duration of stress on the aging venous system from prolonged standing, further contributes to a state of venous hypertension.

Anatomically, with higher pressure, veins become elongated and dilated, tortuous and bulging. Valves become incompetent due to venous hypertension and valvular thickening, decreasing function and causing reflux from deep veins into superficial veins. This low-pressure superficial venous system then transforms into a high-pressure environment, causing vessel dilation and varicose vein formation. Treatment using compression and elevation may help reduce progression. In cases in which venous insufficiency worsens, capillary pressures increase, favoring edema formation and movement of proteins into tissues. This movement can include hemosiderin, which can be deposited in the superficial tissues and cause darkening of the skin in the affected region. More severe manifestations include dermal fibrosis and subcutaneous fat inflammation, referred to as lipodermatosclerosis, and development of skin ulcers[31] (**Figure 9.33**).

Clinical Implications

Understanding risk factors for venous insufficiency is critical in the care of older adults. Risk factors include older age, sedentary lifestyle, tobacco use, family history of chronic venous insufficiency, history of DVT, obesity, diabetes, heart failure, and peripheral vascular disease.

Early development of **venous ulcers** can manifest as stasis dermatitis, characterized by a scaling and

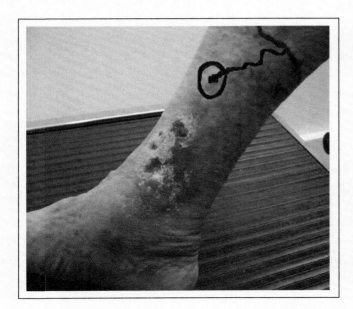

FIGURE 9.33 Leg ulcer secondary to venous insufficiency. Note skin color changes of the affected region.
Source: From Johnson FK, Johnson RA, and Rhodes SA.

reddened skin. Symptoms include leg pain or feelings of limb heaviness; lower extremity edema; pigment changes of brown or yellow color due to hemosiderin, and also purple due to blood leaking into surrounding tissues, with shiny appearance of the skin.

Evaluation includes use of the ABI (described earlier in this chapter) to determine whether arterial insufficiency is also present, Doppler ultrasound, Doppler bidirectional flow studies, and venography. Patient and caregiver education should include daily examination of feet and lower legs for changes in pigment, leg ulcers, or sores; avoidance of prolonged sitting or standing; avoidance of crossing legs while sitting; importance of smoking cessation (tobacco/nicotine increase hypercoagulability); regular elevation of the legs; increase in frequency of activity/exercise, as tolerated; and use of compression stockings (which can be purchased over the counter). Treatment options may include use of compression stockings, endovenous laser ablation, or radiofrequency ablation of affected veins, which will increase blood flow to the affected leg; sclerotherapy for varicosities; and direct open surgical intervention.

CASE STUDY 9.1: A Patient With Hypertension

David A. Roberts and Michelle Zappas

Patient Complaint: *"I was here a couple of weeks ago for a checkup. The nurse said my blood pressure was high. She gave me a machine, and I have been taking my pressures at home since then. I was told to come back today. I feel fine."*

History of Present Illness/Review of Systems: A 43-year-old African American man presents to the office for a blood pressure recheck. On his two previous visits to the office, his blood pressure was 142/88 mm Hg and 154/92 mm Hg, respectively. After the most recent visit, he was sent home with a blood pressure cuff to perform at-home blood pressure monitoring. The results of his home blood pressure readings reveal a mean systolic blood pressure that is 130 mm Hg or higher, and a diastolic pressure that is 80 mm Hg or higher. Based on the home readings, white coat hypertension is ruled out and he is diagnosed with essential hypertension. The review of systems finds no chest pain or shortness of breath. Right knee pain and stiffness are noted, but all other findings are negative.

Past Medical/Family History: The patient's past medical history is significant for obesity and osteoarthritis of his knees. He works a desk job and is sedentary most days. He frequently consumes fast food for convenience. His family history is significant for prostate cancer, hypertension, and hyperlipidemia on his father's side, and hypertension, hyperlipidemia, and type 2 diabetes mellitus on his mother's side. He currently takes naproxen, 500 mg twice a day as needed, for knee pain.

Physical Examination: You observe a well-appearing obese man in no acute distress. His body mass index

(BMI) is 31 kg/m². *General appearance:* The patient is alert and oriented. Funduscopic examination is negative for hemorrhage, papilledema, cotton wool spots, arteriolar narrowing, and arteriovenous nicking. Neck is supple, with no carotid bruits, thyromegaly, or nodules. Cardiovascular examination reveals regular rate and rhythm, with no murmurs, thrills, or gallops. Lungs are clear to auscultation bilaterally. Abdomen is soft, nontender, and nondistended, with no renal masses or aortic or renal artery bruits. Extremities reveal no edema bilaterally, and peripheral pulses are normal. Neurological examination is grossly intact, with no focal weakness.

Laboratory and Diagnostic Findings: You perform baseline tests, including electrolytes and serum creatinine, fasting glucose, urinalysis, CBC, TSH, and lipids; obtain an ECG; and initiate amlodipine, 5 mg by mouth daily. You set a follow-up appointment in 2 weeks to check on this patient's blood pressure and review the laboratory results.

CASE STUDY 9.1 QUESTIONS
- *Amlodipine is a calcium channel blocker. What site of blood pressure regulation does this medication work on, and why does it help?*
- *What vasodilating mediator may be reduced in a patient taking naproxen, a nonsteroidal anti-inflammatory drug?*
- *Long-standing blood pressure control is mediated by endocrine and renal function. Describe the hormones involved and how they contribute to blood pressure control.*

CBC, complete blood count; TSH, thyroid-stimulating hormone.

CASE STUDY 9.2: A Patient With Edema

David A. Roberts and Michelle Zappas

Patient Complaint: *"My legs swell up every day after work. This didn't happen to me until I started that new medication. I was feeling fine before. My blood pressure never made me feel bad."*

History of Present Illness: A 43-year-old African American man was diagnosed with essential hypertension 2 weeks ago at his previous visit (see Case Study 9.1). Amlodipine, 5 mg, was initiated, and he has been taking this daily as prescribed. He has continued to obtain home blood pressure readings: Mean blood pressure values are now <130 mm Hg systolic and <80 mm Hg diastolic. He is feeling well; however, he reports bilateral lower extremity edema and fullness. The swelling is worse in the evening, after standing on his feet most of the day at work. It improves after elevating his legs. Laboratory values obtained at his last visit were all unremarkable, and the review of systems is similarly unchanged.

Past Medical/Family History: His past medical history is significant for obesity and osteoarthritis of his

right knee. His family history, as noted previously, is significant for prostate cancer, hypertension and hyperlipidemia on his father's side, and hypertension, hyperlipidemia, and diabetes mellitus type 2 on his mother's side. He currently takes naproxen, 500 mg twice a day as needed, for knee pain.

Physical Examination: You observe a well-appearing obese man in no acute distress. The patient is alert and oriented, and findings on funduscopic, cardiovascular, pulmonary, abdominal, and neurological examinations are unchanged from his previous visit. However, in contrast to his previous visit, examination of the extremities now reveals +1 pitting edema bilaterally, with normal peripheral pulses.

CASE STUDY 9.2 QUESTIONS
- *What role do calcium channels play in VSM cell function?*
- *How might blocking calcium channels lead to increased capillary filtration manifested as edema?*

VSM, vascular smooth muscle.

BRIDGE TO CLINICAL PRACTICE: Vascular System

Ben Cocchiaro

PRINCIPLES OF ASSESSMENT
History
Evaluate:
- Symptoms of peripheral artery disease: Calf pain with walking, toe pain while lying down
- History of blood clots, hyperlipidemia, syncope
- Smoking status (active habit and total pack-years)
- Diet – Salt, sugar, fruits, vegetables, fats, carbohydrates
- Physical activity – Minutes/day, days/week, how well tolerated
- Family history of hypertension, diabetes, kidney disease, varicose veins, coronary artery disease, stroke

Physical Examination
- *Vital signs:* Know the proper methods for obtaining an accurate blood pressure measurement

- *Observe:*
  - Jugular venous pressure
  - Cyanosis of lips or extremities
  - Clubbing of the fingertips
  - Discoloration of the skin
  - Varicose veins, especially around the umbilicus
  - Nonhealing ulcers or wounds of the lower extremities
- *Auscultate:*
  - Carotid arteries and abdomen for bruits
  - Lung bases for pulmonary edema
  - Liver scratch test for hepatomegaly
- *Palpate:*
  - Blood pressure by palpation
  - Pulses
  - Capillary refill
  - Lower extremities for altered temperature, edema

(continued)

Diagnostic Tools
- *Ankle-brachial index (ABI):* Highly sensitive and specific bedside screening test for peripheral artery disease and stenosis. Patients with decreased ABI should be evaluated with segmental pressure and pulse volume recordings available in most vascular laboratories.
- *Ultrasound:*
  - Lower extremity doppler study to identify deep vein thrombosis (DVT)
  - Pulse wave velocity to measure arterial stiffness and predict atherosclerotic end-organ damage
  - One-time ultrasonographic screening for abdominal aortic aneurysm for men ages 65 to 75 years who have ever smoked
- *Ophthalmoscopic/funduscopic examination:* Allows for direct visualization of small blood vessels and can demonstrate end-organ damage associated with hypertension and atherosclerosis.
- *Coronary angiography:* To assess atherosclerotic coronary artery disease
- *Surrogate measures of vascular disease:* Carotid intima-medial thickness and coronary artery calcification have demonstrated some value in predicting vascular outcomes, but their benefit remains unclear.

Laboratory Evaluation
- *Lipid panel:* Measures total cholesterol, triglycerides, as well as high- and low-density lipoprotein (HDL and LDL)
- *ASCVD score:* A patient's fasting lipid profile can be combined with the age, sex, race, smoking, and hypertensive history to compute their Atherosclerotic Cardiovascular Disease (ASCVD) score. This 10-year estimate of a patient's risk of heart disease or stroke is the basis for lipid-lowering treatment decisions (see also Framingham Risk Score)
- *Inflammatory markers:* C-reactive protein, IL-6, and ESR are nonspecific markers for vascular endothelial damage.

MAJOR DRUG CLASSES
- *Antihypertensives:*
  - Diuretics (thiazide, loop, potassium sparing) – Decrease blood volume
  - Calcium channel blockers – Decrease vascular smooth muscle tone
  - Angiotensin-converting enzyme (ACE) inhibitors and angiotensin receptor blockers (ARBs) – Decrease angiotensin-mediated vasoconstriction and aldosterone release, protect kidneys and heart from hypertensive damage
  - Adrenergic receptor agents (α- and β-blockers, and α_2-agonists) – Decrease vasoconstriction, cardiac output, and sympathetic norepinephrine release, respectively
  - Vasodilators, nitrates – Promote nitric oxide production, directly vasodilate, some risk of postural hypotension
  - Aldosterone receptor antagonists – Reduce aldosterone-mediated sodium retention, decreasing blood volume, potassium-sparing action
- *Antianginals:* Nitrates, β-blockers, and calcium channel blockers – correct myocardial balance of oxygen supply and demand
- *Antiplatelet:* cyclooxygenase inhibitors (aspirin), ADP receptor inhibitors
- *Lipid-lowering agents:* Reduce atherosclerosis progression
- *Vasopressors:* epinephrine, norepinephrine, vasopressin – used to treat hypotension and shock

ABI, ankle–brachial index; ACE, angiotensin-converting enzyme; ARBs, angiotensin-receptor blockers; ASCVD, atherosclerotic cardiovascular disease; DVT, deep venous thrombosis; ESR, erythrocyte sedimentation rate; HDL, high-density lipoprotein; IL, interleukin; LDL, low-density lipoprotein.

KEY POINTS

- The circulatory system consists of two vascular circuits operating in parallel. The pulmonary circulation provides blood to the lungs for addition of oxygen and removal of carbon dioxide. The systemic circulation provides blood to the tissues to bring oxygen and nutrients and to remove carbon dioxide and wastes. The circulatory system also activates and inactivates hormones and vasoactive mediators and regulates body temperature.

- The main focus of this chapter is the systemic circulation, a high-pressure system that receives the cardiac output of the left side of the heart and branches extensively to provide blood flow from head to toe and all of the organs and tissues between.

- Gravity influences pressures in the systemic circulation while in the upright or sitting position, and the systolic pressure in the aorta must be sufficient to propel the blood to all levels of the body and back to the right side of the heart.

- From the aorta, blood flows sequentially through large, then small arteries, arterioles, capillaries, venules, small veins, and large veins, to the superior and inferior vena cava. Each of these segments has unique wall properties and characteristic volumes, pressures, and rates of blood flow that serve its physiological functions. Disorders of the circulation generally affect one vascular segment more than others.

- Large arteries have thicker walls than other vessels in order to withstand the higher hydrostatic pressure generated by left ventricular ejection. Their walls are normally enriched in the protein elastin, enabling them to stretch to receive the ejected volume and then to recoil to provide an additional pumping action, propelling the blood into the smaller vessels.

- Larger and moderate-sized arteries have high rates of blood flow, and the interior walls experience both perpendicular pressure from hydrostatic forces and shear stress of laminar flow within the vessel. This maintains normal health of the endothelial layer lining the vessel and promotes production of the vasodilator nitric oxide and the vasodilator and antithrombotic compound prostacyclin.

- Regions of turbulent flow alter shear stress patterns and contribute to endothelial damage. This is a first step in atherosclerosis—the most common disorder of large arteries.

- The pathogenesis of atherosclerosis involves a series of particles and cells recruited to the intimal layer, beginning with LDL cholesterol particles, followed by monocytes that mature into macrophages. The initial site becomes an inflammatory lesion with recruitment of T lymphocytes, dendritic cells, and mast cells. Cytokines are produced and further activate macrophages. ROS are generated and modify LDL cholesterol. Macrophages express scavenger receptors, ingest modified LDLs, and become immobilized foam cells. VSMs are recruited from the media to the intima and produce extracellular matrix that enlarges the growing plaque. Over time, foam cells die, leaving behind cholesterol crystals, and plaque becomes hardened and calcified.

- The effects of atherosclerosis include tissue ischemia and vulnerability to plaque rupture with formation of an occlusive thrombus producing a myocardial infarction or stroke. Turbulent flow in the region and vascular damage predispose to aneurysm formation adjacent to the plaque.

- Arterioles have abundant VSM cells in their walls that are sensitive to circulating vasoactive mediators. They provide vascular resistance to maintain systemic arterial pressure, particularly while in the upright position.

- At rest, constriction of arteriolar smooth muscle is maintained by intrinsic calcium channels and by tonic sympathetic release of norepinephrine. Simultaneously, endothelial cells produce nitric oxide, giving vasodilator tone to the balance of forces acting on the VSM.

- Several systems regulate VSM in response to physiological and pathophysiological challenges. Inflammatory mediators such as histamine and bradykinin generally produce vasodilation in a region of tissue injury and inflammation. This vasodilation diverts blood flow to the region to begin tissue healing. More global states of hypotension and hypovolemia are compensated for initially by baroreflexes and autonomic adjustments, and later by the RAAS and vasopressin hormone systems.

- Blood pressure restoration requires alterations of cardiac output and peripheral resistance, as well as renal retention of sodium and water to restore circulating fluid volume.

- Although the body is well defended against hypotension and hypovolemia, it is not able to compensate as well for increases in blood pressure. Acute increases in blood pressure stimulate parasympathetic outflow to reduce heart rate and sympathetic vasoconstrictor tone, but chronic elevations in blood pressure (as in hypertension) are not detected by baroreceptors, so there is no compensatory mechanism.

- Hypertension is among the most common of cardiovascular disorders—95% of cases are primary hypertension, the cause of which remains elusive. Management is achieved through lifestyle changes and pharmacological approaches. Adequate control of hypertension is critical to reduce long-term complications that include atherosclerosis, kidney disease, aneurysm formation, stroke, and heart disease.

- Shock is a state of severe hypotension and inadequate cardiac output. Acute systemic vasodilation occurs secondary to histamine release in anaphylactic shock. Septic shock similarly results from systemic inflammation and vasodilation due to overwhelming bacterial infection. Hemorrhagic or hypovolemic shock results from underfilling of the vascular system due to fluid losses. Cardiogenic shock can be caused by massive myocardial infarction with subsequent acute heart failure. Neurogenic shock reflects generalized loss of sympathetic vasoconstrictor tone due to neurological insults.

- The capillaries are responsible for exchange of oxygen, carbon dioxide, small molecule nutrients, and wastes between blood and tissues. Capillary walls are composed of a single layer of endothelial cells. Pores between the cells allow the exchange of fluid and plasma components, but do not generally permit movement of the proteins and cellular elements of blood.

- The forces governing fluid movement across capillary walls are the hydrostatic pressures inside the capillary and in the tissues, and the colloid osmotic pressures in these regions. Fluid movement out of the vascular space is referred to as filtration, while fluid returning to the vascular space is referred to as reabsorption.

- A variety of acute and chronic alterations of pressure in the arteries or veins, as well as the concentration of plasma proteins, influences the likelihood of net filtration that can result in edema formation.

- Veins have thinner walls than arteries and are able to hold about two thirds of the blood volume at a relatively low pressure. Their walls are innervated, and sympathetic venoconstriction can push some of the venous volume toward the heart in states of dehydration and hypotension.

- The volume and pressure of blood in veins are influenced by the pull of gravity. In the upright position, venous pressure increases along the length of the legs between thigh and foot. Walking and other leg muscle activity compresses deep leg veins, pushing the blood toward the vena cava and reducing venous pressure. Superficial leg veins can then transfer some of their volume to the deep veins. Valves within the veins prevent backflow of blood into lower parts of the leg.

- Varicose veins are one result of elevated pressure in the leg veins. With chronic pooling of blood in the legs, the superficial veins widen and become tortuous in shape. This process often causes incompetence of the venous valves, contributing to the swelling and pain experienced by patients.

- Circulatory disorders are rare in children; however, the incidence of hypertension is increasing in children. Blood pressure screening should be done correctly and levels compared with published population norms.

- Older adults have higher prevalence of all disorders of the circulatory system. Aging is associated with degradation of elastin in arterial walls, and increased levels of collagen. Compounding this situation is a relative increase of vasoconstrictor tone over vasodilator tone in older adults. The reduced compliance of arterial walls and increased arteriolar vasoconstriction causes systolic hypertension and increases the work of the heart.

- Aneurysms are more common in older adults and may progress to dissection, in which the vessel wall tears and blood accumulates in the wall, ultimately compressing the remaining lumen.

- Venous insufficiency is more prevalent with age as valves become thicker and more likely to allow reflux into dependent regions. Venous abnormalities may present as varicose veins, skin color changes due to pigment deposition into tissues, or ulcers due to local inflammation.

REFERENCES

1. World Health Organization. Cardiovascular diseases (key facts). http://www.who.int/news-room/fact-sheets/detail/cardiovascular-diseases-(cvds). Accessed January 10, 2019.

2. Fryar CD, Ostchega Y, Hales CM, et al. *Hypertension Prevalence and Control Among Adults: United States, 2015–2016.* NCHS Data Brief No. 289. Hyattsville, MD: National Center for Health Statistics; 2017. https://www.cdc.gov/nchs/data/databriefs/db289.pdf.

3. Roth GA, Johnson C, Abajobir A, et al. Global, regional, and national burden of cardiovascular diseases for 10 causes, 1990–2015. *J Am Coll Cardiol.* 2017;70:1–25. doi:10.1016/j.jacc.2017.04.052.

4. Herrington W, Lacey B, Sherliker P, et al. Epidemiology of atherosclerosis and the potential to reduce the global burden of atherosclerosis. *Circ Res.* 2016;118:535–546. doi:10.1161/CIRCRESAHA.115.307611.

5. National Cholesterol Education Program. *ATP III Guidelines At-A-Glance Quick Desk Reference.* NIH Publication No. 01-3305. Bethesda, MD: National Institutes of Health; May. 2001 https://www.nhlbi.nih.gov/files/docs/guidelines/atglance.pdf.

6. Barnes M, Heywood AE, Mahimbo A, et al. Acute myocardial infarction and influenza: a meta-analysis of case-control studies. *Heart.* 2015;101:1738–1747. doi:10.1136/heartjnl-2015-307691.

7. Bouhairie VE, Goldberg AC. Familial hypercholesterolemia. *Cardiol Clin.* 2015;33:169–179. doi:10.1016/j.ccl.2015.01.001.

8. American Heart Association Statistics Committee and Stroke Statistics Subcommittee. Heart disease and stroke statistics—2017 update. A report from the American Heart Association. *Circulation.* 2017;135:e146–e603. doi:10.1161/CIR.0000000000000485.

9. American Heart Association. High blood pressure redefined for the first time in 14 years: 130 is the new high. http://newsroom.heart.org/news/high-blood-pressure-redefined-for-first-time-in-14-years-130-is-the-new-high. Published November 13, 2017. Accessed March 30, 2019.

10. Kumar V, Abbas AK, Aster JC, eds. *Robbins Basic Pathology.* 10th ed. Philadelphia, PA: Elsevier; 2018.

11. Centers for Disease Control and Prevention. National Diabetes Statistics Report—2017. https://www.cdc.gov/diabetes/pdfs/data/statistics/national-diabetes-statistics-report.pdf. Accessed January 23, 2019.

12. Massaro AF. Approach to the patient with shock. In: Kasper D, Fauci A, Hauser S, et al., eds. *Harrison's Principles of Internal Medicine.* 20th ed. New York, NY: McGraw-Hill; 2018:chap 296.

13. Boulpaep EL. The microcirculation. In: Boron WF, Boulpaep EL, eds. *Medical Physiology.* 3rd ed. Philadelphia, PA: Elsevier; 2017: 461–482.

14. Meissner MH, Moneta G, Burnand K, et al. The hemodynamics and diagnosis of venous disease. *J Vasc Surg.* 2007;46:4S–24S. doi:10.1016/j.jvs.2007.09.043.

15. Hamdan A. Management of varicose veins and venous insufficiency. *JAMA.* 2012;308:2612–2621. doi:10.1001/jama.2012.111352.

16. Bernstein D. History and physical exam. In: Kliegman RM, Stanton BF, St Geme JW, et al., eds. *Nelson Textbook of Pediatrics.* 20th ed. Philadelphia, PA: Elsevier; 2015: 2163–2170.

17. Falkner B. Changes in the 2017 pediatric hypertension clinical guidelines. *Am J Hypertens.* 2017;31:18–20. doi:10.1093/ajh/hpx190.

18. Flynn JT, Kaelber DC, Baker-Smith CM, et al. Clinical practice guidelines for screening and management of high blood pressure in children and adolescents. *Pediatrics.* 2017;140:1–72. doi:10.1542/peds.2017-1904.

19. Litwin M, Feber J, Ruzicka M. Vascular aging: lessons from pediatric hypertension. *Can J Cardiol.* 2016;32:642–649. doi:10.1016/j.cjca.2016.02.064.

20. Paneni F, Diaz Canestro C, Libby P, et al. The aging cardiovascular system. Understanding it at the cellular and clinical levels. *J Am Coll Cardiol.* 2017;69:1952–1967. doi:10.1016/j.jacc.2017.01.064.

21. Dai X, Hummel SL, Salazar JB, et al. Cardiovascular physiology in older adults. *J Geriatr Cardiol.* 2015;12:196–201. doi:10.11909/j.issn.1671–5411.2015.03.015.

22. Donato AJ, Machin DR, Lesniewski LA. Mechanisms of dysfunction in the aging vasculature and role in age-related disease. *Circ Res.* 2018;123:825–848. doi:10.1161/CIRCRESAHA.118.312563.

23. Strait JB, Lakatta EG. Aging-associated cardiovascular changes and their relationship to heart failure. *Heart Fail Clin.* 2012;8:143–164. doi:10.1016/j.hfc.2011.08.011.

24. Savji N, Rockman CB, Skolnick AH, et al. Association between advanced age and vascular disease in different arterial territories. A population database of over 3.6 million subjects. *J Am Coll Cardiol.* 2013;61:1736–1743. doi:10.1016/j.jacc.2013.01.054.

25. Johnston KW, Ritherford RB, Tilson MD, et al. Suggested Standards for Reporting on arterial aneurysms. Subcommittee on Reporting Standards for Arterial Aneurysms. Ad Hoc Committee on Reporting Standards. Society for Vascular Surgery and North American Chapter, International Society for Cardiovascular Surgery. *J Vasc Surg.* 1991;13:452–458. doi:10.1067/mva.1991.26737.

26. Miller AP, Huff CM, Roubin GS. Vascular disease in the older adult. *J Geriatr Cardiol.* 2016;13:727–732. doi:10.11909/j.issn.1671-5411.2016.09.011.

27. Criado FJ. Aortic dissection. A 250-year perspective. *Tex Heart Inst J.* 2011;38:694–700. https://www.ncbi.nlm.nih.gov/pmc/articles/PMC3233335.

28. Hiratzka LF, Bakris GL, Beckman JA, et al. ACCF/AHA/AATS/ACR/ASA/SCA/SCAI/SIR/STS/SVM guidelines for the diagnosis and management of patients with thoracic aortic disease: a report of the America College of Cardiology Foundation/American Heart Association Task Force on Practice Guidelines, American Association

for Thoracic Surgery, American College of Radiology, American Stroke Association, Society of Cardiovascular Anesthesiologists, Society for Cardiovascular Angiography and Interventions, Society of Interventional Radiology, Society of Thoracic Surgeons, and Society for Vascular Medicine. *Circulation*. 2010;121:e266–e369. doi:10.1161/CIR.0b013e3181d4739e.

29. Bergan JJ, Schmid-Schönbein GW, Smith PD, et al. Chronic venous disease. *N Engl J Med*. 2006;355:488. doi:10.1056/NEJMra055289.

30. van Langevelde K, Sramek A, Rosendaal FR. The effect of aging on venous valves. *Arterioscler Thromb Vasc Biol*. 2010;30:2075–2080. doi:10.1161/ATVBAHA.110.209049.

31. Eberhardt RT, Raffetto JD. Chronic venous insufficiency. *Circulation*. 2014;130:333–346. doi:10.1161/CIRCULATIONAHA.113.006898.

SUGGESTED RESOURCES

Klabunde RE. *Cardiovascular Physiology Concepts*. 2nd ed. Philadelphia, PA: Lippincott Williams & Wilkins; 2012.

Kumar V, Abbas AK, Aster JC, eds. *Robbins Basic Pathology*. 10th ed. Philadelphia, PA: Elsevier; 2018.

Libby P. Atlas of atherosclerosis. In: Kasper D, Fauci A, Hauser S, et al., eds. *Harrison's Principles of Internal Medicine*. 20th ed. New York, NY: McGraw-Hill; 2018:chap A10.

Lilly LS, Leonard S. *Pathophysiology of Heart Disease: A Collaborative Project of Medical Students and Faculty*. 5th ed. Philadelphia, PA: Lippincott Williams & Wilkins; 2011.

Morhman DE, Heller LJ. *Cardiovascular Physiology*. 9th ed. New York, NY: McGraw-Hill; 2018.

Preston RR, Wilson TE. *Lippincott's Illustrated Reviews: Physiology*. Philadelphia, PA: Lippincott Williams & Wilkins; 2013.

10

HEART

Fruzsina K. Johnson, Robert A. Johnson, and Spencer A. Rhodes

THE CLINICAL CONTEXT

Heart disease is the leading cause of death in the United States, accounting for one in four deaths. Sixty percent of these deaths result from myocardial infarction.[1] Worldwide statistics are similar: Cardiovascular disease is the number one cause of death globally. Of the 17.9 million deaths worldwide, 85% are caused by myocardial infarction and stroke.[2] In the United States, 85.6 million adults have one or more forms of cardiovascular disease, and there is substantial comorbidity between hypertension, coronary heart disease, heart failure, and stroke. Heart failure is a leading cause of hospitalization and healthcare expense and contributes to one in nine deaths annually. Importantly, the American Heart Association in 2011 developed goals for healthy lifestyle behaviors to improve heart health and reduce cardiovascular risk for people of all ages in the United States. These guidelines include improving diet patterns, increasing physical activity, reducing obesity, and smoking cessation, as well as clinical management to achieve targets for blood lipids, blood pressure, and blood glucose. By providing education and coaching their patients toward optimal lifestyle choices, clinicians can aid in reducing the global toll of cardiovascular morbidity and mortality.[3]

OVERVIEW OF CARDIOVASCULAR STRUCTURE AND FUNCTION

HOMEOSTATIC FUNCTIONS OF THE HEART

As described in Chapter 9, Circulation, the heart is one of the three primary components of the cardiovascular system. The primary homeostatic function of the heart is to generate pressure that drives blood flow through the vasculature serially to the lungs and to the organs and tissues. Achieving this function requires electrical impulses, generated by pacemaker cells at regular intervals and propagated through the heart, and contractile cells that respond to this excitation by generating pressure and ejecting a volume of blood into the pulmonary and systemic circulatory beds.

The cardiac cycle is the sequence of events repeated with each heartbeat. It consists of *diastole*, a resting state during which the heart is filling, and *systole*, an active state of contraction and ejection of blood into the vascular system. This rhythmic activity establishes the cardiac output, the product of heart rate and stroke volume (CO = HR × SV), the total blood flow per minute in the cardiovascular circuit. Cardiac output in adult males averages 5 L/min (approximate range 4 to 8 L/min). The heart can support strenuous exercise by increasing heart rate and stroke volume such that cardiac output increases to four to five times the resting amount. The heart is actually two pumps in one organ, simultaneously driving blood flow in both the systemic and the pulmonary circulations (**Figure 10.1**).

STRUCTURAL ORGANIZATION OF THE HEART

Cardiac Chambers and Valves

The heart has four chambers: two atria (right and left) and two ventricles (right and left). Each atrium is connected to a ventricle via an atrioventricular (AV) valve: The tricuspid valve connects the right atrium to the right ventricle, and the bicuspid (mitral) valve connects the left atrium to the left ventricle. The right atrium, tricuspid valve, and right ventricle form the right side of the heart—the pump that receives mixed venous (deoxygenated) blood from the systemic veins and pumps it into the pulmonary circulation. The left atrium, mitral valve, and left ventricle form the left side of the heart—the pump that receives arterial (oxygenated) blood from the pulmonary veins and pumps it into the

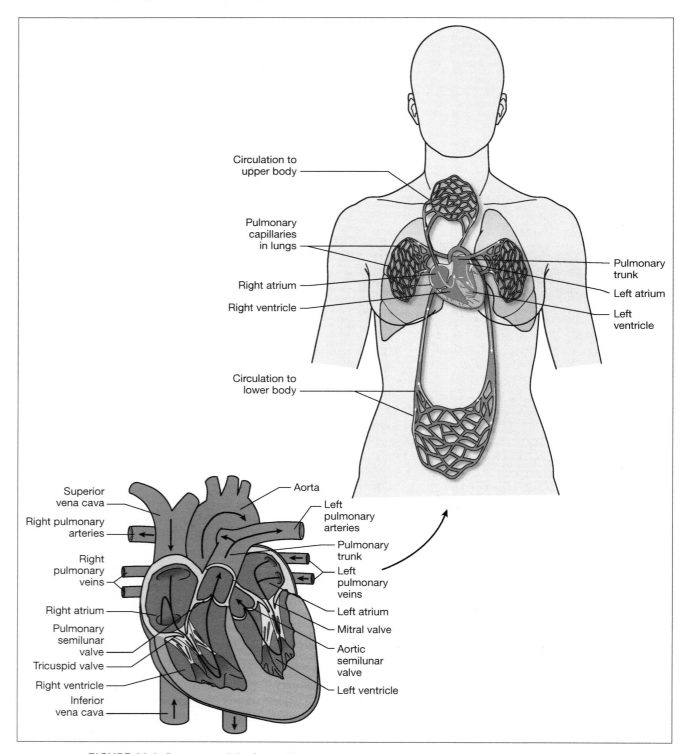

FIGURE 10.1 Structure of the heart. From its entry to the right atrium, blood flows through the tricuspid valve, the right ventricle, and the pulmonary valve, to the lungs. Blood leaving the lungs flows into the left atrium, through the mitral valve, the left ventricle, and the aortic valve on its way to perfuse the body tissues. Thus, the heart consists of four chambers and two circuits, with the right side perfusing the lungs and the left side perfusing the body.

systemic circulation. The two ventricles are connected to their outflow path via semilunar one-way valves: The right ventricle is connected to the pulmonary artery via the pulmonary (pulmonic) valve, and the left ventricle is connected to the aorta via the aortic valve.

Membranes Protecting the Heart

The heart and its connections with the major vessels are surrounded by a multilayered membrane called the pericardium (**Figure 10.2**), forming a compartment referred to as the pericardial sac. The pericardial sac consists of two distinct layers (**Figure 10.2a**): the outer tough fibrous pericardium, and the inner serous pericardium. The serous pericardium has a further two layers: the parietal layer that is connected to the fibrous pericardium, and the visceral layer known as epicardium, which is directly adjacent to the cardiac muscle and forms the outer layer of the heart wall. Between the two layers of the serous pericardium is the pericardial space, which normally contains a small amount of serous fluid that allows for smooth, frictionless movement of the ventricular walls with each contraction. Pathological thickening of the pericardium (constrictive pericarditis) or accumulation of extra fluid in the pericardial space (pericardial effusion and cardiac tamponade; **Figure 10.2b**) can restrict movement of the ventricular walls. Acute, severe tamponade can have high mortality risk due to pulmonary edema and obstructive shock.

Structure of the Heart Wall

The heart wall has three layers (**Figure 10.2a**):

1. *Epicardium*—the visceral layer of the serous pericardium (as previously described)
2. *Myocardium*—the middle and most prominent layer, composed of cardiac muscle
3. *Endocardium*—the layer that lines the cardiac chambers and is continuous with the vascular endothelium

Although myocardium is the dominant layer of the cardiac wall, its thickness varies greatly, depending on the cardiac chamber. Atrial walls are typically thin, as the atria are not designed to generate high pressures. Although they pump the same amount of blood, the left and right ventricles have to generate very different pressures in accordance with the differences in resistance between the systemic and pulmonary circulations. The left ventricle, with thick muscular walls, generates high pressures (normally up to 120 mm Hg) to drive flow in the systemic circulation. In contrast, the thinner, less muscular right ventricle generates lower pressure (normally up to 25 mm Hg) to drive blood flow in the much lower resistance pulmonary circulation (**Figure 10.3**).

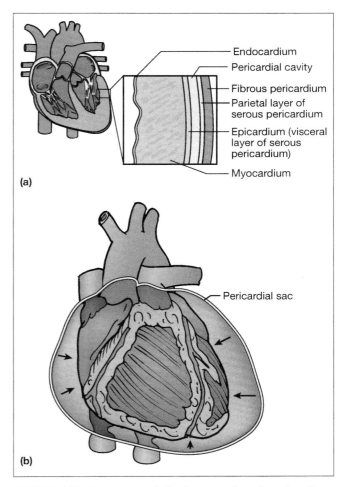

(a)

Endocardium
Pericardial cavity
Fibrous pericardium
Parietal layer of serous pericardium
Epicardium (visceral layer of serous pericardium)
Myocardium

(b)

FIGURE 10.2 Structures of the heart wall and pericardium. **(a)** The walls of the cardiac chambers consist of three layers: inner endocardium, myocardium, and outer epicardium. The epicardium is adjacent to the pericardial space (cavity), the outer boundary of which is the parietal layer of serous pericardium. The fibrous pericardium makes up the outer pericardial layer. **(b)** Buildup of pericardial fluid compresses the heart (*arrows*) and can compromise cardiac filling and cardiac output.

OVERVIEW OF MYOCARDIAL CELL STRUCTURE

Unlike skeletal muscle, which consists of multinucleated long muscle fibers, cardiac muscle cells are relatively short, cylindrical, mononucleated cells (**Figure 10.4**). They have a striated appearance, due to abundant sarcomeres of aligned actin and myosin filaments, and contain many mitochondria, as well as an extensive sarcoplasmic reticulum. Cardiac cells are linked together by desmosomes—clustered proteins in patches that *glue together* adjacent cells for mechanical coupling—and gap junctions—pores made of connexin protein subunits. These pores are nonselective ion channels that permit rapid movement of charges between cells during action potential propagation along the thickness of the atrial and ventricular muscle walls.

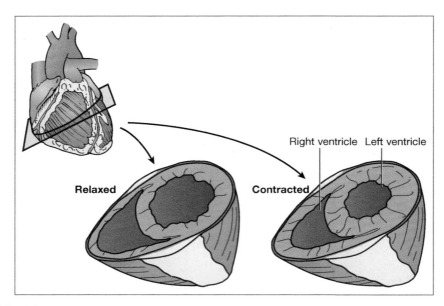

FIGURE 10.3 Ventricular wall structure. The right ventricle pumps blood under low pressure into the low-resistance pulmonary circuit. This requires less force generation such that the right ventricular wall thickness is substantially less than that of the left ventricle. The left ventricle must achieve higher pressure to open the aortic valve (about 70 mm Hg) and must generate substantial pressure (about 120 mm Hg) to eject its stroke volume. As a consequence, the left ventricle has a narrower chamber and a thicker wall.

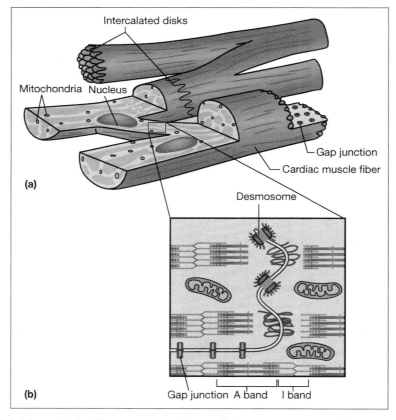

FIGURE 10.4 Myocardial cell structure and intercellular connections. **(a)** Myocardial cells are relatively short and cylindrical and are connected by specialized portions of the plasma membrane called intercalated disks. Their cytoplasm has abundant myofilaments consisting of actin and myosin proteins arrayed in sarcomeres. **(b)** Cardiac cell-cell junctions at intercalated disks include desmosomes that are mechanical links between cells, and gap junctions that are electrical links between cells.

MYOCARDIAL OXYGEN SUPPLY AND DEMAND

Weighing about 300 g, the heart tissue receives blood flow of 84 mL/min/100 g at rest—more than any other organ except the kidney. The heart also has the highest oxygen consumption of any organ, at 9.7 mL/100 g/min at rest (the whole-body average is 0.4 mL/100 g/min).[4] This high consumption is due to the constant workload of rhythmic muscle contractions and the fact that the heart uses aerobic metabolism almost exclusively. The main fuel for the heart is energy-rich free fatty acids. The high myocardial demand for oxygen presents a point of vulnerability: high rates of coronary artery blood flow and turbulent flow dynamics at the origin of the coronary arteries from the aorta predispose to atherosclerosis, and narrowed arteries that reduce blood supply to the oxygen-hungry heart can precipitate myocardial ischemia.

CARDIAC ELECTROPHYSIOLOGY AND PATHOPHYSIOLOGY

MYOCARDIAL CELL ION CHANNELS AND TRANSPORTERS

Electrical and mechanical events of cardiac rhythmic activation and pump function depend on specific ion channels and transporters of the plasma membrane (*sarcolemma*) and sarcoplasmic reticulum membrane (**Figure 10.5**). As with other excitable cells, myocardial cells have a high rate of the active transporter sodium–potassium–adenosine triphosphatase (Na$^+$/K$^+$–ATPase)

activity that establishes and maintains ionic gradients across the plasma membrane: sodium (Na$^+$) predominates in the extracellular fluid, and potassium (K$^+$) in the intracellular fluid. At rest, the membrane is most permeable to K$^+$, thus setting a resting membrane potential—a voltage difference across the membrane in which the intracellular potential is negative relative to the extracellular fluid, as described in Chapter 4, Cell Physiology and Pathophysiology. Voltage-gated ion channels selective for Na$^+$, calcium (Ca^{2+}), and K$^+$ shape action potentials of cardiac cells. Ca^{2+}–ATPase active transport pumps in the sarcolemma and sarcoplasmic reticulum membranes actively transport Ca^{2+} out of the cell and into the sarcoplasmic reticulum, respectively. Ca^{2+} is also removed from the cytoplasm by a secondary active transporter—the Na$^+$–Ca^{2+} exchange protein. The ryanodine receptor of the sarcoplasmic reticulum membrane is a Ca^{2+} ion channel that links Ca^{2+} entry into the cell to additional Ca^{2+} release into the cytoplasm to cause muscle contraction. As previously noted, gap junctions between adjacent cells are ion channels that allow rapid propagation of the action potentials between myocardial cells. The energy demands of Na$^+$/K$^+$ and Ca^{2+} pumps contribute to the high metabolic demands of cardiac tissue.

STRUCTURE OF THE CARDIAC CONDUCTION SYSTEM

The heart has its own impulse generation and conduction system (**Figure 10.6**) that initiates rhythmic beats and coordinates function of the cardiac chambers.

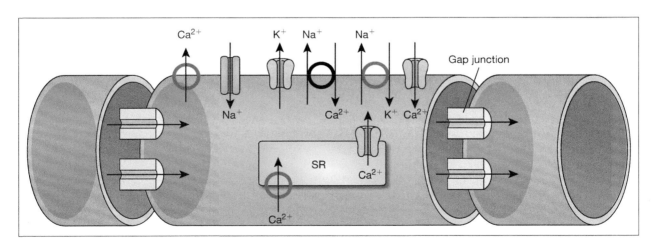

FIGURE 10.5 Cardiac cell membrane proteins. These proteins are responsible for action potential propagation and contractile activity. The sarcolemma contains voltage-gated sodium (Na$^+$), calcium (Ca^{2+}), and potassium (K$^+$) channels that shape the action potentials. Gap junction ion channels allow electrical impulses to be propagated between adjacent cells. The Na$^+$/K$^+$ pump maintains ion gradients and the resting membrane potential, and the Ca^{2+} pump and Na$^+$–Ca^{2+} exchanger contribute to low intracellular Ca^{2+} concentration at rest. The SR membrane contains a Ca^{2+} release channel, also known as the ryanodine receptor, and the sarco-endoplasmic reticulum calcium ATPase (SERCA). SERCA sequesters Ca^{2+} in the SR, causing diastolic relaxation that allows ventricular filling after each contraction.

SERCA, sarcoendoplasmic reticulum Ca^{2+} ATPase (adenosine triphosphatase); SR, sarcoplasmic reticulum.

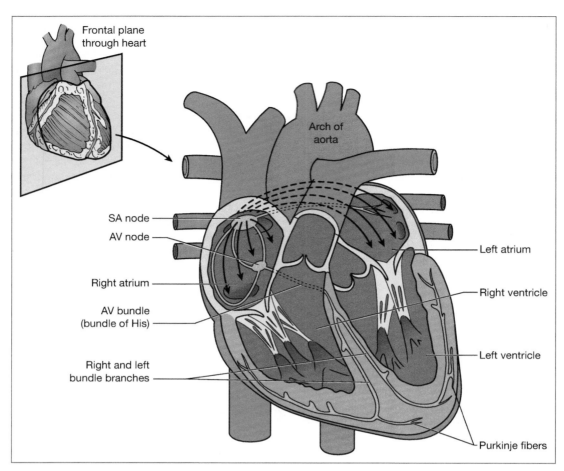

FIGURE 10.6 The cardiac conduction system—anterior view of frontal section. Action potentials are generated at regular intervals by the pacemaker cells of the SA node. The action potentials propagate through pathways to the right and left atria and through specialized internodal pathways to the AV node. Action potential propagation slows briefly as it moves through the AV node cells, then accelerates through the bundle of His, bundle branches, and Purkinje fibers. From the Purkinje fibers the impulse is propagated through the walls of the right and left ventricles.
AV, atrioventricular; SA, sinoatrial.

The conduction system structures are made of modified cardiac muscle cells with electrical properties that differ from those of normal contractile cardiac cells. Under normal conditions, the cardiac atria are almost completely electrically insulated from the ventricles by the fibrous cardiac skeleton that supports the cardiac valves. The two atria and the two ventricles are in direct electrical contact with each other, but normally the only impulse-conducting pathway between the atria and the ventricles is the AV node and the bundle of His (collectively called the *AV junction*).

Typically, the action potential that triggers cardiac contraction is generated in the sinoatrial (SA) node in the wall of the right atrium. The impulse is then conducted via (a) internodal pathways to the AV node (still in the atrial wall) and (b) interatrial pathways to the left atrium, while also propagating throughout the right atrium. The slowest impulse conduction occurs at the AV node, creating the AV nodal delay. This is important for normal cardiac function, as it allows the atria to contract while ventricles are still relaxed at the end of diastole, finishing ventricular filling (sometimes called the *atrial kick*). The impulse is then conducted to the ventricles, causing ventricular contraction during systole. From the AV node, the impulse is conducted via the His (AV) bundle to the septum separating the two ventricles. The His bundle divides into left and right bundle branches that further branch to supply the left and right ventricles. Both bundle branches reach the cardiac apex and connect to very rapidly conducting Purkinje fibers that distribute cardiac impulses to the ventricular muscle cells.

CARDIAC CELL ACTION POTENTIALS

The heart is mostly composed of excitable cardiac muscle cells. Electrical activity (changes in membrane potential) of these cells is vital for (a) action potential generation, (b) action potential conduction, and (c) contraction of cardiac muscle. Spontaneous generation of action potentials by the SA node triggers rhythmic cardiac contractions normally at 60 to 100 beats/min. Conduction pathways ensure highly coordinated sequential activation of the cardiac chambers, optimizing ventricular filling and ejection. Contraction of cardiac muscle generates the force to increase ventricular pressure, providing the driving force for blood flow in the circulatory system.

Cardiac cells can be categorized as one of the two types based on their action potentials (**Figure 10.7**):

- *Nonpacemaker cells* make up the majority (99%) of cells of the atria and ventricles. These cells are specialized to do the work of contraction, leading to pressure development and the pumping action of the heart. Based on their action potential properties, they are also referred to as *fast-response cells*. Their

function and actions are described in **Box 10.1** and **Figure 10.8**.

- *Pacemaker-type cells*, representing about 1% of cardiac cells, are primarily found in the SA and AV nodes. These cells spontaneously generate action potentials at a regular rate and rhythm. Based on their action potential properties, they are also referred to as *slow-response cells*. The rate of action potential generation of these cells is modulated by autonomic nerves, with parasympathetic activity decreasing their firing rate, and sympathetic activity increasing their firing rate.

Refractory Periods in Contractile Cardiac Muscle Cells

Refractory periods refer to time intervals during the action potential when membrane excitability is zero,

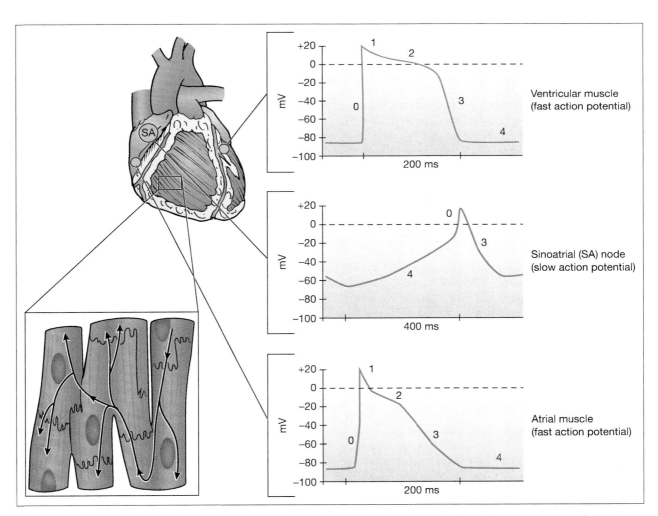

FIGURE 10.7 Action potentials differ in different cardiac regions and cells. Cells of the sinoatrial node, atrial muscle, and ventricular muscle have action potentials with distinctive phases and shapes. Rapid propagation through electrically coupled cells is facilitated by gap junctions and is capable of bidirectional movement.
Source: From Rhoades, Bell. *Medical Physiology.* 5th ed. Figure 12.1 modified by the author, Fruzsina K. Johnson.

BOX 10.1
Phases of Fast-Response Action Potentials in Contractile (Nonpacemaker) Cardiac Muscle Cells

Figure 10.8 illustrates a fast-response action potential seen in typical contractile cardiac muscle cells of the atrial and ventricular walls (99% of cardiac muscle cells). These cells are designed for force generation by contraction. The action potentials trigger contractions (excitation–contraction coupling), and conduct waves of depolarizations to neighboring cardiac muscle cells connected via gap junctions. These action potentials have five phases (numbered 0 to 4), as follows:

- **Phase 0** is *rapid depolarization* caused by opening of fast Na^+ channels and influx of Na^+.

- **Phase 1** is *transient early repolarization*. During this phase, Na^+ channels inactivate and transient outward K^+ channels open briefly and begin to repolarize the membrane. These channels are open only for a brief period.

- **Phase 2** is called the *plateau phase*, because the membrane potential remains fairly stable at a mostly depolarized state. In this phase, Ca^{2+} influx via the slow, long-lasting (L)–type Ca^{2+} channels and K^+ efflux via repolarizing K^+ channels balance each other. Fast Na^+ channels remain inactivated. Ca^{2+} entering the contractile cardiac muscle cells during this phase triggers Ca^{2+} release from the sarcoplasmic reticulum (Ca^{2+}-induced Ca^{2+} release), a vital step in excitation–contraction coupling.

- **Phase 3** is *membrane repolarization*. During this phase, Ca^{2+} channels close but slow K^+ channels remain open, and the K^+ leaving the cells returns membrane potential toward baseline. In this phase, fast Na^+ channel gates progressively reset to their resting position. The

Na^+/K^+ pump and Ca^{2+} transporters reestablish the ion gradients, and the cell membrane returns to resting membrane potential (phase 4).

- **Phase 4** is the *resting membrane potential* (–90 mV). In this phase, K^+ leak channels are open and K^+ is leaking out of the cell; other channels are closed.

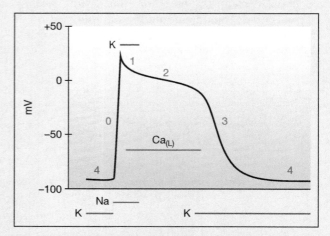

FIGURE 10.8 Fast-response action potential. Nonpacemaker cells have a stable resting membrane potential (phase 4). When a wave of depolarization is propagated from neighboring cells, the resulting depolarization brings the membrane to threshold for opening fast Na^+ channels (phase 0, Na^+ current-mediated upstroke). At the peak of the action potential, the Na^+ channels close and inactivate. Phase 1 is a transient repolarization. During phase 2, voltage-gated Ca^{2+} channels are open and maintain the plateau membrane potential. Ca^{2+} entry is also linked to release of Ca^{2+} from the sarcoplasmic reticulum and muscle tension development. In phase 3, Ca^{2+} channels close and delayed K^+ channels open, repolarizing the membrane back to the resting membrane potential.

or greatly decreased. In most excitable cells, we distinguish two refractory periods (**Figure 10.9**):

1. *Absolute* refractory period—at this point membrane excitability is zero, so another depolarizing stimulus cannot elicit another action potential
2. *Relative* refractory period—when the membrane can produce an action potential, but only in response to larger than typical depolarizing stimulus

Refractory periods are caused by unique two-part gating of fast Na^+ channels. The fast Na^+

channel has two gates that close the ion channel pore: the *activation* gate, which is normally closed during resting membrane potential; and the *inactivation* gate, which is normally open at rest. At resting membrane potential, the activation gate keeps the channel closed, so Na^+ cannot enter the cell. A depolarizing stimulus that reaches the channel's voltage threshold opens the activation gate, enabling Na^+ to enter the cell (because both activation and inactivation gates are open); this creates the upstroke of the action potential. Once the membrane potential becomes positive (at the peak of the action potential), the inactivation gate closes the

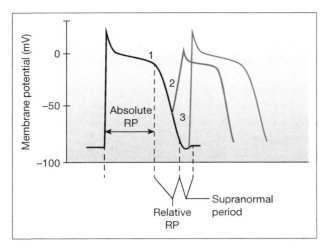

FIGURE 10.9 Nonpacemaker cells have RPs. During the absolute RP **(1)**, the cell cannot be excited to have a second action potential. This is primarily due to continued inactivation of Na⁺ channels that cannot open until the membrane potential is more negative. During the relative RP, an incoming wave of depolarization may cause the cell to have a premature action potential **(2)**, but it may not have the usual height or speed of conduction. After complete repolarization, there is a supranormal period during which the cell is more vulnerable to depolarization producing hyperexcitability **(3)**. RP, refractory period.
Source: From Lilly LS. *Pathophysiology of Heart Disease: A Collaborative Project of Medical Students and Faculty.* 6th ed. Wolters Kluwer; 2015, modified by the author Fruzsina K. Johnson.

channel, preventing further Na⁺ entry (despite the activation gate being still open). In this state, the Na⁺ channels are blocked by the inactivation gate, so further depolarization is not possible; this causes the absolute refractory period.

During the absolute refractory period of a cardiac cell, an action potential propagated from an adjacent cell will not produce another action potential of the refractory cell (identified by [1] in **Figure 10.9**). During repolarization (phase 3), as the membrane potential returns toward resting, the activation gate begins to close, while the inactivation gate begins to open simultaneously. Thus, there is no Na⁺ entry through the channel (one or the other gate is still closing the channel), but the gates reset to their original resting state and the membrane becomes excitable again.

The relative refractory period occurs when some of the Na⁺ channels are recovered (their inactivation gates have opened). During this period, a larger than typical stimulus can cause opening of the already recovered channels, triggering membrane depolarization and a second, smaller action potential following immediately on the first ([2] in **Figure 10.9**). The likelihood that this will happen depends on the slope of phase 3

repolarization. The more rapid it is, the more likely a second action potential can be generated. One class of antiarrhythmic drugs works by blocking K⁺ channels, thereby prolonging the refractory period and making it less likely for an ectopic beat to be propagated to adjacent cells.

Supranormal Period in Contractile Cardiac Muscle Cells

In addition to the refractory periods, cardiac muscle cells also have a supranormal period following the relative refractory period. During the supranormal period, membrane excitability is greater than normal, and the cell can respond to a propagated action potential with a full-sized action potential ([3] in **Figure 10.9**). For some ventricular cells, this period coincides with the peak of the T wave on the ECG and marks the time when a depolarizing stimulus may trigger life-threatening ventricular fibrillation. Synchronized direct-current cardioversion (used as a treatment option for atrial fibrillation) monitors the ECG and ensures that the electric shock is not delivered during this vulnerable period.

Slow-Response Action Potentials in Pacemaker Cardiac Muscle Cells

As previously noted, pacemaker cells are found in the SA and AV nodes and represent about 1% of all cells in the heart. These are modified cardiac muscle cells that have lost their ability to contract but are capable of spontaneous action potential generation. The SA node cells serve as the primary pacemakers of the heart, and the rate of action potentials generated by these cells determines heart rate. The phases of these action potentials are numbered similarly to the fast-response action potentials described in **Box 10.1**, earlier, but phases 1 (rapid repolarization) and 2 (plateau) are missing. Although the rest of the phases are numbered the same as in contractile cells, different ion currents are responsible for the various phases of the action potential. Phases of the slow-response action potential are shown in **Figure 10.10** and described in **Box 10.2**.

 Thought Questions

1. What are the ionic events that shape the action potentials of nonpacemaker cells, and how do they compare with the ionic events shaping the action potentials of pacemaker cells?

2. What membrane proteins are responsible for the ion distributions across the plasma membrane during the resting membrane potential and ion movements making up the action potentials?

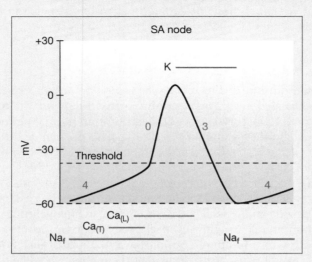

FIGURE 10.10 Pacemaker cells have no resting membrane potential. The ability to generate regular action potentials and serve as a pacemaker requires a source of spontaneous depolarization that continuously brings the membrane to action potential threshold. In pacemaker cells during phase 4, there is a progressive depolarization caused by Na+ entry through hyperpolarization-activated cyclic nucleotide-gated channels, accompanied by a small Ca^{2+} current carried by transient T-type Ca^{2+} channels ($Ca^{2+}_{(T)}$). This continues until the threshold is reached for opening larger voltage-gated L-type Ca^{2+} channels ($Ca^{2+}_{(L)}$). The upstroke (phase 0) mediated by Ca^{2+} entry through L channels does not have the rapid rate of voltage change associated with nonpacemaker cells. Phase 3 repolarization results from K+ efflux through voltage-gated K+ channels, similar to nonpacemaker cells. SA, sinoatrial.
Source: From Klabunde RE. *Cardiovascular Physiology Concepts.* 2nd ed. Lippincott; 2012.

- **Phase 0**, *upstroke*, begins when the spontaneous depolarization reaches the threshold potential. In pacemaker cells, fast Na+ channels are either missing or mostly inactivated (due to the less negative MDP, described later); thus, the upstroke is mediated by Ca^{2+} influx via slow voltage-gated (L-type) Ca^{2+} channels. These are the same types of Ca^{2+} channels that are open during the plateau (phase 2) of the contractile cardiac muscle cell action potential, as outlined in **Box 10.1**. Pacemaker action potentials are referred to as *slow response* in comparison with the contractile cell action potentials,

because the L-type Ca^{2+} channels open more slowly than fast Na+ channels, and the rate of rise of the membrane potential in phase 0 is correspondingly slower.

- **Phases 1 and 2** are missing from the pacemaker cell action potentials.

- **Phase 3**, *repolarization*, is mediated by K+ leaving the cells via voltage-gated K+ channels, similar to the fast-response action potential. Phase 3 ends as the membrane achieves its MDP, at which point most K+ channels close and phase 4 diastolic depolarization begins.

- **Phase 4** is *spontaneous diastolic depolarization*, also called the *pacemaker potential*. In phase 4, cells do not have a stable resting membrane potential because of the actions of unique cation channels, called *funny* channels (f) or HCN channels.
  - The primary current through the HCN channels occurs because of Na+ influx. The *funny* channels are so called because unlike the fast Na+ channels of nonpacemaker cells, which open in response to depolarization, the HCN channels open when the membrane is most (hyper)polarized at the end of repolarization.
  - As a result of these channels, as soon as the pacemaker cells are repolarized at the end of an action potential, they begin to depolarize again. Thus, in these cells, the most negative membrane potential occurs as phase 3 transitions to phase 4. This point is termed the MDP, as these cells do not have a stable resting membrane potential.
  - Na+ influx via the HCN channels is responsible for most of the phase 4 depolarization, but transient (T-type) Ca^{2+} channels also open and contribute to the later part of the pacemaker potential. T-type Ca^{2+} channels are different from the slow L-type Ca^{2+} channels responsible for phase 0. The slope (rate) of this spontaneous depolarization is a very important determinant of heart rate.
  - The combination of decreased K+ permeability at the end of phase 0, Na+ entry through funny channels, and Ca^{2+} entry through T-type Ca^{2+} channels constitutes the upward slope of membrane potential that controls pacemaker cell action potential frequency.

HCN, hyperpolarization-activated cyclic nucleotide-gated; MDP, maximum diastolic potential.

FUNCTIONAL ASPECTS OF CARDIAC ACTION POTENTIALS

Slope of Phase 4 Depolarization in the SA Node Cells Regulates Heart Rate

Under normal conditions, the SA node pacemaker cells provide the impulse for cardiac contractions, and every action potential generated by these cells is propagated through the AV node, resulting in a ventricular contraction (normal sinus rhythm). Thus, the heart rate (beats per minute, also known as *chronotropy*) is determined by the frequency of action potential generation by the SA node pacemaker cells. Once the pacemaker cell membrane depolarizes to threshold potential, the voltage-gated (L-type) Ca^{2+} channels open and a typical action potential is generated. Thus, the SA node firing rate is primarily determined by the duration of phase 4 spontaneous depolarization—the length of time it takes for the cell membrane to depolarize from the maximum diastolic potential to threshold potential. The intrinsic SA node firing rate is approximately 100 beats/min under conditions of no autonomic input to the heart. SA node cells are innervated by both the sympathetic and parasympathetic branches of the autonomic nervous system, and increased activity of sympathetic or parasympathetic cardiac nerves increases or decreases heart rate, respectively.

The duration of phase 4 can be increased by various mechanisms, leading to slower heart rate. **Figure 10.11** illustrates three potential mechanisms:

- *Panel a*: Decreased rate of spontaneous depolarization can result from reductions in the Na^+ *funny* current.
- *Panel b*: Negative shift in maximum diastolic potential (hyperpolarization of the cell membrane) can take the membrane potential farther away from the threshold voltage.
- *Panel c*: Positive shift in threshold potential requires greater time for diastolic depolarization to reach threshold.

These mechanisms alone or combined may result in increased length of phase 4 and decreased firing rate of the SA node.

The vagus nerve (cranial nerve X) innervates the SA and AV nodes. The parasympathetic neurotransmitter acetylcholine activates muscarinic receptors on cells in both regions, reducing both heart rate and AV conduction rate. Several mechanisms explain parasympathetically mediated decreases in heart rate. Activation of muscarinic (M_2) receptors inhibits cyclic adenosine monophosphate (cAMP) production (via G_i protein), which decreases activity of the hyperpolarization-activated, cyclic nucleotide-gated (HCN) channels and slows phase 4 depolarization (**Figure 10.11a**). Inhibition of cAMP formation

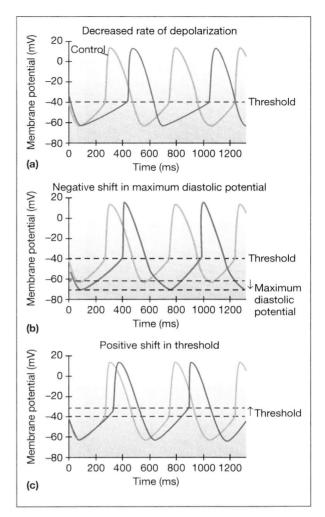

FIGURE 10.11 Parasympathetic activity decreases heart rate by three mechanisms. These changes include **(a)** decreased slope of phase 4 depolarization, **(b)** increased K^+ permeability makes the maximum diastolic potential more negative, and **(c)** inhibiting Ca^{2+} L-type channels raises the threshold.
SA, sinoatrial.
Source: From Boron WF and Boulpaep EL. *Medical Physiology*, 3rd ed, Elsevier 2017.

also decreases L-type Ca^{2+} channel activity, which raises the threshold potential (**Figure 10.11c**). Acetylcholine also promotes opening of muscarinic receptor-sensitive K^+ channels and thus makes maximum diastolic potential more negative, taking it further away from threshold potential (**Figure 10.11b**). All three of these changes contribute to the decrease in pacemaker cell firing rate seen in response to parasympathetic stimulation. Under resting conditions, the SA node is under parasympathetic control, lowering the typical heart rate from the intrinsic rate. In addition, parasympathetic tone varies with the respiratory cycle, so there is variability in the heart rate that is synchronized to the breathing rate. This respiratory sinus arrhythmia and heart rate variability is noticeable on the ECG at slower heart rates, but is generally absent at high heart rates and during conditions of stress and illness.

The sympathetic nervous system increases heart rate. Norepinephrine released from sympathetic nerve terminals and circulating epinephrine released from the adrenal medulla activate β_1-adrenergic receptors in the SA node. This, in turn, leads to activation of the cAMP second messenger system and protein kinase A (PKA). Activated PKA has two primary effects: (a) it increases activity of the HCN (*funny*) channel, and thus increases the slope of phase 4 depolarization and shortens the time to reach threshold, and (b) it increases the rate of opening of the L-type Ca^{2+} channels responsible for the upstroke (phase 0) of the action potential, causing a negative shift in threshold potential (**Figure 10.12**). States that increase sympathetic activity, such as psychological stress or biological stress (e.g., hypotension due to hemorrhage), are associated with sympathetic activation and increased heart rate.

Pharmacological Slowing of the Heart Rate by HCN Inhibition

In various heart diseases (e.g., arrhythmias, ischemic heart disease, and heart failure) and cardiovascular diseases (e.g., hypertension), pharmacological agents may be used to slow heart rate. β_1-Adrenergic

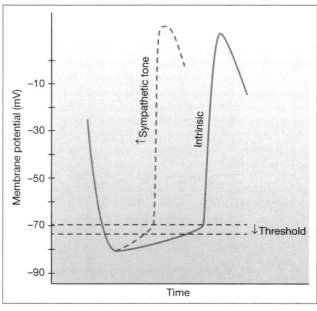

FIGURE 10.12 Sympathetic activity increases heart rate. The neurotransmitter norepinephrine binds to β_1-receptors on sinoatrial node cells, leading to phosphorylation of hyperpolarization-activated cyclic nucleotide-gated and L-type Ca^{2+} channels. These changes increase the slope of diastolic depolarization and lower the threshold for action potential generation, allowing the cell to reach threshold faster.

receptor antagonists (β-blockers) slow heart rate, but also decrease the strength of cardiac contractions. The recently developed medication ivabradine selectively inhibits the HCN channel and thus can slow heart rate without affecting contractile function.[5]

Cardiac Action Potentials Determine Conduction Speed in the Heart

All cardiac muscle cells (pacemaker and contractile) are able to conduct action potentials because they are connected to each other via gap junctions (**Figure 10.13**). Gap junctions are special channels between neighboring cells that allow the passage of ions (such as Na^+) and small molecules from one cell to another (**Figure 10.13a**). From an electrophysiological perspective, gap junctions function as electrical synapses that allow the rapid spread of depolarization from one cell to another. Both pacemaker and contractile cells have gap junctions; thus, the impulse initiated at the SA node can spread to the adjacent atrial contractile cells (**Figure 10.13b**). Conduction speed depends on three parameters: (a) the size and speed of the upstroke (phase 0) of cardiac action potentials, (b) the resting membrane potential (or maximum diastolic potential), and (c) electrical resistance of the gap junctions.

AV Node Conduction Slows Action Potential Propagation to the Ventricles

Cells of the AV node have pacemaker-like characteristics similar to SA node cells, but with a slower intrinsic rate. As in the SA node, the upstroke of the action potential is mediated by Ca^{2+} influx via L-type Ca^{2+} channels. These channels are slower to open than fast Na^+ channels; thus, action potential propagation through the AV node is slower than through the rest of the atrial or ventricular tissue. As a part of the cardiac conduction system, the AV node normally represents the only route of impulse conduction from the atria to the ventricles. Slow conduction in the AV node (i.e., AV node delay) serves a vital function: it allows the atria to contract first and finish ventricular filling before systole (ventricular contraction) during the cardiac cycle. AV node conduction velocity (also known as *dromotropy*) is modulated by the autonomic nervous system. It is increased by sympathetic stimulation and decreased by parasympathetic stimulation. Autonomic influences on AV conduction follow the same general pattern and mechanisms described for the influences on SA node cells.

Alterations of Fast-Response Action Potentials Can Also Influence Action Potential Conduction

Atrial and ventricular contractile cells, as well as the His bundle, bundle branches, and Purkinje fibers, have fast-response action potentials because the upstroke (phase 0) of their action potentials is caused by Na^+

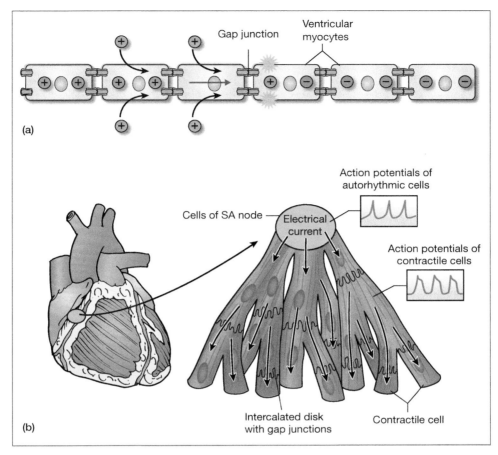

FIGURE 10.13 Spread of depolarization through the myocardium. **(a)** Depolarization spreads quickly through the myocardium, with waves of positive ions moving from cell to cell through gap junctions. **(b)** From the pacemaker cells of the SA node, the current passes through transitional cells to the atrial contractile cells that have a fast Na^+ upstroke. The faster depolarization associated with Na^+ channel activation is more efficient for rapid conduction through the atrium and the ventricle.
SA, sinoatrial.

influx via fast Na^+ channels. Action potential conduction velocity in these tissues is accordingly faster. Relative to the working cells of the ventricles, Purkinje cells have more Na^+ channels and larger diameter gap junctions, making them the fastest conducting cells in the heart. Changes in resting membrane potential, as well as intra- or extracellular Ca^{2+} or K^+ levels, can influence fast Na^+ channel function and action potential conduction velocity in these tissues. Decreased conduction speed can predispose to arrhythmia formation by creating regions of temporary block. Purkinje cells also have T- and L-type Ca^{2+} channels, and can exhibit slower conduction and pacemaker-like activity during pathophysiological conditions such as ischemia.

L-Type Ca²⁺ Channels Play Multiple Roles in Cardiovascular Function

Voltage-gated L-type Ca^{2+} channels play a role in both cardiac and vascular function. In arterioles, L-type Ca^{2+} channels are found in vascular smooth muscle cells and are important in maintaining basal vascular tone (see Chapter 9, Circulation). In the heart, L-type Ca^{2+} channels are found in both contractile and pacemaker cardiac cells. In pacemaker cells, L-type Ca^{2+} channels are responsible for the upstroke (phase 0) of the slow-response action potential. In SA node cells, increased L-type Ca^{2+} current contributes to heart rate acceleration by lowering threshold potential (moving it closer to maximum diastolic potential). In AV node cells, increased L-type Ca^{2+} current causes increased conduction speed. In contractile cardiac muscle cells, L-type Ca^{2+} channels are responsible for the plateau (phase 2) of the fast-response action potential that is a vital step in excitation–contraction coupling. Increased L-type Ca^{2+} current in these cells causes greater Ca^{2+} release from intracellular stores, resulting in a stronger contraction (increased contractility). Cardiac muscle L-type Ca^{2+} channels are stimulated by β_1-adrenergic receptor activation, resulting in increased heart rate, increased AV nodal conduction speed, and increased contractility.

Most clinically used Ca^{2+} channel blocking drugs (e.g., nifedipine and amlodipine) preferentially block L-type Ca^{2+} channels in vascular smooth muscle cells, causing a decrease in arteriolar tone and thus vascular resistance (see Chapter 9, Circulation). These drugs may be used in the treatment of hypertension. However, *cardioselective* Ca^{2+} channel blockers (verapamil and diltiazem) also block L-type Ca^{2+} channels in cardiac muscle cells. Although these drugs can be beneficial in arrhythmias by lowering heart rate and AV nodal conduction speed, they also decrease cardiac contractility and thus should be used cautiously.

Thought Question

3. **What are the cellular mechanisms of heart rate modulation by the parasympathetic and sympathetic nervous systems?**

The ECG: Record of Cardiac Electrical Activity

Waves of depolarization and repolarization moving through cells of the atria and ventricles during the cardiac cycle can be recorded using body surface electrodes, creating the typical ECG. Cardiac action potentials temporarily change the surface charge of cardiac muscle cells. At resting membrane potential, the inside of the cell is negatively charged compared with the relatively positive outside. During depolarization, the inside becomes positively charged and the outside of the cell becomes relatively negative. Because the entire heart is not depolarized at once, differences in surface charge in various locations of the heart create changing electrical vectors that can be recorded using ECG leads placed in various standard orientations on the patient's limbs and the chest. Normal conduction of waves of depolarization of the atria, followed (after a delay in the AV node) by ventricular activation and repolarization, causes typical ECG waves that can be correlated to various phases of cardiac action potentials. **Box 10.3** and **Figure 10.14** outline these events.

The ECG is correlated in time with the electrical events of millions of individual cells as the action potential is propagated along the cardiac conduction system. The SA node action potential (Ca^{2+}-mediated upstroke) excites atrial and internodal pathways and is rapidly propagated through the atrial tissue (Na^+-mediated upstroke). Atrial activation sums to form the P wave. The action potential slows at the AV node (Ca^{2+} mediated), reflected in the PR interval, before accelerating at the His–Purkinje system and spreading through

the ventricular wall, producing the QRS complex. During the ST segment, cells of the ventricle are in the plateau (phase 2) of their action potentials. The ECG in this segment, between ventricular depolarization and repolarization, is at baseline because the ventricular cells are all relatively isoelectric (i.e., having the same membrane potential) with the surrounding cells. Repolarization of ventricular cells is reflected in the T wave. Pathological changes to the ECG waveforms may be (a) caused by primary problems in cardiac electrophysiology that may interfere with pump function (arrhythmias) or (b) secondary to other cardiac diseases (ischemia, hypertrophy). Recording and evaluating ECG waveforms have become a vital diagnostic tool in cardiac diseases.

DISORDERS OF CARDIAC ELECTRICAL ACTIVITY (ARRHYTHMIAS OR DYSRHYTHMIAS)

Typical heart rate at rest in adults is between 60 and 100 beats/min, although lower heart rates are common in trained athletes. A heart rate slower than normal is referred to as *bradycardia*, and a heart rate faster than normal is referred to as *tachycardia*. This determination can be made while taking the pulse manually. Heart rate is also reported by oscillometric blood pressure monitors. **Arrhythmias**, on the other hand, can only be detected by ECG, and can be subdivided by their effect on heart rate as *bradyarrhythmias* (overall slower heart rate) or *tachyarrhythmias* (overall faster; **Table 10.1**).

General Mechanisms of Arrhythmias

Arrhythmias can result from spontaneous impulse generation (**automaticity** or **ectopy**) or abnormal impulse conduction. Although automaticity is most prominent in cells of the SA and AV nodes, other cardiac cells have phase 4 diastolic depolarization and can autonomously generate impulses. These cells are found in a few atrial regions near the SA node, and also within the His-Purkinje system. In addition, most cardiac cells can develop automaticity during hypoxic and ischemic states, producing ectopic beats. Small waves of depolarization during or after an action potential also may trigger abnormal action potential activity. Abnormal impulse conduction is another source of arrhythmias, arising from areas of conduction block due to fibrotic or ischemic tissue changes.

Altered Impulse Formation: Native and Latent Pacemakers, Escape Rhythms

The intrinsic rate of SA node cells is the fastest of all of the potential pacemaker sites in the heart, making the SA node the primary pacemaker of the heart. The SA node also receives the most extensive autonomic innervation, allowing homeostatic modulation of heart rate during normal and pathological challenges. Other

BOX 10.3
Electrocardiographic Events

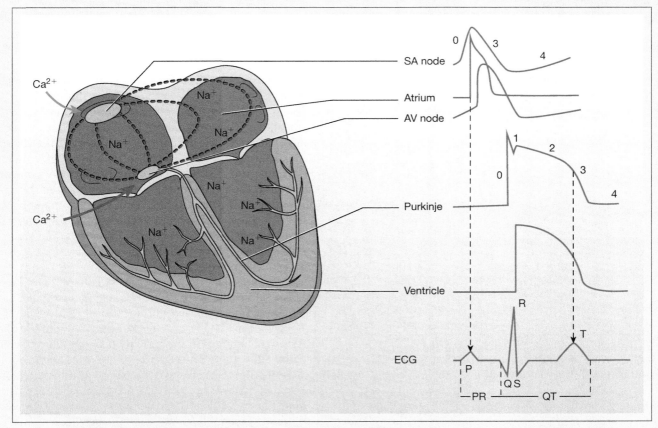

FIGURE 10.14 The ECG. ECG recordings represent the summed electrical activity of many nonpacemaker cells. Calcium-mediated action potentials of SA and AV node cells are not detectable on ECG recordings. As the waves of depolarization from SA and AV node cells moves across the atria and the ventricles, the shifting membrane potentials of many millions of cells generate voltages detectable at the surface of the body. The rapid (sodium-mediated) depolarization of atrial nonpacemaker cells is detected first, noted as a P wave. The delay, or PR interval, reflects conduction delay at the AV node, followed by the QRS complex reflecting (sodium-mediated) depolarization of ventricular nonpacemaker cells. Repolarization of ventricular cells is reflected by the T wave.
AV, atrioventricular; SA, sinoatrial.

The sections and corresponding cardiac events are identified on an ECG as follows:

P wave = atrial depolarization

PR interval = atrial and AV nodal conduction

QRS complex = ventricular wall depolarization

ST segment = ventricular cells isoelectric, plateau region

T wave = ventricular repolarization

cardiac cells, including AV node cells and Purkinje fibers, have action potentials with diastolic depolarization and the potential for spontaneous pacemaker activity. Although they are often called *latent pacemakers*, their pacemaker activity is normally not significant in cardiac function. Under normal conditions, the faster SA node rate generates action potentials that spread to these other cells and depolarize them before they can depolarize on their own (an effect known as overdrive suppression). However, if the SA node is generating impulses too slowly or not at all, other cardiac pacemakers can take over, typically resulting

	Bradyarrhythmias (Heart Rate <60 beats/min)	Tachyarrhythmias (Heart Rate >100 beats/min)
Location		
Sinoatrial (SA) node	Sick sinus syndrome	—
Atria	—	Atrial premature beats (APBs) Atrial flutter Atrial fibrillation Paroxysmal supraventricular tachycardia Focal atrial tachycardia Multifocal atrial tachycardia
Atrioventricular (AV) node	Conduction blocks Junctional escape rhythm	AV nodal reentrant tachycardia
Ventricles	Ventricular escape rhythm	Ventricular premature beats (VPBs) Ventricular tachycardia Torsades de pointes Ventricular fibrillation

TABLE 10.1 Common Arrhythmias

Source: From Lilly LS. *Pathophysiology of Heart Disease: A Collaborative Project of Medical Students and Faculty.* 6th ed. Philadelphia, PA: Wolters Kluwer; 2015.

in bradyarrhythmias according to their own inherent rates (**Figure 10.15**). These rhythms are referred to as escape rhythms. Under other pathological conditions, these latent pacemakers can acquire enhanced automaticity, and if their rates exceed the SA nodal rate they can take over cardiac pacing, resulting in premature beats or tachyarrhythmias.

Ectopic Pacemakers, Triggered Activity, and Premature Beats

Under pathological conditions, even contractile cardiac muscle cells that have fast-response action potentials can spontaneously generate action potentials like pacemaker cells. During conditions such as hypoxia, hypocalcemia, hyperkalemia, or increased sympathetic activity, membrane excitability increases, which can result in generation of action potentials by contractile cardiac muscle cells. This is termed **ectopic pacemaker activity**. Ectopic beats are very common during myocardial ischemia and infarction. The combination of excess extracellular K^+ accumulation, local depolarization, and sympathetic activation occurring secondary to the stress of the infarction increases risk of ectopy. Under these conditions, the resting membrane potentials of all of the cells in the ischemic region are depolarized, bringing them closer to threshold. Also, Ca^{2+} channels have greater permeability owing to sympathetic stimulation. In sum, the probability of ectopic action potential generation and arrhythmias is greatly enhanced by myocardial ischemia and infarction.

Another mechanism of ectopic beat generation occurs when an additional wave of depolarization occurs during a normal action potential in the form of delayed after-depolarization (DAD) or early after-depolarization (EAD). DAD and EAD are known as **triggered activity** because they are depolarization events that occur after an action potential or toward the end of an action potential, respectively (**Figure 10.16**). DADs occur after the cardiac muscle cell has been repolarized and are typically triggered in conditions of increased intracellular Ca^{2+} levels, such as extreme sympathetic stimulation or digitalis toxicity. DADs can cause tachyarrhythmias in hearts with normal structure. EAD can occur during phase 2 or phase 3 of the fast-response action potential and can be mediated by additional Ca^{2+} influx (phase 2) or Na^+ influx

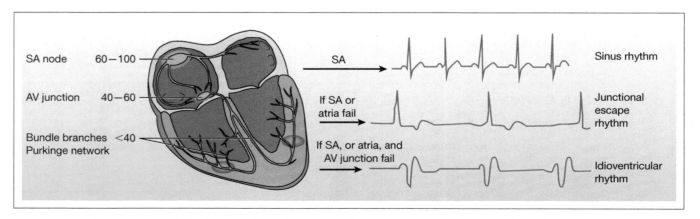

FIGURE 10.15 Latent pacemakers. Cells within the cardiac conduction system have the property of automaticity, the ability to generate rhythmic action potentials. The intrinsic firing rate is slower than the intrinsic rate of SA node pacemaker cells, but if the SA node fails, one of these sites can be the source of excitation to generate a heartbeat and resulting in characteristic ECG changes. Characteristic rates (in beats/minute) are shown for the SA node and latent pacemakers. AV, atrioventricular; SA, sinoatrial.

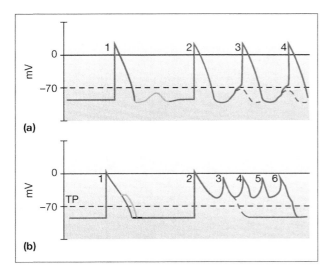

FIGURE 10.16 Triggered activity shown by intracellular recording. **(a)** Premature beats can occur when a spontaneous depolarization reaches a cell immediately after one action potential ends—a DAD. **(b)** Another mechanism of premature beats is a depolarization that reaches a cell during the relatively refractory period—an EAD. Under the proper conditions of excitability, either of these depolarizations may or may not jump-start a tachyarrhythmia.
DAD, delayed after-depolarization; EAD, early after-depolarization; TP, threshold potential.
Source: From Wit AL. Afterdepolarizations and triggered activity as a mechanism for clinical arrhythmias. *Pacing Clin Electrophysiol.* 2018;41:883–896.

(phase 3). EAD is more likely to occur in conditions of prolonged action potential, such as genetic long QT syndrome (LQTS). EADs can trigger life-threatening ventricular tachycardia (see later discussion of tachycardias).

Because of overdrive suppression during normal sinus rhythm, ectopic action potentials have to be generated earlier than the next normal action potential to capture the conduction system and activate an extra beat; when sustained, they typically cause tachyarrhythmias. If they occur intermittently in-between normal sinus beats, the resulting impulse is called a **premature beat** **(Figure 10.17)**. Premature beats always occur early, and often show different ECG wave morphology (due to altered activation sequence in the heart). Ectopic pacemakers can also take over cardiac pacemaker function, typically resulting in atrial (supraventricular) or ventricular tachyarrhythmias. However, many people have sporadic atrial or ventricular premature beats (sometimes sensed as palpitations) without underlying heart disease or progression to tachyarrhythmias.

Conduction Blocks and Reentry

Normal cardiac excitation relies on cell-to-cell conduction of action potentials throughout the heart via gap junctions. The typical conduction pattern relies on forward (anterograde) conduction from the SA node

to the rest of the cardiac muscle (see **Figure 10.14**). However, the presence of gap junctions allows for different conduction patterns, including backward (retrograde) conduction. **Conduction blocks** can be complete (bidirectional), whereby conduction is slowed or blocked in both directions. This typically occurs at the AV node, where conduction is slowest in the first place, and leads to various degrees of AV blocks causing bradycardia.

Conduction blocks may be unidirectional, whereby normal forward conduction is blocked but retrograde conduction is intact, although slower than normal. Myocardial ischemia and infarction are associated with intracellular Ca^{2+} accumulation that blocks gap junctions. This can be a source of focal conduction blocks in the region of ischemia, and can often be detected by ECG (bundle branch blocks, fascicle blocks). If retrograde conduction is sufficiently slowed, a reentry circuit may be established. Reentry circuits are also likely to occur when the conduction pathway is longer than normal (atrial or ventricular enlargement) or when there is an additional conduction pathway between the atria and the ventricles, as in **Wolff–Parkinson–White** **(WPW) syndrome** and other AV reentrant tachycardias, as described in the next sections. Reentry circuits typically cause tachycardias with very high heart rates.

Bradyarrhythmias

There are two general mechanisms of **bradyarrhythmias**: (a) abnormal SA node function and (b) conduction blocks, typically at the AV node. **Table 10.1**, introduced earlier, lists the most common bradyarrhythmias by location. **Figure 10.18** demonstrates the four conditions that must be met for an ECG to demonstrate normal sinus rhythm. Arrhythmias deviate from normal sinus rhythm in various ways. Bradyarrhythmias can be transient or chronic. Pharmacological treatment of bradyarrhythmias is limited; when they are chronic and symptomatic, pacemaker placement is typically warranted.

Sinus Bradycardia and Escape Rhythms

Decreased automaticity of the SA node can result in sinus bradycardia with otherwise normal ECG morphology. Sometimes, sinus tachycardia and bradycardia alternate (**sick sinus syndrome**). If the SA node slows down or fails, latent pacemakers may take over. If the SA node fails, the AV junction usually takes over (junctional rhythm) with an intrinsic rate of 40 to 60 beats/min. In this case QRS complexes are normal (the impulse still originates from a supraventricular common point), but P waves are missing or have abnormal appearance. If the SA node and the AV junction both fail, ventricular pacemakers (bundle branches, Purkinje fibers) may take over (ventricular escape rhythm) at an intrinsic rate of 20 to 40 beats/min. In this case the QRS complexes are wide because of the abnormally

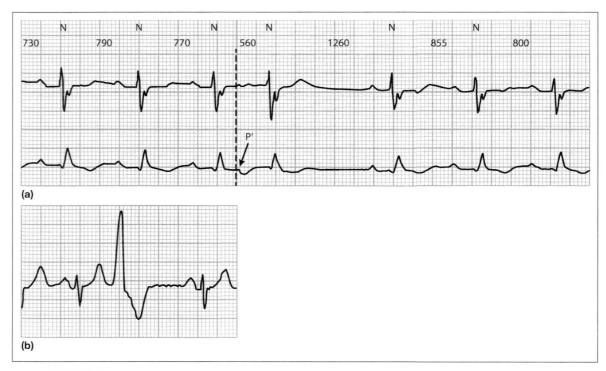

FIGURE 10.17 Premature beats. **(a)** A premature beat arising from an atrial focus has an abnormally shaped P wave (P') and is followed by a pause. The QRS complex has a normal appearance, indicating propagation through the AV node and usual ventricular conduction pathways. **(b)** A premature beat arising from a ventricular focus has a wide and bizarre appearance, indicating an abnormal path of propagation through the ventricle. It is followed by a pause, as it blocked an impulse that would have arrived from the sinoatrial node through the AV node.
AV, atrioventricular.
Source: (a) From Bagliani G, et al. *Cardiac Electrophysiol Clin.* 2018;10:257–275.

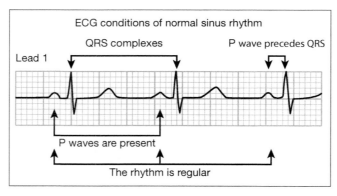

FIGURE 10.18 Characteristics of normal sinus rhythm. The four features listed must be met for electrocardiographic interpretation of normal sinus rhythm.
Source: From Thaler MS. *The Only EKG Book You'll Ever Need.* 9th ed. New York, NY: Wolters Kluwer; 2019:218.

prolonged sequence of ventricular activation. Because these latent pacemakers were previously suppressed by action potentials originating at the SA node, there can be a pause between failure of SA node–generated activity and activity generated by one of the latent pacemakers.

This period of sinus pause or arrest can be long enough to result in brief fainting with loss of consciousness.

AV Conduction Blocks

Conduction blocks at the AV junction may present in three different degrees based on severity of the block (**Figure 10.19**). In **first-degree AV block**, AV conduction is slowed; thus, PR interval is uniformly increased, but every P wave is followed by a QRS complex. In **second-degree AV block**, conduction failure is intermittent, and some P waves are not followed by QRS complexes. In **third-degree AV block**, AV conduction is completely blocked. There are P waves that represent the atrial rate and completely dissociated QRS complexes that may be wide and typically represent a much lower rate (ventricular escape rhythm). Second- and third-degree AV blocks can result in bradycardia. AV conduction blocks can be permanent, as a result of structural defects (infarctions), or reversible, as a result of influences (vagal stimulation) or antiarrhythmic drugs that slow AV nodal conduction, such as β_1-receptor blockers and L-type Ca^{2+} channel blockers. Permanent blocks with significant bradycardia may require pacemaker implantation.

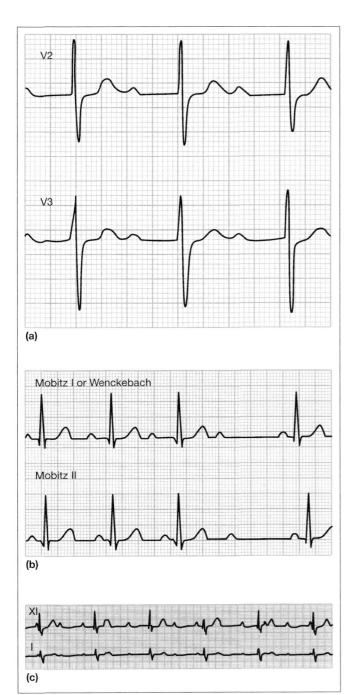

(a)

(b)

Mobitz I or Wenckeback

Mobitz II

(c)

XI

I

FIGURE 10.19 Degrees of AV block. **(a)** First-degree heart block: Each P wave is followed by a QRS complex, but the PR interval is >200 ms. **(b)** Second-degree heart block: Some P waves are not followed by QRS complexes. This may occur with a gradually lengthening PR interval followed by a missed beat (referred to as Wenckeback or Mobitz type I), or in a regular rhythm, such as 4:1 block, or 3:1 block, and so on (referred to as Mobitz type II). **(c)** Complete heart block is characterized by randomly occurring P waves and QRS complexes that have no relationship with respect to timing. AV, atrioventricular.

Tachyarrhythmias

Tachyarrhythmias occur when the heart rate is >100 beats/min. There are three general mechanisms of arrhythmias with increased heart rate: (a) increased automaticity of the SA node or other pacemakers; (b) triggered activity, as previously described; and (c) reentry.

Supraventricular Versus Ventricular Tachycardias

Tachycardias are clinically classified into two major groups: (atrial) supraventricular and ventricular. This distinction is typically made based on the QRS complex being narrow (atrial tachycardia) or wide **ventricular tachycardia** (VT), with some exceptions. In **supraventricular tachycardia**, the QRS is usually narrow because the impulse is conducted through the typical conduction pathways (AV junction) and the ventricles are depolarized in normal sequence. In VT, the QRS is wide because of delayed propagation of the impulse through the ventricles.

The mechanism of reentry is well illustrated by the most common supraventricular tachycardia, **AV nodal reentrant tachycardia** (AVNRT; **Figure 10.20**). In this condition, the AV node itself has two pathways, one fast and one slow, conducting the action potential to the bundle of His. The normal beat generated by the SA node and propagated to the AV node moves quickly along the fast pathway and through to the bundle of His. However, before the next normal beat, a premature beat generated by an atrial ectopic focus arrives during the refractory period of the fast pathway. It therefore is propagated down the slow pathway and to the bundle of His, producing an early beat. At the same time, the premature action potential captures the lower end of the fast pathway (which is no longer refractory) and generates an action potential propagated in the retrograde direction. This wave of excitation continues in the retrograde direction to stimulate atrial cells and also captures the slow pathway, regenerating an action potential there. The circular pattern of activation gives rise to the term *circus movement* for this type of arrhythmia.

Figure 10.21 illustrates the consequences of having an alternative or accessory pathway electrically connecting atria and ventricles. An example is the bypass tract in people with WPW syndrome. This accessory pathway allows a normal beat to reach parts of the ventricle quickly, because the bypass has faster conduction than the slowly conducting AV node. This is reflected in the ECG as a delta wave that quickly transitions to the QRS complex, shortening the PR interval and prolonging the QRS (**Figure 10.21a**). The presence of a bypass tract also promotes reentry when an atrial ectopic beat occurs. As shown in **Figure 10.21b**, a large reentrant circuit can be formed with the AV node forming the

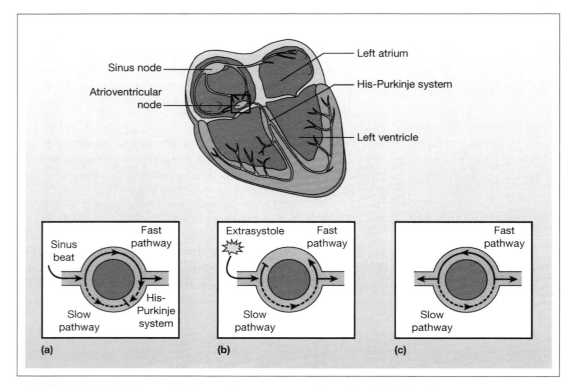

FIGURE 10.20 Atrioventricular nodal reentrant tachycardia (AVNRT). The presence of two pathways within the atrioventricular (AV) node, one of which conducts faster than the other, sets up the conditions for reentry and a circus rhythm within the AV node that can produce tachycardia.

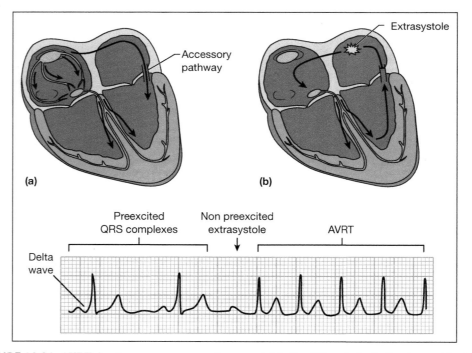

FIGURE 10.21 AVRT due to an accessory pathway outside the AV node, but allowing an electrical connection between atria and ventricles.

AV, atrioventricular; AVRT, atrioventricular reentrant tachycardia.

slow pathway, and the abnormal AV connection, the fast pathway.

In **atrial flutter**, a reentrant circuit traveling up the interatrial septum and down the lateral walls can activate the atria in a regular fashion, commonly at 300 beats/min. The AV node cannot conduct all of these beats, so the ventricles are depolarized at a slower rate (90 to 150 beats/min). In atrial fibrillation, several tiny micro-reentrant circuits can lead to chaotic activation of the atrium. Because impulses are reaching the AV node at irregular intervals, ventricular depolarization is irregular. This is often referred to as irregularly irregular rhythm (absolute arrhythmia), whereby no two R-R intervals are the same.[6]

Atrial Fibrillation

Atrial fibrillation (commonly referred to as *A-fib*) is the most common sustained (chronic) arrhythmia in the United States. It affects over 2.7 million people, and the prevalence is rising.[3] Hemodynamic and thromboembolic complications of atrial fibrillation result in significant morbidity, mortality, and healthcare costs. This is especially true for the elderly, as the prevalence of atrial fibrillation increases with age.

Definition

Atrial fibrillation is a chaotic rhythm in which distinct P waves are not discernible on the ECG owing to the lack of coordinated atrial depolarization. Similar to atrial flutter, many of the atrial impulses arrive during the refractory period at the AV node, because AV nodal conduction is slow and cannot support such high heart rates. As a result, only some of the depolarizations are conducted to the ventricles in a very irregular fashion (indicated by a characteristic *irregularly irregular* rhythm). The typical average ventricular rate in atrial fibrillation without treatment is around 140 to 160 beats/min. The ECG shows baseline low-amplitude undulations punctuated by QRS complexes and T waves at irregular intervals.

Mechanisms of Atrial Fibrillation

The underlying mechanism of atrial fibrillation likely involves multiple wandering small reentrant circuits within the atria. In some patients, the rhythm can repetitively shift between atrial fibrillation and atrial flutter. Atrial fibrillation can be sustained or episodic (paroxysmal). Sudden, unpredictable episodes of paroxysmal atrial fibrillation are often initiated by rapid-firing ectopic foci in sleeves of atrial muscle that extend into the pulmonary veins. Enlarged atria increase the risk of sustained atrial fibrillation, in which only a minimum number of reentrant circuits is needed. Accordingly, diseases that increase atrial pressure and size promote atrial fibrillation, including valvular diseases (e.g., mitral stenosis or regurgitation), heart failure, hypertension, coronary artery disease, and pulmonary disease. Additional predisposing factors include thyrotoxicosis and alcohol consumption. Atrial fibrillation is also a common rhythm disturbance in the elderly, and in many cases no underlying heart disease can be detected.

Functional Consequences of Atrial Fibrillation

Atrial fibrillation leads to three major complications: decreased ventricular filling, tachycardia, and thromboembolic events.

1. *Decreased ventricular filling*: Disorganized electrical activity in the atria translates to lack of organized atrial systole at the end of ventricular filling. This lack of atrial kick typically reduces end-diastolic volume by about 15%. This effect is especially pronounced in patients with reduced ventricular compliance (stiff left ventricle), who are more reliant on the atrial contraction for ventricular filling. This effect alone decreases stroke volume and thus cardiac output.

2. *Tachycardia:* Atrial fibrillation with ventricular rate <100 beats/min may be asymptomatic. Typically, the ventricular rate is faster in untreated atrial fibrillation, and it can further increase when AV nodal conduction is facilitated by elevated sympathetic tone during illness. Rapid ventricular rate shortens the duration of diastole, and thus decreases filling time, further compromising ventricular filling. In addition, shortening the duration of diastole interferes with coronary perfusion, which can compromise ventricular contractility. Both of these effects may compromise cardiac output, resulting in hypotension and pulmonary congestion. Management with cardioversion or antiarrhythmic drugs aims to restore sinus rhythm.

3. *Thromboembolic events:* Atrial fibrillation is also an important cause of stroke and other systemic thromboembolic complications. The absence of organized atrial contraction promotes blood stasis in the atria, increasing the risk of thrombus formation (in the left atrial appendage), which can embolize to the cerebral circulation and other systemic sites. This is an especially dangerous complication in patients with intermittent (paroxysmal) atrial fibrillation, because an atrial thrombus might form during fibrillation and then be ejected into the ventricle and beyond, to the pulmonary or systemic circulation, when normal sinus rhythm restores coordinated atrial contractions. Stroke risk in patients with atrial fibrillation but without valve disease is evaluated—based on age, sex, and history of heart failure, hypertension, diabetes, stroke or transient ischemic attack, or vascular disease—in an assessment with the acronym CHA_2-DS_2-VASc.[7] Management with direct oral anticoagulants is common for patients with high scores.

Ventricular Arrhythmias

VT is a series of three or more consecutive ventricular premature beats. VT is divided arbitrarily into two categories: (a) sustained VT—which persists for more than 30 seconds, produces severe symptoms (such as syncope) or requires termination by cardioversion; and (b) nonsustained VT—shorter, self-terminating episodes of VT. Both forms of VT occur most commonly in patients with structural heart disease, such as myocardial ischemia and infarction, heart failure, ventricular hypertrophy, valvular heart diseases, and congenital cardiac abnormalities. VT can be initiated by reentry, EADs or DADs, as noted above. VT is a life-threatening condition that can also convert to **ventricular fibrillation**. In ventricular fibrillation, the ECG shows fast, low voltage activity but no coordinated waves of excitation. No cardiac contractions are initiated and cardiac output falls to zero. This rapidly results in death if resuscitation measures are not initiated.

Genetic Disorders Associated With Arrhythmias

Primary electrical diseases are due to ion channel mutations, either sporadic or inherited. These occur infrequently, but are important because they can cause life-threatening polymorphic VT or ventricular fibrillation in young, otherwise healthy people without prior warning. These diseases are the primary cause of sudden cardiac death in young people. The most common of these conditions are Brugada syndrome and congenital LQTS.

Brugada Syndrome

Brugada syndrome is caused by inherited, autosomal dominant mutations in the fast Na^+ channel gene (*SCN5A*). A potential clue to the presence of this syndrome is varying forms of ST elevation in leads V_1 through V_3 on the ECG. This pattern may be present chronically or intermittently. The ECG findings may be unmasked by administering Na^+ channel–blocking antiarrhythmic drugs (e.g., flecainide, procainamide).

Brugada syndrome is a potentially fatal condition, and intracardiac defibrillator implantation is the most effective way to prevent an arrhythmic death.

Long QT Syndrome

Long QT syndromes (LQTS) refers to a set of related inherited and acquired disorders that delay phase 3 membrane repolarization in ventricular myocytes and manifest as a prolonged QT interval on the ECG. Prolonged QT interval can lead to a type of life-threatening polymorphic VT called torsades de pointes. Various gene mutations with autosomal dominant and recessive patterns may result in LQTS (**Table 10.2**). Most identified mutations alter ion channel function to either enhance the depolarizing Na^+ current or impair the repolarizing K^+ current, thus increasing excitability as well as increasing the relative refractory period. The most common form of LQTS (LQT1) is caused by K^+ channel gene mutation, which reduces the repolarizing K^+ current during phase 3. LQT3 is a particularly lethal form of LQTS in which mutations prevent the Na^+ channel from inactivating fully during depolarization.[8] Arrhythmic events may be precipitated by a variety of factors, including exercise and abrupt sounds. Patients typically suffer palpitations, syncope, seizures, or sudden cardiac death as a result. Certain medications are contraindicated in some patients with genetically identified LQTS.

Thought Questions

4. What are examples of arrhythmias caused by ectopic beats? What types of factors enhance automaticity of myocardial cells?

5. What portion of the cardiac conduction system is most vulnerable to conduction blocks? How is this condition manifested on the ECG?

	Gene		Mechanism of Prolonged	
Type	(Location)	Protein	Repolarization	Inheritance
LQTS 1	*KCNQ1* (11p15)	KvLQT1 (α subunit of I_{Ks} K^+ channel)	↓ Outward K^+ current	AD or AR
LQTS 2	*KCNH2* (7q35)	HERG (α subunit of I_{Kr} K^+ channel)	↓ Outward K^+ current	AD
LQTS 3	*SCN5A* (3p21)	Nav 1.5 (cardiac fast Na^+ channel)	↑ Inward Na^+ current	AD

TABLE 10.2 Most Common Types of Genetic Long QT Syndrome (LQTS)

AD, autosomal dominant; AR, autosomal recessive.
Source: From Lilly LS. *Pathophysiology of Heart Disease: A Collaborative Project of Medical Students and Faculty.* 6th ed. Philadelphia, PA: Wolters Kluwer; 2015; Box 12-1.

CARDIAC PERFORMANCE PHYSIOLOGY

CARDIAC MUSCLE

Histology

As shown in **Figure 10.4**, cardiac muscle cells are short and contain a single nucleus in the middle. The cells are cylindrical, branch and interdigitate, and are connected to one another by intercalated disks. Intercalated disks contain gap junctions that serve as electrical connections between the cells, allowing transmission of action potentials. Through the gap junctions, the cardiac action potential travels from the SA node to the entire cardiac muscle via cell-to-cell conduction; thus, cardiac muscle works as a single unit (syncytium). Intercalated disks also contain desmosomes—very strong mechanical connections that prevent the cells from being pulled apart during contraction.

Cardiac muscle cells are packed with myofibrils composed of myofilaments arranged in sarcomeres. The plasma membrane (sarcolemma) of cardiac muscle cells includes deep T tubules that transmit the action potential to the interior of the cell close to sarcoplasmic reticulum terminal cisterns. Sarcoplasmic reticulum surrounds myofibrils and T tubules and serves as the intracellular Ca^{2+} store. Cells also contain myoglobin, an oxygen-binding protein, and numerous mitochondria for oxidative energy generation to provide very high oxygen extraction (up to 70% to 75%) to support the regular contractions at 60 to 100 beats/min and higher rates with exercise.

Parameters of Cardiac Function

As previously noted, cardiac output is equal to heart rate times stroke volume (CO = HR × SV). An average adult male may have a cardiac output of about 5.0 L/min, with a heart rate of 72 beats/min and a stroke volume of 70 mL.

Focusing on the systemic circuit, what are the volumes associated with the left ventricle? The ventricle never completely empties; rather, the volume of blood remaining after ventricular contraction is termed the *end-systolic volume*. The volume of blood in the ventricle after filling and just before contraction begins is the *end-diastolic volume*. The stroke volume, then, is the end-diastolic volume minus the end-systolic volume.

An important clinical index is the ejection fraction, the ratio of the stroke volume and the end-diastolic volume. This is usually reported as the percent of end-diastolic volume. A normal ejection fraction is generally between 55% and 70%.

The pumping action of the heart is produced by muscular contraction initiated by the heart's electrical activity in the process of excitation–contraction coupling. Pump effectiveness is stimulated by the sympathetic nervous system and is modulated by the degree of filling, the systemic blood pressure, and the intrinsic contractility of the muscle.

Excitation–Contraction Coupling

In cardiac muscle the link between action potential activity (excitation) and contractile force development (contraction) is referred to as excitation–contraction coupling. Excitation–contraction coupling critically depends on Ca^{2+} entry via L-type Ca^{2+} channels during the plateau (phase 2) of the action potential (**Figure 10.22**). The relatively small amount of Ca^{2+} entering the cell through these channels triggers a sarcoplasmic reticulum ryanodine receptor, leading to a much greater release of Ca^{2+} from the sarcoplasmic reticulum.

Recall from Chapter 4, Cell Physiology and Pathophysiology, the steps in cardiac cell contraction:

1. Ca^{2+} binds to troponin C and shifts the troponin–tropomyosin complex.
2. Myosin-binding sites are exposed on actin filaments.
3. Actin–myosin crossbridges form.
4. Myosin heads pivot, pulling the actin filaments in the direction that leads to cell shortening.
5. This cycle repeats, as long as Ca^{2+} is available to bind to troponin C and adenosine triphosphate (ATP) is available to allow crossbridges to break and new crossbridges to form.
6. Contraction ends when the sarcoendoplasmic reticulum Ca^{2+} ATPase (SERCA) pumps cytoplasmic Ca^{2+} back into the sarcoplasmic reticulum.

Phospholamban is a protein of the sarcoplasmic reticulum membrane that regulates the rate of SERCA activity. When an individual is at rest with a relatively slow heart rate, phospholamban is not phosphorylated, and it inhibits SERCA activity. As a result, when heart rates are relatively slow, the rate of ventricular relaxation (also known as *lusitropy*) is moderate. This is altered when the heart is stimulated by increased sympathetic nervous system activity.

Contractility, Preload, and Afterload: Determinants of Pump Function and Stroke Volume

Sympathetic Activity Increases Force of Contraction and Rate of Relaxation

Sympathetic fibers project extensively throughout the ventricles (**Figure 10.23**), and the sympathetic transmitter norepinephrine is the major regulator of cardiac performance in response to physiological and pathophysiological challenges. During physiological challenges, such as exercise, sympathetic activity increases both heart rate and contractility, providing large increases in cardiac output. Norepinephrine binding to β_1-receptors on ventricular myocardial cells increases intracellular cAMP, followed by activation of PKA. PKA phosphorylates membrane Ca^{2+} channels and phospholamban. The consequences are increased Ca^{2+} influx, stimulating Ca^{2+}-initiated Ca^{2+} release; greater cytoplasmic Ca^{2+} elevations, promoting stronger

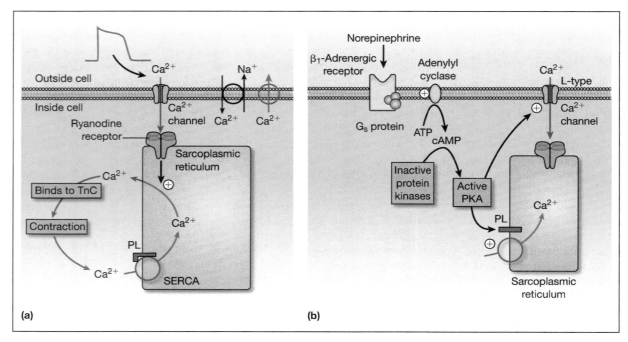

FIGURE 10.22 E-C coupling in myocardial cells. **(a)** E-C coupling and **(b)** sympathetic influences. Ca²⁺ entry through L-type Ca²⁺ channels during the plateau of the action potential initiates E-C coupling. The small initial Ca²⁺ spike triggers the ryanodine receptor to release more Ca²⁺ from SR storage (Ca²⁺-initiated Ca²⁺ release). Ca²⁺ is then available for actin–myosin crossbridge formation until the action potential ends and SERCA pumps Ca²⁺ back into the SR, allowing diastolic relaxation. Norepinephrine binding to β₁-adrenergic receptors activates Gₛ, increasing intracellular cAMP and activating PKA. Ca²⁺ entry is enhanced by phosphorylation of membrane Ca²⁺ channels, and SERCA activity is increased owing to phosphorylation of phospholamban. These actions promote inotropy and lusitropy.

cAMP, cyclic adenosine monophosphate; E-C, excitation–contraction; PKA, protein kinase A; PL, phospholamban; SERCA, sarcoplasmic reticulum Ca²⁺ ATPase (adenosine triphosphatase); SR, sarcoplasmic reticulum; TnC, troponin C.

Source: Adapted from Lilly LS. *Pathophysiology of Heart Disease: A Collaborative Project of Medical Students and Faculty.* 6th ed. Wolters Kluwer; 2015.

contractions; greater amounts of Ca²⁺ stored in the sarcoplasmic reticulum, increasing strength of subsequent contractions; and faster rates of relaxation in diastole. This set of changes contributes to increased stroke volume and is also beneficial, because the increase in heart rate shortens diastolic filling time, which can be partially compensated for by the increased rate of SERCA activity.

Increase in Preload Increases Stroke Volume

Similar to skeletal muscle, cardiac muscle has greater contractile performance when contraction begins from a greater initial length (referred to as the length–tension relationship; **Figure 10.24a**). Based on actin–myosin overlap in the sarcomeres and other factors, an optimal muscle length is defined as the length at which contractile strength is maximal. Cardiac muscle cells at rest (during diastole before ventricular filling)

are shorter than optimal length. As the ventricles fill with blood during diastole, the cardiac muscle cells are passively stretched and get much closer to optimal length. End-diastolic volume in the ventricles sets cardiac muscle length before contraction (*preload*). Thus, the greater the ventricular filling (preload, within normal limits), the closer muscle contraction strength is to maximal. This has been referred to as the Frank–Starling law of the heart, or the Frank–Starling relationship (**Figure 10.24b**).

The exact mechanism underlying this phenomenon remains unknown but likely involves multiple factors. One hypothesis is that increased ventricular loading stretches myofibers, enhancing crossbridge formation by optimizing actin–myosin overlap in the sarcomeres. Another proposed mechanism is that stretching improves Ca²⁺ delivery or increases Ca²⁺ sensitivity of troponin C. It has also been speculated that increased

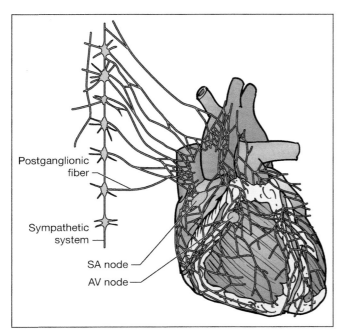

FIGURE 10.23 The heart is abundantly supplied with sympathetic nerves.
AV, atrioventricular; SA, sinoatrial.

volume loading in the ventricles should reduce "slack" between myofibrils. What is clear is that increased ventricular preload reliably increases contractile strength and thus stroke volume. Physiologically, increased preload occurs during exercise because muscle activity squeezes the veins, increasing the volume of venous return to the vena cava and the heart. This mechanism provides a component of the enhanced stroke volume and cardiac output needed to support the body's increased oxygen consumption. Trained athletes develop chronic improvements in cardiac function with increased left ventricular filling and contractile performance. One indication of this change is that a trained athlete will have slower resting heart rate, indicating that cardiac output is being maintained with improved stroke volume.

Increased Contractility Augments Preload Effects on Performance

The positive inotropic effect of sympathetic stimulation is seen at any preload, and increased sympathetic activity shifts the preload/contraction strength curve in the upward direction (**Figure 10.24b**). The result is greater contractile strength and stroke volume at any level of preload. This mechanism complements the stimulatory effects of the sympathetic nervous system on heart rate and AV nodal conduction speed and results in a major increase in cardiac output. The increase, however, comes with a metabolic cost in that it increases

myocardial oxygen demand. In individuals with normal, healthy coronary vessels, blood flow can increase to supply adequate oxygen to meet this increased demand.

Digitalis Increases Cardiac Contractility by Increasing Intracellular Calcium

Cardiac glycosides such as digitalis are sometimes used to increase cardiac contractility in heart failure. Digitalis acts by blocking the Na^+/K^+ pump on cardiac muscle cells (among others). The resulting increase in intracellular Na^+ concentration reverses the action of the $Na^+–Ca^{2+}$ exchanger; thus, instead of removing Ca^{2+} from the cells, it is actually removing Na^+. This effect causes increased intracellular Ca^{2+} concentration after contraction, resulting in increased contractility. Owing to the narrow therapeutic range and widespread toxicity of digitalis, lately its clinical use has become limited.

Increased Afterload Reduces Stroke Volume

Afterload is the force experienced by the ventricle after contraction has started. The most common source of afterload is the aortic diastolic pressure that must be overcome in order for the aortic valve to open and ejection to begin. As aortic diastolic pressure increases (e.g., in a patient with hypertension), myocardial cells must generate greater systolic pressure to initiate ejection. This burden reduces the speed of valve opening and slows the velocity of ejection once the valve is open. Overall, increased afterload reduces stroke volume and increases the work of the heart. In cases of aortic stenosis, the narrowed valve obstructs outflow from the left ventricle, representing another mechanism of increased afterload that reduces stroke volume.

Summary: Determinants of Cardiac Output

To summarize the influences on cardiac output (heart rate times stroke volume), both components of cardiac output—heart rate and stroke volume—are under the control of the autonomic nervous system. Heart rate is decreased (negative chronotropy) by parasympathetic activity and is increased (positive chronotropy) by sympathetic activity. Stroke volume is determined by *preload, afterload,* and *cardiac contractility.* The influence of preload is illustrated in the Frank-Starling law of the heart—greater filling leads to greater stroke volume. Afterload is the force the ventricle must overcome to achieve ejection—greater afterload leads to decreased stroke volume. Finally, cardiac contractility is modulated by the sympathetic nervous system in accordance with the body's needs while at rest or during physical activity, it exerts a positive inotropic effect. Sympathetic activity also accelerates ventricular relaxation, allowing better filling as heart rate increases.

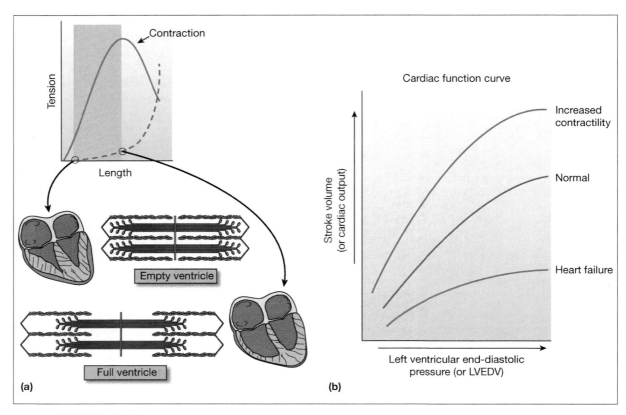

FIGURE 10.24 Basis of the Frank–Starling law of the heart. As with all muscles, the greater the original passive length of the muscle, the greater the force of contraction it can generate. **(a)** The transition from a mostly empty ventricle to a full ventricle increases stretch of the heart before contraction (preload) and results in stronger contractile activity. This is hypothesized to result from a better lineup of actin and myosin filaments as the muscle is stretched. **(b)** Plotting stroke volume against LVEDV illustrates the improved performance achieved as LVEDV increases for the normal heart (*purple line*). Increased contractility that could result from sympathetic stimulation shifts the curve upward, increasing stroke volume at each level of LVEDV (*green line*). The weakened muscle associated with heart failure cannot achieve adequate stroke volume to sustain modest physical activity at any level of preload (*red line*).
LVEDV, left ventricular end-diastolic volume.

Thought Questions

6. Can you trace the relative concentrations and movements of Ca^{2+} as myocardial cells move from their resting membrane potential through the action potential sequence in fast-response cells?

7. What specific membrane channels and transporters are involved in these movements?

8. What is the effect of these changes on myocardial contraction or relaxation?

CARDIAC CYCLE

The heart functions by a cycle of electrical and mechanical events. It alternates between ventricular contraction (systole) and a period of ventricular relaxation (diastole); each of the repeating series is referred to as a cardiac cycle. At resting heart rate, systole typically lasts one third of the cycle and diastole lasts two thirds of the cycle. Typically, the contractile events of the heart predictably follow the electrical events of atrial activation (P wave) and ventricular activation (QRS complex) recorded by the ECG, as shown in **Figures 10.25** and **10.26**. This discussion focuses on events and structures on the left side of the heart, which provides cardiac output to the systemic circulation. However, it should be noted that these events occur simultaneously on the right side of the heart. **Figure 10.26** shows the events of the cardiac cycle correlated with phases numbered 1 through 7, as described in **Box 10.4**.

Viewing the Cardiac Cycle Using Pressure–Volume Loops

The mechanical events of filling, pressure development, ejection, and relaxation during the cardiac cycle can also be illustrated by pressure–volume loops

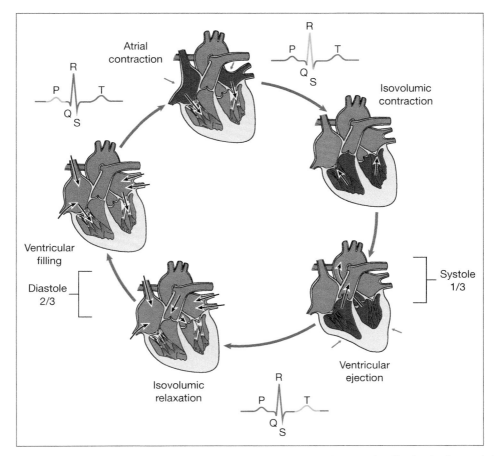

FIGURE 10.25 The ECG and mechanical events of the cardiac cycle. Dark shading of the chambers indicates the contractile state. Systole starts when an action potential is propagated to the ventricles, denoted by the QRS complex. After a brief period of pressure development (isovolumic contraction), aortic and pulmonary valves open and ejection begins. The T wave signifies ventricular repolarization and rapid ventricular relaxation, initiating diastole. After a brief period of isovolumic relaxation, mitral and tricuspid valves open and filling of the ventricles begins. The P wave signifies atrial depolarization and atrial contraction provides the final volume filling the ventricle.

(**Box 10.5** and **Figures 10.27** through **10.29**). These *loops* are a means for expressing the primary relationships between the left ventricular volume and the left ventricular pressure throughout the cardiac cycle, as influenced by the intrinsic properties of the cardiac muscle.

Thought Question

9. What factors increase and decrease stroke volume? For each of those factors, identify one condition under which the factor will increase or decrease, and describe the effect on stroke volume.

CORONARY BLOOD FLOW AND ISCHEMIC HEART DISEASE

CARDIAC VASCULATURE

The cardiac vessels consist of the coronary arteries, veins, and lymphatics. The largest diameter segments of these vessels lie within the loose connective tissue in the epicardial fat.

Coronary Arteries

In the majority of people, oxygen and nutrients are delivered to the heart muscle by a left and a right coronary artery (RCA; **Figure 10.30**). The coronary arteries arise from the root of the aorta. These vessels pass toward the anterior aspect of the heart on each side of the pulmonary artery and branch into smaller

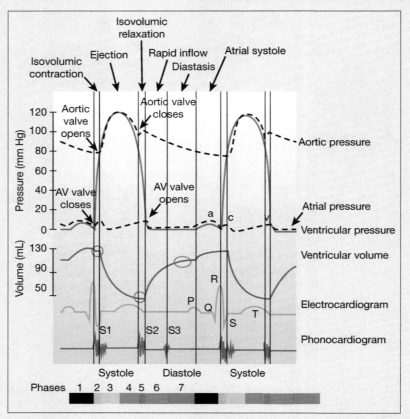

FIGURE 10.26 Phases of the cardiac cycle and their corresponding events. Although many of the variables shown can only be measured invasively, auscultation of heart sounds and inspection of jugular venous waves can be performed during the physical examination. Heart sounds are shown from phonocardiogram data—S1 correlates with closure of the atrioventricular valves (mitral and tricuspid), and S2 correlates with closure of the ventricular outflow valves (aortic and pulmonary). S3 can be heard during rapid ventricular filling in early diastole. Atrial pressures vary during the cardiac cycle and can be deduced from pulsations reflected back to the jugular vein from the right atrium, producing a, c, and v waves. These correspond to atrial contraction (a), ventricular contraction (c), and increased pressure due to atrial filling against a closed atrioventricular valve during systole (v).
AV, atrioventricular.
Source: From Guyton AC, Hall JE: *Textbook of Medical Physiology.* Elsevier, 2006.

1. The P wave, representing atrial depolarization, initiates atrial contraction, which completes ventricular filling. This is the last phase of ventricular diastole.

2. The QRS complex, representing ventricular depolarization, initiates ventricular contraction. The first event of systole is the beginning of ventricular contraction, which immediately generates pressure that closes the mitral valve. As both mitral and aortic valves are now closed, this period of pressure development is referred to as *isovolumic contraction.* On physical examination, this phase is also associated with the S_1 heart sound, due to closure of the mitral and tricuspid valves.

3. As soon as ventricular pressure exceeds aortic diastolic pressure, the aortic valve opens and ejection begins. Left ventricular volume rapidly empties early in the ejection phase even as left ventricular and aortic pressures continue to increase.

BOX 10.4 (*continued*)
Phases of the Cardiac Cycle

4. Late systole is associated with reduced volume in the ventricle, so ejection slows. The T wave represents ventricular cell repolarization and the beginning of relaxation of myocardial cells. As left ventricular pressure falls to a level below aortic pressure, the aortic valve closes. Closure of the aortic and pulmonary valves produces the S_2 heart sound.

5. Isovolumic relaxation occurs at the beginning of diastole. The aortic valve has closed and left ventricular pressure is still higher than left atrial pressure, so this phase of relaxation occurs without a change in left ventricular volume.

6. Once left ventricular pressure is lower than left atrial pressure, the mitral valve opens. This phase is associated with rapid ventricular filling and may sometimes end with a heart sound (S_3), indicating rapid blood entry into an almost full ventricle. S_3 may be heard as a normal variant in young athletes, but it is more likely in older adults with heart failure.

7. The end of the passive filling phase shows little change in ventricular volume and pressure. This stage terminates with the P wave and the beginning of atrial contraction (phase 1).

BOX 10.5
Evaluation of the Cardiac Cycle Using Pressure–Volume Loops

EVENTS COMPRISING THE PRESSURE–VOLUME LOOP

When evaluating a pressure–volume loop (**Figure 10.27**), note that the events in the loop proceed in a counterclockwise direction. At point *A*, the atrial pressure exceeds that in the ventricle to open the mitral valve and permit an initial filling of the still-relaxing ventricle. At point *B*, the ventricle is fully relaxed and fills as the atrium starts to contract. Point *C* is the onset of ventricular contraction when the left ventricular pressure exceeds that of the atrium and the mitral valve closes. At this point, the ventricular pressure rapidly builds, but the volume does not change (isovolumetric contraction) as it has not exceeded the aortic pressure. At point *D*, the left ventricular pressure exceeds aortic pressure, and the aortic valve opens, beginning ejection. The pressure at point *D* corresponds to the diastolic blood pressure. The peak ventricular/aortic pressure noted at point *E*, accordingly, is the systolic blood pressure achieved as ejection/systole is waning.

After the ventricular contraction is maximized (point *E*), the pressure drops with the start of diastole. When the left ventricular pressure is lower than aortic pressure (point *F*), the aortic valve closes. The ventricular pressure then precipitously falls (points *F* to *A*). Because the aortic valve and the mitral valves are both closed, the left ventricular volume cannot change (isovolumetric relaxation)

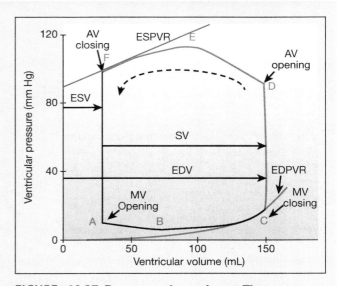

FIGURE 10.27 Pressure–volume loop. The pressure–volume loop describes changes in both pressure and volume as they take place during a cardiac cycle.

until the pressure drops below that of the left atrium with reopening of the mitral valve (point *A*).

Also depicted in **Figure 10.27** is the end-diastolic volume (EDV, achieved at point *C*), which corresponds to the total volume in the ventricle achieved during the diastolic phase. It is easy to determine the difference in ventricular volume between the onset and termination of systole (achieved at point F).

(*continued*)

This volume is also the SV, which is the volume of blood ejected during a single cardiac cycle. A portion of the left ventricular blood remains in the heart after contraction. This residual volume remains as the heart cannot completely empty during a single cycle. The residual volume is normally about 40% of the EDV. A commonly used index of cardiac function is the ejection fraction. It is calculated as the SV/EDV, which is typically around 60%. A decreased ejection fraction that drops below 50% signals compromised cardiac contractility and the development of heart failure.

Diastolic filling generates a pressure within the relaxed ventricle, and the magnitude of that pressure depends on the volume of filling (the greater the volume, the greater the pressure) and on the intrinsic stiffness of the ventricular wall. This relationship is depicted by the EDPVR line. Increased diastolic filling increases ventricular pressure, contributing to the stretch of the ventricle that promotes improved stroke volume by the Frank–Starling relationship. The ability of the ventricle to eject a normal stroke volume is limited by the ESPVR line, which represents a segment of the overall length–tension or Frank–Starling curve for the ventricle.

The pressure–volume loop can also be used to determine the cardiac work, which is the ability of the heart to eject blood against the aortic pressure. The area within the pressure–volume loop correlates with cardiac work and the energy demands of the heart.

CHANGES WITH PRELOAD

Pressure–volume loops show how preload affects cardiac stroke volume and work (**Figure 10.28**). In accordance with the Frank–Starling mechanism, increased preload increases stroke volume. Increased preload also increases cardiac work and metabolic demand. In contrast, the increases in peak systolic pressure are relatively conservative.

CHANGES WITH AFTERLOAD

The effect of changes in afterload can also be depicted in pressure–volume loops (**Figure 10.29**). As aortic pressure increases, the stroke volume decreases. The cross-sectional areas within the

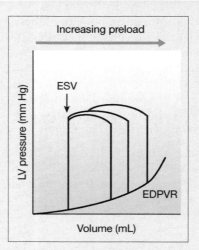

FIGURE 10.28 Pressure–volume loop: changes with preload. Increased preload can increase the SV, as predicted by the Frank–Starling relationship. Note that the widening of the SV suggests that increased preload will also increase cardiac work and metabolic demand.

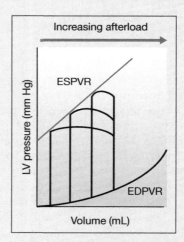

FIGURE 10.29 Pressure–volume loop: changes with afterload. Afterload increases as arterial pressure increases. The ventricle must work harder to overcome high diastolic pressure to open the aortic valve, and must continue to have a stronger contraction to eject the SV against the rapidly rising systolic pressure. These factors result in decreased SV, but an equal amount of cardiac work.

loops are minimally affected by increased afterload. This shows how cardiac work is unaffected by increased afterload, but it can reduce cardiac output. Conversely, vasodilators—which reduce afterload—will increase the cardiac output with minimal effect on the cardiac work.

AV, aortic valve; EDPVR, end-diastolic pressure–volume relationship; EDV, end-diastolic volume; ESPVR, end-systolic pressure–volume relationship; ESV, end-systolic volume; LV, left ventricle; MV, mitral valve; SV, stroke volume.

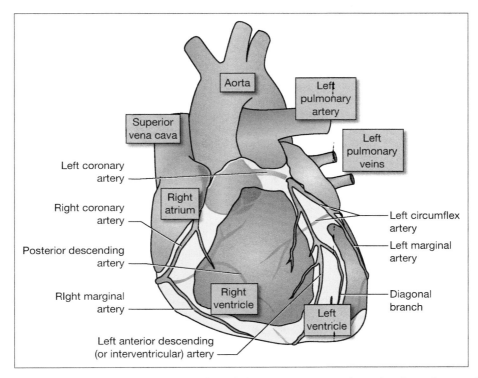

FIGURE 10.30 Coronary arteries. The left and right coronary arteries arise from the proximal aorta, behind the cusps of the aortic valve. They travel in the epicardial layer, giving rise to branches that penetrate the myocardium.

epicardial vessels before dividing into yet smaller vessels that penetrate the thick myocardium to provide a dense capillary supply.

The RCA supplies the entire right ventricle, the inferior and posterior side of the left ventricle, and the posterior one third of the interventricular septum. The RCA also provides the blood to the AV node in 90% of people. The left coronary artery (sometimes referred to as left main coronary artery [LMCA]) branches within 2.5 cm of its origin, giving rise to the left anterior descending (LAD) and the left circumflex (LCX) arteries. The LAD artery provides blood to the anterior wall of the left ventricle, the apex of the heart, and the anterior two thirds of the interventricular septum. The LCX artery provides the blood for the lateral and posterior walls of the left ventricle. The SA nodal artery arises from the RCA in 70% of the population, from the LCX artery in 25% of people, and from both the RCA and LCX arteries in 5% of the population.

From their epicardial locations, the coronary arteries of the epicardium send branches into the ventricular muscle. These vessels are extensively branched, with anastomoses that feed all the layers from epicardium to endocardium. The capillaries form an elaborate network that surrounds each cardiac muscle fiber. Muscle fibers of the inner wall of the endocardium are supplied by terminal branches of the coronary arteries or from *thebesian veins* that tunnel directly from the ventricular cavity. Collateral connections exist at the subarteriolar level between the coronary arteries. In a normal heart, only a small number of these 200-μm diameter collateral vessels may be active. However, when a coronary artery is obstructed, these vessels may dilate to deliver blood from healthy collateral vessels to adjacent regions that are affected by ischemia.

Coronary Veins

The coronary veins are distributed along the major coronary arteries. These vessels return blood from the myocardial capillaries to the right atrium through the coronary sinus. In addition, the thebesian veins provide a very limited return of blood directly through the walls of the chambers.

CARDIAC OXYGEN SUPPLY AND DEMAND

In normal cardiac function, the delivery of oxygen typically matches myocardial oxygen demands. The heart has very high oxygen extraction of 70% to 75% at resting heart rate and contractility; thus, increased oxygen demand due to exertion must be met by an increase in coronary blood flow. If the oxygen needs of the myocardium are not met, ischemia develops, impairing, and sometimes irreversibly injuring myocardial tissues. Thus, as with any tissue, oxygen supply must meet oxygen demand to prevent tissue damage.

Determinants of Cardiac Oxygen Supply

Oxygen delivery requires adequate pulmonary function to oxygenate the blood and clear carbon dioxide, as well as adequate blood flow. Since the coronary oxygen extraction rate is so high, the delivery of oxygen to coronary tissues must be carefully regulated. Coronary blood flow is pulsatile but, in contrast to other organs, has a peak flow during *diastole*. This seemingly contrary pattern is due to the unique anatomy of the coronary vasculature (**Figure 10.31**).

Blood flow to the left ventricle is higher than that to the right ventricle as the former has a higher mass accompanied by greater oxygen demands and a larger vascular network. During systole, the cardiac muscle contracts and *compresses* the coronary vasculature, increasing its local resistance and limiting blood flow. At the onset of diastole, coronary blood flow increases, depending on aortic pressure. As aortic pressure drops during diastole, the ventricles are relaxing, relieving the coronary vessels from compression. This drop in coronary resistance allows the local coronary blood flow to surge. This diastolic surge is also reflected in the right branch but is attenuated due to the relatively smaller and thinner right ventricular wall. Overall, coronary blood flow is maximal during diastole but reduced during systole.

The duration of diastole, then, affects total myocardial blood flow. As noted earlier, diastole during a resting heart rate of 70 beats/min is typically about two thirds of a cardiac cycle. The heart is only actively engaged in contraction about one third of the time, with *recovery* and maximal cardiac perfusion during the remainder. However, as heart rate increases, the duration of diastole shortens, while the duration of systole remains relatively constant (**Figure 10.32**). Shortening of diastole is paralleled by a shortened period of coronary blood flow, reducing blood and oxygen supply just as tissue oxygen demands are increasing because of the faster heart rate. The result is greater vulnerability to ischemia as heart rate increases in patients with compromised coronary arteries due to atherosclerosis.

Coronary blood flow also undergoes autoregulation, as described in Chapter 9, Circulation. This intrinsic property of the heart adjusts coronary vascular resistance to maintain coronary blood flow despite changes in perfusion pressure from 60 to 140 mm Hg. In addition, local endothelial and vascular factors contribute to regulation of coronary blood flow.

Determinants of Cardiac Oxygen Demand

The metabolic demand of the heart varies with the cardiac work. Sympathetic discharge increases heart rate and cardiac contractility, both of which increase myocardial oxygen demand. Simultaneously, reduced duration of diastole decreases oxygen supply. Furthermore, any condition that increases cardiac work, such as increased preload, afterload, or contractility, also increases oxygen demand.

CORONARY ARTERY DISEASE

The major factor limiting cardiac oxygen supply is the presence of atherosclerotic plaque, as described in Chapter 9, Circulation. As noted earlier, **coronary artery disease** resulting in myocardial infarction is the most common cause of death in developed countries. When cardiac oxygen demand is not met by oxygen supply, the resulting cardiac ischemia can produce symptoms of **angina**. Patient-reported symptoms of angina vary greatly. Some patients deny pain but describe pressure or a squeezing sensation or tightness

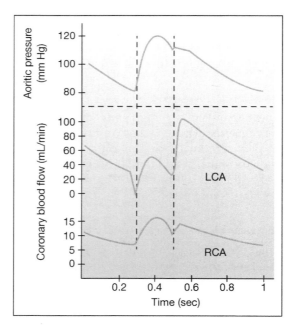

FIGURE 10.31 Myocardial blood flow varies through the cardiac cycle. Total blood flow through the coronary vessels is maximal during diastole. The higher blood flow through the left ventricle is due to its greater mass and higher oxygen consumption than the right ventricle.

LCA, left coronary artery; RCA, right coronary artery.

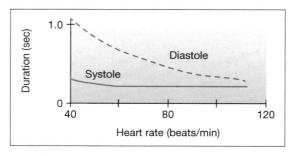

FIGURE 10.32 Diastole shortens as heart rate increases. At faster heart rates, the time for each beat shortens; however, this change arises almost exclusively by shortening the duration of diastole. Because most coronary blood flow occurs during diastole, diastolic shortening can significantly reduce coronary perfusion during tachycardia.

in the chest. Other patients complain of pain that can be severe and may radiate to the shoulders, arms, and neck. Other patient-reported symptoms include nausea, fatigue, and shortness of breath.

In the earliest phases of coronary heart disease, exercise or other physically demanding activities may promote angina symptoms that resolve shortly after stopping the activity. This form is referred to as *exertional angina* but is sometimes also referred to as **stable angina**. Although it is not an acute crisis, this symptom is often the initial clue that cardiac blood flow is not delivering enough oxygen to meet the heart's needs. It can be an early indication of a developing atherosclerotic plaque in the coronary vasculature, which can be confirmed by catheterization, or by monitoring and cardiac imaging during a stress test. Exertional angina may show some acute improvement using a vasodilator such as nitroglycerin. Nitroglycerin has multiple effects that may relieve angina symptoms. Most prominent is that it relaxes smooth muscle in the walls of the veins, increasing blood pooling in these capacitance vessels, which reduces the preload and, consequently, the work of the heart.

Over days, weeks, or months, the intensity of pain of stable angina can increase in severity and take longer to resolve. Eventually the pain may occur more often with elevated intensity and may be accompanied by labored breathing. It can progress to a state where it does not follow a predictable pattern, can arise without physical exertion, and may not be alleviated by medication. The sensation is typically described as *having a house on the chest*. This progression, known as **unstable angina**, is indicative of deterioration of coronary blood flow and should be regarded as an emergency. Because it is associated with atherosclerotic plaque formation, a coronary plaque occlusion >80% is typically symptomatic and may be improved by physical dilation with a cardiac catheter or a bypass procedure using a vascular graft (cardiac bypass surgery).

In contrast, **variant angina**, also known as **Prinzmetal angina**, is a less common condition that does not begin during exertion but characteristically occurs while resting, during the night, or during early morning hours. Pain and nausea are typically severe and are not relieved by rest. Variant angina is triggered by coronary vasospasms and is not indicative of a coronary plaque-based restriction. Fortunately, variant angina can be treated using vasodilators such as nitroglycerin; unfortunately, coronary arterial vasospasms are thought to be the primary event associated with triggering sudden cardiac death.

ACUTE CORONARY SYNDROMES

Patients with **coronary atherosclerosis** often progress along a spectrum from stable angina into unstable angina as coronary blood flows are reduced. The rupture of an atherosclerotic plaque's fibrous cap can promote immediate formation of a thrombus that acutely obstructs coronary blood flow, precipitating cardiac tissue hypoxia and symptoms of ischemia. A partial obstruction can promote *unstable angina* or a **non–ST-elevation myocardial infarction** (NSTEMI) with intermittent chronic tissue damage. In contrast, complete obstruction of a coronary vessel may produce an NSTEMI or may rapidly destroy a greater volume of cardiac tissue, resulting in myocardial necrosis and full-thickness cardiac wall damage; this presents as an **ST-elevation myocardial infarction** (STEMI).

Non–ST-Elevation Myocardial Infarction and Unstable Angina

Reduced coronary artery blood flow decreases the delivery of oxygen-rich blood to cardiomyocytes. During exercise and other increased cardiac activity, metabolic demands may exceed the supply that can be delivered by the coronary circulation. Small arteries and other vessels located along the endocardial membrane lining the inside of the chambers of the heart are subjected to maximal compression during ventricular contraction; consequently, their resistance is high during systole, severely compromising flow. Accordingly, impaired blood delivery produces the highest level of ischemia in the subendocardium **(Figure 10.33)**. This transient cardiac event may result in alterations of the ST segment of the ECG in the form of depression of the ST segment or an inverted T wave. The distinguishing feature between NSTEMI and unstable angina is that NSTEMI has the characteristic elevations in blood levels of troponins and other markers of cardiac cell death, indicating that an infarction has indeed occurred. It is important to

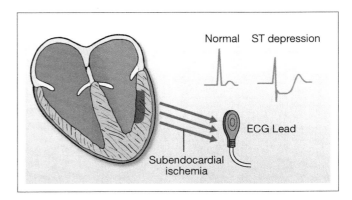

FIGURE 10.33 Manifestations of NSTEMI. During an NSTEMI event, the ischemic region is typically in the subendocardium. Cell dysfunction results in loss of ionic gradients, with extracellular K+ accumulation and loss of membrane potential and an electrical gradient between the ischemic region and normal tissue (arrows directed toward ECG lead). This change alters the electrical dipoles across the heart and is reflected by lower measured potential at the ST segment relative to the rest of the ECG, known as ST-segment depression. NSTEMI, non–ST-elevation myocardial infarction.

note that unstable angina or NSTEMI can occur without ECG manifestations, so monitoring and preparation for intervention should still be conducted.

ST-Elevation Myocardial Infarction

In a patient with preexisting (known or clinically silent) atherosclerosis, acute factors—including hypotension, inflammation, and prothrombotic states—can further reduce coronary flow, resulting in a STEMI. Rupture of an atherosclerotic plaque releases thrombogenic substances, rapidly precipitating formation of a clot that may completely occlude the narrowed vessel. This leads almost immediately to profound tissue hypoxia and ischemia, and cardiomyocyte death that extends fully through the ventricular wall (transmural infarction). This acute injury causes a full-blown *heart attack* and is a medical emergency requiring rapid steps to monitor the patient and restore coronary blood flow. The massive damage to cardiomyocytes causes a *blank* region of conduction that shifts the resting membrane potential observed during the ST segment, relative to the rest of the ECG. This shift is responsible for the observation, during a STEMI, of an elevated ST segment (**Figure 10.34**). The tissue damage arising during a STEMI also causes the release of cardiac cellular enzymes and proteins.

Troponins are regulatory proteins in the thin filaments that are integral to cardiac myocyte contraction. Acutely damaged cardiomyocytes undergo necrotic cell death with swelling and rupture of the plasma membrane, releasing the contents of their cytoplasm into the circulation. Levels of both cardiac-specific *troponin I* and *troponin T* can be detected 6 to 12 hours after the onset of myocardial injury, peaking at about 24 hours. Levels then decline gradually over several days for the following 2 weeks. *Creatine phosphokinase* is found in both skeletal and cardiac muscle but can be also released by damage to either type of tissue. The myocardial band (MB) fraction of

creatine phosphokinase (CK-MB) was previously measured as a marker of myocardial infarction; however, the test has now generally been replaced by troponin measurements.

ECG changes associated with STEMIs can evolve when and if the tissue damage resolves. After the full-wall damage has occurred, the dead tissue is slowly replaced by scar tissue. Gradual resolution of altered electrical activity causes the ST segment to return to the pre-STEMI baseline. The damaged section of the wall is unable to conduct depolarizations, but a downward-reflected Q wave appears, remaining as a permanent marker of the coronary infarction.

Patterns of Ischemic Heart Disease in Women

Women were once thought to be protected from ischemic heart disease; hence, research into pathophysiology, diagnosis, and management focused on men. This focus is gradually changing with the recognition that the burden of ischemic heart disease in women is almost equal to that of men (46% of U.S. patients with coronary heart disease are women), that the mortality rate associated with myocardial infarction is higher in women, and that disease presentation differs between women and men. The evidence basis for management of ischemic heart disease in women is now being investigated with the goal of improving outcomes.

Symptoms of ischemic heart disease differ between men and women, with women more likely overall to report angina. Women are less likely to report exertional angina and more likely to report emotional stress-induced angina and persistent angina, as well as angina at rest. Women are more likely to report that their angina is associated with decreased quality of life. Acute coronary syndrome presentation also varies with sex. Women are less likely to report any chest pain and have higher rates of undetected myocardial infarction. Women with angina are more likely than men to have an array of associated symptoms, including pain in the back, neck, and jaw; shortness of breath; nausea or indigestion; and fatigue.

Pathological analysis of coronary atherosclerosis in women reveals a disconnect between the extent to which the coronary arteries are narrowed and the amount of myocardial ischemia. Although many women have severely narrowed coronary arteries on coronary angiography, other women with severe myocardial ischemia may have no angiographic signs of lumen narrowing. Recent studies have identified coronary microvascular dysfunction in both men and women who have angina and even myocardial infarction without the signs of disease in the large coronary arteries. As shown in **Figure 10.35**, the amount of resistance and mechanisms of flow regulation varies along the segments of the coronary microvasculature.

The coronary arteries travel along the surface of the epicardium, giving off branches that go to three

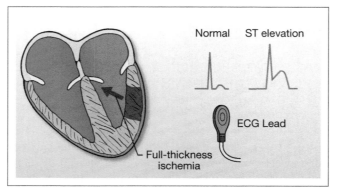

FIGURE 10.34 Manifestations of STEMI. A STEMI produces a full-thickness lesion through the endocardium. This irreversible damage raises the measured potential during the ST portion relative to the remainder of the ECG, as shown by the arrow pointing away from the ECG lead.
STEMI, ST-elevation myocardial infarction.

different depths before branching into smaller arteries, arterioles, and capillaries (see **Figure 10.35**). Each segment of vessel is regulated by different mechanisms, with the large epicardial arteries (representing <10% of the vascular resistance) primarily modulated by shear-activated forces, small arteries (representing ~20% of the resistance) regulated by shear-activated forces, large arterioles (representing ~50% of the resistance) regulated by myogenic mechanisms, and the smallest arterioles regulated by local metabolism. **Coronary microvascular dysfunction** is the term proposed to describe vascular compromise that results in myocardial ischemia in the absence of significant lesions in the large coronary arteries. Factors such as abnormal vascular smooth muscle cell spasticity/reactivity or altered endothelial function can account for compromised blood flow arising from microvascular dysfunction in the presence of coronary arteries that appear normal on angiography.[9]

Shaw and colleagues note that traditional Framingham risk scores may not provide a full picture of risk of coronary artery disease in women and can be strengthened by additional measures. Their model incorporates contributing factors that may account for the varied presentations of ischemic heart disease in women (**Figure 10.36**).[10] Women may have altered levels of gonadal steroids that influence cardiovascular risk. In particular, polycystic ovary syndrome (PCOS) has high comorbidity with the metabolic syndrome and its state of hyperlipidemia, hypertension, and insulin resistance. Women are more likely to have autoimmune disorders and higher levels of inflammatory markers such as C-reactive protein. In addition to vascular changes that may affect medium-sized to small vessels, women are also more likely to have an episode of acute vasospasm, and younger women have a higher risk of acute coronary artery dissection, both of which may lead to myocardial infarction.[10]

Sequelae Associated With Myocardial Infarctions

The damage produced by a full-wall myocardial infarction can initiate a collection of potential complications or sequelae that include cardiogenic shock and arrhythmias.

Cardiogenic shock is the most common cause of death in patients with acute myocardial infarction. Impaired flow into the cardiac tissues produces hypoxia, which promotes local release of cytokines that can impair cardiac contractility. This complication often arises within hours after a myocardial infarction. The reduced blood flow through infarcted tissues also slows the clearance of these cytokines, thus amplifying their effects. The resulting decreased cardiac contractility reduces the stroke volume to decrease cardiac output and lowers systolic blood pressure below 80 mm Hg; this is accompanied by tachycardia and a weak pulse. The fall in blood pressure decreases cardiac

and peripheral perfusion, lowers urinary output, and reduces cranial perfusion. If left untreated, cardiogenic shock leads to terminal circulatory collapse.

Myocardial infarctions damage cardiac conduction, in part, through elevated intracellular Ca^{2+} that blocks gap junctions. Regional blocks can promote unpredictable redirections of currents, causing arrhythmias. Arrhythmias can promote uncoordinated contractions of the cardiac chambers that decrease flow efficiency or promote valvular damage. Lack of effective chamber emptying promotes clot formation that can generate pulmonary emboli (if the right ventricle is affected) or stroke (if the left ventricle is affected).

Postinfarction care encompasses close monitoring and cardiac rehabilitation. Ultimately, some patients may have a complete recovery, while others have subsequent myocardial infarction or may progress to heart failure.

Thought Questions

10. Coronary artery disease is a major killer in the United States and worldwide. Why is this disorder so common? What anatomical features might make the coronary vasculature vulnerable to developing atherosclerotic plaque, and what common behaviors and lifestyle factors foster plaque development?

11. What accounts for the extremely high oxygen demand of myocardial tissue?

HEART FAILURE

Heart failure is a progressive condition in which the heart is unable to pump enough blood to meet the body's needs for blood flow and oxygen delivery. **Table 10.3** contrasts the effects of left-sided versus right-sided heart failure.

LEFT-SIDED HEART FAILURE

The left ventricle is responsible for rhythmic ejection of a stroke volume at a heart rate adequate to support cardiac output sufficient for the needs of all the body's tissues and organs. The workload and vulnerability of the left ventricle to ischemic and other insults makes it more prone to develop heart failure than the right ventricle. The causes of left ventricular failure may be grouped as (a) impairments in cardiac contractility, (b) chronic increases of afterload or restrictions in ventricular relaxation and filling, and (c) chronic increases in tissue/blood flow demands beyond the range of normal cardiac output, as seen in hyperthyroidism and some cases of anemia (also known as **high-output heart failure**).

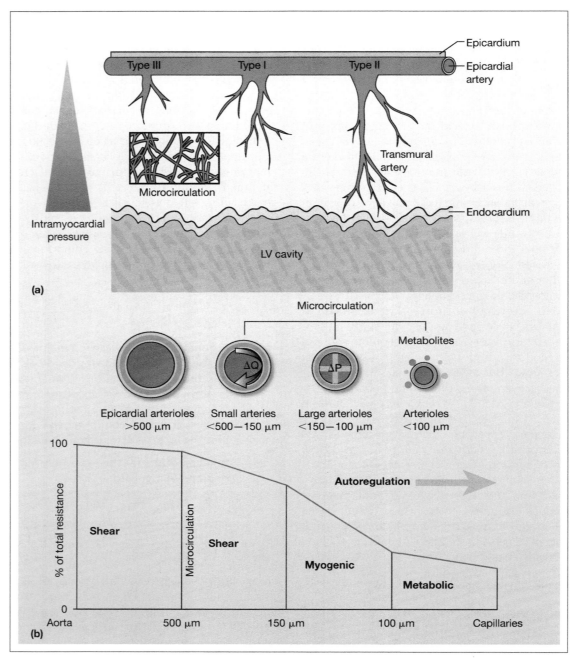

FIGURE 10.35 Coronary microvascular dysfunction. Myocardial ischemia and infarction can occur in the absence of detectable occlusion of the large coronary arteries. **(a)** Three categories of large arteries traveling in the epicardium branch to perfuse different depths of the myocardium and endocardium. Type II vessels branch in the deepest layers, perfusing the microcirculation of the subendocardium. These vessels are subjected to the greatest intramyocardial pressure during systole, and therefore the subendothelial tissue is most vulnerable to ischemia. **(b)** Much of the coronary vascular resistance occurs distal to the coronary arteries, in small arteries with flow regulated by shear stress, and in arterioles smaller than 150 μm that are controlled by myogenic or metabolic autoregulation. Potential mechanisms accounting for myocardial ischemia in the absence of large vessel disease include vasospasm or endothelial dysfunction of small vessels. Coronary microvascular dysfunction is more prevalent in women, and may account for some of the sex differences in angina and myocardial infarction symptoms.

ΔP, changes in pressure contributing to vascular regulation (myogenic); ΔQ, changes in flow contributing to vascular regulation by altering shear stress.

Source: From Camici PG, Rimoldi OE, Crea F. Coronary microvascular dysfunction. In: de Lemos JA, Omland T, eds. *Chronic Coronary Artery Disease: A Companion to Braunwald's Heart Disease*. Philadelphia, PA: Elsevier; 2018.

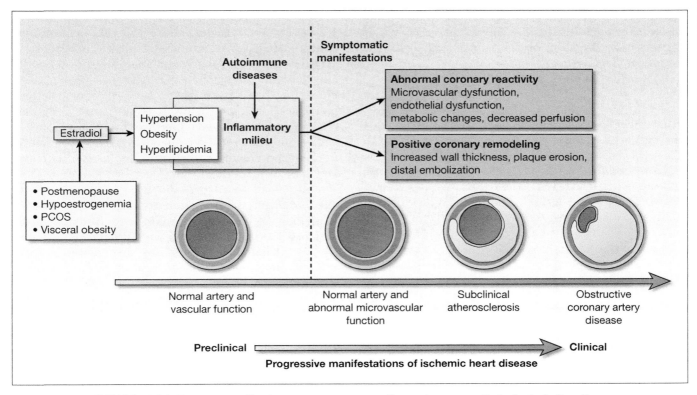

FIGURE 10.36 Factors contributing to coronary artery disease in women. Pathological alterations contributing to myocardial ischemia may accumulate long before visible obstruction of large vessels occurs.

PCOS, polycystic ovary syndrome.

Source: From Shaw LJ, Bugiardini R, Merz NB. Women and ischemic heart disease. *Evol Knowl J Am Coll Cardiol.* 2009;54:1561–1575.

TABLE 10.3 Heart Failure Comparison: Left-Sided Versus Right-Sided Heart Failure

	Left-Sided Heart Failure	Right-Sided Heart Failure
Effects of decreased cardiac output	Fatigue Exercise intolerance Poor capillary refill Cool extremities Peripheral cyanosis Decreased renal perfusion and function Neurohormonal compensatory mechanisms activated	Decreased blood flow through lungs—decreases filling of the left side of the heart, reducing systemic cardiac output Often develops secondary to left-sided heart failure and the associated elevated pulmonary vascular pressures
Effects of elevated filling pressures of the affected ventricle and atrium	Increased pulmonary vascular pressures Dyspnea Orthopnea (dyspnea increases when lying down) Paroxysmal nocturnal dyspnea (severe dyspnea at night due to fluid shifts from legs and feet) Pulmonary edema with hypoxemia and pulmonary crackles Right-sided heart failure	Increased systemic venous pressures Dependent edema, particularly pitting edema affecting ankles and feet Hepatomegaly and ascites Gastrointestinal engorgement Jugular vein distention

Two main forms of heart failure are currently categorized based on the ejection fraction. A patient can be characterized as having **heart failure with reduced ejection fraction** (HFrEF), encompassing characteristics that were formerly termed *systolic failure*. The other form is **heart failure with preserved ejection fraction** (HFpEF), which includes characteristics that were formerly termed *diastolic failure*. The diagnosis of HFpEF is becoming more common as the recognition of this form of heart failure is increasing in clinical practice. However, much of the existing literature and many management strategies focus on HFrEF, as this form of heart failure has been recognized and studied far longer than HFpEF.

Left Ventricular Failure With Reduced Ejection Fraction

When the left ventricle undergoes serious tissue injury, the resulting damage reduces cardiac contractility. This reduces stroke volume at all levels of preload (see **Figure 10.24b**). While the Frank–Starling mechanism remains intact, the curve is shifted downward. Over time, left ventricular end-diastolic and end-systolic volumes gradually increase and the chamber dilates, with thinning of the ventricular wall. The ratio of stroke volume to end-diastolic volume (ejection fraction) decreases, giving rise to the term *HFrEF* (**Figure 10.37**). In addition to STEMI, this form of heart failure can develop from any condition that promotes progressive myocardial damage and deterioration, such as cardiomyopathies and some infectious disorders (e.g., Chagas disease). Chest x-ray can detect cardiac enlargement that develops in many cases of chronic heart failure. Echocardiography is one method of assessment of chamber volume and ejection fraction. In HFrEF, expected findings include an increase in chamber size with wall thinning and ejection fraction <40%.

Heart Failure Stimulates Neurohormonal Compensation

Whatever the initiating mechanism, the reduced cardiac output of heart failure is detected in the periphery as lack of sufficient blood flow and pressure, resulting

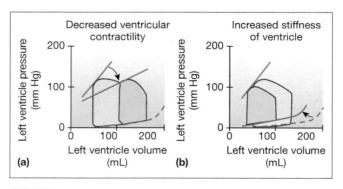

FIGURE 10.37 Two pathways to reduced stroke volume in heart failure are illustrated by pressure-volume loops. **(a)** Weakening of the ventricular wall shifts the ESPVR line down and initially reduces stroke volume and ejection fraction. As greater volumes of blood are retained in the ventricle, preload increases, shifting the pressure–volume relationship to the right and somewhat improving stroke volume, but at the expense of enlarging and dilating the ventricle. **(b)** Increased ventricular stiffness shifts the EDPVR line up and limits ventricular filling, as diastolic pressure rapidly rises with added volume. This limits the diastolic filling, decreasing the amount of blood available for ejection.

in fatigue and decreased physical activity. Homeostatic responses are initiated to restore cardiac output (**Figure 10.38**). The carotid and aortic baroreceptors suppress parasympathetic stimulation of the SA node and activate the sympathetic nervous system, thus increasing heart rate. Sympathetic vasoconstriction increases, helping to maintain blood pressure, but at the expense of increased afterload. Pituitary vasopressin secretion increases, promoting renal water retention, but potentially contributing to vasoconstriction and increased afterload.

Decreased blood pressure due to heart failure also reduces renal perfusion pressure. This works in tandem with increased sympathetic stimulation to activate the renin-angiotensin-aldosterone system (RAAS). Angiotensin II initiates vasoconstriction to raise blood pressure (but also afterload), and aldosterone enhances renal Na^+ retention. Volume expansion is also promoted by vasopressin-mediated water retention. In addition to renal/vascular hemodynamic effects, angiotensin II and aldosterone promote fibrotic changes in the wall of the heart that contribute to cardiac remodeling. Inflammatory mediators are induced by tissue injury in heart failure, and it is likely that members of the IL-1, IL-6, and TNF cytokine families contribute to compensatory and decompensatory responses in the progression of heart failure.

Left-Sided Heart Failure Effect on Lung Vascular Volumes and Pressures

Fluid retention increases cardiac preload, which is predicted to increase cardiac output, but only to a limited degree. The end-diastolic volume continues to increase, but since the cardiac function curve is shifted downward, increased preload does not restore normal stroke volume (see **Figure 10.37a**). The increase in left ventricular end-diastolic pressure requires a similar increase in left atrial pressure needed to fill the left ventricle. A corresponding pressure increase develops in the pulmonary vascular bed that empties into the left atrium. The lung's vast delicate capillary network is highly susceptible to increases in hydrostatic pressure, which promotes migration of capillary fluid into the pulmonary extravascular space. Pulmonary congestion can stimulate lung receptors, producing a sensation of dyspnea. As pressures rise further, pulmonary edema forms and fluid accumulates in the alveoli, impairing lung gas exchange. In addition, the elevated pulmonary vascular pressures impede right ventricular output by increasing right ventricular afterload, while reducing right ventricular stroke volume and cardiac output. Collectively, these events gradually decrease the cardiac output and promote pulmonary edema.

A beneficial effect of increased atrial volume and pressure is to stimulate the release of atrial natriuretic peptide (ANP). In a similar fashion, stretch of the

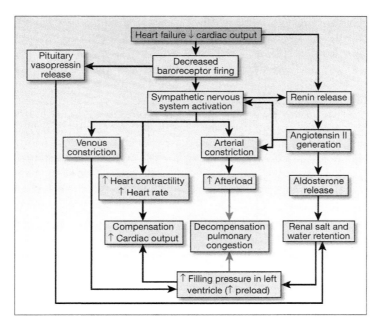

FIGURE 10.38 The vicious cycle that perpetuates heart failure. Decreased cardiac output and blood pressure are signaled via baroreceptors. Compensatory mechanisms include increased sympathetic stimulation of heart rate and contractility, increased RAAS activity, and vasopressin secretion. Fluid retention secondary to aldosterone and vasopressin contributes to preload, but at the risk of further dilating the heart. Venoconstriction also augments preload, and contributes to ventricular enlargement. Sympathetic vasoconstriction is augmented by angiotensin II and vasopressin, increasing blood pressure but also increasing afterload and the work of the heart. Increased ventricular volume and wall distention promote cardiac fibrosis and slippage of fibers, thinning the wall. Fluid retention contributes to elevated pulmonary vascular pressures and dyspnea. ANP and BNP secretion increases but is inadequate to stimulate renal excretion of retained Na⁺ and water.
ANP, atrial natriuretic peptide; BNP, B-type natriuretic peptide; RAAS, renin-angiotensin-aldosterone system.
Source: From Waller DG, Sampson AP. *Medical Pharmacology & Therapeutics.* 5th ed. Elsevier; 2018.

ventricles stimulates the release of B-type natriuretic peptide (BNP). ANP and BNP are peripheral vasodilators, which helps the heart by reducing afterload. In addition, these natriuretic hormones promote renal Na⁺ excretion, reducing total body fluid volume. Plasma BNP and a related peptide, N-terminal pro B-type natriuretic peptide (NT-proBNP), can be assayed and used as markers of heart failure progression. Interestingly, treatment with a combination of valsartan (an angiotensin receptor-blocking drug) and sacubitril has proved beneficial in patients with heart failure. Sacubitril inhibits the enzyme neprilysin, which normally degrades BNP (and bradykinin) in the circulation. The combined treatment is predicted to reduce vasoconstriction and fluid retention caused by angiotensin II while also prolonging the action of the vasodilators BNP and bradykinin to reduce afterload.

Left Ventricular Failure With Preserved Ejection Fraction

If the left ventricle loses the ability to relax normally (because the muscle has become stiff), then the heart cannot properly fill with blood during diastole. Left ventricular end-diastolic volume decreases, reducing stroke volume even if ejection fraction is normal. In HFpEF, the left ventricle is stiffer than normal. Because of that, it cannot relax properly, limiting the volume of filling during diastole, which then reduces the stroke volume (see **Figure 10.37b**). Thus, HFpEF, is distinguished from HFrEF by its etiology—it is caused by loss of compliance of the ventricular wall, which limits filling during diastole. Because contraction and ventricular ejection are starting from a lower end-diastolic volume, stroke volume is below normal even if ejection fraction is normal. Conditions that chronically increase afterload, such as hypertension and aortic stenosis, are common causes of HFpEF. Ongoing studies are directed to understanding facets of HFpEF, including the mechanisms underlying individual risk factors such as obesity, hypertension, diabetes, and female sex.

The functional outcome of HFpEF is similar to that in HFrEF: Reduced cardiac output limits activity and exercise tolerance, and predisposes the individual to fluid retention and pulmonary congestion. HFpEF appears to be more common in older adults, particularly in women, and in those with a history of hypertension. Imaging shows an enlarged heart with a thickened ventricular wall, reduced ventricular volumes, and an ejection fraction about normal at 50%.

RIGHT-SIDED HEART FAILURE

Primary failure of the right ventricle can be caused by chronic lung disease. This disorder, termed **cor pulmonale**, results from hypoxia-mediated pulmonary vasoconstriction (discussed in Chapter 11, Lungs). However, right-sided heart failure commonly develops secondary to left-sided heart failure. The mechanism connecting failure of the two sides of the heart relates to the pulmonary vascular manifestations of left-sided heart failure discussed earlier. Chronic elevations of pulmonary vascular pressures due to poor contractility of the left ventricle create increased afterload for the right ventricle. As the right ventricle is normally responsible for generating relatively low pressures (25 mm Hg systolic pressure) to achieve ejection, this overload can rapidly translate to right ventricular damage and failure.

As occurs with left-sided heart failure, increasing right ventricular end-diastolic volume to achieve increasingly larger preload enlarges the ventricle and elevates filling pressures from the right atrium. Ultimately, the systemic venous pressure rises, promoting peripheral edema that is initially manifested by swelling of the feet and ankles. As the disease progresses, venous congestion can also affect the liver and gastrointestinal structures, manifested by ascites and abdominal discomfort. Right-sided heart failure is imminent when left-sided heart failure is present and further exacerbates the progression of congestive heart failure. **Table 10.3** compares the findings in left-sided and right-sided heart failure.

MANAGEMENT OF HEART FAILURE

Strategies previously employed to manage heart failure were based on promoting cardiac contractility with positive inotropic drugs such as digoxin, while reducing fluid retention with diuretics. These strategies had some effectiveness, but research indicates better maintenance of activity and function in HFrEF through neurohormonal blockade of the RAAS and sympathetic nervous system. Angiotensin-converting enzyme inhibitors and, more commonly, angiotensin receptor antagonists are a mainstay of treatment, and β-blockers are also effective. As mentioned, neprilysin inhibition may be a useful addition to angiotensin receptor antagonism in some patient groups. Aldosterone inhibitors are also effective add-ons to other medications. If cardiac function continues to deteriorate, then heart transplantation can be an option. Ventricular assist devices have also been developed to provide mechanical support, improving cardiac ejection; these devices can be useful for patients whose condition is deteriorating while awaiting heart transplantation.

Management of comorbidities such as hypertension and diabetes is critical. In addition, lifestyle modifications, including reducing salt intake and maintaining physical activity, are of importance in heart failure care.

 Thought Questions

12. What change in the Frank–Starling relationship would be seen in someone who has HFrEF? What is the effect of the altered relationship on cardiac pressure–volume loops?

13. Why is afterload reduction helpful in people with heart failure?

STRUCTURAL CARDIAC DISORDERS

NORMAL STRUCTURE OF THE HEART AND CARDIAC VALVES

Blood flow in the four chambers of the heart is regulated by orchestrated opening and closing of the four cardiac valves (**Figure 10.39a** and **b**). All cardiac valves open and close *passively* in response to pressure differences between cardiac chambers, and normally form a tight seal when closed, preventing backward blood flow (regurgitation). AV valves are located between the atria and corresponding ventricle: The tricuspid valve is on the right side, and the mitral (bicuspid) valve is on the left side of the heart. These one-way valves are anchored by fibers (chordae tendineae) to special sections of cardiac muscle called papillary muscles. Papillary muscles do not open the AV valves; rather, they contract along with the rest of the ventricle and pull down on the valves to counter the effects of increased ventricular pressure and thus prevent valve eversion during systole (**Figure 10.39b**).

The AV valves open and close according to pressure gradients between the two chambers they connect: (a) when atrial pressure exceeds ventricular pressure, the valve opens, allowing blood to flow from the atrium to the ventricle; (b) when ventricular pressure exceeds atrial pressure, the valve closes, preventing blood flow back toward the atria during ventricular contraction. Closure of the mitral and tricuspid valves generates the first heart sound (S₁) during the cardiac cycle and signals the beginning of systole.

The two ventricles are connected to their outflow path by semilunar one-way valves. The right ventricle is connected to the pulmonary artery via the pulmonary valve, and the left ventricle is connected to the aorta via the aortic valve. These are tricuspid valves; however, 1% to 2% of the population has a congenitally bicuspid aortic valve (which is more common in men).

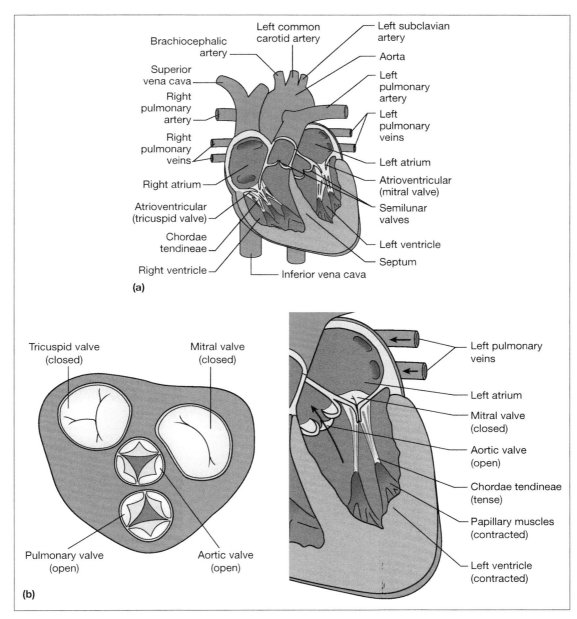

FIGURE 10.39 Valves of the heart. **(a)** The tricuspid and mitral valves separate atria and ventricles on the right and left side, respectively. The semilunar valves separate ventricles from their outflow tracts, the pulmonary and aortic valves for right and left ventricles, respectively. **(b)** During ventricular contraction, papillary muscles contract, pulling the chordae tendineae downward and preventing the mitral valve from being pushed open by the high ventricular systolic pressure.

The aortic and pulmonary valves also operate by pressure gradients. When ventricular pressure exceeds diastolic pressure in the outflow vessel, these valves open and ventricular ejection occurs; when ventricular pressure falls below the pressure in the pulmonary artery or aorta, the valves close and prevent blood flow back to the ventricles during diastole. Closure of the semilunar valves creates the second heart sound (S_2), which signals the end of systole and beginning of diastole in the cardiac cycle. S_2 can sometimes be heard as two sounds for separate closures of the aortic (A_2) and pulmonary

(P_2) valves even under normal conditions (physiological splitting of S_2 during inspiration). Under normal conditions, heart valve openings do not create sounds.

VALVE DISEASES

Cardiac valve diseases have two major hemodynamic phenotypes: (a) *stenosis*, which increases the resistance of the heart valve, requiring higher chamber pressures to maintain flow; and (b) *regurgitation*—backflow due to insufficient closure of the valve. Sometimes, both problems are present at the same time, especially in conditions that cause thickening and distortion of the valves, such as atherosclerotic plaque development or inflammation (bacterial endocarditis, rheumatic heart disease, and some autoimmune diseases). The most common valve disorder is **aortic stenosis**, followed by **mitral regurgitation**. Globally, the most common cause of valve disorders is rheumatic heart disease, which can develop as a consequence of group A β-hemolytic streptococcal pharyngitis. Prevalence of valve disorders is decreasing in resource-rich countries, due to detection and treatment of strep throat. Over time, the physical manifestations of valve disorders grow more severe, necessitating surgical treatment to repair or replace the valve.

Types of Cardiac Murmurs

Blood flow through stenotic or regurgitating (leaky) valves creates turbulence, leading to vibration and murmurs. **Figure 10.40** illustrates that stenotic valves generate murmurs when they are open, while regurgitation due to insufficient valves generates murmurs when the valve is supposed to be closed during the cardiac cycle. Based on the type of valve disease (stenosis or regurgitation or both) and the valve involved, murmurs can be heard during cardiac systole or diastole. In patients with combined valve problems, murmurs may be heard in both phases of the cardiac cycle. Murmurs are typically loudest above the auscultation point for the valve(s) involved (**Figure 10.41**). Typically, aortic valve problems can also be heard over the carotid arteries, while mitral valve murmurs may be heard in the midaxillary line. The shape of the murmur's phonographic appearance depends on the pressure changes during the cardiac cycle, while the intensity of the murmur may be related to the severity of the valve disease. Examples of murmurs can be found online in the University of Michigan's Heart Sound & Murmur Library (www.med.umich.edu/lrc/psb_open/html/repo/primer_heartsound/primer_heartsound.html).

Aortic Valve Dysfunction

Aortic Stenosis

There are three major causes of **aortic stenosis**: (a) degenerative calcification of a previously normal aortic valve, (b) calcification of a congenitally bicuspid aortic valve, and (c) inflammation resulting from rheumatic fever. Degenerative disease of a normal aortic valve increases with aging and shares some pathological features with atherosclerosis, particularly the association with chronic inflammation and Ca^{2+} deposition. Patients with bicuspid aortic valves (1% to 2% of the population, as previously noted) typically develop severe aortic stenosis a decade earlier than patients with normal aortic valve degeneration. Rheumatic aortic valve disease is a less common cause of aortic stenosis and is nearly always accompanied by involvement of the mitral valve.

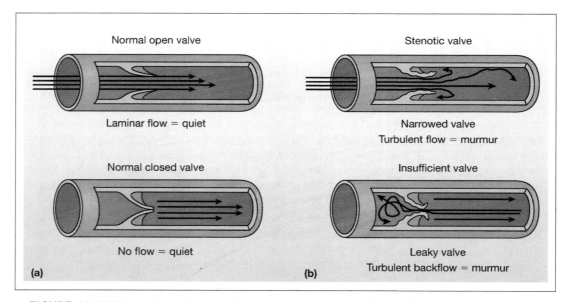

FIGURE 10.40 Blood flow through diseased heart valves produces distinctive murmurs. **(a)** Laminar flow through an open valve does not produce any sound, and a competent valve blocks all flow when closed, also preventing sound production. **(b)** Turbulent flow through a tight, stenotic valve produces a murmur during the associated phase of the cardiac cycle (systolic murmur for ventricular outflow pathways, diastolic murmur for atrioventricular valves). A damaged valve that permits regurgitant flow can produce a murmur during the phase of the cycle when that valve would normally be closed (diastolic murmur for ventricular outflow pathways, systolic murmur for atrioventricular valves).

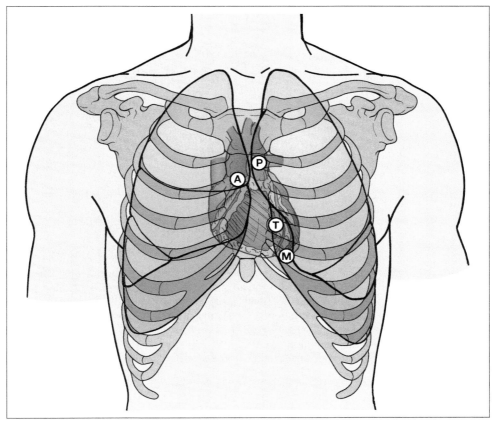

FIGURE 10.41 Anatomical locations for auscultating heart sounds associated with specific valves. A, aortic; M, mitral; P, pulmonary; T, tricuspid.

The impediment to left ventricular outflow in aortic stenosis results in elevated left ventricle pressures and ventricular hypertrophy (**Figure 10.42**). A systolic pressure gradient is present between the left ventricle and aorta, and stroke volume is reduced. The S_2 is diminished in intensity, and there is a crescendo–decrescendo systolic murmur that does not extend beyond S_2. Arterial pressure and pulse pressure are reduced.

There are three major clinical presentations in advanced aortic stenosis:

1. Angina that results from the combination of increased myocardial oxygen demand of the hypertrophied ventricle and decreased perfusion pressure due to lower aortic diastolic pressure
2. Exertional syncope that results from inadequate cardiac output due to reduced stroke volume
3. Heart failure that ultimately results from impaired cardiac output

Over time, elevated left ventricle pressures lead to elevated left atrium pressures, contributing to pulmonary vascular pressure increases and associated symptoms of dyspnea on exertion and, eventually, dyspnea at rest. Inadequate left ventricle relaxation and high end-systolic pressure further increase the demand for late filling by the atrial kick. Elevated left atrium pressures also lead to chamber dilation and increase the incidence of atrial fibrillation. Symptomatic aortic stenosis greatly increases the risk of sudden cardiac death; thus, valve replacement or other surgical treatment is required.

Aortic Regurgitation

Aortic regurgitation may result either from abnormalities of the aortic valve leaflets or from dilation of the aortic root. Primary valvular causes include (a) bicuspid aortic valve (in some patients aortic regurgitation predominates over aortic stenosis), (b) infective endocarditis (due to perforation or erosion of a leaflet), and (c) rheumatic heart disease (due to thickening and shortening of the aortic valve cusps). Aortic root disease results in aortic regurgitation when the aortic annulus dilates sufficiently to cause separation of the leaflets. Examples include age-related degenerative dilation of the aortic root, aortic aneurysms, and aortic dissection.

In aortic regurgitation, abnormal backflow of blood occurs from the aorta into the left ventricle during diastole. Thus, with each contraction, the left ventricle must pump that regurgitant volume plus the normal quantity of blood entering from the left atrium. Hemodynamic

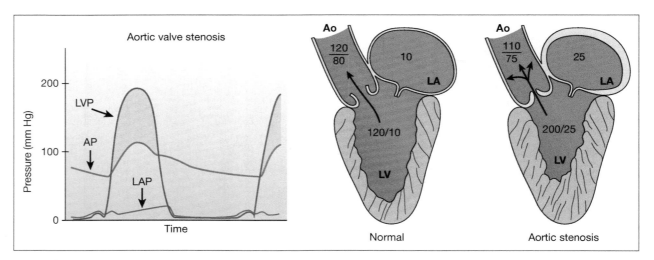

FIGURE 10.42 Cardiac alterations in aortic stenosis. In response to increased afterload, the LV becomes hypertrophied. The pressure gradient across a severely stenotic valve is markedly increased, with elevated LV systolic pressure and aortic pressure normal to low. Chronic elevation of LV diastolic pressure is reflected back to increase LAP, producing atrial dilation and hypertrophy and pulmonary vascular congestion. Numbers refer to pressures in each area, measured in mm Hg. Ao, aorta; AP, arterial pressure; LA, left atrium; LAP, left atrium pressure; LV, left ventricle; LVP, left ventricle pressure; AP, arterial pressure.
Source: From Klabunde RE. *Cardiovascular Physiology Concepts.* 2nd ed. Lippincott; 2012.

compensation relies on the Frank–Starling mechanism to augment stroke volume. Factors influencing the severity of aortic regurgitation are (a) the size of the regurgitant aortic orifice, (b) the pressure gradient across the aortic valve during diastole, and (c) the duration of diastole. Aortic regurgitation typically causes fatigue, dyspnea on exertion, and palpitations due to the increased pulse pressure.

In patients with chronic aortic regurgitation, adaptive enlargement of the left ventricle and atrium has occurred; thus, greater volume of regurgitation can be accommodated with less of an increase in diastolic left ventricle pressure. In these patients, pulmonary congestion is less likely. Acute aortic regurgitation can be an emergent situation due to aortic aneurysm or other cause. The left ventricle is of normal size and relatively low compliance; thus, diastolic pressure rises significantly. Increased left ventricle pressure is reflected back to the left atrium and pulmonary vasculature, resulting in pulmonary congestion or edema. Acute severe aortic regurgitation is usually a surgical emergency, requiring immediate valve replacement.

Mitral Valve Dysfunction

Mitral Stenosis

The most common (50% to 70% of patients) underlying cause of **mitral stenosis** is inflammatory distortion of the mitral valve due to prior rheumatic fever, which may have preceded the valve dysfunction by many years. Other causes include infective endocarditis that can result from implanted medical devices (vascular catheters, implanted valves, and others), intravenous drug use, or congenital valve defects. Acute and recurrent inflammation causes fibrous thickening and calcification of the valve leaflets, fusion of the commissures (the borders where the leaflets meet), and thickening and shortening of the chordae tendineae.

The stenotic valve obstructs flow from the left atrium into the ventricle. As the stenosis progresses, left atrium pressure and volume increase throughout the cardiac cycle, which in turn elevates pressures in the pulmonary circulation (pulmonary hypertension) and the right side of the heart. Retention of volume that cannot be ejected into the left ventricle leads to dilation of the left atrium, predisposing patients to atrial fibrillation. There is a pressure gradient between the left atrium and ventricle during diastole. Abnormal heart sounds are present, consisting of a diastolic opening snap that corresponds to the opening of the mitral valve, followed by a decrescendo murmur. The murmur intensifies just before S$_1$ due to the increased pressure gradient during atrial contraction in sinus rhythm (presystolic accentuation).

Mitral Regurgitation

The mitral valve is a complex structure composed of an annulus, two leaflets, chordae tendineae, and papillary muscles, supported by the adjacent myocardium. Disruption of any of these components can result in abnormal closure of the valve during systole, with ensuing **mitral regurgitation**. Mitral regurgitation can be primary, due to a structural defect of one or more of the valve components. Secondary mitral regurgitation can also occur if the valve is structurally normal but the valve opening is widened by left ventricular enlargement (during heart failure or dilated cardiomyopathy). Mitral regurgitation can also present acutely due to papillary muscle rupture within days of STEMI or chronically due to valve degeneration or inflammation.

In the normal heart, contraction of the left ventricle during systole forces blood exclusively through the aortic valve into the aorta; the closed mitral valve prevents regurgitation into the left atrium. In mitral regurgitation, a portion of left ventricular output is forced backward into the left atrium and thus forward cardiac output into the aorta is decreased. Acute mitral regurgitation can be a complication of myocardial infarction with rupture of the chordae tendineae or papillary muscle, or it can result from mitral valve prolapse (see next section). This is an emergency situation with severe symptoms of pulmonary edema and dyspnea. In acute mitral regurgitation, the left atrium is of normal size and is relatively noncompliant (does not stretch easily); thus, the pressure in the atrium rises significantly, causing pulmonary edema to develop.

In chronic mitral regurgitation, the left atrium adapts to the increased pressure by dilation, so that the pressure in the atrium is less elevated and pulmonary congestive symptoms are less common. During diastole, left ventricular volume increases more than normal as the normal left atrial filling is augmented by the volume of regurgitant flow from the previous systole. This produces enlargement of the left ventricle as well as increased wall thickness from the chronically elevated volume load. A holosystolic murmur is present in chronic mitral regurgitation, beginning at S_1 and continuing through S_2.

Mitral Valve Prolapse

Mitral valve prolapse (Barlow syndrome) occurs in response to degeneration of the mitral valve, causing the leaflets to become *floppy*. It is characterized by abnormal billowing of a portion of one or both mitral leaflets into the left atrium during ventricular systole in the middle of systole when left ventricle pressure peaks. This prolapse creates a characteristic mid systolic click. Mitral valve prolapse is frequently accompanied by mitral regurgitation, leading to a late systolic murmur, and it is often asymptomatic. Mitral valve prolapse may be inherited, or it may accompany certain connective tissue diseases (Marfan or Ehlers–Danlos syndrome). Pathologically, the valve leaflets, particularly the posterior leaflet, are enlarged, and the normal dense collagen and elastin matrix is fragmented and replaced with loose connective tissue. More severe lesions may be present. Mitral valve prolapse occurs in about 2% of the population and

is more common among women. The findings in major valve disorders are summarized in **Table 10.4**.

CARDIOMYOPATHIES

Cardiomyopathies are a diverse set of cardiac muscle disorders that cause mechanical or electrical dysfunction of the myocardium, or both. Excluded from this group of diseases is heart muscle impairment resulting from other specific cardiovascular disorders, such as hypertension, valvular abnormalities, or congenital heart disease. Cardiomyopathies often cause inappropriate ventricular hypertrophy or dilation, resulting in progressive heart failure and cardiovascular death. These conditions can involve the heart alone or may be a component of a systemic disease.

Cardiomyopathies can be classified into three main types:

1. **Dilated cardiomyopathy** is characterized by ventricular enlargement (dilation) with impaired *systolic* contractile function.
2. **Hypertrophic cardiomyopathy** (HCM) manifests as an abnormally thickened ventricular wall with abnormal *diastolic* relaxation but usually intact systolic function.
3. **Restrictive cardiomyopathy** (RCM) is characterized by abnormally decreased ventricular compliance (stiffened myocardium due to fibrosis or an infiltrative process), leading to impaired *diastolic* relaxation, but systolic contractile function is typically normal.

Hypertrophic Cardiomyopathy

HCM occurs in at least one in 500 people in the general population.[11] The disorder is characterized by left ventricular hypertrophy that is not caused by chronic pressure overload (i.e., not the result of hypertension or aortic stenosis). Other terms used for this condition are **hypertrophic obstructive cardiomyopathy** and **idiopathic hypertrophic subaortic stenosis**. In HCM, the systolic contractile function of the left ventricle is increased, but the thickened muscle is stiff, resulting in impaired ventricular relaxation and high diastolic pressures (diastolic dysfunction). Many different gene mutations can lead to HCM, which is often inherited as an autosomal dominant trait. Most of the mutations involve genes coding for components of the contractile apparatus: myosin, actin, troponin, or tropomyosin. HCM is the most common cardiac abnormality found in young athletes who die suddenly during vigorous physical exertion.

Figure 10.43 shows anatomical features of HCM. The left ventricular outflow tract is abnormally narrowed between the hypertrophied interventricular

TABLE 10.4 Characteristics of Valve Disorders

Valve Disorder	Associated Chamber and Pump Alterations	S_1/S_2	Murmurs	Other Manifestations
Aortic stenosis	LV: ↑P, hypertrophy, ↓stroke volume LA: ↑V, P, dilation ↑Pulmonary vascular pressures ↓Aortic mean and pulse pressure	Normal/single or paradoxically split	Systolic murmur–crescendo/decrescendo	Angina Syncope Exercise intolerance Dyspnea Left-sided heart failure
Aortic regurgitation (chronic)	LA: ↑V, normal to ↑P LV: ↑V, normal to ↑P, ↑wall thickness Aortic pressure: normal to ↑, ↓diastolic, ↑pulse pressure	Soft/normal	Diastolic decrescendo	Early compensation often blocks appearance of symptoms Palpitations associated with widened pulse pressure With progression, dyspnea develops
Mitral stenosis	LA: ↑V, P, dilation LV: normal V, P, filling slows	Loud/normal	Opening snap, decrescendo diastolic murmur	Pulmonary pressures increase Atrial enlargement increases risk of atrial fibrillation and stroke Exertional dyspnea Pulmonary hypertension May lead to right-sided heart failure
Acute mitral regurgitation	LA: ↑V, P LV: Initially normal volumes and pressures, ↓forward flow (cardiac output) into the aorta, portion of ejection fraction flows back to LA	Soft/normal or split	Holosystolic murmur	Rapid increase in pulmonary vascular pressures and afterload on RV May develop pulmonary edema
Chronic mitral regurgitation	LA: ↑V, P produce dilation LV: ↑V, chamber dilation, wall thickness increases	Soft/normal or split	Holosystolic murmur	Pulmonary vascular pressures elevated, not as severely as in acute mitral regurgitation

↑, increased; ↓, decreased; LA, left atrium; LV, left ventricle; P, pressure; RV, right ventricle; S_1/S_2, first and second heart sounds: V, volume.

septum and the anterior leaflet of the mitral valve. **Figure 10.44** shows the pathophysiology of signs and symptoms in HCM. The hypertrophied and disarrayed cardiac muscle cells may trigger ventricular arrhythmias that can cause syncope or sudden death. Left ventricular hypertrophy leads to impaired diastolic relaxation, which causes elevated left ventricle filling pressures and dyspnea. If dynamic left ventricular outflow obstruction is present (see earlier discussion), it is often accompanied by mitral regurgitation, which contributes to dyspnea, and exertional syncope due to the impaired ability to raise cardiac output during exercise. The thickened left ventricle wall and increased systolic pressure associated with outflow tract obstruction each contribute to increased myocardial oxygen consumption and can precipitate angina.

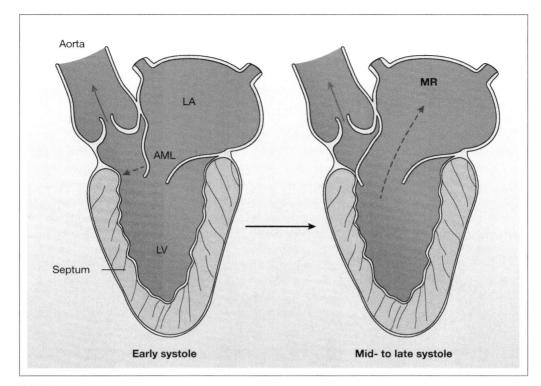

FIGURE 10.43 Cardiac alterations in hypertrophic cardiomyopathy. Pathological hypertrophy of the LV distorts the mitral valve geometry, resulting in obstructed flow through the aortic valve and MR that increases LA volume and pressure. In early systole (left panel) rapid ejection velocity through the narrowed tract draws the anterior leaflet toward the septum (*short dashed arrow*). In mid- to late systole (right panel), as the anterior leaflet abnormally moves toward the septum, outflow into the aorta is transiently obstructed. Because the mitral leaflets do not align normally in systole, MR also occurs (*long dashed arrow*).

AML, anterior mitral leaflet; LA, left atrium; LV, left ventricle; MR, mitral regurgitation.

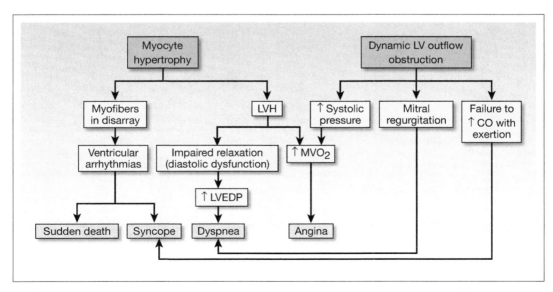

FIGURE 10.44 Pathophysiological cascade leading to clinical manifestations of hypertrophic cardiomyopathy.

CO, cardiac output; LV, left ventricle; LVEDP, left ventricular end-diastolic pressure; LVH, left ventricular hypertrophy; MVO_2, myocardial oxygen consumption.

Source: From Lilly LS. *Pathophysiology of Heart Disease: A Collaborative Project of Medical Students and Faculty.* 6th ed. Wolters Kluwer; 2015.

Fruzsina K. Johnson, Robert A. Johnson, Spencer A. Rhodes, and Mary B. Mehta

NORMAL CARDIAC DEVELOPMENT

During embryonic life, the complex heart structure of four chambers and four valves develops from a single tube (**Figure 10.45**). The septa separating the ventricles and the atria develop gradually until the left and right sides of the heart are almost completely separated from each other. During fetal life, the placenta supplies oxygenated blood and the fetal lungs are not used for gas exchange. Thus, in the fetal circulation (**Figure 10.46**), three adaptations exist that allow blood to be directed away from the nonfunctioning lungs:

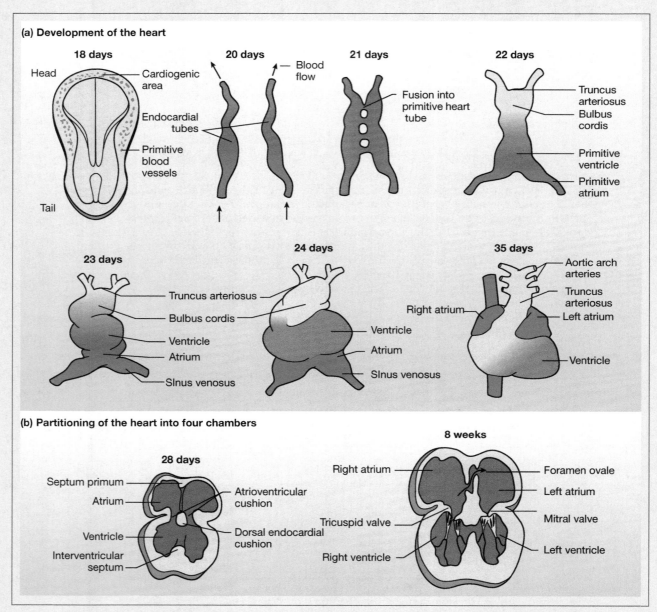

FIGURE 10.45 Embryonic development of the heart from a single tube to a four-chambered structure.

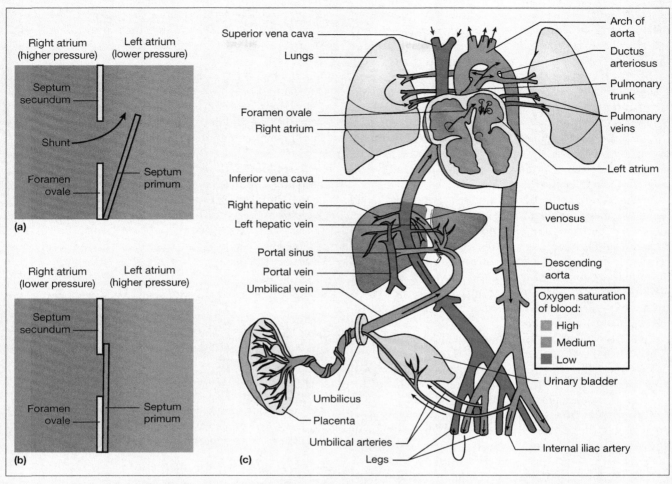

FIGURE 10.46 Fetal circulation. **(a)** The foramen ovale is open during prenatal development. **(b)** Two membranes are responsible for closing the foramen ovale after birth, when the right heart blood flow to the lungs has been established. **(c)** Oxygenated blood from the placenta travels to the fetus through the umbilical vein. The ductus venosus connects to the inferior vena cava, joining systemic venous blood from the lower part of the body. The mixed blood enters the right atrium, much of it flowing through the foramen ovale to the left atrium, and then on to the left ventricle and aorta. Venous blood from the upper body and head enters the right atrium via the superior vena cava. From the right atrium, this deoxygenated blood may flow to the left atrium or may enter the right ventricle to be pumped out via the pulmonary artery. From the pulmonary artery, most blood flows through the ductus arteriosus to the aorta. Thus, the aortic flow in the fetus is relatively low in oxygen, particularly that blood flowing to the lower part of the body. Lower abdominal branches of the aorta form the umbilical arteries taking deoxygenated blood to the placenta for gas exchange. *Source:* From Lilly LS. *Pathophysiology of Heart Disease: A Collaborative Project of Medical Students and Faculty.* 6th ed. Wolters Kluwer; 2015.

1. Fluid-filled fetal lungs have very high vascular resistance.
2. The open foramen ovale in the interatrial septum allows highly oxygenated blood to flow from the right atrium to the left without going through the right ventricle and the pulmonary circulation.
3. Any blood that does enter the pulmonary artery mostly escapes through the ductus arteriosus to the aorta before ever reaching the fetal lungs.

In the fetal circulation the pressure gradients are the opposite of the adult: (a) the systemic circulation has low vascular resistance and pressure due to the presence of the very low-resistance placenta; and (b) the pulmonary circulation has high resistance and pressure, because the lungs are fluid filled and not yet inflated. This pressure gradient creates blood flow from the right atrium to the left, and allows the foramen ovale to remain open. At birth, the first breath of the newborn inflates the lungs and thus lowers pulmonary resistance. Meanwhile the umbilical vessels are closing off, causing an increase in the systemic vascular resistance, and the ductus arteriosus begins to close. These responses transition the pressure gradients to the normal postnatal relationships: The pressure in the left atrium increases while the pressure in the right atrium decreases, allowing the flap (septum primum) to close the foramen ovale. Later, the septum primum adheres to the edges (septum secundum) and the foramen ovale becomes permanently closed, completing the transition to the adult pattern of blood flow.

In a substantial number of infants, the foramen ovale never closes (termed *patent foramen ovale*). This does not create a hemodynamic problem as long as the pressure in the left atrium is greater than that in the right atrium. If the pressure gradient reverses (e.g., due to pulmonary hypertension), blood entering the right atrium can flow to the left atrium through the patent foramen ovale. The greatest danger from the right-to-left flow is that an embolism forming in the venous circulation can bypass the lungs and flow into the left ventricle and systemic circulation. This increases the risk for stroke and other consequences. However, many individuals with patent foramen ovale do not ever require treatment for the condition.

Congenital heart defects are the most common birth defect, occurring in close to 1% of births annually.[12,13] Some are detected prenatally by ultrasound imaging; others are not detected until childhood or later in life. Pulse oximetry screening of newborns can indicate the presence of some heart defects. Findings that raise suspicion of a heart defect include cyanosis, tachypnea, decreased pulses, difference in pulses between upper and lower body, failure to thrive, hepatomegaly, displaced point of maximal impulse, and cyanosis. The most common heart defects are described here. Surgical procedures have reduced mortality rates in children with congenital heart disease. Those with the most severe defects may need multistage operations over the first few years of life. It is important to note that the increased survival rates of children born with congenital heart disorders and undergoing successful procedures necessitate ongoing monitoring and lifelong cardiology care.

PRINCIPLES OF DEVELOPMENTAL CARDIAC ANOMALIES

SHUNTING

After birth, there is no mixing of blood between left and right sides of the heart. **Shunting** is a phenomenon in which blood makes its way from one side of the heart to the other. Shunting typically develops when the isolation of the left and right sides of the circulation is incomplete due to either abnormal cardiac structural

development or fetal adaptations (shunts) that persist after birth (i.e., ductus arteriosus and foramen ovale). There are two possible scenarios:

1. *Right-to-left shunting* allows deoxygenated (venous) blood to mix with oxygenated blood, thus lowering arterial oxygenation (hemoglobin oxygen saturation and partial pressure of oxygen [P_{O_2}]), creating hypoxemia that can lead to **cyanosis**.
2. *Left-to-right shunting* causes the mixing of oxygenated blood with venous blood. This does not create hypoxia, but it does create volume overloading of the pulmonary circulation that eventually causes pulmonary hypertension (due to increased pulmonary vascular resistance), leading to shunt reversal and hypoxemia. This progression is also known as **Eisenmenger syndrome.**

TYPES OF CONGENITAL CARDIAC ANOMALIES

Congenital cardiac anomalies can cause shunting—or not (**Table 10.5**). Within shunting anomalies, we distinguish left-to-right shunting (acyanotic) and right-to-left shunting (cyanotic) conditions. Right-to-left shunting anomalies cause early cyanosis (*blue babies*) and thus must be surgically corrected soon after birth. Left-to-right shunting anomalies do not cause cyanosis initially (acyanotic), but they can do so later in life if right heart pressures increase and the shunt reverses (*blue kids*).

Left-to-Right Shunting Anomalies (Late Cyanosis)

The three most common anomalies that cause left-to-right shunting, in order of prevalence, are (a) **ventricular septal defect** (VSD), (b) **atrial septal defect** (ASD), and (c) **patent ductus arteriosus** (PDA; see **Figure 10.47**). These conditions may remain undiscovered initially, because early on, the left-to-right shunting does not cause major symptoms. Eventually, the volume overloading of the pulmonary circulation can lead to an increase in pulmonary vascular resistance, reversal of the shunt, and cyanosis (Eisenmenger syndrome).

Prostaglandins Regulate Patency of the Ductus Arteriosus

The ductus arteriosus is a fetal vascular structure that connects the pulmonary artery to the aorta and allows shunting of blood flow away from the lungs. During fetal life, the ductus arteriosus is kept open by a vasodilatory prostaglandin—prostaglandin E_2 (PGE_2)—produced by endothelial cyclooxygenase. Typically, decreased PGE_2 formation causes closure of the ductus arteriosus within the first two days after birth. If PGE_2 formation persists, PDA occurs. This condition is sometimes treated with a nonsteroidal anti inflammatory drug (NSAID) that decreases PGE_2 formation. Accidental administration of an NSAID to the mother in late pregnancy can bring about premature closure of the ductus arteriosus, creating an acute fetal emergency.

TABLE 10.5 Types of Congenital Cardiac Anomalies

Type	Shunting Type	Common Anomalies
Non-shunting	None	Coarctation of the aorta Congenital pulmonic stenosis Congenital aortic stenosis
Shunting	Left-to-right shunting (acyanotic or late cyanotic—"blue kids")	Ventricular septal defect (VSD) Atrial septal defect (ASD) Patent ductus arteriosus (PDA)
	Right-to-left shunting (cyanotic or early cyanotic—"blue babies")	Tetralogy of Fallot Transposition of the great vessels Truncus arteriosus Tricuspid atresia

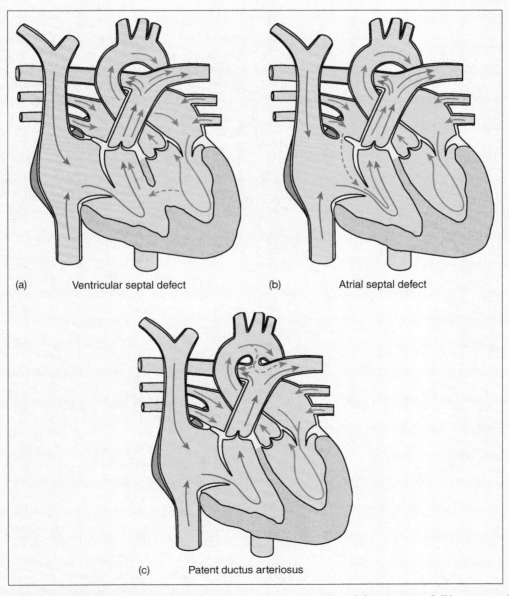

(a)   Ventricular septal defect

(b)   Atrial septal defect

(c)   Patent ductus arteriosus

FIGURE 10.47 Anatomy and flow of oxygenated (*red arrows*) and deoxygenated (*blue arrows*) blood associated with **(a)** ventricular septal defect, **(b)** atrial septal defect, and **(c)** patent ductus arteriosus. Dashed lines indicate the paths of altered flow.

Right-to-Left Shunting Anomalies (Early Cyanosis)

Tetralogy of Fallot

The most common early cyanotic congenital heart defect is **tetralogy of Fallot** (**Figure 10.48**). It is typically an association of four anomalies (*tetra*logy), three of which—VSD, pulmonary outflow obstruction (stenosis), and overriding aorta (only present in 50% of the cases)—occur as a result of developmental defects. The fourth anomaly, right ventricular hypertrophy, develops in compensation for the pulmonary outflow obstruction. Right-to-left shunting occurs via the overriding aorta that originates from both ventricles (if present) and the VSD. Depending on the severity of the condition, surgical correction may be delayed for a few years after birth.

Although VSD alone causes left-to-right shunting, the pulmonary outflow obstruction increases afterload for the right ventricle, causing an increase in right ventricular pressure and reversal of the shunt. The severity of the shunting is directly related to the severity of the right outflow obstruction. Children with tetralogy of Fallot are prone to cyanotic episodes under conditions that require an increase in cardiac output. In these cases, squatting can be used to increase systemic vascular resistance that elevates left ventricular pressure (by increasing afterload) and thus reduces the severity of right-to-left shunting.

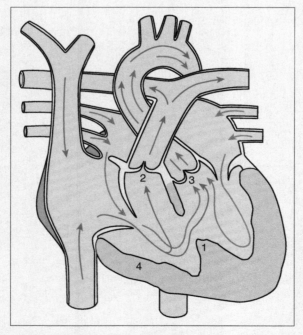

FIGURE 10.48 Anatomy and flow of oxygenated (*red arrows*) and deoxygenated (*blue arrows*) blood associated with tetralogy of Fallot. Areas of abnormalities are: 1. VSD, 2. pulmonary valve stenosis, 3. overriding aorta, 4. right ventricular hypertrophy.

Transposition of the Great Vessels

In **transposition of the great vessels**, the aorta and the pulmonary artery are switched: the aorta originates from the right ventricle, while the pulmonary artery originates from the left ventricle. This causes complete disconnection between the systemic and the pulmonary circulations—they are present in parallel, rather than being coupled in series. This and similar anomalies are compatible with fetal life, because of the PDA, but quickly become incompatible with life after birth if the ductus arteriosus closes. In these patients, infusion of the vasodilatory prostaglandin (PGE_2) can maintain ductus arteriosus patency until surgical correction of the anomaly can be performed.

COARCTATION OF THE AORTA

In **coarctation of the aorta**, the aorta is constricted—most often at the site where the ductus arteriosus closes, just distal to the left subclavian artery. This congenital defect can appear alone or in combination with other abnormalities, such as tetralogy of Fallot. The infant most often presents with poor lower extremity pulses, and with perfusion and hypertension in upper extremities. Infants with coarctation of the aorta can be irritable, are ashy colored, have poor weight gain, and are tachypneic, and usually no murmur is heard. They have higher blood pressure in the arms, particularly the right arm, and low systolic blood pressure in the legs. An older child may complain of pain in the legs with running.

COMPLEX SINGLE VENTRICLE– HYPOPLASTIC LEFT HEART SYNDROME

Complex single ventricle-hypoplastic left heart syndrome is considered one of the most severe congenital heart disorders because of the multiple structures affected. It is rare, occurring in <1,000 infants born in the United States each year.[11] In infants with this condition, almost all left-sided structures (mitral valve, left ventricle, aortic valve, and ascending aorta) fail to develop and therefore are unable to support systemic circulation once the ductus arteriosus closes. Infants are often diagnosed prenatally; if not, they are identified within the first 2 to 3 days of life upon developing severe cyanosis, tachypnea, and shock. Improvements in surgical procedures have greatly reduced the associated mortality rate. Three consecutive procedures rebuild the heart—essentially by connecting the vena cavae to the pulmonary artery, and using the remainder of the heart (primarily the right ventricle) to pump blood through the aorta to the body. A heart transplant is also an option. With improved surgical treatments, many children with hypoplastic left heart syndrome are living through adolescence and into adulthood.

Systolic hypertension, HFpEF, atrial fibrillation, and coronary artery disease all become more common with aging and can lead to cardiovascular disease. However, aging itself leads to changes in the structure and function of the cardiovascular system that, while not a disease state, can lead to decreased functional capacity of the heart when the system is under stress. These changes also lower the threshold for the emergence of heart disease.

These changes do not develop in isolation; as people age, they become less active. Thus, the cardiac changes associated with aging may be related to lifestyle factors as well as other comorbidities rather than purely a result of aging itself. For example, dysfunction in one or more body systems, such as the renal system (e.g., chronic renal insufficiency) or endocrine system (e.g., diabetes), will also have consequences for cardiovascular system function. It is important to understand how the functional impairment of normal physiological responses that accompany aging impacts disease. Studies that aim to define the cardiovascular aging process need to carefully select healthy older individuals who do not have underlying cardiovascular conditions. The Baltimore Longitudinal Study of Aging (www.blsa.nih.gov) and the Framingham Heart Study (www.framinghamheartstudy.org) are examples of large longitudinal studies that have carefully selected participants in an attempt to isolate the changes that are a result of aging rather than comorbidities.

AGE-RELATED CHANGES IN CARDIAC STRUCTURE

MYOCARDIAL CELLS AND CHAMBERS

Age-related changes affect cardiac myocytes, ventricular remodeling, and atrial and ventricular chamber size. The left ventricle undergoes significant remodeling with age—as does the right, but to a lesser degree. The number of cardiac myocytes declines by approximately 35% between the ages of 30 and 70 years due to apoptosis, necrosis, and autophagy from oxidative stress and mitochondrial damage. Stem cells replace the loss, but at approximately half the rate in older adults, compared with their younger counterparts.[14]

The remaining cardiac cells hypertrophy in response to an increased afterload placed on the heart, and the ventricle thickens asymmetrically with a redistribution of cardiac muscle mass to the interventricular septum.

The effect of aging on ventricular chamber size is unclear; some studies have noted a decrease in internal dimensions of the left ventricle, and others have found no change. However, the overall shape of the heart changes and becomes more spherical rather than the elliptical as it is in younger hearts.

The left atrium enlarges and left atrial volume increases significantly from age 30 to 80 years. Atrial dilation is thought to occur in response to the change in diastolic function of the left ventricle. The consequences of enlarging atrial size include atrial fibrillation; further, left atrial size is associated with the age-adjusted risk for stroke and death. Similar changes also occur on the right side of the heart, but to a lesser degree.

CONNECTIVE TISSUE

With age, there is a degradation and stiffening of connective tissue due to deposition of adipose cells and tissue, particularly in the AV groove, and deposits of collagen in the ventricular wall. Nonenzymatic cross-linking creates a less flexible form of collagen, contributing to lower compliance of the connective tissue. The muscle-to-collagen ratio remains relatively stable because of the hypertrophy of the remaining myocytes. Amyloid, uncommon in people younger than 60 years, and lipofuscin, a pigment that accumulates with *wear and tear* or oxidative damage in cells, also accumulate to varying degrees with aging.

VALVES

Age-related degenerative changes affect the aortic valve, mitral valve, and annulus over time. Sclerosis, as result of collagen deposition and degeneration (called myxomatous degeneration), mildly thickens the aortic valve. Eventually, through a process of progressive lipid accumulation, inflammation, and eventually calcification, leaflet motion can become severely impaired and the valve can become stenotic. Aortic valve stenosis can remain asymptomatic for several years, but once symptoms appear, mortality rate may be as high as 50% over a 2-year period. Aortic valve stenosis results in increased afterload due to increased resistance of flow through the narrowed valve orifice.

The mitral valve develops microscopic calcifications as part of a chronic degenerative process that occurs along and below the mitral annulus. This is more common in women than men and occurs typically in people older than 70 years of age. It usually remains asymptomatic but can be associated with mitral regurgitation or, less often, stenosis. Microscopic mitral annular calcification is associated with AV and bundle-branch blocks, including complete heart block, because of the valve's proximity to the conduction system.

CONDUCTION SYSTEM

The number of cells in the SA node decreases with aging by up to 90% by age 75. Cell loss also occurs to a lesser degree at the AV node and bundle of His, and to a greater degree within the bundle branches. Structural changes in the conduction system can produce changes to the ECG (Box 10.6); these have little to no effect on mortality, with the exception of a prolonged QT interval, which may increase risk of death.

The changes within the conduction system and fibrosis and calcification on the left side of the heart (described earlier) can predispose older adults to arrhythmias, including conduction blocks and atrial and ventricular arrhythmias.

BOX 10.6
Changes in the Electrocardiogram With Aging

- Increased P-wave duration
- Prolongation of the PR interval
- Prolongation of the QT interval

- Left shift of the QRS axis
- Decreased QRS voltage
- Decreased T-wave voltage

AGE-RELATED CHANGES IN CARDIAC FUNCTION

CALCIUM HOMEOSTASIS AND AUTONOMIC SIGNALING

Excitation–contraction coupling—the process of pairing myocyte depolarization and muscle contraction—changes as cardiac myocytes age. As noted earlier, myocyte action potentials cause an increase in intracellular Ca^{2+} concentration that initiates the contraction. The force of the contraction is dependent on the concentration of Ca^{2+} released. In aging cells, the action potential is prolonged and the cytosolic Ca^{2+} transient is increased. There is delayed inactivation of L-type Ca^{2+} channels, delayed and decreased uptake of Ca^{2+} by SERCA, and delayed phase 3 repolarization by K^+ efflux, so Ca^{2+} remains in the cells longer. This results in prolonged contraction and impaired diastolic relaxation, contributing to the somewhat small left ventricular chamber size noted with aging.

Sympathetic stimulation of the heart also is altered with aging. Levels of norepinephrine in the plasma are increased; reuptake of catecholamines by transporters in the sympathetic nerve terminals decreases, tissue spillover of catecholamines is increased, and plasma clearance is reduced, all leading to higher levels in the plasma and tissues.[15] Over time, elevated norepinephrine levels produce downregulation of cardiac β-receptors. Receptor desensitization and changes in Ca^{2+} homeostasis cause decreased inotropy and chronotropy of the heart in the aging population.

FUNCTIONAL CHANGES

Although a number of structural changes occur in the aging heart, resting cardiac function remains relatively stable. Despite increases in systemic and pulmonary arterial blood pressure, which increase afterload of the left and right ventricles, cardiac output, stroke volume, heart rate, and ejection fraction remain stable at rest. It is with increased demand on the cardiovascular system that the changes of aging become more clinically significant.

Systolic Function

Resting left ventricular systolic function, stroke volume, and cardiac output are preserved with aging, but overall exercise tolerance declines. During exercise, the heart must be able to deliver blood to meet increased demand. This is measured by maximum oxygen consumption (VO_2 max). It is unclear at what age the decline in exercise tolerance truly begins, but it is reported that VO_2 max begins to decline as early as the second or third decade and continues to decline approximately 10% per decade.[16]

Maximal heart rate during exercise is reduced in older adults, due to decreased responsiveness to sympathetic stimulation, among other factors. Older adults also have smaller exercise-induced increases in stroke volume relative to younger adults. Some ability to increase stroke volume during exercise is maintained, but not by the same mechanisms as in younger people: older hearts rely more on the Frank–Starling mechanism to maintain stroke volume (since contraction is somewhat impaired by age-related changes in Ca^{2+} homeostasis and β-adrenergic signaling). With exercise, venous return increases, improving end-diastolic volume and stroke volume. This ability to increase stroke volume offsets the decrease in maximum heart rate to continue to sustain exercise capacity, albeit at a lower maximal level than in younger individuals.[16]

Diastolic Function

Although resting systolic function is well preserved, diastolic function decreases with age as left ventricular relaxation begins to slow down. The blunted chronotropic modulation induced by decreased β-adrenergic responsiveness and the reduced inotropic effects of changes in Ca^{2+} homeostasis previously described result in a change in the pattern of diastolic filling. Normal diastolic filling is separated into two phases: (a) the early passive phase, during which left ventricular volume rapidly increases, and (b) an active phase, during which the remainder of the ventricle fills through atrial contraction—the so-called atrial *kick*. The normal ratio of filling during these two phases is 2:1 for passive to active. With aging, the rate of passive diastolic filling slows due to the longer isovolumic relaxation time, with a larger contribution from the atrial contraction. Visible on echocardiography, the passive–active ratio is decreased. The active component forces blood into the relatively stiff ventricle, sometimes producing an S_4 heart sound on physical examination—a normal finding in people older than 75 years of age. Ventricular stiffness may also contribute to left atrial enlargement in older adults.

During exercise, the change in the end-diastolic volume is smaller than it is in younger people—a change that is attributed to increased ventricular wall thickness and stiffness. Left ventricular end-diastolic pressure is higher with aging, a major reason that HFpEF is more common in older adults.

HEART RATE AND RHYTHM

Resting heart rate may show mild decreases with aging; however, in response to stress or exercise there is a substantial decrease in the maximal heart rate, contributing to the decrease in cardiac reserve. The intrinsic heart rate (the heart rate without either sympathetic or parasympathetic stimulation) decreases by 5 to 6 beats/min with each decade. Other age-related changes in heart rate include decreased responsiveness to β-adrenergic agonists and parasympathetic antagonists. Heart rate variability also decreases with age—likely due to decreased parasympathetic tone and decreased sympathetic responsiveness. This decline is slower in women than in men.

The prevalence of supraventricular and ventricular arrhythmias increases with aging due to β-receptor downregulation and impairment of signaling.[17] Atrial premature beats are seen on ECG in 5% to 10% of older adults, and short runs of paroxysmal supraventricular tachycardia in 13% to 50%. These arrhythmias are predictors for atrial fibrillation (which has a prevalence of 5.9% in people over 65), but not for coronary events. Atrial fibrillation is more likely to precipitate heart failure in older adults, because there is a greater reliance on filling the ventricle during the active phase of diastole. Ventricular ectopy is common in aging and is found in over 80% of older adults undergoing ambulatory telemetry monitoring.

SUMMARY OF AGE-RELATED CARDIAC CHANGES

The complex cardiac changes attributed to aging are outlined in **Figure 10.49**. Aging of the heart is tightly associated with and related to age-related changes of the vascular system and is characterized by structural, cellular, molecular, and functional changes to the left ventricle, valves, and conduction system. These changes lead to left ventricular hypertrophy, diastolic dysfunction, valvular calcification, regurgitation, and, in some cases, stenosis; and ultimately, decreased cardiac reserve. Decreasing reserve makes the heart more vulnerable to stress and leads to higher rates of cardiovascular disease, including heart failure, atrial fibrillation, and coronary artery disease. A better understanding of the mechanisms underlying age-related changes in heart structure and function may inform future directions for modifying cardiovascular disease trajectories in older adults.

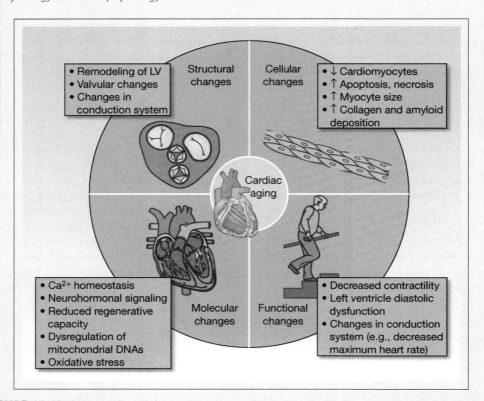

FIGURE 10.49 Structural, cellular, molecular, and functional changes associated with aging of the heart.

Source: From Nakou et al. *Intl J Cardiol.* 2016;209:167–175.

CASE STUDY 10.1: A Patient With Heart Failure Symptoms

Lisa Rathman

Chief Complaint: *"I haven't felt well for the past few weeks. I have no energy, and no appetite. My chest is congested, and I have episodes of wheezing. I get short of breath when I do any activity and can't sleep at night because of the coughing and shortness of breath. I was seen last week at urgent care. They told me I had asthmatic bronchitis. I was given antibiotics, steroids, and breathing treatments. At first, I felt a bit better, but now I feel worse. I can barely make it through the day at work."*

History of Present Illness/Review of Systems: The patient is a 43-year-old obese man who denies any chest pain, but does have occasional chest tightness. He reports shortness of breath with usual activity. He denies any peripheral nerve disease but has been sleeping on the recliner. He does not have any fever, chills, or sore throat. He has a dry cough that seems to be worse at night. He has not noticed any lightheadedness, dizziness, palpitations, or syncope. The patient reports that his appetite is poor. He states that he feels full after eating a small amount of food, and feels bloated in the abdomen. He has noted some swelling in his ankles and calves this week. The patient does not know his weight.

Past Medical/Family Social History: The patient has a history of diabetes and *borderline* high blood pressure. He is taking metformin for his diabetes. He smoked cigarettes for 5 years, quitting in his early 20s. The patient enjoys beer, and notes that he regularly consumes one to two beers (12 oz.) each evening, and more on the weekend. Recently, he has decreased his alcohol intake due to abdominal bloating and poor appetite. He has not noted any improvement in his symptoms. The patient reports that his maternal grandfather had a heart attack. His father died in his sleep in his late 40s from an unknown cause. His mother is alive and well in her 70s.

Physical Examination: You observe a moderately obese, but otherwise healthy-appearing man in no acute distress. He is visibly short of breath after walking to the examination room from the waiting room with the medical assistant. Findings are as follows: temperature of 98°F, blood pressure of 138/90 mm Hg, heart rate of 92 beats/min, respirations of 24 breaths/min, with a pulse oximetry reading of 94% on room air. Body mass index (BMI) is 33 kg/m². Respirations are unlabored at rest. Lung examination reveals crackles at bases bilaterally. Cardiac exam reveals jugular venous pressure of 10 cm H_2O; positive hepatojugular reflex; normal S_1 and S_2 sounds, no S_3 or S_4; normal heart rate and rhythm; and a 2/6 systolic murmur at apex, but no lift or thrill. The patient's abdomen is distended, with normal bowel sounds and no hepatomegaly. Peripheral edema of extremities is present, with 1+ to mid-calf; 2+ peripheral pulses. Skin is warm, dry, and pink, with good coloring, and no cyanosis or bruising.

Laboratory and Diagnostic Findings: The ECG today reveals normal sinus rhythm at 96, with left bundle branch block. There is no previous ECG for comparison. Chest x-ray reveals cardiomegaly and mild interstitial edema. Basic laboratory findings include normal results for thyroid function tests, CBC, and CMP. Cardiac enzymes are normal. BNP is 3,400 pg/mL. An echocardiogram has been ordered.

CASE STUDY 10.1 QUESTIONS
- *What findings from the history, physical, and laboratory and diagnostic testing lead you to suspect that the patient might have heart failure?*
- *What findings on an echocardiogram would provide further evidence that this patient has heart failure?*

BNP, B-natriuretic peptide; CBC, complete blood count; CMP, comprehensive metabolic panel.

CASE STUDY 10.2: A Patient With Angina

David A. Roberts

Patient Complaint: *"I keep having this pressure all over my chest and I feel short of breath. It started while I was raking leaves in the yard this morning. It went on for about 5 minutes before it finally got better. It seemed to help if I sat down for a bit, but it came right back if I tried to rake again."*

History of Present Illness/Review of Systems: The patient is a 54-year-old Hispanic man who presents to the ED with complaints of two episodes of chest pressure and dyspnea on exertion that occurred this morning while working in his yard. He noted some radiation to the left lower jaw. During the episode, his discomfort was a 6 out of 10. The symptoms lasted about 5 minutes and were relieved by rest. He denies any symptoms currently. He has never experienced anything similar before. Chest pain and shortness of breath are reported; all other systems negative.

Past Medical/Family/Social History: The patient has a history of hypertension. He has smoked 1 pack of cigarettes per day for 20 years. He reports a family history of ischemic stroke in his mother at age 62. He takes lisinopril, 5 mg daily.

Physical Examination: You observe a well-appearing adult man in no acute distress. Findings are as follows: temperature of 98.4°F; blood pressure of 138/76 mm Hg, heart rate of 92 beats/min, and respirations of 12 breaths/min. The patient is alert

CBC, complete blood count; CMP, comprehensive metabolic panel.

and oriented. Skin color is normal with no rashes. Head is normocephalic. Pupils are equal, round, reactive to light, and accommodating. Neck is supple with no carotid bruits, jugular venous distention, lymphadenopathy, or tenderness. Oral mucous membranes are moist and without lesions. Lungs are clear to auscultation. Chest is without tenderness to palpation, with no masses. Heart rate is regular, with no murmurs, thrills, or gallops noted. Abdomen is soft, nondistended, and nontender. No peripheral edema is noted, with 1+ radial and pedal pulses.

Laboratory and Diagnostic Findings: The ECG shows normal sinus rhythm at 88, normal axis, but meets criteria for mild left ventricular hypertrophy. No findings indicating ischemia or infarction: there are no ST-T-wave abnormalities, and no abnormal Q waves. Posteroanterior and lateral chest radiographs show no cardiopulmonary abnormalities. Laboratory tests of CBC, CMP, and troponin are unremarkable.

CASE STUDY 10.2 QUESTIONS
- *What aspects of the patient's history, physical, and laboratory and diagnostic findings provide support for a diagnosis of myocardial ischemia?*
- *What are the patient's risk factors for coronary artery disease? What additional tests might the provider request to evaluate this risk?*

CASE STUDY 10.3: A Patient With Atrial Fibrillation

Linda W. Good

Patient Complaint: *"My heart has been racing and thumping for the past few weeks off and on, sometimes at rest—like when I'm trying to fall asleep—and sometimes when I'm active. I tried cutting down on coffee and alcohol, and backing off a bit on my gym workouts, but nothing has helped. I've been consciously avoiding conflicts at school, where I teach a full schedule of classes. I've even been stricter about using my CPAP machine at night for my sleep apnea and taking my blood pressure pills. But I feel dizzy and weak at times, and just getting through each day is tiring. I'm only 62, but maybe I should consider early retirement."*

History of Present Illness/Review of Systems: You observe a moderately obese but otherwise healthy-appearing adult man in no acute distress, but with a discouraged expression. On closer questioning, he reveals that his palpitations last anywhere from minutes to hours, and are not associated with shortness of breath, chest pain, vertigo, presyncope, focal neurological deficits, peripheral edema, or orthopnea. The episodes are getting more frequent and prolonged, and now may be present most of the time.

Past Medical/Family/Social History: The patient has well-controlled high blood pressure, diagnosed 10 years ago, for which he takes a diuretic and ACE inhibitor. He was prescribed a CPAP machine for obstructive sleep apnea 5 years ago. He also takes a statin for elevated cholesterol. He has been followed for prediabetes with serial glycated hemoglobin (HbA_{1c}) measurements that have always been <6.5. He smoked a half-pack of cigarettes a day for 35 years

and quit when he was diagnosed with hypertension. He considers himself a light drinker, with a daily cocktail and glass of wine. His brother and father both had myocardial infarctions in their 50s.

Physical Examination: Findings are as follows: temperature of 97.8°F, blood pressure of 150/90 mm Hg, heart rate of 112 beats/min, and respirations of 20 breaths/min. BMI is 35 kg/m². Heart rate is irregularly irregular. Thyroid is normal size and nontender. Lungs are clear without adventitious sounds. Abdomen is benign. Ankles are significant for +1 edema, but with normal pulses. The patient is neurologically intact with normal strength, sensation, balance, coordination, and reflexes.

Laboratory and Diagnostic Findings: The ECG from a past office visit shows normal sinus rhythm at 80, but meets criteria for mild left ventricular hypertrophy and incomplete left bundle branch block. The current ECG shows irregular R-R intervals, no clear P waves, only fibrillatory waves, and a QRS interval of 0.22 second. Basic laboratory results include normal thyroid function tests, CBC, and CMP. Cardiac enzymes are within normal limits. Results of an echocardiogram and nuclear stress test are pending.

CASE STUDY 10.3 QUESTIONS
- *What are the normal electrical events of SA node pacemaker cells?*
- *How would you describe the electrical events in the atrium in a person with atrial fibrillation, relative to normal heart function?*
- *What are the risks associated with persistent atrial fibrillation?*

ACE, angiotensin-converting enzyme; BMI, body mass index; CBC, complete blood count; CMP, comprehensive metabolic panel; CPAP, continuous positive airway pressure; SA, sinoatrial.

BRIDGE TO CLINICAL PRACTICE

Ben Cocchiaro

PRINCIPLES OF ASSESSMENT
History
Evaluate:
- Chest pain (especially whether or not pain is associated with exertion), palpitations, shortness of breath, peripheral edema, dyspnea on exertion
- History of blood clots, hyperlipidemia, heart arrhythmias, syncope
- Smoking status (active habit and total pack-years), cocaine use
- Diet: consumption of fruits and vegetables, patterns of intake for meat, fish, fatty/fried foods, carbohydrates, salt, sugar
- Physical activity habits: minutes/day, days/week, how tolerated
- Family history of early cardiac death (in parent or sibling prior to age 65)

Physical Examination
- *Vital signs:* Know the proper methods for obtaining an accurate blood pressure measurement
- *Observe:*
  - Jugular venous pressure
  - Cyanosis of lips or extremities
  - Clubbing of the fingertips
- *Auscultate:*
  - In seated and supine positions, listen over each valve for murmurs, pericardial friction rubs, or extra heart sounds; listen for changes with handgrip or Valsalva maneuver
  - Carotid arteries for bruits
  - Lung bases for inspiratory rales indicating atelectasis and potential fluid overload
- *Palpate:*
  - Apical pulse – point of maximum impulse (PMI) – displaced laterally in cardiomegaly
  - Blood pressure by palpation
  - Pulse for irregularity and correspondence with auscultated heart sounds
  - Chest wall for tenderness
  - Lower extremities for pitting edema

Diagnostic Tools
- Chest x-ray study: evaluates heart size, lung congestion, pericardial effusion
- ECG (point-in-time and ambulatory monitoring): indications of arrhythmias, conduction blocks, infarction, axis deviation (altered in ventricular hypertrophy)
- Echocardiography: size and contractility of heart, valve integrity, transvalvular flow

- Stress tests, performed either through exercise or pharmacological challenge; with ECG, echocardiography, or nuclear imaging
- Coronary artery catheterization: images flow, detects obstructions, can be combined with percutaneous coronary interventions (angioplasty, stent placement)

Laboratory Evaluation
- Electrolytes necessary for cardiac conduction: K^+, Ca^{2+}, Mg^{2+}
- Cardiac enzymes that suggest damage to the myocardium: troponin, CK-MB
- Thyroid-stimulating hormone (TSH) – abnormal thyroid function often presents with cardiac manifestations
- Laboratory tests to evaluate the patient with suspected heart failure
  - BNP
  - Creatinine and electrolytes to guide diuretic therapy
  - GGT to evaluate for liver congestion

MAJOR DRUG CLASSES
- *Antiarrhythmics:* Classified into four groups, depending on their site of action
  - Class I—Na^+ channel modifiers
  - Class II—β-blockers
  - Class III—K^+ channel blockers
  - Class IV—Ca^{2+} channel blockers
- *Antihypertensives:*
  - Diuretics (thiazide, loop, K^+ sparing)
  - Ca^{2+} channel blockers
  - Angiotensin-converting enzyme (ACE) inhibitors and angiotensin receptor blockers (ARBs)
  - Adrenergic receptor agents (α- and β-blockers, and $α_2$ agonists)
  - Vasodilators
  - Aldosterone receptor antagonists
- *Heart failure management:* ACE inhibitors, angiotensin receptor blockers, β-blockers, diuretics, afterload-reducing drugs (vasodilators, nitrates)
- *Antianginals:* Nitrates, β-blockers, and Ca^{2+} channel blockers
- *Antiplatelet agents:* Aspirin and adenosine diphosphate (ADP) receptor inhibitors
- *Inotropes:* β-agonist dobutamine, vasopressin, phosphodiesterase inhibitors
- *Lipid-lowering agents: Statins, fibrates, omega-3 fatty acid ethyl esters, PCSK-9 inhibitors*

BNP, B-type natriuretic peptide; CK-MB, creatinine kinase-myocardial band; GGT, gamma-glutamyl transferase.

KEY POINTS

- Cardiovascular disease is the most common cause of death in the world, and much of its morbidity and mortality risks could be reduced by relatively simple lifestyle changes.
- The heart consists of four chambers: the right atrium and ventricle, and the left atrium and ventricle. The right side of the heart pumps blood to the lungs; the left side of the heart pumps blood to the body.
- Myocardial cells have action potentials with characteristics that are determined by their membrane voltage-gated ion channels.
- The coordinated contractions of the heart occur at a rate set by the SA node, the heart's pacemaker. Pacemaker cells have unique action potential characteristics that result in regular depolarization to threshold, typically at a rate of 60 to 100 beats/min in adults. This rate is modulated by the parasympathetic and sympathetic nervous systems.
- A specialized conduction system spreads the action potential to the working muscle cells of the atria, leading to atrial contraction, while also conducting the action potential to the AV node, where there is a brief delay.
- After the AV node, the action potential is rapidly propagated through the rest of the conduction system and to the working cells of the ventricles, producing ventricular contraction. The electrical events of the cardiac cycle are measured with the ECG.
- Rapid action potential propagation is possible through gap junctions providing a low-resistance pathway between cardiac cells, plus a rapid action potential upstroke due to fast Na^+ channels. Ionic imbalances, tissue ischemia, or lengthening of the pathway can reduce conduction speed or result in conduction blocks, resulting in abnormal ECG recordings and generation of arrhythmias.
- Abnormal excitability or conduction can lead to arrhythmias due to action potentials generated from ectopic foci within or without the conduction system.
- The most common sustained rhythm disturbance is atrial fibrillation—a condition of disorganized atrial electrical activity that causes the heartbeat to become irregular. With the loss of regular atrial contractions, there is a danger of clot formation due to stasis of blood in the atria, and cardiac output may be reduced due to the lack of atrial contraction to assist ventricular filling.
- The pump function of the heart depends on the intracellular Ca^{2+} concentration achieved as the ion enters the cell during the action potential plateau phase, releasing additional Ca^{2+} from the sarcoplasmic reticulum and leading to actin–myosin crossbridge formation and cardiac contraction.
- Relaxation occurs when the SERCA pumps Ca^{2+} back into the sarcoplasmic reticulum.
- The cardiac cycle is a depiction of the integrated series of electrical, volume, and pressure changes occurring during one cycle of systole and diastole—reflecting electrical activation, contraction of atria and ventricles, ejection of blood, followed by relaxation, and filling. Among these events are the characteristic heart sounds detected by auscultation.
- Cardiac output is equal to heart rate times stroke volume. Stroke volume (end-diastolic volume minus end-systolic volume) is normally about 60% of end-diastolic volume. The ratio of stroke volume to end-diastolic volume—the ejection fraction—is an indicator of cardiac performance and health.
- Cardiac performance and stroke volume are influenced by three main factors: contractility, preload, and afterload.
- Contractility is an intrinsic property of the ventricle. The major influence on contractility is the sympathetic nervous system, which increases intracellular Ca^{2+} during systole and increases rate of relaxation by accelerating Ca^{2+} pumping by SERCA during diastole.
- Preload is the stretch on the left ventricular wall by diastolic filling. Increased end-diastolic volume increases end-diastolic pressure, which is associated with better contractile function. This relationship between increased filling and increased contraction is known as the Frank–Starling law of the heart. Increased contractility augments this effect, with better contractile function at each level of preload, shifting the Frank–Starling curve in the upward direction.
- Afterload is the pressure the ventricle must counter to begin ejection. It is generally represented by the aortic diastolic pressure. As afterload increases, stroke volume decreases. Aortic stenosis is another source of increased afterload that decreases stroke volume, although in this pathological condition, the aortic diastolic pressure is decreased.
- Ischemic heart disease occurs when there is an imbalance between cardiac tissue oxygen supply and demand. The most common cause for

this is atherosclerotic narrowing of coronary arteries. The heart has highly aerobic metabolism and has the highest oxygen extraction in the body. The coronary arteries have turbulent flow that is affected by the cardiac cycle, being lowest during systole and greatest during diastole.

- Myocardial ischemia ranges in severity from intermittent, exercise-related chest pain (angina) to complete blockage resulting in STEMI. STEMI presents a great risk of immediate cardiogenic shock and arrhythmias, and long-term progression to heart failure.

- Some individuals with angina do not have detectable significant occlusion of large coronary arteries. These individuals are considered to have coronary microvascular dysfunction that produces ischemia at narrower vascular segments like the arterioles. This form of ischemic heart disease is more common in women than in men.

- Heart failure is a condition in which cardiac output is not sufficient to meet the needs of the body. This leads to fatigue and activity intolerance. Adaptation to heart failure can include neurohormonal alterations promoting vasoconstriction, fluid retention, increased heart rate, and sympathetic outflow to the ventricle. These alterations ultimately provide further stress on the heart and accelerate deterioration of cardiac function.

- Two main forms of heart failure are identified: HFrEF and HFpEF. HFrEF is associated with increased heart size and increased ventricular chamber size; ventricular wall thinning often occurs. Stroke volume is maintained through increased preload, but at the cost of chamber dilation and wall weakening. HFpEF is associated with normal or increased heart size with increased ventricular wall thickness. This narrowing of the chamber limits diastolic filling, reducing end-diastolic volume and stroke volume, but ejection fraction is maintained.

- Manifestations of heart failure depend on which side of the heart is more affected. Left ventricular failure is the most common form and presents with symptoms of inadequate cardiac output (fatigue, activity intolerance, neurohormonal compensation) and overfilling of the left ventricle and atrium (dyspnea due to pulmonary vascular congestion, increased risk of pulmonary edema).

- Structural cardiac disorders include degenerative diseases of the valves that result in outflow obstruction (stenosis), or incompetence and inability to close (regurgitation). These present with characteristic clinical signs and murmurs to cardiac auscultation. Management is by surgical replacement. HCM produces abnormal pump function due to poor diastolic filling, as well as outflow obstruction due to blockage before the aortic valve.

- Developmental anomalies of the heart are common, and congenital heart disease is one of the most common birth defects. Some defects are relatively mild and do not impede normal growth and development; others require surgical intervention in infancy or childhood.

- Congenital heart defects that result in right-to-left shunting are associated with cyanosis and need earlier repair. They include tetralogy of Fallot, transposition of the great vessels, truncus arteriosus, and tricuspid atresia.

- Older adults have progressive degenerative changes with decreased numbers of cells in the myocardium and particularly in the sinus node. Valve disorders are relatively common, with aortic stenosis being the most common.

- The major age-related limitations in cardiac function are seen with physical activity, as cardiac performance remains normal while at rest. Factors such as decreased maximal heart rate, impaired sympathetic influence, and reduced diastolic function all contribute to age-related reductions in ability to augment cardiac output during exercise.

REFERENCES

1. Centers for Disease Control and Prevention. Heart disease facts. https://www.cdc.gov/heartdisease/facts.htm. Accessed January 30, 2019.
2. World Health Organization. Cardiovascular diseases. http://www.who.int/news-room/fact-sheets/detail/cardiovascular-diseases-(cvds). Published May 17, 2017. Accessed January 30, 2019.
3. Mozaffarian D, Benjamin EJ, Go AS, et al. Heart disease and stroke statistics—2016 update. A report from the American Heart Association. *Circulation*. 2015;133:e38–e360. doi:10.1161/CIR.0000000000000350.
4. Barrett KE, Barman SM, Brooks HL, et al. *Ganong's Review of Medical Physiology*. 26th ed. New York, NY: McGraw-Hill; 2019.
5. Doig F. Ivabradine: first of a new class for angina. *Prescriber*. 2006;17(15):14–17. doi:10.1002/psb.404.
6. Whinnett ZI, Afzal Sohaib SM, Wyn Davies D. Diagnosis and management of supraventricular tachycardia. *BMJ*. 2012;345:e7769. doi:10.1136/bmj.e7769.

7. Gage BF, Waterman AD, Shannon W, et al. Validation of clinical classification schemes for predicting stroke: results from the National Registry of Atrial Fibrillation. *JAMA.* 2001;285:2864–2870. doi:10.1001/jama.285.22.2864.

8. Nakano Y, Shimizu W. Genetics of long-QT syndrome. *J Hum Genet.* 2016; 61:51–55. doi:10.1038/jhg.2015.74.

9. Camici PG, Rimoldi OE, Crea F. Coronary microvascular dysfunction. In: de Lemos JA, Omland T, eds. *Chronic Coronary Artery Disease: A Companion to Braunwald's Heart Disease.* Philadelphia, PA: Elsevier; 2018:55–68.

10. Shaw LJ, Charney P, Wenger NK. Women and ischemic heart disease: an evolving saga. In: Fuster V, Harrington RA, Narula J, et al., eds. *Hurst's The Heart.* Vol 2. 14th ed. New York, NY: McGraw-Hill; 2017:chap 108.

11. Semsarian C, Ingles J, Maron MS, Maron BJ. New perspectives on the prevalence of hypertrophic cardiomyopathy. *J Am Coll Cardiol.* 2015;65:1249–1254. doi:10.1016/j.jacc.2015.01.019.

12. Centers for Disease Control and Prevention. Heart defects. https://www.cdc.gov/ncbddd/heartdefects/data.html. Accessed February 4, 2019.

13. Bernstein D. Epidemiology and genetic basis of congenital heart disease. In: Kleigman RM, Stanton BF, St Geme JW, Schor NF, eds. *Nelson Textbook of Pediatrics.* 20th ed. Philadelphia, PA: Elsevier; 2016:2182–2187.

14. Bergmann O, Bhardwaj S, Zdunek F, et al. Evidence for cardiomyocyte renewal in humans. *Science.* 2009;324:98–102. doi:10.1126/science.1164680.

15. Paneni F, Diaz Canestro C, Libby P, et al. The aging cardiovascular system: understanding it at the cellular and clinical levels. *J Am Coll Cardiol.* 2017;69:1952–1967. doi:10.1016/j.jacc.2017.01.064.

16. Kappagoda T, Amsterdam E. Exercise and heart failure in the elderly. *Heart Fail Rev.* 2012;17:635–662. doi:10.1007/s10741-011-9297-4.

17. Nakou ES, Parthenakis FI, Kallergis EM, et al. Healthy aging and the myocardium: a complicated process with various effects in cardiac structure and physiology. *Int J Cardiol.* 2016;209:167–175. doi:10.1016/j.ijcard.2016.02.039.

SUGGESTED RESOURCES

Fuster V, Harrington RA, Narula J, Eapen ZJ, eds. *Hurst's The Heart.* 14th ed. New York, NY: McGraw-Hill; 2017.

Issa ZF, Miller JM, Zipes DP. *Clinical Arrhythmology and Electrophysiology.* 3rd ed. Philadelphia, PA: Elsevier; 2019.

Kibble JD, Halsey CR. *Medical Physiology: The Big Picture.* New York, NY: McGraw-Hill; 2009.

Klabunde RE. *Cardiovascular Physiology Concepts.* 2nd ed. Philadelphia, PA: Lippincott Williams & Wilkins; 2012.

Lilly LS, ed. *Pathophysiology of Heart Disease: A Collaborative Project of Medical Students and Faculty.* 6th ed. Philadelphia, PA: Wolters Kluwer; 2016.

Preston RR, Wilson TE. *Lippincott's Illustrated Reviews: Physiology.* Philadelphia, PA: Lippincott Williams & Wilkins; 2013.

University of Michigan Heart Sound & Murmur Library. https://www.med.umich.edu/lrc/psb_open/html/repo/primer_heartsound/primer_heartsound.html. Accessed February 4, 2019.

Zipes DP, Libby P, Bonow RO, et al., eds. *Braunwald's Heart Disease: A Textbook of Cardiovascular Medicine.* 11th ed. Philadelphia, PA: Elsevier; 2018.

11

LUNGS

Nancy C. Tkacs, Charrell S. Porter, and Nicholas A. Barker

THE CLINICAL CONTEXT

The lungs have the central and critical function of oxygen intake and carbon dioxide removal that sustains life. Data from the National Health Interview Survey indicate that lung diseases are common: Asthma affects 8.2% of the adult population, whereas reported rates of emphysema, chronic bronchitis, sinusitis, and hay fever are 1.8%, 4.1%, 13.6%, and 8.6%, respectively.[1] If one combines chronic lower respiratory disease with influenza and pneumonia, then lung diseases are the third leading cause of death in the United States.[2] Worldwide, the burden of lung disease in terms of years lived with disability is almost equal to that of cardiovascular disease, and the prevalence of all chronic respiratory diseases combined is actually higher than that for cardiovascular disease at more than 570 million patients. The greatest contributors to lung disease burden are chronic obstructive pulmonary disease and asthma.[3] Chronic lung disease can impair quality of life and reduce functional status for many years before causing death, which often is due to an acute event such as pneumonia after many years of reduced lung function.

OVERVIEW OF LUNG STRUCTURE AND FUNCTION

To maintain homeostasis and accomplish movement and cellular work requires energy. Energy in the form of adenosine triphosphate (ATP) is derived from dietary nutrients such as sugars and fats, and is released in processes of anaerobic and aerobic metabolism, with the majority of energy derived from oxygen-requiring oxidative metabolism. Metabolic processes also generate carbon dioxide (CO_2)—a gas that causes acidosis and that must be continuously eliminated by the lungs. Average oxygen (O_2) requirements and CO_2 production of an adult human depend on size and activity level. At rest, an adult man may consume 3.5 mL O_2/kg/min, or about 250 mL/min for a 70-kg person. Typically, CO_2 production is about 80% of O_2 consumption. During exercise, O_2 consumption can increase to ten to 15 times the resting level, and the respiratory system must increase O_2 intake and CO_2 elimination accordingly.[4]

Additional lung functions include acid–base balance, immune surveillance and protection from inhaled pathogens, metabolism of certain endogenous and exogenous molecules, and contributing to communication in the form of spoken language. Average respiratory rate in adults is 10 to 16 breaths/min, with average tidal volume of 500 mL at rest. Thus, minute ventilation, stated as respiratory rate multiplied by tidal volume, is about 5 to 8 L/min. Air movement into the lungs (inspiration) and out of the lungs (expiration) is generated by a sequence of contraction and relaxation of the major muscles of inspiration, creating movements of the chest wall and diaphragm surrounding the lungs. The lungs closely follow the movements of these structures due to surrounding negative intrapleural pressure. In this chapter, these processes are described first, followed by descriptions of lung mechanics and disorders of lung mechanics. Processes of alveolar gas exchange are detailed, along with disorders of gas exchange. Finally, unique aspects of the pulmonary vasculature are described, along with disorders of lung circulation.

STRUCTURES OF THE RESPIRATORY SYSTEM

The structures of the respiratory system are shown in **Figure 11.1**. Air enters and exits via the nose and mouth. On inspiration, air is drawn in, primarily via the nose, moving successively through the upper respiratory tract, including the pharynx and larynx, followed by the progressively branching structures of the lower respiratory

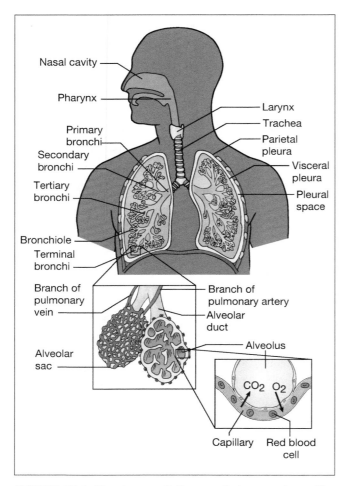

FIGURE 11.1 Structures of the respiratory system. The respiratory system consists of upper airway structures of the nose, mouth, throat, and larynx, and lower respiratory system structures of the trachea, bronchi, and successive airway generations within the lung tissue, ending in the delicate alveoli—sites of gas exchange.

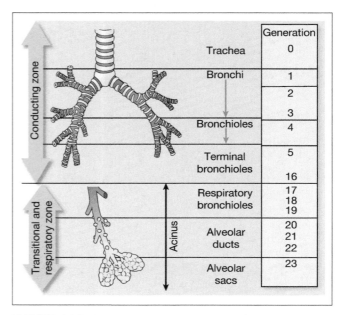

FIGURE 11.2 Branching airways. As the airways branch, total cross-sectional area and surface area increase markedly. The total surface area for gas exchange in the adult lung is estimated to be >70 m², about the size of a tennis court.

tract—trachea, bronchi, bronchioles, alveolar ducts, and alveoli. The successive levels of airway branching are referred to as airway generations (**Figure 11.2**). From the trachea, airways branch repeatedly into smaller tubes. Each level of branching (generation) is smaller in diameter than the previous level, but total cross-sectional area increases dramatically. Within the conducting zone, no gas exchange is possible; thus, this volume is known as the anatomical dead space.

Beginning with generation 17, alveoli are present, budding off from the walls of the respiratory bronchioles and permitting gas exchange. Branching continues until terminating at alveolar sacs, which are clusters of alveoli. Each alveolus is surrounded by a capillary network. This proximity allows rapid exchange of O_2 and CO_2 between the blood flowing in the alveolar capillaries and alveolar air that is refreshed with O_2 and has CO_2 removed with each breath. Each lung has 200 to 300 million alveoli and receives about half the cardiac

output—the output of the right ventricle—via the right and left pulmonary arteries.

MECHANISMS OF RESPIRATION

The major muscles of inspiration are the diaphragm and the external intercostal muscles. (**Figures 11.3** and **11.4**) Contraction of the diaphragm requires activation of phrenic motor neurons found at cervical spinal levels C3–C5. Axons of these neurons travel in the right and left phrenic nerves to innervate the diaphragm. Diaphragmatic contraction results in downward movement and flattening of this arched muscle, enlarging the chest cavity and compressing the abdominal cavity. Simultaneously, the external intercostal muscles (innervated by motor neurons in the thoracic spinal cord) contract, causing the ribs to elevate and move outward, increasing the circumference of the chest.

The increase in thoracic volume pulls the lungs to a more open position, dropping pressure in the airways and alveoli. This causes air to flow in, drawn by a pressure gradient from atmospheric pressure to negative pressure inside the lungs. When strenuous exertion increases body O_2 consumption and CO_2 production, respiratory rate and depth increase. Although the alterations depend on physical training, for an untrained athlete, maximal exercise can be associated with a five- to six-fold increase in both respiratory rate and tidal volume, with minute ventilation increasing about 20 times the resting level.[5] Augmented tidal volume can be achieved by the additional effort of accessory muscles of respiration, including the scalene, sternocleidomastoid,

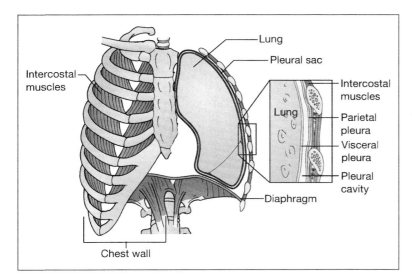

FIGURE 11.3 Major muscles of inspiration. The boundaries of the thoracic cavity are made up of the bones of the spine (posteriorly) and sternum (anteriorly), the ribs and their associated intercostal muscles, and the diaphragm inferiorly. These structures are lined with a membrane termed the *parietal pleura*. A thin virtual space, the pleural cavity, separates the parietal pleura from the visceral pleura, making up the outer covering of the lungs. A small volume of pleural fluid is spread thinly through the pleural space, and the pleural membranes move almost as one structure as the thoracic cavity expands during inspiration and contracts during expiration. This elegant system allows the muscles of inspiration to create lung expansion and filling. During quiet breathing, expiration is passive as the inspiratory muscles relax, returning the thoracic cavity to its preinspiratory size.

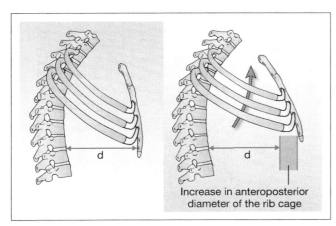

FIGURE 11.4 Rib movements. Contraction of external intercostal muscles lifts the ribs up and out—a movement that has been described as similar to lifting a bucket handle. d, diameter.

and trapezius muscles, which expand the chest cavity in the upward and outward direction. Increased respiratory efforts in many conditions of lung pathology are also associated with recruitment of accessory muscles.

During inspiration, the contraction of the inspiratory muscles stores potential energy in the elastic tissues of the lung. During quiet breathing, expiration occurs when the diaphragm and external intercostal muscles relax, decreasing the volume of the thoracic cavity, and creating positive pressure within the recently expanded lungs (**Figure 11.5**). Lung elastic recoil converts potential energy to kinetic energy, contributing to this positive pressure that drives expiration of the tidal volume. When exercise increases respiratory demands, or during pulmonary function testing, forced (active) expiration occurs. The muscles of forced expiration are the internal intercostal muscles and the abdominal muscles

(**Figure 11.6**). The internal intercostal muscles pull the ribs down and narrow the ribcage and thoracic cavity, compressing the lungs from the circumference. The abdominal muscles compress the abdominal contents, forcing them upward against the diaphragm and causing the diaphragm to move further upward, compressing the lungs within the chest cavity. These combined movements create positive intrapleural pressure that translates to positive pressure inside the airways, increasing expiratory airflow. This maneuver is limited, however, by simultaneous airway compression, as described later in this section.

Similar to the cardiovascular system, breathing is characterized by *automaticity:* Conscious control is not required for regular breathing to occur, although breathing rate and depth can be controlled voluntarily. Neural control of respiration is initiated within the brainstem, primarily from a pattern generator that influences clusters of medullary neurons controlling inspiratory muscles (**Box 11.1** and **Figure 11.7**). These inspiratory neurons project to the spinal cord, where they synapse on phrenic motor neurons, external intercostal motor neurons, and accessory muscle motor neurons. Inspiration ends when the medullary inspiratory neurons cease firing, decreasing the drive to motor neurons and allowing the inspiratory muscles to relax, with expiration occurring passively. In the case of forced expiration, separate medullary expiratory neurons stimulate expiratory motor neurons. The respiratory control system is pathologically disrupted by neurological conditions such as stroke, brainstem or high spinal cord injury, lower motor neuron lesions of the phrenic nerve due to Guillain–Barré syndrome or polio, or prescribed or street drugs that suppress the respiratory centers, such as opioids, alcohol, benzodiazepines, and barbiturates. Hypoventilation or apnea (an absence of inspiratory effort) occurring from any of these causes can be fatal.

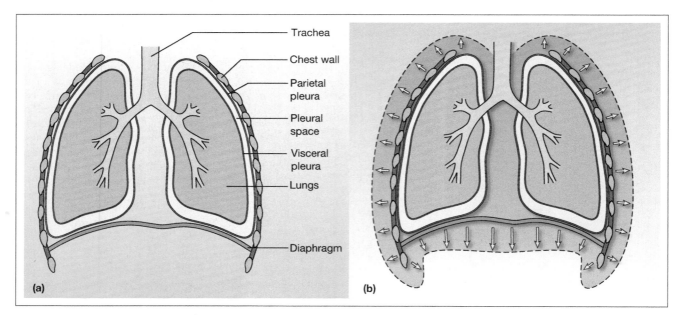

FIGURE 11.5 (a) At rest, the diaphragm and external intercostal muscles are relaxed and lung volume is at functional residual capacity. **(b)** Contraction of the diaphragm and external intercostal muscles increases the total volume of the thoracic cavity, reducing the pressure in the airways and causing inspiration. Relaxation of these muscles at the end of inspiration decreases the volume of the thoracic cavity and passively generates positive pressure within the lungs that causes expiration. This is assisted by elastic recoil of the lungs also exerting pressure on the air held within the air spaces (alveoli and airways).

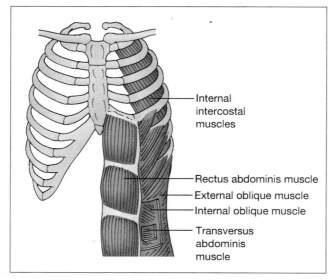

FIGURES 11.6 Muscles of forced expiration. Forced expiration is used during heavy exertion when tidal volume goes up to provide increased oxygen intake and carbon dioxide removal. Measurement of airflow during forced expiration is also part of pulmonary function testing.

ANATOMY AND HISTOLOGY OF AIRWAYS AND ALVEOLI

Air is inhaled first into the upper respiratory structures, beginning with the nose. The nasal epithelium has a folded surface that increases contact between air and tissue; at this level, the inspired air is warmed and humidified. Mucus lining the nasal passages begins to trap particulate matter before it can enter the lungs, and cilia move the mucus toward the oropharynx. The pharynx consists of the nasopharynx, oropharynx, and laryngopharynx, encountered in succession as the inspired air moves to the lower respiratory tract. The pharyngeal structures include tonsils and adenoids—lymphoid tissues able to conduct immune surveillance of the air entering the airways.

Beginning with the trachea, the airways are generally divided between the *conducting zone* that begins with the strong, cartilage-reinforced trachea and progressively divides into smaller bronchi and bronchioles, and the *respiratory zone*, consisting of small bronchioles with alveoli budding off, and ending in alveolar sacs appearing like clusters of grapes. The walls of the airways are lined with epithelial cells that get progressively thinner in the respiratory zone (**Figure 11.8**). In the conducting zone, the walls have abundant goblet cells that produce and secrete mucus. The ciliated epithelial cells have numerous cilia that beat in one direction—toward the mouth, continually moving the mucus layer to the mouth from which it can be swallowed or expectorated. As the airways get smaller, they have less or no supporting cartilage, with two significant consequences: first, the airways are prone to collapse if the pressure surrounding the airway is greater than pressure inside

BOX 11.1
Overview of Neural Control of Respiration

- The medulla contains several clusters of neurons that are the source of rhythmic outputs causing regular contractions of inspiratory muscles and initiating the respiratory cycle. (**Figure 11.7**)

- These brainstem respiratory pattern generator neurons signal spinal cord (and in some cases, cranial) motor neurons that stimulate the primary muscles of inspiration. Motor neurons to accessory muscles of inspiration are recruited upon physiological need.

- Respiratory muscles contract, providing mechanoreceptor feedback to brainstem and spinal cord.

- Alterations in arterial blood gases (O_2 and CO_2) provide chemoreceptor feedback to the brainstem respiratory nuclei.

- Other peripheral receptors detect irritant substances (initiating coughing) or vascular congestion.

- Inputs from higher centers can modify the respiratory pattern for voluntary activities such as speaking and singing. In addition, involuntary actions like belching, swallowing, and vomiting relay through brainstem pathways to alter the pattern of breathing.

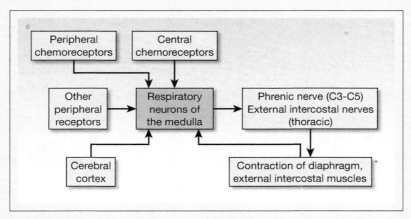

FIGURE 11.7 Overview of neural control of respiration.

the airway; second, bronchial smooth muscle contraction is able to narrow the collapsible airway.

MECHANISMS OF LUNG PROTECTION

Inspiration of 5 to 8 L of air each minute of the day represents a large risk of exposure of the delicate airways to environmental toxins, particulate matter, and pathogens such as bacteria and viruses. The lungs are well protected from larger particles by the mucociliary escalator mechanism described earlier. Epithelial cells of the mucosa are tightly joined and prevent movement of pathogens across that surface lining. Nonspecific defenses such as lysozyme, defensins, and antimicrobial peptides attack many pathogens. Mucosal dendritic cells phagocytose and present antigen to T lymphocytes, activating the adaptive immune system to produce secretory immunoglobulin isotype A (IgA). IgA provides protection against specific invaders by intercepting incoming pathogens and marking them for phagocytosis and destruction. At the level of

alveoli, the final small particles that arrive are phagocytosed by resident alveolar macrophages, in addition to being neutralized by IgG. Once activated, alveolar macrophages secrete cytokines that recruit additional monocytes, neutrophils, and lymphocytes to assist in host defense. Natural killer cells are present in the alveoli and can contribute to a rapid response to invading pathogens. Finally, protective antimicrobial proteins are also components of the surfactant that lines the alveoli.

Cystic Fibrosis: A Genetic Disorder That Compromises Lung Protection

Cystic fibrosis (CF) is a common autosomal recessive genetic disorder among certain populations. The prevalence of CF is highest in people of northern European ancestral descent. CF is screened for at birth in the United States, and neonatal screening results indicate a prevalence of 1:3,500 infants who are Caucasian, 1:7,000 infants who are Latinx, and 1:17,000 in those of African

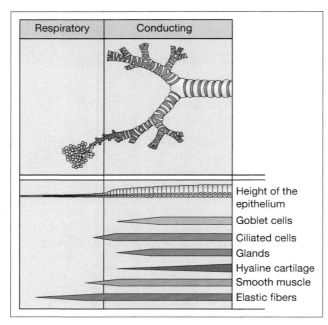

FIGURE 11.8 Characteristics of respiratory tract segments. As airways repeatedly branch from trachea to alveoli, the smaller segments begin to have alveoli capable of gas exchange. The transition from conducting airways to respiratory airways begins at about generation 16 to 17 (as discussed in text). The upper airways have mucus-producing goblet cells and submucosal glands. The lining epithelial cells are ciliated. Protection from inhaled particulate matter is achieved by mucociliary clearance. Smooth muscle cells are responsive to autonomic nervous influences producing dilation (sympathetic control) or constriction (parasympathetic control). Elastic fibers contribute to elastic recoil that drives passive expiration.
Source: Artwork by Holly Fischer.

ancestral origin.[6] There are close to 2,000 mutations in the gene coding for the cystic fibrosis transmembrane conductance regulator (CFTR) channel, a large transmembrane protein found in cell membranes that permits movement of Cl^- and HCO_3^- across an epithelial membrane. Normally, movement of these ions attracts water, resulting in production of fluid secretions, such as that of mucus lining the airways. Most of the known *CFTR* mutations are extremely rare; the most common mutation is present in about 90% of disease alleles globally. This F508del mutation results from a deletion of three nucleotides that code for a phenylalanine at amino acid position 508 within this very large and complex protein. The result is a misfolded protein that accumulates in the endoplasmic reticulum and is targeted for degradation without ever reaching the plasma membrane of the cell.

The pathophysiological consequences of *CFTR* mutations are manifested in tissues that depend on a lining layer of mucus that can support movement of secretions along tubular structures. Thus, these mutations are associated with chronic lung disease, diminished pancreatic enzyme secretion leading to poor digestion and nutrition, abnormalities of bile secretion, and infertility. With respect to lung function, without normal CFTR function, the mucociliary clearance mechanism is severely impaired. Lack of Cl^- transport across the epithelial cell membranes reduces the associated water movement, so the mucus layer is abnormally thin and very viscous, and the cilia are unable to properly move the mucus toward the mouth. Loss of HCO_3^- secretion makes the mucus acidic, reducing effectiveness of white blood cells in attacking pathogens. The function of an associated Na^+ transporter (epithelial sodium channel, or ENaC) is increased, promoting intracellular Na^+ accumulation and water retention, contributing to the thick mucus (**Figure 11.9**). Patients with CF have chronic lung infections that result in localized inflammation, and plug formation that leads to airway dilation, termed *bronchiectasis*.[7,8]

LUNG VOLUMES AND CAPACITIES

Pulmonary function testing is the primary laboratory assessment of lung function in health and disease. In spirometry, an individual is instructed to breath in and out through a tube—normally for several breaths—followed by taking the deepest possible breath (maximal inspiration) and then expiring until all of the air possible has been expelled. The resulting graph of volume of air moved during the time of the test allows calculation of certain lung volumes and capacities (see **Box 11.2** and **Figure 11.10**). In conjunction with this test, either plethysmography or helium dilution are used to measure the *residual volume (RV)*—the amount of air that remained in the lungs after the maximal expiration, which cannot be measured by the spirometer. Once the RV is known, additional measures can be calculated based on the spirometry measurements and the RV. An additional maximal inspiration and expiratory maneuver measures the airflow rate during forced expiration (by contracting abdominal and internal intercostal muscles). Forced expiratory maneuvers are used in assessment of obstructive lung diseases.

Pulmonary function values vary with body size, age, sex, and obesity. Reports will typically include the raw values as well as the percent of predicted values for a person's height, weight, age, and sex.

LUNG–CHEST WALL INTERACTIONS

The pleural space is a virtual space lying between the parietal pleura lining the chest cavity and the visceral pleura, the membrane covering the lungs. Pleural pressure (Ppl) within the space is subatmospheric, at about minus 5 centimeters of water pressure (–5 cm H_2O) at functional residual capacity (FRC). The source of the negative pressure is the competing tendencies of the lung to collapse down versus the chest wall to expand

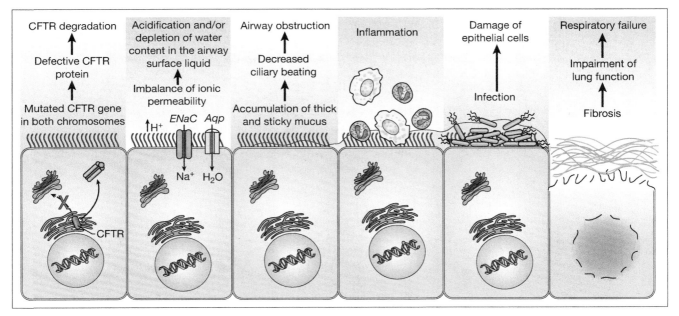

FIGURE 11.9 Cystic fibrosis pathology. Transcription and translation of the *CFTR* gene with the F508 deletion produces a protein that cannot pass through the Golgi apparatus to be inserted in the membrane. Rather, the abnormal protein is moved to the proteasome for degradation. Because Cl⁻, HCO_3^-, and water cannot diffuse across the epithelial barrier, the mucus layer becomes very acidic, viscous, and difficult to move. Abnormally high Na⁺ absorption further depletes water from the mucus layer. Ciliary function is lost, and pathogens begin to accumulate in the mucus lining of the airways. Ultimately, chronic infection and inflammation lead to scarring and obstruction of airways with loss of lung capacity.
Aqp, aquaporin; ENaC, epithelial sodium channel.

BOX 11.2
Key Lung Volume and Capacity Measurements and Their Significance

- *Tidal volume (VT)*—the volume of air inspired and expired during quiet breathing at rest; when multiplied by respiratory rate (breaths/min), resting minute ventilation is calculated.

- *Functional residual capacity (FRC)*—the volume of air in the lungs at the end of each expiration at rest. This represents the resting position of the respiratory system (lungs plus chest wall). At this point, there is an equilibrium between the intrinsic tendency of the lungs to collapse down, and the intrinsic tendency of the chest wall to expand outward. FRC is sensitive to disease processes that alter lung or chest wall mechanical properties.

- *Vital capacity (VC)*—the maximum volume of air that can be exhaled after a maximal inhalation. Depending on the context, this value can also be called forced vital capacity (FVC). This represents the greatest volume of air the respiratory system can move in response to a maximal expiratory effort. VC is sensitive to disease processes affecting the lung, the chest wall, and the neural control of muscles of respiration.

- *Residual volume (RV)*—the amount of air left in the lungs after a maximal expiratory effort. The RV depends on elastic recoil of the lung and is altered by diseases that affect either lung or chest wall compliance. It is measured by helium dilution or plethysmography.

- *Total lung capacity (TLC)*—the total amount of air in the lungs after a maximal inhalation; also equal to VC + RV. TLC is similarly affected by lung and chest wall disorders, as well as neuromuscular disorders affecting the muscles of respiration.

(continued)

BOX 11.2 (*continued*)
Key Lung Volume and Capacity Measurements and Their Significance

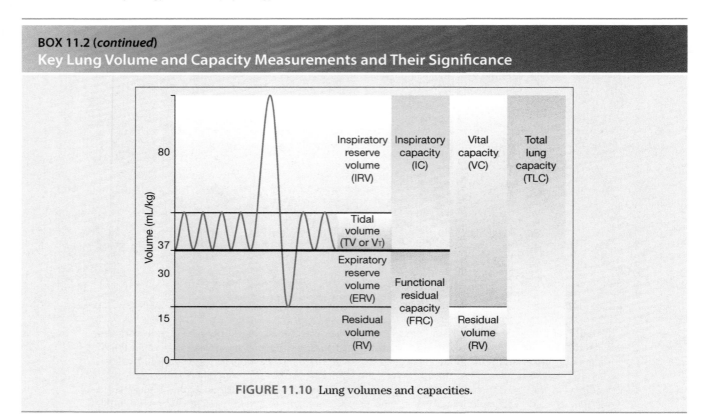

FIGURE 11.10 Lung volumes and capacities.

outward. At FRC, these two forces are balanced, tugging with equal strength in opposite directions. The negative pressure acts like a vacuum, pulling together the surfaces of the parietal and visceral pleural membranes, with the stiffer structures of the chest wall pulling the delicate lungs open (**Figure 11.11**). Another way to think of this relationship is that the lungs are inflated because the pressure inside the lungs (atmospheric pressure at rest) is higher than the surrounding pleural pressure, which is negative. This transpulmonary *pressure gradient* (pressure difference across the lungs—between inside and outside the airways) consists of about 5 cm H_2O, keeping the lungs open.

This relationship is disrupted when a spontaneous **pneumothorax** occurs and air accumulates in the pleural space, allowing the lung to collapse. In a similar fashion, a traumatic or surgical wound through the entire thickness of the chest wall (such as a stab wound, bullet wound, or incision to perform lung surgery) allows the pleural space to equilibrate with atmospheric pressure (defined as 0 cm H_2O with respect to the respiratory system). As soon as this happens, the chest wall expands in the outward direction and the lung collapses down.

The pleural space contains a small amount of pleural fluid that keeps the tissues lubricated and reduces the friction between chest wall and lungs. As inspiration

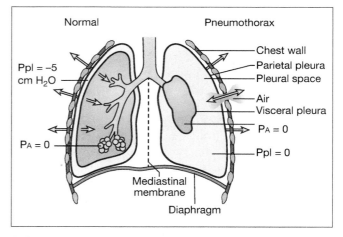

FIGURE 11.11 Lung/chest wall relationships. The volume of air inside the lungs at end-expiration (i.e., the FRC) is determined by two factors: the elastic recoil tendency of the lung to collapse down, and the tendency of the chest wall structures (ribs and intercostal muscles) to expand outward. The balance between these tendencies creates a negative pressure in the pleural space that holds the visceral and parietal pleura together. If a pneumothorax occurs, air enters the pleural space and Ppl equilibrates with atmospheric pressure. Immediately, the lung collapses down and the chest wall expands.
FRC, functional residual capacity; PA, alveolar pressure; Ppl, pleural pressure.

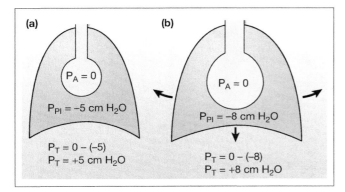

FIGURE 11.12 Lung pressures and relative volumes at the beginning and end of quiet inspiration. **(a)** At the end of a normal expiration, the lung volume is FRC, the diaphragm and external intercostals are relaxed, and Ppl is –5 cm H_2O. Thus, the distending (transpulmonary) pressure holding the lungs open (PT) is the pressure inside the lungs (PA) minus the pressure outside the lungs (Ppl), or +5 cm H_2O. **(b)** At the end of a normal inspiration, the external muscles are contracted, pulling the chest wall upward and outward, and the diaphragm is contracted, descending and lengthening the thoracic cavity between neck and abdomen. Volume is increased to FRC + VT, and the distending pressure on the lung has increased to +8 cm H_2O.

FRC, functional residual capacity; PA, alveolar pressure; Ppl, pleural pressure; PT, transpulmonary pressure; VT, tidal volume.

begins with diaphragm descent and external intercostal muscle contraction, the lungs follow the movements of these surrounding structures, held to them by surface tension—the lungs are pulled to a more open position, and the pleural membranes slide smoothly along one another. At the end of inspiration, Ppl is more negative and the lung has reached its end-inspiratory volume **(Figure 11.12)**. To achieve greater lung volumes if needed, during inspiration, greater action potential firing rates of neurons to inspiratory muscles will result in a more forceful muscle contraction, increasing the tidal volume (VT).

Pleural Effusion

Pleural fluid is produced by capillary filtration, under the influence of Starling forces of capillaries of the visceral and parietal pleura. Pleural fluid is reabsorbed across the visceral pleura and drained by lymph vessels of the lungs. Inflammation of the pleural membranes, or loss of lubricating pleural fluid, can cause pain with each breath. States of systemic fluid imbalance such as pulmonary edema, nephrotic syndrome, or cirrhosis can increase pleural fluid, causing **pleural effusion** by a transudative process. On the other hand, disease processes directly affecting the lungs, such as pneumonia, malignancy, or inflammatory disorders, can increase pleural fluid by an exudative process. Fluid accumulation in the pleural space impinges on the lung, limiting ventilatory capacity.

Symptoms include shortness of breath, cough, and pain that increases with breathing. With larger volumes of pleural fluid accumulation, there may be dullness to percussion and decreased tactile fremitus. A friction rub may be auscultated over the affected area. Treatment is directed to correcting the original cause and draining the excess fluid by thoracentesis.

Thought Questions

1. How is the lung protected against the particulates and pathogens that can enter the airways?

2. How do the structures of the lung and chest wall create lung inflation based on musculoskeletal movements of the chest wall and diaphragm?

3. Which of the lung volumes and capacities cannot be measured by using simple spirometry?

COMPLIANCE OF THE LUNGS AND CHEST WALL IN HEALTH AND DISEASE

The lungs are very compliant, readily stretching to accommodate the addition of the VT and greater inspired volume as needed. By convention, pressure changes during the respiratory cycle are measured in units of centimeters of water pressure (cm H_2O), rather than millimeters of mercury (mm Hg). Because 1 mm Hg pressure equals 1.36 cm H_2O (notice the change in units: 1 cm = 10 mm), increasing the distending lung pressure by 3 cm H_2O to inspire a VT of 500 mL represents about 2 mm Hg pressure, a relatively small amount.

Pathophysiological changes in lung compliance can occur in both acute and chronic lung disorders **(Figure 11.13)**. In pulmonary fibrosis, compliance is chronically decreased, and many acute disorders cause temporary decreases in compliance that are reversible as the condition resolves. Emphysema, discussed in this section, is the most common disease of increased compliance, although degenerative tissue changes with lungs during aging are also associated with increased compliance.

SURFACTANT AND LUNG COMPLIANCE

Surfactant, the fluid that lines the alveoli, is a major factor in lung compliance. The air–alveolar tissue interface is not completely dry; rather, there is a thin layer of liquid at that interface. This aqueous fluid has high surface tension (as described in Chapter 2, Chemical and Biochemical Foundations). Intermolecular attractions

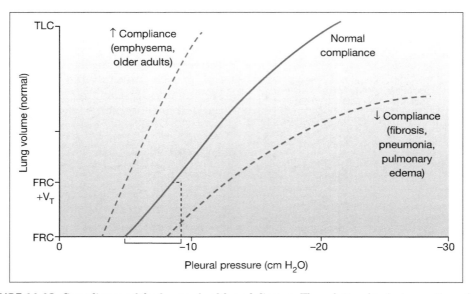

FIGURE 11.13 Compliance of the lung in health and disease. The relationship between the volume change of the lung with the distending pressure is termed the *compliance of the lung*. From FRC, it takes about 3 cm H_2O pressure to inflate the lungs with the usual V_T. In response to physiological needs (e.g., during exercise), the inspiratory muscles are able to create a more negative intrapleural pressure and drive intake of a greater inspired volume. Diseases of decreased lung compliance create a stiffer structure—greater pressure changes are needed to maintain even normal V_T. As a compensation, in certain of these conditions there is an increase in respiratory rate and decreased V_T, creating more work (particularly dead space ventilation), but reducing stress on inspiratory muscles. Diseases of increased lung compliance, primarily emphysema, make it easier to inflate the lungs on inspiration, but also result in a much higher FRC that can limit the maximum inspired volume. FRC, functional residual capacity; TLC, total lung capacity; V_T, tidal volume.

that pull water molecules toward each other contribute to this surface tension that would tend to collapse alveoli and make them quite difficult to inflate.

This problem is solved by a layer of surfactant lining all alveoli under healthy conditions. Type 2 alveolar cells produce this phospholipid/protein solution rich in amphipathic molecules that spread out over the alveolar surface. Surfactant greatly reduces surface tension, making inspiration easier. Think of blowing a soap bubble using a bubble wand: A small amount of air pressure causes slight bowing outward of the bubble fluid, but if you stop blowing, the fluid comes right back to a flat surface, because of the surface tension between the liquid molecules. After blowing with a bit more force, the bubble gets larger, and it takes less force to enlarge it further. Eventually the developing bubble forms a sphere and detaches.

In a similar fashion, from the moment of birth when a full-term newborn takes its first breath, the alveoli require a fair amount of pressure to inflate as the previously liquid-filled lungs fill with air for the first time. The pressure needed is reduced by the fact that fetal surfactant secretion begins during labor and increases with alveolar expansion during the first few breaths. When babies are born prematurely, before surfactant production is adequate, their lungs have low compliance,

which causes *neonatal respiratory distress syndrome*. This condition may require pressure-assisted ventilation to inflate the lungs (see Pediatric Considerations, later in this chapter). Artificial surfactant can be used to replace the endogenous fluid until production begins. Similarly, in adults, critical injuries such as sepsis can damage type 2 alveolar cells and reduce surfactant production, resulting in *acute respiratory distress syndrome (ARDS)*; see later discussion. In either neonates or adults lacking surfactant, lung compliance is greatly reduced, and lung inflation will often require pressure-assisted ventilation.

The inverse of compliance is elastance—the ability to recoil and return to the original size after being stretched. As noted earlier, expiration occurs as the inspiratory muscles relax at the end of inspiration; the lung's elastic recoil and conversion of stored energy generates pressure that drives expiration. For this reason, diseases that alter lung compliance also alter elastic recoil. Diseases of decreased compliance are associated with increased elastic recoil. Although it takes more pressure and effort to inflate the lung during inspiration, expiration occurs quickly and forcefully. Diseases of increased lung compliance reduce elastic recoil; the lungs become floppy and difficult to empty during expiration (**Figure 11.14**). This is manifested

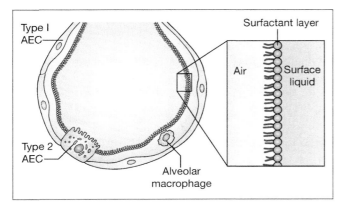

FIGURE 11.14 Surfactant reduces alveolar surface tension. Type 1 AECs are the thin cells making up the majority of the alveolar wall. The interface between alveolar air and tissue fluid lining the alveolar wall is the source of potential surface tension that would oppose alveolar expansion during inspiration (decreasing compliance). Type 2 AECs synthesize and secrete surfactant, a fluid rich in amphipathic phospholipid molecules that spread out on top of the fluid facing the alveolar air, greatly reducing surface tension and making alveolar expansion easier. AEC, alveolar epithelial cell.

by increased RV and FRC, which is particularly evident in emphysema.

Emphysema

Emphysema is, above all, a disease of increased compliance and decreased lung elastic recoil due to an imbalance of forces that damage the structural fibers of the lung and the forces that protect against such damage. Exposure of the lung to repeated insults of cigarette smoke, environmental particulate matter, inflammation, and oxidative stress stimulates the resident alveolar macrophages, recruits additional neutrophils and lymphocytes, and results in the release of proteases and reactive oxygen species. Proteases break down extracellular matrix, and local inflammation perpetuates neutrophil recruitment and induces alveolar epithelial cell apoptosis. This leads to loss of alveolar structure and dilation of air spaces, disrupting lung mechanics and gas exchange surface area. Normally, lung protective mechanisms include antioxidant defenses and antiproteases, particularly circulating α_1–antiprotease (also known as α_1–antitrypsin [AAT]); however, these protections are blunted by smoking. As air spaces enlarge, air trapping occurs in a vicious cycle wherein the enlarged spaces have reduced ability to empty on expiration. Emphysematous effects on pulmonary function are described later in this chapter, in the context of obstructive lung disease pathophysiology.

Emphysema is characterized as an obstructive disorder and overlaps with chronic bronchitis, another chronic obstructive pulmonary disease

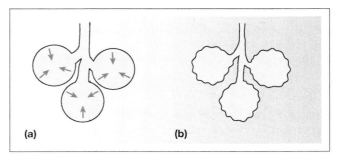

FIGURE 11.15 Elastic recoil of normal alveoli is lost in emphysema. **(a)** Normal alveoli: Elastin fibers in alveolar walls create elastic recoil upon expansion (due to inspiration). Relaxing diaphragm and external intercostal muscles promotes passive expiration proportional to the degree of lung elastic recoil. **(b)** Emphysema: Elastic recoil decreases when elastin fibers are destroyed by the disease emphysema. There is little elastic recoil, and air remains trapped in ever-larger spaces within the lung.

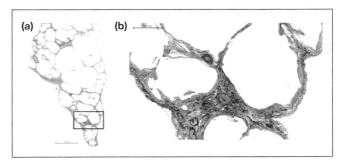

FIGURE 11.16 **(a)** Autopsy specimen of a patient who died of combined pulmonary fibrosis and emphysema, who also had lung cancer. Dilated air spaces with thin walls are characteristic of emphysema. **(b)** Enlargement from panel (a) inset shows a region of fibrotic cyst formation and smooth muscle hyperplasia consistent with pulmonary fibrosis. *Source:* From Inomata M, et al. An autopsy study of combined pulmonary fibrosis and emphysema: correlations among clinical, radiological, and pathological features. *BMC Pulm Med.* 2014;14:104.

(COPD) described later. Further complexity arises when patients have a combination of emphysematous changes (enlargement of air spaces, thinning of extracellular matrix) with fibrotic changes due to chronic inflammation. This combination is common in heavy smokers, leading to mixed findings on pulmonary function tests, imaging, and tissue pathology **(Figures 11.15 and 11.16)**. A major genetic disorder that increases emphysema risk is α_1**-antitrypsin deficiency** (AATD), which is also discussed in Chapter 14, Liver, under Pediatric Considerations. AAT is synthesized by the liver and circulates systemically, counteracting the activity of protease enzymes in many tissues. The lung is particularly dependent on this antiprotease for protection. Individuals with AATD are counseled to avoid cigarette smoking, as the combination greatly accelerates development of emphysema.

DISEASES OF DECREASED LUNG COMPLIANCE

Lung stiffness increases acutely in cases of pneumonia or ARDS, and chronically in many diseases of lung injury, inflammation, and connective tissue accumulation that may affect the lung interstitial tissues. Collectively, these are termed *restrictive* lung disorders, due to the restriction on lung expansion. **Interstitial lung disease** is another term that encompasses many of these conditions. They include idiopathic pulmonary fibrosis (discussed here in detail), sarcoidosis, systemic lupus erythematosus, rheumatoid arthritis, and scleroderma. **Pneumoconiosis** is a similar restrictive disease normally related to occupational exposures to inhaled fine particulates and dusts, including the specific syndromes of silicosis, asbestosis, and coal workers' pneumoconiosis.

Idiopathic Pulmonary Fibrosis

The pathogenesis of progressive lung fibrosis appears to depend on both environmental exposures (particularly cigarette smoke) and genetic predisposition, although it is not a monogenic disorder. Mutations in telomerase genes and mucin genes have been shown to contribute to pulmonary fibrosis susceptibility. **Idiopathic pulmonary fibrosis** (IPF) is diagnosed more often in adults over the age of 50, but it is likely that pathological changes of mild IPF occur before symptoms develop, resulting in delayed detection of the disorder.

In IPF, the tissues around the alveoli accumulate fibroblasts, and formation of extracellular matrix with collagen deposition increases (see **Figure 11.16**). These changes cause generalized stiffening of the normally compliant lung tissue. In addition to the loss of lung compliance, IPF also reduces gas exchange by limiting diffusion across the alveolar membrane. As the fibrosis progresses, it limits lung expansion, and RV, FRC, vital capacity (VC), and total lung capacity (TLC) all decrease, along with the anterior–posterior size of the chest. Greater pressure changes are required during inspiration, leading to a sensation of dyspnea and the appearance of labored breathing. V_T decreases and respiratory rate increases; these adaptations reduce the work of breathing as it is optimal to take more frequent and shallower breaths. Because gas exchange is impaired as well as lung mechanics, an early and prominent finding is dyspnea and hypoxemia on exertion—the system is unable to adequately increase ventilation to keep up with increased oxygen demands. Recent changes in IPF treatment approaches include the use of nintedanib (a tyrosine kinase inhibitor that reduces fibroblast proliferation) and pirfenidone (an antiinflammatory and antioxidant treatment that slows fibrosis progression). Evidence indicates that these medications may reduce progression of the disorder and delay death. Lung transplantation is another treatment, depending on patient characteristics and donor availability.[9,10]

CHEST WALL COMPLIANCE

Although not as common, changes to chest wall properties can also alter compliance of the lung–chest wall unit, resulting in compromised ventilation. Musculoskeletal conditions such as kyphosis and scoliosis can impinge on volume of the thoracic cavity, surgery and trauma to the chest wall can reduce mobility, and obesity can decrease thoracic volume—in part due to increased abdominal fat deposition. In each of these cases, the presentation is as a restrictive defect, and treatment is based on management of the underlying cause of the disorder.

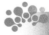

Thought Question

4. **How does smoking-induced damage to lung tissue lead to emphysema?**

AIRWAY RESISTANCE

OVERVIEW OF AIRWAY RESISTANCE

Movement of air or fluid through a cylindrical tube is governed by the pressure difference between the inflow and outflow, and the relative resistance of the tube. The resistance is inversely proportional to the fourth power of the tube's radius; therefore, the smaller the tube, the greater the resistance. The movement of air during respiration is facilitated by the large number and large cross-sectional area of airways. Although the repeated branching pattern means that individual terminal airways have a very small radius, air can flow through so many paths that the total resistance to airflow is very low under normal conditions. The greatest degree of resistance is encountered in the upper airways—generations 1 to 8. Beyond generation 8, total cross-sectional area increases and resistance decreases rapidly. A major determinant of airway resistance is lung volume; from FRC up to TLC, distensible airways progressively fill and their radius increases, reducing airway resistance. Therefore, at TLC, resistance is lowest, while expiration is associated with progressive increases in airway resistance that reaches a maximum at RV.

FORCED EXPIRATORY MANEUVERS ARE USED TO ASSESS AIRWAY RESISTANCE

During pulmonary function testing, the subject's ability to deeply inspire and then forcefully expire a maximal breath is measured. The volume of air (in liters) inspired and then expired is measured, and the rate of airflow (in liters per minute) is determined. These data are then graphically displayed in two ways. One display shows the volume expired during the time of the forced expiration (volume/time analysis) and the other plots the rate of airflow during expiration relative to the volume of air remaining in the lungs (flow/volume analysis). Volume/time analysis in a person without airway disease is shown in **Figure 11.17**. Beginning at TLC, close to 80% of the forced vital capacity (FVC) is expired within the first second. This value is termed the *forced expiratory volume in 1 second*, or FEV_1. Expiration of the remaining volume, down to RV, occupies the remaining time.

Flow/volume analysis is shown in **Figure 11.18**. By convention, the airflow is plotted against the volume in the lungs from RV (on the right) to the TLC (on the left). Forced expiratory flow is associated with a characteristic triangle-shaped flow/volume curve. Maximum expiratory flow (peak flow) is achieved at the beginning of the maneuver, reflecting the fact that airway resistance is lowest at TLC. From that point, airflow steadily decreases until RV is reached. Two factors can explain this decrement: First, as volume in the airways decreases, the radius of each airway also decreases, increasing resistance; second, forced expiration generates positive Ppl that tends to collapse airways. As shown in **Figure 11.19**, the Ppl, which is normally negative and contributes to airway expansion, becomes positive during forced expiration, tending to collapse airways. In this way, forced expiratory testing is able to detect disease processes in which airways are pathologically narrowed. In primary care and home settings, a handheld peak flowmeter can be used to get a quick measurement of forced expiratory flow.

CONCEPTS IN OBSTRUCTIVE LUNG DISEASE

The major obstructive lung diseases are asthma and COPD, which has two major presentations: chronic bronchitis and emphysema. There is some overlap among these three, and some patients have manifestations of

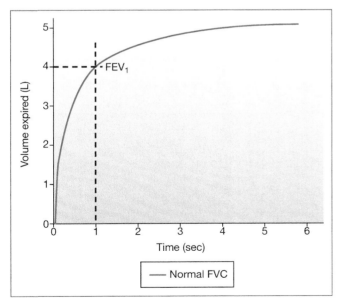

FIGURE 11.17 Plot of the volume of air expired over time during spirometry. The FEV_1 represents the volume of air expired in the first second of a forced expiratory maneuver. This corresponds to the time of minimal airway resistance as the maneuver begins at total lung capacity. FEV_1 is generally 75% to 85% of the FVC.

FEV_1, forced expiratory volume in 1 second; FVC, forced vital capacity.

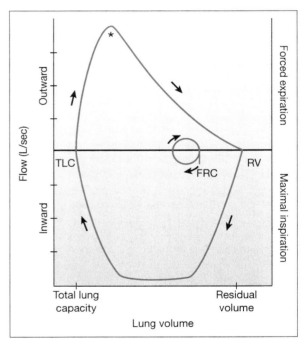

FIGURE 11.18 Spirometry flow/volume analysis. Airflow (with directional arrows) is depicted during a maximal inspiration (*lower box*) and a forced expiration from TLC to RV (*upper box*). Note volumes on *x*-axis are plotted from lowest (RV, on the right) to highest (TLC, on the left). The small circle shows the usual flow/volume relationship during a normal quiet breath—from a volume of FRC to FRC + V_T. Inspiration is associated with increasing flow rate to a maximum, a plateau region at that maximum, and then decreasing flow rate until TLC is reached. Forced expiration, however, is associated with an early increase to *peak expiratory flow (asterisk)* and progressively diminishing flow until RV remains in the lungs. The mechanism is termed *dynamic airway compression*.

FRC, functional residual capacity; RV, residual volume; TLC, total lung capacity.

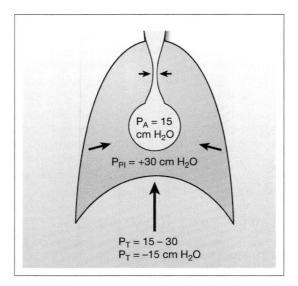

FIGURE 11.19 Lung pressures during forced expiration. During a forced expiration, the abdominal muscles contract, pushing the diaphragm up and compressing the chest cavity from the bottom. Internal intercostal muscles contract, drawing the chest wall down and in. Ppl becomes positive (represented as +30 cm H_2O). Thus, the airways are subjected to greater pressure on the outside (Ppl) than the inside (PA), giving a negative pressure gradient that tends to collapse the airways.

PA, alveolar pressure; Ppl, pleural pressure; PT, transpulmonary pressure.

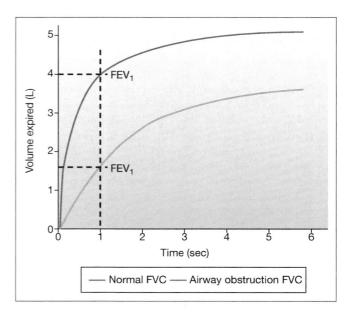

FIGURE 11.20 Obstructive diseases alter the volume/time relationship during forced expiration. Obstructive airway pathology in asthma or COPD limits the rate of expiratory flow and promotes air trapping, increasing residual volume and decreasing FVC. The FEV_1/FVC ratio is about 52%, indicating a moderate to severe degree of obstruction.

COPD, chronic obstructive pulmonary disease; FEV_1, forced expiratory volume in 1 second; FVC, forced vital capacity.

all forms. In all three disorders, when airway resistance increases due to chronic changes or acute exacerbation, pulmonary function is markedly compromised. Airway obstruction and premature airway closure during expiration are manifested by decreased peak flow, and FEV_1 and FVC are both reduced. FEV_1 shows the greatest changes, and the FEV_1/FVC ratio is abnormally low. Following inspiration, air is trapped behind closed airways, often increasing RV, FRC, and TLC. These changes are readily apparent on graphical representations of spirometry data (**Figures 11.20** and **11.21**).

Airway resistance is partly determined by the contractile state of bronchial smooth muscle. The parasympathetic branch of the autonomic nervous system innervates most of the conducting airways of the lung, whereas sympathetic innervation is more limited. The airways also have receptors for systemic and locally generated mediators. It is useful here to briefly review the mechanisms of smooth muscle contraction and relaxation (**Figure 11.22**). As described in Chapter 4, Cell Physiology and Pathophysiology, smooth muscle cells have irregular alignment of actin and myosin, and crossbridge formation leading to cell contraction and shortening is mediated by increases in intracellular calcium. The sequence of events leading to bronchial smooth muscle contraction consists of intracellular calcium accumulation, calcium–calmodulin binding, phosphorylation of myosin light chain kinase (MLCK), and actin–myosin

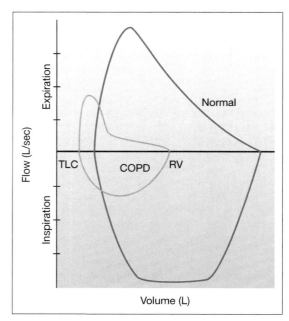

FIGURE 11.21 Obstructive diseases alter the flow/volume relationship during forced expiration. COPD produces marked changes in the flow/volume loop, with reduced peak flow, increased RV and TLC due to air trapping, and a concave "scooped out" appearance of the expiratory flow decline from peak. The concave flow pattern indicates premature airway closure during forced expiration.

COPD, chronic obstructive pulmonary disease; RV, residual volume; TLC, total lung capacity.

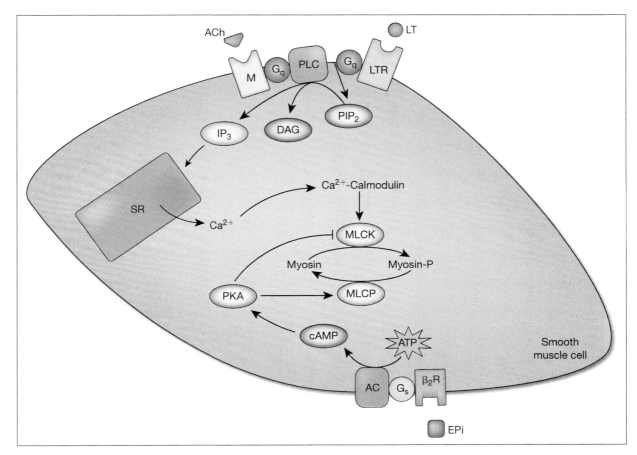

FIGURE 11.22 Neural and humoral control of bronchial smooth muscle. Bronchial smooth muscle contraction is under three major influences. Under normal conditions, there is modest bronchoconstriction due to ACh released from vagal innervation of the airways, acting on bronchial smooth muscle cell muscarinic receptors (M). During exercise or stress, circulating Epi binds to β_2-adrenergic receptors (β_2 Rs), causing bronchodilation. In an acute asthma attack, mast cell–generated LTs bind to LTRs and cause bronchoconstriction. The actions of ACh and LT are mediated by the G_q–phospholipase C system, increasing intracellular DAG, IP_3, and calcium (Ca^{2+}). The Ca^{2+}–calmodulin system phosphorylates MLCK, producing smooth muscle contraction. The action of epinephrine is mediated by the G_s–adenylyl cyclase system, converting ATP to cAMP, and activating PKA. PKA activates MP and inhibits MLCK, producing bronchodilation. These receptor-mediated actions are the targets of many drugs used to manage both asthma and chronic obstructive pulmonary disease.

AC, adenylyl cyclase; ACh, acetylcholine; ATP, adenosine triphosphate; cAMP, cyclic adenosine monophosphate; DAG, diacylglycerol; Epi, epinephrine; IP_3, inositol triphosphate; LT, leukotriene; LTRs, leukotriene receptors; MLCK, myosin light chain kinase; MLCP, myosin light chain phosphatase; MP, myosin phosphatase; PIP_2, phosphatidylinositol-4,5-bisphosphate; PKA, protein kinase A; PLC, phospholipase C; SR, sarcoplasmic reticulum.

crossbridge formation, shortening the cells. Because the airway smooth muscle cells are arranged radially around the airway walls, smooth muscle contraction leads to airway narrowing. Conversely, activation of the enzyme myosin light chain phosphatase, or inhibition of MLCK, produces smooth muscle relaxation and increased airway diameter, or bronchodilation. Under normal conditions, parasympathetic tone prevails, with modest bronchoconstriction. Exercise or the fight-or-flight response increases sympathetic tone to the airways, promoting bronchodilation.

In asthma, local release of histamine and leukotrienes contributes to bronchoconstriction.

Asthma

Asthma is an obstructive airway disease characterized by acute exacerbations with dyspnea, coughing, wheezing, and airflow obstruction measured by spirometry that usually reverts to almost-normal airway function on prompt treatment. Asthma prevalence in adults averages 4.3% worldwide.[11] Asthma attacks often begin in childhood, during which the most common pathogenesis is type 1 hypersensitivity (allergy). The hallmarks of allergic disorders include the following:

- Elevated production of T-helper 2 (Th2)-generated cytokines, including interleukin (IL)-4, IL-5, and IL-13
- Class-switching by B cells that produce IgE rather than IgG
- Binding of IgE to mast cells, thus priming them to respond to allergen exposure by degranulation, releasing histamine and inflammatory prostaglandins
- Recruitment of eosinophils to the affected tissue, perpetuating inflammatory mediator production and releasing eosinophil major basic protein, which further inflames tissues

In adults, other asthma subtypes have been identified, with airway accumulation of both neutrophils and eosinophils, or neutrophil accumulation alone.[11] Some forms of asthma have minimal airway granulocyte colonization. Regardless of the histological profile, all forms of asthma have chronic changes to the airways, including bronchial smooth muscle hypertrophy and hyperresponsiveness, altered goblet cell function with mucus hypersecretion, and airway narrowing due to fibroblast accumulation. Although not often done, airway provocation testing with a muscarinic agonist such as methacholine shows an exaggerated bronchoconstrictor response, whereas inhalation of a β-adrenergic agonist usually improves spirometry measures.[11,12] Thus, even

in the absence of an exacerbation, an individual with chronic asthma often has persistent airway narrowing evidenced by concavity of the expiratory flow/volume curve that becomes more pronounced during an acute asthma attack (**Figure 11.23**).

In addition to allergic causes, other asthma triggers include respiratory infections, exercise (particularly outdoors in cold, low-humidity conditions), aspirin in sensitive patients, and occupational exposures. Initial management generally involves a stepwise approach that includes inhaled corticosteroids to reduce airway inflammation, a long-acting β-agonist drug to promote bronchodilation, while providing a separate rescue inhaler with a short-acting β-agonist drug. If these strategies are not sufficient, leukotriene antagonists and muscarinic receptor blockers are additional options. Omalizumab, a monoclonal antibody to IgE, is an additional treatment option for patients with allergic asthma.

To summarize, the pathophysiology of asthma is characterized by acute but reversible airflow obstruction. In response to allergic and other triggers, mucus secretion increases, the mucosa becomes swollen with inflammatory cells and mediators that cause vasodilation and increased capillary permeability, and bronchial smooth muscle contracts. All three factors contribute to severely constricted airways and limited airflow. Over time, airway changes persist with modest degrees of airway narrowing between acute attacks. These airway changes include continued white blood cell infiltration, particularly with eosinophils and

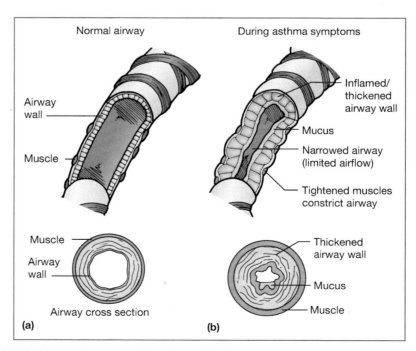

FIGURE 11.23 Airway changes with asthma. **(a)** Cross section of a normal airway. **(b)** Cross section of an airway during asthma symptoms.
Source: United States National Institutes of Health: National Heart, Lung, and Blood Institute.

lymphocytes; bronchial smooth muscle hypertrophy; hyperplasia; and hyperreactivity. With advancing age, asthma can overlap with the development of COPD.

Chronic Obstructive Pulmonary Disease

Chronic obstructive pulmonary disease (COPD) is the third leading cause of death in the United States, with prevalence estimated at 12% of the population, or 30 million people. Globally, COPD is the fourth leading cause of death, and the mortality rate due to COPD is increasing over time.[13] COPD is defined by reduced expiratory airflow (particularly FEV_1 and FEV_1/FVC) that is not reversible (unlike asthma), along with exertional dyspnea, cough, and sputum production. COPD is a complex disorder with overlapping disease processes that include air space enlargement due to tissue destruction (as in **emphysema**), and chronic inflammation with cough and sputum production (**chronic bronchitis**). Most cases are caused by current or former smoking, although environmental exposures (smoking in the environment, cooking indoors with biomass fuel) can also produce these manifestations. Having a history of asthma is a risk factor for later COPD development. Most studies of COPD pathophysiology involve individuals who currently or formerly were smokers, making this the best-understood group regarding pathological mechanisms. Smoking-induced injury of airway epithelial cells recruits white blood cells and initiates local inflammation. Generation of reactive oxygen species and neutrophil proteases damages lung tissues, and chronic inflammation can persist even if the individual stops smoking.[14]

Expiratory airflow limitation in patients with emphysema is due to decreased elastic recoil and occurs simultaneously with the increase in lung compliance (*elastance*, or elastic recoil, is the inverse of compliance). In addition, airways are prone to collapse because of the loss of adjacent tissue that would normally exert a tethering function, helping to keep airways open. Pursed-lip breathing may help to reduce airway collapse and support expiratory flow (**Figure 11.24**). Exhaling through pursed lips creates positive pressure in the mouth and along the airways, maintaining a pressure gradient that holds the airways open and counteracts the tendency of floppy airways to collapse. Using pursed-lip breathing during pulmonary function testing can result in improved measurement of VC, sometimes called *slow vital capacity*, in comparison with the usual forced expiratory measurement.

The diagnosis of chronic bronchitis is based on the clinical history of persistence of productive cough for at least 3 months that is documented in at least 2 consecutive years. Chronic inflammation with neutrophil and macrophage infiltration is similar to emphysema. In addition to increased mucus production, airway mucosal tissue becomes edematous, contributing to airway

narrowing, dyspnea, and cough. Fibrotic changes can also thicken bronchiolar walls and reduce the airway lumen.

Airway obstruction in COPD is associated with air trapping and can chronically increase RV, FRC, and TLC. Chest anterior–posterior dimension may be visibly increased (visible as a barrel-shaped chest) and identifiable on chest x-ray. CT of the chest is able to distinguish features such as bronchiectasis in some cases of COPD. Progression of the disease is associated with development of hypoxia and hypercapnia. Respiratory infections are the most common causes of exacerbations, and vaccinations for pneumococcal pneumonia and influenza are strongly recommended. Management approaches are similar to those used for asthma, including inhaled corticosteroids and long-acting β-adrenergic agonists, but better understanding of subtypes within the broad COPD diagnosis is needed to refine and target treatment options.[15,16]

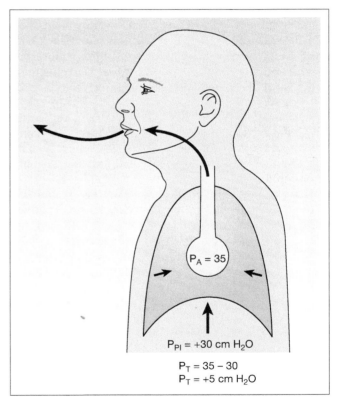

$$P_A = 35$$

$$P_{Pl} = +30 \text{ cm H}_2O$$

$$P_T = 35 - 30$$
$$P_T = +5 \text{ cm H}_2O$$

FIGURE 11.24 Forced expiration with pursed-lip breathing. Individuals with obstructive airway disease can reduce airway collapse during expiration by slowing down expiratory flow and by pursing the lips to create a block to airflow. This maneuver allows airway pressure to increase and reduces the tendency of positive Ppl to collapse the airways. In older adults and those with obstructive disease, airway collapse can even occur in the absence of forced expiration, so the pursed-lip breathing maneuver is helpful for maintaining vital capacity at normal levels and reducing residual volume.
P_A, alveolar pressure; Ppl, pleural pressure; P_T, transpulmonary pressure.

Obstructive Sleep Apnea

Obstructive sleep apnea (OSA) is the most common example of sleep-disordered breathing, a condition of abnormal breathing patterns occurring during sleep. In OSA, the upper airway becomes partly or completely obstructed for 20- to 40-second episodes during sleep, causing apnea (complete airflow cessation despite inspiratory muscle contraction) or hypopnea (decreased depth or duration of a breath). These episodes cause blood oxygen levels to decline and carbon dioxide levels to rise, terminating in (often unconscious and unsuccessful) respiratory efforts, a brief arousal and surge of sympathetic nervous system activity before sleep resumes.

The diagnosis of OSA depends on sleep laboratory documentation of the apnea/hypopnea index (AHI) of greater than five episodes per hour, in conjunction with signs and symptoms of sleep loss, or AHI greater than 15. Using the AHI cutoff of greater than 5 AHI, prevalence varies from 9% to 38%; while using the AHI cutoff of greater than 15, prevalence varies from 6% to 17%. Prevalence is higher in men and increases with age.[17] Some patients with OSA have 100 or more episodes per hour. Findings that confirm an OSA diagnosis in someone with an AHI greater than five include the following[18]:

- Patient complains of sleepiness, fatigue, or insomnia symptoms.
- Patient wakes experiencing breath holding, gasping, or choking.
- Bed partner reports snoring, grunting, or snorting (signs of partial airway obstruction) or breathing interruptions during sleep.
- Patient has a diagnosis of hypertension, mood disorder, cognitive dysfunction, coronary heart disease, stroke, heart failure, atrial fibrillation, or type 2 diabetes mellitus.

The soft tissues surrounding the back of the mouth and extending to the larynx (soft palate, oropharynx, and laryngopharynx) are collapsible and are capable of occluding the open space of the airway. In addition, in the supine position, the tongue tends to relax toward the back of the pharynx, also occluding the airway. The neural circuits controlling inspiratory muscles also control upper airway dilator muscles, thus favoring airway opening during inspiration. The genioglossus muscle that extends the tongue is the best studied of these muscles. Although coordinated activation of upper airway dilation is very effective while awake, activity drops with sleep onset and is particularly low during rapid eye movement (REM) sleep.

Airway obstruction during sleep is not the only factor leading to OSA; rather, conditions that narrow the airway provide the initial risk factor for apnea during sleep. In particular, obesity is associated with fat accumulation in the tissues surrounding the airway, providing the initial narrowing and predisposing to OSA. Obesity is also associated with decreased lung volume (due to increased abdominal contents pushing upward on the diaphragm). As lung volume decreases, airway resistance increases due to loss of tethering pulling airways open. Other factors narrowing upper airways during sleep include dilator muscle dysfunction, abnormal cycling between arousals and sleep that disrupts the usual respiratory cycle, and altered chemoreceptor sensitivity.[19]

During an episode of airway obstruction, blood O_2 levels fall and CO_2 levels rise, stimulating increased inspiratory efforts through chemoreceptor drive. This leads to greater depth of negative pleural pressures as the diaphragm and the external intercostal muscles contract in an attempt to bring air in through the obstructed airway. The more negative Ppl leads to a more negative airway pressure, sucking the soft tissues in and collapsing additional airways. Brief arousal may occur at the time of this activation of inspiratory activity. Pathophysiological consequences of repeated arousals, nocturnal spikes of sympathetic activity, intermittent hypoxia, and oxidative stress include cardiovascular pathology—heart disease, hypertension, and atrial fibrillation. **Excessive daytime sleepiness** can disrupt work and psychosocial functioning. Driving while drowsy can lead to automobile accident–related morbidity and mortality.[20]

OSA management with continuous positive airway pressure (CPAP) has been shown to mitigate some of the cardiovascular consequences of OSA. Nevertheless, adherence has been challenging, and other approaches should be incorporated in the management strategy, including weight loss, regular exercise, avoidance of smoking and alcohol, and avoidance of sleeping in the supine position.

Finally, a subset of patients has **central sleep apnea**, in which there is a failure of brainstem respiratory drive to the inspiratory muscles. Although the consequences of central sleep apnea are similar to those of OSA, the risk factors differ. In particular, patients with heart failure, stroke, and atrial fibrillation have an increased risk of developing central sleep apnea—and sleep apnea can also worsen heart failure and atrial fibrillation.

To summarize, biophysical properties of the respiratory system, compliance and resistance, shape pulmonary function in health and disease. Understanding these general principles provides the foundation for ordering and interpreting diagnostic tests, as well as devising management strategies. **Table 11.1** lists pulmonary function test findings in several pathological states.

TABLE 11.1 Findings in Common Lung Disorders

Disorder	FEV_1/FVC	FVC	RV, TLC, FRC	DL_{CO}
COPD/emphysema	↓	↓	↑	↓
Pulmonary fibrosis	–, ↑	↓	↓	–, ↓
COPD/chronic bronchitis	↓	↓	RV, FRC ↑ TLC –	–
Asthma (acute phase)*	↓	↓	↑	–

*In asthma, most changes are reversible upon recovery from exacerbation or are relieved by acute bronchodilator treatment.
–, no change; ↑, increase; ↓, decrease; COPD, chronic obstructive pulmonary disease; DL_{CO}, diffusing capacity of the lung for carbon monoxide, a measure of gas exchange area and thickness; FEV_1, forced expiratory volume in 1 second; FRC, functional residual capacity; FVC, forced vital capacity; RV, residual volume; TLC, total lung capacity.
Source: From Levitzky MG. *Pulmonary Physiology*. 9th ed. New York, NY: McGraw-Hill; 2018.

Thought Questions

5. **What is the rationale for the use of β-agonist drugs in diseases of increased airway resistance?**

6. **What are the mechanisms linking allergic airway disease and increased airway resistance?**

7. **How is CPAP treatment for obstructive sleep apnea similar to pursed-lip breathing in COPD?**

GAS EXCHANGE IN THE LUNG

OVERVIEW OF GAS EXCHANGE

As previously noted, the main function of the lungs is to provide an interface between alveolar airflow (referred to as *ventilation*) and pulmonary capillary blood flow (referred to as *perfusion*). At this interface, inspired O_2 can diffuse into the blood for transport to tissues, and tissue-generated CO_2 can be removed from the body via the alveolar–capillary membrane. Alveolar surface area is estimated to be at least 75 m^2 in a young adult, although it declines with aging.[21] Each alveolus is surrounded by a dense capillary network. Most of the surface area between the alveolar epithelium and capillary endothelium is a fused basal lamina with a few fibers of elastin, the protein responsible for lung elastic recoil.

Oxygen diffuses across the thin alveolar–capillary interface relatively easily, down its partial pressure gradient from alveolar air to capillary blood plasma.

Simultaneously, CO_2 diffuses in the opposite direction, from capillary blood to alveolar air. Each breath refreshes the alveolar air with fresh O_2 and removes CO_2. Oxygen delivery within the body is accomplished by binding to the oxygen-carrying protein *hemoglobin* (Hb) in red blood cells. Carbon dioxide is carried bound to Hb and also dissolved in blood plasma. The majority of CO_2 travels in the blood in the form of bicarbonate ions (HCO_3^-).

OXYGEN–HEMOGLOBIN DISSOCIATION CURVE

Oxygen is poorly soluble in blood plasma, and dissolved O_2 in the blood is not adequate to supply the body's O_2 needs. To solve this problem, Hb produced in red blood cells works as the major oxygen-carrying protein of the body. From the alveolar air, O_2 molecules diffuse into pulmonary capillary blood and then diffuse across red blood cell membranes, after which they are able to bind to Hb. Hb must bind O_2 efficiently at the partial pressure of the oxygen (Po_2) of the alveolus (referred to as *loading* the Hb with O_2), retain O_2 while in the arteries and arterioles, and release it to tissues at the Po_2 of tissue capillary beds (referred to as *unloading* O_2 from Hb). Each protein chain of the Hb tetramer contains a heme molecule with an attached iron ion (Fe^{2+}). The heme irons are the sites to which O_2 can bind reversibly, at relatively high O_2 partial pressures in the alveoli, and from which O_2 can be released to the tissues, where local Po_2 is lower due to tissue O_2 utilization (**Figure 11.25**).

The relationship between the local Po_2 and percent saturation of hemoglobin (Hb % sat) is a nonlinear relationship graphically depicted in the oxygen–Hb (oxyhemoglobin) dissociation curve (**Figure 11.26**). Oxygen partial pressure (Po_2, in units of mm Hg) is on the *x*-axis as the independent variable, whereas Hb percent saturation with O_2 (HbO_2/total Hb) is on the *y*-axis as the dependent variable. When the surrounding Po_2 is low, Hb is partially deoxygenated. As Po_2 rises, the first O_2 molecule binds to Hb. After this process is initiated, the shape of the Hb molecule changes, its oxygen-binding affinity increases, and the slope of the oxyhemoglobin dissociation curve increases. Once each Hb molecule has achieved 75% saturation (three binding sites are filled with O_2), the curve flattens out. Oxygen binding to Hb reaches close to 100% Hb saturation when the Po_2 reaches about 100 mm Hg, which is the average Po_2 of alveolar air.

A person's oxygen-carrying *capacity* is directly dependent on the amount of Hb in the blood: The greater the Hb concentration, the greater will be the oxygen-carrying capacity. If a person has anemia—decreased Hb concentration—he or she will have lower oxygen-carrying capacity. Oxygenation by the lungs can only increase blood O_2 *content*—the actual amount of oxygen carried—to the extent that Hb is available for loading. A person with anemia may have normal Po_2 and Hb saturation as shown on the oxyhemoglobin dissociation curve; however, if his or her Hb concentration is decreased, O_2 content will be decreased and the tissues may develop *anemic hypoxia*.

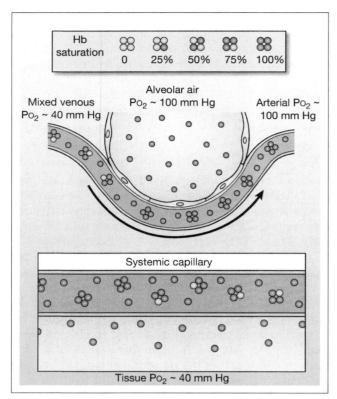

FIGURE 11.25 Qualitative display of Hb loading with oxygen in the alveolar capillaries and unloading in the tissues. In the top panel, blood entering the alveolar capillary has an average Po_2 of 40 mm Hg, corresponding to 75% saturation of Hb with oxygen. Immediately on encountering the alveolar Po_2 of 100 mm Hg, oxygen moves down its partial pressure gradient to equilibrate with capillary blood. Oxygen molecules then enter red blood cells and contribute the final oxygen addition to achieve 100% saturation: On each Hb molecule, all four oxygen-binding sites are occupied. In the bottom panel, oxygen delivery to the tissues is shown. Average tissue Po_2 is 40 mm Hg, so plasma Po_2 rapidly equilibrates to that level, as does the red blood cell cytoplasm. This favors unloading of oxygen from Hb, until the saturation level has reached 75%, the value associated with Po_2 of 40, as seen in the oxyhemoglobin dissociation curve. In tissues with greater rates of oxidative metabolism and CO_2 production, the curve shifts to the right, and greater amounts of oxygen are delivered at the same tissue Po_2 level.

Hb, hemoglobin; Po_2, partial pressure of oxygen.

Cardiorespiratory adaptations to anemic hypoxia include increased cardiac output and respiratory rate. These changes allow faster circulation of the blood through the lungs and back to the body to increase O_2 delivery to tissues. Levels of red blood cell 2,3-diphosphoglycerate (2,3-DPG) increase in anemia, improving O_2 delivery to tissues, as discussed in the next sections.

Influences on the Oxyhemoglobin Dissociation Curve

The affinity of Hb for O_2 is altered by a number of factors. Developmentally, fetal hemoglobin (HbF) consists of two α chains and two γ chains. HbF has greater O_2 affinity than HbA, the most common adult Hb, which

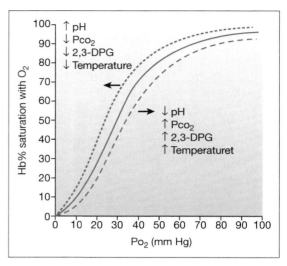

FIGURE 11.26 Oxyhemoglobin dissociation curve. Average mixed venous Po_2 is 40 mm Hg, which corresponds to 75% saturation of Hb (Hb % sat) with oxygen. This is the usual composition of blood entering alveolar capillaries. Average alveolar gas Po_2 is 100 mm Hg, so loading of oxygen onto Hb occurs, up to the usual arterial level of 97.5% Hb sat, with Po_2 averaging 100 mm Hg. Systemic and local factors alter Hb's affinity for oxygen, shifting the curve to the left (greater affinity) or to the right (lesser affinity), as shown. 2,3-DPG, 2,3-diphosphoglycerate; Hb, hemoglobin; Pco_2, partial pressure of carbon dioxide; Po_2, partial pressure of oxygen.

consists of two α chains and two β chains. This facilitates O_2 transfer from maternal blood to fetal blood at the placenta, providing O_2 for fetal development. In addition, HbF concentration is higher than maternal Hb concentration, so fetal O_2 content is predicted to be higher, delivering additional O_2 to the fetus.

Other physiological factors can alter the shape and position of the oxyhemoglobin dissociation curve. These can affect loading of O_2 onto Hb in the lungs and are particularly significant in unloading O_2 from Hb at the tissues. They are described next.

Effects of Partial Pressure of Carbon Dioxide and pH

The influence of pH and partial pressure of CO_2 (Pco_2) on the oxyhemoglobin dissociation curve is referred to as the *Bohr effect*. As pH decreases, the oxyhemoglobin dissociation curve shifts to the right, and oxygen is released from Hb more easily, at a higher Po_2 level. The Bohr effect is a result of a stabilizing effect of protons on deoxyhemoglobin, decreasing its tendency to bind O_2. Note that the pH of blood falls as its CO_2 content and partial pressure increase, which normally occurs in the transit of blood through the tissues. Physiologically this is ideal as Hb will deliver more O_2 in the presence of higher concentrations of CO_2 (and lower pH) in the tissues with the highest oxidative metabolism and CO_2 generation.[22] Conversely, low tissue CO_2 levels in tissues that have lower aerobic activity maintain stable pH, normal Hb affinity for O_2, and O_2 delivery at a lower level consistent with tissue requirements.

Effect of 2,3-Diphosphoglycerate

2,3-DPG (also called 2,3-bisphosphoglycerate, or 2,3-BPG) is produced by red blood cells during the reactions of glycolysis. 2,3-DPG binds to Hb and decreases the affinity of Hb for O_2, such that increased 2,3-DPG levels shift the oxyhemoglobin dissociation curve to the right, favoring O_2 delivery from Hb at higher levels of P_{O_2}. Synthesis of 2,3-DPG is favored in chronic conditions of hypoxia such as high altitude or chronic lung disease.

Effects of Temperature

Body temperature influences the affinity of Hb for O_2, with increased temperature decreasing the affinity and shifting the curve to the right. This effect can be manifested at the organ level. For example, in the heart, the rhythmic muscle contractions and high aerobic metabolic rate combine to increase the temperature. Thus, in the myocardial capillaries, the red blood cell Hb is exposed to conditions of increased temperature, in addition to lower pH and greater P_{CO_2}, with all of these factors assisting with greater O_2 delivery than in other tissues. On the other hand, at low blood temperatures, the curve shifts to the left and Hb has higher O_2 affinity, requiring lower P_{O_2} levels to release its O_2.

HYPOXIA AND HYPOXEMIA

Hypoxia refers to any deficiency of O_2, whereas **hypoxemia** refers to below normal levels of O_2 in arterial blood. Hypoxia of tissues can result from low inspired O_2 (in an airplane or at high altitude), anemia (due to lack of blood oxygen-carrying capacity), lack of perfusion (due to thromboembolic vascular occlusion), or poisoning that prevents cells from using O_2. Here, we focus on hypoxemia, specifically on the relationship between lung disease and decreased arterial O_2 partial pressure.

Although healthy lungs efficiently exchange O_2 and CO_2, hypoxemia can indicate failure of the lungs to provide adequate gas exchange to sustain life. An understanding of how gas exchange occurs and the causes of insufficient gas exchange are vital to caring for patients with lung diseases. Like hypoxia, hypoxemia may occur at high altitudes, as a result of lowered inspired P_{O_2}. The short-term adaptation is through increased rate and depth of breathing, whereas long-term adaptation to high altitude is via increased red blood cell production (polycythemia) and increased 2,3-DPG. For extreme elevations (e.g., climbing Mount Everest and similar peaks), O_2 supplementation is required. Individuals with healthy lung function are able to make these adaptations, but people with preexisting lung disease may not be able to adapt well to high altitude. The common pathological mechanisms of hypoxemia that will be discussed in this book are generalized hypoventilation, ventilation/perfusion mismatch, shunt, and diffusion limitation (Table 11.2).[23]

TABLE 11.2 Mechanisms of Hypoxemia

Cause of Hypoxemia	Such as That Observed in:
Generalized hypoventilation	OSA/OHS Opioid/drug overdose Central nervous system disease Neuromuscular weakness
Ventilation/perfusion mismatch and regional hypoventilation	COPD/asthma Pneumonia Pulmonary embolism Pulmonary fibrosis Pulmonary edema
Shunt	Anatomical: Cyanotic congenital heart defects Physiological: ARDS
Diffusion abnormality	Interstitial lung disease (many types) May also occur in pneumonia—with alveolar fluid accumulation

ARDS, acute respiratory distress syndrome; COPD, chronic obstructive pulmonary disease; OHS, obesity hypoventilation syndrome; OSA, obstructive sleep apnea.
Source: Reproduced with permission from Naureckas ET, Solway J. Disturbances of respiratory function. In: Jameson JL, et al., eds. *Harrison's Principles of Internal Medicine*. 20th ed. New York, NY: McGraw-Hill; 2018.

Generalized Hypoventilation

Alveolar **hypoventilation** is a state in which the breathing depth, rate, or both are inadequate to meet the body's needs, and, for our purposes, it is useful to distinguish **generalized hypoventilation** due to neurological or neuromuscular disorders as a category separate from hypoventilation in lung disease. It is important to note here that not all of the V_T reaches alveoli to refresh alveolar air composition. The conducting airways of the lungs have no alveoli and are unable to conduct gas exchange; thus, they are collectively known as *dead space*. As a general rule, a person's dead space (in milliliters) is about the same as his or her weight (in pounds); thus, a man with average body composition and weighing 150 pounds would have about 150 mL of dead space. The V_T during inspiration, then, consists of the sum of air entering the dead space and air entering alveoli. Calculation of minute ventilation is thus:

$$(V_T \times \text{Respiratory rate}) =$$
$$(V_D \times \text{Respiratory rate}) + (V_A \times \text{Respiratory rate})$$

where V_D refers to the dead space portion of V_T, and V_A refers to the alveolar portion of V_T. Minute ventilation is then made up of dead space ventilation plus alveolar ventilation.

An extreme case of hypoventilation is exemplified by a **traumatic high spinal cord injury** that disrupts neural pathways between the medullary respiratory pattern generators and the spinal cord motor neurons of the phrenic and intercostal nerves. This leaves the accessory muscles of the upper chest as the only inspiratory muscles, while the diaphragm and external intercostals cease activity. In such a case, the V_T is dramatically decreased, perhaps falling from 500 mL to 200 mL.

Table 11.3 shows data that would be consistent with this condition. Immediately after such a traumatic neurological injury, suppose that respiratory rate does not change. That drops minute ventilation by more than half, and alveolar ventilation drops to one-seventh of its previous value. CO_2 retention will be extreme at this level, and arterial O_2 will rapidly drop. These changes will stimulate chemoreceptors, quickly driving an increase in respiratory rate (depth of breathing cannot change because of spinal cord injury). Despite increasing respiratory rate, alveolar ventilation will still be inadequate to meet the body's O_2 needs, even at rest. Furthermore, supplementing O_2 will have only limited usefulness, as CO_2 will continue to build up in the alveolar spaces and in the blood. The only treatment that will be effective is mechanical ventilation.

Clinical manifestations of other, less dramatic hypoventilation syndromes can be nonspecific and variable, depending on factors such as the underlying disorder as well as severity of hypoventilation and the rate at which hypercapnia develops. These syndromes include acute disorders such as acute neurological injury, rapid-onset Guillain–Barré syndrome, or the much more common opioid overdose. Chronic hypoventilation is seen in obesity-related hypoventilation syndrome, restrictive thoracic disorders and rib injuries, degenerative neurological and neuromuscular disorders such as amyotrophic lateral sclerosis and myasthenia gravis, and central sleep apnea syndromes. Symptoms can include daytime somnolence and fatigue, poor-quality sleep, and snoring; these are common among patients with sleep-disordered breathing.

Ventilation/Perfusion ($\dot{V}/\dot{Q}$) Mismatch

Optimal gas exchange depends on both the rate of ventilation reaching the alveoli and the rate of blood flow (perfusion) traveling through the alveolar capillaries (**Figure 11.27**). Atmospheric air has a Po_2 of about 160 mm Hg at sea level, and has minimal CO_2. Upon entering the airways, water vapor is added, humidifying the air and reducing O_2 and CO_2 partial pressures slightly. As the air is breathed in, it meets air in the dead space that was depleted in O_2 and enriched in CO_2 from the previous expiration. At the level of the alveoli, the approximate partial pressures are $Po_2 = 100$ mm Hg and $Pco_2 = 40$ mm Hg. Blood traveling in the pulmonary arteries to the alveolar capillaries has the average composition similar to mixed systemic venous blood, with $Po_2 = 40$ mm Hg and $Pco_2 = 46$ mm Hg. As soon as the blood is exposed to alveolar air, it normally equilibrates to the composition of alveolar air, leaving the lungs through the pulmonary veins with the composition shown in **Figure 11.27**.

In clinical situations, imbalance between ventilation and perfusion of the alveoli (**ventilation/perfusion mismatch**) is the most common cause of hypoxemia in chronic lung disease as well as in acute conditions such as pulmonary edema and pneumonia. Rather than generalized hypoventilation, as described earlier for certain neurological disorders, hypoventilation in many lung disorders is often regional and patchy and blood flow can also be variable, depending on the disease process. Pneumonia, for example, may cause inflammatory exudate in many alveoli of one lung lobe, while the remaining lung may have relatively normal function. Similar uneven pathology can occur in COPD. In these scenarios, perfusion of alveoli in underventilated regions results in the incomplete oxygenation of exiting blood (**Figure 11.28**). When mixed with oxygenated blood coming from areas with a higher $\dot{V}/\dot{Q}$ ratio, the partially oxygenated blood decreases final Po_2 of blood leaving the lungs. Hypoxemia caused by $\dot{V}/\dot{Q}$ mismatch is typically responsive to oxygen therapy as inhalation of supplemental O_2 raises the Po_2, shown in **Figure 11.29**.[24]

TABLE 11.3 Hypoventilation Example: Data From a Hypothetical Patient With Spinal Cord Injury

Variables	Respiratory Rate (breaths/min)	Volumes (mL)			Ventilation: Volume × Rate (mL/min)		
		Tidal	Dead Space	Alveolar Space	Total	Dead Space	Alveolar Space
Before injury	12	500	150	350	6,000	1,800	4,200
Immediately after injury	12	200	150	50	2,400	1,800	600
Shortly after injury	30	200	150	50	6,000	4,500	1,500

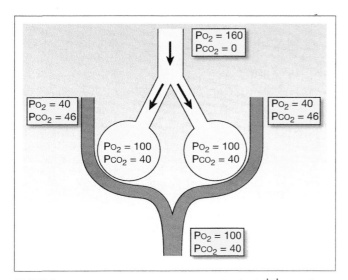

FIGURE 11.27 Arterial blood gases with ideal $\dot{V}/\dot{Q}$ matching. All blood gas pressures are in units of mm Hg. Air entering alveoli from the atmosphere continually replenishes alveolar O_2 and removes CO_2. Blood flowing through alveolar capillaries initially has essentially the same gas composition of O_2 and CO_2 as mixed systemic venous blood, but equilibrates with alveolar air. Alveolar gas exchange results in the average blood gas composition shown leaving the alveolar region to join the pulmonary veins, with $P_{O_2} = 100$ and $P_{CO_2} = 40$. If ventilation increases in rate or depth while perfusion stays the same, P_{O_2} will rise and P_{CO_2} will fall, with a corresponding change in blood gases leaving the lungs. If ventilation decreases in rate or depth while perfusion stays the same, P_{O_2} will fall and P_{CO_2} will rise. If both ventilation and perfusion change simultaneously and in the same direction, there will be little effect on alveolar and arterial blood gas levels.

P_{O_2}, partial pressure of the oxygen; P_{CO_2}, partial pressure of carbon dioxide; $\dot{V}/\dot{Q}$ ventilation/perfusion.

Shunt

In the lungs, **shunt** is usually considered to be an extreme degree of $\dot{V}/\dot{Q}$ mismatch in which blood is flowing by alveoli that are receiving no ventilation at all (**Figure 11.30**). Shunted venous blood decreases the arterial partial pressure of O_2 when mixed with fully oxygenated blood leaving other well-ventilated lung areas. As shunt represents areas where no gas exchange occurs, such hypoxia cannot be treated with 100% inspired O_2. In fact, a poor response to oxygen therapy is a hallmark feature that differentiates shunt from other mechanisms of hypoxemia. Clinically, if giving pure O_2 at 100% for 5 to 10 minutes does not improve arterial O_2 levels, it is evidence that the defect in the lung is due to a pulmonary shunt in contrast with $\dot{V}/\dot{Q}$ mismatch.[24]

As described next, a physiological response to regional hypoxia within the lung is constriction of the pulmonary vasculature. This response is known as **hypoxic vaso-constriction**, and it helps to compensate for areas of shunt and regional hypoventilation by reducing blood flow to the affected areas. This essentially improves $\dot{V}/\dot{Q}$

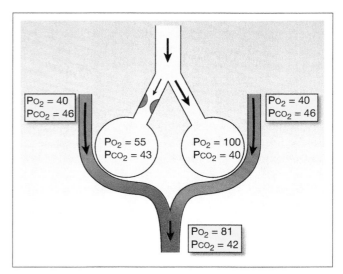

FIGURE 11.28 Ventilation/perfusion ($\dot{V}/\dot{Q}$) mismatch. $\dot{V}/\dot{Q}$ mismatch can be unevenly distributed in different lung regions. All blood gas pressures are in units of mm Hg. Here, the airway on the left is partially blocked, providing a region of low ventilation, whereas adjacent regions have normal ventilation. Blood flowing through the underventilated region is unable to pick up sufficient O_2 or remove sufficient CO_2. When mixed with blood perfusing units with better $\dot{V}/\dot{Q}$ matching, the resulting pulmonary venous blood has lower O_2 and higher CO_2 than normal.

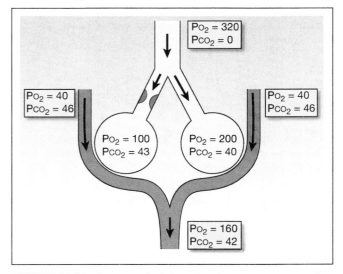

FIGURE 11.29 Oxygen administration improves oxygenation in ventilation/perfusion ($\dot{V}/\dot{Q}$) mismatch with regional hypoventilation. All blood gas pressures are in units of mm Hg. Increasing the fraction of inspired oxygen (F_{IO_2}) generally improves hypoxemia in patients with $\dot{V}/\dot{Q}$ mismatch. The effects on CO_2 levels vary with the degree of regional hypoventilation, but CO_2 and pH levels may remain relatively normal due to stimulation of respiratory rate and depth by CO_2-sensitive central chemoreceptors.

matching toward normal. Without this hypoxic pulmonary vasoconstriction, the effects of shunt and regional hypoventilation would cause progressively greater hypoxemia. This principle is not able to compensate for other situations of anatomical shunting; for example, the type of shunting that occurs in infants with cyanotic congenital heart defects, allowing blood to bypass the lungs and flow to the systemic circulation instead.

Diffusion Limitation

Diffusion limitation is a cause of hypoxemia in which O_2 transport across the alveolar–capillary membrane is impaired. Based on Fick's law of diffusion, gas movement down a concentration gradient is dependent on the properties of the gas, the surface area and thickness of the barrier to movement, and the magnitude of the concentration gradient:

$$J \propto -DA\frac{\Delta c}{\Delta x}$$

where

- J = the rate of movement of the gas, which is a negative value because it moves from higher to lower concentration, thus decreasing the amount on the side with higher concentration from which there is net loss
- D = the diffusing constant of the molecule that reflects the unique properties making it easier or harder to move through a barrier
- A = the surface area for diffusion, maximized in the lungs by the millions of alveoli
- Δc = the concentration difference across the barrier
- Δx = the thickness of the barrier, optimized in the lungs by the thin layers of alveolar epithelium, minimal extracellular matrix, limited interstitial fluid, and endothelial cells making up the alveolar–capillary walls

Diffusion limitation has several potential mechanisms and causes. Decreased surface area can occur with

- Alveolar loss as in emphysema
- Removal of all or part of a lung for cancer surgery
- Atelectasis (complete alveolar collapse)
- Complete alveolar flooding due to pulmonary edema or inflammatory fluid in pneumonia

Thickness of the alveolar–capillary interface may increase due to

- Fibroblast accumulation and collagen deposition due to idiopathic pulmonary fibrosis
- Fluid accumulation along the alveolar walls in early pulmonary edema or pneumonia

Diffusing capacity of the lung is measured during pulmonary function testing, usually by giving a single breath of carbon monoxide and measuring its uptake. The result is reported as $D_{L_{CO}}$ (diffusing capacity of the lung for carbon monoxide). This measurement can be normal in asthma and chronic bronchitis, and is usually

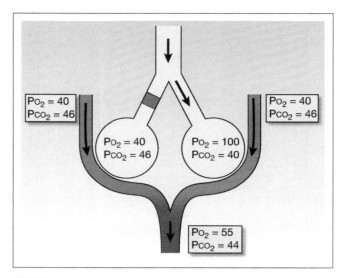

FIGURE 11.30 In shunt, one region of lung is receiving no airflow at all, due to atelectasis, mucus plugging, or flooding due to pneumonia or pulmonary edema. All blood gas pressures are in units of mm Hg. Blood flowing through these lung regions has no addition of O_2 or removal of CO_2, creating more severe hypoxemia and hypercapnia of the mixed pulmonary venous blood. Oxygen administration is ineffective at improving blood gases, as inspired air can never reach the affected regions.

reduced in emphysema, severe fibrotic lung disease, and pulmonary hypertension. Although diffusion limitation can result in hypoxemia, normally it is rare in humans at rest. It is more common in individuals with interstitial lung disease, particularly when they attempt to increase physical activity. As O_2 demands increase, respiratory rate and heart rate increase to optimize O_2 delivery. However, this also decreases transit time for red blood cells in the alveolar capillaries, and O_2 transfer cannot be completed before the blood leaves the capillary. Diffusion limitation responds well to supplemental O_2. As oxygen therapy raises the alveolar P_{O_2}, the partial pressure difference across the membrane barrier increases and promotes greater diffusion rate, as predicted by the Fick equation.

Thought Questions

8. Describe the path of an O_2 molecule entering the nose, traveling down the airways to an alveolus, and traveling in a blood cell for delivery to the tissues. What factors influence that path and the ease of oxygen movement at each transition?

9. What causes of hypoxemia can be treated simply with supplemental O_2? How do those causes compare with hypoxemia treatment that requires other measures?

LUNG VASCULAR CONSIDERATIONS

The pulmonary circulation provides lung perfusion that eliminates CO_2 produced by tissue metabolism and provides O_2 for tissue metabolism. It is astonishing to realize that the lungs, weighing about 850 g, receive the entire output of the right side of the heart, with a flow rate averaging 5 L/min. This cardiac output is equal to that pumped by the left side of the heart through the rest of the body! The blood vessels of the lungs branch extensively, ending in dense plexuses of capillaries that surround each alveolus. Deoxygenated blood is ejected by the right ventricle into the pulmonary arteries, eventually reaching the pulmonary capillary beds where gas exchange occurs. Oxygenated blood then returns to the left atrium via pulmonary veins. Pulmonary vascular resistance is substantially lower than systemic resistance, so pulmonary vascular pressures are much lower than systemic vascular pressures, despite receiving an equal cardiac output. Mean pulmonary artery pressure averages 15 to 20 mm Hg in adults younger than 50 years.[25] Owing to lower pressures, gravity has a substantial effect on blood flow distribution from the top to the bottom of the lungs, with the smallest amount of blood flow reaching the apex of each lung, and the greatest amount of flow to the bases when in the upright posture.

In addition to gravity, lung blood flow is modified by local tissue Po_2. As previously noted, optimal oxygenation is achieved when blood flow (perfusion) matches ventilation at each level of the lung. A vascular adaptation to lung regions that are hypoxic due to poor ventilation is vasoconstriction. This hypoxic vasoconstriction limits blood flow to poorly ventilated alveoli and maximizes blood flow to well-ventilated alveoli.

Although this mechanism is protective in patients with limited, focal areas of consolidation, it is problematic in patients with progressive, generalized lung disease. In such disorders, widespread hypoxia and hypoxic vasoconstriction may be present, leading to chronic elevations in pulmonary arterial pressures, termed **pulmonary arterial hypertension**. Increased pressures in the pulmonary vasculature damage vessel integrity, stress the heart, and spill over into negative effects on the systemic circulation that empties into the right side of the heart.

CARDIAC CONSEQUENCES OF PULMONARY DISEASE

Diffuse lung diseases with low levels of ventilation throughout the lungs have the greatest potential for damaging the right side of the heart. As the lungs become generally hypoxic, pulmonary vascular resistance rises, creating secondary pulmonary hypertension. Elevated pulmonary artery pressures increase afterload on the right ventricle, which ultimately responds by developing right ventricular hypertrophy and, in many cases, right-sided heart failure. Enlargement of the heart secondary to chronic lung disease with pulmonary hypertension is termed **cor pulmonale**. Obstructive and restrictive lung diseases commonly associated with the development of cor pulmonale are COPD, CF, kyphoscoliosis, sarcoidosis, interstitial pulmonary fibrosis, obesity hypoventilation syndrome, and sleep apnea syndrome.[26] Primary pulmonary hypertension, discussed later in this section, is highly associated with cor pulmonale. The progression to right-sided heart failure favors development of increased systemic venous pressures and can precipitate left-sided heart failure as well. Treatments for the underlying lung condition (β_2-receptor agonists, inhaled corticosteroids to reduce airway inflammation) are administered to improve lung oxygenation and relieve hypoxic bronchoconstriction. Other treatments can include diuretics, directed to the fluid-retaining aspects of heart failure.

PULMONARY EMBOLISM

Pulmonary embolism (PE) occurs when a clot or other particulate matter moves from the systemic veins into the pulmonary circulation, causing vascular obstruction. The result is a focal loss of pulmonary blood flow distal to the blockage. Potential causes of PE include thromboembolism, fat, air, amniotic fluid, tumor cells, and septic emboli related to bacteremia. Venous thromboembolism due to deep vein thrombosis is the most common cause of PE, accounting for 90% of cases. There are an estimated 500,000 to 600,000 cases of PE each year in the United States, resulting in 100,000 deaths.[27] Risk factors related to venous thromboembolism are described in Chapter 8, Blood and Clotting, so this section focuses on the consequences of PE for function of the lungs and right side of the heart.

PE is subdivided clinically with respect to anatomical location and presence or absence of hemodynamic stability. Depending on the size of a clot, blood flow may be blocked to a lung subsegment, segment, lobe, or the whole lung. Very large clots called *saddle emboli* may lodge at or near the bifurcation of right and left pulmonary arteries; patients with these clots have a 5% mortality rate. The greater the degree of vessel occlusion, the more likely it is that the right side of the heart will be unable to pump effectively against the increased vascular resistance and the left side of the heart will receive inadequate filling, resulting in systemic hypotension. Recent clinical guidelines include the following stratified definitions of PE:

- Massive PE, characterized as persistent hypotension lasting more than 15 minutes or necessitating inotropic support, with systolic blood pressure <90 mm Hg, heart rate <40 beats/min, or absence of pulse
- Submassive PE without hypotension, but with right ventricular dysfunction based on pulmonary angiography, transthoracic echocardiogram, or biomarker elevation (brain natriuretic peptide, troponin)
- Low-risk PE without hypotension or right ventricular dysfunction

The lung region affected by the embolism will receive no perfusion, but will still continue to be ventilated. This constitutes additional dead space, and if enough lung tissue is affected, it will lead to hypoxia and consequently tachypnea to compensate. The typical patient presentation includes dyspnea, which may be accompanied by chest pain, cough, and hemoptysis. Diagnosis of PE can be difficult and is typically done via imaging (CT angiogram, chest radiograph, and echocardiogram). Treatment modalities include anticoagulation, hemodynamic stabilization, catheter-directed administration of thrombolytics, and thrombectomy.[28]

PULMONARY EDEMA

Pulmonary edema is defined as the accumulation of fluid in the alveoli. Pulmonary edema can be due to cardiac or noncardiac causes. An excess of filtration over reabsorption by alveolar capillaries can be due to alterations in the capillary Starling forces (capillary hydrostatic pressure, capillary oncotic pressure, tissue hydrostatic pressure, tissue oncotic pressure), as noted in Chapter 9, Circulation. Pulmonary edema occurs in three distinct stages, based on the degree of fluid accumulation:

- During stage 1, fluid moves from the capillaries into the interstitial space but is still able to be removed via lymphatic drainage.
- Stage 2 is characterized by maximum lymphatic drainage and increased fluid accumulation in the interstitial space, creating crescentic filling along the alveolar margins.
- Flooding of the alveoli occurs in stage 3, with filling of the air space and disruption of the alveolar membrane.

Cardiogenic pulmonary edema secondary to heart failure or other cardiac pathology is associated with protein-poor fluid accumulation in the alveoli. The increased capillary filtration is caused by an increase in left ventricular filling pressures and left atrial pressures, ultimately increasing alveolar capillary hydrostatic pressure. Although acute decompensated heart failure is the most common cause of pulmonary edema, additional causes of edema include volume overload secondary to blood transfusion, severe hypertension, renal artery stenosis, and severe renal disease in patients with no evidence of heart disease. **Transfusion-associated circulatory overload** (TACO) is a form of volume overload related directly to the amount of volume administered during transfusion of blood products.

Noncardiogenic pulmonary edema is classified based on the radiographic evidence of fluid accumulation without clinical evidence of a cardiac cause. The most common cause is **acute respiratory distress syndrome** (ARDS), which is caused by damage to the alveolar–capillary membrane that greatly increases alveolar–capillary permeability, alters normal alveolar osmotic balance, and promotes capillary filtration at any level of Starling force imbalance. The lung lymphatic system normally clears fluid that leaks out of alveolar capillaries, but in ARDS, the rate of capillary filtration overwhelms the capacity of lung lymphatics to remove the edema fluid. Disease processes most likely to precipitate ARDS are (in descending order of prevalence) sepsis, pneumonia, aspiration, trauma, transfusion, pancreatitis, and drug overdose.[29]

The pathological changes contributing to pulmonary edema in ARDS begin with an escalating inflammatory response that is promoted by alveolar macrophage cytokine production. Neutrophils are recruited into alveoli and become activated, releasing proteases and reactive oxygen species that damage both the primary alveolar epithelial cells (type 1 cells) and type 2 cells that manufacture surfactant (**Figure 11.31**). The inflammatory cascade promotes alveolar–capillary permeability, favoring filtration of fluid into the narrow interstitial space around the alveoli, while loss of type 1 alveolar cells leaves gaps that allow edema fluid to enter and flood the alveoli. Surfactant production stops, increasing alveolar surface tension and promoting collapse. As the numbers of collapsed and fluid-filled alveoli increase, there is increasing shunt, producing severe hypoxemia despite O_2 administration.[30] Estimates of ARDS mortality rate range from 35% to 46%, depending on severity and patient characteristics.[29]

PULMONARY HYPERTENSION

Pulmonary hypertension—defined as the mean pulmonary artery pressure >25 mm Hg and pulmonary capillary wedge pressure <15 mm Hg[31]—is a complex disorder having five major subdivisions and many causes. Common causes are left-sided heart failure (although typically that is associated with increased pulmonary capillary wedge pressure) and chronic lung disease with hypoxic vasoconstriction, as described

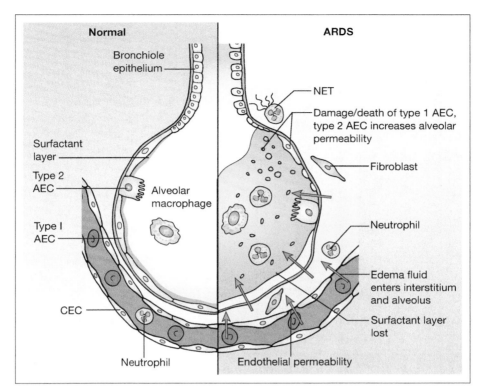

FIGURE 11.31 ARDS produces pulmonary edema due to macrophage and neutrophil recruitment and activation that greatly increase alveolar capillary permeability and damage type 1 and type 2 AECs. Loss of surfactant contributes to alveolar flooding and atelectasis.

AECs, alveolar epithelial cells; ARDS, acute respiratory distress syndrome; CEC, capillary endothelial cell; NET, neutrophil extracellular trap.

earlier. A detailed discussion of other forms of pulmonary hypertension is beyond the scope of this chapter, but it is useful to describe the pathophysiology of **idiopathic pulmonary hypertension** (IPH).

IPH is a rare disorder of the small muscular arteries in the pulmonary circulation. Resistance increases as the smooth muscle layer of the blood vessels become thickened, for reasons that are still unknown. Additional pathological findings can include intimal thickening and complex lesions of both arteries and arterioles. Early symptoms include dyspnea on exertion, chest pain, tachycardia, fatigue, and decreased appetite. Later symptoms may include fainting, lower extremity edema, and cyanosis.

Management of IPH is based on the pharmacology of vascular smooth muscle (VSM) constriction. Nitric oxide and prostacyclins are potent vasodilators, inhibit platelet activation, and are antiproliferative. Nitric oxide activates vascular smooth muscle cyclic guanosine monophosphate (cGMP) production, producing vasodilation. Phosphodiesterase-5 (PDE-5) inhibitors decrease degradation of cGMP, whereas guanylyl cyclase stimulators directly increase cGMP

production. Prostacyclin may be administered intravenously, and prostacyclin-related drugs are available in oral and inhaled forms. Endothelin-1 (ET-1) is a potent vasoconstrictor, and its action is blocked by ET-1 receptor antagonists. These are currently the most commonly used management approaches and have a common endpoint of increasing vasodilation and lowering pulmonary pressures.[32] The pathophysiology of pulmonary hypertension, along with its management, is an important example of the interdependence of cardiovascular and lung function.

Thought Questions

10. What is the major mechanism differentiating heart failure–associated pulmonary edema and ARDS?

11. What is the effect of a relatively large pulmonary embolism on lung ventilation/perfusion relationships?

Randall L. Johnson

LUNG DEVELOPMENT

During embryonic development, the trachea and esophagus are divisions of the foregut that soon diverge. The primordial trachea and lung buds begin to differentiate and later develop into the bronchial tree. Airway branching continues during fetal development, and all airway generations are present by about 25 weeks of gestation. Maturation of type 1 and type 2 alveolar epithelial cells at this time contributes to the beginning of airway surfactant production. Formation and expansion of the gas exchange surface area begin before birth and grow through childhood in the process of *alveolarization*. Pulmonary vascular development parallels alveolar development, with the alveolar capillary bed continuously developing during childhood[33] (**Figure 11.32**). Fetal and early life influences on lung health can have lasting effects on vulnerability to conditions such as asthma, pulmonary fibrosis, and other chronic lung conditions.[34]

Relative to adults, infants and children have significant differences in lung structure and function. Respiratory rate is high at birth (averaging about 40 breaths/min), decreasing throughout childhood to approximate adult rates during the teen years. In early childhood, elastin synthesis is just beginning, so there is reduced elastic recoil, less airway support, and greater tendency to develop airway collapse. The chest wall is more flexible and compliant in young children. Diaphragmatic contractions are stronger than those of the intercostal muscles, so as the diaphragm moves down, making the pleural pressure more negative, the chest wall moves inward, rather than outward. This is referred to as *paradoxical movement*. The diameter of the peripheral airways is much smaller than that of adult airways until 5 years of age, when airway diameter begins to increase and airway resistance decreases. For this reason, children younger than 5 years old have more airway resistance in small airways and have greater respiratory difficulties with small airway diseases such as bronchiolitis, as well as greater vulnerability to airway obstruction due to inhaled small objects such as nuts, candies, and toys.[35]

RESPIRATORY PROBLEMS ASSOCIATED WITH PRETERM BIRTH

Premature birth is associated with a variety of respiratory problems that are most severe in those with the greatest prematurity. As noted, surfactant production begins between 25 and 26 weeks, so very premature infants may develop **neonatal respiratory distress syndrome** and require administration of exogenous surfactant, as well as oxygen and CPAP or mechanical ventilation. Of infants born at or before 28 weeks of gestational age, about 40% go on to develop **bronchopulmonary dysplasia** (BPD).

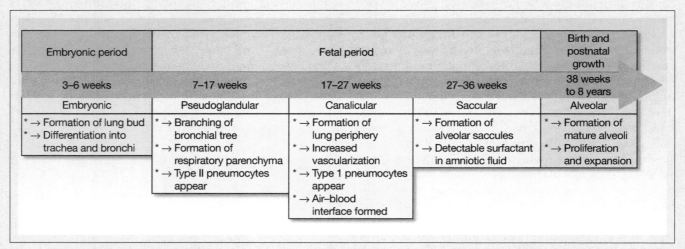

Embryonic period	Fetal period			Birth and postnatal growth
3–6 weeks	7–17 weeks	17–27 weeks	27–36 weeks	38 weeks to 8 years
Embryonic	Pseudoglandular	Canalicular	Saccular	Alveolar
* → Formation of lung bud * → Differentiation into trachea and bronchi	* → Branching of bronchial tree * → Formation of respiratory parenchyma * → Type II pneumocytes appear	* → Formation of lung periphery * → Increased vascularization * → Type 1 pneumocytes appear * → Air–blood interface formed	* → Formation of alveolar saccules * → Detectable surfactant in amniotic fluid	* → Formation of mature alveoli * → Proliferation and expansion

FIGURE 11.32 Milestones of prenatal lung development. Note that surfactant production does not begin until 25 to 27 weeks, after which the level of surfactant production increases in parallel with alveolar saccule formation. Formation of alveoli begins late, at 36 weeks, and continues after birth.
Source: From Hameed A, Sherkheli MA, Hussain A, Ul-haq R. Molecular and physiological determinants of pulmonary developmental biology: a review. *Am J Biomed Res.* 2013;1(1):13–24. https://doi.org/10.12691/ajbr-1-1-3.

Understanding of the pathology of BPD has evolved over the years since it was first described in the 1960s. At that time, infants with neonatal respiratory distress syndrome were treated with positive pressure ventilation and relatively high O_2 pressures, resulting in subsequent lung damage with marked fibrosis. As the standard of care has evolved to focus on surfactant treatment and protective ventilation, including CPAP, BPD is becoming less common in infants born after 32 weeks of gestational age, whereas it remains common in infants born sooner, at 26 to 28 weeks of gestational age. This "new" BPD is associated with the development of abnormally large and simplified alveoli, altered pulmonary capillary development, and some interstitial fibroproliferative changes.

BPD is graded as mild, moderate, or severe, depending on gestational age at birth, oxygen dependency, and need for pressure-assisted ventilation. As previously noted, alveoli are developing both before and after term birth; thus, extremely premature birth disrupts that process much earlier in alveolar development. Exposure before birth to stressors such as intrauterine growth retardation, steroid treatments, and infections can initiate the lung damage of BPD. After premature birth, exposures to ventilator-induced lung injury, oxidative stress, steroid treatments, infections, fluid overload, and nutritional deficits all can produce lung injury and prevent normal lung development. Long-term outcomes of BPD include greater risk for other lung disorders such as severe lung infections, reactive airway disease and asthma, and impaired physical and neurological development.[36,37]

LUNG CONCERNS IN INFANCY

Growth of the lungs and supporting structures during early infancy and into adolescence provides the capacity for full recovery from lung injuries in early life.[33] Within the first year of life, respiratory infections are the most common lung insult because of the relative immaturity of the immune system. Viral infections are the most common, particularly in younger children in daycare settings.

Respiratory syncytial virus (RSV) is the most common cause of pneumonia and bronchiolitis in infants. The pathophysiology of RSV infection involves the surface expression of fusion proteins that cause host cells to cluster, forming giant cells that lose normal function. Severe cases cause respiratory failure requiring hospitalization, and the virus is highly contagious, requiring careful precautions to prevent spread to other hospitalized infants. Older children and adults generally develop colds from RSV, rather than lower respiratory infections. Another point of vulnerability comes at the end of life: Older adults and adults with chronic diseases may also develop lower respiratory infections and pneumonia from RSV. Although some adaptive immunity is stimulated by RSV infection, it is incomplete, so an individual may have more than one RSV infection, and there is currently no RSV vaccine. Laboratory pathogen identification is by rapid antigen testing or nucleic acid amplification.

Bronchiolitis is diagnosed by history and physical examination, based on a history of symptoms of upper respiratory infection (rhinorrhea, fever) followed by development of increased respiratory effort and wheezing. Tissues around the bronchioles are swollen with white blood cells and inflammatory secretions, obstructing the small, delicate airways. Thus, the main airflow defect in bronchiolitis is obstructive, with air trapping and atelectasis. Nutrition suffers as infants are unable to feed normally. Care is supportive, and usually only brief hospitalizations are needed, with recovery in about 2 weeks. Preexisting conditions such as BPD, congenital heart disease, and family history of asthma or smoking all are associated with greater risk of bronchiolitis infection. Bronchiolitis in early life can also be a risk factor for later development of asthma, particularly in those with a family history of asthma.[38]

CHILDHOOD ASTHMA

Asthma is a common childhood illness; in the United States one in 12 children from birth to 17 years had asthma in 2016. Of these children, asthma is seen more frequently in boys, non-Hispanic black children, Puerto Rican children, and children from lower-income households. Although asthma prevalence is high, the number of asthma attacks per year decreased significantly from 2001 to 2016. This may be attributed to the finding that 50.8% of children with asthma had an asthma action plan that included education about asthma and early interventions.[39]

As previously noted, many cases of asthma result from allergy associated with IgE production. Although this is true for children older than 5 years of age, below that age infections are the most common causes of asthma. Other nonallergic causes of asthma in children from birth to 4 years are drug sensitivity to aspirin and other nonsteroidal antiinflammatory drugs and environmental irritants such as air-polluting particulates, smoke, and cold air. Neutrophils are the main airway white blood cell in nonallergic asthma. Rates of wheezing are high, probably due to the fact that airways are smaller and more easily obstructed in children. Bronchial smooth muscle may develop hypertrophy and hyperreactivity, as in adults. Although recurrent RSV infections may trigger asthma and airway obstruction, they may also strengthen Th1 lymphocyte responses and ultimately reduce the incidence of allergic asthma. Treatment of asthma in children is similar to that in adults, with particular emphasis on an asthma action plan that involves parents and school nurses as well as the child.[40]

Ingrid Deming and Alison Fife

Respiratory changes in older adults include greater vulnerability to lung disease and decreased lung capacity (functional reserve) to adapt to challenges such as exercise, altitude, and disease processes. Sustaining a lifetime of insults arriving with the inhaled air takes its toll in terms of oxidative stress, smoking, occupational and other environmental exposures, and sporadic respiratory infections. Advancing age is associated with progressive changes to the structures of the lungs and the chest wall that alter compliance, resistance, gas exchange, and neural control. In addition, prevalence of many chronic and acute lung disorders—including COPD, pulmonary fibrosis, and pneumonia—increases with advancing age.

Alveolar changes with aging are similar to those observed in emphysema, but without the inflammatory infiltrate and elastin destruction. Pertinent age-related changes include increased alveolar size and modestly reduced alveolar elastic recoil. Increased lung compliance means that the chest wall can exert greater pull in the outward direction, resulting in air space enlargement and greater TLC. Contrasting with the lung tissue's greater compliance, the chest wall becomes stiffer with aging from the calcification of the ribs and ossification of cartilage. This causes a stiffening of the thoracic cavity and inhibits the ability for expansion during inspiration. These changes, along with vertebral distortion by kyphosis, can increase the anterior–posterior diameter, producing a characteristic barrel-shaped thorax. Decreased muscle strength and increased chest stiffness promote an overall decrease in TLC, whereas the loss of elastic recoil and alveolar enlargement promote increased TLC. The result in healthy

aging is usually little change in TLC, accompanied by a decrease in VC.

Decreased elastic recoil and structural airway support contributes to a modest but progressive decline in airway patency. This is manifested as an increase in alveolar units that are distal to blocked airways, increasing RV and decreasing surface area for gas exchange. FEV_1 is reduced and the expiratory flow/volume curve assumes more of the convex "scooped out" appearance associated with obstructive disorders (see **Figure 11.21**). With increased air trapping, FRC also increases and FVC decreases. FEV_1 decreases to a greater extent than FVC, so the FEV_1/FVC ratio decreases with aging, consistent with a modest obstructive defect. Loss of alveolar surface area also changes the area of gas exchange, which decreases with aging and limits the overall diffusing capacity of the lungs.[40] Structural and functional alterations in the pulmonary system with aging are summarized in **Box 11.3** and **Table 11.4**.

There are moderate decreases in respiratory muscle strength with aging, but it appears that in healthy older adults the continuous activity of breathing maintains a good degree of overall respiratory muscle function. Age-related calcification and stiffening of the chest wall, ribs, and muscles, and kyphosis, may prevent full lung expansion with inspiration (because of decreased chest wall compliance), altering the curvature of the diaphragm, thereby inhibiting the diaphragm from having an optimal force of contraction. The pulmonary system may function normally at rest but may be impaired in its ability to increase rate and depth of breathing to enable increased physical activity. Some of these structural changes can

---

BOX 11.3

Normal Age-Related Pulmonary Physiological Changes in Older Adults

Loss of lung elastic recoil, increased airway resistance	→	Decreased expiratory flow
Premature airway closure	→	Reduced functional alveolar surface area Reduced gas exchange
Calcification of ribs and ossification of cartilage	→	Increased chest anterior–posterior diameter Flattened diaphragm Decreased overall pulmonary compliance
Muscle atrophy/sarcopenia	→	Decreased strength of diaphragm, intercostal muscles, and accessory muscles Decreased endurance and exercise tolerance

TABLE 11.4 Age-Related Changes in Pulmonary Function Tests

Pulmonary Function Parameter	Changes With Age	Mechanisms, Observations
FRC	Increase	Premature airway closure, air trapping
RV	Increase	Premature airway closure, air trapping
TLC	Unchanged	
Lung compliance	Increase	Alveoli and airway increase in diameter
FEV$_1$	Decrease	Peaks around 20–36 years old and declines with age
FVC	Decrease	Declines later in life and at slower rate than FEV$_1$
Lung diffusing capacity	Decrease	Loss of alveolar surface area
Diaphragm strength	Decreased	13% decrease in older adults

FEV$_1$, volume of expired air in 1 second; FRC, functional residual capacity; FVC, forced vital capacity; RV, residual volume; TLC, total lung capacity.

also impair the ability to efficiently expectorate and clear the airways during an acute or chronic infection.[41,42]

Neural control of breathing is somewhat impaired with aging, with decreased responsiveness to chemoreceptor activity signaling either hypoxemia or hypercapnia. Older adults are more likely to describe dyspnea at rest and particularly with exertion.

PNEUMONIA

A more detailed discussion of **pneumonia** in older adults appears in Chapter 5, Infectious Disease. Here, it is important to note that age-related changes in upper airway tone, control, and cough and swallowing reflexes lead to increased frequency and severity of aspiration, and subsequently aspiration pneumonia, with age. Lung factors contributing to the greater incidence of pneumonia in older adults include decreased effectiveness of cough and mucociliary clearance, decreased secretory IgA in airways, and decreased chest compliance and respiratory muscle strength.[43] In addition, the presenting signs and symptoms of pneumonia may be blunted or altered in older adults, obscuring the diagnosis. Above all, in clinical practice, it is important to reinforce the available vaccines for pneumococcal pneumonia and influenza, as these infections are the common causes of community-acquired pneumonia in older adults.

Older adults at risk for aspiration include those who are immobile or have alterations in posture (cervical hyperextension due to degenerative spine disease) or neuromuscular conditions. Additionally, older adults with dysphagia secondary to a new or previous stroke and poor oral health or dentition are also at risk. Clinical manifestations of aspiration pneumonia appear within 24 to 48 hours after aspiration and include dyspnea, fever, tachycardia, decreased oxygen saturation, increased serum leukocyte count, and mental status changes such as acute confusion. Treatment includes appropriate antibiotic selection. The most common organism in aspiration pneumonia is *Pseudomonas aeruginosa*.

CHRONIC OBSTRUCTIVE PULMONARY DISEASE (CHRONIC BRONCHITIS AND EMPHYSEMA)

As noted earlier in the chapter, **chronic obstructive pulmonary disease** (COPD) encompasses both chronic bronchitis and emphysema, and refers to conditions with a resistance to airflow at any level by a partial or complete obstruction. The disease is common in older adults, particularly those with a history of smoking.[44] The chemicals and particles inhaled with smoking cause lung cell damage and chronic inflammation.

Although aging does not directly affect the underlying pathophysiology of COPD, the presentation in older adults may be complicated by some of the previously described changes (e.g., diaphragmatic and accessory muscle atrophy, ossification and calcification of ribs, loss of alveolar elastic recoil). As life expectancy increases, the number of older adults with chronic bronchitis also increases, and a lower threshold for impaired lung function makes them more prone to exacerbations. These exacerbations can be significantly worse, especially in patients who continue to smoke or those exposed to environmental toxins. COPD may progress faster in older adults due to physical deconditioning, decreased mobility, fragile state, and immobility. These conditions, superimposed on the damage and chronic inflammation of the lung parenchyma and loss of ciliary protection, place older adults at an even greater increased risk of airway infections.

CASE STUDY 11.1: A Child With Asthma

Stephanie L. Carper

Patient Complaint: An 8-year-old boy reports: *"I had a runny nose and it felt like it was harder to take a breath 2 days ago, then yesterday I started coughing."* His father adds, *"My son has asthma, and he's been coughing almost nonstop for the last day. He brings up yellowish stuff most of the time, and I can hear him wheezing when he takes a breath."*

History of Present illness: The patient is an 8-year-old boy who came to the clinic today with his father because of respiratory symptoms. As reported by the child and his father, he has been afebrile, with no sore throat, chills, rash, abdominal pain, vomiting, or diarrhea. He has had slightly decreased food and fluid intake, but normal urine output. The boy and father both feel that his respiratory symptoms are worsening, and he stayed home from school today. The boy had been previously diagnosed with asthma and his medications include daily fluticasone and (as needed) albuterol. Over the last 24 hours, the boy has been taking fluticasone as directed, and has been requiring albuterol every 4 hours for cough. His last dose of albuterol was 3 hours ago. The father states that his son has asthma exacerbations with cold weather, strenuous physical activity, and illness, most notably upper respiratory infections.

Review of Systems, Past Medical/Social History: The patient has moderate, persistent asthma that is currently being treated with fluticasone (44 mcg, two puffs twice daily via metered dose inhaler [MDI] with spacer, daily) and albuterol (90 mcg/actuation, two puffs via MDI with spacer, every 4 hours, as needed). His father reports that his son is a curious and active child who has no health issues other than asthma. The patient is a second grader at a nearby elementary school. He lives at home with his mother, father, two sisters, brother, and dog.

Physical Examination: Findings are as follows: temperature of 99.0°F, blood pressure of 105/78 mm Hg, heart rate of 100 beats/min, respirations of 36 breaths/min. O_2 saturation is 93% on room air. The patient is alert, afebrile, and well appearing. On examination, his skin is warm and dry, with no lesions. Head is normocephalic and atraumatic. Sclerae and conjunctivae are clear, with no active discharge; pupils are equal, round, and reactive to light and accommodation (PERRLA), and extraocular movements are intact. Nasal cavity has a scant amount of clear rhinorrhea. Oral cavity has moist mucous membranes, pharynx without injection, and no tonsillar hypertrophy or exudative tonsils. The neck and upper extremity examination is normal. Lung examination reveals diffuse inspiratory and expiratory wheezes throughout, positive tachypnea, and mild subcostal retractions. Heart rate and rhythm are regular, S_1 and S_2 are present, and there are no murmurs. Abdomen is soft, nontender, and nondistended, with no hepatosplenomegaly. Lower extremities show full range of motion. On neurological exam, the patient is alert and oriented appropriately for age and development, and cranial nerves II to XII are intact, with normal tone for developmental age and normal gait for development.

Additional Testing: Peak flow by handheld meter is reduced from previous visits; no other laboratory tests are indicated in this case (stable asthma with a superimposed respiratory infection).

CASE STUDY 11.1 THOUGHT QUESTIONS
- *What factors contribute to decreased peak flow in the context of a respiratory infection in a patient with chronic asthma?*
- *What environmental factors in the home should be assessed in a child who has chronic asthma?*

CASE STUDY 11.2: A Patient With Chronic Bronchitis

Linda W. Good

Chief Complaint: *"I just can't catch my breath sometimes for all the coughing fits these last 4 months. I'm tired all the time because I wake up at night coughing. I have trouble getting through my workday as a painter because I'm exhausted. My work mates call me 'old man' even though I'm only 57. I stopped smoking 6 months ago and this is the thanks I get. I got this albuterol inhaler from the urgent care doctor and it's worthless."*

History of Present Illness/Review of Systems: The primary care provider observes an anxious man appearing slightly older than his stated age, speaking in full sentences without laboring to breathe. The interview is disrupted by several paroxysms of coughing that produce clear mucus. The patient comments that he has tried over-the-counter remedies, including dextromethorphan, guanfacine, pseudoephedrine, and diphenhydramine. In addition, he used various home remedies including hot tea and honey, cough drops, and gargles. He also stated that he had a previous prolonged coughing episode 1 year ago that eventually was treated with several courses of antibiotics, which did not seem to help, but he gradually improved with codeine cough syrup. The patient denies chest pains, palpitations, orthopnea, fevers, discolored sputum, wheezing, and hemoptysis. He admits to gradually reduced exercise tolerance, some achy chest tightness especially after coughing spells, and low mood.

Past Medical History: The patient states that he has sinus infections two to three times per year, and had one episode of pneumonia associated with

FEV$_1$, forced expiratory volume in 1 second.

influenza. He has had allergic rhinitis symptoms in the spring and fall. He stopped smoking 6 months ago after smoking a pack of cigarettes a day from age 17, and has had work-related exposure to paint fumes for almost 40 years.

Physical Examination: Findings are as follows: temperature of 98°F, blood pressure of 150/85 mm Hg, heart rate of 88 beats/min, and respirations of 20 breaths/min. Body mass index (BMI) is 32 kg/m^2. Throat exam revealed a red oral pharynx with cobblestoning on the posterior pharyngeal wall. Sinuses are nontender and nasal turbinates are not enlarged. There is no cervical adenopathy or thyroid hypertrophy. Heart tones are slightly muffled but regular in rate and rhythm, without murmur or gallop. Lung fields are clear with symmetrical, slightly coarse breath sounds and no wheezes, rhonchi, or rales. When asked to accentuate his exhalation, the patient develops a prolonged coughing paroxysm and appears to have difficulty catching his breath.

Additional Testing: Laboratory tests are normal except for an elevated eosinophil count in the white blood cell differential. Chest radiograph is within normal limits. Spirometry is significant for mildly reduced FEV$_1$, but otherwise normal flows and volumes.

CASE STUDY 11.1 THOUGHT QUESTIONS
- *What risk factors for chronic bronchitis does this patient have?*
- *What is the pathogenesis of chronic bronchitis in a patient with a smoking history?*

BRIDGE TO CLINICAL PRACTICE

Ben Cocchiaro

PRINCIPLES OF ASSESSMENT

History and Physical Examination

- *Dyspnea:* Ask about duration, triggers, co-occurring symptoms, and functional limitations imposed by shortness of breath.
- *Cough:* Note the duration of any cough, presence of sputum, and any acute changes in sputum color. Ask about hemoptysis and clarify its amount and appearance. Examine the posterior oropharynx for signs of cobblestoning or postnasal drip, which might indicate a diagnosis of upper airway cough syndrome.
- *Physical appearance:* Look for digital clubbing, pallor, cyanosis, nicotine stains on the teeth or fingernails, use of accessory respiratory muscles, tracheal deviation, jugular venous distention, and large neck circumference.
- *Auscultation:* Breath sounds are best auscultated in the posterior intercostal spaces over the apices, superior and inferior lobes, and the lung bases. Unilateral inspiratory rales or crackles may indicate pneumonia, whereas similar sounds found at both lung bases could indicate pulmonary edema and fluid overload.

Diagnostic Tools

- *Spo$_2$ (oxygen saturation):* This test is an inexpensive proxy for oxygenation. Notable shortcomings include failure to account for hypercapnia, inability to distinguish between oxygen and carbon monoxide hemoglobin binding, and limited correlation with arterial Po$_2$.
- *PFTs:* These tests include spirometry, which measures respiratory flow loops, differentiating obstructive lung diseases such as asthma and COPD from restrictive conditions such as interstitial lung disease or sarcoidosis.
- *CXR:* Quick and inexpensive, CXR is a useful first-line study in the diagnosis of pneumonia, pleural effusion, pneumothorax, tuberculosis, and some malignancies.
- *Lung CT:* More sensitive than CXR (at the cost of exposing the patient to 70× more radiation), chest CT with intravenous contrast agent is the first-line test in the emergent evaluation of suspected pulmonary embolism.
- *Bronchoscopy:* This diagnostic and therapeutic procedure, performed by pulmonologists, visualizes the endobronchial tree and allows for both bronchial and transbronchial biopsies to be obtained.

Laboratory Evaluation

- *Thoracentesis:* This invasive procedure is used to remove fluid from the intrapleural space. Laboratory evaluation of extracted fluid can differentiate malignant, infectious, and cardiac causes.
- *D-dimer:* This sensitive though nonspecific quantitation of fibrin degradation products occasionally is used to rule out deep vein thrombosis and pulmonary embolism when pretest probability is low.
- *Sputum culture:* This test is used in the diagnosis of hospital-acquired lower respiratory tract infections. Normal respiratory flora is often a contaminant, making diagnosis by culture of expectorated sputum difficult unless samples are obtained by bronchoscopy.

MAJOR DRUG CLASSES AND THERAPEUTIC MODALITIES

- *Steroids:* Both oral (e.g., prednisone) and inhaled (e.g., fluticasone, mometasone) steroid preparations are used in the treatment of inflammatory lung conditions. Inhaled corticosteroids are preferred due to the adverse effects associated with systemic corticosteroid therapy.
- *Bronchodilators:* These medications include long-acting (e.g., formoterol) and short-acting (e.g., albuterol) β-receptor agonists as well as anticholinergic agents (e.g., tiotropium, ipratropium). They are mainstays in treating asthma and COPD, and are often administered in combination with inhaled corticosteroids.
- *Antitussives:* Both central (dextromethorphan, codeine) and peripherally acting (benzonatate) agents have been employed in the symptomatic treatment of cough.
- *Oxygen:* Oxygen is used in the treatment of both acute and chronic hypoxemia secondary to pulmonary disease. The risks of oxygen-induced hypercapnia in patients with COPD and oxygen-induced free radical damage are often overlooked.
- *CPAP:* This modality is used in the management of obstructive sleep apnea.

COPD, chronic obstructive pulmonary disease; CPAP, continuous positive airway pressure; CXR, chest x-ray exam; PFTs, pulmonary function tests.

KEY POINTS

- The respiratory system encompasses lungs and the surrounding structures of the pleural space, chest wall, and diaphragm. Lung inflation depends on an intact nervous system and connections with spinal and brainstem motor neurons innervating the muscles of respiration, particularly the diaphragm and external intercostal muscles.

- Several mechanisms, including a mucus blanket over the ciliated airway epithelium, protect the lungs from inhaled particulate matter and pathogens.

- Lung and chest wall properties and neuromuscular strength of respiratory muscles determine the capacity for airflow and volume inspired and expired. Pulmonary function testing reports these volumes and capacities as part of lung assessment.

- The lungs are highly compliant, easily expanding during inspiration and recoiling during expiration with appropriate volume changes driven by relatively small pressure gradients.

- Pathophysiological loss of lung compliance limits the lungs' ability to expand, requiring extra effort to inflate the lungs and decreasing measured lung volumes. This is characteristic of acute surfactant deficiency or chronic fibrotic or infiltrative lesions of lung tissue.

- In emphysema, breakdown of lung elastin and other connective tissue fibers increases lung compliance and enlarges lung air spaces, hampering gas exchange. Inflation of the lungs is very easy, but elastic recoil is poor and emptying the lungs is difficult. Air trapping enlarges lung volumes.

- The airways are relatively low-resistance passageways and only small pressure changes are needed to move air in and out with normal quiet breathing. The main measure of airway function is the volume of air exhaled in the first second of a maximal expiratory effort (called a forced expiratory maneuver). The FEV_1 stresses the airways by surrounding them with positive pleural pressure. This tends to collapse the airways as lung volume decreases. Disorders of airway resistance are known as obstructive diseases.

- Airway smooth muscle is controlled by the autonomic nervous system, with sympathetic stimulation causing bronchodilation via β-adrenergic receptors, and parasympathetic stimulation causing bronchoconstriction via muscarinic receptors.

- Asthma is the principal acute obstructive disorder. It usually results from type 1 hypersensitivity (IgE/mast cell mediated), with airway narrowing after antigen exposure caused by mast cell degranulation, leukocyte recruitment, and prostaglandin and leukotriene production. Mucosal swelling, excess mucus production, and bronchoconstriction cause airway obstruction in the acute phase. A late phase may be refractory to pharmacological management. Between asthma attacks, the airways may still be hyperresponsive to bronchoconstricting stimuli.

- COPD is the principal chronic obstructive disorder. In COPD with emphysema, airflow obstruction occurs from premature collapse of weak airways and loss of elastic tethering by surrounding alveoli. In chronic bronchitis, bronchial mucus production is excessive, and small airways have reactive bronchial smooth muscle.

- First-line management strategies in obstructive diseases include inhaled corticosteroids to suppress inflammatory responses and long-acting bronchodilators.

- OSA is the most common form of sleep-disordered breathing. It is more common in those who are obese and in older adults. Repeated episodes of apnea and hypoxia during the night cause recurrent spikes of sympathetic nervous system activity, blood pressure, and heart rate. These episodes, in turn, increase cardiovascular morbidity and mortality risks.

- Alveolar ventilation is the process of air entry during inspiration, refreshing the alveolar P_{O_2}. Air exit during expiration reduces the alveolar P_{CO_2}. The continual renewal of O_2 and removal of CO_2 create a partial pressure gradient between alveolar air and blood perfusing the alveolar capillaries. Diffusion of the gases across the alveolar–capillary membrane causes the blood gas composition leaving the alveolar capillary to be higher in O_2 and lower in CO_2 as it leaves the lungs.

- As oxygen diffuses from alveolar air to pulmonary capillary blood, it binds to red blood cell Hb for transport to the tissues. The match of alveolar ventilation to blood perfusion determines the alveolar P_{O_2}, which in term determines the percent saturation of Hb with oxygen and the arterial P_{O_2}.

- Lung disease can result in low blood O_2 levels in a variety of ways. Some of these are failure of adequate neuromuscular activation of muscles of respiration, alveolar–capillary membrane thickness increasing and reducing gas diffusion, shunt-like regions of lung that receive no ventilation but still receive blood flow, and ventilation/perfusion mismatching, with some alveolar units and lung regions receiving too little ventilation for the amount of blood flow they receive, and others having too much ventilation in poorly perfused alveoli.

- The lung vasculature is a richly branched bed that accommodates the entire cardiac output of the right side of the heart, surrounding each of the millions of alveoli with blood flow for oxygenation and CO_2 removal. Regional lung blood flow is sensitive to local Po_2, with hypoxia leading to vasoconstriction, and to gravity, with the greatest flow going to the dependent lung regions.
- Pulmonary vascular pressures are substantially lower than systemic vascular pressures, and the right side of the heart has a thinner wall consistent with its lighter workload. Increased pulmonary vascular pressures can result from heart failure, leading to pulmonary congestion and ultimately pulmonary edema. On the other hand, increased pulmonary vasoconstriction due to hypoxic lung disease can cause secondary heart failure.
- The lung circulation is vulnerable to blockage by emboli, usually arising from deep vein thromboses that embolize. Pulmonary emboli can be small and spontaneously resolving, whereas others are large and lead to hypoxemia and cardiovascular instability.
- The two major forms of pulmonary edema are cardiogenic and noncardiogenic. The cardiogenic form is secondary to heart failure with elevated left-sided heart pressures that subsequently elevate pulmonary capillary hydrostatic pressure, promoting edema formation. The noncardiogenic form is associated with sepsis and the acute respiratory distress syndrome, in which excessive release of inflammatory mediators increases pulmonary capillary permeability and destroys alveolar integrity, leading to alveolar flooding even at normal alveolar capillary hydrostatic pressures.
- Pulmonary hypertension is a common finding in several lung diseases because of hypoxic vasoconstriction. Idiopathic pulmonary hypertension is a rare, disabling disease of unknown mechanism. It is treated with vasodilators.
- Although much lung development occurs prenatally, extensive alveolization occurs postnatally. Infants born preterm have very underdeveloped lungs, and those born at or before 25 weeks of gestational age will also lack surfactant, with very low lung compliance. These infants have a high risk of BPD that can predispose them to later life lung dysfunction.
- Infant bronchiolitis is generally infection-related and usually resolves spontaneously.
- Asthma often begins in childhood, and can have greater airflow limitations owing to the smaller airways in children.
- Older adults have normal age-related reductions in compliance, resistance, alveolar recoil, and chest wall compliance. Those factors, combined with increased aspiration and decreased mucociliary clearance and cough efficacy, predispose to greater risk of pneumonia and greater pneumonia-associated morbidity and mortality.

REFERENCES

1. National Center for Health Statistics. National Health Interview Survey 2017. Public-use data file and documentation. https://https://www.cdc.gov/nchs/nhis/nhis_2017_data_release.htm. Accessed January 4, 2020.
2. Murphy SL, Xu JQ, Kochanek KD, Arias E. *Mortality in the United States, 2017 [NCHS Data Brief No. 328].* Hyattsville, MD: National Center for Health Statistics; 2018. https://www.cdc.gov/nchs/data/databriefs/db328-h.pdf.
3. GBD 2016 Disease and Injury Incidence and Prevalence Collaborators. Global, regional, and national incidence, prevalence, and years lived with disability for 328 diseases and injuries for 195 countries, 1991–2016: a systematic analysis for the Global Burden of Disease Study 2016. *Lancet.* 2017;390:1211–1259. doi:10.1016/S0140-6736(17)32154-2.
4. Jetté M, Sidney K, Blümchen G. Metabolic equivalents (METS) in exercise testing, exercise prescription, and evaluation of functional capacity. *Clin Cardiol.* 1990;13:555–565. doi:10.1002/clc.4960130809.
5. Dempsey JA, Jacques AJ. Respiratory system response to exercise in health. In: Grippi MA, Elias JA, Fishman JA, et al., eds. *Fishman's Pulmonary Diseases and Disorders.* Vol 1. 5th ed. New York, NY: McGraw-Hill; 2015:219–232.
6. Baby's First Test. Cystic fibrosis. https://www.babysfirsttest.org/newborn-screening/conditions/cystic-fibrosis-cf. Accessed July 28, 2019.
7. Derichs N. Targeting a genetic defect: cystic fibrosis transmembrane conductance regulator modulators in cystic fibrosis. *Eur Respir Rev.* 2013;22:58–65. doi:10.1183/09059180.00008412.
8. Lopes-Pacheco M. CFTR modulators: shedding light on precision medicine for cystic fibrosis. *Front Pharmacol.* 2016;7:275. doi:10.3389/fphar.2016.00275.

9. Plantier L, Cazes A, Dinh-Xuan AT, et al. Physiology of the lung in idiopathic pulmonary fibrosis. *Eur Respir Rev.* 2018;27:170062. doi:10.1183/16000617.0062-2017.

10. Richeldi L, Collard HR, Jones MG. Idiopathic pulmonary fibrosis. *Lancet.* 2017;389:1941–1952. doi:10.1016/S0140-6736(17)30866-8.

11. Papi A, Brightling C, Pedersen SE, Reddel HK. Asthma. *Lancet.* 2018;391:783–800. doi:10.1016/S0140-6736(17)33311-1.

12. Erle DJ, Sheppard D. The cell biology of asthma. *J Cell Biol.* 2014;205:621–631. doi:10.1083/jcb.201401050.

13. Global Initiative for Chronic Obstructive Lung Disease. Global strategy for the diagnosis, management, and prevention of chronic obstructive pulmonary disease: 2019 report. https://goldcopd.org/wp-content/uploads/2018/11/GOLD-2019-v1.7-FINAL-14Nov2018-WMS.pdf. Published 2019. Accessed July 28, 2019.

14. Rabe KF, Watz H. Chronic obstructive pulmonary disease. *Lancet.* 2017;389:1931–1940. doi:10.1016/S0140-6736(17)31222-9.

15. Riley CM, Sciurba FC. Diagnosis and outpatient management of chronic obstructive pulmonary disease. A review. *JAMA.* 2019;321:786–797. doi:10.1001/jama.2019.0131.

16. Duffy SP, Criner GJ. Chronic obstructive pulmonary disease. Evaluation and management. *Med Clin North Am.* 2019;103:453–461. doi:10.1016/j.mcna.2018.12.005.

17. Senaratna CV, Perret JL, Lodge CJ, et al. Prevalence of obstructive sleep apnea in the general population: a systematic review. *Sleep Med Rev.* 2017;34:70–81. doi:10.1016/j.smrv.2016.07.002.

18. Berry RB, Wagner MH. Fundamentals 19: diagnosis of obstructive sleep apnea syndromes in adults. In: Berry RB, Wagner MH, eds. *Sleep Medicine Pearls.* 3rd ed. Philadelphia, PA: Saunders/Elsevier; 2014:208–214.

19. Eckert DJ, Malhotra A. Pathophysiology of adult obstructive sleep apnea. *Proc Am Thorac Soc.* 2008;5:144–153. doi:10.1513/pats.200707-114MG.

20. Javaheri S, Barbe F, Campos-Rodriguez F, et al. Sleep apnea: types, mechanisms, and clinical cardiovascular consequences. *J Am Coll Cardiol.* 2017;69:841–858. doi:10.1016/j.jacc.2016.11.069.

21. Mescher AL. *Junquieira's Basic Histology Text & Atlas.* 15th ed. New York, NY: McGraw-Hill; 2018.

22. Woodworth A. The respiratory system. In: Laposata M, ed. *Laboratory Medicine: The Diagnosis of Disease in the Clinical Laboratory.* New York, NY: McGraw-Hill; 2014:317–326.

23. Naureckas ET, Solway J. Disturbances of respiratory function. In: Jameson JL, Fauci AS, Kasper DL, et al., eds. *Harrison's Principles of Internal Medicine.* 20th ed. New York, NY: McGraw-Hill; 2018:chap 279.

24. Rodriguez-Roisin R, Ferrer A. Effect of mechanical ventilation on gas exchange. In: Tobin MJ, ed. *Principles and Practice of Mechanical Ventilation.* 3rd ed. New York, NY: McGraw-Hill; 2013:851–868.

25. Taichman DB, Mandel J, Smith KA, Yuan JX-J. Pulmonary arterial hypertension. In: Grippi MA, Elias JA, Fishman JA, et al., eds. *Fishman's Pulmonary Diseases and Disorders.* Vol 1. 5th ed. New York, NY: McGraw-Hill; 2015:1064–1109.

26. Weitzenblum E, Chaouat A. Cor pulmonale. *Chron Respir Dis.* 2009;6:177–185. doi:10.1177/1479972309104664.

27. Giordano NJ, Jansson PS, Young MN, et al. Epidemiology, pathophysiology, stratification, and natural history of pulmonary embolism. *Tech Vasc Interv Radiol.* 2017;20:135–140. doi:10.1053/j.tvir.2017.07.002.

28. Essien EO, Rali P, Mathai SC. Pulmonary embolism. *Med Clin North Am.* 2019;103:549–564. doi:10.1016/j.mcna.2018.12.013.

29. Yang CY, Chen CS, Yiang GT, et al. New insights into the immune molecular regulation of the pathogenesis of acute respiratory distress syndrome. *Int J Mol Sci.* 2018;19:588. doi:10.3390/ijms19020588.

30. Huppert LA, Matthay MA, Ware LB. Pathogenesis of acute respiratory distress syndrome. *Semin Respir Crit Care Med.* 2019;40:31–39. doi:10.1055/s-0039-1683996.

31. Foshat M, Boroumand N. The evolving classification of pulmonary hypertension. *Arch Pathol Lab Med.* 2017;141:696–703. doi:10.5858/arpa.2016-0035-RA.

32. Dodson MW, Brown LM, Elliott CG. Pulmonary arterial hypertension. *Heart Fail Clin.* 2018;14:255–269. doi:10.1016/j.hfc.2018.02.003.

33. Schittny JC. Development of the lung. *Cell Tissue Res.* 2017;367:427–444. doi:10.1007/s00441-016-2545-0.

34. Hameed A, Sherkheli MA, Hussain A, Ul-haq R. Molecular and physiological determinants of pulmonary developmental biology: a review. *Am J Biomed Res.* 2013;1:13–24. doi:10.12691/ajbr-1-1-3.

35. Ochs M, O'Brodovich H. The structural and physiologic basis of respiratory disease. In: Wilmott RW, Deterding R, Li A, et al., eds. *Kendig's Disorders of the Respiratory Tract in Children.* 9th ed. Philadelphia, PA: Elsevier; 2018:63–100.

36. Davidson LM, Berkelhamer SK. Bronchopulmonary dysplasia: chronic lung disease of infancy and long-term pulmonary outcomes. *J Clin Med.* 2017;6:4. doi:10.3390/jcm6010004.

37. Greenberg JM, Haberman B, Narendran V, et al. Neonatal morbidities of prenatal and perinatal origin. In: Resnik R, Lockwood CJ, Moore TR, et al., eds. *Creasy and Resnik's Maternal–Fetal Medicine: Principles and Practice.* 8th ed. Philadelphia, PA: Elsevier; 2018:1309–1333.

38. Øymar K, Skjerven HO, Mikalsen IB. Acute bronchiolitis in infants, a review. *Scand J Trauma Resusc Emerg Med.* 2014;22:23. doi:10.1186/1757-7241-22-23.

39. Zahran HS, Bailey CM, Damon SA, et al. Vital signs: asthma in children—United States, 2001–2016. *MMWR Morb Mortal Wkly Rep.* 2018;67:149–155. doi:10.15585/mmwr.mm6705e1.

40. Skloot GS. The effects of aging on lung structure and function. *Clin Geriatr Med.* 2017;33:447–457. doi:10.1016/j.cger.2017.06.001.

41. Campbell EJ. Aging of the respiratory system. In: Grippi MA, Elias JA, Fishman JA, et al., eds. *Fishman's Pulmonary Diseases and Disorders.* Vol 1. 5th ed. New York, NY: McGraw-Hill; 2015:233–244.

42. Lalley PM. The aging respiratory system—pulmonary structure, function and neural control. *Respir Physiol Neurobiol.* 2013;187:199–210. doi:10.1016/j.resp.2013.03.012.

43. El Chakhtoura NG, Bonomo RA, Jump RLP. Influence of aging and environment on presentation of infection in older adults. *Infect Dis Clin North Am.* 2017;31:593–608. doi:10.1016/j.idc.2017.07.017.

44. Centers for Disease Control and Prevention. Chronic obstructive pulmonary disease among adults—United States,2011.*MMWR Morb Mortal Wkly Rep.*2012;61:938–943. https://www.cdc.gov/mmwr/preview/mmwrhtml/mm6146a2.htm.

SUGGESTED RESOURCES

Global Initiative for Chronic Obstructive Lung Disease (GOLD-COPD). https://goldcopd.org.

Heckman EJ, O'Connor GT. Pulmonary function tests for diagnosing lung disease. *JAMA.* 2015;313:2278–2279. doi:10.1001/jama.2015.4466.

Johnson JD, Theurer WM. A stepwise approach to the interpretation of pulmonary function tests. *Am Fam Physician.* 2014;89:359–366. https://www.aafp.org/afp/2014/0301/p359.html.

Levitzky MG. *Pulmonary Physiology.* 9th ed. New York, NY: McGraw-Hill; 2018.FVC, forced vital capacity.

12

KIDNEYS

Connie B. Scanga and Nancy C. Tkacs

THE CLINICAL CONTEXT

The worldwide and U.S. incidence and prevalence of kidney disease are very high and encompass these variations: (a) chronic kidney disease (CKD), comprising five stages from mild disease to kidney failure; (b) end-stage renal disease (ESRD)—stage 5 of the CKD continuum, requiring treatment by dialysis or transplantation; and (c) acute kidney injury (AKI).

A recent report of the U.S. Renal Disease System (www.usrds.org), which tracks statistics on kidney disease in the United States, found the prevalence of CKD (all stages) to be 15%, with 7% of patients in stages 3 (moderate) to 5 (kidney failure). Stage 3 kidney disease is by far the most common, affecting about 6% of the U.S. population. Most deaths in patients with CKD occur before they reach ESRD, and the most common causes of death are cardiovascular disease and cancer. ESRD prevalence in the United States was relatively low at about 726,000 cases at the end of 2016.[1] AKI is increasing in developed countries and is generally managed by hospitalization and inpatient care. In community settings, AKI prevalence that leads to hospital admission is estimated at 4.3%; however, this may not capture all patients sustaining AKI.[2] In critical care patients, AKI prevalence is estimated at 60%. Many acute conditions can precipitate AKI, including severe myocardial infarction, shock, adverse drug effects and drug interactions, and radiocontrast dye–initiated reactions.

Older adults and individuals with CKD are vulnerable to AKI secondary to drug-induced kidney injury or critical illness. Monitoring and appropriate care and medication choices are the best prevention strategies against kidney injuries in vulnerable patients.

OVERVIEW OF KIDNEY STRUCTURE AND FUNCTION

THE KIDNEY AND HOMEOSTASIS

The kidneys play essential roles in maintaining homeostasis. In young adults, each kidney has about 1 million nephrons, and the presence of two kidneys provides a redundancy that makes it possible to donate a kidney and still maintain near-normal renal function for the rest of one's life. Although there is a normal, progressive loss of nephrons with aging, the ability of healthy adults to donate a kidney, even up to the age of 70, indicates that there is substantial reserve capacity in renal function. Loss of nephrons is generally compensated by hypertrophy and increased activity of the remaining nephrons. In certain conditions, such as diabetes mellitus and hypertension, this increase in individual nephron activity may ultimately provoke a cycle of nephron damage and loss leading to greater vulnerability of the remaining nephrons.

The kidneys regulate the volume of water in the body as well as the composition of body fluids. In this chapter, we review key information about body fluid compartments, the kidneys' role in maintaining fluid and solute homeostasis, and renal pathophysiology underlying common clinical conditions.

A prominent role of the kidney is to help maintain fluid balance by varying urine output. This activity is coupled with and dependent on regulated secretion and reabsorption of solutes, which maintains normal osmolarity and electrolyte concentrations in the blood. The kidney excretes nitrogenous wastes and acid generated by protein metabolism. It also helps to regulate blood pH through its handling of hydrogen (H^+) and bicarbonate (HCO_3^-) ions during urine production. The renal tubules are enriched in membrane transport proteins that reabsorb filtered nutrients needed for body metabolism, and transporters that add metabolic wastes (creatinine, uric acid, conjugated bilirubin, conjugated steroid hormones, and sulfuric acid) and drug metabolites to the urine for excretion. Several tubular transporters are the targets of diuretic drugs as well as drugs used to treat diabetes and gout.

The kidneys play a key role in calcium homeostasis. It is in the kidneys that vitamin D is converted to its biologically active form, calcitriol, which is an important hormone regulator of bone remodeling and calcium absorption in the small intestines. Parathyroid hormone increases the rate of vitamin D activation and also regulates calcium and phosphate transport in the kidney, further ensuring normal blood calcium levels are maintained. The kidneys are also the primary regulator of red blood cell production (erythropoiesis). In response to hypoxia, kidney cells release erythropoietin, the hormone that stimulates erythropoiesis in the bone marrow. Last, and certainly not least, the kidneys secrete the enzyme renin. The renin-angiotensin-aldosterone system (RAAS) plays a key role in blood pressure and blood volume regulation.

OVERVIEW OF BODY FLUID COMPARTMENTS

Water: The Solvent of Body Fluids

Water fulfills varied roles in the body and is essential for life. Many of the body's key metabolic reactions unfold in an aqueous environment, with water participating in the biochemical reactions (e.g., hydrolysis of large organic molecules) or being produced by chemical reactions (e.g., water production in the mitochondria at the end of the electron transport chain), or both. Water is an excellent solvent and transports nutrients, waste products, blood gases, electrolytes, hormones, and other essential solutes through the body. It serves as a lubricant, reducing friction between adjacent tissues and organs and in the joints. Water has a high specific heat, which means that it can resist temperature changes; this helps us maintain a core temperature ideally suited to human metabolism.

Various factors—including sex, age, body mass, and body composition—determine one's total body water (TBW). Water accounts for over half of the total body mass of most adults. Adipose tissue is a hydrophobic

tissue and contains the least water of all body tissues, while skeletal muscle contains the most. As a result, the relative adiposity of an individual is the main determinant of his or her TBW. Women tend to have less muscle and more adipose tissue than men, so the average woman has less TBW than the average man. Older adults tend to lose muscle mass and accumulate adipose tissue, so the average TBW may decrease with age.

Distribution of Fluids in the Body

Water is dispersed through the cells, tissues, and organs of the body, with the notable exception of fat cells, which contain very little water. For practical purposes, however, it is considered to be contained within two main aggregate compartments, intracellular and extracellular, which are separated by physical barriers (e.g., plasma membranes) and have unique solute compositions (**Table 12.1, Figure 12.1**).

Intracellular fluid (ICF), body water contained within the body cells, represents approximately two thirds of the TBW. Extracellular fluid (ECF), all the body fluid outside the cells, constitutes approximately

TABLE 12.1 Main Electrolytes of the Body Fluid Compartments

Electrolytes	ICF (mOsm/L H_2O)	ECF (mOsm/L H_2O) Plasma Fluid	ECF (mOsm/L H_2O) Interstitial Fluid
Cations			
Sodium (Na^+)	14	142	139
Potassium (K^+)	140	4.2	4.0
Calcium (Ca^{2+})	0	1.3	1.2
Magnesium (Mg^{2+})	20	0.8	0.7
Anions			
Chloride (Cl^-)	5	106	108
Bicarbonate (HCO_3^-)	10	24	28.3
Mono- and dihydrogen phosphate (HPO_4^{2-}, $H_2PO_4^-$)	11	2	2
Proteins	4	1.2	0.2

ECF, extracellular fluid; ICF, intracellular fluid.
Source: Adapted with permission from Hall JE, ed. *Guyton and Hall Textbook of Medical Physiology.* 13th ed. Philadelphia, PA: Saunders Elsevier; 2016.

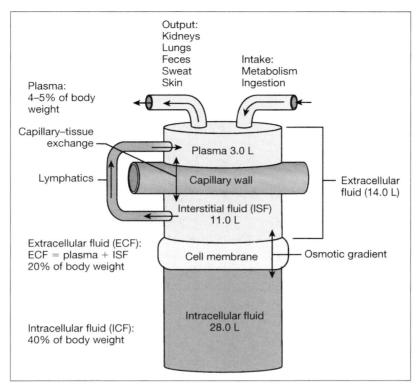

FIGURE 12.1 Body fluid distribution. Water and solutes make up 55% to 60% of body weight in adults. The aqueous compartments are made up of ECF (including plasma and interstitial fluid) and ICF. ECF moves between the plasma and interstitial space by filtration and reabsorption across the capillary membrane and via the lymphatics. Movement of water between the ICF and ECF compartments involves osmosis across cell plasma membranes.

one third of the TBW. The ECF is itself subdivided into discrete compartments: interstitial fluid, blood plasma, and transcellular fluids. Interstitial fluid (the fluid that surrounds and bathes the body cells) and blood plasma (the fluid portion of the blood) constitute approximately 80% and 20% of the ECF, respectively.

Transcellular fluid is actively secreted by cells and contained within epithelium-lined spaces in the body. Examples of transcellular fluids are cerebrospinal fluid; aqueous humor of the eye; synovial fluid; serous fluids filling the pleural, peritoneal, and pericardial cavities; lymph; and fluids in the urinary and gastrointestinal tracts. Transcellular fluids vary dramatically in their composition and function. They represent 1% to 3% of TBW and are typically not included in discussions of normal body fluid homeostasis.

The body fluids are a soupy solution of electrolyte and nonelectrolyte solutes. There are notable differences in composition of the ECF and ICF. Specifically, the ICF has high concentrations of potassium (K^+) and magnesium (Mg^{2+}) cations and relatively low concentrations of sodium (Na^+) and chloride (Cl^-) ions, while in the ECF Na^+ and Cl^- are in high concentration and K^+ and Mg^{2+} are low. The one notable difference in solute composition of the ECF subcompartments is the presence of plasma proteins. Plasma proteins are not normally able to leak out of the vascular space; thus, there is virtually no accumulation of protein molecules in interstitial fluid.

Water Movement Between Fluid Compartments

Within the body, fluid moves freely in and out of compartments along osmotic and hydrostatic pressure gradients. Osmosis, the net movement of water from one fluid compartment to another, occurs when there is a difference in solute concentration (i.e., osmolarity) between the compartments. The range of normal plasma ECF osmolarity is about 280 to 295 mOsm/L. Because the plasma membranes of cells are freely permeable to water, any change in blood plasma osmolarity creates an osmotic gradient that will draw water from one side of the plasma membrane to another (see **Figure 12.1**). For example, intravenous infusion of a hypotonic saline solution will cause solutes to be less concentrated in the plasma, creating a difference in osmolarity between the ECF and ICF. As a result, water will be drawn across the plasma membrane into cells, attracted to the hypertonic ICF. The net movement of water from the ECF to the ICF will continue until the osmolarities of the two fluid compartments are again equal; at this point there will be no further net movement of water between compartments. Note that as a result of the hypotonic infusion, the *volume* of both the ECF and ICF will increase while the *osmolarity* of both compartments decreases.

KIDNEY STRUCTURE

The kidneys are bilateral bean-shaped organs positioned in the retroperitoneal space against the posterior wall of the abdominal cavity on either side of the vertebral column. They extend from approximately the 12th thoracic to the third lumbar level, and the right kidney is usually slightly inferior to the left owing to the presence of the liver in the right upper quadrant of the abdominal cavity. The renal hilum, an indentation on the medial side of the kidney, opens into the renal sinus and is the site where the renal artery and veins, ureter, nerves, and lymphatics enter and leave the kidney (**Figure 12.2**).

Internally, there are three distinct regions in the kidney: cortex, medulla, and sinus. The outermost region, the renal cortex, has a grainy appearance and is densely packed with small blood vessels and renal glomeruli. Deep to the renal cortex is the renal medulla, composed of a variable number (seven to 18) of conical structures, called the renal pyramids and the renal columns. Renal tubules fill the pyramids; the distal structures of the renal tubular system are ducts

that empty urine into minor calyces. Renal columns, extensions of the renal cortex that pass between the pyramids, anchor the pyramids and provide passages for blood vessels supplying the nephrons. Each renal pyramid empties urine into a minor calyx. Minor calyces converge to form major calyces, which in turn converge to form the renal pelvis. Urine drains out of the pelvis of the kidney to a ureter. The renal calyces and pelvis occupy the innermost region of the kidney, the renal sinus.

NEPHRON STRUCTURE

At birth, each kidney contains approximately 1 million nephrons; from this maximum, the number slowly decreases as we age. Nephrons are the microscopic *workhorses* of the kidney. Each nephron consists of two main parts, the glomerulus and the renal tubule (**Figures 12.3** and **12.4**). The glomerulus is a vascular structure with an afferent arteriole that brings blood from a small interlobular artery; a tuft of glomerular capillaries with high permeability, specialized to produce the glomerular filtrate; and an efferent arteriole with high vascular resistance that maintains high glomerular capillary hydrostatic pressure to promote filtration. The glomerulus is surrounded by an area called Bowman's space, which is further bounded by Bowman's capsule. Bowman's capsule is the starting point for the nephron tubule, consisting of a proximal tubule (PT); loop of Henle (LOH), with a thin descending limb and an ascending limb that has an initial thin

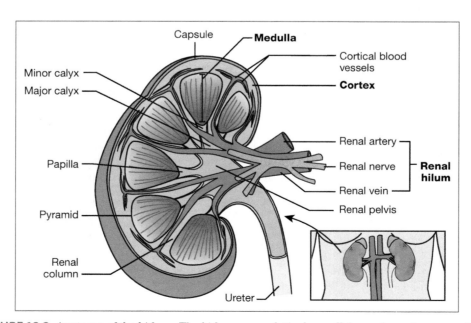

FIGURE 12.2 Anatomy of the kidney. The kidneys are relatively small, bean-shaped organs with an outer cortex, inner medulla, and hilum—the point of entry and exit for renal artery, vein, and nerve.

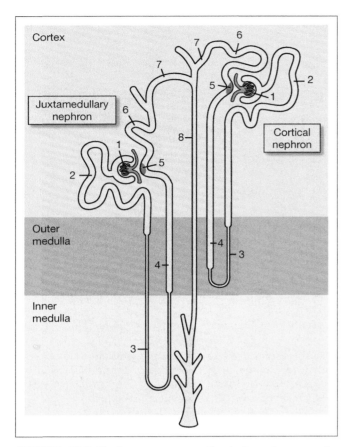

FIGURE 12.3 Nephron structure. Cortical nephrons make up 85% of the nephrons of the kidney and much of the cortical volume. Juxtamedullary nephrons have long loops of Henle that descend deep within the renal medulla, making a hairpin turn before ascending back to the glomerular region. (**1**) Glomerulus; (**2**) proximal tubule; (**3**) loop of Henle, thin descending and ascending limbs; (**4**) thick ascending limb of Henle's loop; (**5**) macula densa of the juxtaglomerular apparatus; (**6**) distal tubule; (**7**) connecting tubule; (**8**) collecting duct.

segment transitioning to the thick ascending limb (TAL); distal tubule (DT); and connecting tubule. The TAL segments contain cells that are enriched in mitochondria for oxidative energy production and use for active ion pumping. The connecting tubules of a number of nephrons drain into a single collecting duct in the cortex. Collecting ducts converge to form papillary ducts, which drain urine into a minor calyx.

Nephrons are classified as either cortical nephrons or juxtamedullary nephrons (see **Figure 12.3**). Cortical nephrons, which are the predominant nephron type, have glomeruli located in the outer cortex and a relatively short LOH that extends only into the superficial medulla. Most of the secretory and reabsorptive activities required for urine production are conducted by cortical nephrons. Juxtamedullary nephrons have

glomeruli located near the corticomedullary junction and long LOHs that dip deep into the medulla. Although they make up only 15% of all nephrons, the juxtamedullary nephrons confer the essential ability to vary urine concentration and volume.

GLOMERULAR FUNCTION

Glomerular Vascular Structure and Glomerular Filtration Barriers

The kidneys are highly vascular organs, receiving over 1 L/min of blood (20% to 25% of resting cardiac output), carried from the abdominal aorta into the organs via the renal arteries. Inside the kidney, the renal artery branches into successively smaller arteries, the smallest of which are the interlobular arteries that extend outward through the renal cortex. Afferent arterioles branch off interlobular arteries and carry blood into the glomerulus. Blood leaves the glomerulus through an efferent arteriole; the short efferent arteriole branches almost immediately to form a network of peritubular capillaries that surround the proximal and distal convoluted tubules of the nephron. After percolating slowly through peritubular capillaries, blood is carried into interlobular veins in the renal cortex and from there flows through successively larger veins, ultimately leaving the kidney to flow into the inferior vena cava via the renal vein. The efferent arterioles of juxtamedullary nephrons branch to form the vasa recta capillaries perfusing the LOH and collecting ducts of the medulla.

The glomerulus is the site where urine formation begins (**Figure 12.5**). Here, fluid and small solutes are forced out of the blood into the capsular space, forming filtrate that will subsequently be modified to become urine in the renal tubule (**Figure 12.5a**). Glomerular filtration occurs across the *filtration membrane*, a functional barrier consisting of three layers (**Figures 12.5b** and **12.6**). Innermost are the endothelial cells forming the glomerular capillary wall; outermost are the podocytes composing the visceral layer of Bowman's capsule. Sandwiched between them is the glomerular basement membrane, which anchors the two cell layers together and helps regulate solute movement across the filtration membrane.

The glomerular capillaries are fenestrated (i.e., there are large gaps between endothelial cells that facilitate solute movement out of the capillaries), making the glomerular capillaries much more permeable to solutes than the continuous capillaries found in most other parts of the systemic circulation. The basement membrane surrounding the capillaries is rich in negatively charged molecules that repel passage of many of the larger negatively charged plasma proteins. The outermost layer of the filtration

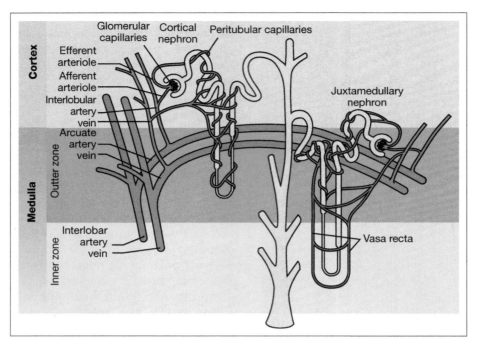

FIGURE 12.4 Nephron-associated blood vessels. Each nephron is supplied by an afferent arteriole that gives rise to the glomerular capillary cluster, ending in an efferent arteriole that gives rise to the peritubular capillaries. The glomerular capillaries are the site of filtration—movement of water and solutes out of the vascular space and into Bowman's space. The peritubular capillaries are the site of reabsorption of water and solutes transported across the tubular epithelium to the interstitial space, followed by bulk flow into capillaries. The vasa recta are specialized peritubular capillaries of juxtamedullary nephrons.

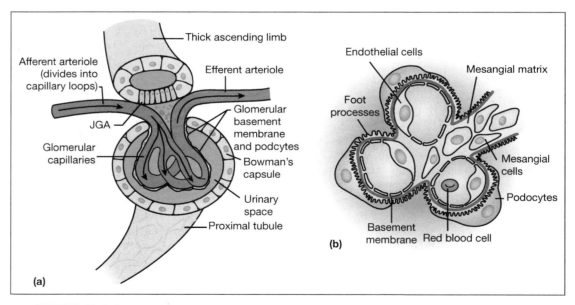

FIGURE 12.5 Glomerular structure. (**a**) The glomerular capillary loops are the major functional components of the glomerulus. They are surrounded by mesangial cells and Bowman's space. As the glomerular filtrate forms, pressure in Bowman's space rises, pushing the filtrate into the proximal tubule and down the remaining nephron tubule. At the junction of the afferent and efferent arterioles, the thick ascending limb of the nephron passes between the two vessels, forming the JGA. The JGA cells monitor nephron processing of the filtrate and initiate homeostatic adjustments. (**b**) A cross section through a capillary loop shows the glomerular capillary filtration barrier, composed of endothelial cells, basement membrane, and foot processes of adjacent podocyte cells. Mesangial cells provide the supporting structure for the capillaries and podocytes. JGA, juxtaglomerular apparatus.

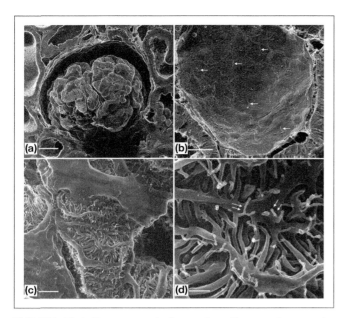

FIGURE 12.6 Structure of glomerulus, Bowman's capsule, and podocytes. **(a)** Electron micrograph shows the capillary tuft in Bowman's capsule. **(b)** After glomerular capillaries are removed, epithelial cells of Bowman's capsule are visible, with cilia indicated by arrows. **(c)** View of podocytes with extensive processes wrapping around glomerular capillaries. **(d)** Close-up view of podocyte foot processes separated by fine slits that form the final filtration barrier to fluid entering the tubule system. Arrows indicate protrusions from podocytes into Bowman's space. Scale bars in each panel indicate the following dimensions: (a) 20 μm, (b) 10 μm, (c) 2 μm, and (d) 0.5 μm.

Source: From Rice WL, et al. High resolution helium ion scanning microscopy of the rat kidney. *PLoS One.* 2013;8(3):e57051. https://doi.org/10.1371/journal.pone.0057051

membrane is also quite porous. The cells of this layer (podocytes) are characterized by cellular extensions, called foot processes, that wrap around the capillary–basement membrane structures, leaving narrow filtration slits between adjacent cell processes that block the filtration of all but the smallest proteins.

Glycoproteins cross the openings of the capillary fenestrations and filtration slits, restricting the size of molecules that can move through the filtration membrane. These glycoproteins carry a negative charge, which helps to restrict movement of similarly charged plasma proteins (e.g., albumin) into the filtrate. Of the three layers of filtration barrier, the filtration slits are the smallest and represent the major barrier to protein movement into the urine space. Compared with continuous capillaries found elsewhere in the body, the relatively permeable nature of all of these structures promotes a high rate of glomerular filtration needed for renal function.

Mesangial cells are found between loops of glomerular capillaries. These cells are able to synthesize extracellular matrix, to conduct phagocytosis, and to contract and alter the glomerular capillary resistance and surface area. These cells and capillary endothelial cells may proliferate in response to glomerular insults, contributing to glomerular fibrosis and reducing glomerular filtration. The high pressure and blood flow rates expose the delicate filtration barrier to damage due to loss of negative charges or deposition of antigen–antibody complexes. Such pathological changes damage the filtration barrier and allow proteins to leak into the urine. Clinically, the measurement of urine proteins is one of the most important tests of kidney function.

Filtration in the glomerulus, like filtration in the systemic capillaries, occurs because the interaction of hydrostatic and colloid osmotic pressures across the capillary wall favors an outward movement of fluid (**Figure 12.7**). The forces, called *Starling forces*, and their interaction to produce net filtration pressure are described in detail in Chapter 9, Circulation. Glomerular filtration rate (GFR) is a measure of the total filtrate formed per minute in both kidneys. GFR varies with age, sex, and body size. A normal young adult value is 90 to 120 mL/min/1.73 m^2 of body surface area, or 150 to 180 L/day. The rate of filtration is much higher than that of any other vascular bed, due to the high rate of renal blood flow (RBF) and the large surface area and high permeability of the filtration membrane in the kidneys, and is directly proportional to net filtration pressure in the glomerulus (**Figure 12.7a**).

As in the systemic capillaries, net filtration pressure represents the difference between Starling forces promoting fluid filtration and those promoting fluid reabsorption. However, net filtration pressure is much greater in the glomeruli than in the systemic capillaries because of high glomerular hydrostatic pressure. Unlike a systemic capillary bed, which lies between an arteriole and a postcapillary venule, the glomerulus is positioned between two arterioles. The efferent arteriole, which carries blood out of the glomerulus, has a smaller diameter than does the afferent arteriole carrying blood in. As a result, there is resistance to blood flow into the efferent arteriole, which maintains a high hydrostatic pressure in the glomerulus; constriction of the efferent arterioles only increases this resistance and further increases glomerular hydrostatic pressure. Both arterioles can constrict or dilate to alter their diameters and adjust blood flow into and out of the glomerulus. Afferent arteriole constriction or dilation allows the kidneys to maintain a fairly constant glomerular hydrostatic pressure despite physiological fluctuations in RBF

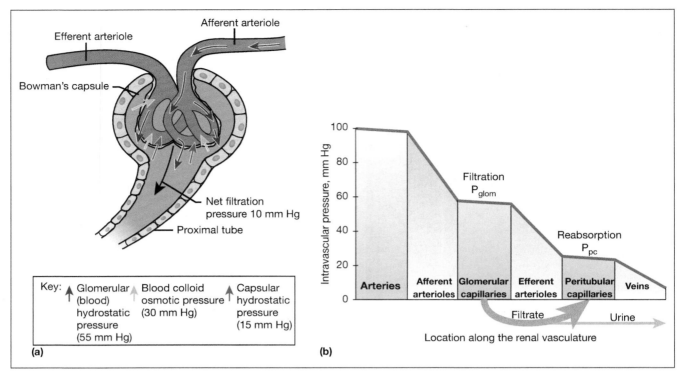

FIGURE 12.7 Renal vascular pressures promote filtration in the glomerular capillaries and reabsorption in the peritubular capillaries. **(a)** Net filtration pressure in the glomerular capillaries is dominated by high capillary hydrostatic pressure, due to the resistance posed by the efferent arteriole (*purple outward arrows*). Opposing the capillary hydrostatic pressure is the oncotic pressure, which rises along the capillaries due to filtration of water and solutes that concentrates proteins within the vessels (*tan inward arrows*). Capsular hydrostatic pressure also opposes filtration (*blue inward arrows*), but in addition provides a driving force for the fluid moving down the nephron. **(b)** In contrast to systemic capillaries in other organ systems, the hydrostatic pressure changes in the renal vessels affect two capillary beds. The first of these, the glomerular capillary bed, has higher-than-normal capillary hydrostatic pressure (P_{glom}), promoting production of the glomerular filtrate that enters the nephron tubule. The peritubular capillaries have lower-than-normal hydrostatic pressure (P_{pc}), aiding reabsorption of more than 99% of the glomerular filtrate. The remaining tubular fluid is excreted as urine.

and blood pressure. The filtration fraction (i.e., the amount of renal plasma flow that becomes filtrate) is typically about 20%, which means that about 80% of the plasma entering the glomerulus flows through the efferent arteriole and into the peritubular capillaries. In healthy kidneys, the filtration membrane effectively prevents loss of plasma proteins from the blood while permitting this high rate of fluid filtration.

Peritubular Capillary Reabsorption and Secretion

Hydrostatic pressure along the renal vessels is determined by resistance in the afferent arterioles and the efferent arterioles. As previously noted, the resistance in the efferent arteriole creates high glomerular capillary hydrostatic pressure that promotes filtration.

The job of the rest of the nephron and postglomerular capillaries (peritubular capillaries and vasa recta) is to reabsorb more than 99% of the filtered fluid back into the blood in order to maintain fluid balance. This is facilitated by the relatively low peritubular capillary hydrostatic pressure created by the additional pressure drop across the efferent arteriole (**Figure 12.7b**). Therefore, the capillary Starling forces at the postglomerular capillaries include high oncotic and low hydrostatic pressure, strongly favoring fluid reabsorption. Reabsorption by the peritubular capillaries and vasa recta occurs as fluid and solutes move down osmotic and electrochemical gradients from the nephron tubular lumen to the interstitial space, and then into the adjacent capillaries.

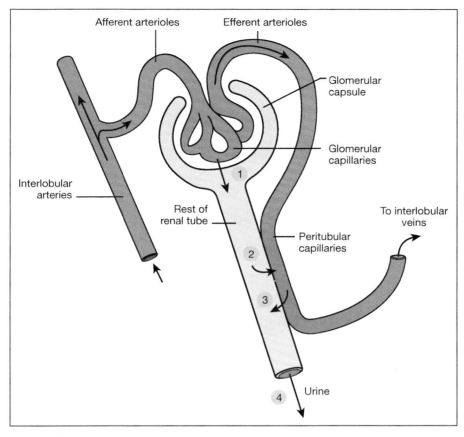

FIGURE 12.8 Overview of nephron processes. **(1)** Filtration occurs at the glomerulus, where about 10% of the renal blood flow enters the tubular space. **(2)** More than 99% of filtered water, electrolytes, and small molecules (glucose, amino acids) is reabsorbed by the tubules and peritubular capillaries. **(3)** Wastes are secreted from the peritubular capillary blood into the tubule for excretion in the urine **(4)**.

The role of the tubules and peritubular capillaries in processing the glomerular filtrate and producing urine is the focus of the next sections. After filtration (**Figure 12.8, step 1**), any solute (ion or molecule) entering the nephron can follow one of three paths.

- The solute may be reabsorbed by tubule cells and pass into the peritubular capillary blood, leaving the urine space and returning to the circulation (as is true for filtered glucose; **Figure 12.8, step 2**).
- The solute may be enriched in the urine space by transporters secreting additional molecules from the peritubular blood across the tubular cell layer and into the lumen (as is true for many antibiotic drugs; **Figure 12.8, step 3**).
- The solute may remain in the tubule, with its absolute amount unchanged by reabsorption or secretion until it is excreted in the urine (**Figure 12.8, step 4**).

Understanding Renal Clearance and Glomerular Filtration Rate

Healthy kidneys not only help maintain the body's fluid balance but are also responsible for removing various metabolic wastes, medications, and toxins from the blood, effectively clearing a solute from the blood. *Clearance* is defined as the volume of blood plasma that is cleared of a certain solute in a given period of time, usually 1 minute. The renal clearance of any solute depends on its properties and tubular handling. Glucose is freely filtered, but at normal plasma concentrations it is completely reabsorbed by tubular transporters, giving it a renal clearance of zero. Proteins and solutes bound to proteins are generally not filtered; however, protein-bound molecules may be picked up by tubular basolateral membrane transporters and enter the urine by secretion. Penicillin and many other antibiotics that are not filtered are secreted into the urine by tubule cells, so they have a high clearance rate and can readily be excreted from the body by the kidneys.

Creatinine is a waste product produced as a breakdown product of the high-energy compound, creatine phosphate, during muscle metabolism. It is usually produced at a fairly constant rate at a level proportional to the body's muscle mass. Although creatinine is present in the blood, its concentration is maintained within a narrow range because the kidneys continuously remove creatinine from the blood through a combination of filtration and tubular secretion. Thus, the renal clearance for creatinine is essentially determined by the GFR. When GFR decreases because of acute or chronic kidney dysfunction, creatinine builds up in the blood, despite a compensatory increase in renal tubular creatinine secretion. Serum creatinine levels are routinely used to estimate GFR using equations that take into account age, sex, body size, and ethnic ancestral descent. Measured or estimated GFR (eGFR) is the primary indicator of kidney function in health and disease. Knowledge of a patient's eGFR is essential prior to prescribing many medications, particularly those that are generally cleared by the kidneys, as a reduction in GFR will delay drug clearance and could result in toxic levels building up at otherwise normal doses.

Thought Questions

1. What properties of the glomerular capillary filtration barrier and glomerular Starling forces contribute to the high rate of glomerular filtration?

2. What properties of the glomerular capillary filtration barrier prevent most plasma proteins from leaving the capillary space and entering Bowman's space?

GLOMERULAR INJURIES

Permeability, blood flow, and capillary hydrostatic pressures are higher in glomerular capillaries than in other organ beds. These factors combine to make the glomeruli particularly vulnerable to damage from vascular sources. Some of these disorders are primary to the kidney and target only the glomerulus, while others are systemic and can affect the glomerulus, tubules, and interstitial cells of the kidney. Although some disorders begin at the level of the glomerulus, many progress to involve the tubules as they transition to chronic kidney disease (CKD).

GLOMERULAR INJURY BY IMMUNE MECHANISMS

The high permeability of the glomerular filtration barrier is associated with certain acute and chronic kidney disorders, in particular disorders involving immune activation. Autoantibodies and antigen–antibody complexes are able to leave glomerular capillaries and bind to targets in the basement membrane or on podocytes, precipitating **immune-mediated kidney injury**. This initiates the immune cascade, consisting of innate and adaptive immune responses (see Chapter 6, The Immune System and Leukocyte Function). The innate immune response activates complement, which directly attacks glomerular structures. Macrophages are attracted to the inflammatory site and secrete inflammatory mediators that recruit additional immune cells. Increased blood flow elevates glomerular pressure to damaging levels, while inflammatory debris blocks filtration and reduces GFR. B and T lymphocytes may enter the region, perpetuating the inflammatory response and worsening antibody accumulation. Antibodies and antigen–antibody complexes can be deposited within the glomerular filtration barrier, impeding filtration. Nonspecific agents of tissue injury and inflammation accumulate along with lymphocytes, causing progressive injury to the glomerular tissue.[3]

Biopsy specimens of affected glomeruli often demonstrate the presence of antigens, antibodies, and immune complexes consisting of both antigens and antibodies in the glomerulus (**Figures 12.9** and **12.10**). The resulting damage may be transient, occurring after an acute infection and then subsiding. But other glomerular disorders have a progressive course, resulting in chronic renal failure. **Box 12.1** lists some of the disorders associated primarily with glomerular injury. The acute presentation of glomerular disorders may include proteinuria, hematuria, oliguria, blood urea and creatinine elevations, hypertension, and edema. In addition to autoimmune disorders that specifically involve the kidney, other systemic disorders may damage the kidney through glomerular antibody deposition; these include systemic lupus erythematosus, scleroderma, and multiple myeloma.[4,5]

DIABETIC NEPHROPATHY

Diabetes is the most common cause of CKD in the United States and worldwide. Manifestations of **diabetic nephropathy** include progressive decreases in GFR and increase in proteinuria. Spot measurements of the urinary albumin/creatinine ratio (ACR) are often used for screening. The normal ratio is <30 mg albumin per gram of creatinine (g Cr), and the test should be

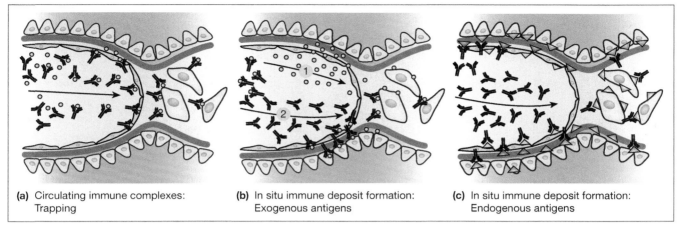

(a) Circulating immune complexes: Trapping

(b) In situ immune deposit formation: Exogenous antigens

(c) In situ immune deposit formation: Endogenous antigens

FIGURE 12.9 Targets and pathways of immune-mediated glomerular damage. **(a)** Preformed immune complexes can be filtered and deposited in the mesangium, promoting the local inflammatory response. Antibodies are shown as black Y-shaped structures and antigens as pink circles. **(b)** Antigens (*pink circles*) may first deposit in the mesangium **(1)**, where circulating antibodies then bind **(2)** to initiate the inflammatory response. **(c)** Endogenous substances recognized as antigens (*shown as triangles*) can be located on glomerular capillary cells (*tan*), basement membrane (*purple*), podocytes (*blue*), or mesangial cells (*green*), attracting antibodies that promote the immune response.

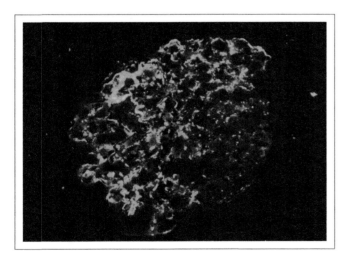

FIGURE 12.10 Glomerulonephritis resulting from a disseminated gonococcal infection. Immunofluorescence detects mesangial and glomerular capillary deposits of complement protein C3 (bright green) in a biopsy specimen.
Source: From Noor A, et al. Acute infection-related glomerulonephritis with disseminated gonococcal infection in a 13-year-old girl. *BMJ Case Rep.* 2018;2018:bcr-2018-225371.

confirmed by one or two repeat measurements as factors such as dehydration, recent exercise, infection, fever, and hypertension can alter the ratio. An ACR between 30 and 300 mg/g Cr is considered microalbuminuria, while a ratio greater than 300 mg/g Cr is considered proteinuria. Diagnostic findings in diabetic kidney disease include a history of type 1 or type 2 diabetes, presence of

retinopathy (another microvascular complication of diabetes), decreased eGFR, and proteinuria.[6] Glomerular injury predominates in diabetic nephropathy, although tubular injury can also occur.

Hyperglycemia is the primary culprit in diabetic nephropathy, and intensive management of blood glucose (and blood pressure) reduces progression of the disorder. Glucose plays an important role in part due to the formation of advanced glycation end products in the glomerulus, as well as the increase in oxidative stress accompanying excess glucose. Immune activation can contribute, as well as the elevated levels of transforming growth factor-beta. Inflammation and hypertension are also implicated in diabetic nephropathy. The RAAS may contribute by promoting fibrosis, and treatment with angiotensin-converting enzyme (ACE) inhibitors or angiotensin receptor blockers (ARBs) can be protective. Pathological changes in the glomerulus in patients with diabetes include thickening of the glomerular basement membrane, expansion of the mesangial matrix and extracellular matrix, loss of basement membrane negative charges, endothelial dysfunction, and vascular fibrosis. The vascular alterations may increase glomerular capillary hydrostatic pressure, contributing to tissue deterioration. Hyperfiltration—due to enlargement of the kidneys from elevated insulin-like growth factor-1—leads to increased filtration across all functioning glomeruli and is thought to be damaging over the long term due to tubular overload and fibrotic changes to peritubular capillaries and tubules.[7,8]

BOX 12.1
Histological Categories of Major Glomerular Disorders

- Minimal change disease (often occurring in children)

- Focal segmental glomerulosclerosis

- Membranous nephropathy

- Acute postinfectious glomerulonephritis

- Membranoproliferative glomerulonephritis

- Immunoglobulin A nephropathy

- Dense deposit disease

- Chronic glomerulonephritis

Source: Modified from Kumar V, Abbas AK, Aster JC, eds. *Robbins Basic Pathology.* 10th ed. Philadelphia, PA: Elsevier; 2017.

HYPERTENSIVE NEPHROPATHY

Hypertension is the second most common cause of CKD, and persistent elevations in blood pressure produce pathological alterations of renal arterioles characteristic of **hypertensive nephropathy**. Hypertension promotes hyperfiltration, causing slow deterioration of nephron function. In addition, wall thickening and protein deposition (called hyaline arteriosclerosis) contributes to hypertensive glomerular damage. As previously noted, hypertension commonly co-occurs with diabetes, and the combination of these disorders synergistically increases the risk of developing CKD.

Thought Questions

3. What types of pathological conditions damage the renal glomeruli?

4. How does the glomerular damage resulting from immune-mediated disorders differ from the damage resulting from diabetes?

REGULATION OF RENAL BLOOD FLOW AND GLOMERULAR FILTRATION RATE

GFR is a measure of renal function that is dependent on RBF, net filtration pressure, permeability of the filtration membrane, and total surface area of filtration membrane, which in turn depends on the number of functional nephrons in the kidneys. Maintaining a fairly constant RBF and GFR ensures that the kidneys adequately clear the blood of metabolic wastes and maintain homeostasis of the ECF. Regulation of RBF and GFR is accomplished through renal autoregulation—mechanisms intrinsic to the kidneys themselves. The ability to maintain constant blood flow and GFR across a wide range of arterial pressures is important to prevent overloading of the nephron, with subsequent hyperfiltration (**Figure 12.11**). Extrinsic regulation provided by the endocrine and sympathetic nervous systems also indirectly affects RBF and GFR through their influence on systemic blood pressure and on afferent and efferent arterioles.

AUTOREGULATION OF RENAL BLOOD FLOW

The kidney employs two different intrinsic mechanisms to maintain RBF at a relatively constant level despite fluctuations in mean arterial pressure (MAP) at the renal artery. One, called the *myogenic mechanism*, depends on the inherent property of vascular smooth muscle cells to contract in response to stretch. As a result of the myogenic response, when arterioles in the kidneys are stretched by an increase in systemic blood pressure, the vascular smooth muscle responds by contracting, much the way a rubber band that is pulled open resists the pull of your fingers. The resulting vasoconstriction decreases blood flow into the glomerulus, thus preventing the increase in glomerular hydrostatic pressure that might have otherwise occurred. The myogenic effect is most pronounced in preglomerular blood vessels (e.g., the interlobular artery and afferent arteriole) and, within normal physiological ranges, helps to prevent alterations in RBF and GFR in response to variations in systemic blood pressure (see **Figure 12.11**)—note the change in diameter associated with renal blood vessels as pressure goes from low (dilated) to high (constricted).

The kidneys' ability to maintain fluid and electrolyte balance is negatively impacted when RBF and GFR are extremely high or low. Tubuloglomerular feedback is a negative feedback mechanism that serves to *notify* the afferent arteriole of downstream alterations in tubular flow associated with

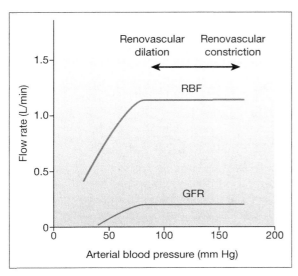

FIGURE 12.11 Renal autoregulation. RBF and GFR are relatively constant over a wide range of perfusion pressures, between mean arterial pressures of about 80 and 160 mm Hg. One autoregulatory mechanism (myogenic) is indicated by a change in average blood vessel diameter that occurs inversely to pressure: As arterial pressure increases, blood vessel diameter decreases, maintaining flow at a relatively constant level. If renal vessels are damaged, autoregulation may be lost, allowing RBF and GFR to increase as pressure increases, and overloading the nephrons.
GFR, glomerular filtration rate; RBF, renal blood flow.

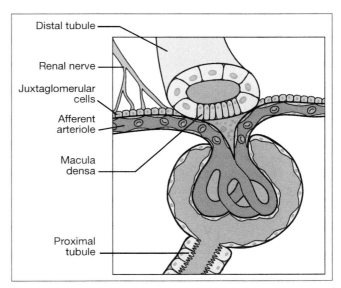

FIGURE 12.12 The juxtaglomerular apparatus is found at the junction of a nephron's afferent and efferent arterioles and the TAL just before the junction with the distal tubule. In this region, specialized *macula densa* cells of the TAL wall contact the afferent arteriole. Adjacent afferent arteriole granule cells synthesize the hormone renin. As concentrations of sodium and chloride in the TAL are sensed by the macula densa cells, an increase in flow or NaCl concentration causes constriction of the afferent arteriole, reducing the glomerular filtrate entering that nephron. A decrease in flow or NaCl concentration causes afferent arteriole vasodilation and release of renin. This is, therefore, a mechanism of renal autoregulation of renal blood flow and GFR, as well as a long-term mechanism of body sodium content through the RAAS.
GFR, glomerular filtration rate; NaCl, sodium chloride; RAAS, renin-angiotensin-aldosterone system; TAL, thick ascending limb.

fluctuations in GFR, resulting in alterations in afferent arteriole diameter that lead to adjustments in GFR. The macula densa is a spot of densely packed tubular cells at the end of the TAL, just before it joins the DT (**Figure 12.12**). The transition between these two regions of the renal tubule occurs at a site where the tubule itself passes between the afferent and efferent arterioles of the nephron and the tubule is in close proximity to the arteriole walls. The macula densa responds to changes in tubular flow rate or NaCl concentration of the filtrate flowing from the TAL into the DT as an indicator of GFR. When GFR falls, as would happen with a decrease in systemic arterial pressure, filtrate flow into the DT decreases, and the NaCl concentration of the filtrate drops. The macula densa responds to this change by releasing less vasoconstrictor substances near the afferent arteriole, resulting in vasodilation of the vessel, increased blood flow into the glomerulus, and a subsequent increase in net filtration pressure and GFR. This regulation sequence is reversed when GFR is high: increased filtrate flow or NaCl concentration of the filtrate, or both, leads to increased vasoconstrictor release by the macula densa; the afferent arteriole constricts and, as a result, GFR decreases.

EXTRINSIC REGULATION OF RBF AND GFR

Extrinsic regulation of RBF and GFR is provided by endocrine and sympathetic nervous system signals and is especially important in preventing and reversing extreme decreases of systemic blood pressure. Endocrine regulation is provided primarily through the RAAS via mechanisms that begin with the juxtaglomerular apparatus (JGA) of the nephrons. The JGA is the specialized region of the nephron that comprises the macula densa; juxtaglomerular (JG) cells, also called *granular cells*; and extraglomerular mesangial cells, located near the glomerulus where the macula densa lies between the afferent and efferent arterioles of the nephron. The location and role of the macula densa in tubuloglomerular feedback have been described. The JG cells are modified smooth muscle cells in the wall of the afferent arteriole that produce renin and store it in cytoplasmic granules prior to release. The stimuli that trigger renin release are: sympathetic nerve release of norepinephrine, which activates β_1-adrenergic receptors on the JG cells; reduced blood pressure in the afferent arteriole; and stimulation by activated macula densa cells.

Finally, when arterial pressure drops below the autoregulatory range (<80 mm Hg MAP), sympathetic nerves stimulate vasoconstriction of the afferent arterioles, which subsequently reduces RBF. This is a short-term compensatory mechanism that decreases the normally abundant RBF to preserve flow to the heart and brain under low-pressure/low-volume states such as hemorrhage and extreme dehydration. Although effective in the short term, this mechanism can precipitate AKI.

IMPORTANCE OF eGFR AS THE INDICATOR OF RENAL FUNCTION

As previously noted, serum creatinine concentration is used to estimate GFR by several empirically derived equations, and eGFR is reported along with the serum creatinine. In CKD arising from any cause, GFR is progressively reduced, indicating the cumulative loss of functioning nephrons. Clinical staging of CKD is based on measures of eGFR, with additional diagnostic indicators such as degree of proteinuria also influencing staging and management, as described later in this chapter.

FACTORS REDUCING RBF AND GFR IN DISEASE STATES

Although blood flow to the renal cortex is abundant, blood flow and oxygen tension drop in the renal medulla (**Figure 12.13**).[9] The vasa recta are a subset of postglomerular capillaries. Although they represent only about 10%–15% of renal capillaries, they provide the majority of blood flow to the renal inner medulla. The looped structure of the vasa recta preserves osmotic concentration in the medullary interstitium that is required for

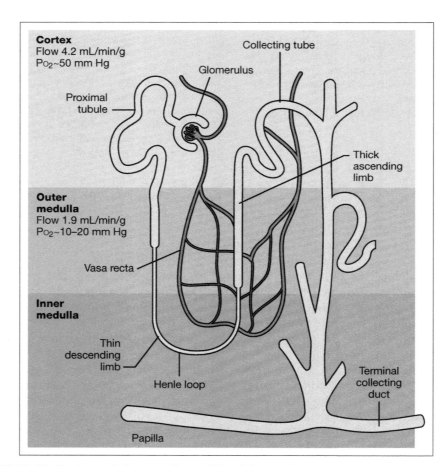

FIGURE 12.13 Corticomedullary gradient of blood flow and oxygen tension. Blood flow to the renal cortex is very high, perfusing the glomerular capillaries of the approximately 1 million nephrons per kidney. The juxtamedullary nephrons, representing about 15% of all nephrons, have specialized peritubular capillaries called *vasa recta* that descend to the inner medulla and make a U-turn, ascending back to the cortex. Oxygen leaves these capillaries along their length, creating relative hypoxia deep in the renal medulla. This creates a vulnerable region that can sustain hypoxic damage during systemic hypotension and hypoxemia.

concentrating the urine. A consequence of the close association between descending and ascending vasa recta is that oxygen can shunt from the arterial side to the venous side before reaching the very tips of the vessels in the inner medulla, leaving both outer and inner medulla relatively hypoxic. In addition, the high metabolic rate of cells in the distal portion of the PT and the thick ascending LOH drives greater oxygen demand in these tubular structures of the outer medulla.[9] Thus, there is a delicate balance between oxygen supply and demand and high vulnerability to renal medullary hypoxic injury.

Hypoxic renal damage causes **prerenal failure**, commonly seen in critical illness involving hypotension and hypovolemia, with hypoxic injury leading to rapid loss of renal function in patients with sepsis, trauma, myocardial infarction, and other critical illnesses. The risk of kidney injury is further increased in patients who have taken nonsteroidal anti inflammatory drugs (NSAIDs), as prostaglandin E_2 is a major vasodilating mediator in RBF. In some cases, patients can be managed with renal replacement using dialysis on a temporary basis until the acute injury resolves. A history of AKI is one risk factor for later development of CKD.

Thought Questions

5. What mechanisms can explain renal autoregulation, defined as the ability to maintain relatively constant blood flow to the kidneys despite changing pressures of blood entering the renal arteries? What happens when blood pressure drops below the autoregulatory range?

6. What region of the kidney receives the smallest amount of blood flow, and what is the reason for the relative lack of blood flow to this region?

STRUCTURE AND FUNCTION OF THE RENAL TUBULE

Filtrate quickly passes from the capsular space into the renal tubule where, through the processes of tubular secretion and reabsorption, its volume and solute composition are dramatically modified. The end result of tubular processing is urine.

TUBULAR TRANSPORT OVERVIEW

The renal tubule is composed of simple epithelium a single cell layer thick. In all segments of the tubule system, specialized membrane proteins move solutes across the wall of the tubule.

Below is a summary of renal membrane transport mechanisms:

- *Active transport:* Conducted by ATPase pumps, allows solute movement against a concentration gradient (uphill)
- *Secondary active transporter:* Allows solute movement against a concentration gradient when accompanied by movement of another solute (usually sodium) downhill
- *Cotransport:* Movement of two solutes in the same direction
- *Countertransport (or exchange):* Movement of two solutes in the opposite direction
- *Facilitated diffusion:* Movement of a solute down a concentration gradient (downhill) through a membrane transport protein
- *Ion channel:* Permits movement of an ionic solute down a concentration gradient through a selective pore
- *Reabsorption:* Movement of a solute from the tubular lumen across the tubule wall to the peritubular capillary
- *Secretion:* Movement of a solute from the peritubular capillary across the tubule wall to the tubular lumen
- *Apical transporters:* Proteins found in the tubular cell membrane facing the lumen
- *Basolateral transporters:* Proteins found in the tubular cell membrane facing the interstitial space and peritubular capillary

The function of each region of the tubule is defined by its characteristic profile of channels and transporters. In most parts of the tubule, reabsorption and secretion are only possible via a transcellular route (through cellular apical and basolateral membranes) because tight junctions between epithelial cells prevent the leakage of solutes. In some portions of the tubule, tight junctions are looser and allow leakage of water or solutes or both between adjacent cells, permitting paracellular (between adjacent tubular cells) reabsorption.

Na^+ ions are the most abundant ions in the ECF and, as a result, sodium is the most abundant ion in the filtrate. Most of the adenosine triphosphate (ATP) expended by the nephron in active transport is used in Na^+ reabsorption. Tubular transport depends on the *continuous* activity of Na^+/K^+ pumps in the basolateral membrane of all tubule cells. The pumps, found in all segments of the renal tubule, move two ions of K^+ into the tubule cell and return three Na^+ to the blood per molecule of ATP expended. Leak channels for K^+ in the lateral walls of the tubule cells allow K^+ to diffuse back into the interstitial fluid and tubular lumens, preventing excessive buildup of K^+ in the tubule cells. The Na^+/K^+ pumps maintain an electrochemical gradient that allows Na^+ to move across the apical membrane of the tubule cells via facilitated diffusion or secondary active transport. Reabsorption of Na⁺ is important in its own right, and also contributes to the reabsorption of other solutes and water.

Water reabsorption is always passive, occurring by osmosis through specialized water channels called *aquaporins (AQP)*, and follows the osmotic pull based on reabsorption of solutes. The AQP family of water channels is large, and the profile of AQP expression varies significantly along the tubule. AQP1, for example, is expressed at significant levels in the apical and basolateral membranes of the PT and thin descending limbs of the LOH; as a result, water reabsorption is highly efficient. In contrast, the apical expression of AQP2 by collecting duct cells is regulated by the hormone vasopressin; in the absence of vasopressin, virtually no water can be reabsorbed in the collecting ducts.

SEGMENTAL TUBULAR PROCESSING

Proximal Tubule

The PT is located in the cortex and extends from Bowman's capsule to the LOH. Its cells have a dense brush border in the initial portions (which thins in the later PT) and numerous infoldings of the basolateral membrane. Internally, large numbers of mitochondria fill the basal regions of the cytoplasm. These cellular characteristics—significantly increased surface area of the cells and capacity to produce large amounts of ATP—contribute to efficient reabsorption in this portion of the tubule.

Reabsorption in the PT is *driven* by the rate of Na⁺ reabsorption by the Na⁺/K⁺ pumps in the basolateral membrane (**Figure 12.14a**). At the apical surface, Na⁺ enters the tubule cells via cotransporters that reabsorb glucose, amino acids, or other solutes, or countertransporters linked to secretion of H⁺ or other wastes. Basolateral transport mechanisms completing the reabsorption processes include facilitated diffusion, secondary active transport, active transport, and ion channels. Small proteins that escape through the filtration membrane into the filtrate are taken up by pinocytosis and digested within PT cells; the amino acids produced are reabsorbed into the blood. Reabsorption of electrolytes and other solutes promotes reabsorption of water by AQP1 and solvent drag (reabsorption of water and electrolytes) by the paracellular route. Approximately 120 to 125 mL/min of iso-osmotic filtrate flows from the capsular space into the PT. By the time the filtrate reaches the end of the PT, all organic nutrient molecules (i.e., glucose and amino acids), 85% of filtered HCO_3^-, and approximately 70% of other electrolytes have been reabsorbed from the filtrate through active transport, secondary active transport, facilitated diffusion, cotransport, and countertransport. At the end of the PT, tubular fluid is still iso-osmotic with the interstitial space.

PT glucose reabsorption is worthy of extra attention for its clinical relevance. Apical membrane secondary active transport linked to sodium entry mediates glucose uptake from the lumen, and facilitated diffusion across the basolateral membrane moves glucose to the tubular interstitium for uptake into the peritubular capillary. Ninety percent of this uptake occurs early in the PT by means of SGLT2, one of two key sodium–glucose cotransporter proteins. The remaining 10% is reabsorbed in the late PT by means of SGLT1. SGLT2 is the target of drugs used to treat type 2 diabetes mellitus. Blocking SGLT2 reduces postprandial swings of blood glucose by causing urinary excretion of excess glucose. This has been found to be effective, along with other drug classes, in improving outcomes in patients with diabetes.

Renal regulation of calcium (Ca^{2+}) and phosphate balance is integral to calcium homeostasis, which is needed for bone formation and maintenance, blood clotting, membrane excitability of neurons and muscles, and numerous cellular actions. Most filtered Ca^{2+} is passively reabsorbed in the PT by diffusion and solvent drag. A small fraction of PT Ca^{2+} reabsorption is an active process, mainly stimulated by parathyroid hormone. Approximately 80% of filtered phosphates are reabsorbed in the PT. The amount of phosphate reabsorption is determined by the number of sodium–phosphate cotransporters expressed by the cells. A major regulator of phosphate transport is fibroblast growth factor-23 (FGF-23), which depends on a local cofactor, Klotho, for its action. FGF-23/Klotho reduces the expression and action of PT phosphate transporters, resulting in greater phosphate excretion.[10]

PT bicarbonate (HCO_3^-) reabsorption is coupled to H⁺ secretion and is made possible by the enzyme carbonic anhydrase (see **Figure 12.14b**). Carbonic anhydrase catalyzes the interconversions of carbon dioxide and water with the dissociated ions of carbonic acid. The reaction sequence is:

$$CO_2 + H_2O \Leftrightarrow H_2CO_3 \Leftrightarrow H^+ + HCO_3^-$$

Carbonic Anhydrase

PT cells secrete H⁺ across their apical border by Na⁺-H⁺ countertransport or H⁺-ATPase (adenosine triphosphatase). Secreted H⁺ combines with filtered HCO_3^- in the lumen of the tubule to form H_2CO_3. The presence of carbonic anhydrase in the brush border catalyzes the rapid dehydration of H_2CO_3 to $H_2O + CO_2$. Inside the cell, carbonic anhydrase catalyzes formation of H_2CO_3, which quickly dissociates into $H^+ + HCO_3^-$. The HCO_3^- is moved across the basolateral membrane by either Na⁺-HCO_3^- cotransport or HCO_3^--Cl⁻ countertransport and diffuses into the peritubular capillaries. Note that for every HCO_3^- that is reabsorbed, one H⁺ is secreted; each secreted H⁺ combines with a filtered HCO_3^- to generate CO_2, which can reenter the tubule cell to generate another HCO_3^-. The process is so effective that 80%

to 85% of filtered HCO_3^- can be reabsorbed in the PT. Factors that enhance HCO_3^- reabsorption are increased concentration of HCO_3^- in the filtrate, increased partial pressure of carbon dioxide (P_{CO_2}), and angiotensin II. In the PT and elsewhere in the nephron, additional H^+ can be excreted in the form of ammonium ion (NH_4^+) generated from glutamine metabolism, or can be buffered by binding to urinary phosphate ions. Binding to either of these molecules buffers the change in urinary pH and prevents the rapid acidification that would result from secretion of free H^+.

Finally, PT secretion of organic anions and cations is responsible for renal clearance of many endogenous compounds and water-soluble drugs (see **Figure 12.14c**).[11] The high rate of PT reabsorption decreases filtrate volume by about 70%, while concentrating substances such as drugs that are destined for urinary excretion. Reabsorptive processes in the PT decrease filtrate volume by nearly 75% through the osmotic gradient created by solute reabsorption; these actions concentrate drugs in the lumen.

Loop of Henle

The second segment of the renal tubule, the LOH (also known as the nephron loop), begins in the renal cortex and descends into the medulla (the descending limb), where it makes a U-turn that brings it back to the renal cortex (the ascending limb). Initially, the LOH is continuous with the PT and, like the PT, consists of simple cuboidal epithelium. As the tubule moves into the medulla, the epithelium changes to simple squamous tissue, forming the thin portion of the descending limb. This simple epithelium continues after the U-turn as the thin ascending limb and soon after the turn becomes cuboidal or columnar, increasing the height of the epithelial layer. Thus, it is the thickness of the epithelium and not changes in lumen diameter, that create the thick and thin portions of the LOH.

Functionally, the LOH and later segments of the renal tubule are quite different from the PT. The descending limb of the LOH is freely permeable to water and impermeable to solutes. Thus, as filtrate passes through the descending limb, water is reabsorbed by osmosis, and solutes—which are trapped in the tubule—become more concentrated. The ascending limb, however, is impermeable to water, but it does have transport mechanisms for several ions, including Na^+, Cl^-, K^+, and Ca^{2+}. As a result, while filtrate volume is not further decreased in the ascending limb, the reabsorption of NaCl results in the filtrate becoming increasingly dilute (i.e., hypo-osmotic) as it passes through the ascending limb.

Although NaCl is reabsorbed along the length of the ascending limb, the mechanism by which the reabsorption occurs varies. The thin ascending limb is permeable to Na^+ and Cl^-, and because the filtrate arriving from the descending limb is hyperosmotic, these ions are able to be reabsorbed passively via the paracellular route. NaCl reabsorption in the TAL is an active process involving secondary active transport by the $Na^+/K^+/2\ Cl^-$ cotransporters in the luminal membrane (see **Figure 12.14d**). These cotransporters are blocked by the *loop* diuretic drugs such as furosemide. LOH sodium reabsorption accounts for about 25% of all sodium reabsorbed by the nephron.

Distal Tubule

The DT, the shortest segment of the renal tubule, is positioned between the ascending limb of the LOH and the collecting duct. Its wall is simple cuboidal epithelium. It is now recognized that the DT is uniform in neither structure nor function along its length—the distal end of the DT is a transitional region, called the connecting tubule, where tubule characteristics become quite similar to those of the collecting ducts and less like the earlier portion of the DT.

Electrolyte reabsorption is the primary activity of the DT (see **Figure 12.14e**). Along the length of this segment, Na^+-Cl^- cotransporters in the apical membrane function in secondary active reabsorption of these electrolytes, allowing them to move down the electrochemical gradient created by the action of Na^+/K^+-ATPase pumping in the basolateral membrane. The Na^+-Cl^- cotransporter is blocked by thiazide diuretics. Na^+ reabsorption in this part of the nephron accounts for about 5% of total nephron sodium absorption. Although most filtered Ca^{2+} is reabsorbed in the PT and additional Ca^{2+} reabsorption occurs in the ascending LOH, the DT is an important site for parathyroid hormone–regulated reabsorption of Ca^{2+}. In response to parathyroid hormone, DT cells upregulate Ca^{2+} channels in the apical membrane of the cells. Ca^{2+} flows passively through these channels down an electrochemical gradient and binds to the carrier protein calbindin in the cytoplasm. Ultimately, the Ca^{2+} ions leave the DT cells across the basolateral membrane by Na^+-Ca^{2+} antiporters and Ca^{2+}-ATPase (secondary and primary active transport, respectively).

Late Distal Tubule and Collecting Duct

Two important cell types become increasingly numerous in the later portion of the DT, connecting tubule, and collecting duct: principal cells and intercalated cells. Principal cells, named because they are the primary cell type in the connecting tubule and collecting duct, are target cells for the hormones aldosterone and vasopressin (**Figure 12.14f**). Aldosterone stimulates increased production and insertion of Na^+ and K^+ channels in the apical membrane and increases activity of basolateral membrane Na^+/K^+-ATPase.

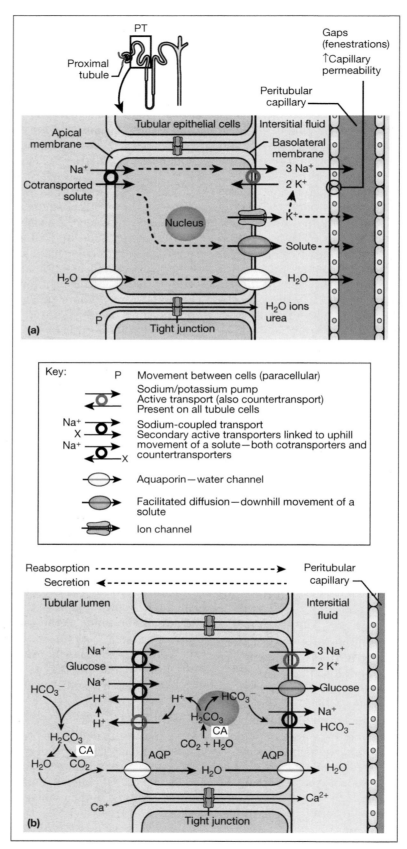

FIGURE 12.14 Tubular cell transport processes by segment (processes are described in the text). (*continued*)

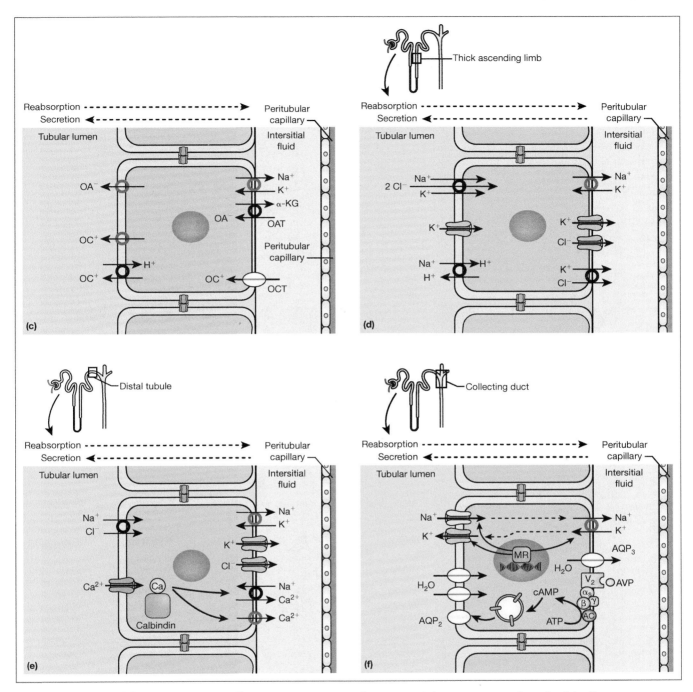

FIGURE 12.14 Tubular cell transport processes by segment (processes are described in the text). (**a**), (**b**), (**c**) General and proximal tubule processes; (**d**) Thick ascending limb processes; (**e**) Distal tubule processes; (**f**) Collecting duct processes. α-KG, α-ketoglutarate; AQP, aquaporins; ATP, adenosine triphosphate; ATPase, adenosine triphosphatase; CA, carbonic anhydrase; cAMP, cyclic adenosine monophosphate; DT, distal tubule; MR, mineralocorticoid receptor; PT, proximal tubule; OA⁻, organic anion; OAT, organic anion transporter; OC⁺, organic cation; OCT, organic cation transporter; TAL, thick ascending limb.

This has the effect of increasing Na⁺ reabsorption and increasing K⁺ secretion in this segment of the tubule, consistent with the role of aldosterone as a sodium-retaining and potassium-secreting hormone. The hormone vasopressin increases AQP2 production and insertion in the apical membrane by principal cells. Without vasopressin, the distal nephron would be virtually impermeable to water; vasopressin, then, allows water reabsorption (passive reabsorption) in this part of the tubule. It should be noted that the direct effect of aldosterone is to increase the osmolarity of the blood; vasopressin increases blood volume by enabling water diffusion down its osmotic gradient.

Intercalated cells of the late DT and collecting ducts exert the final control of acid–base balance. Type A intercalated cells use a carbonic anhydrase mechanism similar to that described for the PT to secrete H$^+$ into the tubule and to absorb HCO$_3^-$, which acidifies the urine and provides the final opportunity to remove H$^+$ from the body. In cases of alkalosis, type B intercalated cells secrete HCO$_3^-$ and reabsorb H$^+$, creating alkaline urine and restoring normal body pH. Thus, through actions in both the PT and other nephron regions, renal control of acid–base balance can compensate for body states of either acidosis or alkalosis.

Tubular segmental transport functions are briefly summarized in **Table 12.2**.

Thought Questions

7. What is the general pattern of solute movements between tubular fluid and peritubular capillary blood? What is the energy source for this movement?

8. How do the processes of the PT differ from the processes of the late DT and collecting duct in volume of solute and water transported, types of solutes transported, and modulation of transport?

TABLE 12.2 Tubular Segmental Transport

Tubule Segment	Major Processes	Additional Comments
Proximal tubule	Na$^+$, Cl$^-$, Ca^{2+}, phosphate, and water are reabsorbed in bulk and high capacity Glucose and amino acids are 100% reabsorbed HCO$_3^-$ is 85% reabsorbed Hydrogen ions are secreted – linked to HCO$_3^-$ reabsorption Organic anions, cations, and many drugs are secreted	Water and ions move between cells (paracellular path) Isoosmotic processing – water follows bulk flow of solutes via transcellular and paracellular pathways SGLT2 glucose transporter is the target of antidiabetic drugs
Descending loop of Henle	Water is reabsorbed into the hypertonic medullary interstitium	The osmotic gradient is created by buildup of Na$^+$, Cl$^-$, and urea
Thick ascending limb of Henle's loop	Na$^+$/K$^+$/2 Cl$^-$ (NKCC) transporter provides secondary active transport of K$^+$ and downhill movement of Na$^+$ and Cl$^-$ High rate of ion reabsorption ensures that fluid entering distal tubule is hypotonic	High activity of Na$^+$/K$^+$ pump in this segment increases oxygen demand, worsening medullary hypoxia Ion pumping contributes to hypertonic medullary interstitium NKCC protein is the target of loop diuretic drugs
Distal tubule	High rate of water reabsorption down the osmotic gradient from hypotonic tubule fluid to isotonic interstitium Apical membrane Na$^+$/Cl$^-$ cotransport to reabsorb these major extracellular ions Ca^{2+} reabsorption regulated by parathyroid hormone	Na$^+$/Cl$^-$ cotransport is blocked by thiazide-type diuretics
Late distal tubule/collecting duct	Apical Na$^+$ and K$^+$ channels facilitate Na$^+$ reabsorption and K$^+$ secretion AQP are inserted under control of vasopressin, promoting water retention and concentrating the urine	Fine-tuning of Na$^+$ and K$^+$ levels, acid/base balance, and water reabsorption Hormonal regulation by aldosterone (blocked by potassium-sparing diuretics) and by vasopressin

REGIONAL KIDNEY FUNCTION

CORTICOMEDULLARY OSMOLARITY GRADIENT

If we were to summarize the role of the kidney tubules in renal processing of glomerular filtrate, we could correctly say that:

- The PT's main functions are (a) bulk reabsorption of solutes and water, (b) secretion of major wastes and toxins, and (c) reduction of the volume of tubular fluid by about two thirds. PT processing is high volume without fine-tuning the composition of the tubular fluid.
- The DT and collecting duct are the sites where, under hormonal regulation, solute concentration of the urine is refined and urine volume adjusted in response to homeostatic needs of the body.
- The LOH serves two closely aligned functions: (a) reabsorption of 25% of filtered sodium and chloride and (b) generation of the concentrated medullary interstitium, which enables the formation of concentrated urine to conserve body water and fluid volume. It accomplishes these goals through a looped structure in which the descending limb is primarily permeable to water and the ascending limb is impermeable to water but is able to move sodium chloride from the lumen to the interstitial space.

Differential movements of water, sodium, and chloride along the LOH descending and ascending limbs ultimately create a gradient such that the interstitial fluid and tubular fluid are extremely concentrated at the inner medullary tips of the loops of Henle, relative to the rest of the kidney. As shown in **Figure 12.15**, there is a gradient of osmotic strength from the isotonic renal cortex with increasing osmotic strength moving inward to the most hypertonic point in the inner medulla.

Medullary hypertonicity is further sustained by the vasa recta—the U-shaped blood vessels running parallel to the loops of Henle. Blood flows through the vasa recta at a relatively slow rate and the walls of the vasa recta are very permeable to water and solutes. Water and solutes freely move into and out of the blood along the entire length of the vasa recta. As a result, blood in the vasa recta remains iso-osmotic with the surrounding medullary interstitium. This mechanism provides a way to ensure continuous blood flow and the return of reabsorbed solutes and water to the general circulation while not diluting or destroying the medullary osmotic gradient.

Urea movements in the nephron are quite complex (see **Figure 12.15**). Urea is produced by the liver to detoxify ammonia generated from amino acid metabolism. It is freely filtered and osmotically active, but is ultimately a waste product and must be excreted daily in amounts equal to the amount generated. Still, urea is an important factor helping the kidney to concentrate the urine to avoid excessive urinary water losses. The PT reabsorbs about half of filtered urea. Thin segments of the LOH are permeable to urea, and the urea concentration in the medullary interstitium is usually higher than in the filtrate of the LOH; this allows some urea to be secreted into the filtrate in the thin LOH. The TAL, DT, and outer (cortical) collecting duct are impermeable to urea. However, the inner (medullary) portion of the collecting duct is permeable to urea. The concentration of urea is very high in this portion of the collecting duct because the urine is becoming concentrated here. Thus, the conditions favor urea reabsorption, and about 55% of the filtered urea remaining in the urine in this portion of the tubule is normally reabsorbed in the inner medulla. Vasopressin also impacts urea reabsorption. When vasopressin is present, it causes expression of urea transporters in the medullary portion of the collecting duct, enhancing urea reabsorption even further.

A small portion of the urea reabsorbed by the medullary collecting duct is carried back into the blood of the vasa recta. A larger part is *recycled* by being secreted into the thin segment of the LOH. Recycled urea increases the urea concentration in the filtrate entering the collecting duct, helping ensure urea reabsorption in the inner medullary collecting ducts. As urea is recycled, its presence in the medullary interstitial fluid constitutes about 50% of the medullary osmotic gradient in the presence of vasopressin.

PRODUCTION OF CONCENTRATED URINE AND HOMEOSTATIC REGULATION OF URINE COMPOSITION AND OSMOLARITY

A large proportion (85%) of all nephrons are cortical nephrons. These nephrons, owing to their sheer number, are responsible for much of the reabsorption that occurs to reduce filtrate flow into the DT and return filtered solutes to the general circulation. Although much smaller in number, juxtamedullary nephrons play the important role of creating and maintaining the medullary osmotic gradient, making it possible to vary the composition and volume of urine produced by the kidneys. The DTs of both cortical and juxtamedullary nephrons empty urine into collecting tubules, which converge to form larger collecting ducts.

Adjustments to urine concentration and volume occur as urine flows through the collecting ducts. As noted earlier, the main cell type of this distal part of the tubule is the principal cell. Principal cells are a target for the action of vasopressin. When vasopressin is absent, the collecting duct is impermeable to water.

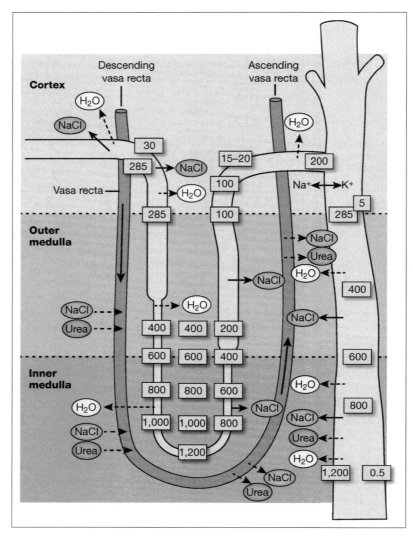

FIGURE 12.15 Corticomedullary osmotic gradient. Production of concentrated urine depends on osmotic equilibration between urine in the collecting duct and the concentrated medullary interstitium. The numbers show the osmotic strength at each location of tubules and interstitium, in mOsm/L. Factors contributing to the buildup of osmolarity in the medulla include movement of more sodium and chloride than water over the entire LOH, lack of water permeability of the ascending LOH, vasopressin-dependent reabsorption of water and urea at the collecting duct, recycling of urea between descending and ascending loops of vasa recta, and urea reabsorption in the collecting duct.
LOH, loop of Henle.

As a result, as urine passes through the collecting duct its osmolarity decreases as solute is reabsorbed, and large quantities of dilute urine are produced. With vasopressin, principal cells become more permeable to water and the solute concentration of the urine increases as it flows through the collecting ducts. At maximal levels of vasopressin, passive water reabsorption will be at its highest and urine osmolarity will equal the osmolarity of the medullary interstitial fluid, resulting in a small volume of highly concentrated urine (**Figure 12.16**).

CONCEPTS IN FLUID, ELECTROLYTE, AND ACID–BASE BALANCE

The kidneys play an essential role in regulating body fluid volume and composition. Maintaining water balance requires that the volume of water gained per day in the body equal the volume lost (**Figure 12.17**). On average, approximately 2.0 L/day of water is taken into the body from foods and beverages. Approximately 0.6 L/day of water is output from the body via the skin

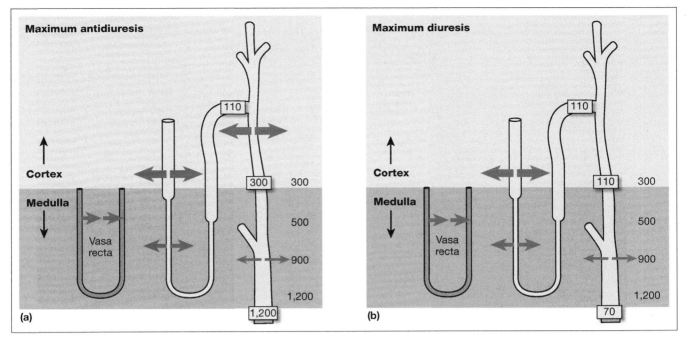

FIGURE 12.16 Vasopressin regulation of urine osmolality. **(a)** Under conditions of dehydration, vasopressin levels and collecting duct water reabsorption (blue arrows) increase, resulting in decreased urine volume (antidiuresis) and increased urine osmolality up to a maximum of 1,200 mOsm/L. **(b)** When fluid intake is normal or high, vasopressin secretion is inhibited, collecting duct water reabsorption is inhibited, and increased amounts of dilute urine (diuresis) are excreted.

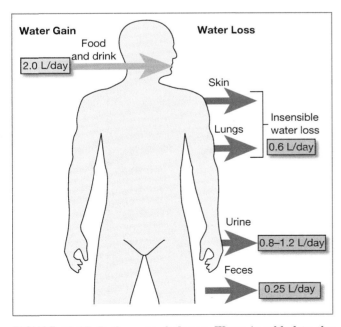

FIGURE 12.17 Daily water balance. Water is added to the body through ingestion and cellular metabolism and is then removed by insensible water loss, sweat, urine, and feces. To prevent fluid overload or depletion, intake must equal output. Renal control of water excretion, regulated by vasopressin, is the main point of control of water retention or removal. Thirst, regulated by angiotensin II and blood osmolality, is the main point of control of water intake.

and mucosa of the airways (insensible water loss), and 250 mL or less in feces. On average, urine output is approximately 800 to 1,200 mL/day, although urine production is quite variable and depends on intake. The kidneys require a minimum amount of urine production of about 300 mL/day to excrete daily wastes. Above that, urine output provides a net balance of zero of intake and output, given all the sources of fluid intake and fluid losses.[12]

Dietary intake of food and beverages is absorbed by the gastrointestinal tract, adding to the body glucose, amino acids, lipids, sodium, chloride, potassium, calcium, phosphate, and myriad minerals, vitamins, and chemicals. To maintain homeostasis, equal amounts of these substances or their metabolic end products must be excreted through renal, biliary/fecal, or respiratory routes. As described earlier, the fine-tuning of renal excretion of water, sodium, potassium, acid, calcium, and phosphate, among other substances, is largely handled by the distal portions of the nephron. States of imbalance can result from disrupted kidney function and loss of renal processing due to decreased GFR. More often, states of fluid imbalance result from pathological processes arising outside the kidney. These can arise acutely in clinical scenarios, such as trauma with hemorrhage, severe dehydration due to gastrointestinal fluid losses in diarrhea or vomiting, or severe exertion in extreme heat. Chronic disorders that produce fluid imbalance states include heart failure, severe liver disease, and endocrine disorders such as diabetes insipidus or Addison disease. Acid–base imbalances can occur in diabetes and in chronic lung disease. Renal compensation is essential to survival in the face of these and other acute and chronic fluid and electrolyte disorders.

RENAL COMPENSATION IN STATES OF HYPOVOLEMIA AND HYPOTENSION

Long-term regulation of blood volume and pressure is dependent on the kidneys, as noted in Chapter 9, Circulation. High-pressure baroreceptors in the carotid sinus and aortic arch and low-pressure volume receptors in the atria and veins sense arterial blood pressure and blood volume, respectively. The outputs of these sensors impact autonomic cardiovascular responses acutely while simultaneously initiating endocrine responses. **Hypotension** and **hypovolemia** are detected and linked to these compensatory responses:

- Increased sympathetic vasoconstrictor activity, as well as increased sympathetic outflow to the kidneys, stimulates renin secretion and renal Na+ retention.
- Renin secretion is further stimulated by macula densa activation of the juxtaglomerular apparatus granular cells (see **Figure 12.12**).
- Increases in circulating renin lead to angiotensin I production and conversion to angiotensin II. In addition to increasing vasoconstriction, angiotensin II stimulates thirst, tubular sodium reabsorption, adrenal aldosterone secretion, and posterior pituitary vasopressin secretion, and promotes increased sympathetic activity.
- Aldosterone acts on distal nephron structures to promote sodium reabsorption.
- Baroreceptor signaling of hypotension is also linked through neural pathways to increased pituitary vasopressin secretion, reinforcing the actions of angiotensin II.
- Vasopressin acts on the distal nephron to promote water reabsorption.
- All of these responses promote water acquisition (through thirst → drinking), water retention, and sodium retention, restoring ECF volume and blood pressure over the longer term than the rapidly acting baroreflexes.

Although these compensatory mechanisms are necessary and restorative in states of acute volume loss, they are not as useful in certain chronic disease states. In heart failure, for example, inadequate cardiac output resulting in low blood pressure initiates this process of fluid retention that ultimately worsens the load on the failing heart. Management strategies include blocking the compensatory mechanisms through administration of a variety of drug classes including β-blocking drugs, angiotensin blockade (via ACE inhibitors or ARBs), aldosterone antagonists, and diuretics.

Edema occurring in heart failure, liver failure, and other states also can be treated with diuretic drugs. As noted earlier, renal transport mechanisms targeted by diuretic drugs include the TAL Na+/K+/2 Cl− cotransporter blocked by furosemide and other loop diuretics, and the DT Na+/Cl− cotransporter blocked by thiazides. Aldosterone antagonists (spironolactone) can also be used as diuretics, as they reduce sodium absorption in the distal nephron. The relative potency of diuretics relates to the amount of sodium normally reabsorbed in the target segment. The LOH reabsorbs about 25% of filtered Na+ and Cl− and contributes to the generation of the hyperosmolar medullary interstitium; thus, loop diuretics produce a very potent diuresis. The DT reabsorbs about 5% of filtered Na+ and Cl−; thus, the diuretic effect of thiazide diuretics is not as strong as that of loop diuretics.

RENAL COMPENSATION IN STATES OF HYPERVOLEMIA AND HYPERTENSION

States of fluid and volume overload are less common than the deficit states. Upon ingestion of a large, salty meal accompanied by a large beverage, the ECF volume will transiently expand. This could result in a mild increase in blood pressure while also swelling the venous capacitance vessels and being detected by both baroreceptors and volume receptors, as well as intrarenal sensors. Such a state would suppress the RAAS and vasopressin secretion, and increase secretion of atrial and B-type natriuretic peptides. The natriuretic peptides, in addition to causing vasodilation to reduce blood pressure, act to suppress sodium reabsorption in the distal nephron, leading to natriuresis and accompanying diuresis (assisted by reduced vasopressin levels), until body fluid and sodium balance returns to normal.

Unfortunately, chronic hypertension is associated with resetting of arterial baroreceptors, such that these compensatory mechanisms are no longer activated and renal compensation does not occur. The drug classes mentioned earlier, particularly ARBs and diuretics, are useful in management of hypertension.

Thought Question

9. What are the mediators that alter renal electrolyte and water transport to maintain systemic homeostasis? What are the cellular mechanisms of actions of those mediators?

ACUTE KIDNEY INJURY–CHRONIC KIDNEY DISEASE CONTINUUM

As noted in the chapter introduction, kidney disease encompasses several entities, including **acute kidney injury** (AKI), which is often, but not always, reversible, and **chronic kidney disease** (CKD), which tends to progress through several stages until ending at stage 5 (also known as **end-stage renal disease** [ESRD]). The definitions of these terms and stages usually depend on laboratory assessments of kidney function, evaluation of the history and physical findings, and presence of comorbidities. For the CKD-ESRD continuum, global prevalence is estimated at 13.4%. Prevalence by stage was determined based on the eGFR and ACR (Table 12.3). CKD staging has evolved to include consideration of both eGFR and ACR, as some individuals have eGFR within the normal range but demonstrate renal impairment in the form of excessive urinary albumin excretion.[13]

ASSESSMENT OF KIDNEY FUNCTION

Laboratory assessment in suspected kidney disease involves tests of the blood and the urine. The hallmark of acute or chronic kidney dysfunction is an increase in blood levels of urea (blood urea nitrogen [BUN]) and creatinine, indicating loss of the clearance function of the kidneys. Blood creatinine levels are used to estimate GFR, with several equations available to make this estimation. Among the existing equations, which include the Cockcroft–Gault, Modification of Diet in Renal Disease (MDRD), and Chronic Kidney Disease Epidemiology Collaboration (CKD-EPI), the CKD-EPI is often recommended as calculating an eGFR closest to a measured GFR (mGFR).

In addition to estimating equations, 24-hour urine collections can be used to calculate creatinine clearance, a more precise GFR measure than those provided by a single plasma sample for creatinine.

Nephrology laboratory-based mGFR determinations use infusions of iothalamate or iohexol to determine glomerular clearance. Although their use is not common clinically, mGFR is considered the *gold standard* of GFR measurements, and estimating equations are generally validated by comparison with mGFR. Serum measurement of the protein cystatin C has also been proposed as a measure of GFR; however, this test has not been widely adopted for clinical use. Finally, as previously noted, the urinary ACR is a common test of renal function, with the normal level being <30 mg albumin/g Cr.

Patients with AKI may present with or develop oliguria or anuria, and urinalysis may show red blood cells, tubule cells, or casts (urine particles containing proteins often consolidated around red blood cells or tubule cells that have sloughed off in the process of kidney injury). Proteinuria can occur during acute glomerular injury states, in the context of nephrotic syndromes with little tubular damage, or in the context of CKD. Although several different proteins may be present in urine, the most common assay is to measure the urine albumin and to report it as a ratio with the urine creatinine concentration. Patients with CKD do not generally present with oliguria or anuria. Either AKI or CKD can have manifestations of altered kidney maintenance of fluid and electrolyte homeostasis, including hypertension, edema, and acidosis. Long-standing CKD causes other homeostatic imbalances including anemia, hyperphosphatemia, and associated bone abnormalities.

MECHANISMS AND MANIFESTATIONS OF ACUTE KIDNEY INJURY

AKI is a common complication of critical care, with sepsis the most common cause. AKI is also relatively common in patients hospitalized for heart failure, as a consequence of inadequate renal perfusion due to low cardiac output. However, AKI can also occur in at-risk patients within community settings, so a careful history is important to evaluate the likelihood of this diagnosis

TABLE 12.3 Estimated Global Prevalence of Chronic Kidney Disease by Stage		
Stage and Definition	Mean (%)	Range (%)
Stage 1: eGFR >90, ACR >30	3.5	2.8–4.2
Stage 2: eGFR 60–89, ACR >30	3.9	2.7–5.3
Stage 3: eGFR 30–59	7.6	6.4–8.9
Stage 4: eGFR 15–29	0.4	0.3–0.5
Stage 5: eGFR <15	0.1	0.1–0.1

ACR, albumin/creatinine ratio; eGFR, estimated glomerular filtration rate, stated in mL/min/1.73 m². *Source:* Derived from Hill NR, et al. Global prevalence of chronic kidney disease—a systematic review and meta-analysis. *PLoS One.* 2016;11. https://doi.org/10.1371/journal.pone.0158765.

in patients entering the clinic. AKI is defined clinically by rise in serum creatinine or decrease in eGFR, as well as changes in urine output. Rapidly rising serum creatinine and falling eGFR, as well as urine output, are best monitored in inpatient settings, so hospitalization is appropriate for patients with suspected AKI entering a primary care setting.

Historically, AKI has been subdivided by cause into prerenal, intrarenal, and postrenal. **Prerenal kidney damage** results from inadequate RBF that could occur in a variety of low flow states such as cardiogenic shock, hemorrhagic shock, or sepsis. Treatment must be directed at the initial cause while carefully monitoring to assess whether acute renal replacement therapy by dialysis is needed. **Postrenal kidney damage** results from obstruction within the renal tubular system, ureters, bladder, or urethra. In the case of a kidney stone, blockage of one ureter may not manifest as AKI, because of function of the remaining kidney, but can cause an abrupt change in eGFR.

AKI due to **intrarenal kidney damage** can result from pathological dysfunction of the glomerulus, tubule, interstitium, or renal vasculature.[2] Sources of glomerular injury were previously discussed. Damage to the tubules can result from direct injury by endogenous substances such as myoglobin and hemoglobin released during rhabdomyolysis or hemolysis, respectively. Nephrotoxic drugs, including several antibiotics, chemotherapy drugs, and radiographic contrast media, are a common source of kidney injury due to altered hemodynamics, tubular cell damage and death, or tubule occlusion due to crystal formation. Examples of nephrotoxic drugs are listed in **Table 12.4**.[14] Finally, hypoxia and ischemia during low flow states, in addition to causing prerenal AKI, can precipitate **acute tubular necrosis** and tubule cell damage and death. In all of these tubular insults, cells can slough off the basement membrane, obstructing the tubular lumen and acutely reducing GFR and urine output. The renal interstitium can also be the target of damage by hypoxia, nephrotoxic drugs, and viral and bacterial infections. Finally, the highly vascular kidneys are particularly vulnerable to generalized vascular disorders such as vasculitis, microangiopathic thrombotic states (hemolytic uremic syndrome [HUS], thrombotic thrombocytopenic purpura), and thrombi or emboli.

AKI is generally managed with fluid replacement, correction of acid and base imbalances or alkalinization to assist with clearance of a toxic substance, and dialysis in some cases. Recovery may be complete after the original event, but AKI predisposes to later development of CKD.[15] Knowing individual risk factors (patient age, presence of diabetes and hypertension, prior eGFR measurements) should guide drug prescribing to prevent precipitating AKI.

TABLE 12.4 Drugs Associated With Kidney Injury

Mechanism	Examples
Altered hemodynamics	ACE inhibitors ARBs Antihypertensives Diuretics Laxatives NSAIDs
Tubular toxicity	Aminoglycoside antibiotics Amphotericin Calcineurin inhibitors (cyclosporine, tacrolimus) Cisplatin Proton pump inhibitors Radiographic contrast media Vancomycin
Luminal crystal formation	Acyclovir Statin-induced rhabdomyolysis Sulfonamides Tricyclic antidepressants

ACE, angiotensin-converting enzyme; ARBs, angiotensin receptor blockers; NSAIDs, nonsteroidal anti inflammatory drugs.
Source: Synthesized from Cervelli MJ, Russ GR. Principles of drug therapy, dosing, and prescribing in chronic kidney disease and renal replacement therapy. In: Feehally J, Floege J, Tonelli M, Johnson RJ, eds. *Comprehensive Clinical Nephrology.* 6th ed. Philadelphia, PA: Elsevier; 2019:chap 74, 870–879.

Kidney Stones

Nephrolithiasis is another term for formation of **kidney stones**, also known as **renal calculi**. Kidney stones are common; in the United States the adult prevalence is 10.6% in men and 7.1% in women. Stone formation is more common in individuals with obesity and diabetes. Up to 40% of those who present with kidney stones will have recurrent stone formation within 15 years.[16] Stone formation starts with a supersaturated solution of crystal-forming molecules in the renal calyces. Thus, having maximally concentrated urine increases risk of stone formation. On a Western diet that favors urine acidity, most stones are formed from calcium oxalate or uric acid. Calcium phosphate stone formation is promoted by urine alkalinity and is also more common during pregnancy.

Not all stones lodge in the ureters. Some remain in the kidney or are excreted painlessly. However, when a stone lodges and blocks the ureter, it is associated with intense pain. Once a stone has formed, it cannot be dissolved. If it does not pass spontaneously, then a variety of invasive and noninvasive methods are employed for its removal. Prevention of stone formation includes increasing water intake, reducing intake of meats and poultry while increasing vegetable intake, and avoiding soda beverages.[17]

10. What is the most common setting in which AKI occurs? What are the short-term and long-term outcomes of AKI?

MECHANISMS AND MANIFESTATIONS OF CHRONIC KIDNEY DISEASE

The prevalence of **chronic kidney disease** (CKD) in the United States is estimated at almost 15% of the adult population, while self-reports of a diagnosis of CKD are far lower at 3%, indicating a low degree of awareness of this disorder.[1] This lack of awareness is likely due to the asymptomatic nature of CKD before it reaches stage 5 or ESRD. Unfortunately, the disease will continue to progress in the unaware patient, who might otherwise, upon diagnosis, be monitored closely and managed for conditions, such as diabetes and hypertension, that accelerate CKD. Criteria for the diagnosis and staging of CKD involve laboratory measurements of eGFR, often using the previously mentioned CKD-EPI estimating equation, as well as laboratory measurement of the urinary ACR.

As noted earlier and in **Table 12.3**, most patients with CKD are in stage 3, and stages 1 through 3 are often asymptomatic. Stage 5, the most severe grade of CKD, is associated with an eGFR of <15 mL/min/1.73 m² body surface area. It should be noted that ESRD is a *diagnosis based on patient management*.[18] Although there is a large overlap between ESRD and stage 5 CKD, the diagnosis of ESRD implies that a patient cannot survive without receiving renal replacement therapy (either hemodialysis or peritoneal dialysis) or kidney transplantation. Without such treatments, ESRD will be fatal.

Mechanisms of CKD begin at birth. The number of nephrons at birth depends on intrauterine factors, such as growth restriction with low birth weight, as well as prematurity. Both of these conditions reduce the initial nephron number.[19] Because new nephrons do not develop after birth, the infant with a lower number of nephrons is predisposed to later life CKD.[20] The kidneys can compensate for decreased nephron number, whether due to fetal influences or even kidney donation, by growing in size (kidney enlargement and nephron hypertrophy) and by increasing filtration rate by remaining nephrons (hyperfiltration). Kidney donors undergo screening to ensure optimal functioning, as determined by mGFR and absence of risk factors, before receiving permission to donate.

As previously noted, diabetes mellitus is the most common cause of CKD. This is due, in part, to the effects of elevated blood glucose on proteins of the glomerulus, including basement membrane, podocytes, and mesangial cells.[8] In addition, increased tubular glucose tends to promote hyperfiltration, increasing stress on the glomerulus.[21,22] Other causes of CKD range from genetic disorders such as polycystic kidney disease to the glomerular disorders listed in **Box 12.1**, and include a history of AKI, nephrotoxic events, and obesity. The final common pathway to progressive CKD often involves loss of glomerular function and the pathological appearance of **glomerulosclerosis** (scarring and loss of surface area of glomerular capillaries), along with capillary volume shrinkage in Bowman's space, even as there is expansion and fibrosis of the surrounding mesangial tissue. **Tubular atrophy** ensues as glomerular function is lost and tubule cells undergo apoptosis. **Interstitial fibrosis** is often seen, as fibrotic tissue replaces some of the kidney tissue after nephron death.

Loss of normal podocyte structure and function has been proposed as an initiating mechanism in development of glomerulosclerosis (**Figures 12.18** and **12.19**). After an initial insult, the glomerular capillary forms scar tissue and adheres to the wall of Bowman's space, after which the space fills, initially with hyaline fluid that is then displaced by expansion of the mesangial matrix. Thus, capillary loops progressively drop out of function until the entire unit (glomerulus + nephron tubules) degenerates and is reabsorbed.[19] For reasons that are not completely understood, there is a prominent relationship between CKD and cardiovascular disease, and most patients in stages 3 and 4 are more likely to die of cardiovascular disease than ESRD. Dyslipidemia is common in CKD and may be a major predisposing factor in cardiovascular mortality risk.[20,23]

END-STAGE RENAL DISEASE

Beginning with stage 4, and continuing through stage 5 CKD, fluid and electrolyte homeostasis becomes progressively more disordered, requiring regular dialysis treatments. **Anemia** is very common, resulting from shorter red blood cell life span as well as lack of erythropoietin. **Hypertension** and **metabolic acidosis** are also common. **Chronic kidney disease mineral and bone disorder** (CKD-MBD) is associated with dysregulation of calcium and phosphate metabolism characterized by hyperphosphatemia, decreased 1,25-dihydroxy vitamin D, and elevated parathyroid hormone. The result is bone demineralization that helps to maintain normal blood calcium levels, but predisposes to fractures.[24]

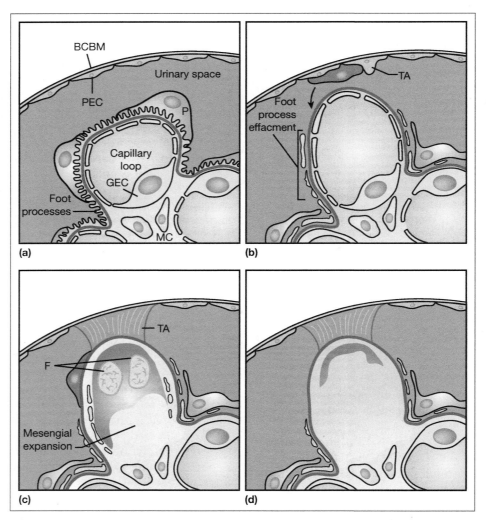

FIGURE 12.18 Glomerulosclerosis pathology. (**a**) Normal appearance of glomerular capillary surrounded by basement membrane and podocytes' foot processes separated by small filtration slits. (**b**) Podocyte damage initiates degenerative changes—foot processes are effaced, exposing glomerular basement membrane, which forms abnormal attachments to the PECs lining Bowman's capsule. (**c**) PECs deposit matrix on the outside of the glomerular capillary, while the mesangial matrix expands within the capillary. The capillary fills with hyaline fluid and foam cells. (**d**) The glomerular capillary collapses with fibrotic changes, surface area for glomerular filtration in this loop is completely lost, contributing to an overall decrease in glomerular filtration rate.

BCBM, Bowman's capsule parietal cell basement membrane; F, foam cell; GEC, glomerular endothelial cell; MC, mesangial cell; P, podocyte; PEC, parietal epithelial cell; TA, tuft adhesion.

 Thought Questions

11. What is nephron hyperfiltration? What conditions promote hyperfiltration, and what are the consequences?

12. How is the GFR measured? What are the strengths and limitations of methods of determining GFR?

13. What is a normal urinary ACR, and what disorders alter this ratio?

APOL1 AND CKD PROGRESSION

Studies evaluating racial differences in CKD outcomes have identified a racial difference in rate of progression of CKD as well as prevalence of individuals with ESRD. Specifically, Americans with African ancestral descent have a greater prevalence of ESRD, are more likely to have advanced kidney disease at a younger age, and are more likely to be on dialysis. In addition, African American patients are less likely than Whites to have rapid declines in eGFR and more likely to have proteinuria, suggesting a potentially different

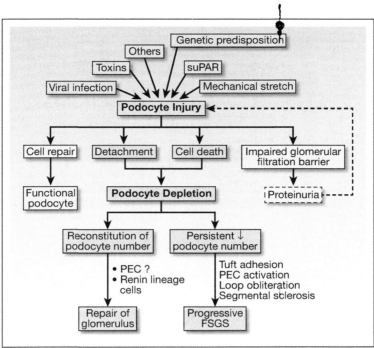

FIGURE 12.19 Proposed pathogenesis of FSGS originating with podocyte dysfunction. Different insults can lead to the common point of podocyte injury. If the inducing agent is removed and supportive care is given, the nephron may recover. If not, ongoing insults will end in progressive glomerulosclerosis, decreased glomerular filtration rate, and chronic kidney disease progression.

FSGS, focal segmental glomerulosclerosis; PEC, parietal epithelial cell; suPAR, soluble urokinase-type plasminogen activator receptor.

Source: From Jefferson JA, Shankland SJ. The pathogenesis of focal segmental glomerulosclerosis. *Adv Chronic Kidney Dis.* 2014;21:408–416.

pathophysiological process of CKD in this group. In recent years, there has been accumulating evidence of two high-risk mutations in the gene coding for APOL1, a protein associated with high-density lipoprotein, and kidney disease progression. The relationship is complex, in that being heterozygous or homozygous for a high-risk allele either may directly increase development of CKD or may predispose to CKD development after a second *hit*, such as infection with HIV or other infections. APOL1 mutations may be evolutionarily favored because they are protective against certain trypanosome infections, which are mainly found in various countries in Africa. The mechanisms linking these mutations to accelerated CKD and other kidney diseases have not yet been identified, but this finding has important implications for the screening and kidney status monitoring of patients with a high degree of African ancestral descent.[25,26]

PEDIATRIC CONSIDERATIONS

Theresa Kyle

URINARY SYSTEM DEVELOPMENT

The embryonic kidneys develop from the urogenital sinus, with the nephrons developing specifically from the intermediate mesoderm and ureteric bud throughout gestation until about 29 weeks. In the full-term newborn, the kidney is approximately 6 cm in length and weighs 24 g. During the first decade of life, as the kidneys functionally mature, the length increases to at least 12 cm and weight increases to 150 g (in the adult).[27]

NEPHRON DEVELOPMENT

Nephron development is complete by 36 to 40 weeks of gestation and does not continue after birth. As noted earlier in this chapter, the kidneys contain on average approximately 1 million nephrons. However, the number of nephrons at birth can vary from 250,000 to 1.1 million—a difference that is strongly associated with birth weight: low birthweight infants have fewer nephrons. Premature birth is also associated with lower nephron numbers. Thus, the life span risk of CKD can potentially be influenced by prenatal factors that reduce nephron number at birth. Similarly, childhood overweight and obesity can increase blood pressure and nephron hyperfiltration, predisposing to later life progression to CKD.[28,19]

GLOMERULAR FILTRATION

Around the sixth week of fetal life, glomerular filtration begins.[27] The term newborn exhibits a GFR of 17 to 60 mL/min/1.73 m², which increases over the first 2 to 3 years of life to adult levels. Development of the concentrated medullary interstitium is delayed, with a corresponding delay in the ability to concentrate urine, placing neonates and young children at increased risk for dehydration as compared with the older child and adult.

URINE PRODUCTION

In the term newborn, the normal rate of urine flow is 1 to 3 mL/kg/h.[29] As the renal system matures and urine concentrating abilities are increased, expected urine output is about 1 to 2 mL/kg/h. Oliguria is defined as urine output <1.0 mL/kg/h in the infant and <0.5 mL/kg/h in the child.[30]

PEDIATRIC DISORDERS OF URINARY TRACT AND KIDNEYS

CONGENITAL ANOMALIES OF THE URINARY TRACT

Several urinary tract anomalies may manifest as congenital findings at birth. Each of these **congenital urinary anomalies** is believed to be a result of aberrant formation during the embryonic stage. The obstructive uropathies often lead to hydronephrosis, which may be diagnosed by prenatal ultrasound. Table 12.5 summarizes several of these anomalies and their clinical implications.

VESICOURETERAL REFLUX

Often an incidental finding during a urinary tract infection workup, in **vesicoureteral reflux** (VUR) urine flows from the bladder back up the ureters. Reflux is most often congenital (primary VUR) and can result from abnormal development of the ureteral orifice, as well as higher-than-normal bladder pressure. VUR is common in infants but gradually resolves, with few children manifesting the condition past age 5. Before the age of 6 months, VUR is more common in boys than girls, by a 3:1 ratio. After that age, the ratio gradually changes until prevalence equalizes at 20 to 24 months, with female predominance thereafter.[31] VUR is graded according to the amount of dilation that results in the collection system. Grade 1 is reflux into the ureter without dilation; in grade 2, the reflux extends into the upper collecting system without dilation. Grade 1 or 2 VUR may resolve spontaneously. Grades 3, 4, and 5 result in dilation of the ureter(s) and collecting system(s); grade 5 is often associated with a prolonged time course of resolution, recurrent urinary tract infections, hydronephrosis, and subsequent kidney damage. Antibiotic prophylaxis is sometimes indicated for recurrent infections in all grades of VUR, while severe grades are generally managed surgically.[32]

ACUTE KIDNEY INJURY

As discussed earlier in this chapter, AKI in adults commonly accompanies critical illness. In a similar fashion, critically ill neonates, infants, and children have high rates of AKI that can result in prolonged kidney dysfunction, even after hospitalization. AKI risk is increased by cardiac surgery to correct congenital heart disease, and by necrotizing enterocolitis, diabetes mellitus, and sickle cell disease.[33]

TABLE 12.5 Congenital Anomalies of the Kidney, Ureter, and Bladder

Anomaly	Description	Clinical Implications
Bladder exstrophy	Bladder is open and exposed outside the abdomen	Requires surgical correction
Hypospadias	Urethral meatus is on ventral side of penis rather than center of glans	Requires surgical correction
Epispadias	Urethral meatus is on dorsal side of penis rather than center of glans	Requires surgical correction
Horseshoe kidney	Fusion of lower poles of kidney resulting from contact between metanephric blastemas	Adequate (usually) kidney and ureter function; increased incidence of urinary tract infection or obstruction
Obstructive Uropathies		
UPJ obstruction	Narrowing of UPJ	Results in hydronephrosis on affected side
UVJ obstruction	Narrowing at UVJ	Results in dilated ureter and hydronephrosis on affected side
Posterior urethral valves (only in males)	Flaps of tissue in proximal urethra	Results in distended proximal urethra, bladder, and ureters, and hydronephrosis
Ureterocele	Ureter swells into bladder causing a cystic pouch where ureter inserts	Results in dilated ureter and hydronephrosis on affected side

UPJ, ureteropelvic junction; UVJ, ureterovesicular junction.
Source: From Cadnapaphornchai MA, Lum GM. Kidney and urinary tract. In: Hay WW, et al., eds. *Current Diagnosis and Treatment Pediatrics.* 23rd ed. New York, NY: McGraw-Hill; 2016:710–734; Gaylord NM. Genitourinary disorders. In: Burns CE, et al., eds. *Pediatric Primary Care.* 6th ed. St. Louis, MO: Elsevier; 2017:911–946; Hill MA. Lecture: renal development. https://embryology.med.unsw.edu.au/embryology/index.php/Lecture_-_Renal_Development. Updated August 28, 2018.

ACUTE POSTSTREPTOCOCCAL GLOMERULONEPHRITIS

Acute poststreptococcal glomerulonephritis (APSGN) follows a respiratory or skin infection with a nephritogenic strain of group A β-hemolytic streptococcus. An immune-mediated response to the bacteria causes inflammation of glomeruli, resulting in mesangial cell proliferation, polymorphonuclear leukocyte infiltration, and enlargement of the kidneys. It occurs most commonly in children ages 5 to 12 years, and usually presents with hematuria and hypertension. The natural history of APSGN ranges from spontaneous resolution within 6 to 8 weeks to (uncommonly) renal failure.[34]

HEMOLYTIC UREMIC SYNDROME

Hemolytic uremic syndrome (HUS) is identified by three concurrent features: microangiopathic hemolytic anemia, thrombocytopenia, and acute renal failure. In 85% to 90% of patients, HUS follows an antecedent diarrheal illness with shiga toxin–producing *Escherichia coli* (STEC), particularly *E. coli* O157. Watery diarrhea is followed by hemorrhagic crisis and then renal failure. Hemorrhagic crisis results from renal microvascular injury and endothelial cell damage caused by the shiga toxin. This leads to thrombosis in the glomeruli, which decreases the GFR. Platelet aggregation in areas of microvascular injuries causes thrombocytopenia. Renal arteries and arterioles can become completely occluded, causing acute ischemic necrosis of the cortex and complete loss of GFR. Many children with HUS require dialysis, and the prognosis is improved with early recognition and treatment. Long-term outcome can include progression to CKD.[35,36]

MINIMAL CHANGE DISEASE/NEPHROTIC SYNDROME

Minimal change disease/nephrotic syndrome is a relatively rare condition, occurring in two to seven per 100,000 children.[37] Nephrotic syndrome refers to excretion of large amounts of protein in the urine, resulting from increased permeability of the glomerular basement membrane and leading to a deficit of plasma proteins. The term *minimal change* was based on early evidence that individuals with this form of proteinuria do not have any glomerular pathology that is visible under light microscopy. Rather, electron microscopy shows abnormal podocyte structure, which is the source of the loss of glomerular barrier function. Children with minimal change disease present most often by age 6 years with proteinuria, hypoalbuminemia, and edema. As albumin is lost during glomerular filtration, a shift in capillary oncotic pressure occurs, promoting widespread capillary filtration and edema. Loss of vascular volume triggers endocrine compensation that stimulates the kidneys to conserve water and sodium, perpetuating the edematous state. The liver increases production of lipoproteins, resulting in hyperlipidemia as well.

Urinary losses of immunoglobulins and properdin factor B, as well as defective cell-mediated immunity and other factors, place children at increased risk of significant infection with *Streptococcus pneumoniae*. In most cases, steroid administration reverses the nephrotic state, but children with steroid-resistant nephrotic syndrome may progress to ESRD requiring dialysis or renal transplantation.[37,38]

POLYCYSTIC KIDNEY DISEASE

Autosomal dominant polycystic kidney disease (ADPKD or PKD) is the most common disorder of renal structure and function, affecting one in 400 to 1,000 live births.[39] Global prevalence is 4 to 7 million.[40] Two different genes, *PKD1* and *PKD2*, can cause the disorder. These genes code for polycystin proteins 1 and 2, respectively. The polycystin proteins are part of a protein complex that forms cilia on the tubular epithelial cells and regulates intracellular calcium signaling. The mechanisms by which these alterations predispose to cyst formation are not well understood. Over time, epithelial cells form cysts that grow and crowd out the normal nephrons, progressing to ESRD.

ADPKD is 100% penetrant but has variable expressivity, and a second hit to a normal gene allele is required to produce the phenotype, so the age at which altered kidney function develops is quite variable. In the past, it was thought that ADPKD did not develop until adulthood. Now, it is clear that some affected individuals begin to develop cystic kidneys and loss of GFR in childhood (termed very early onset [*VEO*] *PKD*), while others may not have these manifestations until well into adulthood. Variable expressivity in individuals with ADPKD gene mutations is manifested, in part, by age of onset and rate of progression to requiring renal replacement therapy (RRT). Some mutations are embryonic lethal and others have VEO kidney manifestations. Most people do not have clinically detectable CKD until adulthood, and some are quite slow to progress. Some have intermediate forms, with some evidence of decreased GFR in late childhood and requiring RRT by the age of 40. ESRD results when virtually all of the kidney tissue has been replaced by cystic tissue. As with other kidney disorders in children and adults, progression is associated with risk factors such as low birthweight and high body mass index, and presentation may include hypertension, urinary infections, proteinuria, and decreased GFR.[39]

Autosomal recessive PKD is much less common than the autosomal dominant form, occurring in one in 20,000 live births.[41] Kidney abnormalities are present before birth, and are often diagnosed by prenatal ultrasound. The perinatal mortality rate due to this disease is about 30%. Other aspects of the phenotype include liver abnormalities with dilated bile ducts, liver fibrosis, and portal hypertension; systemic hypertension; and cognitive deficits. *PKHD1* is the gene mutated in this form of PKD. It encodes a membrane protein associated with cilia and apical membranes of tubule cells in the kidney. This is a large gene with a range of mutations, some of which have more severe clinical consequences than others. The age of onset and progression to ESRD is also variable, depending on the severity of the syndrome. Kidney transplantation is a treatment option and can be combined with liver transplantation to treat the manifestations of kidney and liver failure.[41]

Ryan Prince

AGE-RELATED CHANGES IN THE KIDNEY

Age-related changes in the kidney include changes in organ size, number of nephrons, GFR, vasculature, and metabolism. Knowledge of age-associated changes in kidney function and histology has been greatly informed by studying tissue biopsies from healthy kidney donors of different ages (Box 12.2).[42]

CHANGES IN KIDNEY MASS AND VOLUME

The kidneys start to decrease in both weight and volume starting at about the fourth decade of life.[43,44] Loss of mass occurs mainly in cortical tissue owing to reduction in number and function of nephrons, while medullary mass is generally preserved.

CHANGES IN RENAL BLOOD FLOW AND GLOMERULAR FILTRATION RATE

In the adult, RBF is about 1,000 to 1,200 mL/min in the absence of kidney disease, and GFR is about 10% of that. Each decade after age 40, RBF is reduced by about 10% and average GFR decreases by about 8 mL/min/1.73 m^2.[44] The reduction in GFR and RBF are interconnected and primarily involve structural changes within the kidney and its vasculature. As noted earlier, studies such as the one described in Box 12.2 have shown that many of these processes will occur independently of comorbid pathological processes. However, metabolic syndromes such as diabetes and hypertension, as well as pathological processes such as atherosclerosis and vasculitis, correlate with more pronounced structural changes and decreases in kidney function. Finally, muscle mass and creatinine production can decline with aging, so serum creatinine may remain normal despite reduced GFR.[44]

CHANGES IN NEPHRON NUMBERS AND FUNCTION

At approximately age 40, the number of nephrons begins to decrease by more than 6,000 per kidney per year, partially explaining the decreased RBF and GFR described earlier.[43] Because nephron number at birth

---

BOX 12.2

Relationship Between Age and Nephrosclerosis in Older Adults

A cross-sectional study of more than 1,200 living kidney donors examined directly mGFR as well as eGFR estimates (using the MDRD equation), urine 24-hour albumin and protein measurements, blood pressure monitoring, and blood glucose measurements to learn whether abnormalities in the kidney are more prevalent with age, and whether these findings are explained by age-related differences in kidney function or by CKD risk factors.[42]

Among these healthy donors, mGFR had a significant relationship with age, showing a decrease with aging. Tissue biopsies were analyzed for nephrosclerosis, which was defined as having signs of two or more of the following histological changes: glomerulosclerosis, tubular atrophy, arteriolar narrowing, and interstitial fibrosis. Although nephrosclerosis increased with age, the relationship between mGFR and age was not influenced by degree of nephrosclerosis. Thus, the relationship between histological findings and their functional implications remains unclear. Key findings were as follows:

- Nephrosclerosis was significantly associated with 24-hour urine albumin, nocturnal systolic and diastolic blood pressure, and hypertension (defined as use of antihypertensive medications).

- Kidney donors aged 18 to 29 years had mGFR of 114 ± 19 mL/min/1.73 m^2, whereas donors aged 60 to 69 years old had mGFR of 90 ± 12 mL/min/1.73 m^2.

- Prevalence of nephrosclerosis was 2.7% in the younger age group and 58% in the older age group.

This suggests that, although GFR declines with normal healthy aging, histological changes may occur to a greater extent and may not produce a direct impact on GFR. It is important to note, however, that prospective kidney donors were selected for healthy kidney function and absence of diabetes. Across the entire population of older adults, it is very likely that average GFR is lower than that observed in this study.[42]

CKD, chronic kidney disease, eGFR, estimated glomerular filtration rate; GFR, glomerular filtration rate; MDRD, Modification of Diet in Renal Disease; mGFR, measured glomerular filtration rate.

varies greatly, the loss of nephrons with age is predicted to have the greatest impact in individuals who started life with fewer nephrons due to premature birth or other prenatal influences. General nephron changes associated with aging include thickened basement membrane; dilation, atrophy, and fibrosis of tubules; and degenerative changes in renal vessels. Decreased tubular regulation of sodium and potassium homeostasis has been reported with aging.[45]

MECHANISMS OF ON KIDNEY FUNCTION ALTERATIONS WITH AGING

A number of identified age-related changes at the molecular, cellular, and tissue level have particular significance for age-associated declines in kidney function, as described here.

Arteriosclerosis

Arteriosclerosis, an increase in vascular stiffness, occurs in aging arteries and arterioles. **Hyaline arteriosclerosis** is identified by the presence of clear deposits that thicken the walls of arteries and arterioles. This form is common with aging and is more severe in older adults with hypertension. **Hyaline arteriolosclerosis** of the afferent arterioles can reduce glomerular blood flow and can become severe enough to lead to shunting of blood from afferent to efferent arterioles, completely bypassing some glomeruli.[46]

Different signaling pathways and feedback mechanisms play a role in arteriosclerosis, some of which are specific to the kidney. Total renin and aldosterone levels fall during aging as the RAAS is less active. Studies show, however, that the renal response to angiotensin receptor activation is actually increased. ACE inhibitors and ARBs have been shown to reduce the age-related decline in kidney function. Sex hormones and their effect on the RAAS may play a role in renal preservation with aging. Androgens have been shown to upregulate RAAS activity, whereas estrogen, by suppression of tissue levels and activity of angiotensin II and ACE, downregulates it. Women tend to have slower progression of CKD than men, potentially reflecting this protective effect of estrogen.[44]

Glomerulosclerosis

Glomerulosclerosis is identified histologically, in part, as the presence of shrunken glomerular capillaries that detach from the surrounding Bowman's capsule. Glomerulosclerosis contributes to age-related nephron loss, in combination with arteriosclerosis, tubular atrophy, and interstitial fibrosis.

Tubular Atrophy and Interstitial Fibrosis

Tubular atrophy and interstitial fibrosis are likely the final steps in nephron death and are preceded by glomerular collapse. Tubular atrophy is evident by overall loss or collapse of visible tubules in biopsy specimens. Interstitial fibrosis involves the deposition into the tubule walls of extracellular proteins that are filtered due to glomerular injury.

CLINICAL CONSIDERATIONS IN OLDER ADULTS

MEDICATION DOSING

Reductions in nephron number and GFR impact renal drug clearance in older adults. One study examining medication use in older adults showed that adverse drug reactions correlated inversely and exponentially with declining kidney function.[47] Both direct and indirect changes in the aging kidney can account for this, including many of the changes discussed earlier.

Direct Mechanisms

Decreases in GFR and in PT drug transport capacity increase the risk for reduced drug clearance, allowing accumulation of drugs and their active metabolites. These changes can allow drugs, especially those with narrow therapeutic indexes, to reach toxic levels in the serum and exhibit deleterious effects.

Indirect Mechanisms

Renal pharmacokinetic alterations in older adults compound the changes in other systems, particularly declining liver blood flow and reduced stage I biotransformation. Most drugs have higher bioavailability as GFR and liver metabolism decrease. Given the changes in pharmacokinetics in CKD, it is important to dose medications according to the manufacturer guidelines based on GFR. Unfortunately, the estimating equations based on serum creatinine have not been fully validated across all age ranges. As previously noted, older adults have reduced muscle mass, which decreases creatinine production and influences eGFR as calculated by the MDRD and CKD-EPI equations. Recent efforts have been directed at developing eGFR estimating procedures that better reflect alterations with age and sex.[48] Additionally, medications with narrow therapeutic indexes and known risk of nephrotoxicity can be monitored routinely with serum level measurements.

OTHER CONSIDERATIONS

Other clinical considerations related to declining kidney function in older adults include a greater probability of AKI given declining renal reserves. Older adults with or without CKD are still at risk of AKI and of drug-induced kidney injury, and prescribing must take these factors into consideration, along with any comorbidities. Hypertension management that reduces blood pressure and flow could have negative effects if it further reduces renal perfusion.

SUMMARY OF AGE-RELATED CONCERNS

To conclude, the kidneys have tremendous capacity, filtering about 150 to 180 L/day in healthy young adults and maintaining homeostasis of body fluid volume and composition, acid–base balance, endogenous waste excretion, and elimination of drugs and toxins. Losses with aging often do not correlate with any manifestations of CKD, and homeostasis appears to be maintained. Many instances of AKI can be managed and do not result in long-term loss of renal function. Nevertheless, the high rate of kidney blood flow and high glomerular capillary hydrostatic pressure represent a risk of nephron, and particularly glomerular,

damage in the context of diabetes, hypertension, autoimmune disease, and infections. When the glomerular barriers are breached, the tubules can be exposed to damage from inflammatory cells and mediators. If some nephrons become completely nonfunctional, the remaining nephrons receive excess blood flow and are subject to hyperfiltration. This sets up a vicious cycle of further nephron damage and progression of CKD. The challenge to clinicians is to use protective strategies such as angiotensin blockade in patients at risk for kidney disease; to avoid inducing kidney injury in patients by careful attention to risk factors, including CKD and aging, when prescribing drugs; and to conduct appropriate monitoring based on comorbidities, age, and known risk factors.

CASE STUDY 12.1: A Patient With Chronic Kidney Disease

Kim Zuber and Jane S. Davis

Patient Complaint: *"My wife made me come in because I've never had a physical. I'm really healthy, and have never needed to see a doctor since I tore my ACL in college. My wife worries because I get up to urinate a few times at night and that wakes her up, but all guys do that, don't they?"*

History of Present Illness/Review of Systems: The patient is a 47-year-old Black man who works as a supervisor in an office environment. He tries to keep active, although his job involves significant sedentary time on a computer, but has noticed some recent fatigue. He is often thirsty and has been awakening to urinate several times each night. He has had no other symptoms. The patient states that he considers himself to be *pretty healthy*; he denies changes in vision, appetite, bowel habits, sensation, or coordination, and reports no episodes of dizziness, faintness, palpitations, or dyspnea.

Past Medical/Family/Social History: He has no past medical history but admits he has not been seen by a healthcare practitioner since he tore his ACL in college. His father died at age 61 of a heart attack after having high blood pressure for many years. His mother is still alive at age 70 years and has diabetes. His sister (age 45) is overweight, and his brother (age 42) has multiple orthopedic complaints but still plays basketball or tennis each week. The patient denies ever using cigarettes. He drinks a can of beer one to two times per week and denies use of illicit drugs. He reports occasional

use of over-the-counter ibuprofen for joint pain and stiffness.

Physical Examination: You observe a healthy-appearing patient in no acute distress. Vital signs are as follows: temperature of 97.6°F, blood pressure of 148/92 mm Hg, heart rate of 68 beats/min, and respirations of 20 breaths/min. His BMI is 27 kg/m². Upon auscultation, his heart appears to have a regular rate and rhythm, no murmurs are noted, no jugular vein distention is seen, lungs are clear, and abdomen is soft without tenderness or rebound. He has a scar on his left knee that corresponds to ACL reconstruction, and trace pedal edema bilaterally. His neurological function is intact, with normal strength, sensation, and reflexes. His pulses are intact and equal bilaterally. Pupils are equal, round, and reactive to light.

Laboratory and Diagnostic Findings: Laboratory tests reveal the following data: serum creatinine: 1.6 mg/dL; eGFR: 59 mL/min/1.73 m²; BUN: 12 mg/dL; potassium: 4.5 mEq/dL; calcium: 9.8 mg/dL; bicarbonate: 22 mmol/L; glucose: 132 mg/dL; sodium: 136 mEq/dL; hemoglobin A_{1c}: 7.4% (laboratories automatically run A_{1c} if random glucose is high); and urine ACR: 32 mg/g.

CASE STUDY 12.1 QUESTIONS
- *What major risk factors for kidney disease does this patient have?*
- *Explain the significance of increased serum creatinine and urine ACR.*

ACL, anterior cruciate ligament; ACR, albumin/creatinine ratio; BMI, body mass index; BUN, blood urea nitrogen; CKD, chronic kidney disease; GFR, glomerular filtration rate.

CASE STUDY 12.2: A Patient With a Kidney Stone

Kim Zuber and Jane S. Davis

Patient Complaint: *"I was in agony. I woke up in the middle of the night with such a terrible pain in my side and back that I fell out of bed. Then the pain eased up, and I got up to use the bathroom. My urine was pink, then turned red, so I got dressed and came to the emergency room right away. I haven't had any more pain, but I'm worried about what would cause my urine to be red."*

History of the Present Illness/Review of Systems: The patient is a 53-year-old White man who appears well, but worried. He presents to the ED complaining of an episode of pain that went away, followed by bloody urine. During the episode, the pain was 9/10, which he describes as *the worst pain I have ever felt.* He denies excessive thirst or urination, burning, urgency, or difficulty with urination. He reports that he has no joint pain or difficulty with movement or walking. He states that he has generally been in good health, with no distress, until he experienced the acute pain in his lower abdomen.

Past Medical/Family History: The patient has a history of hypertension (currently well controlled) and mild obesity. He had an attack of gout a few years ago, but has had no recurrences since he started treatment with allopurinol. In addition to

OTC, over-the-counter.

allopurinol 100 mg once daily, he takes amlodipine 10 mg once daily, and occasional OTC naproxen. His mother and brother have hypertension, and his father has gout.

Physical Examination: During your examination, the patient is diaphoretic and short of breath. Just as fast as the pain occurred, it is gone. Blood pressure is 158/98 mm Hg, respirations are 35 breaths/min, heart rate is 100 beats/min, and lungs are clear to auscultation. On examination, the abdomen is soft, without rebound but with slight tenderness in the left lower quadrant. Both rectal and hernia examinations are negative.

Laboratory and Diagnostic Findings: Serum creatinine is 1.3 mg/dL, uric acid is elevated at 8.5 mg/dL, and urine shows 2+ blood on dipstick, with many red blood cells on microscopic inspection. The complete blood count is normal. A flat-plate abdominal x-ray study of the kidneys, ureters, and bladder shows a small white calculus in the left ureter.

CASE STUDY 12.2 QUESTIONS
- *What are kidney stones made of?*
- *What are the risk factors for stone formation, and how can patients avoid a recurrence of stones?*

BRIDGE TO CLINICAL PRACTICE

Ben Cocchiaro

PRINCIPLES OF ASSESSMENT
History and Physical Examination
- *Renal/Urologic History:* Assess frequency and volume of urination, urgency, hesitancy (difficulty initiating urination), continence, dysuria, odor, and menstrual patterns. Hypertension, diabetes, autoimmune conditions, and smoking all negatively impact renal health. Review all medications taken for potential nephrotoxicity.
- *Pain:* Assess for suprapubic pain and tenderness indicative of inflammation of the urinary bladder (cystitis); dull, constant flank pain at the costovertebral angle suggests renal inflammation or distension. The ureteric pain of nephrolithiasis

is sharp and colicky, coincident with peristalsis of the ureter around an obstructing stone.
- *Urine Color:* Darkened urine may indicate dehydration. Red-brown urine may indicate the presence of red blood cells, or of myoglobin. Various dyes, medications, and foods are capable of altering urine color. Persistently frothy urine may indicate the presence of protein (usually albumin), while cloudy urine is sometimes seen in urinary tract infections.
- *Uremia:* Indicative of end-stage renal disease, uremia is the result of the accumulation of waste products. Symptoms include altered mental status, fatigue, nausea, pruritis, and bleeding.

(continued)

Diagnostic Tools
- *Renal Ultrasound:* Noninvasive study useful in the diagnosis of urinary obstruction, renal vascular flow, and some masses.
- *Computed Tomography:* Noncontrast low-dose CT scans are the gold standard for the diagnosis of renal calculi. Standard CT with contrast is more sensitive than ultrasonography in the evaluation of renal masses.
- *Cystoscopy:* An invasive procedure for the evaluation of obstructive and hematuric complaints performed by a urologist in which a camera is passed through the urethra and the inside of the bladder is visualized.
- *Biopsy:* A percutaneous, invasive process, renal biopsy can help establish definitive diagnoses in patients with renal masses, idiopathic nephrotic and nephritic syndromes, and unexplained acute renal failure.

Laboratory Evaluation
- *Urinalysis:*
  - *Dipstick:* Includes qualitative and semi-quantitative measures of leukocytes and nitrites (useful in the diagnosis of urinary tract infections), urobilinogen, protein, pH, hemoglobin, specific gravity, bilirubin, ketones, and glucose.
  - *Laboratory:* Formal urinalysis provides quantitative analysis of the above parameters, as well as squamous epithelial cells (indicative of a contaminated sample),
  - *Microscopic:* Microscopic urinalysis reveals and characterizes crystals, bacteria, and glomerular casts useful in the differentiation of nephritides.

- *Metabolic Panel:* Decreased renal function will increase plasma levels of potassium, phosphate, and magnesium, and often decreased levels of sodium, calcium, and albumin. Creatinine can be used to estimate the glomerular filtration rate, or GFR.
- *FeNa:* A comparison between urine and plasma creatinine and sodium concentrations is useful in differentiating pre-renal etiologies of acute kidney injury.
- *CBC:* Blood counts may demonstrate anemia in the setting of renal blood loss or through chronic renal damage resulting in decreased secretion of erythropoietin.

MAJOR DRUG CLASSES AND THERAPEUTIC MODALITIES
- *ACE Inhibitors and ARBs:* Through inhibition of the renin-angiotensin-aldosterone system, ACEs and ARBs have a vasodilatory effect, decreasing systemic vascular resistance and reducing glomerular capillary pressure. These properties protect against the nephropathies of both hypertension and diabetes mellitus.
- *Phosphate Binders:* Toxic levels of phosphate accumulate in the body during ESRD. Phosphate binders prevent GI absorption of this electrolyte.
- *rhEPO:* In anemia of chronic kidney disease, rhEPO is often given with ferrous sulfate to increase hemoglobin.
- *Hemodialysis:* Used in ESRD, severe cases of acute renal failure, and in some poisonings; employs an extracorporeal filtration system to replace lost renal function.

ACE, angiotensin-converting enzyme; ARBs, angiotensin receptor blockers; CBC, complete blood count; ESRD, end-stage renal disease; FeNa, fractional excretion of sodium; rhEPO, recombinant human erythropoietin.

KEY POINTS

- The kidney has several functions that contribute to homeostasis, but the primary role of the kidney is to maintain fluid and electrolyte balance over a wide range of body states and varying intake of water, electrolytes, and nutrients.
- The kidney has several endocrine roles, including production of erythropoietin, which stimulates red blood cell production, activation of vitamin D, and production of renin.

- The body is 50% to 60% water, depending on sex, age, and body composition, and the kidneys regulate the amount of body water as well as its composition.
- The functional unit of the kidney is the nephron, and each kidney contains about 1 million nephrons. There is considerable functional reserve; therefore, someone with healthy kidney function can donate a kidney and still maintain normal kidney function.
- The kidney receives a far greater blood flow (20% of cardiac output) than its size and weight

- (~0.5% of body weight) would dictate. High RBF enables a high rate of glomerular filtration (referred to as the GFR).
- The high rate of glomerular filtration is enabled by two principal factors:
  - Net filtration pressure in glomerular capillaries is much higher than in other capillary beds, primarily because of a high glomerular capillary hydrostatic pressure.
  - Glomerular capillary permeability is much higher than in other capillary beds, with a three-layer structure that promotes a high rate of fluid movement while restricting filtration of proteins.
- As filtered fluid (water and small molecules and electrolytes of the plasma, generally without the plasma proteins) enters the nephron, it is processed by the cells of the nephron tubules where more than 99% of the filtrate is reabsorbed and the volume is reduced to <1% of the original filtered volume, which is excreted as urine.
- Reabsorption of most filtered substances is a carrier-mediated process of movement from the lumen of the tubule to the interstitial space. Abundant transporters, ion channels, and water channels in the apical and basolateral membranes of tubule cells conduct this movement across the tubular membrane. From the interstitial space, the reabsorbed substances then move passively into peritubular capillaries.
- Metabolic waste products, toxins, neurotransmitters, hormones, and drugs are enriched in the urine by the process of tubular secretion. Transporters carry these substances from the interstitial space around the peritubular capillaries into the lumen to clear them from the blood by urinary excretion.
- The bulk of renal processing in the PT reabsorbs about 70% of filtered water, sodium, and chloride; 100% of glucose and amino acids; and 85% of bicarbonate. The PT is also a major site of secretion of wastes, drugs, and drug metabolites.
- The remainder of the nephron—LOH, DT, and collecting duct—primarily focuses on retention of sodium, chloride, and water; fine tuning of potassium, acid, calcium, and phosphate levels by reabsorption or secretion; and final processing to produce a concentrated urine, excreting wastes without excessive loss of water. These processes are moderated by hormones to maintain systemic fluid and electrolyte homeostasis.

- The most common causes of kidney disease are systemic:
  - CKD is a common consequence of diabetes mellitus (up to 50% of all CKD cases), hypertension (25% of CKD), or both.
  - AKI is most common in critical care settings as a consequence of hypovolemia and hypotension from causes such as sepsis, trauma, and acute heart failure. Nephrotoxicity from medications, hemolysis, or rhabdomyolysis is an additional source of AKI. Urine blockage from kidney stones or neoplasms is the third source of AKI.
  - AKI may resolve with treatment but is a risk factor for later CKD development.
  - CKD is also a risk factor for subsequent AKI.
- The glomerulus is the primary site of injury in patients with diabetes and hypertension, although disease progression later extends to tubular dysfunction.
- The glomerulus is further vulnerable to immune-mediated injury, principally due to the ability of antibodies and antigen–antibody complexes to pass through the highly permeable glomerular capillary walls to be deposited in Bowman's space. Immune activation in the glomerulus can be accompanied by complement-mediated tissue destruction, further damaging the filtration barrier or completely blocking filtration and acutely or chronically reducing GFR.
- Proteinuria is present in many cases of declining kidney function and is routinely monitored in patients at risk for kidney disease due to diabetes or hypertension. In nephrotic syndrome, proteinuria is the major manifestation and may present with resulting fluid losses and peripheral edema due to loss of plasma proteins, while aspects of tubular function may be maintained.
- On the other hand, chronic loss of kidney function in patients with diabetes and hypertension is characterized by the combination of nephron losses with increased glomerular permeability of the remaining nephrons. The combination is manifested by decreased eGFR accompanied by proteinuria.
- Staging of kidney disease involves eGFR values and the urine ACR.
- For reasons that are not completely clear, CKD at any level increases atherosclerosis and cardiovascular disease.
- ESRD is treated with dialysis or kidney transplantation when they are available; there are no other therapies at this time. ESRD is manifested

with the consequences of the loss of all short- and long-term kidney functions: increased BUN and creatinine, hypertension, hyperkalemia, acidosis, anemia (due to loss of erythropoietin), and CKD-MBD due to loss of calcium and phosphate homeostasis and metabolic acidosis.

- The kidney is the target for many drugs, some of which may increase kidney vulnerability to damage.
- Nephron development is complete by 36 weeks of gestational age. Prematurity and low birth weight are associated with reduced nephron numbers at birth and may predispose individuals to development of hypertension and kidney disease later in life.
- Pediatric urinary disorders include both malformations of urogenital structures and abnormalities of nephron function. Minimal change disease often has pediatric onset and results in nephrotic syndrome.
- Older adults have progressive renal tissue alterations, including loss of nephrons with glomerulosclerosis. They also have progressive reductions in estimated and measured GFR that may not be proportional to the histological changes. With sarcopenia in advanced age, creatinine production decreases, and it is not certain whether current estimating equations for GFR from serum creatinine accurately reflect GFR in older adults.
- Owing to altered RBF, urine concentrating ability, nephron number, and polypharmacy, older adults are at higher risk of AKI, particularly drug-induced kidney injury.

REFERENCES

1. United States Renal Data System. *2018 USRDS Annual Data Report: Epidemiology of Kidney Disease in the United States*. Bethesda, MD: National Institutes of Health, National Institute of Diabetes and Digestive and Kidney Diseases; 2018. https://www.usrds.org/2018/view/Default.aspx.
2. Makris K, Spanou L. Acute kidney injury: definition, pathophysiology, and clinical phenotypes. *Clin Biochem Rev*. 2016;37:85–98. https://www.ncbi.nlm.nih.gov/pmc/articles/PMC5198510.
3. Couser WG. Basic and translational concepts of immune-mediated glomerular diseases. *J Am Soc Nephrol*. 2012;23:381–399. doi:10.1681/ASN.2011030304.
4. Heher EC, Rennke HG, Laubach JP, Richardson PG. Kidney disease and multiple myeloma. *Clin J Am Soc Nephrol*. 2013;8:2007–2017. doi:10.2215/CJN.12231212.
5. Kurts C, Panzer U, Anders H-J, Rees AJ. The immune system and kidney disease: basic concepts and clinical implications. *Nat Rev Immunol*. 2013;13:738–753. doi:10.1038/nri3523.
6. American Diabetes Association. 11. Microvascular complications and foot care: *Standards of Medical Care in Diabetes–2019. Diabetes Care*. 2019;42(suppl 1):S124–S138. doi:10.2337/dc19-S011.
7. Magee C, Grieve DJ, Watson CJ, Brazil DP. Diabetic nephropathy: a tangled web to unweave. *Cardiovasc Drugs Ther*. 2017;31:579–592. doi:10.1007/s10557-017-6755-9.
8. Papadopoulou-Marketou N, Paschou SA, Marketos N, et al. Diabetic nephropathy in type 1 diabetes. *Minerva Med*. 2018;109:218–228. doi:10.23736/S0026-4806.17.05496-9.
9. Brezis M, Rosen S. Hypoxia of the renal medulla—its implications for disease. *N Engl J Med*. 1995;332:647–655. doi:10.1056/NEJM199503093321006.
10. Blaine J, Chonchol M, Levi M. Renal control of calcium, phosphate, and magnesium homeostasis. *Clin J Am Soc Nephrol*. 2015;10:1257–1272.
11. Ivanyuk A, Livio F, Biollaz J, Buclin T. Renal drug transporters and drug interactions. *Clin Pharmacokinet*. 2017;56:825–892. doi:10.1007/s40262-017-0506-8.
12. Neal MD. Fluid and electrolyte management of the surgical patient. In: Brunicardi FC, Andersen DK, Billiar TR, et al., eds. *Schwartz's Principles of Surgery*. Vol 1. 11th ed. New York, NY: McGraw-Hill Education; 2019: 83–102.
13. Hill NR, Fatoba SF, Oke JL, et al. Global prevalence of chronic kidney disease—a systematic review and meta-analysis. *PLOS ONE*. 2016;11(7):e0158765. doi:10.1371/journal.pone.0158765.
14. Cervelli MJ, Russ GR. Principles of drug therapy, dosing, and prescribing in chronic kidney disease and renal replacement therapy. In: Feehally J, Floege J, Tonelli M, Johnson RJ, eds. *Comprehensive Clinical Nephrology*. 6th ed. Philadelphia, PA: Elsevier; 2019:870–879.
15. Chawla LS, Eggers PW, Star RA, Kimmel PL. Acute kidney injury and chronic kidney disease as interconnected syndromes. *N Engl J Med*. 2014;371:58–66. doi:10.1056/NEJMra1214243.
16. Ziemba JB, Matlaga BR. Epidemiology and economics of nephrolithiasis. *Investing Clin Urol*. 2017;58:299–306. doi:10.4111/icu.2017.58.5.299.
17. Khan SR, Pearle MS, Robertson WG, et al. Kidney stones. *Nat Rev Dis Primers*. 2016;2:16008. doi:10.1038/nrdp.2016.8.
18. Levin A, Stevens PE. Summary of KDIGO 2012 CKD guideline: behind the scenes, need for guidance, and a framework for moving forward. *Kidney Int*. 2013;85: 49–61. doi:10.1038/ki.2013.444.
19. Luyckx VA, Bertram JF, Brenner BM, et al. Effect of fetal and child health on kidney development and long-term risk of hypertension and kidney disease. *Lancet*. 2013;382:273–283. doi:10.1016/S0140-6736(13)60311-6.
20. Romagnani P, Remuzzi G, Glassock R, et al. Chronic kidney disease. *Nat Rev Dis Primers*. 2017;3:17088. doi:10.1038/nrdp.2017.88.
21. Jefferson JA, Shankland SJ. The pathogenesis of focal segmental glomerulosclerosis. *Adv Chronic Kidney Dis*. 2014;21:408–416. doi:10.1053/j.ackd.2014.05.009.

22. Tuttle KR. Back to the future: glomerular hyperfiltration and the diabetic kidney. *Diabetes*. 2017;66:14–16. doi:10.2337/dbi16-0056.

23. Stenvinkel P, Herzog CA. Cardiovascular disease in chronic kidney disease. In: Feehally J, Floege J, Tonelli M, Johnson RJ, eds. *Comprehensive Clinical Nephrology*. 6th ed. Philadelphia, PA: Elsevier; 2019:942–957.

24. Seifert MA, Hruska KA. The kidney-vascular-bone axis in the chronic kidney disease-mineral bone disorder. *Transplantation*. 2016;100:497–505. doi:10.1097/TP.0000000000000903.

25. Freedman BI. APOL1 and nephropathy progression in populations of African ancestry. *Semin Nephrol*. 2013;33:425–432. doi:10.1016/j.semnephrol.2013.07.004.

26. Nally Jr JV. Chronic kidney disease in African Americans: puzzle pieces are falling into place. *Cleve Clin J Med*. 2017;84:855–862. doi:10.3949/ccjm.84gr.17007.

27. Pan CG, Avner ED. Introduction to glomerular diseases. In: Kliegman RM, Stanton BF, St. Geme JW, et al., eds. *Nelson Textbook of Pediatrics*. 20th ed. Philadelphia, PA: Elsevier; 2016:2490–2494.

28. Bertram JF, Douglas-Denton RN, Diouf B, et al. Human nephron number: implications for health and disease. *Pediatr Nephrol*. 2011;26:1529–1533. doi:10.1007/s00467-011-1843-8.

29. Smith D, Grover TR. The newborn infant. In: Hay WW, Levin MJ, Deterding RR, Abzug MJ, eds. *Current Diagnosis and Treatment Pediatrics*. 23rd ed. New York, NY: McGraw-Hill Education; 2016:10–70.

30. Shaw K. Nephrology. In: Enghorn B, Flerlage J, eds. *The Harriett Lane Handbook*. 20th ed. Philadelphia, PA: Elsevier Saunders; 2015:438–466.

31. Edwards A, Peters CA. Managing vesicoureteral reflux in children: making sense of all the data. *F1000Res*. 2019;8(F1000 Faculty Rev):29. doi:10.12688/f1000research.16534.1.

32. Tullus K. Vesicoureteric reflux in children. *Lancet*. 2015;385:371–379. doi:10.1016/S0140-6736(14)60383-4.

33. Selewski DT, Hyatt DM, Bennett KM, et al. Is acute kidney injury a harbinger for chronic kidney disease? *Curr Opin Pediatr*. 2018;30:236–240. doi:10.1097/MOP.0000000000000587.

34. Pan CG, Avner ED. Acute poststreptococcal glomerulonephritis. In: Kliegman RM, Stanton BF, St. Geme JW, et al., eds. *Nelson Textbook of Pediatrics*. 20th ed. Philadelphia, PA: Elsevier; 2016:2498–2501.

35. Fakhouri F, Zuber J, Frémeaux-Bacchi V, et al. Haemolytic uraemic syndrome. *Lancet*. 2017;390:681–696. doi:10.1016/S0140-6736(17)30062-4.

36. Karpman D, Loos S, Tati R, Arvidsson I. Haemolytic uraemic syndrome. *J Intern Med*. 2017;281:123–148. doi:10.1111/joim.12546.

37. Vivarelli M, Massella L, Ruggiero B, et al. Minimal change disease. *Clin J Am Soc Nephrol*. 2017;12:332–345. doi:10.2215/CJN.05000516.

38. Pais P, Avner ED. Nephrotic syndrome. In: Kliegman RM, Stanton BF, St. Geme JW, et al., eds. *Nelson Textbook of Pediatrics*. 20th ed. Philadelphia, PA: Elsevier; 2016:2521–2527.

39. De Rechter S, Bammens B, Schaefer F, et al. Unmet needs and challenges for follow-up and treatment of autosomal dominant polycystic kidney disease: the paediatric perspective. *Clin Kidney J*. 2018;11(suppl 1):i14–i26. doi:10.1093/ckj/sfy088.

40. Akoh JA. Current management of autosomal dominant polycystic kidney disease. *World J Nephrol*. 2015;4:468–479. doi:10.5527/wjn.v4.i4.468.

41. Hartung EA, Guay-Woodford LM. Autosomal recessive polycystic kidney disease: a hepatorenal fibrocystic disorder with pleiotropic effects. *Pediatrics*. 2014;134:e833–e845. doi:10.1542/peds.2013-3646.

42. Rule A, Hatem A, Cornell L, et al. The association between age and nephrosclerosis on renal biopsy among healthy adults. *Ann Intern Med*. 2010;152:561–567. doi:10.7326/0003-4819-152-9-201005040-00006.

43. Hommos MS, Glassock RJ, Rule AD. Structural and functional changes in human kidneys with healthy aging. *J Am Soc Nephrol*. 2017;28:2838–2844. doi:10.1681/ASN.2017040421.

44. Weinstein J, Anderson S. The aging kidney: physiological changes. *Adv Chronic Kidney Dis*. 2010;17:302–307. doi:10.1053/j.ackd.2010.05.

45. O'Sullivan ED, Hughes J, Ferenbach DA. Renal aging: causes and consequences. *J Am Soc Nephrol*. 2017;28:407–420. doi:10.1681/ASN.2015121308.

46. Rosner MH, Abdel-Rahman E, Pani A. Geriatric nephrology. In: Feehally J, Floege J, Tonelli M, Johnson RJ, eds. *Comprehensive Clinical Nephrology*. 6th ed. Philadelphia, PA: Elsevier; 2019:1028–1035.

47. Cantú T, Ellerbeck E, Yun S, et al. Drug prescribing for patients with changing renal function. *Am J Hosp Pharm*. 1992;49(12):2944–2948. doi:10.1093/ajhp/49.12.2944.

48. Werner K, Pihlsgård M, Elmståhl S, et al. Combining cystatin C and creatinine yields a reliable glomerular filtration rate estimation in older adults in contrast to β-trace protein and β2-microglobulin. *Nephron*. 2017;137:29–37. doi:10.1159/000473703.

SUGGESTED RESOURCES

Alpers CE, Chang A. The kidney. In: Kumar V, Abbas AK, Aster JC, eds. *Robbins and Cotran Pathologic Basis of Disease*. 9th ed. Philadelphia, PA: Elsevier; 2015:897–957.

Feehally J, Floege J, Tonelli M, Johnson RJ. *Comprehensive Clinical Nephrology*. 6th ed. Philadelphia, PA: Elsevier; 2019.

Hall JE. *Guyton and Hall Textbook of Medical Physiology*. 13th ed. Philadelphia, PA: Saunders Elsevier; 2016:chaps 25–32.

13

GASTROINTESTINAL TRACT

Wilson Crone

THE CLINICAL CONTEXT

The gastrointestinal (GI) tract is the body's point of entry for nutrients, including fluids and electrolytes needed to sustain life. The GI tract is also the route of most medications that are administered, including prescribed, over-the-counter, and many street drugs. GI functions are complex, and clinicians must appreciate the varied components of those functions and implications for nutritional homeostasis, immune function, and quality of life.

GI disorders are common in the United States and globally. Abdominal pain is estimated to account for 27 million annual office visits in the United States. Common conditions, such as gastroesophageal reflux (7 million diagnoses annually), hemorrhoids (4 million diagnoses annually), constipation, diarrhea, and nausea and vomiting, are often self-diagnosed and managed (although this may not be appropriate!).[1] Although GI drugs such as proton pump inhibitors and laxatives are not prescribed with the frequency of medications for chronic disorders such as diabetes and hypertension, over-the-counter sales of these and other GI drugs constitute more than 15% of the retail market. Sales for heartburn products alone totaled $3.23 billion in 2018, indicating that many people experience occasional or frequent heartburn and self-medicate.[2]

Disorders of the GI tract are often grouped into the following categories: alteration of digestive function, absorptive function, immunologic function, and neuroendocrine function. Some disorders are organic, whereas others are functional disorders. Many acute GI disorders result from infections with bacteria, viruses, or parasites.

These can be self-limiting or can progress to chronic infections such as *Helicobacter pylori* and *Clostridioides difficile*. Chronic inflammatory bowel diseases such as Crohn disease and ulcerative colitis cause significant disability including intestinal failure. Cancer of the colon and rectum ranks third in prevalence among all cancer cases in the United States, and pancreatic cancer deaths rank third among all deaths due to cancer. This chapter reviews the structure, function, and regulation of the GI tract and the most common disorders associated with each site.

OVERVIEW OF GASTROINTESTINAL STRUCTURE AND FUNCTION

The GI tract is surprising in its complexity, functioning as:

- The gateway to oral nutrient, drug, and toxicant access to the rest of the body
- The most critical site of fluid and electrolyte homeostasis outside the kidneys
- The site of digestion and absorption of nutrients
- The route of excretion of insoluble dietary fiber, products of liver transformation of endogenous compounds and xenobiotics, and cholesterol

Beyond these well-known functions, there are several other important characteristics of the GI tract.

- It is the body's largest immune organ, with cells and tissues of both innate and adaptive immunity.
- It is the only organ with a freestanding nervous system, the enteric nervous system.

- It has a high concentration and variety of neurotransmitters, modulators, and hormones, greater than most other organs outside the brain.
- Its mucosal epithelial cells have a high cell turnover rate, potentially removing cells that have sustained damage (but also associated with vulnerability to malignant transformation).

The major function of the gut is to mechanically and chemically process materials (digestion) for absorption. In particular, the process of chemical digestion depends on hydrolysis, or the breaking down of dietary macromolecules into their components: starches into monosaccharides (sugars), proteins into peptides and amino acids, and lipids into fatty acids, monoglycerides, and cholesterol. This breakdown is followed by transport of these components across intestinal epithelial cells (IECs) that line the lumen. Accessory organs such as salivary glands, liver and gallbladder, and pancreas supply digestive fluids such as saliva, bile, and digestive enzymes, respectively.

To place these processes and functions into context, this chapter provides a proximal to distal survey of the organs of the GI tract, from the mouth and salivary glands, through the esophagus, stomach, small intestine, pancreas, and large intestine, highlighting their contributions to nutritional processing, and also providing examples of pathological processes that can arise. Included is an overview of general organizing principles of digestion.

Many viral or bacterial infectious disorders cause acute, self-limited GI dysfunction, including vomiting and diarrhea. Chronic GI disorders may present with pain, diarrhea, or constipation, as well as signs and symptoms of malabsorption and critical nutrient deficiencies. Some chronic conditions improve upon identification and remediation of dietary and lifestyle triggers, whereas others (e.g., type 3 intestinal failures) require chronic treatment.

ALIMENTARY CANAL STRUCTURE AND MOTOR ACTIVITY

The different segments of the alimentary canal have characteristic contributions to digestion and absorption, including motor activity, secretions, and transit time (average duration from entry to exit) as listed here and shown in **Figure 13.1**.

- *Mouth:* Chewing begins food breakdown, swallowing moves food to esophagus; 10 seconds to 2 minutes transit time; secretions are saliva, amylase (begins starch digestion), and lingual lipase (initiates fat digestion)

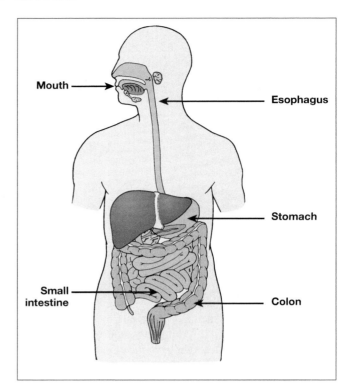

FIGURE 13.1 Gastrointestinal tract overview.

- *Esophagus:* Peristalsis quickly moves food to stomach; transit time is less than 30 seconds; mucus secretion
- *Stomach:* Grinds and mixes food with secretions, peristalsis moves food to small intestine; 15 minute to 3 hour transit time; secretes hydrochloric acid (HCl), pepsin to initiate protein digestion, lipase to continue fat digestion, and intrinsic factor to aid in vitamin B12 absorption
- *Small intestine:* Segmentation contractions mix food with digestive enzymes and improve absorption, peristalsis to move food along length; 2-5 hour transit time; secretions from pancreas (enzymes and bicarbonate), bile from liver and gallbladder, mucus secretion
- *Large intestine:* Segmentation contractions and peristalsis; 12-24 hour transit time; mucus secretion

Structurally, the alimentary canal is a single tube from the mouth to the anus, consisting of four layers with specific functions (**Figure 13.2** and **Box 13.1**). The muscle layer (muscularis) of the GI tract consists of smooth muscle cells with the mechanisms of contraction described in Chapter 4, Cell Physiology and Pathophysiology. Contractions of the circular smooth muscle layer squeeze the intestinal contents, whereas contractions of the longitudinal muscle layer propagate action potentials along the length

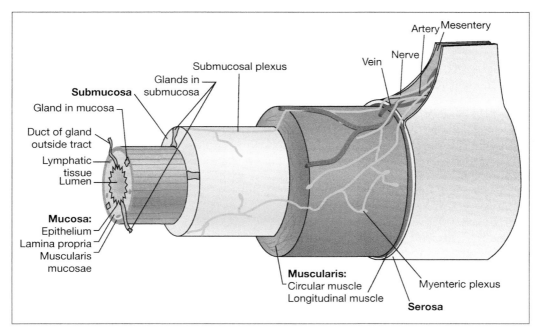

FIGURE 13.2 The general structure of GI tract components surrounding the lumen. These layers include the *mucosa*, the layer of epithelial cells over connective tissue and a thin muscle layer; *submucosa*, containing blood vessels, glands, lymphoid tissues, and a nerve plexus; *muscularis*, layers of circular and longitudinal smooth muscle separated by blood and lymph vessels and a nerve plexus; and *serosa*, connective tissue and covering epithelial layer.

BOX 13.1
Structure of the Gastrointestinal Tract

From the luminal side to the serosa, the layers of the alimentary canal are as follows:

1. ***Mucosa:*** The mucosal epithelium varies, depending on its location in the GI tract. In the mouth and esophagus, the epithelium consists of a nonkeratinizing stratified squamous epithelium. In the rest of the tract for the stomach and intestines, the epithelium consists of simple columnar epithelium. Loose connective tissue—the lamina propria— underlies the epithelium. Regional specializations can be seen along the length of the mucosa. Examples include gastric pits in the stomach and the projections of villi in the small intestine. The mucosa is delineated from the submucosa by a thin muscle layer, the muscularis mucosae, which is innervated by the submucosal plexus.

2. ***Submucosa:*** Additional dense connective tissue with an extensive vascular supply distinguishes the submucosa from the mucosa. A notable feature is the submucosal glands (Brunner glands) in the duodenal region that secrete bicarbonate-rich fluid to neutralize acidic chyme exiting from the stomach.

3. ***Muscularis (externa):*** This tissue consists of internal circular and external longitudinal smooth muscle layers that perform the primary actions of peristalsis and segmentation. These two layers are joined in the stomach by an additional oblique layer of musculature, contributing to the churning activities of the stomach. In the colon, the longitudinal muscles are separated out as teniae coli that, at the cecum, converge at the base of the vermiform appendix. The muscle is innervated by the myenteric plexus. Each gut region has specific motility patterns of muscle contraction that contribute to moving the food bolus through and onto the next region.

4. ***Adventitia/serosa:*** This outer layer is either a collection of loose connective tissue, as an adventitia that attaches the intestines to the dorsal wall of the abdomen, or as a squamous cell–covered serosal layer that allows the abdominal organs to slide against each other. This serosal layer is continuous with the visceral peritoneum that extends from the posterior abdominal wall in a dorsal mesentery pattern.

of the tract and also shorten the tract. Three major types of motor activity characterize GI motility:

1. *Peristalsis* moves GI tract contents away from the mouth, toward the anus (called *aboral* movement), caused by contractions that progress from one segment to the next segment of the tract.
2. *Segmentation contractions* mainly occur in the small intestines. Alternate rings of intestine contract, then relax, without an appreciable wave sweeping from one segment to the next. These contractions aid in mixing the gut contents to optimize the exposure of dietary macromolecules to digestive enzymes and the exposure of products of digestion (monomers) to the absorptive brush border of the mucosa. Periodically peristalsis will occur, moving intestinal contents in the aboral direction. A similar type of activity is found in the colon and promotes exposure of the colon contents to the mucosal surface responsible for fluid reabsorption that reduces fecal volume and fluidity.
3. The *migrating motor complex* is a wave of contractions that occurs every 1 to 2 hours between meals, propelling any GI tract contents from the stomach through the end of the small intestine.

NEURAL, HUMORAL, AND IMMUNE REGULATION OF GASTROINTESTINAL FUNCTION

The principal functions of the gut to digest and absorb ingested food require intermittent changes in motor activity, the nature of which varies depending on the gut segment, and release of secretions (saliva, gastric juice, bile, pancreatic fluid) that are also segment specific and time dependent. Mediators synthesized and secreted by neurons, endocrine cells of the gut, and other specialized cell types contribute to coordinated regulation of GI motor and secretory function. Optimal digestion and absorption are achieved by integrated signals during the progress of a meal as foodstuffs proceed longitudinally along the tract.

Gastrointestinal Innervation

The innervation of the gut has two components: the extrinsic nervous system and enteric (intrinsic) nervous system (**Figure 13.3**). Extrinsic input is via the autonomic nervous system, providing sympathetic and parasympathetic control. Sympathetic innervation reflects the embryological formation of the alimentary canal, with its developmental regions of foregut (associated with celiac arterial blood supply and sympathetic ganglia), midgut (associated with the superior mesenteric artery and ganglia), and

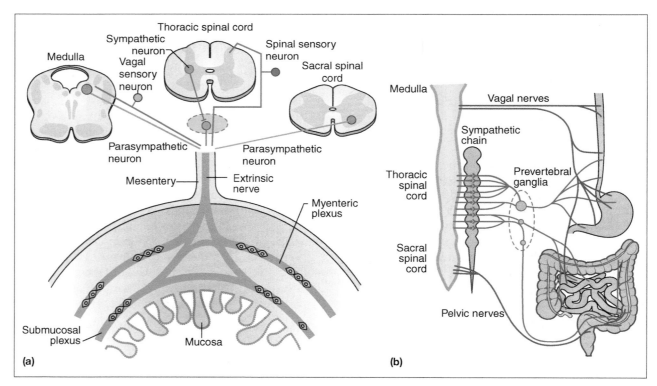

FIGURE 13.3 Overview of GI innervation. (**a**) Neurons in the two plexuses of the enteric nervous system have sensory and motor connections with the autonomic nervous system. Parasympathetic efferent supply comes from the brainstem dorsal motor nucleus of the vagus and sacral parasympathetic nuclei, vagal afferents project to the brainstem. Sympathetic supply comes from preganglionic neurons in the thoracic spinal cord that relay via sympathetic ganglia, accompanied by spinal afferent fibers. (**b**) Overview of anatomical arrangement of extrinsic GI innervation.

hindgut (associated with the inferior mesenteric artery and ganglia). In contrast, the parasympathetic supply for most of the alimentary tract consists of the vagus nerve (cranial nerve [CN] X), which supplies the proximal GI tract through the ascending colon. The parasympathetic pelvic autonomic nerves supply the distal colon. Although most of the parasympathetic nerve supply is afferent (sensory), there is also efferent tone. This circuit facilitates vagovagal reflexes that stimulate smooth muscle activity and release of digestive secretions.

Autonomic control of the gut is by parasympathetic neurons of the vagus nerve and sympathetic neurons from the spinal cord (**Figure 13.4**). Cell bodies of vagal neurons projecting to the GI tract via the vagus nerve (X) are located in the medullary dorsal motor nucleus of the vagus nerve (DMV). Sympathetic preganglionic neurons (spinal sympathetic neurons [SSNs]) projecting to the GI tract have cell bodies in the thoracic spinal cord relaying

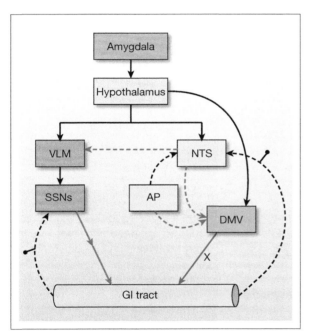

FIGURE 13.4 Brainstem control of the GI tract. Vagal parasympathetic neurons (blue) are located in the DMV, with efferent fibers carried by the vagus nerve (cranial nerve X—identified by X in the figure). Gut afferents (sensory fibers indicated by projections from the GI tract back to the brain) relay sensations of stretch, pressure, irritation, and pain via autonomic nerves. Vagal sensory fibers terminate in the NTS. Neurons of the VLM regulate the activity of SSNs (red), which also receive spinal sensory inputs. Within the brainstem, the area postrema (AP—chemoreceptor trigger zone) and NTS modulate both parasympathetic and sympathetic outflows. Higher centers, particularly limbic cortex, interact via multiple pathways (not shown) that project through the amygdala to the hypothalamus to influence GI activity via autonomic nerves. These centers (purple) contribute to stress-induced alterations in GI signaling and disorders.
DMV, dorsal motor nucleus of the vagus nerve; NTS, nucleus of the tractus solitarius; SSNs, spinal sympathetic neurons; VLM, ventrolateral medulla.

to postganglionic neurons in the sympathetic ganglia listed earlier. Sensory fibers travel in the vagus nerve to the nucleus of the tractus solitarius (NTS) in the medulla. The NTS then can relay impulses to the DMV. Vagal activity can also be modulated by impulses from the area postrema (chemoreceptor trigger zone, discussed later). Some GI sensory neurons travel with sympathetic fibers, providing reflex input to SSNs. Higher centers alter GI activity during acute and chronic stress states by stimulating the amygdala and subsequently the hypothalamus. The hypothalamus can modulate DMV activity and activity of the ventrolateral medulla (VLM), a region of sympathoexcitatory pathways.

In contrast, neurons of the intrinsic (enteric) nervous system can independently control contractile, secretory, and endocrine functions of the GI tract, although modulated by autonomic system input. Of all the internal organs, the GI tract is unique in the number and roles of neurons that mainly function independently of the central nervous system. As noted, the neurons of the enteric nervous system are found in two layers of the gut wall: Neurons in the submucosal plexus principally regulate GI secretions and the microcirculation; neurons in the myenteric plexus regulate motility by stimulating or inhibiting circular and longitudinal smooth muscle contraction. This intrinsic behavior can be seen causing peristaltic contraction of the small intestine. The presence of the semidigested chyme from the stomach within the lumen triggers an ascending/excitatory pathway of neurons to stimulate depolarization and subsequent contraction of the muscle behind the bolus, whereas a descending/inhibitory pathway causes the muscle in front of the bolus to hyperpolarize and to relax.

Gastrointestinal Hormones and Mediators Modulate Gastrointestinal Function

Peptide hormones (e.g., those made by GI endocrine cells) and paracrine signaling agents synthesized and secreted within the mucosa interact with membrane G-protein–coupled receptors and typically trigger rapid responses from stimulation of second messenger systems. Gut hormones allow signaling from one segment of the GI tract to distant segments, gallbladder, and pancreas, to coordinate responses in successive phases of meal digestion and absorption. Unlike classical hormones secreted by endocrine glands and tissues, gut hormones are secreted by a variety of enteroendocrine cells interspersed among the cells of the stomach and IEC layer.

Four major peptide hormones assist in coordinating the digestive activities of the stomach, small intestine, liver (bile), and pancreas. Gastrin is secreted by G cells of the stomach and stimulates parietal cells to secrete hydrochloric acid (HCl) and intrinsic factor. Cholecystokinin (CCK) is secreted by I cells of the small intestine in response to nutrient sensing and stimulates gallbladder contraction and pancreatic enzyme secretion, as well as slowing gastric emptying. Secretin is secreted by S cells of the small intestine and stimulates pancreatic

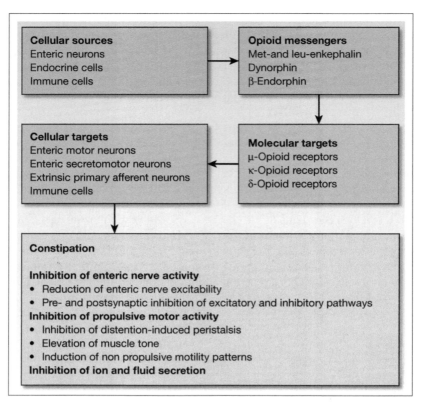

FIGURE 13.5 Endogenous opioids regulate GI function through opioid receptors. Their actions are inhibitory, thus promoting constipation. Exogenous opioids used for pain management often cause severe constipation.

GI, gastrointestinal.

Source: From Holzer P. Opioid receptors in the gastrointestinal tract. *Regul Pept.* 2009;155:11–17.

secretion of water and bicarbonate. There is also glucose-dependent insulinotropic peptide (GIP), secreted by K cells of the duodenum; it inhibits gastric acid secretion and enhances insulin response to oral glucose.

In addition to hormones, several classes of gut peptides act in a hormone- or neurotransmitter-type fashion. These include paracrine peptides secreted by endocrine cells of the GI tract with an intended local action, such as somatostatin, a peptide that inhibits many GI functions. Other gut peptides act as hormones on other target tissues, including glucagon-like peptide 1 (GLP-1), released from the distal small intestine, which decreases stomach motility in addition to stimulating pancreatic insulin secretion. Peptide YY, also released from the distal small intestine and the colon, acts on the brain as a satiety signal.

Peptides that are present in the gut may serve primarily as neurotransmitters, modulating enteric neuron activity or directly targeting gut motility and secretion. Vasoactive intestinal peptide, a vasodilator, also serves as a gut transmitter, causing smooth muscle relaxation and increasing intestinal secretions. Substance P is an excitatory neurotransmitter in the gut. The gut is also richly endowed with opioid receptors (primarily the μ type, although δ and κ opioid receptors are also present), and several opioid

transmitters have been localized to the gut. Stimulation of gut opioid receptors inhibits gut neurotransmission, motility, and secretion. Thus, morphine and other opioid drugs used for pain management or taken as drugs of abuse have the significant side effect of constipation. Therapeutically, these actions of opioids, such as loperamide (which does not cross the blood–brain barrier), are the basis of their use as antidiarrheal agents (**Figure 13.5**).

Gastrointestinal Amine Neurotransmitters and Mediators

Acetylcholine is the neurotransmitter of the parasympathetic nervous system that increases gut motility and secretion. Norepinephrine is the sympathetic neurotransmitter that decreases gut motility and secretion. The mediators, histamine and serotonin, which function in inflammation and blood clotting, have these and other actions in the GI tract. In fact, the GI tract contains 90% of the serotonin in the body.[3] Enterochromaffin-like cells in the wall of the stomach produce histamine as a mediator that stimulates gastric acid secretion. Similar cells in the intestinal mucosa produce serotonin as an excitatory mediator promoting intestinal motility through its actions on the enteric nervous system and gut afferents.

This multitude of mediators in GI physiology and pathophysiology provides the rational basis for pharmacological management of GI disorders. As new mediators are identified, additional therapies are developed, allowing people who suffer from disabling functional gut disorders to have improved activity levels and quality of life. Major peptides, transmitters, and other factors influencing GI activity are listed in **Table 13.1**.

Gastrointestinal Immunology

Ingestion of food and beverages required for nutritional and metabolic support and fluid and electrolyte homeostasis also represents a threat to the organism, as environmental toxins and pathogens are internalized through this route. Furthermore, the gut microbiota, resident bacterial species that have a commensal role in human physiology, stimulate immune defenses that prevent systemic invasion. The gut has a variety of structural protective mechanisms as well as surveillance by cells of innate and adaptive immunity to resist infectious diseases. Many of these mechanisms are summarized in **Figure 13.6**. Immune cells (B cells, T cells, macrophages, dendritic cells) are distributed in many gut-associated lymphoid tissues

TABLE 13.1 Gastrointestinal Tract Hormones and Modulators

Hormone, Neurotransmitter	Secretion Site	Functions
Peptides		
Gastrin	Stomach antrum, duodenum	Stimulates acid and histamine secretion; promotes mucosal growth
Cholecystokinin	Duodenum, jejunum, ileum	Stimulates gallbladder contraction, pancreatic enzyme secretion, and pancreatic bicarbonate secretion; inhibits gastric emptying, satiety
Secretin	Duodenum, jejunum	Stimulates bicarbonate secretion from pancreas and bile, pancreatic growth, and insulin secretion; inhibits gastrin and gastric acid secretion
GIP	Small intestine	Promotes glucose-stimulated insulin secretion
Motilin	Duodenum	Stimulates motility, including the migrating motor complex
Somatostatin	Pancreas, throughout GI tract	Inhibits gastric acid secretion, insulin and glucagon secretion, and gut motility and secretion
Ghrelin	Stomach	Stimulates gastric motility and sensation of hunger
GLP-1	Pancreas, ileum	Signals satiety; decreases gastric motility; stimulates insulin secretion
GLP-2	Ileum, colon	Promotes growth of mucosal cells
Peptide YY	Ileum, colon	Inhibits gastric secretion and emptying, and intestinal motility; signals satiety
Classical and Peptide Neurotransmitters		
Acetylcholine	Parasympathetic and enteric neurons	Stimulates motility and secretions; relaxes sphincters
Norepinephrine	Sympathetic neurons	Decreases motility and secretions; constricts sphincters; stimulates vasoconstriction of GI vasculature
Dopamine	Sympathetic neurons	Has mixed effects of stimulation and inhibition of motility
Serotonin	Enteric neurons	Stimulates sensory neurons to increase motility and secretions; involved in nausea and emesis
Enkephalin	Enteric neurons	Inhibits motility
Substance P	Enteric neurons	Increases motility and neurogenic inflammation
Vasoactive intestinal peptide	Enteric neurons	Inhibits motility; stimulates fluid and electrolyte secretion from epithelium and bile duct cells
Nonpeptide Modulators		
Histamine	Stomach, small intestine	Stimulates gastric acid secretion and inflammatory responses
Nitric oxide	Enteric neurons	Generally inhibitory

GIP, glucose-dependent insulinotropic peptide; GLP, glucagon-like peptide.

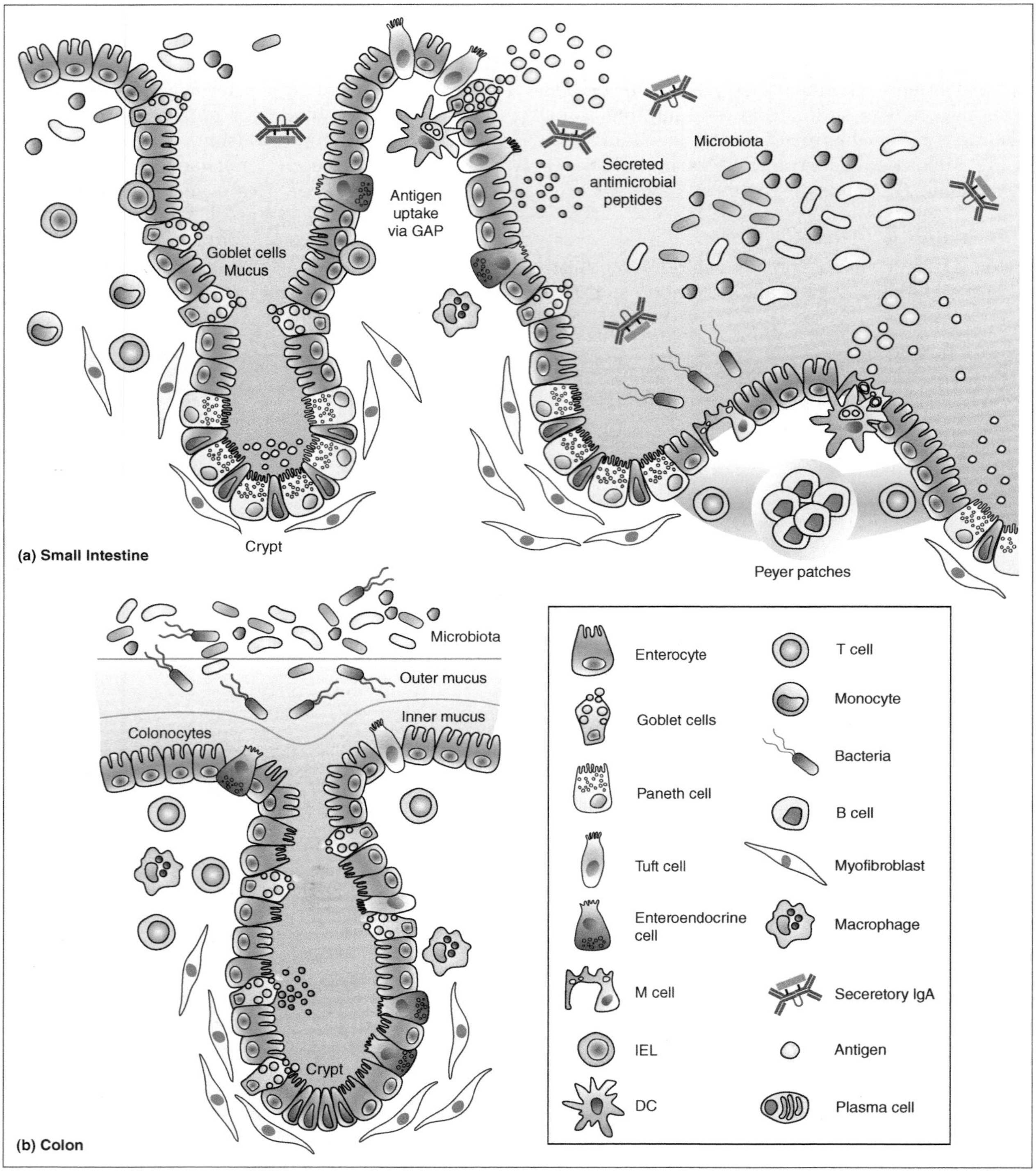

FIGURE 13.6 Bacteria are found in both (**a**) the small intestine and (**b**) colon. These gut microbiota are usually nonpathogenic and contribute to normal gut function. To protect against overgrowth of normal microbiota as well as ingested pathogens, the gut epithelial layer and submucosa have extensive immune surveillance and effector functions, including antimicrobial-secreting Paneth cells, plasma cells that secrete IgA, colonic goblet cells that secrete mucin and protective proteins, M cells that take up antigens and interact with immune cell clusters in the submucosa, gut-associated lymphoid tissues such as Peyer patches, and freely moving DCs, macrophages, and T and B lymphocytes.

DC, dendritic cell; IEL, intraepithelial lymphocyte; IgA, immunoglobulin A.

Source: From Allaire JM, et al. The intestinal epithelium: central coordinator of mucosal immunity. *Trends Immunol.* 2018;39:677–696.

(GALT)—clusters of lymph cells called Peyer patches in the lamina propria beneath the epithelial cell layer. Peyer patches are found throughout the small intestine and are particularly numerous in the ileum. In the epithelial layer itself, cells contributing to immunity include intraepithelial lymphocytes, Paneth cells, and M cells.

IECs lining the small and large intestine are linked by tight junctions that resist the movement of bacteria between cells. IECs also express Toll-like receptors, enabling them to recognize pathogens. Goblet cells secrete mucus that presents an additional barrier to bacterial movement. In the small intestine, Paneth cells in the base of the crypts secrete antimicrobial peptides that directly attack pathogenic bacteria. Several of the other cell types also secrete a variety of antimicrobial substances. B cells secrete immunoglobulin A (IgA), which moves across the epithelial barrier to neutralize pathogens within the gut lumen. M cells are specialized to take up antigens from the lumen and transfer them to antigen-presenting cells such as dendritic cells within the mucosal layer. M cells are found above the Peyer patches, forming a route of communication between the lumen and the immune defense system. Different types of lymphocytes are found in the mucosal region and interspersed between IECs. Absorptive enterocytes at the tips of the villi can, if infected, undergo breakdown and move into the gut lumen for excretion in the feces, removing pathogens from the body. Macrophages beneath the epithelial layer can phagocytose pathogens and initiate an inflammatory response to mobilize other phagocytes to clear invading organisms.[4]

Thought Questions

1. What are the overall functions of the GI tract, and how does the general gut structure contribute to these functions?

2. What is the significance of having multiple levels of regulation of gut function, from neural and endocrine to paracrine regulation?

3. Why is it so important to have extensive representation of immune cells within the gut wall?

PROPERTIES AND DISORDERS OF DIGESTIVE TRACT ORGANS

MOUTH

Ingestion and mechanical processing of food occur in the mouth, with mastication driven by teeth and jaw muscles. Secretion of saliva assists with lubrication of the food for improved mixing by mastication. Some chemical digestion also occurs here, particularly in the form of salivary amylase, which triggers initial carbohydrate breakdown.

Swallowing is an initially voluntary process in the mouth that shifts to involuntary pharyngeal and esophageal phases. Involuntary propulsion, mediated by branches of the vagus nerve as controlled by a swallowing center in the medulla, sets up a peristaltic wave that moves the food down the esophagus to the stomach. The upper esophageal sphincter (UES) opens to allow the bolus of food to pass from the pharynx to the esophagus, while the epiglottis closes across the trachea to protect the airway.

SALIVARY GLANDS

There are three major pairs of salivary glands: sublingual, submandibular, and parotid. Their relative contributions of mucus and watery secretions vary, depending on the histology of the different organs. Their connection to the mouth can affect the pathophysiology associated with them, as the shorter parotid (Stensen) duct is not as prone to sialolithiasis (salivary stones) as the long, winding path of the submandibular (Wharton) duct.

Saliva contains water and mucus to help moisten food, the digestive enzyme α-amylase (ptyalin) to begin carbohydrate digestion, antimicrobial agents such as lysozyme that help to break down bacterial cell walls, and electrolytes such as calcium and fluoride (to help maintain enamel) or bicarbonate (to help buffer regurgitated stomach contents). Both parasympathetic and sympathetic neurons stimulate salivary secretion, although parasympathetic activity predominates.

The **loss of salivary gland function**, as occurs with aging, radiation exposure, or with immunological conditions such as Sjögren syndrome, can result in an increase in *dental caries*, from the lack of enamel maintenance; increased *regurgitatory damage*, from the loss of buffering; or *dysphagia*, from the loss of moistening.

ESOPHAGUS

The esophagus acts as a conduit from the pharynx to the proximal stomach. This collapsible muscular pipe is usually kept mildly sealed by means of an upper and a lower esophageal sphincter (LES). There are three relative compression points in the esophagus: (a) the esophageal–pharyngeal junction, (b) the point where the left mainstem bronchus and aortic arch cross over it, and (c) the gastroesophageal junction that occurs through the esophageal hiatus of the diaphragm. Each of these points can be damaged by ingestion of caustic substances, leading to narrowing. Esophageal motility consists of peristalsis of the bolus of swallowed food, whereas the LES stays in a state of contraction until the food bolus reaches it, when relaxation allows movement into the stomach.

Disorders of the Esophagus

Esophageal Obstruction

Esophageal obstruction is typically caused by mechanical stenosis, most commonly from inflammation, such as by chronic gastroesophageal reflux. In contrast, achalasia is a condition of esophageal obstruction due to the loss of inhibitory neuron function in the myenteric ganglia. The loss of inhibition leads to increased LES tone and the inability of peristalsis to move a food bolus into the stomach. Achalasia manifests with progressive dysphagia and a classic radiographic "bird's beak" presentation of esophageal dilation proximal to narrowing at the affected region.

Esophageal Varices

Esophageal varices are dilated veins in the esophageal submucosa that are the result of a portacaval shunt secondary to portal hypertension. Varices are a common feature of portal hypertension given the proximity of the left gastric vein or the short gastric vein to esophageal veins. With this additional load of blood flow through small vessels, varices can bleed profusely if ruptured.

Esophagitis and Gastroesophageal Reflux Disease

Esophagitis may spring from many conditions, for example, radiation in cancer patients, cytomegalovirus (CMV) or candidiasis in immunocompromised patients, or atopic eosinophilic esophagitis. **Gastroesophageal reflux disease** (GERD) is the most common cause in the United States. GERD esophagitis initially triggers hyperemia, with ongoing inflammation leading to leukocyte recruitment and infiltration.

Because of the underlying issue of reflux in GERD, anything that increases the laxity of the LES, or that increases abdominal pressure driving fluid back through the sphincter into the esophagus, can increase the risk of GERD (**Figure 13.7**). These can include smooth muscle relaxants such as β_2-adrenergic agonists or calcium channel antagonists, the laxity of a hiatal hernia, or the increased abdominal pressure associated with obesity or pregnancy. Chronic GERD may also lead to a change in the esophageal epithelium from stratified squamous epithelium to simple columnar epithelium. This metaplasia is known as **Barrett esophagus**. Most patients with esophageal adenocarcinoma have a precursor Barrett esophagus, although most patients with Barrett esophagus will not develop esophageal cancer.

Esophageal Cancer

Esophageal cancer is more common in men than in women. **Adenocarcinoma** typically originates in the distal third of the esophagus and is associated with Barrett esophagus. In contrast, **squamous cell carcinoma** (more common worldwide) occurs more

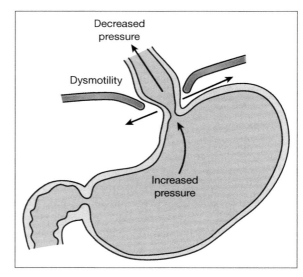

FIGURE 13.7 Factors contributing to GERD include dysfunction of esophageal motility, decreased integrity of the lower esophageal sphincter, decreased intrathoracic pressure, increased gastric pressure, and increased gastric acid production.

GERD, gastroesophageal reflux disease.

often in the mid esophagus. Esophageal squamous cell cancer tends to be associated with exposure to alcohol, with a synergistic effect from tobacco. The alcohol can solubilize tobacco carcinogens, promoting penetration of these carcinogens into the luminal epithelium.

STOMACH

The stomach is the most distensible and muscular part of the GI tract. It stores and grinds food, initiates protein digestion, kills bacteria with gastric acid, and dispenses food particles into the small intestine as chyme. The pouched shape of the stomach can be defined as different regions: the cardia, proximal to the esophagus; the dome-shaped fundus, projecting above the body; the corpus, or body, forming the main portion of the stomach; and an antral region reaching the pyloric sphincter (**Figure 13.8**). The stomach is shaped like a backward-facing "C" with a lesser and a greater curvature. The walls are highly vascularized with anastomosing vessels, such that the stomach is considered to be at less risk for ischemia compared with the intestines. The rich vascular supply helps to supply the mucosa of the stomach, which is shaped into large folds called rugae.

Within the mucosa are numerous gastric pits, about $60/mm^2$ in depth (**Figure 13.9**). The cellular composition and secretions of these pits varies depending on whether they are located in the fundus or body of the stomach or the antral region.

In the fundus and body, the gastric pits are dominated by three main cell types: (a) mucous neck cells,

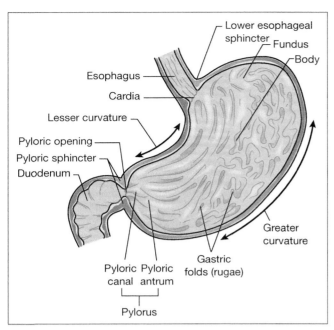

FIGURE 13.8 Anatomy of the stomach highlighting the four main regions: cardia, fundus, body (corpus), and antrum.

which secrete a protective, bicarbonate-rich mucus; (b) chief cells, which secrete pepsinogen, a precursor that is activated to the proteolytic enzyme pepsin when it enters the acidic lumen; and (c) parietal cells. Activated parietal cells expend large amounts of adenosine triphosphate (ATP) on active transport, by H^+/K^+–ATPase, also known as the "proton pump." This transport moves hydrogen ions (protons) into the stomach lumen in exchange for potassium ions. Chloride ions move through an ion channel into the lumen. This secretion of HCl into the lumen decreases the stomach pH to the low levels needed for pepsin activation (pH 1–2). Parietal cells also secrete intrinsic factor, a glycoprotein carrier for the uptake of vitamin B12 (cobalamin) via receptors located in the ileum.

In contrast, in the antrum, the predominant cells are G cells that secrete gastrin, a hormone that triggers enhanced gastric mucosa development. As part of this enhanced mucosal activity, gastrin builds up new parietal cells.

Acid secretion by parietal cells is stimulated by neural, endocrine, and paracrine mediators that are stimulated by meal ingestion (**Figure 13.10**). As food

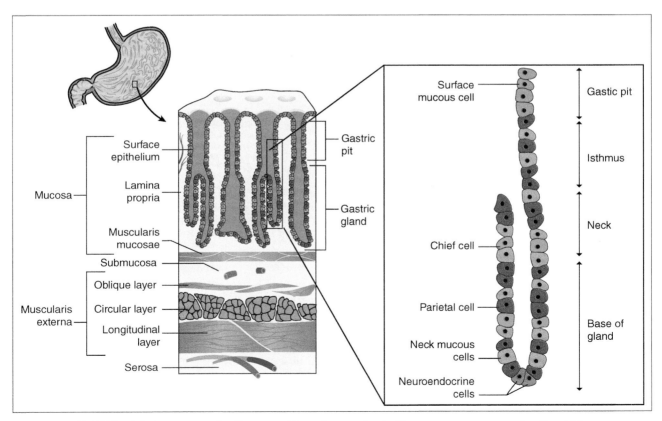

FIGURE 13.9 Location and cell composition of a gastric pit. There are numerous such pits within the mucosa.

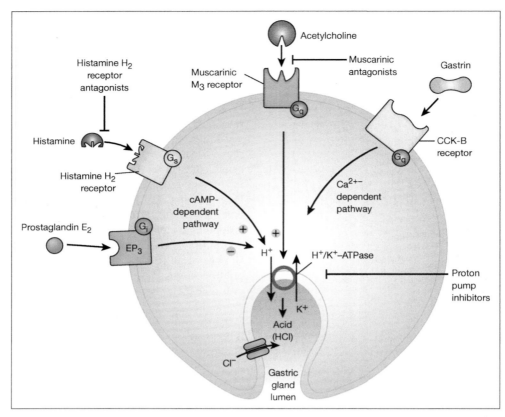

FIGURE 13.10 Parietal cell acid secretion is mediated by the active transporter H^+/K^+–ATPase, also known as the proton pump. Chloride ion moves to the stomach lumen through an ion channel. Proton pump activity is strongly regulated by neural, endocrine, and paracrine signals acting on G protein–coupled receptors. The major factors stimulating acid secretion are acetylcholine (neural), gastrin (endocrine), and histamine (paracrine), which act through G_q and G_s as shown. Prostaglandin E_2 inhibits the proton pump through a G_i-linked receptor. Pharmacological targets of H_2-blocking drugs and proton pump inhibitors are shown.

ATPase, adenosine triphosphatase; cAMP, cyclic adenosine monophosphate; CCK, cholecystokinin; HCl, hydrochloric acid.

intake begins and throughout a meal, the vagus nerve releases acetylcholine, stimulating parietal cell muscarinic (M_3) receptors via G_q and initiating acid secretion. As food components reach the antrum, gastrin secretion from G cells provides endocrine stimulation via CCK_B receptors, also G_q linked. Gastrin and acetylcholine activate enterochromaffin-like cells to secrete histamine, a paracrine mediator that stimulates acid secretion via H_2 receptors linked to G_s. In contrast, the peptide somatostatin and locally produced prostaglandins are linked to G_i and inhibit acid secretion.

Thus, there are three major phases of acid production:

1. The *cephalic phase*, representing a third of acid production, precedes food in the stomach, as the vagus nerve is stimulated by the act of eating and "jump-starts" the acid secretion process.

2. About 60% of acid production occurs in the *gastric phase*, where the presence of food and protein digestion products in the stomach trigger gastrin release, until low pH (<2) inhibits the gastrin-secreting G cells.

3. The remaining acid production occurs in the *intestinal phase*, when chyme enters the intestine. As the stomach empties, acid secretion diminishes, owing to decreased levels of the above stimulating mediators and rising inhibition by prostaglandins and other mediators.

Although the acidic and proteolytic environment of the stomach is helpful for digestion and to kill bacteria ingested in and on foods, it presents a risk to the stomach mucosa. Several protective factors help to maintain gastric integrity against acid- and enzyme-induced damage. The mucous cells produce adherent mucus, which is bicarbonate rich, in response to prostaglandin stimulation. The gastric epithelial cells are held together by tight junctions to minimize acid diffusion to the submucosa. These cells also undergo rapid turnover, quickly replacing damaged cells. Gastric mucosal blood flow is high and is maintained at that level by local prostaglandin production. This high rate of blood flow quickly removes any acid that leaks through the tight junction barrier and promotes repair of damaged tissue.

Disorders of the Stomach

Peptic Ulcers

Peptic ulcer formation, erosion of the mucous membrane of the stomach or more commonly the duodenum, can stem from many causes that lead to an imbalance between damaging and protective forces (**Table 13.2**). Stomach acid and pepsin can directly damage the mucosa. Stress can help to trigger the inflammatory response, and so enhance histamine release, whereas increased sympathetic activity can reduce blood flow. Smoking stimulates vasoconstriction, and smoke-related irritants can trigger neutrophil activity that generates reactive oxygen intermediates. Nonsteroidal anti inflammatory drugs (NSAIDs) inhibit prostaglandin production, reducing parietal cell inhibition and gastric blood flow. A gastrin-producing tumor can lead to excessive acid secretion, in the pattern known as **Zollinger–Ellison syndrome.**

The single largest risk factor for ulceration, however, is the activity of the gram-negative bacterium *Helicobacter pylori*. *H. pylori* is unique in its ability to survive in acidic environments. This is partly due to its production of the enzyme urease, which converts urea to ammonia (NH_3) to neutralize gastric acid, allowing a local buffering effect. The cytotoxins released by *H. pylori* can then break down the

mucosal cells, causing gastritis. Histamine from the subsequent inflammatory response increases acid secretion, perpetuating the damage. Management strategies must eradicate the *H. pylori* infection to prevent ulcer recurrence. Untreated chronic gastritis is the most common risk factor for gastric cancer, which is less common in the United States than in other countries, particularly those in Asia.

Gastroparesis

Motility of the stomach consists of powerful contractions that squeeze the contents, mechanically breaking down the food and mixing it with stomach secretions. This can take 2 to 4 hours after a meal, during which small amounts of chyme are propelled at intervals through the pyloric valve into the duodenum (**Figure 13.11**).

Gastroparesis is a state of decreased stomach motility that results in slower gastric emptying, nausea, vomiting, abdominal pain, and premature satiety. The most common causes are diabetic, idiopathic, and postsurgical. In the context of diabetes, gastroparesis results from diabetic neuropathy. Diabetic gastroparesis complicates blood glucose control due to the unpredictability of meal absorption and postprandial hyperglycemia. Potential mechanisms involved in gastroparesis include altered autonomic neural regulation of motility and loss of intrinsic cells of Cajal that function as the pacemaker of stomach motility. Treatment of gastroparesis includes altering dietary intake to small frequent meals. Agents that increase gut motility (prokinetic drugs) are also used, although some of the current agents have intolerable adverse effects or are only safely used for brief periods of time.

Vomiting

Vomiting is an activity that empties the stomach and upper small intestine of irritating or potentially dangerous compounds or is initiated by a variety of other sensory inputs. Vomiting requires coordinated activation of abdominal muscles (increasing intraabdominal pressure), diaphragmatic contraction (decreasing intrathoracic pressure and pausing breathing during expulsion), and gut smooth muscles (promoting reverse peristalsis). The vomiting center of the medulla coordinates the various efferent signals to skeletal and smooth muscles. Inputs to the vomiting center include the chemoreceptor trigger zone—a brainstem region with a leaky blood–brain barrier that recognizes toxins and some drugs (including many cancer chemotherapy agents). Other inputs include vestibular signals, intracranial sources (including increased intracranial pressure), and peripheral signals from the gut (**Figure 13.12**). Stomach irritation and toxins released by pathogens can cause vomiting in the case of viral or bacterial gastroenteritis. Neurotransmitters involved in vomiting initiation include central or peripheral

TABLE 13.2 Gastric Acid–Induced Damage to the Esophagus, Stomach, and Duodenum: Protective and Exacerbating Factors

Protective Factors	Exacerbating Factors
• Normal tone of the lower esophageal sphincter (protects the esophagus) • Mucus and bicarbonate layers • Epidermal growth factor (promotes regeneration) • Gastric emptying (reduces stimulation) • Prostaglandins (inhibit parietal cell secretion, increase bicarbonate secretion, and promote high blood flow)	• Gastric acid and pepsin • *Helicobacter pylori* infection • Smoking • Stress-mediated vasoconstriction • Nonsteroidal anti inflammatory drugs inhibit prostaglandin formation • Bile acids • Pancreatic enzymes

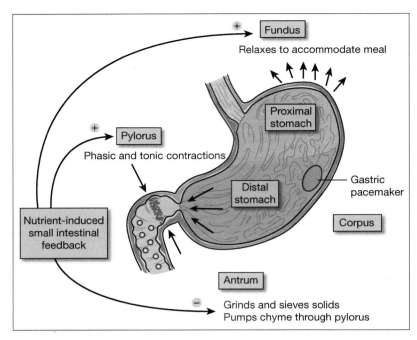

FIGURE 13.11 Gastric motility consists of fundic relaxation early in meal consumption, and strong phasic and tonic contraction of corpus (body) and antrum to pulverize meal contents and promote mixing with gastric secretions. Pacemaker cells (interstitial cells of Cajal) set the frequency of gastric smooth muscle activity. Antral contractions move chyme to and through the pyloric valve into the duodenum.

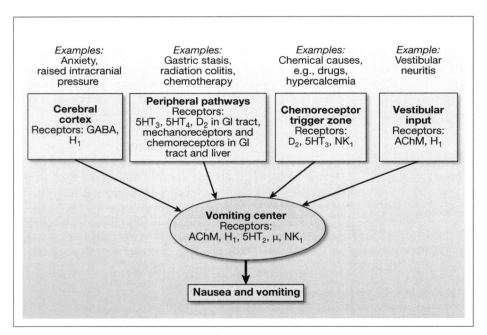

FIGURE 13.12 Signals as varied as motion sickness, acute gastroenteritis, increased intracranial pressure, and chemotherapy drugs can produce nausea and vomiting. Several neurotransmitters have been identified in peripheral or central vomiting circuitry, and antiemetic drugs target their receptors with clinical success.

AChM, muscarinic acetylcholine receptor; D_2, dopamine type 2 receptor; GABA, gamma-aminobutyric acid; GI, gastrointestinal; H_1, histamine type 1 receptor; NK_1, neurokinin type 1 receptor; $5HT_2$, 5-hydroxytryptamine type 2 receptor; $5HT_3$, 5-hydroxytryptamine type 3 receptor; μ, mu opioid receptor.

Source: From Harris DG. Nausea and vomiting in advanced cancer. *Br Med Bull.* 2010;96:175–185. https://doi.org/10.1093/bmb/ldq031.

serotonin and dopamine, substance P acting on neurokinin type-1 receptors, muscarinic acetylcholine receptors, and histamine type 1 (H_1) receptors. These are the targets of the different classes of antiemetic drugs.

Thought Questions

4. How would you summarize the functions of the upper portions of the GI tract, from mouth through stomach?

5. What are the stimuli to the multiple substances that coordinate control of gastric acid secretion? What risks result from having strong acidity in the stomach?

SMALL AND LARGE INTESTINES

The length of the small intestine in adult humans is about 3 to 5 m, and the large intestine is <2 m long. The absorptive surface area of the small intestine is estimated to be 30 m², and the surface area of the large intestine is estimated to be 1.9 m².[5] The duodenum is the initial, and shortest, segment of the small intestine. From the stomach, chyme exits through the pyloric valve and enters the duodenum, a U-shaped loop of gut surrounding the head of the pancreas (**Figure 13.13**). The major duodenal papilla is the site of entry of bile (from the liver and gallbladder) and pancreatic juice, rich in proenzymes that will be activated in the gut to functional enzymes that digest carbohydrates, proteins, and fats. This combination of solutions rich in emulsifying agents, bicarbonate, and proenzymes is the primary source of chemical digestion for the GI tract. Enterokinase enzyme in the small intestine brush border activates the most abundant protease, trypsin, which subsequently cleaves and activates other pancreatic enzymes. Submucosal glands (Brunner glands) add additional bicarbonate-rich mucus to neutralize the acidic chyme.

The main activities of digestion and absorption occur along the length of the small intestine, beginning in the duodenum, reaching their greatest extent in the jejunum, and finishing in the ileum. Villi within the small intestinal mucosa increase surface area to optimize digestion and absorption (**Figure 13.14**). Villi are covered in epithelial cells (enterocytes) and goblet cells (mucus-producing). The core of each villus is made up of connective tissue and a dense vascular network to return absorbed nutrients to the general circulation (**Figure 13.14a**). A central lymphatic vessel (lacteal)

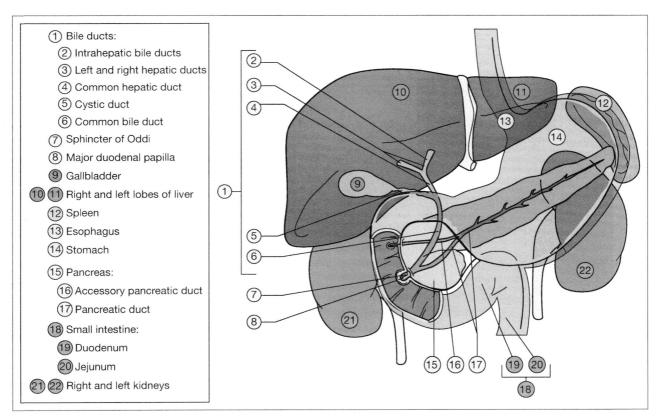

Bile ducts:
1. Bile ducts:
2. Intrahepatic bile ducts
3. Left and right hepatic ducts
4. Common hepatic duct
5. Cystic duct
6. Common bile duct
7. Sphincter of Oddi
8. Major duodenal papilla
9. Gallbladder
10. 11. Right and left lobes of liver
12. Spleen
13. Esophagus
14. Stomach
15. Pancreas:
16. Accessory pancreatic duct
17. Pancreatic duct
18. Small intestine:
19. Duodenum
20. Jejunum
21. 22. Right and left kidneys

FIGURE 13.13 Anatomic orientation of stomach, pylorus, duodenum, liver, gallbladder, and pancreas, with the associated bile and common ducts draining into the duodenum. (See inset key for specific structures.)

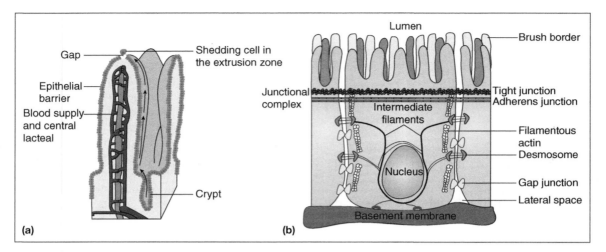

FIGURE 13.14 The small intestine has abundant surface area for nutrient absorption, owing to the folding of the mucosa into villi—finger-like projections into the lumen (**a**)—and the brush border of microvilli projecting from each absorptive epithelial cell (**b**). Small molecule digestion products of carbohydrate and protein cross the epithelial cell layer and basement membrane to be absorbed into the capillaries immediately beneath. Fat digestion products are packaged into chylomicron lipoprotein particles and released from epithelial cells to the lacteal (lymph vessel) for uptake and transport to the systemic circulation.
Source: From Williams JM, et al. Epithelial cell shedding and barrier function: a matter of life and death at the small intestinal villus tip. *Vet Pathol.* 2014;52:445-455. https://doi.org/10.1177/0300985814559404

within the villi picks up large chylomicrons, lipoproteins made up of triglycerides, cholesterol esters, and phospholipids absorbed from digested dietary fats. The mucosal barrier is maintained by tight junctions linking adjacent epithelial cells (**Figure 13.14b**), and the absorptive surface area is enhanced by the finger-like plasma membrane extensions of each enterocyte (brush border).

Membrane transporters of the enterocytes differ between apical and basolateral membranes that face the lumen and the submucosa, respectively (**Figure 13.15**). The basolateral membrane has many sodium–potassium pumps, creating a sodium gradient from the gut lumen to the intracellular fluid. Apical membrane secondary active transporters cotransport sodium with monosaccharides, amino acids, and other digestive products and ions. These substances then leave the cell through basolateral membrane–facilitated diffusion proteins. Most drugs enter gut absorptive cells by simple diffusion. Upon entering the cell, they may leave by a basolateral transporter, but in some cases they are removed from the cell by an apical membrane efflux pump, reducing their bioavailability. Although the majority of drug bioconversion occurs in the liver, enterocytes also have some enzymes for drug bioconversion, in which case the drug metabolites cross the basolateral membrane to enter the bloodstream.

The mucosal regions between the villi are the crypts. Cells of the villi focus on absorption; cells of the crypts are foci for secretion and cell division that regenerates epithelial cells lost daily from the villi. Cell types in the

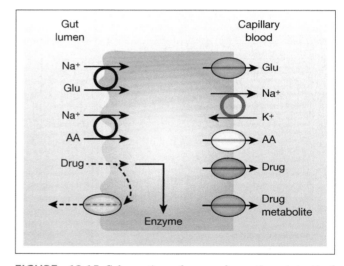

FIGURE 13.15 Schematic of an absorptive intestinal epithelial cell. The general strategy in absorption of products of digestion and orally administered drugs is shown. Hexose sugars (Glu) and amino acids (AA) are taken up by secondary active transport with sodium (circles), while facilitated diffusion transporters mediate their movement across the basolateral membrane to the submucous layer and capillary blood. The sodium gradient is maintained by the basolateral sodium–potassium (Na^+/K^+) pump. Many drugs enter the cell by simple diffusion, where they meet three possible fates: (1) transport via diffusion or facilitated diffusion across the basolateral membrane; (2) metabolism by enzymes of biotransformation in the cytoplasm, followed by metabolite transport across the basolateral membrane; (3) transport back to the GI lumen by efflux transporters, reducing drug bioavailability.

crypts include mucus-producing cells, enteroendocrine cells that secrete hormones such as CCK and secretin, stem cells that regenerate cells of the villi, and Paneth cells that support the health of stem cells and secrete antimicrobial peptides.

The absorptive epithelial cells have further finger-like projections called microvilli (brush border). The microvilli on the simple columnar epithelium add to the surface area and are the source for brush border enzymes that serve to complete digestion of proteins and carbohydrates (**Figure 13.14b**). Of these enzymes, two have distinctive roles. One is enterokinase (also known as enteropeptidase), which cleaves and activates the proenzyme trypsinogen. A second is lactase, responsible for breaking down the milk sugar lactose into the absorbable monosaccharides of glucose and galactose. In some individuals, the lactase gene is not expressed, either from birth or beginning after childhood; thus, they have **lactose intolerance**. The absence of lactase leads to osmotic diarrhea when dairy foods are ingested. Undigested lactose cannot be absorbed; its osmotic strength retains fluids in the lumen of the gut, and it also serves as a food source for gas-producing colonic bacteria, leading to an additional sensation of bloating.

The activity of absorption along the length of the intestines is not uniform (**Table 13.3**). The greatest

TABLE 13.3 **Absorption of Selected Nutrients in the Gastrointestinal Tract**

Nutrient	Absorption Site			
	Duodenum and Jejunum	Proximal Ileum	Distal Ileum	Colon
Sugars	++	+++	++	0
Amino acids	++	++	++	0
Water- and fat-soluble vitamins (except B12)	+++	++	0	0
Long-chain fatty acid absorption and con-version to triglyceride	+++	++	+	0
Bile acids	+	+	+++	+
Vitamin B12	0	+	+++	0
Iron	+++	+	+	?
Calcium	+++	++	+	?

Source: Adapted from Barrett KE, Barman SM, Brooks HL, Yuan J, eds. *Ganong's Review of Medical Physiology.* 26th ed. New York, NY: McGraw Hill; 2019.

absorption of nutrients occurs in the jejunum. The terminal ileum contains receptor sites for bile salt uptake and recycling, driven by sodium–bile salt cotransporters, and receptors for intrinsic factor–vitamin B12 complexes. Inflammation or surgery in the terminal ileum can, therefore, trigger fat malabsorption as well as pernicious anemia.

Normally, the presence of chyme in the terminal ileum stimulates the relaxation of the ileocecal valve. Chyme is slowly propelled forward through the large intestine. The main function occurring within the large intestine is water absorption in the distal colon. The large intestine receives about 1 L of fluid and reabsorbs all but 100 mL. The remaining fecal material travels to the rectum, where it stimulates relaxation of the internal anal sphincter and an urge to defecate. Under proper conditions, the external anal sphincter is relaxed under conscious control, allowing feces to be expelled.

PANCREAS

The exocrine pancreas contains secretory units of acini and ducts that are under parasympathetic (stimulatory) and sympathetic (inhibitory) stimulation (**Figure 13.16**). The acini secrete protein-digesting enzymes (trypsinogen, procarboxypeptidase, and others) in the form of inactive precursors known as zymogens. These proenzymes and other digestive enzymes are stored in zymogen granules within acinar cells. The brush border enterokinase activates the secreted trypsinogen into trypsin, which then triggers activation of other pancreatic proteases. It should not be a surprise that the pancreas produces a trypsin inhibitor (a serine protease inhibitor) as an additional protective strategy. Pancreatic duct cells produce bicarbonate-rich fluid for buffering the chyme delivered to the duodenum. Enzymatic and aqueous portions of the secretion are regulated by means of different pathways, with stimulation of enzymatic secretion through the phospholipase C/diacylglycerol/inositol triphosphate (PLC/DAG/IP$_3$) second messenger system and stimulation of aqueous secretion through the adenylyl cyclase/cyclic adenosine monophosphate (cAMP) system.

Acute Pancreatitis

Acute pancreatitis is a relatively uncommon disorder with potentially high rates of morbidity and mortality (40–50 cases per year per 100,000 in the United States). It is associated with a high rate of hospitalization, among the highest for GI disorders.[6] The most common causes of acute pancreatitis are gallstones, alcohol use, and drug reactions. The pathogenesis of alcohol-induced pancreatitis has been reviewed by Apte and colleagues.[7] Factors include blockage of pancreatic ducts; increased digestive enzyme synthesis; decreased membrane stability of zymogen granules and lysosomes;

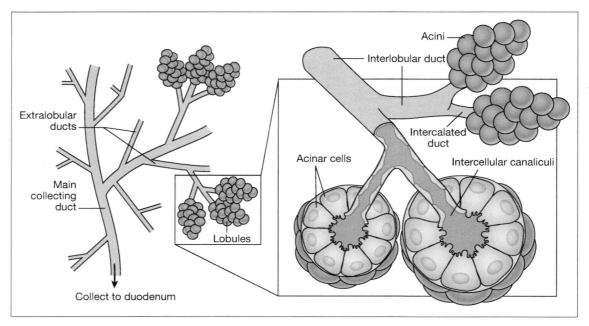

FIGURE 13.16 Pancreatic acinar cells produce and secrete digestive enzymes in the form of proenzymes (so they do not digest acinar cell components). Acinar cell secretions are joined by bicarbonate-rich secretions produced by the epithelial cells of the ducts. All of the pancreatic ducts converge into a common pancreatic duct that joins the bile duct, coming to the duodenum at the ampulla of Vater, and emptying into the duodenum at the major duodenal papilla. Epithelial cell bicarbonate secretion depends on the membrane transport protein CFTR, and patients with cystic fibrosis often have pancreatic dysfunction requiring oral enzyme replacement.
CFTR, cystic fibrosis transmembrane conductance regulator.

pancreatic alcohol metabolism, producing damaging acetaldehyde and reactive oxygen species while reducing glutathione; and stimulation of nuclear factor-kappa B (NF-κB), which stimulates cytokine activation and inflammation. Local stellate cells also contribute to cytokine production and promote tissue inflammation and progression to necrosis (**Figure 13.17**).

Intraacinar activation of digestive enzymes contributes to acute pancreatitis, in which there is potentially fatal autodigestion of the pancreas and surrounding tissues. This leads to inflammation that can be severe, the worst cases triggering systemic inflammation and multisystem organ failure. Repeated episodes may result in chronic pancreatitis and parenchymal fibrosis, leading to loss of exocrine function.

DIGESTION AND ABSORPTION

The small intestine is responsible for digestion and absorption of macronutrients and most micronutrients. As noted, products of digestion are absorbed across intestinal epithelial cells and into the bloodstream through the abundant capillaries of the villi (**Figure 13.18**). As the osmotically active molecules are absorbed, water follows via paracellular pathways.

OVERVIEW OF MACRONUTRIENT DIGESTION AND ABSORPTION

The breakdown products of a mixed meal include monosaccharides, amino acids, monoglycerides, fatty acids, and cholesterol. Monosaccharides and amino acids are transported across the small intestine epithelium to blood vessels of the mucosa for ultimate distribution via the portal vein to the liver and then throughout the body. The general processes of digestion and absorption are similar for carbohydrates and proteins. Polysaccharides are broken down by salivary and pancreatic amylase into disaccharides and monosaccharides (**Figure 13.19a**). Disaccharidase enzymes of the brush border (sucrase, lactase, and maltase) split sucrose into glucose and fructose, lactose into glucose and galactose, and maltose into two glucose molecules. Glucose and galactose are taken up into enterocytes via apical membrane sodium–glucose transporter 1 (SGLT1), a secondary active transport protein driven

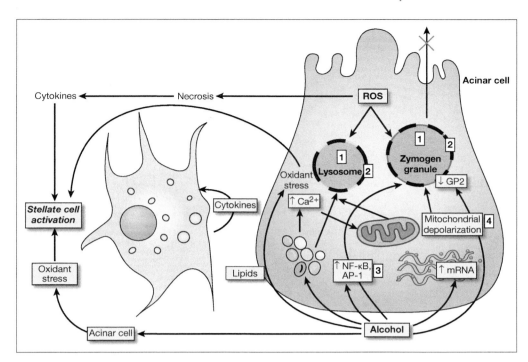

FIGURE 13.17 The pathogenesis of alcoholic pancreatitis involves direct damage to acinar cells and activation of neighboring stellate cells, promoting inflammation due to cytokine secretion and oxidative stress. Within acinar cells, alcohol increases enzyme content of lysosomes and zymogen granules (step 1); while also reducing levels of GP2, a protein thought to stabilize granules to prevent autodigestion (step 2); activates inflammatory pathways through NF-κB and AP-1 (step 3); increases intracellular calcium and lipids and depolarizes mitochondria (step 4). The consequences can be as severe as widespread necrotic cell death of acinar cells and critical illness.

AP-1, activator protein 1; GP2, glycoprotein 2; mRNA, messenger RNA; NF-κB, nuclear factor-kappa B; ROS, reactive oxygen species.

Source: From Apte MV, Pirola RC, Wilson JS. Mechanisms of alcoholic pancreatitis. *J Gastroenterol Hepatol.* 2010;25:1816–1826. https://doi.org/10.1111/j.1440-1746.2010.06445.x.

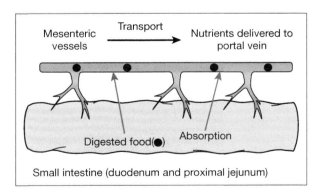

FIGURE 13.18 Absorption of the products of digestion along the small intestine depends on the uptake into adjacent blood vessels along the length of the tract that converge to form the superior mesenteric vein. The superior mesenteric vein joins the portal vein, perfusing the liver prior to returning to the vena cava.

by the sodium gradient created by the basolateral membrane sodium–potassium pump. Fructose is taken up from the lumen by facilitated diffusion via the GLUT5 glucose transporter. All three monosaccharides (glucose, fructose, and galactose) leave the basolateral membrane via GLUT2 to be absorbed into the circulation (Figure 13.20). Sodium–glucose uptake promotes water absorption, following the osmotic pull of sodium and glucose movements from the lumen to the circulation. This is the basis for oral rehydration therapy used for fluid replacement in resource-poor settings. For example, diarrhea associated with *Vibrio cholerae* infection causes profound dehydration that can be managed by oral rehydration therapy that includes sodium, chloride, additional electrolytes, and glucose or a carbohydrate source of glucose.

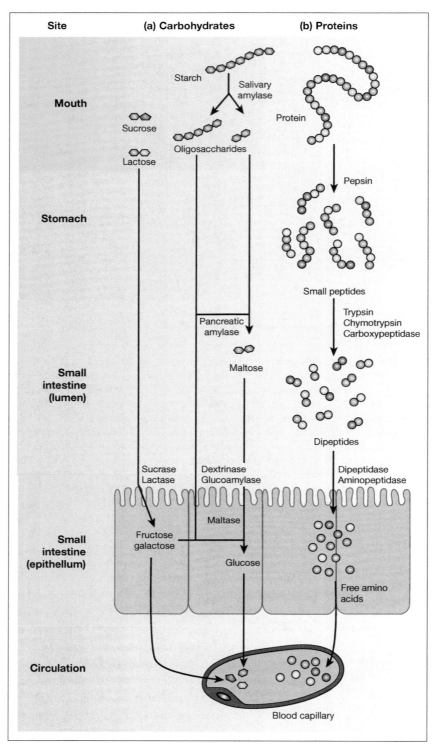

FIGURE 13.19 Digestion and absorption of **(a)** carbohydrates and **(b)** proteins. Carbohydrates are polymers of monosaccharides, and proteins are polymers of amino acids. Digestive enzymes break down these macromolecules into smaller fragments, including di- and trisaccharides, and di- and tripeptides. Brush border disaccharidases and peptidases further break down these molecules into monosaccharides and single amino acids. These monomers move by facilitated diffusion and secondary active transport across the apical membranes of gut epithelial cells. Movement of these products of carbohydrate and protein digestion across the basolateral membrane of the epithelial cells is usually by facilitated diffusion transporters.

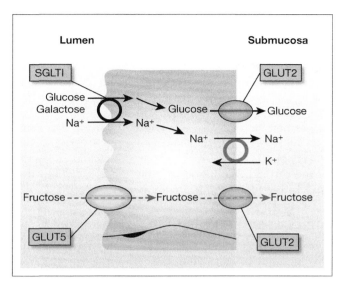

FIGURE 13.20 The monosaccharides glucose and galactose enter the gut epithelial cells by an apical membrane sodium-coupled secondary active transporter, SGLT1. Fructose enters via GLUT5. Galactose is converted to glucose inside the epithelial cell, then glucose and fructose exit the epithelial cell by the basolateral membrane GLUT2-facilitated diffusion protein. GLUT, glucose transporter; SGLT1, sodium–glucose-linked transporter 1.

Protein digestion begins in the stomach with pepsin (**Figure 13.19b**). In the brush border of the small intestine, trypsinogen is converted to trypsin in the presence of enterokinase to begin the bulk of protein digestion. Trypsin can then activate additional proteases like chymotrypsin, carboxypeptidase, and elastase. The different pancreatic proteases hydrolyze peptide bonds at different amino acid sequences. Protease action produces amino acids, dipeptides, and tripeptides. Amino acids and small peptide chains enter the enterocytes via secondary active transport. Dipeptides and tripeptides are hydrolyzed into individual amino acids that are transported out of the cell by facilitated diffusion transporters.

Lipid digestion begins in the mouth and stomach with small contributions from lingual and gastric lipase, respectively. The churning action of the stomach breaks lipids into small droplets that increase the surface area of the fats to be digested, and then slowly releases them into the small intestine. As fat droplets arrive in the duodenum and mix with bile, they are coated with amphipathic bile salts. This emulsification prevents small fat droplets from reaggregating into larger droplets in the aqueous solution of the gut. Pancreatic lipase and its cofactor, colipase, attach to the droplets and break down dietary lipids into their components: Triglycerides release monoglycerides and free fatty acids, phospholipids release lysophospholipids and fatty acids, and cholesterol esters release cholesterol and fatty acids. These small

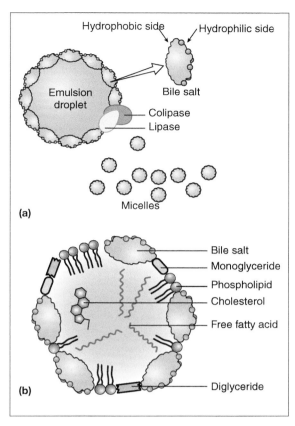

FIGURE 13.21 Fat digestion and absorption is a multistep process requiring bile salts that enter the duodenum from the liver and gallbladder via the bile duct, as well as pancreatic lipase and colipase. **(a)** Large fat droplets are emulsified by bile salts, producing smaller fat droplets. **(b)** Fats in small fat droplets are digested by lipase and their breakdown products are packaged in micelles, also coated by bile salts. The micelle stage allows diffusion to the brush border and absorption of small lipid molecules.

hydrophobic particles are then packaged into much smaller micelles coated with bile salts for movement to the epithelial cell layer and absorption into the enterocytes (**Figure 13.21**).

Once inside the enterocytes, the lipid components are reesterified, regenerating triglycerides, phospholipids, and cholesterol esters. Enterocytes package these lipids, along with fat-soluble vitamins, into chylomicrons. The chylomicrons are coated with a layer of amphipathic phospholipids and apolipoproteins and are released by exocytosis. Chylomicrons enter the lacteals, traveling through the lymphatic system to the circulation. Digestion and absorption of fats are more complicated and vulnerable to disease processes than digestion of carbohydrates and proteins. Optimal fat digestion and absorption require the normal healthy function of the liver (for synthesis and secretion of bile), pancreas (for production of lipase and colipase), and enterocytes (for reesterification of lipid breakdown products and chylomicron packaging and exocytosis). **Steatorrhea** (fat in the stools) and deficiencies of fat-soluble vitamins A, D, E, and K can result from diseases at any of the sites participating in fat digestion and absorption. Absorption of several dietary nutrients is summarized in **Table 13.3**, earlier.

Thought Questions

6. How do the organs of digestion collaborate to break down and absorb carbohydrates, proteins, and fats?

7. What are the consequences of disorders that disrupt function of the pancreas and small intestine?

PRINCIPLES OF MICRONUTRIENT ABSORPTION

Although a complete discussion of micronutrient absorption is beyond the scope of this book, a few principles are highlighted here. Sodium-dependent cotransport molecules absorb water-soluble vitamins, for example, B vitamins (except vitamin B12) and vitamin C, throughout the small intestine. Fat-soluble vitamins (A, D, E, and K) are absorbed with lipids. In contrast to those, vitamin B12 (cobalamin) binds to intrinsic factor in the small intestine, with the complex binding to a receptor in the terminal ileum. There, the absorbed vitamin B12 binds to transcobalamin in the cytosol, is exocytosed to the plasma, and is transported throughout the body, and particularly to the bone marrow for red blood cell production or the liver for storage. Dietary iron can be ingested in the form of heme iron—bound to hemoglobin or myoglobin in meats—or free iron from vegetables. GI iron absorption is poor, averaging 5% to 10% of dietary intake. Fifteen percent to 30% of iron is stored as ferritin in many cells, with the majority of storage in the liver. Absorbed iron is bound to the carrier protein transferrin and transported through the blood to bone marrow, where it is used for red blood cell hemoglobin production.

PRINCIPLES OF FLUID AND ELECTROLYTE ABSORPTION

The small intestine is a site for both fluid secretion and absorption. The fluid volume that enters the gut daily totals almost 10 L, coming from dietary fluids, saliva, gastric juice, pancreatic fluid, bile, and water secreted by small intestinal crypt cells. The secretory activity of the crypt enterocytes is mainly driven by cAMP–stimulated cystic fibrosis transmembrane conductance regulator (CFTR) channels through which chloride ion enters the lumen, followed by sodium ions and water (**Figure 13.22**). This addition of water helps decrease osmotic strength and liquefies food components to optimize digestive enzyme activity. However, crypt secretory activity is also a target of enterotoxins such as cholera toxin that cause persistent cAMP production, leading to profuse secretory diarrhea.

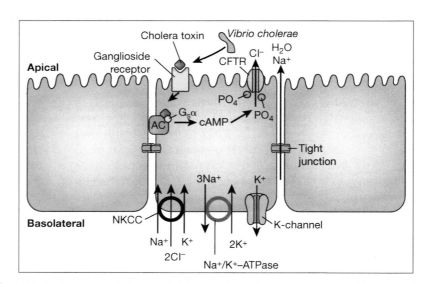

FIGURE 13.22 Water moves into the gut lumen following the osmotic pull of chloride moving across the apical membrane through the CFTR. Chloride secretion is promoted by several paracrine and neurocrine signals in the postprandial state, some of which signal through increased cAMP to trigger channel opening. Cholera toxin A subunit inhibits $G_s\alpha$ GTPase activity, promoting continual adenylyl cyclase activity and cAMP production. This is the mechanism of the profuse secretory diarrhea associated with cholera.

AC, adenylyl cyclase; cAMP, cyclic adenosine monophosphate; CFTR, cystic fibrosis transmembrane conductance regulator; GTPase, guanosine triphosphatase; Na+/K+-ATPase, sodium–potassium pump; NKCC, sodium-potassium-2chloride cotransporter.

Most of the secreted and ingested fluid is absorbed by the small and large intestines. Only a small volume of fluid is ultimately excreted in feces (100–200 mL), so even slight disturbances in the absorption can lead to excessive fluid loss and diarrhea. Mechanisms of fluid and electrolyte absorption vary, depending on location, resulting in varying NaCl concentrations at different intestinal segments. In the absorptive small intestine, the active transport of sodium via Na^+/K^+–ATPase creates a sodium gradient that can then be used to absorb sodium along with glucose and other nutrients by secondary active transport. Absorption of these osmotic substances provides a gradient for water to follow. There are slight differences along the length of the small intestine with respect to the absorption of electrolytes. The main difference is a net absorption of sodium bicarbonate ($NaHCO_3$) in the jejunum and of sodium chloride (NaCl) in the ileum, accompanied by water drawn by osmotic forces. Calcium absorption is under the influence of vitamin D and parathyroid hormone. Phosphorus in the form of phosphate is mainly absorbed in the duodenum and upper jejunum.

In the colon, reabsorption of water follows sodium reabsorption, and the colon contributes about 15% of total GI fluid absorption. **Diarrhea** is excessive fluid excretion with the feces. Fine tuning of bicarbonate and potassium levels is also accomplished in the colon: bicarbonate can be secreted along the intestine, and there is colonic excretion of K^+ under the control of aldosterone, to maintain normal potassium balance. The fluid loss during diarrhea can, therefore, lead to metabolic acidosis and hypokalemia. The small intestine has a greater capacity for absorption/secretion than does the large intestine, so it can be a significant contributor to diarrheal issues. Diarrhea is characterized by these four subtypes: secretory, malabsorptive, osmotic, and inflammatory (**Table 13.4**).

Contaminated food and water are common risks for diarrhea. Protections against invaders include the following mechanisms:

- Bacteria ingested in food usually are killed by low gastric pH.
- Organisms are swept along by gut motility too quickly to multiply.
- The healthy microbiota suppresses the growth of pathogenic bacteria.

Gut immunity also plays a significant role in preventing GI infections and related diarrhea through secretion of IgA and mucosal immune surveillance. Acute infectious diarrhea can be caused by viruses (rotavirus, norovirus), bacteria (*Escherichia coli*, *Salmonella typhi*, *Vibrio* spp.), fungi, or parasites. Globally, infectious diarrhea is associated with a high degree of morbidity and mortality, particularly in children.

Diarrhea may be promoted by the organism itself, or by an exotoxin (such as cholera toxin). Enterotoxins secreted by enterotoxigenic *E. coli* (ETEC) cause secretory diarrhea similar to cholera. Other bacterial cytotoxins targeting gut epithelial cells cause cell death with inflammatory, bloody diarrhea known as **dysentery**. Shiga toxins from *Shigella* and Shiga-related toxins in some *E. coli* species produce diarrhea, and in some cases, this diarrhea is followed by acute hemolyticuremic syndrome. In contrast to diarrhea, constipation is defined as infrequent and hard stools, caused by lack of stool bulk, decreased peristalsis, or mechanical obstruction.

A history of travel or exposure to other individuals known to have experienced the same symptoms is informative when evaluating suspected causes of diarrhea. In some cases, stool culture or identification of pathogen antigen or nucleic acid is used for diagnosis. Assessment

TABLE 13.4 Types of Diarrhea			
Category	Disease Example	Mechanism	Clinical Presentation
Secretory	Cholera from *Vibrio cholerae*, traveler's diarrhea from enterotoxigenic *Escherichia coli*	Enterotoxin stimulates chloride transport out of the cell via increased cAMP activity, with water following	Profuse, watery diarrhea
Malabsorptive	Celiac sprue (gluten sensitivity)	Autoimmune damage to the intestinal lining in response to wheat protein components, with villus atrophy and loss of surface area	Gluten intolerance coupled with steatorrhea
Osmotic	Lactase deficiency	Increased osmolarity of luminal contents, with undigested lactose that then can be a nutrient for colonic bacteria	Diarrhea with bloating
Inflammatory	Inflammatory bowel disease	Direct damage to the mucosa or intestinal wall	Bloody diarrhea, fever, abdominal pain

cAMP, cyclic adenosine monophosphate.

of body fluid balance and hydration status is appropriate to determine the need for parenteral fluids replacement to prevent severe hypovolemia, but most cases in the United States are self-limited and resolve within days.

IMMUNE-RELATED GASTROINTESTINAL DISORDERS

As the recipient of all orally ingested substances, the GI tract is exposed to dietary allergens, pathogen-contaminated foods, and toxins. In addition, the GI tract has an extensive microbiome—a resident bacterial population that functions to maintain healthy gut activities, to aid digestion, and to provide specific nutrients. Protection from potentially damaging substances arises from immune cells of the gut. However, these defenses can contribute to a variety of GI disorders. Celiac disease and inflammatory bowel disease are examples of immune-mediated GI disorders in which both innate and adaptive immune responses are increased, causing loss of normal GI structure and function.

CELIAC DISEASE

Celiac disease is a relatively common disorder worldwide. It appears to result from a combination of genetic and environmental variables. In particular, among the genes coding for major histocompatibility complex II proteins, expression of subtypes HLA-DQ2 and HLA-DQ8 increase the risk of developing celiac disease. However, only a small fraction of individuals with these proteins actually develop celiac disease, so it is clear that other factors are involved. Additional genetic factors, prior viral gastroenteritis infection, and microbiome changes may also contribute to celiac disease development.

In vulnerable persons, exposure to gluten proteins found in wheat, barley, and rye initiates an innate immune response in the gut wall. Tissue transglutaminase 2 (tTG2) removes amine groups from gluten breakdown products, increasing their antigenicity. Mucosal antigen-presenting cells present these antigens to local CD4$^+$ T-helper 1 (Th1) cells, generating an adaptive immune response that reinforces the innate response. Intraepithelial lymphocytes become activated, contributing to the attack on epithelial cells. The mucosal barrier becomes leaky, allowing further penetration of peptide products of gluten digestion into the mucosa to interact with resident immune cells. The initial laboratory test is the evaluation of blood titers for IgA to tTG2. A positive test may be followed by endoscopy with biopsy for definitive diagnosis. Histologically, the gut immune pathology is positive for reactive CD4$^+$ T cells and activated intraepithelial lymphocytes (**Figure 13.23**). The consequence of gluten ingestion is the activation of both acute inflammation and

perpetuation of adaptive immune responses, including activation of T-helper cells and secretion of interleukin (IL)-15, IL-21, tumor necrosis factor alpha (TNF-α), and interferons alpha and gamma (IFN-α and IFN-γ).

The effect of the inflammatory cascade and activation of cytotoxic lymphocytes on the small intestine includes denuding the gut epithelial layer, with extensive villus atrophy and hyperplasia of crypts. This combination results in malabsorption that can be severe. Celiac disease in children can result in slowed growth, whereas in adults, weight loss, chronic diarrhea, and manifestations of malabsorption (anemia, osteoporosis) can occur. There is a high rate of comorbidity between celiac disease and autoimmune disorders such as type 1 diabetes mellitus and Hashimoto thyroiditis. Progression of the disorder increases the risk of developing GI cancer. Maintaining a strict gluten-free diet reverses most of the gut pathology and consequences thereof.

INFLAMMATORY BOWEL DISEASE

Inflammatory bowel disease (IBD) includes **ulcerative colitis** (UC)—which tends to involve only the mucosa and submucosa in the colon, progressing proximally from the rectum—and **Crohn disease** (CD), which can generate transmural lesions, preferentially in the ileum, and potentially throughout the GI tract. Although definitive identification of associated genes is lacking, UC and CD have high familial prevalence.

Both disorders are associated with immune dysregulation that includes impaired tolerance to normal microbiota and hyperactive immune responses that result in inflammation of the mucosa, progressing through deeper layers of the gut wall in CD. The healthy gut barrier of mucus, antimicrobial peptides, and tight junctions between enterocytes is breached, and bacteria enter the mucus layer. In CD, Th1 cells are strongly activated, producing many cytokines that maintain a vicious cycle of inflammation. The cytokines IFN-γ and TNF-α play prominent roles in this cycle.

Genetic influences play a more significant role in CD than in UC. Hundreds of genes have been associated with CD. One of the most significant of these is *NOD2*, a pattern recognition receptor sensitive to muramyl dipeptide, a bacterial cell wall constituent. Other categories of genes that are associated with CD risk include genes that regulate autophagy, cytokine receptors, and intestinal barrier function.

The pattern of enhanced inflammation in CD involves the formation of granulomas that extend deep into the intestinal wall, thus generating the characteristic transmural lesions. This predisposes to the formation of fissures and fistulas that connect the bowel lumen with the peritoneal space or to other abdominal organs, producing scarring and adhesions. In UC, the surface area of inflammation is much greater but is restricted to the

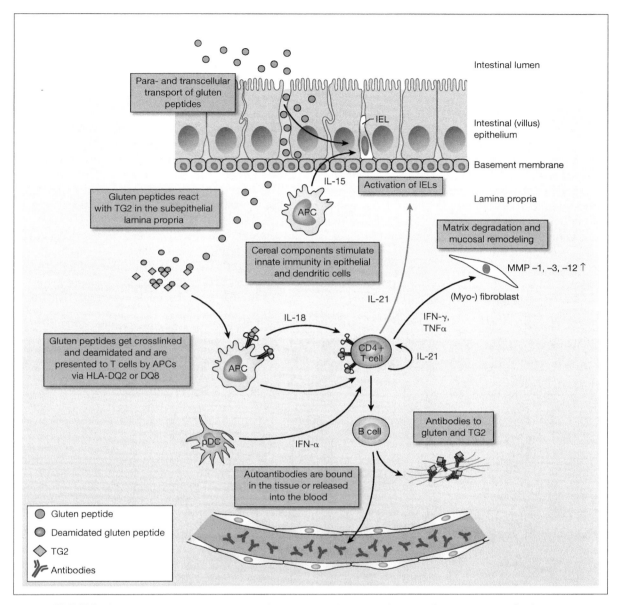

FIGURE 13.23 Pathogenesis of celiac disease includes contributions from innate and adaptive immune systems of the lamina propria beneath the epithelial layer. Gluten peptides are the breakdown products of gluten that may cross the epithelial barrier to initiate an immune response. Deamidation of the peptides increases their antigenicity, particularly when presented on MHC subtypes HLA-DQ2 or HLA-DQ8. Circulating antibodies to gluten and tissue transglutaminase are diagnostic indicators of the disease.

APC, antigen-presenting cell; IEL, intraepithelial lymphocyte; IFN, interferon; IL, interleukin; MHC, major histocompatibility complex; MMP, matrix metalloproteinase; TG2, transglutaminase 2; TNF, tumor necrosis factor.

mucosal layer and does not involve deeper structures of the gut wall. Blood loss is more severe in UC than in CD. Both disorders exhibit patterns of exacerbation and remission, although increased immune activation is evident systemically and in the intestine, even during remission. Finally, both disorders have a high degree of comorbidity with other immune disorders. For example, patients with IBD often exhibit skin lesions such as pyoderma gangrenosum or erythema nodosum, liver disorders such as primary sclerosing cholangitis or pericholangitis, and musculoskeletal inflammatory conditions such as seronegative arthritis or ankylosing spondylitis.

Imaging by endoscopy and noninvasive techniques and biopsies are used for diagnosis. Management of IBD involves immunosuppression by corticosteroids and other antiinflammatory agents. Moderate to severe disease is usually managed with biological agents, including monoclonal antibodies that block cytokines or integrins.

ABDOMINAL PAIN PATTERNS

Abdominal pain is a common and sometimes severe symptom of acute and chronic GI diseases and often presents diagnostic challenges (Table 13.5). Visceral pain fibers travel with autonomic fibers to the gut, and have cell bodies in the nodose ganglion of the vagus nerve (pain fibers from upper GI structures) or in spinal dorsal root ganglia (pain fibers from mid- and hindgut). GI tract structures and the parietal peritoneum contain nociceptors that are sensitive to chemical irritation, inflammatory mediators, distention, and ischemia. Referred pain is that pain appearing in areas of the body surface that send sensory impulses to the same segments of the spinal cord that receive the visceral sensory impulses from the diseased organ. Different structures of the GI tract have different pain referral patterns, based on embryonic development and innervation of these regions:

- The *foregut*, comprising the esophagus, stomach, proximal duodenum, liver, and pancreas
- The *midgut*, comprising the distal duodenum, jejunum, ileum, and proximal to mid-colon
- The *hindgut*, comprising the rest of the colon and gut up to the proximal portion of the anal canal

As a result, one would expect epigastric pain for structures innervated by the celiac artery and ganglion, periumbilical pain for structures innervated by the superior mesenteric artery and ganglion, and lower abdominal pain for structures innervated by the inferior

TABLE 13.5 Common Acute Abdomen Pain Categories

Condition	Classical Presentation	Underlying Pathophysiology
Acute appendicitis	Initial periumbilical pain followed by localized tenderness in right lower quadrant (RLQ)	Initial distention of inflamed appendix, with subsequent involvement of the local parietal peritoneum
Perforated peptic ulcer	Sudden, severe, burning midepigastric pain that can involve entire abdomen	Entrance of acidic stomach contents into peritoneal cavity and subsequent extensive involvement of parietal peritoneum
Acute cholecystitis	Severe RUQ pain associated with nausea and vomiting	Distention/involvement of biliary tree from an inflammatory process
Acute pancreatitis	Deep-seated epigastric pain, radiating to the back	Location of organ and its retroperitoneal position
Acute small intestinal obstruction	Peristaltic pain, epigastric and umbilical regions	Reflective of obstruction process and referred pain locations of duodenum–ileum
Mesenteric infarct	Initial presentation of poorly localized pain that is disproportional to clinical findings on abdominal examination	Branches of superior mesenteric artery supply regions of bowel in segmented fashion, such that small areas can become painfully ischemic Involvement of parietal peritoneum with subsequent necrosis or perforation
Acute diverticulitis	Intermittent LLQ pain that may be cramping	Diverticula are sac-like outward projections of mucosa through muscle and adventitia layers; most common in the colon
Large bowel obstruction	Gradual onset of lower abdominal cramping pain with abdominal distention	The distal location of large intestine will typically lead to a slower presentation than with small bowel
Inflammatory bowel disease	CD: RLQ pain with fever UC: LLQ pain with bloody diarrhea	CD often occurs in the ileocecal region UC has rectal/distal colon predominance and mucosal involvement

CD, Crohn disease; LLQ, left lower quadrant; RLQ, right lower quadrant; RUQ, right upper quadrant; UC, ulcerative colitis.

mesenteric artery and ganglion. These sensations are generally associated with the midline. In contrast, renal pain patterns typically lateralize to the different flanks, given their retroperitoneal development. As disease spreads to involve the parietal peritoneum and its innervation by spinal nerves, localization improves. One can also have a somatic origin of referred pain, as the phrenic nerve (C3-C4-C5) is sensory from the diaphragm, and subsequently, diaphragmatic irritation can trigger shoulder pain.

In addition to pain pattern, the types of pain can offer clues as to the type of involvement. Cramping or colicky pain is characteristic of the distention or obstruction of hollow structures, such as the intestine, biliary tree, or ureters. Tearing pain would be consistent with the rupture or dissection through hollow structures, such as the esophagus or abdominal aorta. Burning pain would be consistent with active peptic ulceration.

IRRITABLE BOWEL SYNDROME

Irritable bowel syndrome (IBS) is a heterogeneous disorder in which abdominal pain presents with alterations of defecation (either constipation or diarrhea). The pain may be relieved by defecation, or the pain onset may coincide with a change in stool characteristics. IBS is very common, affecting more than 10% of people worldwide.[8] Based on the presentation, IBS subtypes are classified as IBS-C, associated with constipation; IBS-D, associated with diarrhea; and IBS-M, associated with mixed stool types. There is some overlap between patients with IBD or celiac disease and those with IBS. One hypothesis is that visceral pain fibers become hypersensitive during IBD exacerbations, such that abdominal pain persists, even after most of the inflammatory manifestations have remitted. IBS is sometimes referred to as a functional disorder, as there are few structural manifestations on biopsy or other imaging results that correlate with the episodes of pain.

In addition to visceral hypersensitivity, hypotheses of IBS include abnormal gut motility, increased inflammation, and stress. In particular, early life events and other preexisting sources of stress are implicated in altered pain thresholds. Some genetic and epigenetic alterations may be associated with IBS, but these possibilities are still under study. Finally, a history of prior gut infectious disease (bacterial or viral) or inflammatory disease (Crohn or celiac disease) is a significant risk factor for IBS development. Ultimately, alterations of the brain–gut relationship underlying IBS may be multifactorial, as shown in **Figure 13.24**. Management can target the specific bowel changes (constipation or diarrhea) as well as lifestyle alterations (smoking cessation, identifying and avoiding food triggers). Empirical evidence suggests that a diet low in fermentable oligo-di-mono-saccharides and polyols (FODMAPs) is often helpful.

HEMORRHOIDS

Hemorrhoids affect the vascular structures of the anus that cushion the anal canal and facilitate defecation by sensory detection of stool quality (loose, hard, relative volume). Pathology of hemorrhoids includes swelling and protrusion into or external to the rectal canal (internal and external hemorrhoids, respectively). Hemorrhoids are often asymptomatic, but swelling can be associated with localized pain and bleeding. Bleeding from hemorrhoids and stool leakage can cause pruritus. The prevalence of pathological hemorrhoids is estimated at 1% to 5% of the population, but many cases are self-managed; hence, underreporting is common. Low-fiber diets and chronic constipation may contribute to hemorrhoid formation and progression, and prevalence increases with age.

INTESTINAL FAILURE AND SHORT BOWEL SYNDROME

Intestinal failure is a syndrome of inability to digest and absorb sufficient nutrients to maintain health and homeostasis. Causes of intestinal failure can include immune-related destruction, neoplastic damage, and ischemia/infarction. Pathophysiologic processes vary, and include short bowel syndrome, intestinal fistulae, dysmotility, mechanical obstruction, and extensive mucosal loss. Intestinal failure can be acute and resolve after weeks to months, or chronic, lasting months to years. Chronic (type 3) intestinal failure presents the greatest clinical challenge, as it requires prolonged parenteral nutrition support, increasing risk of thromboembolic phenomena, and catheter-associated infections.[9]

One cause of intestinal failure is **short bowel syndrome**, in which there is insufficient length of small intestine, and sometimes colon, to maintain nutritional homeostasis and fluid and electrolyte balance. Short bowel syndrome is the result of disease processes or necessary surgical resection that reduces intestinal length below a critical level of 50% of normal. Patterns of pathophysiological alterations depend on the segments affected: Loss of the duodenum and proximal jejunum results in defective iron and calcium absorption, whereas loss of the ileum results in defective vitamin B12 absorption and bile salt recirculation. Each of these comes with a host of other manifestations and management challenges. Regrowth of small intestine is promoted by a GLP-2 agonist, and other aspects of management include careful monitoring and balance of enteral and parenteral nutrition to reduce the pathophysiological consequences.

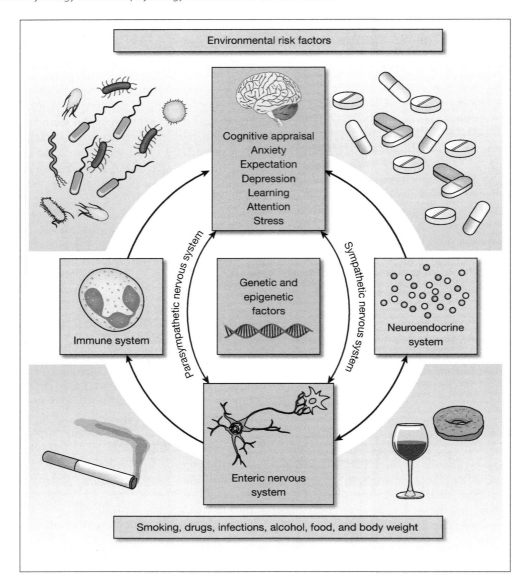

FIGURE 13.24 Proposed multifactorial contributors to irritable bowel syndrome include the brain and learned responses to stress, enteric and other neuroendocrine mediators, genetics, environmental and lifestyle exposures, particularly smoking and gastrointestinal infections, and immune responsiveness.
Source: From Enck et al., Functional dyspepsia. *Nature Reviews Disease Primers*, Volume 3, Article number: 17081 (2017). doi:10.1038/nrdp.2017.81

Thought Questions

8. Compare the causes and consequences of chronic disorders that primarily affect the small versus large intestine. How will this anatomical distinction affect the patient presentation?

9. What are the potential causes of an acute onset of abdominal pain? What features might help to distinguish between these causes?

MALNUTRITION AND OBESITY

Malnutrition is increasingly appreciated as a significant global health issue. Malnutrition can include both undernutrition and overnutrition—in the latter case, the total intake may be greater than normal but diet quality is poor, resulting in specific deficiencies that compromise health and homeostasis. The World Health Organization noted in 2018 that worldwide, 462 million adults were underweight, and 1.9 billion adults were overweight or obese. Statistics for children include the following: 52 million suffer from wasting, with 17 million having severe wasting; 155 million have stunted growth; and 41 million are overweight or obese. Forty-five percent of deaths in children younger than 5 years of age are associated with undernutrition, with the greatest rates in underresourced countries.[10]

Several national and international organizations have extensively reviewed the topic of malnutrition and provided a consensus on clinical identification and definition.[11] At this time, assessment is based on phenotypic findings of any one of the following:

- Nonvolitional weight loss
- Low body mass index (BMI)
- Reduced muscle mass, accompanied by etiological identification of either reduced food intake or assimilation, or known disease burden/inflammatory condition

Inflammation is associated with an increased catabolic state, often increasing energy requirements while reducing appetite. The consensus report concludes that a diagnosis of malnutrition requires the presence of at least one of the phenotypic criteria *plus* one of the etiological criteria. Malnutrition can further be staged for severity based on the phenotypic criteria.

Causes of malnutrition range from food inadequacy/starvation to acute disorders or chronic diseases with a high inflammatory component. Development of consistent diagnostic criteria is a necessary first step to improve identification and developing evidence-based management approaches. Malnutrition causes and presentation differ between acute and chronic healthcare settings, with acute injuries and diseases rapidly altering nutritional state followed by resolution once recovery occurs, while consequences of chronic malnutrition may develop slowly and be refractory to management.

Obesity, as measured by the BMI—calculated as weight in kilograms divided by height in meters squared—is ultimately caused by an imbalance of energy intake and expenditure. Prevalence of overweight (BMI between 25 and 30) and obesity (BMI >30) is increasing in the United States and worldwide, and affects all age groups. Obesity is a chronic inflammatory state and is a significant risk factor for type 2 diabetes mellitus, hypertension, cardiovascular disease morbidity and mortality, cancer, degenerative joint disease, and neurodegenerative disorders, among other consequences.

Although obesity has multifactorial causes, GI-associated function and hormones are involved. The GI tract contributes to energy intake by absorbing most of the available nutrients that are ingested and digested, without regard for the biological necessity for the calories. When calories ingested and absorbed are consistently greater than calories expended, body weight increases with accumulation of fat mass. Physiological

regulation of appetite and energy balance involves several hormones and neurotransmitters, with central processing by the hypothalamus. Many hormones and GI peptides released by the presence of products of food digestion or signals of nutrient adequacy trigger a sense of satiety. These include leptin, produced by adipose tissue; insulin, from the endocrine pancreas; and CCK, GLP-1, and peptide YY, from the intestine. In contrast, ghrelin, produced by the nondistended stomach, stimulates appetite.

Management of obesity and its associated complications by lifestyle changes has varied success rates. Similarly, pharmacological management has mixed results, with some weight-loss medications discontinued due to toxicity and others having limited efficacy. Bariatric surgery for weight loss has had a good degree of success, particularly for short-term outcomes of weight reduction and improvement or resolution of comorbidities such as type 2 diabetes mellitus, metabolic syndrome, and nonalcoholic fatty liver disease. Bariatric surgery involves significant rearrangement of GI structure and function, including major reduction in stomach volume, as performed in sleeve gastrectomy. Greater physiological disruption occurs with procedures such as the roux-en-Y bypass, which combines reduced stomach volume with bypass of lengths of duodenum and jejunum. As the number of bariatric surgeries performed worldwide continues to increase, there will be opportunities to better understand the associated alterations in gut hormones, brain–gut signaling, microbiota alterations, and other potential mechanisms that contribute to postsurgical clinical improvements.[12]

LYNCH SYNDROME

Colorectal cancer (CRC) was the fourth most common cancer in the United States during the years 2012 to 2016.[13] As with most cancers, most cases result from sporadic rather than inherited mutations. Approximately 3% of CRC cases in the United States are attributable to **Lynch syndrome**, also known as **hereditary nonpolyposis colon cancer**, an autosomal dominant disease. Cases are often identified by family history of CRC and other cancers, and are then verified by genetic testing. The mutations responsible for Lynch syndrome involve genes coding for DNA mismatch repair proteins. In addition to CRC, individuals with Lynch syndrome have rates of endometrial and ovarian cancer (in women), gastric cancer, and other cancers that are higher than those of the general population. Rates of cancer in the hepatobiliary system, small intestine, renal pelvis, and ureter are also increased in patients with this syndrome. Once identified, patients are managed by earlier and more frequent screenings, such as colonoscopy.

Randall L. Johnson

GASTROINTESTINAL DEVELOPMENT AND FUNCTION IN CHILDHOOD

The GI tract originates from the endoderm beginning at the third week of embryological development. Over the next several weeks, differentiation takes place involving the original tube of endodermal origin, and influenced by the adjacent mesoderm to form the various segments of the GI tract and the associated liver and pancreas. Neural crest cells originating from the ectoderm move into the developing gut wall, finally forming the enteric nervous system. As the GI tract develops throughout fetal growth, these segments develop the functional systems of digestion and absorption.

At full term, the GI tract is fully formed in infants; however, secretion of enzymes of digestion and absorptive properties are not fully developed. In addition, the epithelial barrier function is not intact, and exposure to diarrhea-causing pathogens can result in severe consequences of diarrhea, fluid loss, and dehydration. Development of GI functional capacity varies with dietary intake, differing in breastfed compared with formula-fed infants. As solid foods are introduced, further developmental changes occur, dependent on diet. Finally, although the gut microbiome is minimal at birth, it develops quickly postnatally, varying by delivery route (vaginal versus cesarean). Establishing the normal gut flora contributes to gut maturation, particularly of gut immune function. Premature infants will have slight deviations and are at greater risk for absorptive issues, particularly affecting very low birthweight infants.[14–16]

During early childhood development, the pancreas increases functional capacity for digestive enzyme production and secretion, and the microbiome continues to approach the composition of an adult. Introduction of new foods should be gradual and employ a systematic approach that includes addition of foods one at a time. The clinician should also ensure that dentition is sufficient for solids. Throughout childhood, GI concerns are often what bring a child to the healthcare setting. It is important to understand some of the more common and life-threatening illnesses that are seen in infants and children.

GASTROENTERITIS

Gastroenteritis is an inflammation of the structures within the GI tract, including the stomach and the small and large intestines. It is the most common condition that brings a child into the healthcare system. Often,

the condition has progressed rapidly, leading quickly to a point of volume depletion of the child. Therefore, immediate medical intervention is necessary. The younger the infant, the greater the possibility of developing gastroenteritis due to immature function of GI tract immune components as well as greater permeability of the mucosal lining. There are two major mechanisms of infectious diarrhea:

1. Tissue invasion denuding the villus epithelium of the small intestine, resulting in acute malabsorptive diarrhea
2. Production of a toxin that stimulates chloride secretion into the gut, producing secretory diarrhea

Globally, gastroenteritis results in 533,800 deaths annually in children younger than 5 years of age.[17,18] Pediatric gastroenteritis can result from viral, bacterial, and parasitic pathogens, in descending order of frequency. Each of these infection types is identified by specific diagnostic techniques and requires specific management. The gravest concern is the potential for dehydration, which is more severe in younger children and those with longer duration of the illness. Rehydration is the foundation of initial acute management. Either intravenous or oral fluids are used, depending on the severity. Globally, oral rehydration therapy (ORT) that provides fluid, electrolytes, and glucose has saved many millions of lives at a very low cost. The physiological basis for ORT is stimulation of sodium and glucose absorption through SGLT1, providing osmotic drive for the absorption of water.

VIRAL GASTROENTERITIS

Viral infections are the most frequent causes of gastroenteritis in children. The most common pathogens causing **viral gastroenteritis** are norovirus and rotavirus, followed by astrovirus and adenovirus, with other viruses occurring much less frequently. Cases of rotavirus infection have declined worldwide since the widespread implementation of rotavirus vaccine. Administration of intravenous or oral fluids to prevent dehydration is the only treatment implemented, as the infections are self-limited, generally lasting several days.

BACTERIAL GASTROENTERITIS

In high-resource settings such as the United States, bacterial causes represent 10% or fewer pediatric

TABLE 13.6 Common Gastrointestinal Tract Bacteria and Diarrhea Pathogenesis

Bacteria	Mechanisms
Salmonella, Campylobacter	Invade mucosa
Shigella, Escherichia coli	Invade mucosa Enterotoxin production
Clostridioides difficile	Invade mucosa Enterotoxin production Exotoxin production

gastroenteritis cases. The most common pathogens causing **bacterial gastroenteritis** are *Campylobacter*, *Salmonella*, *Shigella*, and enterohemorrhagic *E. coli*. However, children treated with broad-spectrum antibiotics may also develop *C. difficile* diarrhea. Bacterial gastroenteritis can be differentiated from other causes by severity, presence of fever, blood or mucus in the stool, and stool positive for fecal leukocytes. Stool culture or nucleic acid testing can confirm the organism. The pathogenic processes for each of these common organisms are listed in **Table 13.6**.

PARASITIC GASTROENTERITIS

The most common causes of **parasitic gastroenteritis** are *Giardia* and *Cryptosporidium*. These organisms may be acquired through direct contact with contaminated individuals, or contaminated water from surface water, wells, or municipal supplies. In young children, transmission occurs frequently at daycare centers where hygienic interventions are not followed carefully. **Giardiasis** is most commonly transmitted through contaminated water during summer recreational activities. Suspicion of parasitic diarrhea arises based on a prolonged course of diarrhea and a history of travel to regions where these infections are endemic.[17]

COMMON SYMPTOMS OF GASTROENTERITIS

In all cases, diarrhea is the most common and often the most life-threatening symptom of gastroenteritis. Other symptoms may include nausea, vomiting, dehydration, fever, and signs of gastric distress such as bloating and gas production. Early recognition of these symptoms will allow for rapid intervention, reduction of distress, and possible interruption of the hypovolemic processes taking place. In addition to the fluid losses, electrolyte imbalances can occur, including hypokalemia and hyponatremia—especially during rehydration, if hypotonic solutions are used.

GASTROESOPHAGEAL REFLUX

Gastroesophageal reflux is a common occurrence in developing children. Clinicians distinguish between *gastroesophageal reflux* (GER), which occurs frequently during infancy (reported as a topic of discussion at 25% of routine 6-month well-baby visits[19]), and **gastroesophageal reflux disease** (GERD), introduced earlier in this chapter, which is also reported in both infants and children. The principal distinction between GER and GERD is the age of primary occurrence: GER is very common in infants and gradually improves by the age of 6 months to 1 year, whereas GERD can manifest within the first year of age or at any time throughout childhood or adolescence. In addition, GER is usually associated with painless, immediate vomiting of an overly large meal, whereas patients with GERD present with complaints of pain, dysphagia, food refusal, poor weight gain, and recurrent vomiting.

GER is managed conservatively with transition to smaller and more frequent meals. Breastfeeding mothers can be encouraged to alter their diet to see if that reduces the infant's symptoms; formula-fed infants may require a change of formula. Placing the infant in an upright position during and for a period after feeding also reduces GER.

GERD in children is similar to the condition in adults and is managed by the same mechanisms, with the caveat that most medications (antacids, H_2 antagonists, and proton pump inhibitors) have not been validated for use in infants or children, particularly for prolonged treatment. GERD in older adults is discussed later in this chapter, in Gerontological Considerations.

HYPERTROPHIC PYLORIC STENOSIS

Hypertrophic pyloric stenosis can be diagnosed as early as the first 2 to 12 weeks after birth on the basis of repeated vomiting, weight loss, and dehydration due to the inability of meal contents to pass through the pylorus to the duodenum. Both circular and longitudinal muscle layers are hypertrophied, and an olive-shaped pylorus is often palpable on physical examination and detectable on ultrasound (**Figure 13.25**). The prevalence is two to four cases per 1,000 children, with a male/female ratio of approximately 4:1. Prevalence is greatest among those of European descent. The causes are thought to be multifactorial, including genetic influences with familial risk, hyperacidity, exposure of infant or breastfeeding mother to macrolide antibiotics, and abnormalities of the nitric oxide system that promote muscle relaxation. Early diagnosis is critical to obtaining surgical treatment and resolution.[20]

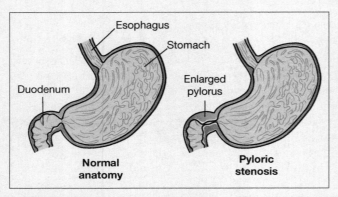

FIGURE 13.25 Normal pylorus (left) and pylorus with hypertrophic stenosis (right).

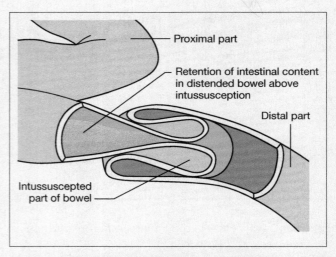

FIGURE 13.26 Intussusception of the bowel occurs when a distal segment of the intestine telescopes over a more proximal segment.

INTUSSUSCEPTION

Intussusception is the telescoping of a distal segment of the intestine over a proximal segment (**Figure 13.26**). It is the most common cause of bowel obstruction in children and occurs most often between the ages of 6 months and 3 years of age. Compression of the bowel and blockage of blood flow results in ischemia of the constricted segment of intestine and obstruction of flow through the intestine. If not treated and resolved, intussusception leads to gangrene and potential for perforation of the bowel.

In 90% of cases, intussusception is idiopathic; in the remaining 10%, it is secondary to anatomical variants, including Meckel diverticulum, tumors and polyps, genetic disorders, and other causes, including viral enteritis. Intussusception is seen slightly more frequently in boys. The symptoms include sudden onset abdominal pain, often identified as colic in infants. Symptoms are often cyclical, with periods of no pain and then extreme pain. Eventually, as the ischemia progresses, pain becomes constant and more severe. Diagnosis is confirmed through ultrasound and air enema, which often reduces the telescoping segment or pushes it back into place, thus resolving the problem. If the enema does not reduce the intussusception, then surgery must be performed emergently to resect the segment of intestine affected.[21,22]

HIRSCHSPRUNG DISEASE

Hirschsprung disease is a rare condition (one in 5,000–10,000 live births) but is notable as the major disorder resulting from abnormal migration of enteric neurons during embryonic development. The defect most commonly affects distal structures, including the sigmoid colon and rectum, but can extend proximally. Identification can be made soon after birth based on failure to defecate meconium for 24 hours or more after birth and development of abdominal distention and vomiting. Peristalsis is blocked due to failure of relaxation of the segment lacking innervation. Diagnosis requires imaging and also biopsy that demonstrates lack of ganglion cells of the enteric nervous system. Treatment is surgical resection of the affected bowel segment.[23]

Rosanna Reda

AGE-RELATED CHANGES OF THE GASTROINTESTINAL TRACT

The GI health of older adults is a concern that requires special attention from healthcare providers. Direct age-related changes in the GI tract may be modest in healthy older adults; however, other health and dental conditions, polypharmacy, and lifestyle changes lead to a high incidence of GI disorders with aging. These include dysphagia, atrophic gastritis, GERD, intestinal obstruction, chronic constipation, and diverticular disease. Decreased motility and sensory function, particularly visceral pain sensation, contribute to atypical presentation of GI disorders in older adults, and disorders can rapidly worsen before coming to the attention of providers and being accurately diagnosed.

Research shows that age-related changes in the anatomy and physiology of the GI tract, summarized in **Box 13.2**, lead to a higher incidence of disorders that can negatively affect the health of older adults. Owing to the complex overlap of disorders, medication use, and behavioral changes, older adults are more likely to be negatively impacted by the damaging effects of GERD, peptic ulcer disease, dysphagia, diverticulosis, and IBD. The combination of these disorders with the heightened inflammatory state in older adults (inflammaging) contributes to malnutrition, loss of lean muscle mass, and frailty.

AGE-ASSOCIATED ALTERATIONS IN MASTICATION

Chewing is the initial step of physical breakdown of food. Older adults frequently experience tooth loss and decay, caused by decreased calcium absorption, poor maintenance, periodontal disease, smoking, and other lifestyle factors. Ill-fitting dentures can create oral ulcerations, making chewing painful and decreasing meal size. Motor activity of the tongue and muscles of mastication also weaken with age. Diseases that affect cognition or neuromuscular coordination of older adults can make chewing and swallowing difficult. Older adults often complain of dry mouth, which is a common side effect of many medications frequently prescribed to them. Some studies also show age-associated decline in the secretion of saliva, a condition known as xerostomia. All of these oral health challenges increase the incidence of **indigestion** in older adults.

DYSPHAGIA

The incidence of **dysphagia** (difficulty with swallowing) is high in older adults, arising from dysfunction of the oral, pharyngeal, and esophageal phases of swallowing. Anatomical and physiological changes associated with aging include weakness of the tongue and associated muscles of the mouth, impaired function of the UES, weakening of the pharyngeal wall, and decreased esophageal peristalsis. Dysphagia can result from or accompany neuromuscular or central nervous system diseases such as stroke, Parkinson disease, and dementia. **Oropharyngeal dysphagia** can be caused by decreased resting pressure, or incomplete relaxation of the UES. Pulmonary aspiration can occur if saliva, food, or emesis is inhaled into airways and into the lungs, providing a medium for bacterial growth, including normal oral flora that can produce bacterial pneumonia. **Zenker diverticulum**, a pouch-like

---

BOX 13.2
Changes in the Gastrointestinal Tract With Aging

- Tooth loss and decay
- Decreased saliva secretion
- Decreased resting pressure of UES
- Incompetence of LES
- Reduced motility
- Delayed gastric emptying

- Slower regeneration of gastric mucosa
- Decreased secretion of digestive enzymes
- Weakening of intestinal walls
- Slower colonic transit
- Decreased tone of external and internal anal sphincter

LES, lower esophageal sphincter; UES, upper esophageal sphincter.

weakening of the pharyngeal wall above the UES, can contribute to dysphagia.

Esophageal dysphagia results in food getting caught en route to the stomach. It is caused by declining motility and peristalsis with aging or common medications. Age-related changes are attributed to the degeneration of neurons and glia in the enteric nervous system, and reduced cholinergic stimulation of esophageal smooth muscle.[24,25] Anticholinergic, antispasmodic, and calcium channel blocker medications often prescribed to older adults interfere with the motility of the GI tract and contribute to dysphagia.

GASTROESOPHAGEAL REFLUX DISEASE IN OLDER ADULTS

GERD, introduced earlier in this chapter, is a chronic disease that leads to complications such as heartburn, regurgitation, and chest pain, the consequences of which are especially harmful to older adults who are at higher risk for developing esophagitis, esophageal strictures, Barrett esophagus, and esophageal cancer. The LES becomes incompetent with age, and thus places older adults at risk for developing reflux. In addition, decrease in gastric motility results in delayed gastric emptying, thus extending exposure of the LES to gastric contents. Older adults may have reduced production and secretion of saliva, which contains bicarbonates that neutralize acids in refluxed gastric contents. Medications such as anticholinergics, antispasmodics, and calcium channel blockers may promote LES incompetence and weaken peristalsis, exacerbating GERD in older adults.

ALTERED DIGESTION

GI secretions, including digestive enzymes, decline with aging, contributing to symptoms of indigestion (heartburn, dyspepsia). Digestion can be further compromised in older adults by a decline in secretion of pancreatic enzymes, which then contributes to impaired digestion of lipid-rich foods, and can lead to a feeling of prolonged satiety. Gastric acid secretion does not decrease significantly with age; however, older adults are more frequently diagnosed with *H. pylori* infection and atrophic gastritis, accompanied by decreased gastric acid secretion.

PEPTIC ULCER DISEASE

Older adults are more commonly hospitalized for **gastric and duodenal ulcers**, owing to age-related physiological changes and frequent use of medications

that exacerbate **peptic ulcer disease**. Older adults are frequently prescribed NSAIDs as an analgesic for musculoskeletal issues, orthopedic procedures, and management and prevention of cardiovascular and cerebrovascular diseases. NSAIDs diminish prostaglandin-mediated protection of the mucosal lining, inhibiting mucus and bicarbonate production. Delayed emptying and slow transit add to the erosive effect of NSAIDs on gastric mucosa. *H. pylori* infection is more prevalent in older adults and can lead to formation of ulcers. In younger adults, gastric mucosa readily regenerates and repairs but this process may be reduced in older adults, especially in those with low calorie intake. Growth-promoting messengers such as gastrin have less effect in the aging gastric mucosa, possibly due to loss or insensitivity of receptors.[26]

CONSTIPATION

Constipation is a symptom complex that consists of at least two of the following complaints:

- Fewer than three bowel movements in a week
- Straining during defecation
- Hard stools
- Sensation of block or incomplete defecation
- Manual maneuvering required to defecate

Constipation becomes increasingly common with aging due to physiological changes in colonic transit and lifestyle factors. Fewer neurons in the myenteric plexus result in slower colonic transit. Behaviors such as sedentary activity level, low fluid intake, low-fiber diet, inadequate chewing, and medication use can cause constipation in older adults. Constipation can be a side effect of other diseases (diabetes mellitus due to gastroparesis, hypothyroidism, uremia) as well as a symptom of IBS.[26] Red flag causes of constipation would be blockage by a neoplastic growth, volvulus, or other structural alteration or paralytic ileus. Many medications cause constipation, including anticholinergics, opioids, calcium channel blockers, and several psychotropic drugs. Chronic use of laxatives can also lead to decreased colonic motility and decreased laxative effectiveness.

Management is first directed at improving intake of fluid and fiber and increasing physical activity, as able. If chronic constipation persists without resolution for several months, additional studies may be warranted. Colorectal motility can be evaluated with lower GI endoscopy and measurements of colonic transit time and rectal motor and sphincter function. Thyroid function should be assessed, as hypothyroidism can cause constipation.

DIVERTICULAR DISEASE

Diverticular disease is extremely common, and incidence increases with age. This age-related increase may stem from thinning of the colon wall, combined with greater incidence of chronic constipation and straining with defecation. The hallmark of diverticular disease is the development of deep pouches in the wall of the large intestine (**Figures 13.27** and **13.28**). Diverticula form when high pressure against the mucosa of the colon leads to herniation in the weaker portions of the intestinal wall, often where blood vessels are entering and exiting. Diverticulitis occurs when these diverticula become inflamed or infected. Decreased motility and slower transit may increase pressures against colon walls. Low-fiber diets therefore contribute to the formation of diverticula because of smaller stools and longer transit times.[27]

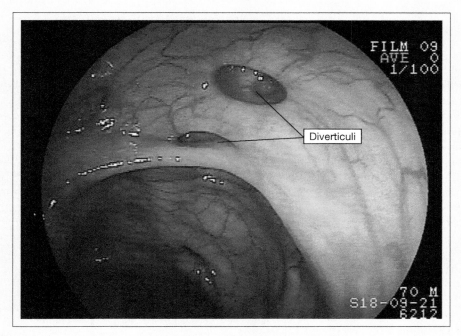

FIGURE 13.27 Appearance of diverticula on colonoscopy.

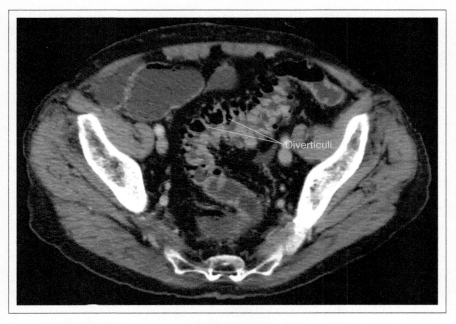

FIGURE 13.28 Appearance of multiple diverticula on CT scan.

CASE STUDY 13.1: A Patient With Peptic Ulcer Disease

Amanda Chaney and Michelle Zappas

Patient Complaint: *"I've been having a hard time lately after I eat. I get this really bad belly pain in the middle of my stomach. Sometimes it burns and feels like it's going up the back of my throat. OTC antacids used to help. But now it hurts and burns every day."*

History of Present Illness/Review of Systems: You observe a healthy-appearing 52-year-old man who appears in no acute distress. He reports epigastric, midsternal, burning pain that worsens with eating. He states that the pain is worse with very fatty foods, such as cheeseburgers. It is associated with early satiety, nausea, and eructation. He denies vomiting. At its worst the pain is a 7 out of 10, and it usually lasts for about 2 hours after eating. He has tried OTC regimens for "heartburn" containing calcium carbonate (Tums) and bismuth subsalicylate (Pepto-Bismol). Although he reports that they used to help, they do not help anymore. He denies fever, chest pain, shortness of breath, or any other symptoms. He denies changes in bowel habits, diarrhea, constipation, or hematochezia. He reported one episode of blackish-colored stool 2 days ago. His last bowel movement was yesterday, and was brown and soft. He reports that he sustained a knee injury a few years ago, and over the past few months the knee pain has gotten worse. He has been taking ibuprofen, 800 mg every 4 hours daily, for the last 2 to 3 weeks with good pain relief. He also takes a baby aspirin once a day. He denies any other OTC or herbal supplement medications.

Past Medical/Family/Social History: The patient's past medical history is significant for a right knee injury in 2012 from a skiing accident, hypertension (for which he takes metoprolol), and a tonsillectomy as a child. He reports occasional alcohol consumption socially, when he will have one or two beers. He denies intravenous or intranasal drug use, recent tattoos, or recent travel. He is a nonsmoker.

Physical Examination: Findings are as follows: temperature of 98.6°F, blood pressure of 135/90 mm Hg, heart rate of 76 beats/min, and respirations of 18 breaths/min. Abdominal pain to the midepigastric area is 7 out of 10. The patient is alert and oriented to person, place, and time. Skin is warm. S_1/S_2 heart sounds are present, and the heart rate and rhythm are regular. Lungs are clear to auscultation bilaterally. Normoreactive bowel sounds are present in all four quadrants of the abdomen, with tenderness in the midepigastric region. No masses are palpable, and there is no rebound or guarding.

Laboratory and Diagnostic Findings: Laboratory data reveal mild anemia (Hb of 9.0 g/dL), guaiac stool positive, and negative urea breath test. An EGD showed two clean-based gastric ulcers. Biopsy samples also were obtained to check for *Helicobacter pylori*, and results were negative.

CASE STUDY 13.1 QUESTIONS
- *What is the rationale for* H. pylori *testing in this patient?*
- *How do NSAID medications alter and impair the gastric mucosa?*
- *What are some additional tests and imaging studies that the provider could perform?*

EGD, esophagogastroduodenoscopy; Hb, hemoglobin; NSAID, nonsteroidal antiinflammatory drug; OTC, over-the-counter.

CASE STUDY 13.2: A Teenage Boy With Celiac Disease

Amanda Chaney and Michelle Zappas

Patient Complaint: "*My stomach has been upset off and on for the past few months. I feel really bloated, especially after I eat, and sometimes my stomach makes really loud noises followed by a lot of gas. I've lost a few pounds and I have been really tired. I never seem to have enough energy. I think I'm just really stressed out about starting college next year.*"

History of Present Illness/Review of Systems: You observe a healthy-appearing, 17-year-old boy, who reports fatigue, some intermittent nausea, and occasional vomiting. He notes that he has had loose, foul-smelling "floating" stools, usually three to four times per day. He denies taking any OTC or herbal supplement medications, with the exception of one iron supplement daily. He does report some intermittent, vague, generalized abdominal pain that comes and goes. He denies fever or any other acute complaints.

Past Medical/Family/Social History: The patient's past medical history is notable for iron deficiency anemia. His weight has been fluctuating over the past year, with weight loss of 10 lb in the past 2 months. With the exception of a tonsillectomy at age 7, he has had no surgeries, hospitalizations, or other chronic illnesses. His social history is negative for use of tobacco, alcohol, or other drugs. He indicates that his mother has autoimmune thyroiditis, which is well controlled; his father is alive and well, with a medical history of diabetes. He has a sister with celiac disease.

Physical Examination: Findings are as follows: temperature of 98.6°F, blood pressure of 110/72 mm Hg, heart rate of 60 beats/min, and respirations of 20 breaths/min. BMI is 20.8 kg/m²; abdominal pain is generalized, 2 out of 10. The patient is alert and oriented, and is a healthy-appearing teenager. Skin is dry and warm, with multiple pruritic papules and vesicles grouped on elbows, knees, and back. Eyes show no scleral icterus. Mouth has moist mucous membranes. S_1/S_2 heart sounds are present, with regular rate and rhythm. Lungs are clear to auscultation bilaterally. Abdomen is flat, soft, and nontender, with hyperreactive bowel sounds in all four quadrants. The liver edge is palpable just below the costal margin, soft and smooth. The spleen is not palpable. No other masses are palpable, and there is no rebound or guarding.

Laboratory and Diagnostic Findings: Laboratory data reveal mild anemia (Hb of 12.2 g/dL). AST, ALT, alkaline phosphatase, glucose, cholesterol, and thyroid levels are all normal; IgA tissue transglutaminase is elevated. EGD shows flattened villi, and a small bowel tissue biopsy sample is positive for IgA-tTG. Additional testing shows low levels of iron, folic acid, and vitamins B12 and D.

CASE STUDY 13.2 QUESTIONS
- *In a patient with celiac disease, what is the effect of exposure to dietary gluten on small intestine structure and function?*
- *Why is the blood tested for IgA-tTG when testing for celiac disease?*
- *When should the provider be concerned about malabsorption in this patient?*

ALT, alanine aminotransferase; AST, aspartate aminotransferase; BMI, body mass index; EGD, esophagogastroduodenoscopy; Hb, hemoglobin; IgA, immunoglobulin A; OTC, over-the-counter; tTG, tissue transglutaminase.

BRIDGE TO CLINICAL PRACTICE

Ben Cocchiaro

PRINCIPLES OF ASSESSMENT

History

- *History:* Assess usual frequency and character of stools, use of dietary supplements (fiber, probiotics) and OTC medications.
- *Symptoms and signs:* Assess heartburn; abdominal pain; nausea; anorexia; vomiting; diarrhea; constipation; change in frequency, character, or color of stool; bloating; flatulence; unintended weight loss; and relationships between symptoms/signs and ingestion of specific foods.

Physical Examination

- *Abdomen:* Inspect; auscultate for bowel sounds and abdominal bruits; percuss for tympanic sounds and shifting dullness; light and deep palpation for diffuse or focal tenderness, guarding, and rebound tenderness.
- *Inspection:* Include mouth and anus.

Diagnostic Tools

- Radiography—abdominal flat plate, abdominal series, emptying studies. These studies are becoming less common as use of CT and MRI increases.
- Abdominal ultrasound, computed tomography (CT), magnetic resonance imaging (MRI) scans are used to assess all regions of the GI tract, as well as liver and pancreas.
- Esophageal pH monitoring for GERD.
- Endoscopy/colonoscopy allows direct visualization of upper GI and lower GI structures, respectively, and can be combined with biopsy to evaluate for Barrett esophagus, *H. pylori* infection, small intestine villus atrophy (as in celiac disease), polyps (cancer or precancer of the colon), lesions characteristic of inflammatory bowel disease.

Laboratory Evaluation

- Urea breath test for *H. pylori*.
- PCR or immunoassay identification of *H. pylori* and its antigen in biopsy or other sample.
- Tissue transglutaminase (tTG) IgA titer for celiac disease.

- Amylase, lipase assays for pancreatitis
- *Complete blood count with differential:* White cell count is elevated in pancreatitis, some cases of appendicitis, other inflammatory disorders; red cell count is decreased in nutritional anemias including iron, vitamin B12, and folate deficiency.
- *Comprehensive metabolic panel:* BUN and other indices are abnormal in acute inflammation, protein is altered in malnutrition and malabsorption, nausea/vomiting/diarrhea alter fluid and electrolyte balance.
- Serum assays of vitamins and minerals as indicated by diagnosis (iron, vitamin B12, etc.).
- Stool culture and examination for pathogens.

MAJOR DRUG CLASSES

- *Acid-reducing drugs:* H_2 antagonists, proton pump inhibitors, antacids (neutralizing agents).
- *Antiemetic drugs:* dopamine antagonists, antihistamines, serotonin (5-HT_3 receptor) antagonists, anticholinergics, neurokinin-1 receptor antagonists—act peripherally and within central nervous system to reduce vomiting center activity.
- *Antidiarrheals:*
  - Opioids reduce GI motility and secretions, forms used for diarrhea do not have central nervous system actions
  - Bismuth compounds have antisecretory and some antimicrobial effects
  - Telotristat reduces serotonin synthesis, decreasing GI stimulation
- *Drug classes for constipation:*
  - Bulk forming, fiber based: psyllium, bran
  - Stool softeners: docusate
  - Lubricants: rectal glycerin
  - Prokinetics: prucalopride
  - Prosecretory: lubiprostone, linaclotide
  - Stimulants: bisacodyl, cascara, senna
  - Osmotics: polyethylene glycol, magnesium sulfate, magnesium citrate
  - Guanylate cyclase agonists: linaclotide

BUN, blood urea nitrogen; IgA, immunoglobulin A; OTC, over-the-counter; PCR, polymerase chain reaction; tTG, tissue transglutaminase.

KEY POINTS

- The GI tract is the route of ingestion of food and water needed to sustain life.
- The process of physically and chemically breaking down complex components of a mixed diet into small molecules suitable for absorption occurs over many centimeters of gut length and square meters of surface area.
- Specialized secretions and smooth muscle motility patterns characterize the segments of the GI tract—mouth, pharynx, esophagus, stomach, duodenum, jejunum, ileum, colon, rectum, and anus. However, there is an underlying similarity among most structures: They are hollow tubes with an inner lining (mucosa), surrounded by smooth muscle layers, and finally wrapped in an outer adventitia layer.
- Regulation and coordination of activity along the GI tract include neural, hormonal, and local influences.
- The enteric nervous system allows some functions to proceed autonomously, independent of control by the parasympathetic and sympathetic branches of the autonomic nervous system.
- Endocrine regulation links sensory signaling from distal segments to release of hormones that coordinate activity in proximal segments according to state of digestion and absorption of a meal.
- The gut is particularly rich in amine and peptide mediators, including serotonin, dopamine, and opioid peptides. Receptors for these mediators are the target of drug classes used to treat GI disorders.
- Gut immune signaling protects against invading pathogens ingested with contaminated food; however, it may predispose patients with certain genetic vulnerabilities to inflammatory and hypersensitivity-related disorders.
- Chronic GERD is a common disorder caused by a combination of LES weakness and gastric hyperacidity, among other factors.
- Stomach function is characterized by intense muscular grinding of ingested food, and the secretion of hydrochloric acid, intrinsic factor (required for vitamin B12 absorption), and pepsinogen, a protein-digesting enzyme precursor.
- Gastric acid can contribute to damage and ulcer formation of the stomach mucosa or, more commonly, the duodenal mucosa. Ulcer formation results from an imbalance of protective forces and damaging forces. The most significant factor in recurrent ulcer formation is infection by *Helicobacter pylori*.
- Pathological alterations in stomach motility include gastroparesis and vomiting.
- The small intestine is the primary site of food digestion and absorption. Absorption is facilitated by an extensive surface area facing the lumen, consisting of mucosal folds (villi), coated with epithelial cells that have additional plasma membrane finger-like projections (brush border).
- The pancreas secretes fluid rich in bicarbonate and digestive enzymes.
- Acute pancreatitis can result from gallstones, alcohol ingestion, and other causes. Although rare, pancreatitis can be very severe, necessitating hospitalization and critical care.
- Digestion reduces large, complex dietary components to small molecules that are then absorbed. Proteins are broken down to amino acids and small peptides, and carbohydrates are broken down to simple sugars.
- Fat digestion and absorption is the most complex process, with hydrolysis of triglycerides, phospholipids, and cholesterol esters to their component molecules, assisted by bile salts provided by the liver. Bile salts secreted by the liver and gallbladder are required for fat digestion and absorption.
- Body fluid balance depends on the absorption of liquid from the diet. In the course of each day's meals, many liters of fluid are secreted by the GI tract segments and are then reabsorbed. Small intestine water secretion involves the cAMP-regulated chloride channel CFTR.
- Diarrhea results from excess GI secretion, hypermotility, presence of undigested osmotically active particles, and malabsorption. Diarrhea with bleeding is also associated with certain GI infections and IBD.
- Celiac disease is an immune disorder characterized by sensitivity to dietary gluten—a protein found in wheat, barley, and rye. Omitting all gluten from the diet restores normal gut structure and function.
- IBD includes Crohn disease and ulcerative colitis. These are painful disorders that present with intermittent diarrhea, malabsorption, blood loss, and structural abnormalities. Family history of IBD is common, as well as comorbidity with other immune disorders.
- Abdominal pain is a common reason for seeking medical treatment, and specific syndromes have characteristic pain patterns that inform follow-up testing and management.

- IBS presents with recurring pain in combination with altered defecation patterns. The pathogenesis of IBS is not fully understood, but the disorder is functional, without structural markers.
- Total body metabolic homeostasis is intimately related to the ingestion, digestion, and absorption of food. Disrupted bowel function in the form of short bowel syndrome and intestinal failure often require parenteral nutrition support due to inability to have sufficient GI function to maintain healthy digestion and absorption.
- Malnutrition is a common concern globally and can encompass undernutrition manifested by underweight or overweight with nutritional deficiencies.
- Obesity has a number of associated health risks, including type 2 diabetes mellitus, metabolic syndrome, and nonalcoholic fatty liver disease. Obesity management strategies include lifestyle changes, weight-loss drugs, and bariatric surgery. Although rates of obesity are increasing worldwide, some regions appear to have reached a plateau.
- The GI tract, particularly the colon, is a common cancer site. Although most lower GI cancer (CRC) is sporadic, some gene mutations are known to be associated with familial risk. Lynch syndrome, associated with mutations in mismatch repair genes, increases the risk for CRC and other cancers associated with abdominal organs.
- The most common disorders of the GI tract in infants and children are infectious gastroenteritis and, in infants, gastroesophageal reflux.
- Pyloric stenosis results from hypertrophic growth of muscle layers of the pylorus. It prevents the ingested food from progressing to the duodenum, resulting in vomiting and dehydration. Bowel intussusception can create complete bowel obstruction that requires immediate treatment, including surgery. Hirschsprung disease results from failure of neural crest cells to migrate to their proper locations in the distal colon and rectum. Despite the differing causes, management of all three conditions may require surgical correction.
- Normal function of the GI tract is maintained throughout the lifetime in many people. Disorders affecting the teeth, oral muscles, and LES can increase the incidence of swallowing difficulties and GERD in older adults.

- Sedentary lifestyle and lack of dietary fiber can lead to chronic constipation, a common complaint in older adults. Medications taken by older adults for chronic health conditions can have GI side effects, including constipation with difficulty passing stool. Finally, diverticular disease becomes more common with age.

REFERENCES

1. Peery AF, Crockett SD, Barritt AS, et al. Burden of gastrointestinal, liver, and pancreatic diseases in the United States. *Gastroenterology*. 2015;149:1731–1741. doi:10.1053/j.gastro.2015.08.045.
2. Consumer Healthcare Products Association. OTC sales by category, 2015–2018. https://www.chpa.org/OTCsCategory.aspx. Accessed January 6, 2020.
3. Bohorquez DV, Liddle RA. Gastrointestinal hormones and neurotransmitters. In: Feldman M, Friedman LS, Brandt LJ, eds. *Sleisenger and Fordtran's Gastrointestinal and Liver Disease*. 10th ed. New York, NY: Saunders/Elsevier; 2016:36–54.
4. Allaire JM, Crowley SM, Law HT, et al. The intestinal epithelium: central coordinator of mucosal immunity. *Trends Immunol*. 2018;39:677–696. doi:10.1016/j.it.2018.04.002.
5. Helander HF, Fändriks L. Surface area of the digestive tract—revisited. *Scand J Gastroenterol*. 2014;49:681–689. doi:10.3109/00365521.2014.898326.
6. Tang JCF. Acute pancreatitis. In: Anand BS, ed. *Medscape*. https://emedicine.medscape.com/article/181364-print. July 25, 2019. Accessed.
7. Apte MV, Pirola RC, Wilson JS. Mechanisms of alcoholic pancreatitis. *J Gastroenterol Hepatol*. 2010;25:1816–1826. doi:10.1111/j.1440-1746.2010.06445.x.
8. Enck P, Aziz Q, Barbara G, et al. Irritable bowel syndrome. *Nat Rev Dis Primers*. 2016;2:16014. doi:10.1038/nrdp.2016.14.
9. Allan P, Lal S. Intestinal failure: a review. *F1000Res*. 2018;7:85. doi:10.12688/f1000research.12493.1.
10. World Health Organization. Malnutrition. https://www.who.int/en/news-room/fact-sheets/detail/malnutrition. Updated February 16, 2018. Accessed March 27, 2019.
11. Cedarholm T, Jensen GL, Correia MITD, et al. GLIM criteria for the diagnosis of malnutrition—a consensus report from the global clinical nutrition community. *Clin Nutr*. 2019;38:1–9. doi:10.1016/j.clnu.2018.08.002.
12. Angrisani L, Santonicola A, Iovino P, et al. IFSO worldwide survey 2016: primary, endoluminal, and revisional procedures. *Obes Surg*. 2018;28:3783–3794. doi:10.1007/s11695-018-3450-2.
13. Centers for Disease Control and Prevention. United States cancer statistics: data visualizations. Leading cancer cases and deaths, male and female, 2016. https://

gis.cdc.gov/Cancer/USCS/DataViz.html. Accessed January 7, 2020.

14. Liacouras CA. Normal development, structure, and function. In: Kliegman RM, Stanton BF, St Geme JW, Schor NF, eds. *Nelson Textbook of Pediatrics*. 20th ed. Philadelphia, PA: Elsevier; 2016:1796–1797.

15. Bäckhed F, Roswall J, Peng Y, et al. Dynamics and stabilization of the human gut microbiome during the first year of life. *Cell Host Microbe*. 2015;17:690–703. doi:10.1016/j.chom.2015.04.004.

16. Xu H, Ghishan FK. Molecular physiology of gastrointestinal function during development. In: Said HM, Ghishan FK, Kaunitz JD, et al., eds. *Physiology of the Gastrointestinal Tract*. 6th ed. Philadelphia, PA: Elsevier; 2018:236–272.

17. Levine AC. Pediatric gastroenteritis in emergency medicine. In: Bechtel KA, ed. *Medscape*. https://emedicine.medscape.com/article/801948-overview. Updated November 25, 2018. Accessed January 7, 2020.

18. Bhutta ZA. Acute gastroenteritis in children. In: Kliegman RM, Stanton BF, St Geme JW, Schor NF, eds. *Nelson Textbook of Pediatrics*.Vol 2. 20th ed. Philadelphia, PA: Elsevier; 2016:1854–1875.

19. Lightdale JR, Gremse DA. Gastroesophageal reflux: management guidance for the pediatrician. *Pediatrics*. 2013;131:e1684–e1695. doi:10.1542/peds.2013-0421.

20. El-Gohary Y, Abdelhafeez A, Paton E, et al. Pyloric stenosis: an enigma more than a century after the first successful treatment. *Pediatr Surg Int*. 2018;34:21–27. doi:10.1007/s00383-017-4196-y.

21. Pepper VK, Stanfill AB, Pearl RH. Diagnosis and management of pediatric appendicitis, intussusception, and Meckel diverticulum. *Surg Clin North Am*. 2012;92:505–526. doi:10.1016/j.suc.2012.03.011.

22. Hunter AK, Liacouras CA. Pyloric stenosis and other congenital anomalies of the stomach. In: Kliegman RM, Stanton BF, St Geme JW, Schor NF, eds. *Nelson Textbook of Pediatrics*.Vol 2. 20th ed. Philadelphia, PA: Elsevier; 2016:1797–1800.

23. Gfroerer S, Rolle U. Pediatric intestinal motility disorders. *World J Gastroenterol*. 2015;21:9683–9687. doi:10.3748/wjg.v21.i33.9683.

24. Phillips RJ, Powley TL. Innervation of the gastrointestinal tract: patterns of aging. *Auton Neurosci*. 2007;136:1–19. doi:10.1016/j.autneu.2007.04.005.

25. Salles N. Basic mechanisms of the aging gastrointestinal tract. *Dig Dis*. 2007;25:112–117. doi:10.1159/000099474.

26. Grassi M, Petraccia L, Mennuni G, et al. Changes, functional disorders, and diseases in the gastrointestinal tract of elderly. *Nutr Hosp*. 2011;26:659–668. doi:10.1590/S0212-16112011000400001.

27. Comparato G, Pilotto A, Franzè A, et al. Diverticular disease in the elderly. *Dig Dis*. 2007;25:151–159. doi:10.1159/000099480.

SUGGESTED RESOURCES

Barrett, KE. *Gastrointestinal Physiology*. 2nd ed. New York, NY: McGraw-Hill; 2014.

Feldstein R, Beyda DJ, Katz S. Aging and the gastrointestinal system. In: Fillit HM, Rockwood K, Young J, eds. *Brocklehurst's Textbook of Geriatric Medicine and Gerontology*. 8th ed. Philadelphia, PA: Elsevier; 2017:chap 21.

Gallegos-Orozco JF, Foxx-Orenstein AE, Sterler SM, Stoa JM. Chronic constipation in the elderly. *Am J Gerontol*. 2012;107:18–25. doi:10.1038/ajg.2011.349.

Johnson, LR. *Gastrointestinal Physiology*. 9th ed. Philadelphia, PA: Elsevier; 2019.

Margolis KG, Gershon MD. Enteric neuronal regulation of intestinal inflammation. *Trends Neurosci*. 2016;39:614–624. doi:10.1016/j.tins.2016.06.007.

Rémond D, Shahar DR, Gille D, et al. Understanding the gastrointestinal tract of the elderly to develop dietary solutions that prevent malnutrition. *Oncotarget*. 2015;6:13858–13898. doi:10.18632/oncotarget.4030.

Said HM, ed. *Physiology of the Gastrointestinal Tract*. 6th ed. San Diego, CA: Elsevier; 2018.

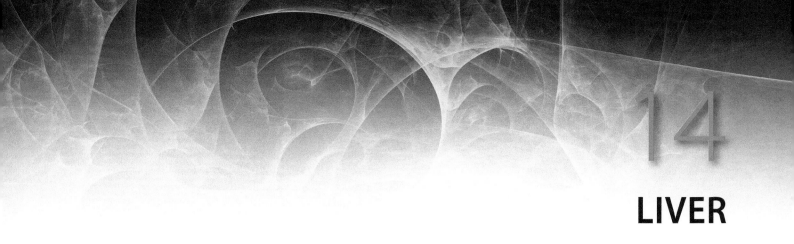

14

LIVER

Jennifer Andres, Adam Diamond, Kimberly A. Miller, Nicole E. Omecene, and Dusty Lisi

THE CLINICAL CONTEXT

The liver is a complex organ with many contributions to homeostasis that are often not appreciated until liver function declines. The liver has the capacity to rebound and regenerate after a variety of acute chemically or virally induced insults, but it is vulnerable to chronic chemical or infectious damage. Liver diseases span a spectrum of severity from acute self-limited episodes like some hepatitis A virus infections or mild drug-induced liver injury, to chronic insults that result in cirrhosis and require liver transplantation. The most common causes of chronic liver disease in the developed world are alcohol-induced liver disease, nonalcoholic fatty liver disease (NAFLD), and hepatitis C. These disorders may progress to hepatocellular carcinoma, or may be cured by abstinence from alcohol, weight loss, and antiviral therapy, respectively.

The rate of deaths due to liver disease increased from 11.3 to 17.8 per 100,000 population between 1950 and 1970, before falling to a low of 8.9 per 100,000 in 2005.[1] Since then, the death rate from chronic liver disease and cirrhosis has once again been rising in the United States; 1.9% of adults reported receiving a diagnosis of liver disease in the 2016 National Health Interview Survey.[2] Much of this increase is attributed to the obesity epidemic and the associated rise in nonalcoholic fatty liver disease (NAFLD) and nonalcoholic steatohepatitis (NASH). Primary care providers are ideally positioned to counsel patients about management of lifestyle factors (alcohol intake, obesity) to reduce liver disease prevalence and about screening for silent hepatitis C.

Management of liver disease is often supportive, as many chronic, progressive liver disorders can only be cured by liver transplantation. The development of effective treatments for hepatitis C virus (HCV) infection is one of the few exceptions to this challenging clinical scenario. Clinicians are best positioned to deliver patient teaching regarding HCV screening and appropriate follow-up.

OVERVIEW OF LIVER STRUCTURE AND FUNCTION

The liver is the largest solid internal organ in the body and is located in the right upper quadrant (RUQ) of the abdomen. The primary cell types of the liver are hepatocytes, sinusoidal endothelial cells, Kupffer cells, stellate cells, and cholangiocytes. The liver receives dual blood flow: 25% of the blood is fully oxygenated blood provided by the hepatic artery. The remaining 75% comes from the portal vein, which combines the relatively deoxygenated venous drainage of the intestines, pancreas, and spleen. This arrangement makes the liver literally the "portal," or gate, between the intestines and the systemic circulation. The liver is connected back to the intestines through the production and secretion of bile, which is delivered to the duodenum via the bile duct. Thus, the liver is uniquely positioned to

- Absorb the primary products of carbohydrate and protein digestion and absorption
- Use the abundant amino acid supply to synthesize a large number of proteins of different classes, including most plasma proteins
- Regulate glucose homeostasis under the influence of insulin or glucagon, enriched by the blood draining the pancreas

- Be the first line of immune defense against bacteria that enter the blood across the intestinal wall
- Detoxify or metabolize drugs and toxins ingested orally
- Synthesize and secrete bile acids needed for fat digestion and absorption
- Secrete detoxified endogenous and exogenous compounds into the bile for eventual fecal excretion

LIVER STRUCTURE

The liver has four lobes: right, left, caudate, and quadrate. Each lobe is made up of lobules, and lobules are made up of hepatocytes, sinusoids, and a central vein. The structures of a segment of a liver lobule and a representative sinusoid are depicted in **Figure 14.1**. The liver accounts for only 2.5% of the body's total weight but receives nearly a quarter of the cardiac output. This abundant

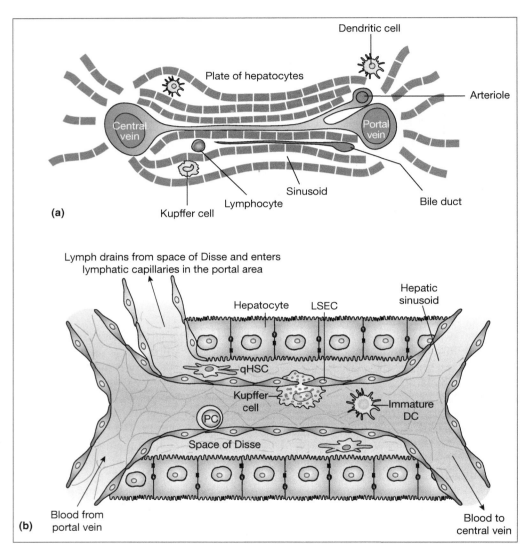

FIGURE 14.1 **(a)** Detail of the structure of the liver. The liver is made up of lobules in which blood flows from branches of the portal vein and arterioles from the hepatic artery, to the central vein, through large modified capillaries (sinusoids). **(b)** Sinusoid structure. Sinusoid walls are made up of specialized LSECs. Rather than a basement membrane, the sinusoid is separated from the surrounding plate of hepatocytes by a space of Disse, which is directly connected to lymph drainage. The immune and reticuloendothelial function of the liver is conducted by Kupffer cells, resident macrophages residing in the sinusoids, as well as lymphocytes called PCs and DCs. These cells provide constant immune surveillance for molecules and pathogens entering the body through the gut wall and traveling through the portal vein, capturing them before they can enter the systemic circulation. Stellate cells in the space of Disse are normally quiescent (qHSCs), but can become activated in response to liver damage and contribute to liver fibrosis.

DC, dendritic cell; LSEC, liver sinusoid endothelial cell; PC, pit cell.

blood supply is integral to the liver's complex metabolic functions. Liver blood flow is approximately 800 to 1,200 mL/min.[3]

The structure of a liver lobule is shown in **Figure 14.2**, including branches of the hepatic artery, portal vein, and bile duct. Blood from the hepatic artery and portal vein meets in the sinusoids. The sinusoids are surrounded by plates of hepatocytes, allowing robust exchange of compounds between blood and liver cells. The sinusoids coalesce to form the central vein of each hepatic lobule. Blood flows from the central veins to one of three hepatic veins and ultimately empties into the inferior vena cava. Blood flow to the liver is shown in **Figure 14.3**.

The biliary tree is crucial to liver function (see **Figures 14.4** and **14.5**). Each hepatocyte has apical membranes with direct secretory sites to microscopic bile canaliculi (**Figure 14.4**). Bile canaliculi coalesce into bile ductules and increasingly larger channels, finally coming together as the right and left hepatic ducts, which merge and become the common hepatic duct. The cystic duct connects the hepatic duct to the gallbladder, where bile is stored between meals. Bile then flows into the bile duct, which joins the pancreatic duct, and through the sphincter of Oddi into the duodenum (**Figure 14.5**). Bile and blood flow in opposite directions and in separate tracts between hepatocyte plates of the lobule.

Liver Cells

Hepatocytes are the functional cells of the liver and are the most abundant cell type. Hepatocytes perform metabolic, storage, and synthetic processes. They surround sinusoids that are specialized capillaries with high permeability. In order to protect the liver from

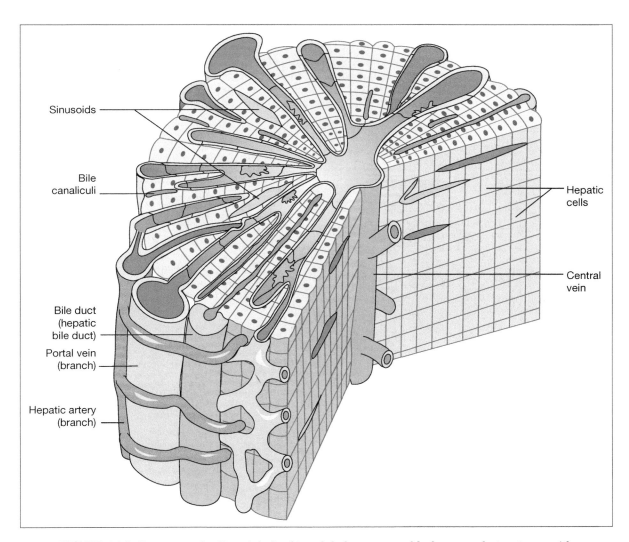

FIGURE 14.2 Structure of a liver lobule. Liver lobules are roughly hexagonal structures with corners demarcated by the "portal triad" made up of branches of the hepatic artery, portal vein, and bile duct. Blood flows in through the sinusoid to the central vein of the lobule, while bile flows out to the bile duct branch.

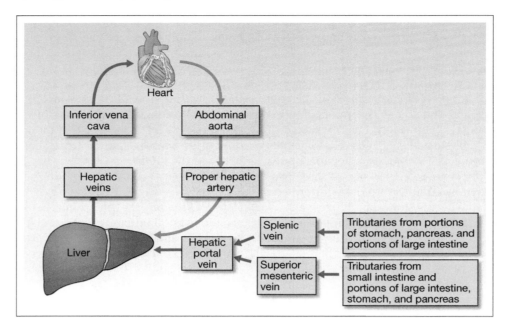

FIGURE 14.3 Hepatic blood flow. Two vascular streams supply the liver with blood. The hepatic artery branches from the abdominal aorta, providing fully oxygenated arterial blood to the liver. The portal vein combines the venous drainage from many of the abdominal organs, making up 75% to 80% of the liver blood flow with blood that is rich in nutrients after meals, but is oxygen poor.
Source: From Tortora GJ, Derrickson BH. *Principles of Anatomy & Physiology.* Hoboken, NJ: Wiley; 2011:862.

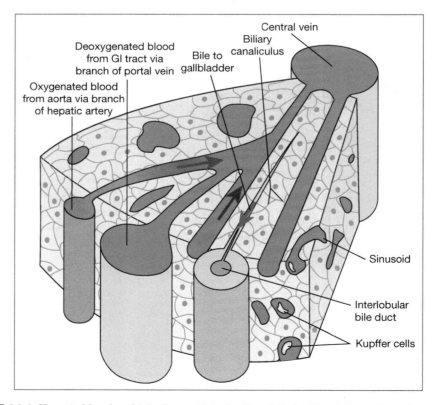

FIGURE 14.4 Hepatic blood and bile flow within the liver lobule. Blood flows from the periphery of the lobule toward the central vein, while bile flows in the opposite direction, to the periphery of the lobule.
GI, gastrointestinal.

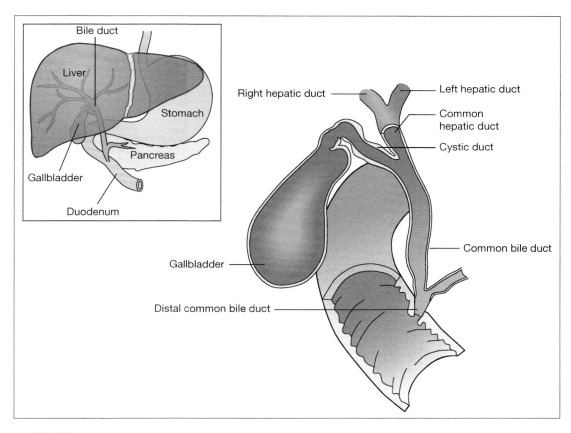

FIGURE 14.5 The biliary tree is formed as small bile canaliculi draining plates of hepatocytes coalesce to progressively larger channels. Ultimately, these vessels form the bile duct that drains bile from the liver and gallbladder into the duodenum.

potential foreign pathogens, sinusoids contain many Kupffer cells, tissue macrophages that destroy foreign pathogens. The space of Disse, between sinusoids and hepatocytes, contains hepatic stellate cells (see **Figure 14.1b**). Stellate cells store vitamin A, and are normally inactive, but become activated as a consequence of liver inflammation. When activated, they contribute to the fibrosis and cirrhosis associated with chronic liver disease.

Hepatocytes have a distinct polarity, with basolateral surfaces facing the space of Disse and sinusoid, and apical surfaces adjacent to bile canaliculi (**Figure 14.6**). The apical surfaces of adjoining cells are sealed with tight junctions that prevent the leakage of damaging bile away from the canaliculi. Hepatocytes have abundant smooth endoplasmic reticulum (SER) and rough endoplasmic reticulum (RER). SER contains many enzymes for drug detoxification and for cellular metabolism; RER is the site of synthesis of proteins that will be secreted. There are many mitochondria, as well as stores of glycogen, fat droplets, iron, and vitamin B12. Large fenestrations (pores) between sinusoidal endothelial cells allow free interchange of molecules between plasma and hepatocytes. This is critical for the ability of plasma proteins synthesized in hepatocytes to make their way to the circulation.

Thought Questions

1. How do the vascular input and output pathways of the liver differ from those of most other organs?

2. What are some of the functional consequences of these differences?

LIVER FUNCTION

Energy Metabolism

The liver is the main organ of energy metabolism of carbohydrates, lipids, and amino acids as shown in **Figure 14.7**. After meals, the portal vein blood is rich in absorbed nutrients from the gastrointestinal (GI)

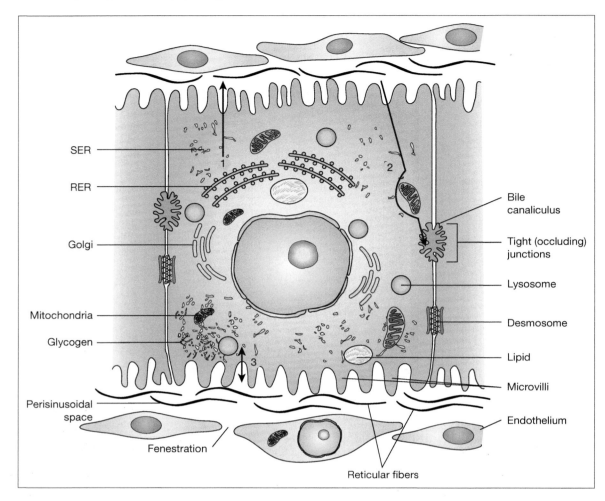

FIGURE 14.6 Hepatocyte structure and function. The microscopic hepatocyte structure gives clues to the varied processes carried out by these cells. There are abundant RER and Golgi apparatus for protein synthesis and secretion (**1**). Protein transfer is assisted by large gaps (fenestrations) between liver sinusoidal endothelial cells. Apical membranes of adjacent hepatocytes are sealed with tight junctions around the site of bile secretion into the canaliculus to prevent toxic bile components from damaging the hepatocytes or leaking into the blood (**2**). SER contains enzymes of drug metabolism and metabolic processes. Fuels are stored in the form of glycogen deposits and lipid droplets. The cells are polarized, with basolateral surfaces enriched by folds where they contact the space of Disse for interchange of proteins between blood and hepatocyte (**3**).

RER, rough endoplasmic reticulum; SER, smooth endoplasmic reticulum.

tract and pancreatic hormones, positioning the liver to conduct the reactions allowing energy storage for times of fasting. Although a more detailed description of the processes of energy metabolism appears elsewhere in this book, an overview is included here. Carbohydrate metabolism aimed at maintaining stable blood glucose is a key responsibility of the liver. The liver regulates blood glucose by controlling the uptake, production, and release of glucose. In periods of excess glucose (high blood sugar), it sequesters glucose as glycogen (glycogenesis). During fasting, glycogen is broken down (glycogenolysis), releasing glucose for use by the body. The liver also has the ability to synthesize glucose from amino acids and other precursors during periods of low blood glucose through the process termed *gluconeogenesis*.

The liver is the dominant organ of lipid metabolism. When it has stored sufficient glucose, excess glucose is converted to triglycerides, which are then packaged as very low-density lipoproteins (VLDLs) to travel through the bloodstream. The triglycerides are broken down by capillary lipase, and the free fatty acids (FFAs) are then re-formed into triglycerides and stored in adipose tissue. The liver can also use glucose to synthesize

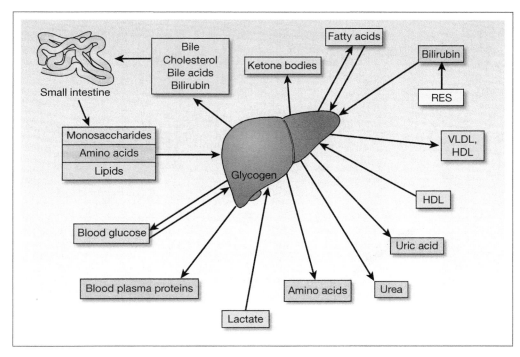

FIGURE 14.7 Principal metabolic liver functions.
HDL, high-density lipoprotein; RES, reticuloendothelial system; VLDL, very low-density lipoprotein.

cholesterol, which is essential for the production of plasma membrane components, bile, hormones, and certain vitamins. The liver takes up low-density lipoproteins (LDLs) and intermediate-density lipoproteins (IDLs) that are formed after tissues remove triglyceride from VLDLs. The liver also synthesizes high-density lipoproteins (HDLs) that are integral to cholesterol distribution and uptake throughout the body and return to the liver.

Synthetic Processes of the Liver

The liver synthesizes and breaks down amino acids in support of protein synthesis and in the process of gluconeogenesis, respectively. Hepatocyte processes of metabolic homeostasis, drug metabolism, and bile salt production require an extraordinary number of intracellular, membrane, and secreted proteins. Liver ranks third in the number of tissue-enriched messenger ribonucleic acids (mRNAs) and proteins, behind brain and testis.[4] Additionally, the liver synthesizes and secretes the majority of plasma proteins (**Table 14.1**).

Dietary fat absorption depends on the fat-solubilizing properties of bile, which is synthesized in the liver, secreted into the biliary tree, and stored in the gallbladder. Bile is composed of water, bile salts, phospholipids, conjugated bilirubin, and other compounds detoxified by the liver and destined for fecal excretion. Bile serves two main functions: fat digestion and toxin excretion. Bile salts are amphipathic molecules, containing both hydrophobic and hydrophilic parts,

synthesized from cholesterol. Bile salts are required for digestion of fats through emulsification and for absorption of fat digestion products and fat-soluble vitamins from the intestines. Bile is also a route of excretion for bilirubin, xenobiotics, and endogenous compounds that have been detoxified by liver enzymes. Bile is the major route of excretion for potentially detrimental lipophilic substances, and the major elimination route for cholesterol. Additionally, bile may protect against intestinal infections through the secretion of immunoglobulin A and stimulation of cytokine release. Approximately 500 to 600 mL of bile is produced per day.

The liver is responsible for detoxifying ammonia through the synthesis of urea, producing a compound that is readily cleared by the kidneys. Ammonia produced by gut bacteria reaches the liver through the portal vein. The liver also forms ammonia through amino acid metabolism. In the urea cycle, chemical reactions occur in the mitochondria and cytosol of the hepatocytes to convert ammonia to urea, which improves water solubility for ease of renal excretion. Ammonia is toxic to the brain and can impair brain function, leading to a change in mental status that can eventually result in seizures and coma. When the liver is unable to detoxify ammonia, as in chronic liver disease, the result is central nervous system dysfunction. Excess levels of ammonia are thought to contribute to hepatic encephalopathy. Consequently, management of hepatic encephalopathy typically aims to reduce ammonia levels. This is often achieved with the administration of

TABLE 14.1 Major Proteins Secreted by the Liver

Protein Category	Proteins	Function
Plasma proteins	Albumin	Maintains colloid osmotic pressure, carrier protein
Acute phase proteins	C-reactive protein	Enhances endogenous immune responses, marker of inflammation and illness
Coagulation cascade proteins	Prothrombin (factor II) and factors V, VII, VIII, IX, X, XI, XIII; fibrinogen; α_2-antiplasmin	Hemostasis, prevention of blood loss
Regulators/inhibitors of coagulation proteins	Protein C, protein S, antithrombin III, plasminogen	Prevent excessive clotting, clot lysis
Stimulator of platelet production	Thrombopoietin	Stimulates bone marrow to increase platelet synthesis and release
Complement cascade proteins	C1–C9	Host defense, innate immunity
Carrier proteins	Transferrin, transcobalamin, transcortin, thyroxine-binding globulin, sex hormone–binding globulin, others	Transport of lipid-soluble or toxic substances, extends half-life of steroid and thyroid hormones
Protective proteins, antioxidants, other roles	α_1-Antitrypsin, glutathione, angiotensinogen	Diverse roles in homeostasis

lactulose, a disaccharide that is retained in the gut. Lactulose reduces pH, increases stool production, and lowers the levels of gut nitrogenous compounds that increase circulating ammonia.

Thought Questions

3. What are the major synthetic reactions carried out by the liver?

4. How do these reactions contribute to homeostasis?

Liver Clearance Mechanisms

The liver has a wide range of protective and clearance functions. As mentioned, it is responsible for the metabolism of xenobiotics, including drugs and toxins. The passage of blood from intestines through the portal vein to the liver allows the liver to process and absorb ingested substances before they reach the systemic circulation by removing unwanted compounds.

Metabolism of Bilirubin

The liver is responsible for the conjugation of bilirubin and its excretion via bile ducts. As red blood cells are broken down in the spleen, the heme component of hemoglobin is released. Heme is metabolized into biliverdin, which is subsequently converted to bilirubin. Bilirubin, a nonpolar substance, is released into the bloodstream and binds with albumin. This form is called unconjugated or indirect bilirubin. When this compound reaches the liver, it is taken up and conjugated in hepatocytes. As with other drugs and substances discussed previously, the addition of glucuronide makes the bilirubin molecule polar, water soluble, and able to be excreted.

Conjugated bilirubin is also referred to as direct bilirubin and can freely travel through the bloodstream to the kidneys for excretion. Conjugated bilirubin can also be secreted into the bile and eventually excreted in feces. While the kidney can excrete excess levels of conjugated bilirubin, most is excreted through the feces after reduction to urobilinogen and stercobilin in the intestine. **Figure 14.8** summarizes the production, metabolism, and excretion of bilirubin. **Hyperbilirubinemia** produces the characteristic yellowing of the skin termed **jaundice**. Such elevations can be caused by excess production of bilirubin, decreased uptake by liver cells, decreased conjugation, decreased secretion into the canaliculi, and bile duct obstruction. Hemolytic anemia is a common cause of excess production of bilirubin. Laboratory measurements of conjugated and unconjugated bilirubin are used to determine the cause of jaundice and the site of liver impairment (**Table 14.2**).

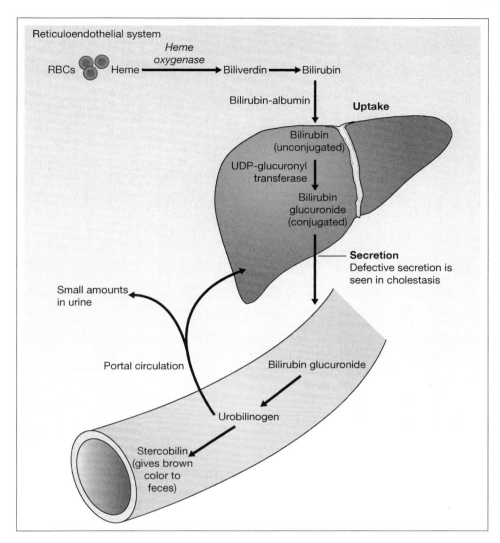

FIGURE 14.8 Bilirubin metabolism. Bilirubin is constantly generated from heme released upon breakdown of aging RBCs by the reticuloendothelial system. Unconjugated (indirect) bilirubin is initially hydrophobic and nonpolar, and travels in the circulation bound to albumin. Hepatocytes take up bilirubin and conjugate it to glucuronic acid. Conjugated (direct) bilirubin glucuronide is hydrophilic and is secreted into the bile. In the gut, bacteria further metabolize bilirubin to urobilinogen, a fraction of which is reabsorbed and ultimately excreted by the kidneys. Much of the remaining urobilinogen is converted to stercobilin and is excreted in the feces, adding the characteristic brown color.
RBCs, red blood cells; UDP, uridine 5'-diphospho-glucuronosyltransferase.

TABLE 14.2 Patterns of Bilirubin Elevation in Hepatic Injury			
Assay Component	Bile Duct Obstruction	Hemolytic Anemia	Liver Failure
Total bilirubin	↑	↑	↑
Direct bilirubin	↑	WNL	↑
Indirect bilirubin	WNL	↑	↑

↑ indicates that the level will be increased.
WNL, within normal limits.

Hormone and Drug (Xenobiotics) Metabolism

Endogenous hormones and xenobiotics (exogenous compounds foreign to the human body) are detoxified and excreted by the liver. The outcome of hepatic metabolism is to make a substance easier to excrete. In general, this occurs by making a product more water soluble. **Figure 14.9** shows the basics of drug metabolism and excretion. Metabolism occurs through microsomal oxidase enzymes, such as the highly active cytochrome P450 (CYP) system, or through enzymatic conjugation that makes the compound or its metabolite more hydrophilic for renal

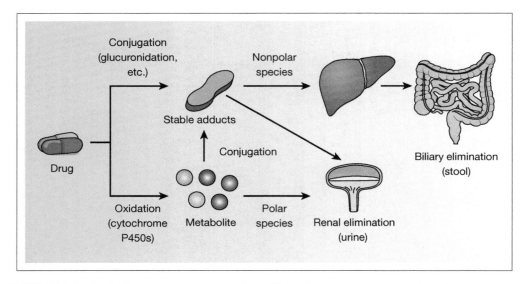

FIGURE 14.9 Metabolism of an exogenous drug. Phase 1 reactions are carried out by enzymes of the cytochrome P450 (CYP) class. These reactions add a hydroxyl or other chemically reactive, oxygen-containing group to the drug. Phase 2 reactions conjugate the drug or its phase 1 metabolite with a larger hydrophilic group, increasing water solubility and renal elimination. Compounds with nonpolar metabolites are usually eliminated by the biliary–fecal route.

excretion, or both. The SER in hepatocytes contains most of the enzymes responsible for drug and hormone metabolism.

Most substances are metabolized in two processes, referred to as phase 1 and phase 2 reactions. Some substances may be metabolized by only one of the phases. CYP enzymes conduct phase 1 metabolism, converting their substrates through oxidation, reduction, or hydrolysis reactions. Many exogenously administered drugs are lipid soluble, which facilitates absorption and distribution, but reduces excretion. In phase 1 metabolism, a polar functional group, most often a hydroxyl group, is added to the parent compound to make the product polar and hydrophilic and thus easier to excrete. There are several potential outcomes of phase 1 metabolism. In some cases, the intermediate metabolite can be toxic, such as with ethanol and acetaminophen, and can cause hepatic injury. In other cases, the administered compound is a prodrug, and phase 1 metabolism converts it to an active drug. Finally, some drug metabolites may be physiologically active, prolonging the time of drug effect on the body.

In the case of a toxic metabolite, phase 2 metabolism will often detoxify the metabolite and allow it to be excreted. If phase 2 metabolism is altered, these toxic intermediates can build up and cause hepatic damage. Phase 2 reactions, or conjugation reactions, result in the covalent attachment of a water-soluble group, such as glucuronic acid, to the drug compound in order to further increase the metabolite's water

solubility and renal excretion. If the metabolite is unable to be excreted by the kidneys, it can also be eliminated through bile.

There are 57 identified CYP enzymes in humans. Five of these enzymes are responsible for the majority of drug metabolism, with 3A4 metabolizing the largest number of drugs (**Table 14.3**).[5] Metabolism varies from person to person owing to a number of factors. Genetic polymorphisms cause differences in CYP enzyme functionality; enzyme induction or inhibition can be caused by other prescribed or over-the-counter drugs or supplements, and comorbidities can alter drug metabolism.

Genetic polymorphisms that alter drug metabolism are the focus of pharmacogenomic research. Polymorphisms in the genes coding for phase 1 enzymes may alter these proteins, causing a patient to

TABLE 14.3 Common Cytochrome P (CYP) Enzymes Contributing to Drug Metabolism

CYP Enzyme	Drug Metabolized (%)
1A2	5
2C9	15
2C19	7–9
2D6	20–30
3A4	40

be a poor metabolizer or a rapid metabolizer, and leading to changes in drug effective concentrations or half-life of elimination. Induction increases the amount of a CYP enzyme, thus increasing the metabolism of its substrate drugs, and resulting in lower drug levels and reduced effectiveness. Inhibition decreases the activity of a CYP enzyme, thus decreasing the metabolism of the substance, resulting in higher drug levels and increasing risk of toxicity. Enzyme induction and inhibition are common sources of drug interactions. Phase 2 metabolism can also be affected by genetic polymorphisms. The phase 2 enzyme *N*-acetyltransferase catalyzes the addition of an acetyl group to a drug or its phase 1 metabolites. Some patients have a genetic polymorphism that reduces *N*-acetyltransferase activity, with a phenotype described as "slow acetylator." They are at increased risk of toxic effects from drugs requiring acetylation for elimination. Genetic tests are available to assess phase 1 and phase 2 enzyme polymorphisms; however, such tests are not widely used in clinical practice. Drug metabolism is altered in patients with liver or kidney disease, or both; in these patients, dosages must be adjusted to reduce adverse drug events.

Liver metabolism may diminish the blood levels of drugs administered orally, through the first-pass effect. Once a drug is absorbed from the GI tract, the portal vein delivers the drug to the liver. The liver can metabolize some of the drugs before it exits through the hepatic vein to systemic circulation, as shown in **Figure 14.10**. This first-pass effect can reduce the amount of active drug available to the body for pharmacologic action as well as delaying the onset of drug effect. This drug has lower bioavailability than a drug that does not undergo this initial metabolism. Drugs administered through the intravenous route do not undergo absorption through the GI tract, and thus will not undergo first-pass effect, leading to higher levels of the active drug, and high bioavailability. Drug absorption through the GI tract and hepatic metabolism takes time, so drugs administered intravenously reach effective blood levels almost immediately, far more quickly than drugs administered orally. Other routes can also bypass the first-pass effect. For example, orally administered nitroglycerin has a high rate of hepatic metabolism that substantially reduces bioavailable drug. Sublingual administration provides rapid absorption and avoids the first-pass effect.

Thought Question

5. How is the way the liver processes bilirubin similar to the way it processes drugs, and how do these processes differ?

Other Functions of the Liver

Reticuloendothelial System

As part of the reticuloendothelial system, the liver contains the largest number of fixed tissue macrophages, also known as Kupffer cells, making it an important component of the immune system. Kupffer cells are responsible for the clearance of gut bacteria and foreign proteins. If the liver is damaged, then the immune system may be unable to defend against foreign proteins and bacteria. This is evident with the high rate of infection in patients with acute liver failure.

Vitamin and Mineral Storage

The liver can store iron in the form of ferritin and can store several vitamins, including A, E, and B12. The liver is responsible for maintaining systemic iron homeostasis by producing the iron transport protein transferrin, storing excess iron as ferritin, and mobilizing iron from hepatocytes to the circulation in times of need. The liver also synthesizes hepcidin, a plasma protein that blocks cellular transport of stored iron back to the circulation, thus decreasing circulating iron levels. Hereditary hemochromatosis, discussed later in this chapter, is a disorder of abnormal hepcidin.

Regenerative Capacity

The liver has the ability to regenerate after an acute injury. In instances of hepatocyte necrosis from acute

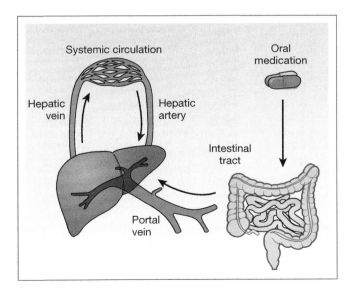

FIGURE 14.10 First-pass effect. Oral medications absorbed in the gastrointestinal tract circulate via the portal vein to the liver prior to entering the systemic circulation. Liver metabolism may either activate a prodrug or inactivate a portion of administered drug, reducing the amount of active drug that reaches the circulation.

pathological processes, the hepatocytes can regenerate. Unfortunately, once a patient has severe liver disease, or cirrhosis, the liver loses this ability. If a person has a partial hepatectomy, as in the case of living liver donors, after removal of a portion of the liver, that donor liver will then regrow in another region and restore normal levels of liver tissue and function.

LIVER DISORDERS

Concerns in patients with liver disorders include abnormalities in blood glucose, lipid, and protein levels; the inability to detoxify and excrete drugs and endogenous toxins such as ammonia and bilirubin; and abnormal clotting. In severe and chronic disorders, blood flow through the sinusoids is restricted, leading to portal hypertension. The development of portal hypertension produces manifestations of decompensated liver disease, including ascites, esophageal varices, and increased risk of infection.

MEASURES OF LIVER FUNCTION AND DYSFUNCTION

Laboratory evaluation can be performed to determine the function and health of the liver. Evaluation techniques encompass methods that assess damage to hepatocytes or indicate loss of liver homeostatic functions. Often the levels of enzymes, results of other tests, and clinical findings are pathognomonic for type of liver disease.

As hepatocytes are damaged, enzymes of liver function are released into the systemic circulation, allowing for quantification in the serum. Elevation of these enzymes is a marker for hepatocyte damage or death, and not necessarily liver function. Examples of these enzymes are aspartate aminotransferase (AST), alanine aminotransferase (ALT), gamma-glutamyl transferase (GGT), and alkaline phosphatase (ALP). Of these tests, ALT is the most specific marker for liver damage because it is found mainly in hepatocytes. AST is found in multiple organs and tissues, including the liver, cardiac and skeletal muscle, and kidney. AST is released from cellular and tissue damage in amounts proportional to the amount of injury that has occurred. GGT is sensitive to hepatocellular damage caused by alcohol ingestion, but is nonspecific. ALP comprises many different isoenzymes produced by the bile canalicular membrane of hepatocytes, but it is also found in bone. Levels of ALP serve as a marker for cholestasis and bone turnover. In chronic end-stage liver disease, fewer hepatocytes are dying and enzymes may return toward normal levels.

In order to assess protein synthesis and detoxification functions, levels of albumin and bilirubin are measured in the serum. As hepatocytes are damaged, the liver's protein-synthesizing capacity is reduced, lowering blood levels of albumin and clotting factors. As hepatic damage worsens, prothrombin time and international normalized ratio (INR) increase. As previously discussed, bilirubin can be measured as direct bilirubin, indirect bilirubin, and total bilirubin. Differential diagnosis is aided by patterns of bilirubin elevation. Increases in indirect bilirubin are usually related to hemolytic anemia. Increases in direct bilirubin are a result of the inability of hepatocytes to eliminate bilirubin or of blockage of the bile ducts. Total bilirubin is the sum of indirect and direct bilirubin.

Ultrasonography, MRI, CT, and elastography are noninvasive ways to assess the level of **liver fibrosis**. Liver biopsy is the gold-standard diagnostic tool to evaluate tissue injury and fibrosis; however, this is an invasive procedure. Biopsy may be required for diagnosis in a person who has hepatomegaly but has discordant clinical findings.[6]

ACUTE LIVER DISORDERS

Many cases of acute liver disease are mild and self-resolve. Symptoms of acute liver disease are typically nonspecific and may include fatigue, malaise, nausea, and loss of appetite. Patients may experience RUQ pain and weight loss. Symptoms such as jaundice may prompt a patient to seek medical attention. Supportive care techniques are usually employed for symptomatic management. Acute liver failure, in contrast, has more severe symptoms and can be defined as the abrupt start of symptoms such as jaundice, coagulopathy, and encephalopathy in a patient who was previously healthy. Acute liver failure due to viral hepatitis is more common in developing countries. In developed countries, **drug-induced liver injury** (DILI) is the most common cause of acute liver failure.[7]

Acute Liver Toxicity and Failure

DILI causes up to 50% of cases of **acute liver failure** in the United States. Additionally, DILI is responsible for most withdrawals of medication from the U.S. market.[7] Thus, when a patient presents with acute liver failure, the patient's drug history should immediately be reviewed.

In order to accurately diagnose DILI, exposure to toxins or drugs must be confirmed. Drugs can cause hepatic damage by direct toxicity or by an idiosyncratic reaction. Direct toxicity caused by drugs is predictable and usually has a dose-dependent response. The larger the dose of the agent, the more likely and more severe the liver damage. Direct toxicity can occur from the parent drug or from a toxic metabolite. With idiosyncratic reactions, the reaction is rare, unpredictable, and dose independent, making diagnosis and prevention more challenging. More than 1,000 drugs can cause DILI, potentially leading to acute liver failure. **Box 14.1** lists some drugs known to cause acute liver toxicity.

> **BOX 14.1**
> **Some Drugs Known to Cause Liver Toxicity**
>
> - Acetaminophen
> - HMG-CoA (β-hydroxy β-methylglutaryl coenzyme A) inhibitors
> - Isoniazid
>
> - Oral contraceptives and anabolic steroids
> - Phenytoin
> - Some herbal supplements
> - Valproic acid

Continuous exposure to some medications may also lead to cumulative hepatic injury. Special concerns related to DILI in older adults are discussed later in this chapter, under Gerontological Considerations.

Acetaminophen is a classic example of a drug with a metabolite that can directly injure the liver. Acetaminophen is found in over-the-counter and prescription products around the world, as a single medication or in combination with other medications. Excessive ingestion of acetaminophen can cause acute self-limiting hepatitis or fulminant liver failure requiring transplantation. Likely because of its availability, acetaminophen is responsible for most cases of acute liver failure in the Western world. Acetaminophen can cause damage by a single toxic ingestion (i.e., an overdose, unintentional or intentional) or by chronic ingestion over a period of days.

Acetaminophen is metabolized primarily through phase 2 reactions (over 80%); however, approximately 20% of acetaminophen is metabolized in a phase 1 reaction by CYP2E1. The product of this phase 1 metabolism is a toxic metabolite, N-acetyl-p-benzoquinone-imine (NAPQI). NAPQI is detoxified by binding to glutathione to become a water-soluble nontoxic metabolite, which can be excreted renally. However, excessive amounts of NAPQI can be formed from ingestion of high levels of acetaminophen, or from acetaminophen administration concomitant with chronic alcohol use that induces CYP2E1. Normal glutathione concentrations are inadequate to detoxify these elevated levels of NAPQI, leading to liver damage. Similarly, if glutathione levels are low, as in malnutrition or in the presence of preexisting severe liver disease, NAPQI will not be detoxified, and liver damage will ensue.

Acetaminophen toxicity follows four stages, as outlined in **Box 14.2**. Identification of acetaminophen overdose is crucial, so the antidote, N-acetylcysteine (NAC) can be administered. NAC increases glutathione levels, allowing NAPQI to be converted to a nontoxic substance that can be eliminated by the body. Severe insults that do not respond to NAC treatment may necessitate acute liver transplantation.[9]

Acute Cholestasis

Cholestasis is a state of interruption of bile secretion caused by intrinsic liver dysfunction or processes outside the liver. Bile is normally secreted from the hepatocytes into bile canaliculi that coalesce into the hepatic duct (within the liver) and finally form the bile duct. Bile enters the gallbladder, where it is stored and concentrated through water absorption. Bile leaving the gallbladder or the liver travels through the bile duct to empty into the duodenum. The bile duct can be blocked by gallstones, neoplasms, or pancreatic inflammation, resulting in cessation of bile flow. Certain medications disrupt bile secretion at the hepatocyte/canalicular interface, stopping bile flow. Finally, spontaneous cholestasis is an occasional complication of pregnancy. The diagnosis of cholestasis is made based on physical and laboratory findings indicating buildup of bilirubin (usually conjugated) and bile salts in the systemic circulation. These findings are accompanied by laboratory measurements indicating increased levels of ALP and of the enzymes 5′-nucleotidase and GGT. Excess bilirubin leads to the hallmark signs of jaundice, dark urine, and light-colored stools. Pruritus is a common manifestation of cholestasis, which may be due to increased bile salt levels in the circulation and in tissues. Drug-induced cholestasis should be considered in a patient presenting with the listed signs and symptoms, as a wide array of agents can cause cholestasis. Antibiotics are the most common cause of drug-induced cholestasis.[10]

Viral Hepatitis

Hepatitis is a general term for the state of liver inflammation that can be acute or chronic. **Acute hepatitis** is defined as inflammation of the liver lasting less than 6 months. **Chronic hepatitis** is defined as inflammation of the liver lasting more than 6 months. Hepatitis can result from liver-damaging processes such as DILI, fatty liver disease, and autoimmunity. Infectious hepatitis is acquired through a viral infection. Hepatitis viruses are not always directly hepatotoxic; however, the liver's inflammatory response to infection leads to hepatocyte dysfunction and death. Chronic hepatitis from a variety

BOX 14.2
Stages of Acetaminophen Toxicity

STAGE 1 TOXICITY

- Nonspecific symptoms, including nausea, vomiting, malaise, lethargy, and diaphoresis, occurring within the first 24 hours of ingestion.

- AST and ALT values are usually normal.

- Patients with severe overdose may have AST and ALT elevations within 8 hours.

STAGE 2 TOXICITY

- Nonspecific symptoms begin to resolve within 24 to 72 hours.

- Elevations of AST and ALT begin.

- Patients with severe overdose can present with right upper quadrant pain, hepatomegaly, jaundice, and coagulopathy.

STAGE 3 TOXICITY

- Nonspecific symptoms return with jaundice, encephalopathy, coagulopathy, and lactic acidosis within 72 to 96 hours after the initial insult.

- AST and ALT are markedly elevated.

- Maximal liver injury is evident in this stage. This stage has the highest risk of death due to multiorgan failure.

STAGE 4 TOXICITY

- Recovery follows stage 3 and usually lasts between 1 and 2 weeks.

- Duration can be prolonged depending on the severity of the ingestion as well as the preparation of acetaminophen ingested.

ALT, alanine aminotransferase; AST, aspartate aminotransferase.

---

of sources (chronic viral infection, alcoholic liver disease, nonalcoholic liver disease) increases the risk of **hepatocellular carcinoma**.

Viral hepatitis is differentiated into several forms, lettered A through E. Of the hepatitis viruses, those causing hepatitis A, B, and C are most commonly encountered. **Table 14.4** provides a description of these viruses. Hepatitis A does not cause chronic infection or long-term hepatic damage. Hepatitis B can be an acute liver disease or chronic disease, depending on the response of the patient's immune system and the age of the infected patient. Hepatitis C is most likely to become a chronic disease leading to cirrhosis and hepatocellular carcinoma. Hepatitis D requires concomitant infection with hepatitis B. Hepatitis E is transmitted via the fecal–oral route and is mainly seen outside the United States. All hepatitis viruses can be assessed using serologic testing for viral antigens and antibodies to viral antigens. Serologic testing can help determine whether disease is acute or chronic, and the time elapsed since exposure.

TABLE 14.4 Commonly Seen Hepatitis Viruses

Features	Hepatitis A Virus (HAV)	Hepatitis B Virus (HBV)	Hepatitis C Virus (HCV)
Transmission route	Fecal–oral	Blood-borne	Blood-borne
Type of virus	RNA virus (Picornaviridae)	DNA virus (Hepadnaviridae)	RNA virus (Flaviviridae)
Time course of infection	Acute	Acute and chronic	Acute and chronic
Serologic detection	HAV antibody	HBs antibody HBV DNA	HCV antibody HCV RNA

HBs, hepatitis B surface.

Hepatitis A

Hepatitis A virus (HAV) infection is a common self-limiting disease in the developing world, where most children have been infected with HAV by the age of 10 years.[11] The infection can be prevented through vaccination with the hepatitis A vaccine. HAV infections are less common in the United States, although sporadic outbreaks occur that can sicken hundreds of people in a given region. The virus is spread via the fecal–oral route; infection requires direct contact with an HAV-infected person or consumption of contaminated food or water. The virus replicates preferentially within hepatocytes and GI epithelial cells and is then released into the bile, where it is excreted into the feces. Exposure to HAV is likely in regions with poor sanitation where water may be contaminated. Consequently, travel to developing countries without vaccination is a major risk factor for acquisition of HAV infection.

Once a patient has been exposed to HAV, incubation can last up to 4 weeks. This is referred to as the preicteric or prodromal phase. During the incubation period, a large amount of HAV is shed into the feces and if tested, HAV RNA will be detected. Clinical, nonspecific symptoms do not begin until after peak viral shedding. Acute hepatitis follows, lasting approximately 1 week. Nonspecific symptoms, such as fatigue, weakness, anorexia, nausea, vomiting, abdominal pain, and, less commonly, fever, can occur with headache, arthralgias, myalgias, rash, or diarrhea following. ALT levels increase, usually peaking at this time, 4 weeks after infection. In the icteric phase, patients may develop jaundice and dark urine from elevated levels of conjugated bilirubin. Jaundice and other symptoms are more common in adults than in children. Children can increase the spread of the virus as they are often asymptomatic and anicteric (lack jaundice) during infection. Even in adults, peak infectivity can occur before the presence of jaundice. Immunoglobulin M (IgM) anti-HAV is detectable 5 to 10 days before symptomatic HAV infections in the majority of patients. Blood levels of immunoglobulin G (IgG) anti-HAV increase following the early IgM peak, indicating host immunity following the acute phase of the infection. Once infected with HAV or immunized, patients are immune to repeat infection.

Hepatitis B

An estimated 257 million people worldwide have chronic **hepatitis B** virus (HBV) infection.[12] The largest numbers of infected individuals are in Africa and Asia, where the infection is acquired at a young age. When the infection is acquired perinatally or as an infant, chronic infection is likely (90%) due to immaturity of the immune response. If acquired later in life, hepatitis B is less likely to become a chronic infection, with only up to 10% of acute cases converting to chronic. In the United States, the incidence of chronic HBV infection is relatively low (0.4%), which is likely due to routine vaccination and increased screening. Similar to HAV infection, a significant decline has been observed in HBV infections owing to routine administration of HBV vaccine to children beginning in 1991. Once an HBV infection becomes chronic, total viral eradication is rare. HBV may remain latent within the nucleus of the hepatocyte for many years, only to reappear with high levels of HBV DNA and hepatic damage. Chronic HBV infection can cause fibrosis, cirrhosis, and hepatocellular carcinoma.

HBV is the only DNA-containing hepatitis virus. The DNA is in the form of a small circular molecule that is only partly double stranded. Replication is similar to that of the retroviruses, with formation of a covalently bonded, closed, circular DNA (cccDNA) that is highly stable and can persist for prolonged periods of time. Hepatitis B virions have three protein antigens that form the basis for serologic testing: a surface antigen (HBsAg), a core antigen (HBcAg), and an additional antigen, HBeAg (**Figure 14.11**). The HBs and HBe antigens themselves, as well as host antibodies against all three antigens, are used for serologic evaluation to determine the chronicity of the infection or the immune status of the subject (**Table 14.5**).

HBsAg is the first hepatitis B protein marker detected after infection and is detectable at the start of clinical symptoms. If HBsAg is present for longer than 6 months, the patient is diagnosed as having chronic HBV infection. If a person is able to mount an appropriate immune response to HBV, he or she will develop an antibody to the HBsAg, denoted as anti-HBs. The development of this antibody indicates immunity to HBV and clearance of the virus. A component of HBsAg is used in HBV vaccination, so if a person has adequately responded to vaccination, then he or she will have detectable anti-HBs titers. The HBc antigen is contained within the viral envelope and is not generally detected in serum. However, anti-HBc can be detected prior to the appearance of anti-HBs. As with anti-HBs, levels of anti-HBc IgM predominate in early weeks to months after infection, after which anti-HBc IgG predominates. A secretory protein, HBeAg, can be detected soon after infection, and is a marker of more severe acute infection. Persistence or reappearance of HBeAg indicates chronic and active infection. Anti-HBe persists for the duration of chronic HBV infection.

HBV infection can be prevented through vaccination. In patients who develop chronic infection, treatment with antiviral agents is recommended if patients have active HBV, evidenced by an elevated viral load, signs of histological liver disease, or ALT more than two times the upper limit of normal.[13] Once a patient develops chronic infection, it is likely that treatment will be lifelong as seroconversion does not typically occur.

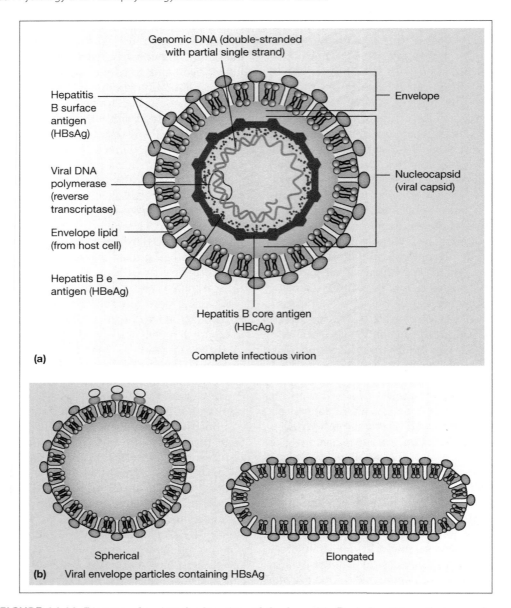

FIGURE 14.11 Diagram showing the location of the hepatitis B viral antigens that provoke an immune response and are the basis of serologic testing.

TABLE 14.5 Serologic Markers Used in Diagnosis of Hepatitis B Virus Infection

HBsAg	Anti-HBsAg	HBcAg	Anti-HBcAg	HBeAg	Anti-HBeAg	Interpretation
+	−	+	−	+/−	+	Acute HBV infection
+	−	+	+	+/−	+	Chronic HBV infection
−	+	−	−	−	−	Immune due to HBV vaccination
−	+	−	+	−	+	Immune due to prior HBV infection

+ denotes presence of serologic marker; − denotes absence of serologic marker; cAg, core antigen; eAg, e antigen; sAg, surface antigen; HBV, hepatitis B virus.

Hepatitis C

Hepatitis C virus (HCV) infection is the primary cause of liver transplantation in the United States. Approximately 3.5 million Americans have HCV infection, with a large number of these cases undiagnosed. A one-time screening test is recommended for individuals born between 1945 and 1965 (baby boomers), who have the highest rates of undiagnosed infections. Screening is also recommended in patients with risk factors for HCV exposure, for example, intravenous drug users, patients who received blood transfusions prior to 1992, and men who have sex with men, among others.[14] Because of its prevalence among older adults, HCV infection is introduced here in detail and then revisited later in this chapter (see Gerontological Considerations).

Most patients with acute HCV infection are asymptomatic and undiagnosed. If symptoms occur, they are mostly self-limiting and nonspecific. Chronic infection can lead to cirrhosis and hepatocellular carcinoma. Patients may be asymptomatic for many years before developing symptoms related to liver disease. Liver biopsy results can generate ratings, such as the Histologic Activity Index (HAI) and the Metavir score, that stage the progression of fibrosis in patients with HCV infection and other patients with chronic hepatitis.

Exposure and acute infection results in chronic infection in 80% of patients. Chronic HCV infection is defined as the presence of HCV RNA for more than 6 months. Approximately 20% of people with hepatitis C will develop cirrhosis after 20 years.[15] The risk of developing cirrhosis increases as long as the infection is present. Progression to cirrhosis is also associated with additional risk of end-stage liver disease and hepatocellular carcinoma. Successful treatment of HCV infection is now possible through one of several recently developed drug regimens, and eradication of the virus minimizes the risk of cirrhosis and long-term complications.

Thought Questions

6. What blood tests are appropriate to order in a patient with suspected acute liver injury?

7. Explain the rationale for ordering these tests, and patterns of results that you might see in a patient with acute HAV infection.

CHRONIC LIVER DISORDERS

Chronic liver disease is defined as liver disease lasting longer than 6 months. Most chronic liver disease processes include inflammation, which is promoted by the high number of Kupffer cells. Chronic inflammation leads to hepatocyte death, release of proinflammatory cytokines, and activation of hepatic stellate cells, resulting in **fibrosis** (**Figure 14.12**). Activated stellate cells secrete extracellular matrix components, including collagen, creating scar tissue in the space of Disse. As this process continues, hepatic endothelial cells lose their normal structure and function. As a result, hepatic sinusoids are transformed into narrower capillaries with low permeability and high resistance. Intrahepatic shunts can be formed due to angiogenesis and loss of parenchymal cells. Often described as scarring of the liver, **cirrhosis** is characterized by dysfunction or degeneration of hepatic cells, inflammation, and fibrous thickening of tissue in the liver. Once it develops, cirrhosis is progressive and irreversible, starting from a compensated stage and progressing to terminal decompensation.[16]

Complications of cirrhosis affect many organs and include hepatic encephalopathy, hepatorenal

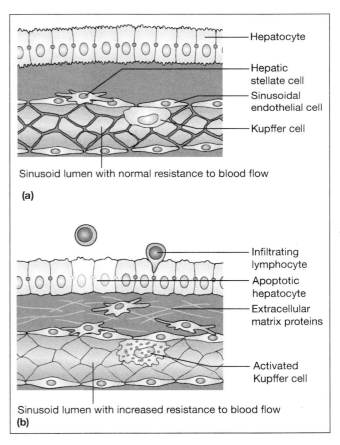

FIGURE 14.12 Comparison of tissue structure within (**a**) the normal liver and (**b**) the liver with advanced fibrosis. Ongoing inflammation promoted by activated Kupffer cells and lymphocytes stimulates stellate cells, which increase production of extracellular matrix, particularly collagen. Thickening and hardening around the sinusoids restrict their diameter, increasing vascular resistance and contributing to portal hypertension. Sinusoidal endothelial cells lose their large fenestrations, decreasing capillary permeability.

syndrome, portal hypertension, jaundice, hyperammonemia, coagulopathy, splenomegaly, hypoglycemia, and infections such as bacterial peritonitis in ascites fluid. The most common causes of cirrhosis include chronic viral hepatitis (discussed earlier), alcoholic liver disease (ALD), and nonalcoholic fatty liver disease (NAFLD).[15]

Portal hypertension results from the increased hepatic resistance to portal blood flow that commonly accompanies cirrhosis. Hepatic resistance increases because of narrowing of the normally large-diameter sinusoids. Upstream from the portal vein, splanchnic vessels become engorged and dilated, giving rise to collateral vessels that bypass the liver to return to the systemic circulation—a mechanism termed **porto-systemic shunting**. The mechanisms of portal hypertension and porto-systemic shunting are presented in **Box 14.3** and **Figure 14.13**. Its consequences include:

- Blood pooling in the spleen, leading to breakdown of platelets and leukocytes, with subsequent thrombocytopenia and leukopenia.

BOX 14.3
Portal Hypertension and Porto-Systemic Shunting

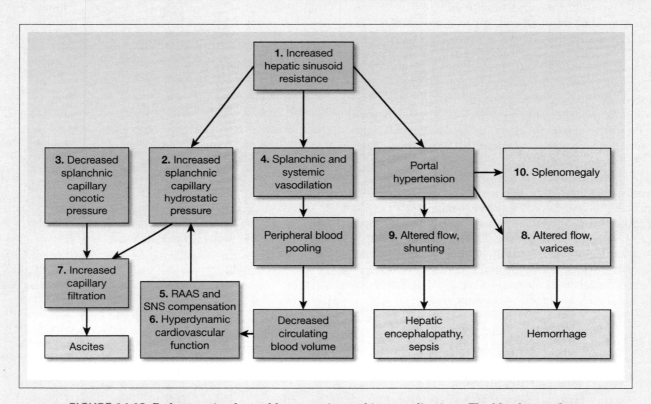

FIGURE 14.13 Pathogenesis of portal hypertension and its complications. The blue boxes show the sequential changes occurring because of increased hepatic sinusoid resistance. The pink boxes show the final consequences of these changes.
RAAS, renin-angiotensin-aldosterone system; SNS, sympathetic nervous system.

Multiple factors and pathways lead to pathophysiological consequences of increased hepatic sinusoid resistance owing to fibrosis and cirrhosis.

1. Activated hepatic stellate cells promote fibrosis around sinusoids, increasing resistance in this region.

2. Splanchnic capillaries draining to the portal vein develop increased hydrostatic pressure.

3. Capillary oncotic pressure decreases because of decreased liver synthesis of plasma proteins, particularly albumin.

(continued)

BOX 14.3 (*continued*)

Portal Hypertension and Porto-Systemic Shunting

4. Splanchnic and other vessels vasodilate because of increased sinusoid resistance and concentration of vasodilating mediators.

5. Decreased circulating blood volume promotes fluid retention and compensation by the renin-angiotensin-aldosterone system (RAAS) and sympathetic nervous system (SNS).

6. RAAS and SNS promote hyperdynamic cardiovascular function.

7. Splanchnic capillary–altered Starling forces promote filtration and ascites formation.

8. Portal hypertension promotes alternate paths of blood flow from the splanchnic circulation to the vena cava, creating varices in the esophagus and other vessels.

9. Blood traveling through shunts and bypassing the liver escapes the liver protective and clearance functions; bacteria and toxins enter the circulation, contributing to encephalopathy and sepsis.

10. Splenic engorgement with blood increases breakdown of leukocytes and platelets, producing leukopenia and thrombocytopenia.

- Diversion of substances absorbed from the GI tract around the liver. This can produce infections and sepsis due to absorption of gut bacteria, and alterations in blood metabolite levels. Glucose, in particular, may reach higher postprandial levels due to lack of liver clearance and fall to lower fasting levels due to lack of liver glycogen storage.
- Increased pressure in liver and splanchnic capillaries promotes excessive capillary filtration and ascites formation, particularly in the context of decreased albumin secretion and plasma colloid osmotic pressure.
- Some of the collaterals form gastroesophageal varices at the junction of the esophagus with the stomach and are prone to dangerous bleeding.

Hepatic encephalopathy, with clinical features ranging from behavioral abnormalities to somnolence and coma, is a late manifestation of chronic liver disease. It is thought to result from a combination of ammonia elevations with altered hepatic clearance of neurotransmitters and their metabolites. Management is directed to reducing gut ammonia production, by administration of lactulose or antibiotics targeting gut bacteria.

Hepatorenal syndrome is the end-stage manifestation of renal dysfunction secondary to liver disease. Portal hypertension results in dilation of splanchnic blood vessels, in part due to elevated nitric oxide. Pooling of splanchnic blood and excessive filtration into the peritoneal space results in decreased effective arterial blood volume and systemic hypotension. Compensatory mechanisms for this apparent lack of blood volume and pressure include the sympathetic nervous system, renin-angiotensin-aldosterone system, and vasopressin. These systems promote sustained systemic and renal vasoconstriction that ultimately damages the kidney, as evidenced by progressive increases in blood creatinine.

Alcoholic Liver Disease

Alcoholic liver disease (ALD) is a major cause of chronic liver disease worldwide. ALD can significantly raise mortality as a result of end-stage liver disease. Risk factors for progressive liver damage as a result of excessive alcohol ingestion include male sex, genetic factors, nutritional status, and HBV and HCV infections. Because of its prevalence among older adults, ALD is also discussed later in this chapter under Gerontological Considerations.

Excessive alcohol consumption has been implicated in approximately 60% to 80% of liver-related deaths. Liver cirrhosis is the cause of death from alcohol in 70% to 80% of reported cases, with alcohol remaining the second most common cause for liver transplantation (accounting for 25% of all liver transplantations in the United States and 40% in Europe). Various complications can result from excessive alcohol consumption; of these, steatosis (infiltration of fat within the liver) is present in nearly all cases in which an excess of 40 g of alcohol per day is routinely consumed. (One standard drink is equivalent to approximately 14 g of alcohol.[17]) ALD progresses in stages from fatty liver, through hepatitis and progressive fibrosis, to cirrhosis. Abstinence in early stages may reverse the liver damage; however, once cirrhosis is present, the pathological changes are poorly reversible. Cirrhosis has been reported to develop in approximately 10% to 15% of heavy drinkers. Hepatocellular carcinoma is of particular concern because of the increasing annual incidence of 1% to 2% reported in patients with alcoholic cirrhosis.[18,19]

The primary insult in ALD is the direct toxicity of the first metabolite of alcohol degradation, acetaldehyde. Alcohol is metabolized to acetaldehyde by two major enzymatic pathways in the liver, alcohol dehydrogenase and CYP 2E1. Alcohol metabolism by CYP2E1 generates reactive oxygen species (ROS), which can contribute to further hepatocyte damage. ROS contribute to progressive liver injury through permanent changes to DNA structure, lipid peroxidation, and enzyme inhibition. Acetaldehyde also stimulates stellate cells that are implicated in fibrosis and progression to cirrhosis. Decreased levels of fat-derived mediators, such as adiponectin and leptin, contribute to fat accumulation, oxidative damage, and progression of ALD, whereas proinflammatory cytokines tumor necrosis factor-α and interleukin-6 levels increase, worsening the inflammatory state.[18]

A diagnosis of ALD is made based on presenting symptoms, clinical history of the patient, and laboratory testing in addition to specific histological markers identified on liver biopsy. Findings consistent with ALD can be similar to those of nonalcoholic liver disease, thus making the clinical history of the patient pertinent to the diagnosis and therapeutic management. Alcohol abuse in addition to existing ALD can lead to alcoholic hepatitis, which is defined as a clinical syndrome of new-onset jaundice or ascites, or both, in this setting. This acute-on-chronic disease is diagnosed based on clinical presentation and history of excessive alcohol abuse.

Nonalcoholic Fatty Liver Disease

Nonalcoholic fatty liver disease (NAFLD) which comprises nonalcoholic fatty liver (NAFL) and nonalcoholic steatohepatitis (NASH), is defined as fat deposition into the liver. Obesity and insulin resistance are major factors leading to accumulation of lipids within liver tissue. The incidence of NAFLD is estimated to be approximately 20% to 30% in Western countries and 5% to 18% in Asia. Poor diet, uncontrolled diabetes, metabolic syndrome, and inactive lifestyle have been found to be significant contributors to the development of NAFLD. NAFLD can lead to the development of advanced liver disease and can result in treatment requiring liver transplantation. A similar pathway in the development of advanced liver disease exists in patients with NAFLD and ALD. Development of steatosis can lead to fibrosis, cirrhosis, and possibly hepatocellular carcinoma. Diet and lifestyle changes, including enhanced physical activity and smoking cessation, are imperative in reversing disease and controlling progression of disease.[20] Because NAFLD affects individuals of all ages, it is introduced here in detail, and touched on again later in this chapter (see sections Pediatric Considerations and Geriatric Considerations).

FFAs from accelerated lipolysis are a major source of hepatic fat accumulation in NAFLD. Insulin resistance in peripheral adipose tissue contributes to elevated FFA levels. FFA accumulation in hepatocytes can impair oxidization and promote formation of triglycerides and other lipids, resulting in damaging fat accumulation and mitochondrial dysfunction. Altered insulin-to-glucagon ratios further propagate insulin resistance within the liver, leading to buildup of FFAs within hepatocytes. Buildup of FFAs, triglycerides, and other lipids within hepatocytes is the source of steatosis.

Steatosis is a hallmark sign of NAFLD. Fats such as fatty acids, diacylglycerol, oxysterols, cholesterol, triglycerides, and phospholipids can all be associated with hepatocyte injury. Triglycerides are of particular concern and are used in grading the severity of NAFLD. Fat-induced cell damage (lipotoxicity) results from several pathways. ROS generated from mitochondrial and peroxisomal fatty acid oxidation can be toxic to hepatocytes on their own but can also lead to depletion of antioxidant reserves, leading to enhanced oxidative stress and further injury. Ultimately, steatosis can damage hepatocytes, sparking the regeneration process of the liver to repair the damaged cells.[21]

Thought Questions

8. What histological changes in the liver account for the development of portal hypertension?

9. How does the development of portal hypertension connect to the manifestations and complications of end-stage liver disease?

HEREDITARY HEMOCHROMATOSIS

One of the most common inherited diseases in the United States, type 1 **hereditary hemochromatosis** is an autosomal-recessive disorder with incomplete penetrance. It is the most common genetic liver disorder in patients of northern European ancestry but is rare in other ancestral lineages. Hereditary hemochromatosis is associated with chronic elevation of circulating and tissue iron levels that can result in hepatotoxicity, heart disease, diabetes, and other end-organ manifestations. The toxic accumulation of iron can have an insidious onset, and patients with hereditary hemochromatosis vary greatly in the severity of their presentation. Type 1, the most common form of hereditary hemochromatosis, accounts for nearly 90% of cases; however, less than 10% of homozygotes develop the complete phenotypic manifestations of the syndrome. The disorder results from a mutation in the *HFE* gene resulting in substitution of cysteine for tyrosine at amino acid 282 of the protein product (C282Y).[22]

The pathogenesis of type 1 hereditary hemochromatosis originates with decreased function of the *HFE* gene protein product, a transmembrane protein that suppresses hepatocyte production of hepcidin, the iron-regulating hormone discussed earlier in this chapter. The two major sources of iron entry into the blood are duodenal enterocytes (bringing iron from dietary absorption) and splenic macrophages (bringing iron from breakdown of aging red blood cells). Iron efflux from both of these cell types uses the transmembrane transport protein ferroportin. Hepcidin decreases iron efflux by binding to and marking ferroportin for intracellular degradation. Iron homeostasis is regulated by a variety of factors, including erythropoiesis rates, inflammation, iron storage, and oxygenation; however, hepcidin plays a key role in the body's iron regulation. Excess hepcidin production resulting from loss of normal *HFE* signaling in type 1 hereditary hemochromatosis promotes increased entrance of iron into the body from gut absorption, and increases macrophage release of iron, elevating circulating levels of iron and ferritin (**Figure 14.14**).[23]

Under normal circumstances, iron is transported throughout the body by transferrin and delivered to the liver, which is the major site of iron storage. With excess iron available in the case of hereditary hemochromatosis, transferrin binding is saturated, causing an increase in free circulating iron, which is readily taken up by hepatic, endocrine, and cardiac parenchymal cells. The excess of free iron within these cells overwhelms their

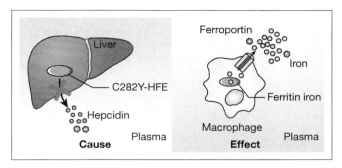

FIGURE 14.14 Type 1 hereditary hemochromatosis results from a mutation (C282Y) in the *HFE* gene regulating hepcidin production. Lack of hepcidin removes inhibition of the iron transporter ferroportin. Ferroportin is found on many cells; however, the key cells affected in hereditary hemochromatosis are splenic macrophages that degrade red blood cells, and absorptive cells of the small intestine. Increased export of iron from these cells leads to chronically high blood iron levels, and can be associated with damaging iron accumulation in the liver and the heart.

ability to export iron, leading to accumulation. Inside the cell, iron catalyzes the production of free radicals, thereby promoting lipid peroxidation and protein damage, cell injury, and death. To summarize, iron-induced damage of parenchymal cells occurs through increased oxidative stress, resulting in an increase in the production of fibrotic tissue.

Mariah Morris and Nicole E. Omecene

FETAL AND CHILDHOOD LIVER DEVELOPMENT

ANATOMICAL AND FUNCTIONAL DEVELOPMENT OF THE LIVER

Formation of the liver begins around gestational week 3 with the formation of a liver bud from endoderm and continues throughout gestation (**Figure 14.15**).[24] Endothelial cells from the mesoderm play a critical role in development of sinusoid structure and formation of lobules. Bile duct development begins in the hilar region in the second month and may not be complete in the liver periphery until after birth. Liver hematopoiesis begins at weeks 4 to 5 of gestation and peaks early in the third trimester, decreasing rapidly in the first 2 months after birth.

Many liver functions during prenatal development are conducted by the maternal liver and the placenta. The fetal liver produces immature bile acids that are not fully functional, and secretion into canaliculi is not fully developed until late in the first year of life. Enterohepatic circulation of bile acids is also developed during this first year. Biliary excretion of drug

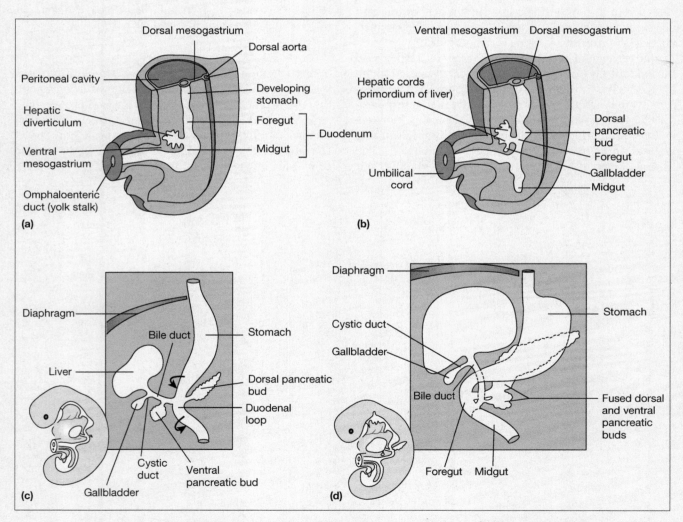

FIGURE 14.15 Liver development at (**a**) week 4 of gestation; (**b**) and (**c**) week 5 of gestation; and (**d**) week 6 of gestation.

metabolites is not well developed at birth, and neonates are vulnerable to cholestatic liver damage.

Developmental changes in liver metabolic pathways involve carbohydrates, proteins, and fats. Fetal carbohydrate metabolism includes production of a large amount of liver glycogen prenatally, which is then used during the early postnatal period to maintain blood glucose. The enzymes of gluconeogenesis are fully functional by the time of term delivery, but premature infants are susceptible to hypoglycemia because of reduced glycogen stores and capacity for gluconeogenesis. Liver protein synthesis begins during fetal development with production of the carrier protein α-fetoprotein. Shortly before and continuing after birth, production of albumin begins, although normal adult levels are not produced until about 1 year of age, thereby increasing free levels of unconjugated bilirubin and many drugs. Coagulation factors are produced at normal adult levels by the time of birth, and are maintained after birth if a vitamin K injection is given soon afterward. Shortly after birth, the liver maintains energy levels by oxidizing fatty acids, and also has the ability to produce ketones. Cholesterol synthesis begins in utero, although mature levels may not be reached until 1 year of age.[25]

DRUG METABOLISM IN INFANCY AND EARLY CHILDHOOD

Infants and children younger than 2 years of age have decreased drug clearance and longer drug half-lives, making them highly susceptible to drug toxicity.[26] A neutral gastric pH, delayed gastric emptying, immature bile production and transport, and reduced renal clearance all result in decreased drug metabolism for infants and children younger than 2 years of age. Starting at ages 2 to 4 years, children begin to metabolize drugs at about the same rate as adults.[27]

HYPERBILIRUBINEMIA

NEONATAL JAUNDICE

Neonatal hyperbilirubinemia is classified as plasma bilirubin level above 1.2 mg/dL. Hyperbilirubinemia in the neonate can be unconjugated or conjugated and is caused by impaired bilirubin uptake and conjugation. In the newborn, serum bilirubin levels are usually between 5 and 10 mg/dL before jaundice is noticeable.

During fetal development, unconjugated bilirubin produced by red blood cell breakdown and heme metabolism crosses the placenta and is metabolized by the maternal liver. The neonatal liver does not have sufficient ability to transport and conjugate bilirubin, predisposing newborns to jaundice. Extreme or prolonged hyperbilirubinemia in the newborn is dangerous because it can lead to brain damage (kernicterus). For a full-term infant physiological jaundice is rarely an issue, and most serum bilirubin levels will return to normal within 5 to 8 days of life. Premature infants are more susceptible to jaundice and take longer to recover; their bilirubin levels return to normal by day 14 of life.

Unconjugated Hyperbilirubinemia

The most common type of unconjugated hyperbilirubinemia is neonatal physiological jaundice due to overproduction of bilirubin secondary to increased fetal red cell count and decreased red blood cell life span. Unconjugated hyperbilirubinemia can be caused by excess hemolysis as seen with sepsis, drug reactions, Rh/ABO incompatibility, or delayed clamping of the cord. Impaired transport of bilirubin can also cause unconjugated hyperbilirubinemia in the newborn. Impaired hepatic uptake or conjugation of bilirubin and abnormal enterohepatic circulation of bilirubin are additional causes of unconjugated hyperbilirubinemia.

Conjugated Hyperbilirubinemia

Conjugated hyperbilirubinemia (cholestatic jaundice) is always pathological in infants and is often caused by an anatomical abnormality of the bile duct or by damage to the hepatocyte membrane. Conjugated hyperbilirubinemia can be acquired (e.g., sepsis, TORCH [toxoplasmosis, other, rubella, cytomegalovirus, herpes] infections, drug induced) or idiopathic (e.g., neonatal hepatitis or biliary atresia). Finally, conjugated hyperbilirubinemia may also result from inherited conditions such as galactosemia, cystic fibrosis, glycogen storage disease, or other inborn errors of metabolism. Rapid determination of the cause is essential in order to initiate appropriate treatment.

JAUNDICE IN THE OLDER CHILD

Unconjugated Hyperbilirubinemia

Hyperbilirubinemia also can occur in children beyond the period of infancy (birth to 1 year of age). In older children, hyperbilirubinemia is seldom pathological and can fluctuate. Nonpathological hyperbilirubinemia is not well understood, but the condition may occur after prolonged fasting. Conditions such as Gilbert syndrome, sickle cell disease, or spherocytosis can also cause unconjugated hyperbilirubinemia in older children.

Conjugated Hyperbilirubinemia

Conjugated hyperbilirubinemia is similarly not very common. It is typically caused by viral hepatitis, most often infection with HAV. Other possible causes of conjugated hyperbilirubinemia in the older child are immunodeficiency disorders such as AIDS or infectious diseases such as mononucleosis, both of which can result in hepatic inflammation. Although rare, cholecystitis in adolescents (mainly female) can also cause conjugated hyperbilirubinemia. Finally, exposure to certain drugs (e.g., some anticonvulsants and antibiotics) can cause hyperbilirubinemia with either a hepatitis- or cholestatic-type pattern.

OTHER LIVER DISORDERS PRESENTING IN CHILDREN

LIVER DAMAGE SECONDARY TO α_1-ANTITRYPSIN DEFICIENCY

α_1-Antitrypsin (AAT) is a protease inhibitor synthesized by the liver and secreted into the blood. AAT protects against tissue damage initiated during inflammatory responses by blocking the action of endogenous proteases released from macrophages and neutrophils. In the most common form of α_1-**antitrypsin deficiency** (AATD), the gene coding for fully functional AAT, known as the M allele, is replaced by the mutant Z allele. Homozygotes (ZZ) produce an abnormal form of the protein that cannot be secreted by hepatocytes. Thus, the liver cells become overloaded with mutant protein, while the circulating levels of AAT are too low to protect other tissues. AATD can present as early-onset emphysema due to lack of AAT protection against damaging effects of lung alveolar macrophage activation. AATD can also present as liver disease resulting from accumulation of the abnormal protein, resulting in hepatocyte cell death and tissue inflammation. Disease presentation is quite variable in homozygous children and adults, ranging from mild elevations of liver enzymes to development of hepatitis, fibrosis, cirrhosis, and hepatocellular carcinoma. Severe cases can be cured by liver transplantation, but most patients do not progress rapidly and do not require transplantation. About 2% of the population of the United States and much of Europe are heterozygotes who do not develop any disease manifestations.[28]

BILIARY ATRESIA

Biliary atresia is a rare, life-threatening disorder involving structural abnormalities of the intrahepatic and extrahepatic bile ducts, which leads to obstructive cholioangiopathy in infants. It is the most common cause of neonatal cholestasis and occurs in approximately one in 12,000 infants in the United States, one in 18,000 infants in Europe, and one in 5,000 in Taiwan.[29] Infants may be classified as having acquired (perinatal) or congenital (embryonic) biliary atresia; the latter may

be accompanied by other types of congenital anomalies or syndromes, such as cardiovascular malformations. The cause remains mostly unclear and is likely multifactorial; however, several theories have been implicated, including perinatal viral infection, autoimmune destruction of the bile duct, morphogenesis, and environmental toxin exposure.

Most cases of biliary atresia are the acquired, nonsyndromic type, in which the child is born with an intact biliary system that undergoes inflammation and fibrosis in early infancy, typically within the first month of life. Without intervention, biliary atresia will progress to end-stage liver disease in early childhood, resulting in death. Thus, affected children often require liver transplantation for long-term survival.

The inflammatory process causes progressive fibrosis and occlusion, or obliteration, of one or more of the bile ducts.[30] Once this occurs, bile is no longer able to flow out of the liver, resulting in cholestasis and accumulation of bile components in the liver and blood. Elevated direct, or conjugated, bilirubin is the principal laboratory finding in an infant with cholestasis because the conjugation of bilirubin continues but the elimination is reduced. Hyperbilirubinemia is sufficient to present as jaundice, often accompanied by dark urine and pale stools. Retention of bile salts in the liver causes direct injury to the hepatocytes, which leads to progressive fibrosis and eventual cirrhosis of the liver. Biliary atresia requires early detection and intervention to prevent devastating effects to newborns. With prompt identification, surgical intervention can improve outcomes and prevent rapid progression to end-stage liver disease.

NONALCOHOLIC FATTY LIVER DISEASE

The prevalence of NAFLD is increasing in children as in adults, paralleling the higher rates of obesity and type 2 diabetes mellitus in children and adolescents. NAFLD is the most common pediatric liver disease, and is often undiagnosed as there are no associated signs and symptoms. As in adults, untreated NAFLD may progress to more severe NASH. Genetic links to NAFLD are currently being explored as there is a high rate of familial clustering. Although candidate genes and single-nucleotide polymorphisms (SNPs) have been identified, these are numerous and risk of NAFLD is likely to be multigenic. Children of Hispanic ancestry have the highest rate of NAFLD (36%), followed by those of Afro-Caribbean (14%) and Asian (10.2%) ancestry. The lowest prevalence (8.6%) is in children with non-Hispanic White ancestry.[31] Treatment is aimed at lifestyle modifications to reduce weight and increase physical activity.

Heather Givans

Age-related changes in the liver affect its size, perfusion, metabolism of medications, and composition. These changes include a 25% to 35% reduction in the size of the liver and a 40% reduction in blood flow in older adults.[32] Reduction in the size of the liver depends on age, sex, body size, and shape. These changes may affect drug metabolism, decrease first-pass metabolism, and decrease phase 1 metabolic reactions in older adults. Consequently, pharmacokinetics of many medications used by older adults is altered. The liver's regenerative capacity is reduced, and the risk of DILI is increased in older adults. However, liver function test values in older adults do not differ from those in younger and middle-aged adults. The primary diseases of the liver in the geriatric population are viral hepatitis, NAFLD, ALD, **autoimmune hepatitis** (AIH), **primary biliary cholangitis** (PBC), and hepatocellular carcinoma.[32–34]

AGING AND HEPATITIS C

Hepatitis C is the most important type of chronic hepatitis in the elderly. In the United States, baby boomers (Americans born between 1945 and 1964) constitute the largest proportion of HCV-infected individuals. HCV-related liver disease progresses more quickly, and hepatic manifestations are worse, in older adults. This may be due to a longer duration of infection, during which other complications may have already developed, or patients may not have been referred for evaluation because they were asymptomatic. Although the pathophysiology of HCV infection in older and younger adults is similar, older adults have more severe initial symptoms and progress more rapidly to cirrhosis and hepatocellular carcinoma. Thus, the complications of HCV infection in older adults are often the first manifestations of the disease. They include ascites, bleeding, jaundice, and hepatocellular carcinoma. Other clinical manifestations include abnormal liver function tests, abdominal pain, edema, and pruritus.[35]

Management of HCV infection in older adults is complex, because of likely comorbid conditions and quality-of-life issues. Treatment is challenging because patients progress rapidly to cirrhosis and are more likely to suffer from extrahepatic manifestations, such as fatigue and neuropsychological disorders. HCV infection can be treated with a combination of antiviral drugs, but the risk and benefit of antiviral therapy should be assessed on an individual basis. Older adults with increased risk for progression to cirrhosis and carcinoma should be treated.

ALCOHOLIC LIVER DISEASE

ALD, introduced earlier in this chapter, is a consequence of excessive alcohol consumption, which can be common in older adults and is exacerbated by social isolation. The pathways from excessive alcohol ingestion to ALD are similar to those in younger adults. However, alcohol has greater toxicity with age because of changes in liver blood flow and metabolism. A reduction in total body water leads to increased serum concentration of water-soluble substances, including alcohol (ethanol). Older patients with ALD usually present with disease at a more advanced stage than younger patients. Alcohol withdrawal in older adults may present as delirium or agitation and can progress to seizures and changes in mental status. As in younger adults, abstinence can often reverse liver damage that has not progressed to cirrhosis.

NONALCOHOLIC FATTY LIVER DISEASE

NAFLD was defined earlier in this chapter as a spectrum of liver abnormalities ranging from steatosis and NASH to fibrosis, cirrhosis, and hepatocellular carcinoma. Progression of NAFLD may be accelerated with advancing age because of reduced blood flow and hepatocyte function, and greater insulin resistance with aging, leading to a worse prognosis than in younger adults. As in younger adults, older adults with NAFLD are usually asymptomatic. Symptoms of advanced NAFLD include fatigue, weakness, loss of appetite, weight loss, abdominal pain, telangiectasia, jaundice, peripheral edema, ascites, and confusion. The clinical presentation of NAFLD in older adults is usually associated with—and at times complicated by—dementia, sarcopenia, autonomic dysfunction, aortic valve sclerosis, and autonomic changes predisposing them to fatigue, falls, and arrhythmia. NAFLD is usually suspected when the results of liver function tests are abnormal, especially with increased serum ALT, GGT, and serum ferritin—findings that are similar in older and younger adults.[36]

DRUG-INDUCED LIVER INJURY

DILI, mentioned earlier in this chapter, is the most common cause of acute liver failure in older adults in the United States. The most significant pharmacokinetic change with aging is the impaired clearance of medications and their metabolites. Factors affecting susceptibility to DILI include age, gender, genetics, metabolism, immunological response, absorption/distribution, inflammation, and nutritional status. Older adults are at increased risk of hepatic injury because of decreased clearance, drug-to-drug interactions, reduced hepatic blood flow, decrease in renal function, variation in drug binding, and lower hepatic volume. Age-related changes in the liver cause variability in therapeutic response to medications in older adults, making them more susceptible to the toxic effects of medications. Hence, the importance of starting with lower doses and slowly titrating upward as needed becomes paramount in older adults. Liver injury can also be caused or exacerbated by self-administered herbal and dietary supplements or xenobiotics. Some of these products lead to abnormal liver function tests or hepatic dysfunction that cannot be explained.

Clinical manifestations of DILI in older adults vary and are nonspecific. Similar to younger adults, older adults present with mild elevation in aminotransferase or ALP enzymes, and are usually asymptomatic. They can have nonspecific symptoms such as anorexia, nausea, vomiting, RUQ pain, skin rash, or itching. Hepatocellular jaundice, ascites, or encephalopathy can be seen, depending on the medication involved. The diagnosis of DILI is usually based on a history of drug consumption and is a diagnosis of exclusion. In older adults, AST and bilirubin levels are the most important predictors of death or the need for liver transplantation. DILI can progress to chronic liver damage even after the offending medication has been discontinued. Treatment of drug-induced liver damage consists of removing the offending agent. Corticosteroid treatment may be considered if liver function tests do not return to normal levels within 4 to 6 weeks.

AUTOIMMUNE HEPATITIS

Autoimmune hepatitis (AIH) is a form of chronic hepatitis that occurs in adults >60 years of age. It is found in all ethnic groups, and is more prevalent in older women. As with other autoimmune disorders, there are genetic influences and comorbidity with other autoimmune disorders. AIH is underdiagnosed in the older population. It is characterized by a loss of immune tolerance to antigens on hepatocytes, leading to destruction of the hepatic parenchyma by autoreactive T cells. Triggering factors that may be involved in the pathogenesis of AIH include viruses, xenobiotics, and drugs. AIH has immunological and autoimmunological features, including high serum globulin concentrations and the presence of autoantibodies. There are two main types of AIH. Type 1, which is most common, is seen in middle-aged and older adults, and is characterized by the presence of circulating antinuclear antibodies (ANAs) and anti-smooth muscle actin (ASMA). Type 2, seen in children and adolescents, is characterized by the presence of antibodies to liver or kidney microsomes or to a liver cytosol antigen, or both.

Older adults with AIH may be asymptomatic or have typical manifestations, including jaundice, fatigue, lethargy, malaise, anorexia, nausea, abdominal pain, pruritus, hepatosplenomegaly, and arthralgias. Diagnosis of AIH in older adults is based on presenting clinical signs and symptoms, abnormal liver function tests, increased total IgG levels, and antibody titers to the previously noted targets. Patients can also present with elevated prothrombin time and aminotransferase levels. A liver biopsy can be obtained if the diagnosis is unclear. In some cases, AIH-induced liver damage progresses more rapidly in older adults than in younger adults, perhaps related to "inflammaging"—enhanced innate immunity with aging. Immunosuppressive therapy is often effective in preventing progression and reversing the autoimmune-induced liver damage.

PRIMARY BILIARY CHOLANGITIS (PRIMARY BILIARY CIRRHOSIS)

Primary biliary cholangitis (PBC) formerly referred to as primary biliary cirrhosis, is a slowly progressive autoimmune liver disease in which the targets of immune damage are the small and medium-sized bile ducts. Onset is usually between the ages of 30 and 70 years, and the condition is more common in women (9:1 female/male ratio) and in individuals in northern latitudes, particularly in the United States and Europe.[37] The major diagnostic laboratory finding is the presence of antimitochondrial antibodies (AMAs) reactive to the pyruvate dehydrogenase complex protein E2, but confirmation of diagnosis requires a liver biopsy. Histologically, autoreactive T cells can be observed clustered around bile ducts. PBC is associated with hepatomegaly, a distinguishing feature relative to other chronic progressive liver disorders that result in shrinking and cirrhosis.

Major laboratory findings include elevated levels of serum transaminase, ALP, and AMAs, and hyperlipidemia. The goal of treatment in PBC is to relieve symptoms, prevent disease progression, and reverse injury from bile duct inflammation. The treatment of choice for PBC has been ursodeoxycholic acid (UDCA), although newer treatments are being investigated. PBC can demonstrate relatively slow progression, and patients who are managed symptomatically and with UDCA may have a prolonged period before developing end-stage liver disease. For PBC patients in whom the disease progresses rapidly, liver transplantation is the definitive treatment.

HEPATOCELLULAR CARCINOMA

Hepatocellular carcinoma (HCC) is common in older adults as it is the final stage for many chronic disorders, including HBV and HCV infection, ALD, NAFLD, and autoimmune disease. Age is a risk factor for developing HCC, and the incidence is on the rise. Older adults with HCC are more likely to be female, which may be due to their longer life expectancy.

HCC in older adults is frequently characterized by one or a few tumors, is often encapsulated, has a lower incidence of vascular invasion, and is associated with greater differentiation. The clinical manifestations of HCC are similar in older and younger adults. They include anorexia, unintended weight loss, RUQ pain, worsening ascites, hepatic encephalopathy, and GI bleeding. Imaging studies and biopsy are the most useful diagnostic tools. Well-localized HCC is often managed with directed, minimally invasive treatments.

CASE STUDY 14.1: A Patient With Hepatitis A Virus Infection

Amanda Chaney and Michelle Zappas

Patient Complaint: *"I haven't been able to keep anything down for the past 3 days since I got back from Mexico. We were there about 3 weeks ago. My stomach hurts, and I noticed my urine is really dark. Also, I have been so tired. I thought that it was because of our traveling, but now with the abdominal pain and fever, I'm wondering if it's something else. And I've been itching all over like crazy!"*

History of Present Illness/Review of Systems: You observe a healthy-appearing 27-year-old woman who appears fatigued. The patient reports nausea, vomiting, and anorexia for the past 72 hours. She tells you she has tried to drink Gatorade and water, and to eat some bland food, but cannot tolerate either. She has had clear or bilious-appearing emesis two to three times per day for the past 3 days. She denies coffee-ground or bloody-appearing emesis. When questioned further about her bowel movements, she reports loose, frequent stools that are pale in color, and not bloody. Her urine has an odor and is very dark. The abdominal pain started about 1 week ago and has progressively worsened. She has taken acetaminophen for the pain, which has not helped. She also reports fatigue and a mild fever for the past week. She began experiencing pruritus 3 or 4 days ago. Other than intermittent acetaminophen, she denies any over-the-counter or herbal supplement medications.

Past Medical/Family/Social History: The patient's past medical history is significant for asthma as a child. She denies alcohol use, intravenous drug use, or recent tattoos, and is a nonsmoker. She reports recent travel to Mexico with her husband on a cruise.

Physical Examination: Findings are as follows: temperature of 100.8°F, blood pressure of 110/80 mm Hg, heart rate of 105 beats/min, and respirations of 14 breaths/min. Severity of abdominal pain to RUQ is 8 out of 10. The patient is alert and oriented to person, place, and time, and appears fatigued. Skin is dry and jaundiced, eyes show scleral icterus, and mucous membranes of the mouth are dry. S_1/S_2 heart sounds are present, and the heart rate is tachycardic, with regular rhythm. Lungs are clear to auscultation bilaterally. Hyperactive bowel sounds are present in all four quadrants of the abdomen, with tenderness in the RUQ. The liver edge is palpable just below the costal margin, soft, and smooth. The spleen is not palpable. No masses are palpable, and there is no rebound tenderness or guarding.

Laboratory and Diagnostic Findings: Laboratory data reveal several significant findings, including elevations of ALT/AST (350/300 U/L) and hyperbilirubinemia (total bilirubin 2.9 mg/dL). The patient is anti-HAV IgM positive. Alkaline phosphatase and INR are normal.

CASE STUDY 14.1 QUESTIONS
- *What types of insult can cause acute onset of liver injury?*
- *Which immunoglobulin fraction is elevated in a first attack of HAV infection?*
- *What additional testing and imaging could the provider perform?*
- *What information is pertinent for other members of this person's household regarding her potential diagnosis?*

ALT, alanine aminotransferase; AST, aspartate aminotransferase; HAV, hepatitis A virus; IgM, immunoglobulin M; INR, international normalized ratio; RUQ, right upper quadrant.

CASE STUDY 14.2: A Patient With Nonalcoholic Fatty Liver Disease

Michelle Zappas and Amanda Chaney

Patient Complaint: *"I'm here for my annual physical exam. I've been feeling well for the past few months. I was told that I have diabetes last year and have been trying to keep it under control with my diet. But I just can't seem to lose any weight. I know I could lose some weight, but I've been big-boned my whole life."*

History of Present Illness/Review of Systems: You observe a healthy-appearing, obese 40-year-old woman. She is here for her annual physical examination and has expressed interest in wellness coaching and weight loss. The patient denies fatigue, nausea, vomiting, or changes in bowel habits but has had some intermittent, vague RUQ abdominal pain that comes and goes. She does not take any over-the-counter or herbal supplement medications. She denies fever or any other acute complaints. She tells you that she has been checking her blood pressure periodically at the local grocery store and it has been high (range 120 to 150s/80 to 90s mm Hg).

Past Medical/Family/Social History: Her past medical history is notable for diabetes (diagnosed 1 year ago—diet controlled), and obesity since age 12 years; her BMI has fluctuated between the high 30s and low 40s kg/m² for the past few years. She has had no surgeries, hospitalizations, or other chronic illnesses. Her social history is negative for use of tobacco, alcohol, or other drugs. She reports that her mother and father are overweight and have issues with hypertension and diabetes. She has a brother who has diabetes and high cholesterol. Her grandfather is deceased from a myocardial infarction.

Physical Examination: Findings are as follows: temperature of 98.6°F, blood pressure of 145/90 mm Hg, heart rate of 78 beats/min, and respirations of 20 breaths/min. BMI is 38.5 kg/m². Severity of abdominal pain to RUQ is 4 out of 10. The patient is alert and oriented to person, place, and time. Skin is dry and warm. Eyes show no scleral icterus. Mucous membranes of the mouth are moist. S_1/S_2 heart sounds are present, and the heart rate and rhythm are regular. Lungs are clear to auscultation bilaterally. Abdomen is protuberant with normoreactive bowel sounds all four quadrants and slight tenderness in the RUQ. The liver edge is palpable just below the costal margin, soft, and smooth. The spleen is not palpable. No other masses are palpable, and there is no rebound tenderness or guarding.

Laboratory and Diagnostic Findings: AST and ALT are moderately elevated, fasting glucose is 140 mg/dL, and triglycerides are 210 mg/dL. Results for all other laboratory tests, including complete blood count, plasma iron, and anti-HCV antibody, are negative. The patient has been vaccinated and is immune to HAV and HBV. Ultrasound examination, performed because of the patient's report of vague RUQ abdominal pain, shows hyperechoic liver with blurring of the vascular margins; these findings may be consistent with fatty liver disease.

CASE STUDY 14.2 QUESTIONS
- *What is a common progression of NAFLD?*
- *What other diseases commonly coexist with this disorder?*

ALT, alanine aminotransferase; AST, aspartate aminotransferase; BMI, body mass index; HAV, hepatitis A virus; HBV, hepatitis B virus; HCV, hepatitis C virus; NAFLD, nonalcoholic fatty liver disease; RUQ, right upper quadrant.

BRIDGE TO CLINICAL PRACTICE

Ben Cocchiaro

PRINCIPLES OF ASSESSMENT

History

- *Medication history:* At every patient visit, review use of all prescription and over-the-counter medications, alcohol, and street drugs.
- *Symptoms and signs:* RUQ pain, nausea, anorexia, fatigue, pruritus, anorexia, jaundice, ascites, right shoulder pain (referred from phrenic nerve irritation in cholecystitis).

Physical Examination

- Hepatomegaly can be both palpated and auscultated: liver edge protruding more than 2 cm beyond the right costal margin.
- Signs of portal hypertension include caput medusae, internal hemorrhoids, abdominal distention with fluid thrill or shifting dullness.
- Murphy sign of cholecystitis—A sharp pain that stops the breath while palpating under the costal margin of the right upper quadrant.

Diagnostic Tools

- *Ultrasonography:* first-line imaging modality for biliary tract abnormalities including cholecystitis and cholelithiasis, as well as liver masses and fibrosis/cirrhosis; Doppler ultrasonography adds the ability to assess portal vein function as well as large tumor vascularity.
- *CT:* CT imaging of the liver can identify and further characterize liver masses and structural abnormalities.
- *MRI:* MRI of the liver includes including magnetic resonance cholangiopancreatography (MRCP).
- *Elastography:* Assessment of liver fibrosis, useful in determining the severity and prognosis of chronic liver disease. Obtained either ultrasonographically or through MRI.
- *Endoscopy:* Used to inspect for varices, and endoscopic retrograde cholangiopancreatography (ERCP) is an invasive diagnostic and therapeutic procedure used in suspected biliary and pancreatic duct obstruction.
- *Liver biopsy:* An invasive test for diagnosing focal liver lesions and assessing hepatic parenchymal damage, biopsy is particularly useful in the assessment of liver cancers and metastases as the results often guide staging and treatment.

Laboratory Evaluation

- *Transaminases:* ALT and AST are intracellular enzymes released into the blood when hepatocytes and some extrahepatic tissues are damaged.
- *Tests of liver synthetic function:* Although transaminases are good indicators of hepatocyte damage and death, true liver function tests assess metabolic functions including:
  - Albumin—Representing more than half of all protein found in blood plasma, albumin acts as a transport protein, sets the plasma oncotic pressure, and is frequently decreased in liver disease.
  - Coagulation studies—In addition to being the site of clotting factor production, the liver also serves an endocrine function, synthesizing and releasing thrombopoietin, which stimulates proliferation of platelet-producing megakaryocytes. As such, coagulation markers such as platelet count and prothrombin time are useful tools in diagnosing and monitoring liver disease.
  - Bilirubin—A degradation product of heme, bilirubin, is conjugated with glucuronic acid in the liver, rendering it soluble in water. Blood concentrations of conjugated and unconjugated bilirubin can indicate liver pathology as well as help clinicians identify extrahepatic causes of hyperbilirubinemia.
- *Markers of cholestasis:* ALP and GGT are important enzymes in the catabolism of waste products in the liver and their flow through biliary system. Increased serum levels of these enzymes can indicate both hepatic and extrahepatic biliary flow obstruction and are often elevated in alcoholic liver disease.

MAJOR DRUG CLASSES

Drugs used for:

- *Acetaminophen overdoses:* Activated charcoal reduces gut acetaminophen absorption, and *N*-acetylcysteine increases the liver's ability to metabolize absorbed acetaminophen into less toxic byproducts.
- *Hepatic encephalopathy:* Rifaximin and lactulose reduce gut ammonia absorption and increase stool ammonia excretion.

(continued)

(*continued*)

- *Ascites:* Diuretics to reduce total body fluid retention; antibiotics to prevent spontaneous bacterial peritonitis; albumin to restore blood protein levels after paracentesis.
- *Portal hypertension/varices:* Nonselective β-blocking drugs may enhance α-adrenergic-mediated mesenteric vasoconstriction, reducing inflow to the portal vein.
- *Hepatitis B:* Nucleoside reverse transcriptase inhibitors, interferons.
- *Hepatitis C:* Direct-acting antivirals, ribavirin.

ALP, alkaline phosphatase; ALT, alanine aminotransferase; AST, aspartate aminotransferase; GGT, gamma-glutamyl transpeptidase; RUQ, right upper quadrant.

KEY POINTS

- The liver is the largest solid organ in the body. It is highly vascular and receives about 25% of the cardiac output, with approximately 25% of its blood flow supplied by the hepatic artery, and the remainder from the portal vein. The portal vein combines the venous outflows from most of the abdominal organs, including stomach, pancreas, spleen, small intestine, and much of the large intestine. Thus, the liver receives blood enriched in the products of digestion and absorption, as well as relatively high concentrations of the pancreatic hormones insulin and glucagon.
- The functional unit of the liver is the lobule, a roughly hexagonal structure consisting of plates of hepatocytes surrounding large permeable capillaries called sinusoids. Blood flows from branches of the hepatic artery and portal vein at the periphery of the lobule, through the sinusoids, to the central vein.
- Hepatocytes are polarized cells with surfaces facing the sinusoids, and other surfaces facing bile canaliculi—the sites of bile secretion. Bile flows outward between hepatocytes to the perimeter of the lobule, to enter branches of the biliary tree.
- Kupffer cells are the resident macrophages of the liver, conducting surveillance for foreign proteins and organisms entering from the GI tract.
- The liver is the major organ of metabolic homeostasis, regulating levels of circulating glucose over daily cycles of feeding and fasting, and responsible for production and uptake of several lipoproteins.
- The liver produces bile, fluid enriched in salts needed for fat digestion and absorption, and providing a route for excretion of waste products such as bilirubin. It also synthesizes urea, reducing buildup of toxic ammonia.
- The liver prepares hydrophobic endogenous and exogenous compounds (xenobiotics) for excretion by phase 1 and phase 2 chemical reactions. Phase 1 reactions modify the parent compound, generally adding an oxygen-containing moiety that is chemically reactive. Phase 2 reactions conjugate a small hydrophilic molecule to the modified parent compound, increasing its hydrophilicity and facilitating renal excretion.
- Some compounds, such as bilirubin, only undergo conjugation reactions that facilitate their excretion in the bile and by the kidneys. The fate of heme groups released on breakdown of red blood cells and from other body sources is conversion to unconjugated bilirubin that travels to the liver for conjugation and excretion.
- Assessment of liver function includes plasma measures of enzymes released from damaged and dying hepatocytes, measures of plasma proteins synthesized by the liver (including clotting assays), and assays for hepatitis virus–associated antigens and host antibodies to hepatitis antigens. Noninvasive imaging and invasive biopsy techniques are used to measure liver fibrosis and cirrhosis.
- Acute liver disorders such as HAV infection and DILI may be time-limited and result in complete recovery and regrowth of normal tissue.
- Chronic liver disease can result from infections with HBV or HCV, from chronic alcohol ingestion, or from obesity-associated NAFLD.
- Chronic HBV and HCV infections may be managed (in the case of HBV) or cured (in the case of HCV) by antiviral drugs.
- Liver damage associated with chronic liver disease is attributed to local inflammatory responses to insults, potentiated by cytokines released from resident Kupffer cells. Activation of local stellate cells, also known as lipocytes, promotes increased extracellular matrix deposition in the space of Disse

surrounding sinusoids. Sinusoidal endothelial cells develop reduced permeability, these normally wide vessels narrow, and hepatic vascular resistance increases.

- Cirrhosis progression results in portal hypertension, with a host of consequences, including splanchnic vascular engorgement, splenomegaly, development of shunt flow bypassing the liver, hepatic encephalopathy, and ascites formation.
- Hereditary hemochromatosis is a genetic disorder of body iron handling with elevated levels of circulating iron and ferritin. The disorder has variable severity of presentation, but serious cases are characterized by cellular accumulation of iron that leads to toxicity that particularly affects liver and cardiac cells.

- Liver metabolism of drugs and toxins is not fully developed until the age of 2 years, making infancy and early childhood a time of greater risk of drug-induced injury.
- Genetic and developmental abnormalities such as AATD and biliary atresia are rare but account for some childhood liver disorders.
- NAFLD is increasing in children and adolescents.
- Healthy older adults do not have systematic patterns of altered liver function; however, they are more susceptible to DILI.
- Immune-mediated liver damage can be more extensive in older adults, as well as vulnerability to ALD and NAFLD.
- Hepatitis in older adults is under-recognized and can progress more rapidly to hepatocellular carcinoma.

REFERENCES

1. Centers for Disease Control and Prevention, National Center for Health Statistics. Health, United States, 2017- data finder. https://www.cdc.gov/nchs/hus/index.htm. Accessed October 9, 2018.
2. Centers for Disease Control and Prevention. National health interview survey, 2016. https://cdc.gov/nchs/nhis/index.htm. Accessed October 9, 2018.
3. Eipel C, Abshagen K, Vollmar B. Regulation of hepatic blood flow: the hepatic arterial buffer response revisited. *World J Gastroenterol*. 2010;16:6046–6057. doi:10.3748/wjg.v16.i48.6046.
4. Uhlén M, Fagerberg L, Hallström BM, et al. Proteomics. Tissue-based map of the human proteome. *Science*. 2015;347(6220):1260419. doi:10.1126/1260419.
5. Cedarbaum AI. Molecular mechanisms of the microsomal mixed function oxidases and biological and pathological implications. *Redox Biology*. 2015;4:60–73. doi:10.1016.j.redox.2014.11.008.
6. Castera L. Noninvasive methods to assess liver disease in patients with hepatitits B or C. *Gastroenterology*. 2012;142:1293–1302. doi:10.1053/j.gastro.2012.02.017.
7. Bernal W, Wendon J. Acute liver failure. *N Engl J Med*. 2013;369:2525–2534. doi:10.1056/NEJMra1208937.
8. Reuben A, Koch DG, Lee WM. Drug-induced acute liver failure: results of a U.S. multicenter, prospective study. *Hepatology*. 2010;52:2065–2076. doi:10.1002/hep.23937.
9. Yoon E, Babar A, Choudhary M, et al. Acetaminophen-induced hepatotoxicity: a comprehensive update. *J Clin Transl Hepatol*. 2016;4:131–142. doi:10.14218/JCTH.2015.00052.
10. Sundaram V, Björnsson ES. Drug induced cholestasis. *Hepatol Commun*. 2017;1:726–735. doi:10.1002/hep4.1088.
11. Jacobsen KH, Wiersma ST. Hepatitis A virus seroprevalence by age and world region, 1990 and 2005. *Vaccine*. 2010;28:6653–6657. doi:10.1016/j.vaccine.2010.08.037.

12. World Health Organization. Hepatitis B. http://www.who.int/news-room/fact-sheets/detail/hepatitis-b. Accessed August 15, 2018.
13. Lok ASF, McMahon BJ, Brown RS, et al. Antiviral therapy for chronic hepatitis B viral infection in adults: a systematic review and meta analysis. *Hepatology*. 2016;63:284–306. doi:10.1002/hep.28280.
14. Centers for Disease Control and Prevention. Testing recommendations for hepatitis C virus infections. https://www.cdc.gov/hepatitis/hcv/guidelinesc.htm. Accessed July 2, 2018.
15. Bataller R, Brenner DA. Liver fibrosis. *J Clin Invest*. 2005;115:209–218.
16. Zhou W, Zhang Q, Qiao L. Pathogenesis of liver cirrhosis. *World J Gastroenterol*. 2014;20:7312–7324. doi:10.3748/wjg.v20.i23.7312.
17. National Institute on Alcohol Abuse and Alcoholism. What is a standard drink? https://www.niaaa.nih.gov/alco-hol-health/overview-alcohol-consumption/what-standard-drink. Accessed July 2, 2018.
18. Farooq MO, Bataller R. Pathogenesis and management of alcoholic liver disease. *Dig Dis*. 2016;34:347–355. doi:10.1159/000444545.
19. Stickel F, Datz C, Jampe J, et al. Pathophysiology and management of alcoholic liver disease: update 2016. *Gut Liver*. 2017;11:173–188. doi:10.5009/gnl16477.
20. Neuschwander-Tetri BA. Non-alcoholic fatty liver disease. *BMC Med*. 2017;15:45. doi:10.1186/s12916-017-0806-8.
21. Machado MV, Diehl AM. Pathogenesis of nonalcoholic steatohepatitis. *Gastroenterology*. 2016;150:1769–1777.
22. Bacon BR, Adams PC, Kowdley KV, et al. Diagnosis and management of hemochromatosis: 2011 Practice Guideline by the American Association for the Study of Liver Diseases. *Hepatology*. 2011;54:328–343. doi:10.1002/hep.24330.
23. Pietrangelo A. Hepcidin in human iron disorders: therapeutic implications. *J Hepatol*. 2011;54:173–181.

24. Bedard MP. Embryology, anatomy, and normal findings. In: Coley BD, ed. *Caffey's Pediatric Diagnostic Imaging.* 12th ed. Philadelphia, PA: Elsevier/Saunders; 2013:845–855.

25. Harpavat S, Mclin VA. Developmental anatomy and physiology of the liver and bile ducts. In: Wylie R, Hyams JS, Key M, eds. *Pediatric Gastrointestinal and Liver Disease.* 5th ed. Philadelphia, PA: Elsevier; 2016:811–822.

26. Lu H, Rosenbaum S. Developmental pharmacokinetics in pediatric populations. *J Pediatr Pharmacol Ther.* 2014;19:262–276. doi:10.5863/1551-6776-19.4.262.

27. Fernandez E, Perez R, Hernandez A, et al. Factors and mechanisms for pharmacokinetic differences between pediatric population and adults. *Pharmaceutics.* 2011;3:53–72. doi:10.3390/pharmaceutics3010053.

28. Teckman JH, Mangalat N. Alpha-1 antitrypsin and liver disease: mechanisms of injury and novel interventions. *Expert Rev Gastroenterol Hepatol.* 2015;9:261–268. doi:10.1586/17474124.2014.943187.

29. Mack CL, Feldman AG, Sokol RJ. Clues to the etiology of bile duct injury in biliary atresia. *Semin Liver Dis.* 2012;32:307–316. doi:10.1055/s-0032-1329899.

30. Hartley JL, Davenport M, Kelly DA. Biliary atresia. *Lancet.* 2009;374:1704–1713. doi:10.1016/S0140-6736(09)60946-6.

31. Temple JL, Cordero P, Li J, et al. A guide to non-alcoholic fatty liver disease in childhood and adolescence. *Int J Mol Sci.* 2016;17:947. doi:10.3390/ijms17060947.

32. Kim H, Kissleveva T, Brenner D. Aging and liver disease. *Curr Opin Gastroenterol.* 2015;31:184–191. doi:10.1097/MOG.0000000000000176.

33. Floreani A. Liver disorders in the elderly. *Best Pract Res Clin Gastroenterol.* 2009;23:909–917. doi:10.1053/bega.2002.0271.

34. Tajiri K, Shimizu Y. Liver physiology and liver diseases in the elderly. *World J Gastroenterol.* 2013;19:8459–8467. doi:10.3748/wjg.v19.i46.8459.

35. Davis G, Alter M, El-Serag H, et al. Aging of hepatitis C virus (HCV)-infected persons in the United States: a multiple cohort model of HCV prevalence and disease progression. *Gastroenterology.* 2010;138:513–521. doi:10.1053/j.gastro.2009.09.067.

36. Targher G, Bellis A, Fornengo P, et al. Prevention and treatment of nonalcoholic fatty liver disease. *Dig Liver Dis.* 2010;42:331–340. doi:10.1016/j.dld.2010.02.004.

37. Hohenester S, Oude-Elferink RPJ, Beuers U. Primary biliary cirrhosis. *Semin Immunopathol.* 2009;31:283–707. doi:10.1007/s00281-009-0164-5.

SUGGESTED RESOURCE

Theise, ND. Liver and gallbladder. In: Kumar V, Abbas AK, Aster JC, eds. *Robbins Basic Pathology.* 10th ed. Philadelphia, PA: Elsevier; 2016:637–677.

15

NERVOUS SYSTEM

Nancy C. Tkacs, Peggy A. Compton, and Kara Pavone

THE CLINICAL CONTEXT

The nervous system is arguably the most complex system in the body and many mechanisms of higher order brain functions are still not well understood. Nevertheless, the human toll and medical costs associated with nervous system–associated disorders in the United States and globally is considerable. Researchers studying the Global Burden of Disease reported the following top five causes of years lost to disability in 2016:

1. Low back pain
2. Migraine
3. Age-related hearing loss
4. Iron-deficiency anemia
5. Major depressive disorder

Of these, four out of five are associated with altered nervous system function.[1] The annual economic cost of neurological disorders in the United States ranges from $243 billion for Alzheimer and other dementias to $15 billion dollars for Parkinson disease.[2] There are 610,000 new strokes every year, resulting in 140,000 deaths, and stroke is a leading cause of disability in the United States.[3]

In the ambulatory setting, the combination of disorders of neurological function, sense organs, and mental health accounts for the largest category of diagnoses noted at primary care office visits. Chronic depression alone was reported by 9.3% of patients during office visits. Analgesics (no. 1), antidepressants (no. 5), and anxiolytics, sedatives, and hypnotics (no. 8) are among the top 20 most frequently discussed medications during office visits.[4]

OVERVIEW OF NERVOUS SYSTEM FUNCTION AND NEUROANATOMY

NERVOUS SYSTEM FUNCTION

The brain serves complex functional, regulatory, and integrative roles that underlie pragmatic functions that maintain the body as well as providing identity, personality, and relational capacity. The nervous system is responsible for taking in external sensory information, monitoring internal processes, and, in turn, directing motor and behavioral responses. The brain exhibits plasticity—the ability to adapt to altered internal or external signals in ways that can be either positive or negative for functional status. Plasticity also underlies the capacity for learning. The nervous system regulates general homeostasis, both through the autonomic nervous system (parasympathetic and sympathetic divisions) and by neuroendocrine control via hypothalamic-pituitary-target gland axes. The brain is responsible for states of consciousness, mood, learning, memory, cognition, and higher executive functions. Diseases of the brain and brain trauma can cause deficits ranging from loss of perception, strength, and coordination to permanent vegetative states, as well as profound alterations of personality and lost or diminished social abilities. The biological basis of mental health disorders is challenging to study, but advances in functional imaging are beginning to shed some light on these topics.

ANATOMY OF THE NERVOUS SYSTEM

The brain consists of neurons and glial cells, along with supporting structures and blood vessels, with an outer protective membrane coat consisting of the meninges. Neurons have axons, short or long projecting structures that make synaptic contacts with target neurons. The brain can be divided into regions associated with specific properties and that have specific connections to functionally related areas within the brain, brainstem, and spinal cord. For that reason, a review of neuroanatomy is a critical introduction to the topic of the brain (**Figure 15.1**). The forebrain consists of the cerebral cortex and deeply embedded white matter (made up of axons), basal ganglia, thalamus, hypothalamus, hippocampus, and amygdala. Moving in the ventral and posterior direction, the forebrain connects to the brainstem, consisting of midbrain, pons, and medulla. The cerebellum overlies the brainstem and has white matter bundles connecting it to various brainstem levels. The medulla connects with the spinal cord, which extends toward the sacral region within the bony vertebral column.

The surface of the cerebral cortex is made up of gray matter—neuron cell bodies organized in layers. The surface area of the cortex is maximized by tissue folding that produces gyri and sulci, giving the brain its characteristic appearance (**Figure 15.1a**). Beneath the superficial gray matter of the cortex is white matter consisting of bundles of axons, many of them thickly myelinated, giving these tracts and pathways a lighter appearance than the gray matter. The medial view of the brain hemisphere also shows the corpus callosum, a thick white matter bundle that connects the right hemisphere to the left (**Figure 15.1b**). The brainstem is also seen on the medial view, connected to the forebrain at the region of the midbrain. The cerebellum overlies the brainstem and has a surface structured with layers and folds, similar to the cortex.

Cortical Anatomy and Functional Regions

The four lobes of the cerebral cortex are the frontal, parietal, temporal, and occipital lobes. Within these lobes are motor regions and sensory regions that are further subdivided into primary and secondary regions. Primary motor cortex encompasses the precentral gyrus in the frontal lobe posterior to the premotor cortex and anterior to the central sulcus that divides the frontal and parietal lobes. Anterior to premotor cortex is the large prefrontal region. Primary somatosensory cortex encompasses the postcentral gyrus, in the parietal lobe immediately posterior to the central sulcus. The secondary somatosensory cortex, or association area, makes up much of the dorsolateral parietal lobe.

Primary visual cortex is found on the medial surface of the occipital lobe, and secondary visual cortex wraps laterally around to the posterolateral occipital lobe and adjoining ventrolateral parietal lobe. Primary auditory cortex is located in a small region of the posterior part of the superior temporal gyrus, surrounded by the auditory association area. A large region encompassing the remaining ventral parietal lobe, posterior temporal lobe, adjoining the visual association area is considered multimodal association cortex, capable of integrating information from several sensory modalities. Cortical regions are interconnected, with specific regions of association cortex having reciprocal connections and most regions of the right and left hemispheres connected by the corpus callosum, the largest white matter bundle in the brain.

Basal Ganglia and Thalamus

Deep structures within the forebrain include the basal ganglia—consisting of caudate and putamen (grouped

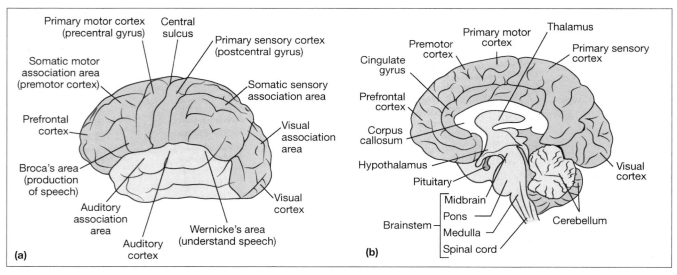

FIGURE 15.1 Surface anatomy and major functional designations of the human brain. (**a**) Lateral view. (**b**) Medial view.

together in the term *striatum*) and globus pallidus—and the thalamus, with relative positions as shown in **Figure 15.2**. The basal ganglia play an important role in motor control and coordination, as described later. All sensory modalities except olfaction relay information to the cortex from relay nuclei in the thalamus. In addition, each cortical region has reciprocal connections with a specific thalamic nucleus, and ongoing thalamocortical activity shapes overall brain activity and motor activity. The nucleus accumbens is an anterior extension of the striatum.

Limbic System

The limbic system is a general term for several structures that have been implicated in emotion perception and regulation (**Figure 15.3**). These include the amygdala and hippocampus, with cell bodies located in the medial temporal lobe and projections to the

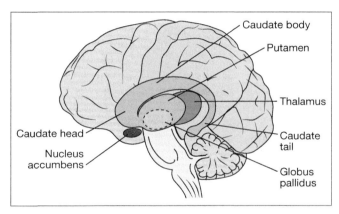

FIGURE 15.2 Basal ganglia and thalamus. The basal ganglia (caudate, putamen, and globus pallidus), nucleus accumbens, and thalamus are buried deep within the forebrain.

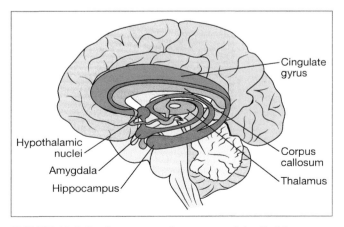

FIGURE 15.3 Limbic system. Structures of the limbic system include the amygdala (anterior to the hippocampus), the hippocampus that circles the thalamus, nuclei within the hypothalamus, and the cingulate gyrus that surrounds the corpus callosum.

hypothalamus; the cingulate gyrus, which circles the corpus callosum; and structures within the hypothalamus. Other brain regions that are interconnected with limbic structures and are sometimes grouped in this designation include the nucleus accumbens, entorhinal cortex, orbitofrontal cortex (OFC), and olfactory cortex.

Connections Between the Central Nervous System and the Periphery

The brain connects to peripheral tissues (skin, muscles, joints, internal organs, glands) through the peripheral nervous system. Cell bodies of sensory neurons and autonomic neurons are found in ganglia clustered outside the brainstem and spinal cord. All other connections of the peripheral nervous system are made by long axons that reach from brainstem and spinal cord to and from peripheral structures. Information enters the spinal cord and brain from the periphery through sensory (afferent) axons. Information from the spinal cord and the brain is carried to peripheral muscles, organs, glands, and blood vessels through somatic or autonomic efferent motor fibers.

Structural Brain Protection

The brain and spinal cord are encased in rigid bony structures of the skull and vertebral column, a first line of protection against traumatic injury. Within these bony structures, the brain and spinal cord are also surrounded by three meningeal layers—the dura, arachnoid, and pia mater, from outer to inner, respectively. Finally, between the arachnoid and pia mater is cerebrospinal fluid that further cushions the brain and reduces brain injury after trauma. The cerebrospinal fluid also circulates internally in the ventricles of the brain: two lateral ventricles and the third and fourth ventricles. Additional protection from circulating systemic toxins is provided by the blood–brain barrier (BBB). Endothelial cells of cerebral capillaries are joined with tight junctions that prevent blood-borne substances from reaching the brain tissue without specific transmembrane transport mechanisms. A few brain regions are free of a BBB, and they are specialized to detect toxins and other circulating substances monitored by the brain that link detection to homeostatic responses.

NEURONS
The Functional Units of the Brain

The adult human brain makes up about 2% of body weight and contains an estimated 100 billion neurons and twice as many glial cells. A typical neuron receives 1,000 to 10,000 synapses, and the total number of synapses in the cerebral cortex is estimated to be more than 100 trillion, which gives the brain excellent

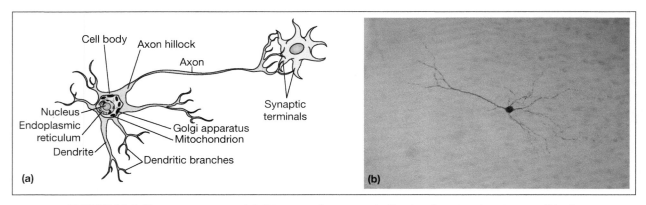

FIGURE 15.4 Neuron structure. **(a)** Diagram of a neuron indicating functional regions: cell body and dendrites, axon hillock and axon, and axon terminals forming synaptic contacts on target postsynaptic cell. **(b)** Photomicrograph of a neuron in rat cerebral cortex. The neuron is labeled with an antibody to HSP 72.
HSP, heat shock protein.

processing power. The structural components of a neuron are the cell body (soma), dendrites, axon, and axon terminal (**Figure 15.4**).

The cell body of the neuron contains much of the cytoplasm and many of the organelles, including the nucleus, endoplasmic reticulum, Golgi apparatus, ribosomes, and mitochondria. Extensions from the cell body comprise the dendritic tree. The dendrites have small projections termed *dendritic spines*, which are the site of many synaptic inputs. Each neuron also has a single axon, an output pathway that branches as it projects to target regions. At the end of each axon branch is the axon terminal, containing synaptic vesicles filled with neurotransmitters. Interneurons have short axons that make local projections. The axons of projection neurons can be a few feet long, for example, motor neurons that project from the spinal cord to the feet. Neuronal communication is both electrical and chemical, beginning with action potentials generated at the cell body and propagated to axon terminals, whereupon chemical transmitters are released.

The long axons of projection neurons are wrapped with myelin, an insulating membrane that supports propagation of the action potential. The myelin coat is interrupted by structures called nodes of Ranvier, where ion channels regenerate the action potential down the length of the axon. At the axon terminal, the cytoplasm contains many vesicles of transmitter, ready for exocytosis into the synapse when an action potential reaches the terminal.

Electrically Excitable Cells

The electrical activity of neurons reflects the properties and activities of proteins of the neuronal plasma membrane (**Figure 15.5**). This electrical activity consists of a negative resting membrane potential (RMP) interspersed with action potentials. The RMP is produced by (a) differing ionic composition of intracellular and extracellular fluids; (b) selective permeability of the neuron membrane, which at rest is more permeable to potassium than to any other ion; and (c) the sodium–potassium (Na^+/K^+) pump, which maintains the ionic composition of intracellular and extracellular fluid. At the resting potential, the cell interior of the neuron is negative with respect to the exterior. This is primarily due to the large concentration gradient favoring outward movement of potassium and the selective permeability of the membrane to potassium. Potassium moves out of the cell through potassium leak channels until the inside becomes negative enough to counteract the force of the concentration gradient that favors this outward movement. The voltage difference between the excess intracellular negative charges and the extracellular fluid can reach up to –90 mV (inside negative with respect to outside of the cell).

The negative RMP is necessary for the neuron to respond to stimuli and conduct impulses. Membrane voltage-gatedion channels can detect depolarization—a shift of the membrane potential toward a less negative value. If the membrane is sufficiently depolarized by synaptic or sensory inputs, a *threshold* voltage will be reached at which *fast* sodium channels open to initiate the action potential. Sodium channel opening allows sodium ions to rapidly enter the cell down their concentration gradient, depolarizing the membrane to a peak of approximately +20 mV. At the peak of this action potential upstroke, the sodium channels close and are briefly inactivated. Simultaneously, *delayed* voltage-gated potassium channels reach their fully open state. Potassium

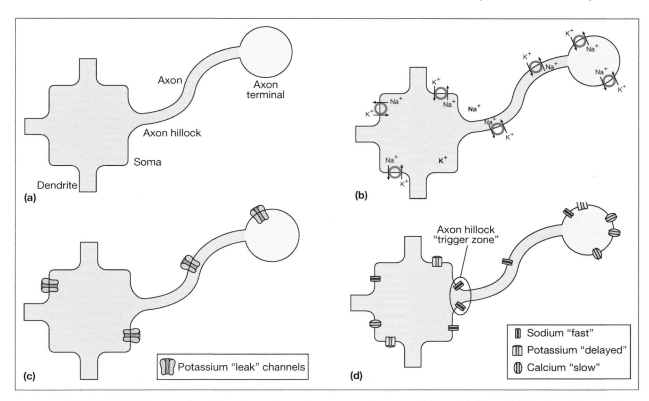

FIGURE 15.5 Neuron functions depend on plasma membrane proteins. **(a)** The distribution of characteristic membrane proteins to specific portions of the neuronal membrane is responsible for the functional properties of each part of the neuron. **(b)** The sodium–potassium pump (Na^+/K^+) is found in the membrane of every part of the neuron, and it is responsible for generating the differential distribution of ions that contribute to the resting membrane potential. **(c)** The presence of potassium leak channels gives neuronal membranes their highest permeability to potassium while they are at rest; thus, the resting membrane potential is close to the potassium equilibrium potential. **(d)** The three voltage-gated ion channels labeled at lower right shape most of neuronal function. **(1)** *Fast sodium channels* are responsible for the upstroke of the action potential. The great density of sodium channels at the axon hillock cause the action potential to be generated here for most neurons (except for sensory neurons). **(2)** *Delayed potassium channels* open as sodium channels are inactivating. These two events (delayed potassium channel opening plus sodium channel inactivation) lead to repolarization of the membrane back toward the resting membrane potential. **(3)** *Slow calcium channels* are found at axon terminals. When the action potential arrives at the axon terminal, opening of calcium channels allow calcium entry that directly leads to exocytosis of vesicles of neurotransmitter.

flows out, repolarizing and eventually reestablishing the negative RMP (**Figure 15.6**). Repolarization also resets the sodium channels so they are ready to be activated upon depolarization to threshold.

To summarize, the neuron membrane is enriched with proteins, including the sodium–potassium pump, potassium leak channels, and voltage-gated sodium and potassium channels. The negative RMP keeps voltage-gated sodium and potassium channels in a state of quiescence until some external input leads to a small level of membrane depolarization. Once membrane depolarization achieves a threshold level, voltage-gated sodium channels open rapidly, producing the upstroke of the action potential. After the action potential peak, sodium channels close, potassium channels open, and the membrane repolarizes and returns to the RMP. Neuronal action potential duration is <2 msec, and many neurons are capable of very rapid bursts of action potential firing—up to 200 action potentials per second. Calcium channels found in the membrane at axon terminals link the electrical depolarization of the action potential to calcium entry. Increased intracellular calcium levels cause release of vesicles of transmitter, converting an electrical signal to a chemical message in the process of synaptic transmission.

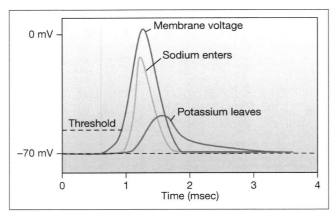

FIGURE 15.6 The neuronal action potential. The action potential consists of a brief depolarization from the RMP, sufficient to open voltage-gated "fast" sodium channels. Sodium channel opening leads to the upstroke of the action potential. As the membrane potential rises to 0 mV and beyond, the neuron membrane is briefly positive on the inside with respect to the outside. At the peak of the action potential, sodium channels close and inactivate, and "delayed" potassium channels open, leading to repolarization and restoration of the RMP.

RMP, resting membrane potential; msec, milliseconds; mV, millivolts.

 Thought Questions

1. How is the RMP established? What membrane proteins participate in establishing the RMP?

2. What additional membrane proteins does a neuron need to generate an action potential?

3. What sequence of events make up the neuronal action potential?

SYNAPTIC TRANSMISSION

Synapse Structure

A synapse is a point of contact between the presynaptic terminal of one neuron's axon and a postsynaptic membrane of the target neuron (**Figure 15.7**). The axon terminal is a swelling at the end of the axon, containing small transmitter-filled synaptic vesicles and mitochondria. The terminal is separated from the postsynaptic membrane by a narrow synaptic cleft. The presynaptic membrane is dense with proteins needed for exocytosis of transmitter vesicles, transporters, and receptors. The postsynaptic membrane also has a specialized dense region that is enriched in receptor proteins. Release of transmitter and diffusion across the synapse provides a brief synaptic delay between the presynaptic action potential and the electrical response of the postsynaptic membrane.

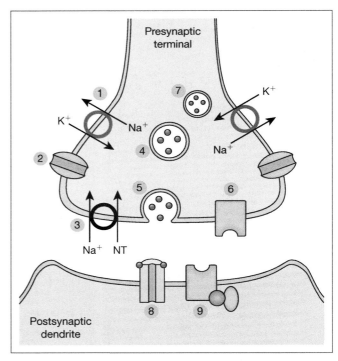

FIGURE 15.7 Components of a central nervous system synapse. (**1**) Sodium–potassium pump on the membrane, to maintain proper ion gradients and membrane potential. (**2**) Voltage-gated calcium channels that open when the action potential reaches the terminal; calcium entry signals for release of transmitter vesicles by exocytosis into the synaptic cleft. (**3**) Secondary active transport protein for the uptake of transmitter into the terminal prior to degradation or repackaging into vesicles. (**4**) Vesicles of transmitter. (**5**) Docking sites for vesicle exocytosis. (**6**) Presynaptic autoreceptors, or heteroceptors, that modulate the amount of transmitter released. (**7**) Enzymes for transmitter synthesis, breakdown, or both. (**8**) Postsynaptic ionotropic receptors, also known as ligand-gated ion channels. (**9**) Postsynaptic metabotropic receptors, also known as G-coupled receptors, shown with the associated G protein and enzyme.

NT, neurotransmitter.

Membrane proteins of the presynaptic membrane include the following:

- The sodium–potassium pump, to maintain normal ion gradients
- Voltage-gated sodium and potassium channels, for action potential propagation
- Voltage-gated calcium channels, to allow calcium entry as the signal for regulated exocytosis of transmitter
- Docking sites for vesicle exocytosis
- Secondary active transport proteins to remove transmitter from the cleft and return it to the cytoplasm of the terminal

Membrane proteins of the postsynaptic membrane include the following:

- Ionotropic receptors
- Metabotropic receptors
- Degradative enzymes to break down neurotransmitter—this is particularly common at synapses using the transmitter acetylcholine. These postsynaptic membranes are enriched in the enzyme acetylcholinesterase, which rapidly breaks down and inactivates acetylcholine.

Electrical and Chemical Events of Synaptic Transmission

Neurons communicate by the process of synaptic transmission. At any given time, if the inputs to a neuron provide sufficient excitation, that neuron will reach threshold to have one or more action potentials. The action potential of a presynaptic neuron results in release of a neurotransmitter—a chemical signal that excites or inhibits its postsynaptic target. If the postsynaptic neuron achieves sufficient excitation, it reaches threshold for its own action potential, and the resulting chain of signals culminates in a change of state, behavior, or movement.

Box 15.1 and Figure 15.8 outlines the process of synaptic transmission. At the cellular level, the effect of chemical synaptic inputs is to create small changes in membrane voltage termed *postsynaptic potentials* (PSPs). Excitatory chemical transmitters produce *excitatory* postsynaptic potentials (EPSPs). Inhibitory chemical transmitters produce *inhibitory* postsynaptic potentials (IPSPs). Threshold is reached when EPSPs exceed IPSPs.

Suppose the intracellular activity of a postsynaptic neuron is recorded during stimulation of excitatory and inhibitory inputs. A single firing of an excitatory synapse results in a modest depolarization, an EPSP, which is

---

BOX 15.1

Sequence of Synaptic Transmission

- The postsynaptic neuron reaches threshold when the number and frequency of EPSPs are greater than IPSPs (**Figure 15.8**).

- Electrical activity of a neuron in response to fast synaptic inputs depends on the nature of the chemical transmitter (excitatory or inhibitory). The neuron in **Figure 15.8** has excitatory inputs A and B (+) and inhibitory input C (−).

- Initially the neuron is at RMP of −70 mV.

- If input A is stimulated one time, the postsynaptic cell will have a brief depolarization (the EPSP), followed by a return to RMP.

- If input A is stimulated two times in close succession, or if inputs A and B are stimulated close together in time, the EPSPs may summate such that the depolarization reaches threshold voltage (V_{Thr}) to open fast sodium channels, and a neuronal action potential results.

- Stimulation of input C alone produces a hyperpolarization—called the IPSP.

- Finally, near-simultaneous stimulation of inputs A, B, and C shows the ability of the inhibitory synapse to prevent the neuron from reaching threshold; thus, no action potential results.

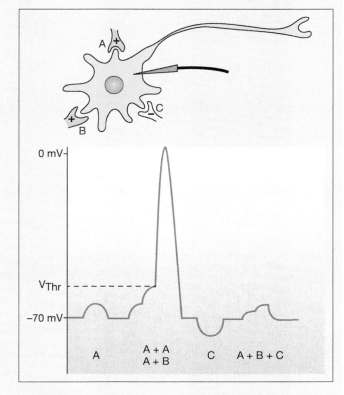

FIGURE 15.8 The basis of synaptic transmission. A and B = excitatory inputs; C = inhibitory input; V_{Thr}, threshold voltage.

EPSPs, excitatory postsynaptic potentials; IPSPs, inhibitory postsynaptic potentials; RMP, resting membrane potential.

not sufficient to reach threshold. If the excitatory input is stimulated two or more times in rapid succession, the EPSPs will build upon each other, and the neuron will achieve threshold and generate an action potential. This is referred to as temporal summation of activity. Another way to have sufficient postsynaptic excitation to reach threshold is to have stimulation of multiple excitatory inputs. Stimulation in close succession of several excitatory inputs to a single neuron will also bring a neuron to threshold for action potential generation, by the process of spatial summation. Inhibitory transmitters hyperpolarize the membrane potential, which makes it more difficult for the membrane to reach threshold. Stimulation of inhibitory inputs as excitatory impulses are occurring may prevent the neuron from reaching threshold.

To summarize, the changes in membrane potential created by synaptic transmitters can either create excitation, favoring action potential generation, or they can create inhibition, inhibiting action potential generation. The language that the nervous system uses is the generation of action potentials, depending on millions of ongoing EPSPs, IPSPs, and action potentials in a multitude of circuits. This activity is constant, even during sleep, and is monitored by the electroencephalogram (EEG).

Neurotransmitter Receptors

Two major classes of transmitter receptors are found on neuronal membranes: ionotropic receptors and metabotropic receptors (**Figure 15.9**).

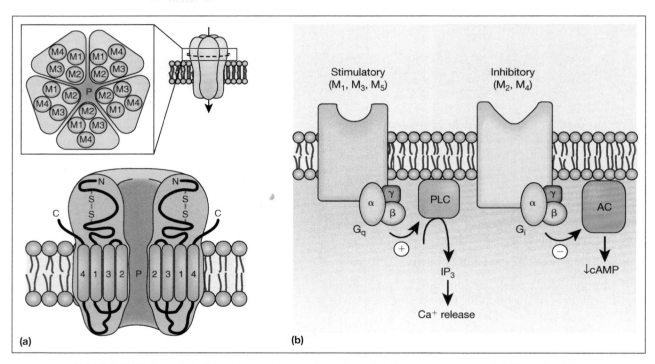

FIGURE 15.9 Acetylcholine acts at ionotropic and metabotropic receptors. (**a**) The nicotinic acetylcholine receptor is a pentameric protein. The five subunits all span the membrane and are arranged around the central pore (P). Each subunit has an extracellular amino end (N), carboxyl end (C), and an intrachain disulfide bond (S-S). There are two acetylcholine binding sites, and when both are occupied with transmitter, the pore opens to allow the movement of sodium and potassium ions. This produces membrane depolarization, sufficient to bring the neuron to threshold for action potential initiation. All ionotropic neurotransmitter receptors have similar structures. (**b**) There are five subtypes of metabotropic AC receptors. These are named muscarinic receptors (M), M_1 through M_5. M_1, M_3, and M_5 receptors are linked to G_q, and ligand binding results in activation of PLC with subsequent production of DAG and IP_3. IP_3 then releases calcium (Ca^{2+}) from the endoplasmic reticulum. Overall, this subgroup of receptors produces slow neuronal excitation. M_2 and M_4 receptors link to G_i, inhibiting adenylyl cyclase and reducing cAMP formation. These receptors are associated with slow neuronal inhibition.

AC, adenylyl cyclase; cAMP, cyclic adenosine monophosphate; DAG, diacylglycerol; IP_3, inositol triphosphate; PLC, phospholipase C.

Ionotropic receptors are also known as ligand-gated ion channels. They are multimeric proteins surrounding a central pore typical of ion channels, and they are selective in their ion permeability. In the extracellular portion of the protein, there are one or two binding sites for the neurotransmitter ligand. Binding of transmitter to that recognition site opens the ion channel, allowing ion movements that either depolarize or hyperpolarize the membrane. The bulk of rapid neuronal signaling involves EPSPs and IPSPs due to ionotropic receptor activation. Excitatory ionotropic receptors have selectivity for sodium, as well as potassium or calcium, or both. Inhibitory ionotropic receptors are selective for chloride.

Metabotropic receptors are G protein–coupled receptors that create slower changes in membrane potential through second messenger cascades and indirect opening or closing of ion channels. Signaling by metabotropic neurotransmitter receptors can be thought of as slow modulation of ongoing activity, rather than rapid signaling that characterizes ionotropic receptor function. Virtually all ionotropic receptors are found at synapses, whereas there is a wider distribution of metabotropic receptors. Many metabotropic receptors are located at synapses, while others are found on cell bodies and axon terminals at some distance from the site of transmitter release. Some of these extrasynaptic receptors are autoreceptors and heteroceptors that inhibit release of their own ligands or other transmitters, respectively. This finding particularly applies to transmission by neuropeptides.

The first identified neurotransmitter, acetylcholine, has both nicotinic (ionotropic) receptors and muscarinic (metabotropic) receptors that illustrate general properties of these receptor types. The names of the receptors are based on pharmacology experiments that demonstrated the ability of nicotine or muscarine to activate the receptors. The nicotinic acetylcholine receptor is found in the brain, in autonomic ganglia, and at the neuromuscular junction. The nicotinic receptor is a multi-subunit transmembrane protein. The quaternary structure has five membrane-spanning regions surrounding a central pore that is permeable to sodium and potassium. When acetylcholine binds, the pore opens, and there is a large influx of sodium, with a much smaller efflux of potassium. As a result, the postsynaptic membrane depolarizes to threshold and has an action potential. Similar excitatory ligand-gated ion channels are responsible for many of the neuronal EPSPs that lead to action potential generation. The nicotinic receptor of the neuromuscular junction is the target of antibodies in the autoimmune disease *myasthenia gravis.*

Muscarinic acetylcholine receptors are found in the brain and in peripheral organs and glands that are modulated by the parasympathetic nervous system. These metabotropic receptors are serpentine, G protein–coupled receptors, as described in Chapter 4, Cell Physiology and Pathophysiology. As with all serpentine receptors, muscarinic receptors have seven membrane-spanning regions. There are five muscarinic receptor subtypes, labeled M_1 through M_5. Within this family, M_1, M_3, and M_5 are coupled to G_q and to activation of phospholipase C. They may also open calcium channels and close potassium channels, resulting in slow neuronal excitation. In contrast, M_2 and M_4 receptors couple to G_i, inhibiting adenylyl cyclase. They may also close calcium channels and open potassium channels, resulting in slow neuronal inhibition. In addition to electrophysiological changes, these serpentine receptors also produce intracellular changes such as altered gene expression, creating prolonged changes in neuron function.[5]

To summarize, the effect of a given neurotransmitter on its postsynaptic target may be excitatory or inhibitory, and the effect may have short or long duration. All of these possibilities depend on the specific receptors for that transmitter that are present on the postsynaptic membrane. The vast repertoire of ionotropic and metabotropic receptors available creates the richness of options for neuron signaling and function, and are the basis of many pharmacological interventions.

Termination of Synaptic Transmission

As in all biological systems, for every *on* switch, there is at least one *off* switch. What are the mechanisms by which transmitter action is terminated, allowing the neuron's return to its original resting state?

There are three principal ways that transmitter action is terminated: (a) uptake into the presynaptic terminal, (b) enzymatic transmitter breakdown, and (c) diffusion away from the synapse (**Figure 15.10**). The most common mechanism of transmitter inactivation is the removal of transmitter from the synapse by a secondary active transport protein on the presynaptic terminal. This process is sometimes referred to as *reuptake* and depends on the favorable concentration gradient for sodium to enter the cell, owing to the action of the sodium–potassium pump. For each molecule of transmitter removed from the synapse, a sodium ion enters the cell, down its concentration gradient. As the transmitter moves away from the receptor sites, back into the synaptic cleft, the presynaptic transporter returns the transmitter molecule to the axon terminal where other proteins package it into synaptic vesicles. This mechanism gives the efficiency

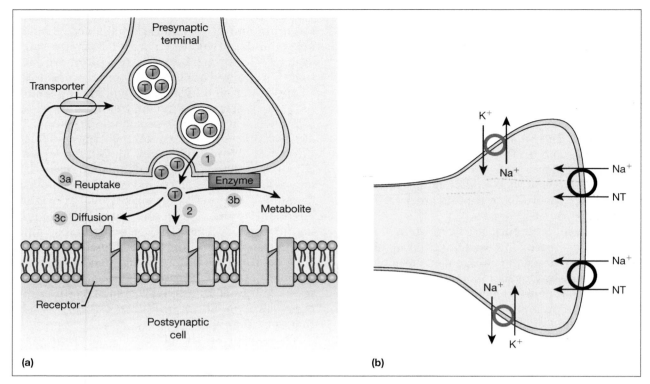

FIGURE 15.10 Termination of transmitter action. **(a)** Neurotransmitter molecules (T) are released into the synaptic cleft **(1)**, reversibly bind to receptors on the postsynaptic cell **(2)**, and are removed from the cleft by transporter-mediated reuptake into the presynaptic nerve terminal **(3a)**, enzymatic degradation **(3b)**, or diffusion **(3c)**. **(b)** Reuptake is a form of secondary active transport. Perpetual activity of the sodium–potassium pump maintains a high concentration gradient for sodium (Na^+) across the cell membrane. Movement of sodium "downhill" (i.e., into the cell) is linked to the "uphill" movement of a molecule of NT *against* its concentration gradient. This allows the removal of most of the neurotransmitter molecules out of the synaptic cleft and back into the axon terminal, where they will be repackaged into vesicles.
NT, neurotransmitter.

of recycling molecules of transmitter, reducing the amount of time and energy needed to synthesize new transmitter. Presynaptic transporters can be the target of pharmacological modulation of neurotransmission in the form of drugs that inhibit reuptake. One of the most famous of these is the selective serotonin reuptake mechanism, which is the target of the antidepressant drug class known as selective serotonin reuptake inhibitors (SSRIs). These agents target and block this transporter protein, increasing the half-life of serotonin in the synapse.

The second way that neurotransmission is terminated is by enzymes that break down the transmitter in the synaptic cleft. The main example of this mechanism is the breakdown of acetylcholine by the enzyme acetylcholinesterase. There are several cholinesterase enzymes, and they are abundant in the brain and at the neuromuscular junction, because acetylcholine is the neuromuscular transmitter. As acetylcholine diffuses away from its postsynaptic receptor sites, it is immediately degraded into a free acetyl group and a molecule of choline. Choline is then selectively transported into the presynaptic terminal, where it is used to synthesize new acetylcholine. Enzymatic breakdown is also the target of drug actions; for example, some drugs used in the treatment of myasthenia gravis and Alzheimer disease block acetylcholinesterase. Certain antidepressants block the enzyme monoamine oxidase (MAO), which breaks down dopamine, norepinephrine, and serotonin.

The third method of transmission termination is by diffusion of the transmitter away from the synaptic cleft. For example, peptide transmitters are generally too large for membrane transporters, and their action ends when they diffuse away from the synapse and are degraded by extracellular proteases.

Thought Questions

4. How does an ionotropic receptor work?

5. Excitatory ionotropic receptors are permeable to which ions? What is the principal ion associated with inhibition?

6. Would a protective reflex (such as rapid withdrawal of your hand after touching a flame) be more likely to involve ionotropic or metabotropic receptors? Why?

7. How is neurotransmitter action terminated? Give examples of proteins involved in terminating transmitter activity.

NEUROTRANSMITTERS

TWO MAIN TRANSMITTER FAMILIES

There are two main families of neurotransmitters, differentiated by their speed of signaling, functions, chemistry, and anatomy (**Figure 15.11**). The major amino acid transmitters, glutamate and gamma-aminobutyric acid (GABA), are the most prominent rapid transmitters and are present in the brain in the greatest concentration (**Figure 15.12**). These transmitters are the workhorses of organized, continual brain function in the processes of sensory and motor activity, reflex and voluntary movements, and learning and cognition. The rapid actions of glutamate and GABA are mediated by

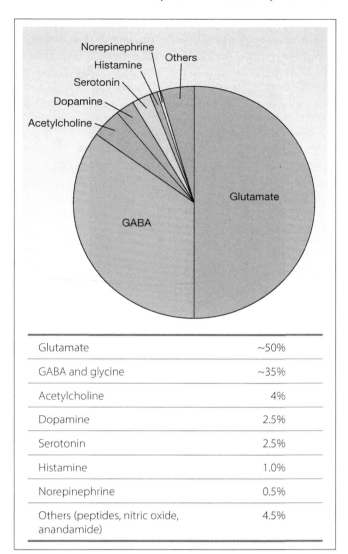

Glutamate	~50%
GABA and glycine	~35%
Acetylcholine	4%
Dopamine	2.5%
Serotonin	2.5%
Histamine	1.0%
Norepinephrine	0.5%
Others (peptides, nitric oxide, anandamide)	4.5%

FIGURE 15.12 Relative abundance of neurotransmitters in the brain. Percentages are approximate. GABA, gamma-aminobutyric acid.

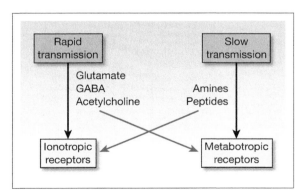

FIGURE 15.11 Modes of neurotransmission differ between neurotransmitter families. Glutamate, GABA, and acetylcholine have rapid actions mediated by ionotropic receptors, with additional actions mediated by metabotropic receptors. Amines (such as dopamine, norepinephrine, and serotonin), as well as peptides (such as orexins and enkephalins), have slower actions mediated almost exclusively by metabotropic receptors. The major exception is the type 3 serotonin receptor (5-HT$_3$ receptor), which is an ionotropic receptor. GABA, gamma-aminobutyric acid.

ionotropic receptors, although each of these transmitters also has metabotropic receptors. Glutamate and GABA-containing neurons are distributed across virtually all brain regions.

Transmission by small molecule amines and larger peptides is more diffuse and modulatory in character. These transmitters usually target metabotropic receptors, having relatively slow and prolonged synaptic effects on postsynaptic targets. Cell bodies of neurons containing amine and peptide transmitters are characteristically found in tight cell clusters in the brainstem or hypothalamus. The axon terminal morphology of amine neurons differs from classic synaptic morphology. Many amine axons have varicosities along the axon, each of which contains vesicles of transmitters. This method of neurotransmission can be thought of as functioning like a garden *soaker* hose that distributes water over a wider region of garden than a traditional hose. Through this method of transmission, a relatively small number of amine neurons can modulate activity in large regions of cerebral cortex. Peptides also have greater anatomical spread in their effects; as they diffuse away from the terminals where they are released, they can bind to receptors at a distance from that site. In the nomenclature of neuroscience, neurons and synapses are named based on the principal neurotransmitter that they contain: glutamate—glutamatergic neurons; GABA—GABAergic; acetylcholine—cholinergic; dopamine—dopaminergic; and so on.

Glutamate

Glutamate is the principal excitatory transmitter of the brain. As an amino acid, glutamate is found in all cells and tissues. Glutamate can be taken into cells by a specific amino acid transporter, or it can be produced intracellularly by addition of an amine group to α-ketoglutarate, a Krebs cycle intermediate. In glutamatergic neurons, much of the glutamate comes from removal of an amine group from glutamine. Vesicular transporters package glutamate into synaptic vesicles for release as a neurotransmitter.

Release of glutamate into the synaptic cleft is followed by binding to one or more types of postsynaptic glutamate receptors (**Figure 15.13**). There are two major types of ionotropic glutamate receptors: they are distinguished by their sensitivity to the selective pharmacological agonists α-amino-3-hydroxyl-5-methyl-4-isoxazole-propionate (AMPA receptors) and *N*-methyl-D-aspartate (NMDA receptors). Binding of glutamate to these receptors opens ion channels permeable to sodium and potassium (AMPA receptors) or to sodium, potassium, and calcium (NMDA receptors); both receptors produce postsynaptic EPSPs. The significant difference between AMPA receptor activation and NMDA receptor activation is that opening NMDA receptor channels increases intracellular *calcium* in postsynaptic neurons. Transient calcium elevation in postsynaptic cells is the key to the long-term consequences of NMDA receptor activation, including a role in learning and memory formation.

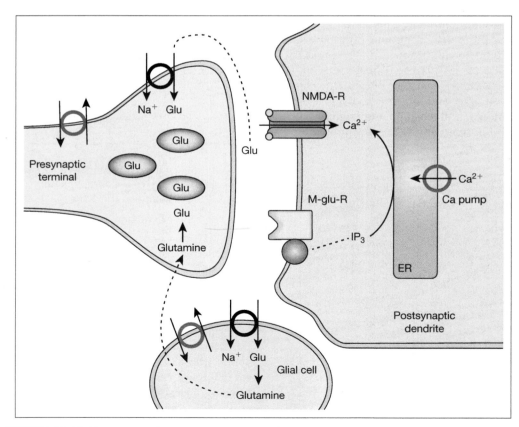

FIGURE 15.13 Events at a glutamatergic synapse. See text for details.
Ca^{2+}, calcium; ER, endoplasmic reticulum; Glu, glutamate; M-glu-R, metabotropic glutamate receptor; IP_3, inositol triphosphate; Na^+, sodium; NMDA-R, *N*-methyl-D-aspartate receptor.

There are several subtypes of metabotropic glutamate receptors, and their action on postsynaptic cells is slow and modulatory, unlike the effects of AMPA and NMDA activation. Some of the metabotropic glutamate receptors link to G_q proteins, thereby increasing postsynaptic inositol triphosphate (IP_3) and inducing release of calcium from the endoplasmic reticulum. Thus, glutamate transmission has at least two potential pathways by which it can increase intracellular calcium.

Termination of glutamate signaling occurs when glutamate diffuses away and is cleared from the synapse by transporters on glial cells surrounding the synapse and into the presynaptic terminal. Glutamate that enters glial cells is converted to glutamine. After this conversion, glutamine is transported out of the glial cell and returns to the presynaptic terminal of the glutamatergic neuron. In the neuron's terminal, the amine is removed by glutaminase, regenerating glutamate that can be repacked into vesicles. **Box 15.2** summarizes the steps in glutamatergic transmission.

It is significant that removal of glutamate from the synapse indirectly requires adenosine triphosphate (ATP), as does the glial conversion of glutamate to glutamine. The principal pathophysiological condition associated with glutamate neurotransmission is *excitotoxicity*, in which neurons are literally excited to death by excess glutamate transmission. Conditions associated with **excitotoxic neuron death** include states of hypoxia and ischemia, such as stroke and traumatic brain injury. In these conditions, excess glutamate is released due to local depolarization causing repeated action potentials (**Figure 15.14**). The lack of oxygen causes mitochondrial ATP production to fail; this is rapidly followed by failure of the membrane sodium–potassium pump. Sodium builds up intracellularly, and potassium leaks into the extracellular fluid, depolarizing the membrane. With the loss of the normal sodium gradient, the sodium–glutamate uptake transporter fails, and glutamate cannot be cleared from the synapse. In addition, glutamate accumulates intracellularly and extracellularly as a result of the inability of glial cells to convert it to glutamine.

The consequence of excessive glutamate transmission is the buildup of calcium in neurons, secondary to excessive activation of both NMDA and metabotropic glutamate receptors. Depletion of ATP means the endoplasmic reticulum calcium pump is unable to restore the normally low intracellular calcium concentration. Intracellular calcium overload activates enzymes that degrade cell components. These degradative enzymes—phospholipases, proteases, and endonucleases—break down plasma membrane, cell proteins, and nucleic acids, resulting in neuron death.

Excitotoxic neuron death is thought to be a major mechanism of irreversible brain injury after stroke and trauma. Excitotoxic neuron death is also hypothesized to contribute to neurodegenerative disorders such as Alzheimer disease and amyotrophic lateral sclerosis. The NMDA receptor blocker memantine is sometimes used in these conditions, in an attempt to reduce NMDA stimulation, neuronal calcium overload, and neuron death.

Gamma-Aminobutyric Acid

Balancing the excitatory actions of glutamate is GABA, the principal inhibitory transmitter of the brain. GABA is widely distributed in all brain regions, primarily in local interneurons. GABA is synthesized from glutamate by glutamate decarboxylase (GAD). GABA transmission is terminated by secondary active transport into the presynaptic terminal. There

---

BOX 15.2
Summary of Glutamatergic Transmission

1. Synthesis of glutamate in the axon terminal, and packaging into vesicles

2. Release of synaptic vesicles when the action potential reaches the terminal

3. Diffusion across the synaptic cleft and binding to ionotropic and metabotropic glutamate receptors

4. Excitation of the postsynaptic cell, with depolarization and increased intracellular calcium

5. Diffusion of glutamate away from the receptor, and uptake by secondary active transport, either into a nearby glial cell or to the presynaptic terminal

6. Glial cell conversion of glutamate to glutamine

7. Glutamine release from the glial cell and return to the glutamatergic neuron terminal

8. Conversion of glutamine to glutamate and repackaging into vesicles

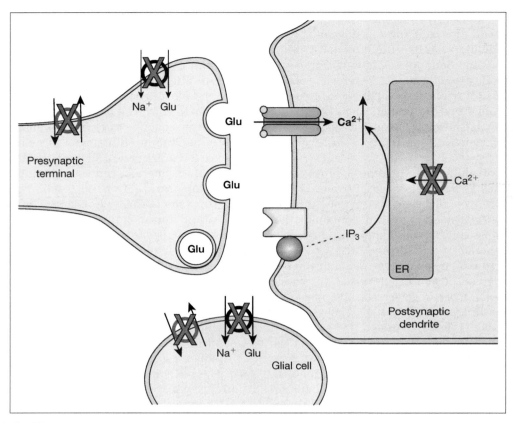

FIGURE 15.14 Glutamate excitotoxicity. Red Xs indicate loss of active transport (sodium/potassium and calcium ATPases) and secondary active transport activities owing to lack of ATP production. Glutamate builds up in the synapse, continually stimulating calcium influx through NMDA receptors and ER calcium release by metabotropic glutamate receptors. Calcium overload initiates degradative enzyme activity that leads to neuron death.

Ca^{2+}, calcium; ER, endoplasmic reticulum; Glu, glutamate; IP_3, inositol triphosphate; Na^+, sodium.

are two major GABA receptors, both of which have inhibitory postsynaptic effects: the ionotropic $GABA_A$ receptor, and the metabotropic $GABA_B$ receptor (**Figure 15.15**).

The $GABA_A$ receptor pore is selective for chloride. When GABA binds to the receptor and the pore opens, chloride enters the postsynaptic neuron and causes hyperpolarization of the postsynaptic membrane, producing an IPSP. The $GABA_A$ receptor is modulated by a variety of drugs of the barbiturate and benzodiazepine classes, as well as by ethanol. Although these agents are not sufficient to open the channel in the absence of GABA, their presence synergizes with GABA and increases the amount of chloride that enters the pore, strengthening inhibitory transmission. Drugs that enhance GABA transmission are indicated as treatments for epilepsy, anxiety, and insomnia. Sedation, drug tolerance, and dependence are adverse effects of $GABA_A$ agonists.

The $GABA_B$ receptor is a metabotropic receptor. When GABA binds to the $GABA_B$ receptor, the cascade of intracellular signals opens potassium channels, closes calcium channels, and inhibits adenylyl cyclase, reducing cyclic adenosine monophosphate (cAMP). Overall, this results in slow inhibition. The antispasticity drug baclofen is an agonist at $GABA_B$ receptors.

Epilepsy Results From Excessive Excitation or Insufficient Inhibition

The contribution of ion channels, glutamate, and GABA to normal neuron function can be seen when studying the pathophysiology and pharmacology of **epilepsy**. Epilepsy syndromes are defined as disorders in which recurrent and unpredictable seizures occur. Seizures are episodes of highly synchronized action potential activity by large numbers of cortical neurons. Such activity can be detected as bursts of high-voltage electrical depolarizations and repolarizations on the EEG. Recording during a focal seizure may show only a few leads with synchronized waves; recording during a generalized seizure shows widespread synchronized activity (**Figure 15.16**). Seizures are usually time limited, lasting <2 minutes, but the worst-case scenario is status epilepticus, an unremitting seizure state that requires prompt, aggressive treatment.

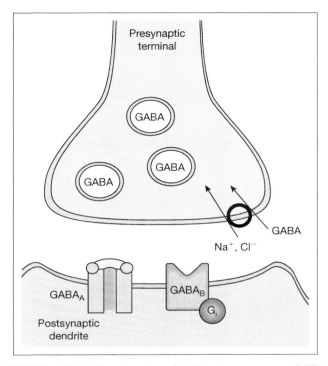

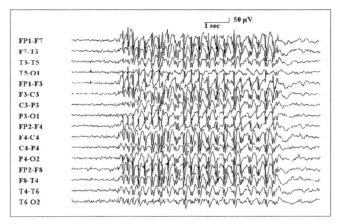

FIGURE 15.16 EEG recorded during a seizure of a patient with absence epilepsy. Synchronized electrical activity is seen across all leads of the EEG, indicating simultaneous electrical discharges in large numbers of cortical neurons. Successive waves of depolarization and repolarization of many cells lasts for several seconds before spontaneously ending.
Source: From Sheth RD, Benbadis SR. EEG in Common Epilepsy Syndromes. https://emedicine.medscape.com/article/1138154-overview#a5.

FIGURE 15.15 Events at a GABAergic synapse. GABA transmission is characterized by two major inhibitory receptors. The GABA_A receptor is an ionotropic receptor. When two molecules of GABA bind, the pore opens and permits chloride (Cl⁻) to diffuse from the extracellular fluid into the cell, rapidly hyperpolarizing the membrane and producing an IPSP. The GABA_B receptor is a metabotropic receptor. When GABA binds, it activates the G_i protein, inhibiting adenylyl cyclase and reducing the levels of cAMP in the cell. In addition, activation of the GABA_B receptor is linked to opening of potassium channels and closing of calcium channels. All of these actions result in a slow inhibitory effect. Termination of GABA signaling is by the presynaptic GABA transporter, a secondary active transport protein that cotransports GABA with sodium (Na⁺), or chloride, or both.
cAMP, cyclic adenosine monophosphate; GABA, gamma-aminobutyric acid; G_i, inhibitory G protein; IPSP, inhibitory postsynaptic potential.

In many cases, the cause of epilepsy is unknown. Epilepsy can show familial clustering, but often a single causative gene has not been identified. Brain trauma, stroke, and tumors, among other causes, can precipitate epilepsy, while alcohol and drug withdrawal may be associated with isolated, but not recurrent, seizures. The relationship between age and epilepsy is U-shaped: onset of epilepsy is most common in childhood, new epilepsy diagnosis is at the lowest levels from ages 20 to 60, and epilepsy incidence increases after age 60. (Seizure disorders in children are discussed in more detail later in this chapter.)

Genetic disorders producing epilepsy present in childhood, and sometimes give clues as to the nature of changes in neuronal function that may underlie idiopathic epilepsy. Monogenic causes of epilepsy can result from mutations of protein subunits of sodium, potassium, or calcium channels. Recall that the upstroke of the action potential is due to sodium channel activation that depolarizes the cell, and repolarization of the action potential is due to opening of potassium channels. Based on these mechanisms, mutations that increase sodium channel excitability or function or mutations that decrease potassium channel excitability or function are expected to promote neuronal hyperexcitability and seizures. Mutations that disrupt function of GABA_A receptors also cause epilepsy by reducing the effectiveness of GABA inhibition.

Pharmacological management of epilepsy is through antiepileptic drugs that target ion channels and transmitter receptors to decrease excitation or increase inhibition. Phenytoin, one of the first antiepileptic drugs to be widely used, blocks fast sodium channel activity, inhibiting action potential formation. Valproic acid blocks both sodium and calcium channel activity. Topiramate and felbamate block glutamate receptors, reducing activity of this main excitatory transmitter. Benzodiazepines and barbiturates enhance the activity of GABA_A receptors, promoting generalized inhibition. Antiepileptic drugs as a class have many drug interactions as well as predictably having sedative effects, yet they are generally effective and are often required lifelong by the person with epilepsy.

Thought Questions

8. What are the rapid-acting transmitters, and what is the cellular mechanism of action of each?

9. Excessive amounts of glutamate can damage and kill neurons. What are the normal mechanisms protecting neurons from glutamate excitotoxicity? How are these mechanisms disrupted during a stroke?

NEUROMODULATORY TRANSMITTERS: AMINES

The remaining transmitters are distinctive in that the overwhelming majority of their receptors are metabotropic, having slow effects on membrane potentials and exerting other second messenger–mediated postsynaptic effects. Many of these transmitters are associated with changes of behavioral state, including sleep, waking, and alerting; hunger and satiety; emotional responses; and pleasure and motivation. Such changes do not appear to require the rapid-acting transmission of glutamate and GABA; rather, they can be accomplished by slower synaptic transmission and other slow changes in neuron structure and function. Examples of long-lasting postsynaptic effects include changes in gene expression, in numbers of synapses, and in types and distributions of receptors.

These neurons using small molecule transmitters differ from glutamatergic and GABAergic neurons in their anatomy, histology, and physiology. Their cell bodies are found in distinct clusters, usually in the hypothalamus or brainstem. An exception is the acetylcholine system, which has cell clusters in the basal forebrain as well as the brainstem and numerous interneurons in the striatum. Histologically, the synaptic structures of neuromodulatory transmitters differ from classic synapses in that their axons have several swellings along their length in target regions, resembling beads on a string. Neurotransmitter vesicles can be found in each of these swellings (also called varicosities). Action potentials propagated down these axons release transmitter from each swelling, and the synaptic clefts are wider than those of classic synapses. In this manner, the neuromodulatory transmitters can easily diffuse to many target neurons in a region, having regional effects rather than discrete inputs to a small number of target cells. Release of these transmitters from their presynaptic terminals is the target of negative feedback in the form of presynaptic autoreceptors that inhibit further transmitter release. The cell bodies and presynaptic terminals of these neurons are also modulated by heteroceptors—receptors for one or more modulatory transmitters. Through this modulation, overall tone of

the modulatory systems can be upregulated or downregulated, globally changing behavioral state.

Scores, if not hundreds, of drugs work on one or more of these transmitter systems, targeting pre- and postsynaptic receptors, uptake mechanisms, vesicular packaging transporters, or degradative enzymes. The relationship between the biological mechanisms of action (determined in lab-based research) and resulting clinical efficacy (determined by clinical trials) is not always clear. It is important to note that, despite this lack of clarity, these psychoactive agents have proved useful for many patients with disabling conditions, including depression, anxiety, and related diagnoses.

Acetylcholine

Acetylcholine was identified as a neurotransmitter in 1915 by Henry Dale, who demonstrated that this compound was capable of slowing the rate of beating of frog hearts. This was subsequently confirmed by Otto Loewi in Germany. This was the first demonstration of chemical synaptic transmission, and the experiments of Dale and Loewi explained the mechanism of action of vagal nerve stimulation to slow the heart rate. Acetylcholine is abundant in the peripheral nervous system as the neurotransmitter of the neuromuscular junction, of all autonomic preganglionic neurons, and of all parasympathetic and some sympathetic postganglionic neurons. As a consequence, the peripheral actions of acetylcholine were the first to be identified for any neurotransmitter. Acetylcholine is also a relatively abundant central neurotransmitter.

Acetylcholine is synthesized from acetyl coenzyme A and choline by choline acetyltransferase. As previously noted, acetylcholine can act at metabotropic muscarinic and ionotropic nicotinic receptors, whose names are derived from naturally derived compounds that were shown to activate such receptors. There are five subtypes of muscarinic receptors, all of which are G protein–coupled receptors. M_1, M_3, and M_5 produce postsynaptic excitation, M_2 and M_4 produce postsynaptic inhibition. Cholinergic transmission is terminated with synaptic degradation by acetylcholinesterases, a highly active family of enzymes found in both brain and periphery. After acetylcholinesterase splits acetylcholine into choline and acetate, the choline is returned to the presynaptic terminal by an uptake transporter, where it can be used to regenerate acetylcholine (**Figure 15.17**).

Cholinergic neurons in the brain are found in clusters in the basal forebrain and in the brainstem. The forebrain nucleus basalis of Meynert and other forebrain cholinergic neurons project widely throughout the cerebral cortex and to the hippocampus, and have a role in alerting and in learning and memory. Cholinergic neurons in the brainstem are implicated in the initiation of rapid eye movement (REM) sleep

in Parkinson disease, and the motor manifestations of the disorder are primarily due to this loss. The second main cluster of dopamine neurons is found in the midbrain ventral tegmental area (VTA). Dopamine neurons of the VTA project to the basal forebrain and to limbic structures such as the hippocampus, amygdala, medial prefrontal cortex (PFC), and other limbic regions of the cerebral cortex. A general function of the dopamine pathways from the VTA appears to be to facilitate motivated behaviors.

One specific basal forebrain structure innervated by VTA dopamine neurons is the nucleus accumbens. This input to the nucleus accumbens is thought to contribute to the sensation of pleasure, while also providing a neural substrate for **addiction** and addictive behaviors. The third cluster of dopamine neurons is in the hypothalamus, where short projection neurons located close to the pituitary stalk provide dopamine to the pituitary. Upon reaching the anterior pituitary gland, dopamine functions to inhibit pituitary prolactin secretion. Dopamine is also enriched in the gut, as a signaling agent in the enteric nervous system. Dopamine antagonists can be used to treat nausea.

There are at least five dopamine receptors, labeled D_1 through D_5. Receptors D_1 and D_5 act through the G_s protein to stimulate adenylyl cyclase and cAMP formation. Receptors D_2, D_3, and D_4 act through G_i and are sometimes inhibitory. Some dopaminergic synapses have D_2 inhibitory autoreceptors (**Figure 15.19**).

In addition to Parkinson disease, mentioned earlier, pathological states of dopaminergic transmission include schizophrenia, and addiction. **Parkinson disease** occurs when substantia nigra dopamine neurons degenerate, depleting the striatum of dopamine. This disrupts motor-processing circuits, producing tremor, rigidity, bradykinesia, and postural instability, as discussed later in this chapter. Some characteristics of Parkinson disease, particularly tremor, are due to relative overactivity of striatal cholinergic transmission—an imbalance resulting from the lack of the normally opposing dopamine tone. Thus, pharmacological management of Parkinson disease can include antagonists of cholinergic transmission.

The pathogenesis of **schizophrenia** is not known at this time; however, it has been well established that the positive signs of schizophrenia (delusions, hallucinations, and mania) are reduced or abolished by first-generation (typical) antipsychotics as well as second-generation (atypical) antipsychotics. The hallmark of these drugs is usually an ability to block D_2 receptors. Most hypotheses of addiction invoke a role for the dopaminergic projection from the VTA to the nucleus accumbens.

Norepinephrine

Norepinephrine is abundant in the periphery, as it is the transmitter of most sympathetic postganglionic neurons. Within the brain, norepinephrine

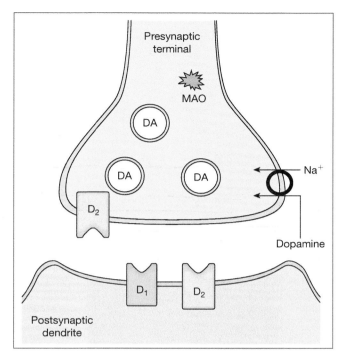

FIGURE 15.19 Dopaminergic synapse. DA is synthesized in a two-step process. In the first step, the amino acid tyrosine is converted to dopa by the enzyme tyrosine hydroxylase. In the second step, a carboxyl group is removed by the enzyme dopa decarboxylase, producing DA. DA is packaged into vesicles and released into the synapse, where it diffuses to the postsynaptic membrane and can bind to excitatory D_1 or inhibitory D_2 receptors, as well as other DA receptor subtypes. DA release can be regulated by presynaptic D_2 inhibitory receptors. The DA transporter is responsible for uptake of DA to the presynaptic terminal, where some of the transmitter will be repackaged into vesicles, and other molecules will be degraded by the enzyme MAO.

DA, dopamine; MAO, monoamine oxidase; Na+, sodium.

neurons are clustered in the locus ceruleus—a small nucleus in the rostral pons (see **Figure 15.18a**). The total number of locus ceruleus neurons bilaterally is approximately 25,000 norepinephrine neurons. Additional norepinephrine neurons occur in cell clusters in the pons and brainstem, and these clusters play a role in autonomic control. However, as modulators of behavioral brain function, the locus ceruleus neurons are primary, projecting widely to distribute norepinephrine throughout the cerebral cortex and the cerebellum.

A general function of cerebral norepinephrine is to set the tone of behavioral arousal and responsiveness. Locus ceruleus neurons are active during waking, with decreased activity during slow-wave sleep, but are completely silent during REM sleep. In animal models, the rate and pattern of action potentials in the locus ceruleus also relate to behavioral state. Focused attention is associated with neuron bursts of action potentials, while stress and hyperactivation are associated with a faster and more continuous rate of action potential firing. Norepinephrine also influences motivation, mood, and affect, and descending norepinephrine pathways to the spinal cord also modulate pain transmission. Central norepinephrine transmission also stimulates sympathetic nervous system outflow, increasing heart rate and blood pressure.

Norepinephrine receptors include β-adrenergic receptors that link through G_s to adenylyl cyclase, and α-adrenergic receptors that link through G_q to phospholipase C. Norepinephrine release is decreased by presynaptic $α_2$-receptors that are the targets of drugs such as clonidine. Certain antidepressants nonselectively (tricyclic antidepressants [TCAs]) or selectively (selective norepinephrine reuptake inhibitors) decrease the activity of norepinephrine, increasing the synaptic concentration of this neurotransmitter (**Figure 15.20**).

Pathological norepinephrine transmission is hypothesized to play a role in **post-traumatic stress disorder** (PTSD) and in **attention-deficit/hyperactivity disorder** (ADHD). In both of these conditions, patients present with deficits in focused attention, while having increased arousal and hyperactive emotional responsiveness to stimuli. Some pharmacological approaches to these conditions include drugs, such as amphetamines, that release norepinephrine from synaptic terminals. However, both amphetamines and methylphenidate (Ritalin) also release dopamine from terminals, so the beneficial effects of these medications may be due to altered norepinephrine or dopamine synaptic levels.

Serotonin

Serotonin was first identified in the gut and in platelets. The role of platelet serotonin is to promote vasoconstriction. In the brain, the chemical structure, anatomy, and synaptic function of serotonin are conceptually similar to dopamine and norepinephrine. However, serotonin is derived from the amino acid tryptophan, rather than tyrosine. Its chemical name is 5-hydroxytryptamine, so serotonin is abbreviated as 5-HT. Tryptophan hydroxylase converts tryptophan to 5-hydroxytryptophan, which is subsequently converted to 5-hydroxytryptamine. In the pineal gland, an additional enzyme converts serotonin into melatonin, which is a cue for sleep onset. Serotonin is broken down by MAO. Serotonin neurons are found in discrete clusters, termed the *raphe nuclei*, within the brainstem. Projections from these nuclei are widely distributed within the brainstem and throughout the cerebral cortex (see **Figure 15.18c**).

Serotonin neurons are implicated in sleep–wake transitions, in arousal and motivated behaviors, in appetite regulation, and in pain modulation. Serotonin may inhibit aggressive behaviors. The efficacy of SSRI

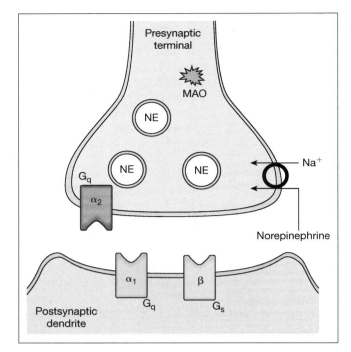

FIGURE 15.20 Noradrenergic synapse. NE is synthesized from dopamine. In addition to the enzymes tyrosine hydroxylase and dopa decarboxylase, NE neurons contain the enzyme dopamine β-hydroxylase, which converts dopamine to NE. NE binds to postsynaptic α or β receptors, or both. α-Adrenergic receptors are coupled to the G_q protein, and β-adrenergic receptors are coupled to G_s. Presynaptic $α_2$-receptors are inhibitory autoreceptors. The NE transporter is responsible for the uptake of NE, terminating transmission. NE returned to the presynaptic terminal is either repackaged into vesicles or degraded by MAO.

MAO, monoamine oxidase; Na$^+$, sodium; NE, norepinephrine.

drugs in alleviating depression and anxiety points to a role for serotonin in mood regulation.

At least 14 subtypes of serotonin receptors have been identified in the human brain, organized in several families including 5-HT_{1A-F}, 5-HT_{2A-C}, 5-HT_3, 5-HT_4, 5-HT_{5A-B}, 5-HT_6, and 5-HT_7. All are metabotropic except 5-HT_3, which is an ionotropic receptor. The 5-HT_1 family members inhibit adenylyl cyclase and generally produce postsynaptic inhibition; some 5-HT_1 receptors are inhibitory autoreceptors (**Figure 15.21**). The 5-HT_2 family members link to the G_q protein and can produce postsynaptic excitation; they are the target of the hallucinogen lysergic acid diethylamide (LSD). The 5-HT_3 receptor is an ionotropic receptor that produces postsynaptic excitation; 5-HT_3 receptors in the brain and gastrointestinal tract contribute to emesis, and antagonists at this receptor (such as ondansetron) are used to treat nausea and vomiting. Several of the 5-HT receptors are the targets of agents to treat migraine, likely through their vascular effects.

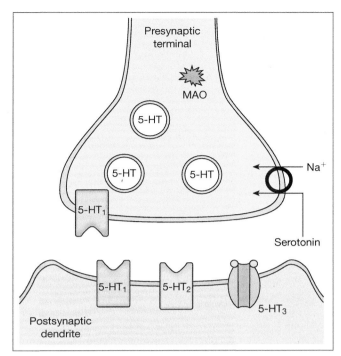

FIGURE 15.21 Serotonergic synapse. The serotonin synapse is similar to the catecholamine synapses; however, at certain sites in the brain, there are 5-HT$_3$ ionotropic receptors. This is the one exception to the principle that amine neurotransmitters have only metabotropic receptors. 5-HT$_3$ receptors are found in the gut and in medullary regions controlling vomiting, and they are the target of antiemetic drugs such as ondansetron. Some serotonergic synapses have presynaptic inhibitory autoreceptors, and all have the selective SERT. Serotonin can be broken down presynaptically by MAO.

MAO, monoamine oxidase; Na$^+$, sodium; SERT, serotonin transporter.

Histamine

Histamine is a multifunctional physiological mediator, serving as a locally active agent of inflammation, a modulator of gastric acid secretion, and a central neurotransmitter. Histamine is produced in one step by decarboxylation of the amino acid histidine. Within the brain, the sole region of histamine neurons is the tuberomammillary nucleus in the posterior hypothalamus (see **Figure 15.18d**). Along with acetylcholine, norepinephrine, dopamine, and serotonin, histamine neurons are active during wakefulness, with decreased activity during slow-wave sleep. The well-known sleep-inducing effects of nonselective histamine antagonists, such as diphenhydramine, are an indication that histamine contributes to the state of waking.

Box 15.3 summarizes key points about the neuromodulatory transmitters.

NEUROMODULATORY TRANSMITTERS: PEPTIDES

Many peptides are found in neurons, and these signaling molecules serve roles similar to the small molecule neuromodulators. Some neuropeptides are also found in the periphery, where they may function in endocrine pathways, the gastrointestinal tract, or both. The multipurpose nature of peptides, as well as their location and action in the periphery, often led to their discovery outside the nervous system before identification of their location and roles inside the nervous system.

Peptides are short proteins, chains of amino acids that can be from three to 40 or more amino acids long. These transmitters are synthesized by the process of transcription and translation in the neuron cell body. Translation results in a large proprotein that is

---

BOX 15.3
Features of Neuromodulatory Amine Transmitters

- Restricted anatomical location of the neurons, primarily in the brainstem and hypothalamus

- Widespread projections to brainstem, thalamus, and cortex

- Wide synaptic clefts around axon varicosities that widely distribute transmitter

- Extensive subtypes of receptors, all of which are metabotropic except for the acetylcholine nicotinic receptor and the serotonin 5-HT$_3$ receptor

- Modulation of transmitter release and neuronal excitation by autoreceptors and heteroceptors

- Termination of transmission by selective transport mechanisms

- Enzymatic breakdown by acetylcholinesterase (acetylcholine) or monoamine oxidase (dopamine, norepinephrine, serotonin)

- Modulatory roles in states of waking, appetite, aggression, mood changes, learning, and cognition, as well as sensory function and motor activity

- An abundance of pharmacological targets and drugs that alter mood, arousal, anxiety, sleep, appetite, learning, and memory

subsequently cleaved, releasing one or more active peptides. After translation and post-translational processing, the peptides are packaged into large vesicles and are transported down the axon to the terminal to be released into the synapse. Some of the classical transmitters described earlier are co-localized in nerve terminals along with the peptide transmitters. In such cases, action potentials release separate vesicles of small molecule transmitters and peptide transmitters.

Receptors for peptide transmitters are all metabotropic, having slow postsynaptic effects. Similar to the small molecule neuromodulators, neuropeptides tend to be involved in slow neuronal responses and modulation of behavioral states, rather than rapid motor activity or reflexes. Table 15.1 lists examples of common neuropeptides and their functions. Several inhibitory peptide receptors are found on presynaptic terminals, where they act as heteroceptors and inhibit transmitter release.

Opioid Peptides

The prototype family of peptide transmitters described here is the endogenous opioid family. Crude extracts from the poppy have been used for more than two millennia for the relief of pain and to achieve sedation. When the active compound morphine was purified from opium, it was used for its analgesic properties, as it is to this day. Morphine and the opioid analgesics are the most effective medications for severe pain, but their use is accompanied by the risk of tolerance and substance use disorders. The search for biological mechanisms of opioid action led in the 1970s and 1980s to the identification of three types of opioid receptors: μ, δ, and κ. Analgesia results from stimulation of μ or κ receptors; pleasure-inducing and addictive properties are primarily due to activation of μ receptors.

Following the identification of opioid receptors, three broad types of endogenous opioid peptides were discovered in mammalian brains: met- and leu-enkephalin, coded by the proenkephalin (*Penk*) gene; dynorphin A and B, coded by the prodynorphin (*Pdyn*) gene; and β-endorphin, coded by the proopiomelanocortin (*POMC*) gene. These three families exemplify the peptidergic property of synthesis by proprotein cleavage (Figure 15.22). Cell bodies expressing *Penk* are the most numerous and are widely distributed in cortex, basal forebrain, thalamus, amygdala, and brainstem. Cell bodies expressing *Pdyn* are less numerous, but show a similar distribution to *Penk* cell bodies. Cell bodies expressing *POMC* are only found in three brain locations: hypothalamic arcuate nucleus, brainstem nucleus of the solitary tract, and pituitary anterior and intermediate lobes. *POMC*-expressing neurons project widely to limbic brain regions as well as to brainstem and spinal cord.

Opioid peptides and receptors are found throughout the cortex, thalamus, basal forebrain, and brainstem. Interestingly, there is not always a close correlation between brain regions that express opioid receptors and regions containing the opioid peptides themselves. This mismatch may indicate that the peptides are able to diffuse away from their sites of synaptic release to have actions a distance away. This mechanism of signaling is possible as there are few degradative enzymes for peptide neurotransmitters in the brain.[6]

Opioid functions are inferred from the known actions of opioid drugs prescribed for their clinical efficacy. The ability to reduce pain and provide analgesia without suppressing other sensory modalities is the central functional consequence of opioid administration, and its primary clinical use. Other well-known actions leading from opioid administration include the perception of pleasure/reward, mild sedation and neurological depression (leading to respiratory depression, if severe), decreased bowel motility leading to constipation, and cough suppression. The intestinal effects of opioids are mediated by abundantly distributed opioid receptors in the gut, including distribution on enteric neurons. This action leads to the constipating effects of opioids, as well as underlying the mechanism of action of opioid derivatives used to treat diarrhea.

Several central nervous system sites are targets of either endogenous opioid peptides or opioid drugs given for pain. These include the periaqueductal gray (PAG) region of the midbrain; the thalamus and limbic system structures; the noradrenergic locus ceruleus and serotonergic raphe magnus; and the spinal cord dorsal horn. Functional imaging of the brain during placebo-induced analgesia combined with either saline or naloxone administration implicates the endogenous opioid system in reducing pain perception during treatment with placebo. The brain regions participating in placebo-induced analgesia include limbic cortex, hypothalamus, PAG, and rostral ventromedial medulla.[7]

TABLE 15.1 Examples of Neuropeptides and Their Functions

Neuropeptide	Proposed Functions
Opioid peptides: enkephalins, dynorphin, β-endorphin	Pain modulation, pleasure/reward, sedation, gut motility modulation
Corticotropin-releasing hormone	Stress, anxiety, fear, withdrawal
Oxytocin	Attachment, bonding
Vasopressin	Affiliative behavior
Orexins A and B	Sleep–wake transitions, feeding, reward
Neuropeptide Y	Feeding initiation

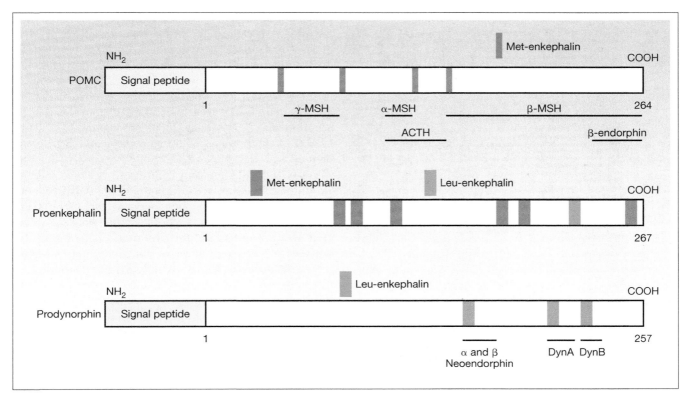

FIGURE 15.22 Opioid peptide synthesis. As peptides, the opioids are synthesized by transcription and translation. Three genes code for the three different opioid families: enkephalin, endorphin, and dynorphin. All are derived from large proproteins that are subsequently cleaved by protease enzymes to release biologically active short peptides. POMC is the proprotein that releases MSH peptides (α-, β-, or γ-MSH). In some cells, alternate processing of this proprotein releases ACTH and β-endorphin. POMC also contains several copies of the met-enkephalin opioid sequence. Enkephalin is a pentapeptide (five amino acids long) that has two biologically active forms: Met-enkephalin ends in methionine, whereas leu-enkephalin ends in leucine. The initial four amino acids are identical: tyrosine-glycine-glycine-phenylalanine. Cleavage of proenkephalin produces six copies of met-enkephalin and one copy of leu-enkephalin. Cleavage of prodynorphin usually produces dynorphins A and B (Dyn A, Dyn B), but can produce the other cleavage products shown. ACTH, adrenocorticotropic hormone; MSH, melanocyte-stimulating hormone; POMC, proopiomelanocortin.

Source: From Pasternak G, Neilan C. Neuropeptides; overview. In: *Encyclopedia of the Neurological Sciences.* Elsevier; 2014:516–519. doi:10.1016/B978-0-12-385157-4.00043-9.

Orexins

Orexin A and orexin B are chemically similar peptides found in neurons in the lateral hypothalamus. Orexin neurons project to neuron groups associated with waking from sleep, including the locus ceruleus, raphe, and tuberomammillary histamine neurons. Thus, orexin is implicated in initiating arousal from sleep and stabilizing the state of waking. Clinically, loss of brain orexin neurons can be caused by autoimmune processes.

APPLICATION OF NEUROTRANSMITTER CONCEPTS

States of sleep and waking, and the transitions between these states, exemplify interactions between the different classes of neurotransmitters. Multicellular organisms, from the worm *Caenorhabditis elegans* to humans, have periodic states of dormancy with reduced motor and sensory function, alternating with times of arousal and movement. Human have several cycles of sleep and wake during their sleep time (Figure 15.23). The waking state is characterized by low-voltage, high-frequency EEG waves indicating widely distributed electrical activity that is not synchronized. Transition into sleep shows slowing of EEG activity and progressive synchronization, indicating depolarizations and repolarizations of large regions of cortex. The deepest stage was previously termed slow-wave sleep, and is now referred to as *nonrapid eye movement* (NREM stage 3, or N3). After varying amounts of time, there is a brief return to a lighter NREM sleep stage before progression into REM sleep.

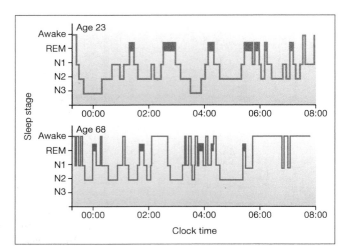

FIGURE 15.23 Sleep cycles during the night in a young adult and an older adult. The cycles usually begin with the transition from wake to NREM sleep, descending to the deepest stage, N3, before ascending through N2 and N1 and into REM sleep. This cycle repeats several times during the night. In young adults, the deepest NREM sleep occurs earliest in the night. In older adults, little or no time is spent in N3, and sleep is more fragmented with frequent awakenings.

NREM, non REM; REM, rapid eye movement.

Source: From Kasper D, et al. Sleep disorders. In: *Harrison's Principles of Internal Medicine.* 19th ed. New York, NY: McGraw-Hill; 2015, part 2, sec. 3, chap. 38, fig. 38-01—Wake-Sleep Architecture.

Muscle tone in most muscles of the body is lowest during REM, although brief twitches can occur. The extraocular muscles are active and produce eye movements, characteristic of this stage. EEG activity in REM returns to low-voltage, unsynchronized activity, similar to the waking EEG. REM episodes terminate with an abrupt change to a brief period of wakefulness, or to a lighter stage of NREM sleep, before the next stage of NREM sleep. Sleep becomes lighter and more fragmented with aging.[8]

Activity in brainstem centers increases during waking, in several of the chemically identified neuron groups: norepinephrine cells in the locus ceruleus, serotonin cells in the dorsal raphe, acetylcholine cells in the brainstem, and glutamate neurons in the pons. These groups comprise the ascending reticular-activating system (ARAS), which projects to the hypothalamus, basal forebrain, thalamus, and cortex. Within the hypothalamus, axons from orexin cells of the lateral hypothalamus and histamine cells in the tuberomammillary nucleus add to the ARAS projection to the basal forebrain arousal region. Within the basal forebrain, acetylcholine, glutamate, and GABA neurons are intermixed. These neurons have cortical projections that initiate and maintain waking[9] (**Figure 15.24**).

The transition from wakefulness to sleep is promoted by neurons in the anterior hypothalamus, specifically, the ventrolateral preoptic and median

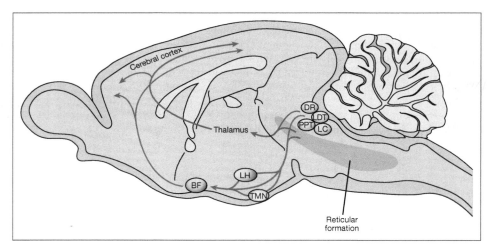

FIGURE 15.24 Brain arousal pathways shown on a rat brain schematic. The primary brain arousal pathway, shown in red, includes brainstem acetylcholine, dopamine, norepinephrine, glutamate, and serotonin neurons that project to the hypothalamus and basal forebrain. Hypothalamic orexin neurons in the LH and histamine neurons in the TMN join the pathway to the BF. Dopamine, norepinephrine, serotonin, and histamine axons continue on to cortex, where they contribute to cortical stimulation. In the basal forebrain, acetylcholine, GABA, and glutamate neurons project to the cortex to provide the major stimulus to awakening. An additional pathway from the brainstem to the cortex via the thalamus, shown in blue, may contribute to the initiation or maintenance of waking.

BF, basal forebrain; DR, dorsal raphe; GABA, gamma-aminobutyric acid; LC, locus ceruleus; LDT, lateral dorsal tegmental nucleus; LH, lateral hypothalamus; PPT, pedunculopontine tegmental nucleus; TMN, tuberomammillary nucleus.

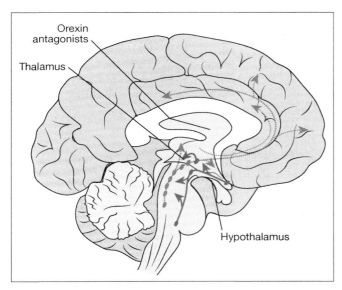

FIGURE 15.25 Pathways of sleep initiation. GABA neurons in the anterior hypothalamic region (blue) project to hypothalamic (orexin, purple) and brainstem nuclei of the ascending arousal system (red dotted), resulting in sleep initiation. GABA, gamma-aminobutyric acid.

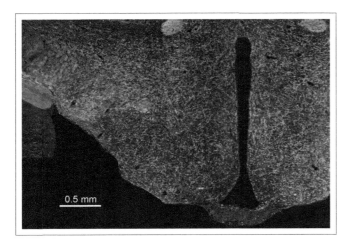

FIGURE 15.26 Photomicrograph of oxexin neurons in the lateral hypothalamus. Orexin cells (red fluorescent stain) have extensive hypothalamic projections, in addition to the ascending cortical projection that contributes to stabilizing the wake state.
Source: Photomicrograph courtesy of Dr. Leszek Kubin, University of Pennsylvania.

preoptic nuclei, source of GABA neurons that project to and inhibit all of the arousal-related cell groups (**Figure 15.25**). The orexin neurons of the lateral hypothalamus (**Figure 15.26**) are strongly implicated in stabilizing the wake state, as autoimmune destruction of these cells results in **narcolepsy**, in which episodes

of sleep occur throughout the day and night. As our understanding of the complex neuroanatomy and neurochemistry of sleep–wake transitions deepens, it is clear that interactions between rapid-acting glutamate and GABA transmission, modulated by slower-acting small molecule transmitters and peptides, shape sleep homeostasis as well as sleep disruptions.[10]

SUMMARY OF NEUROTRANSMITTER CONCEPTS

All 100 billion neurons develop from precursor cells of the embryonic ectoderm that collect to form the neural tube. The precursor cells that will develop into neurons must migrate to their final position in the nervous system, send out dendrites and a branching axon, and make all the correct synaptic connections, receiving perhaps thousands of synapses. In addition to all of these actions, each neuron must turn on a specific array of genes coding for enzymes that synthesize their small molecule transmitter, or genes that code for transcription and translation of peptide transmitters. Genes associated with all other transmitter systems must be turned off.

This differentiation is based on chemical signals in the specific brain and peripheral nervous system regions where certain clusters of neurons are found. For example, the genes for the enzymes tyrosine hydroxylase and dopa decarboxylase are expressed in neurons of the substantia nigra and VTA that make the transmitter dopamine. In the locus ceruleus, both of these enzymes are present *plus* dopamine β-hydroxylase—so the transmitter norepinephrine is made. Differentiation of peptide neurons includes expression of the genes coding for their specific peptide and silencing of genes that code for other neuropeptides.

Finally, once a neuron's transmitter is decided, that neuron must turn on a host of other genes—for synthetic and degradative enzymes, vesicular packaging transporters, uptake transporters, presynaptic receptors, and more. The genes that relate to the remaining neurotransmitters must be shut off. For proper synaptic function, that neuron must also express particular receptors that will be targeted to its dendritic spines and other sites at which it is the recipient of synaptic inputs.

It is difficult to overestimate the complexity of the development and ongoing function of the brain and the number of disordered processes that could potentially underlie neurological and behavioral disorders. Knowing the vocabulary and concepts of neurotransmission and these major neurotransmitters is a critical foundation for clinicians. Key information about the neurotransmitters is summarized in **Table 15.2.**

TABLE 15.2 Summary of Neurotransmitters

Name	Anatomy	Physiology	Pathophysiology
Glutamate	Widely distributed in projection pathways and interneurons	Rapid excitation by ionotropic receptors: AMPA, NMDA Slower effects through metabotropic receptors **Presynaptic and glial uptake** *Tonic activity underlying many brain functions*	Excitotoxicity: neuron death after stroke, brain injury, and neurodegenerative disorders
GABA	Widely distributed, cortical and subcortical projection and interneurons	Rapid inhibition by ionotropic GABA$_A$ receptors Slow inhibition by metabotropic GABA$_B$ receptors **Presynaptic uptake** *Tonic activity prevents seizures, suppresses extraneous activity*	Inadequate inhibition can predispose to seizures/epilepsy Deficits could contribute to anxiety disorders
Acetylcholine	Peripheral: motor neurons, preganglionic parasympathetic and sympathetic neurons, postganglionic parasympathetic neurons Central: basal forebrain nuclei, including nucleus basalis of Meynert, interneurons in striatum, brainstem sleep-regulating nuclei	Rapid excitation by ionotropic nicotinic receptors Mixed excitation or inhibition by muscarinic receptors (five subtypes) **Action rapidly terminated by synaptic acetylcholinesterase** *Muscle contraction* *Autonomic activity, parasympathetic actions* *Learning, memory* *Opposes striatal dopamine, modulating basal ganglia function* *REM sleep initiation*	Neuromuscular: myasthenia gravis Basal forebrain: Alzheimer disease Striatum: Parkinson disease, nicotine addiction
Dopamine	Substantia nigra: projects to motor striatum Ventral tegmental area: projects to limbic cortex and nucleus accumbens Tuberal hypothalamus: projects to pituitary	Mixed excitation or inhibition by dopamine receptors (five subtypes) **Presynaptic DAT and intracellular monoamine oxidase** *Basal ganglia motor refinement* *Motivation/pleasure/reinforcement* *Prolactin suppression*	Parkinson disease Addiction Schizophrenia ADHD Hyperprolactinemia
Norepinephrine	Locus ceruleus Medullary nuclei Postganglionic sympathetic neurons	Primarily excitatory via α_1 and β_1 receptors Inhibition by presynaptic α_2-autoreceptors **Presynaptic NET and intracellular MAO** *Arousal, alerting, stress signaling* *Pain suppression* *Sympathetic autonomic activity*	Mood disorders Stress and anxiety PTSD ADHD Orthostatic tachycardia syndrome
Serotonin (5-HT)	Brainstem raphe nuclei	Mixed excitation or inhibition by metabotropic 5-HT receptors; 5-HT$_3$ receptor is ionotropic **Presynaptic 5-HT transporter (selective serotonin transporter) and intracellular MAO** *Mood, gut activity and vomiting, vasoconstriction, arousal, pain suppression*	Mood and anxiety disorders Vomiting Migraine pain pathway

Note: In the Physiology column, receptor mechanisms are shown in regular type. Mechanisms of termination are shown in **bold**. Functions are shown in *italics*.

ADHD, attention-deficit/hyperactivity disorder; AMPA, α-amino-3-hydroxyl-5-methyl-4-isoxazole-propionate; DAT, dopamine transporter; GABA, gamma-aminobutyric acid; 5-HT, serotonin; MAO, monoamine oxidase; NET, norepinephrine transporter; NMDA, N-methyl-D-aspartate; PTSD, post-traumatic stress disorder; REM, rapid eye movement.

Thought Questions

10. How would you compare the signaling roles of amino acid transmitters glutamate and GABA with the transmitters norepinephrine, dopamine, and serotonin? What particular characteristics of neurotransmission by these different molecules are distinctive to each group?

11. What are some behavioral actions of small molecule and peptide transmitters? How are these actions terminated?

12. What is the difference between an autoreceptor and a heteroreceptor? Where are these membrane proteins found, and how do they work?

SENSORY NEUROPHYSIOLOGY

OVERVIEW OF SPINAL CORD ANATOMY

Sensory and motor functions associated with the arms, trunk, and legs are conducted by neurons in and projecting to the spinal cord. The spinal cord has 31 levels: eight cervical, 12 thoracic, five lumbar, five sacral, and one coccygeal, and at each level there is a single organizational pattern. The central core of the spinal cord, surrounding a central canal filled with cerebrospinal fluid, is gray matter, composed of cell bodies of projection neurons and interneurons. This central core is surrounded by white matter, made up of myelinated and unmyelinated axons of ascending and descending tracts. The dorsal region of the spinal cord consists of dorsal columns (white matter) and dorsal horns of gray matter. This region primarily serves sensory functions. The ventral region of the spinal cord consists of ventral white matter and ventral horns of gray matter. This region primarily serves motor functions. The lateral white matter contains both sensory and motor tracts, and the lateral gray matter at the thoracic and sacral levels contains sympathetic and parasympathetic preganglionic neurons, respectively (**Figure 15.27**).

The diameter and circumference of the spinal cord are greater at the cervical and lumbar enlargements, which are associated with innervation of the arms and legs, respectively. At each level, axons of entering sensory fibers make up dorsal roots, entering at the tip of the dorsal horn. Similarly, at each level, axons of exiting motor and autonomic fibers make up ventral roots. Each dorsal root has a swelling called the dorsal root ganglion, which is the location of cell bodies of sensory fibers. Beyond the dorsal root ganglion, dorsal and ventral roots join to form the spinal nerve that projects through openings between adjacent vertebrae of the vertebral column. After exiting the vertebral column, axons of the spinal nerves separate and continue as components of various peripheral nerves (**Figure 15.28**).

SOMATIC SENSORY FUNCTION

Peripheral sensory fibers respond to external and internal stimuli such as touch, vibration, cold and warm temperature, and pain, and, through ascending pathways and synaptic relays, bring those stimuli to conscious awareness in the sensory cortex. Other stimuli, such as muscle stretch and tension, are not consciously perceived but are conveyed to brain regions where this information is critical for motor control. In each case, the sensory division of the nervous system depends on neurons with specialized receptors found in peripheral tissues that generate action potentials in response to their specific stimuli and relay those action potentials to the central nervous system. Superficial and deep sensations from arms, legs, and trunk are relayed by these peripheral sensory axons to the spinal cord dorsal horn. Sensations from head and neck are relayed to brainstem nuclei. In both cases, the sensory neurons have cell bodies in ganglia outside the central nervous system, with axons that project to target regions in the spinal cord or brain. Sensory neurons are also referred to as *afferent* neurons because they are bringing information into the nervous system.

Sensory neurons differ from other neurons in the way that they reach threshold to generate action potentials. Rather than excitatory synaptic inputs, sensory neurons are depolarized by sensory inputs at specialized nerve endings. Examples of sensory inputs include pain and touch sensation from the skin, muscle stretch and tendon tension that contribute to proprioception (position sense), and the special senses of vision, hearing, smell, and taste. In this section, the focus is on modalities of somatic sensation, emphasizing peripheral sensations with segmental inputs through spinal cord dorsal roots.

Sensory neurons are the exceptions to the principle that neuronal action potential generation begins at the neuron cell body. Rather, specialized sensory nerve endings come to threshold in response to their specific stimuli, generating action potentials that are propagated to the cell body and into the central nervous system. The peripheral sensing region of a somatic sensory cell can be located in the skin, in a muscle, in a joint, or in an organ. These nerve endings are specialized for one modality only, which could be touch, vibration, stretch, temperature, or chemical signals of inflammation and tissue damage. Proprioception, the sense of the location and movement of muscles and joints, is an essential part of motor control and is discussed later in this chapter.

When a specialized sensory ending is stimulated to action potential threshold, the action potential is propagated along the peripheral axon to a cell body in

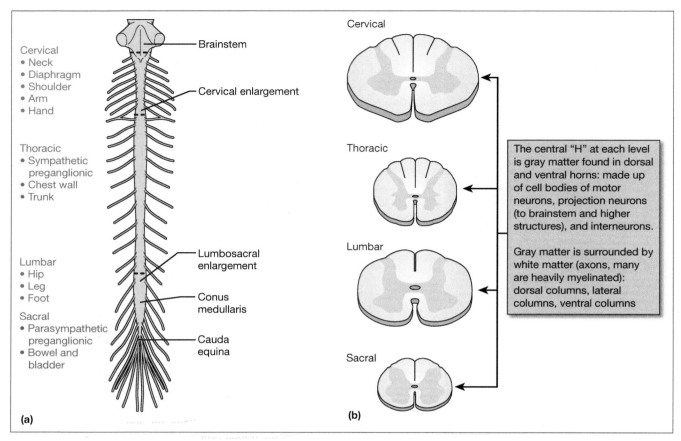

The central "H" at each level is gray matter found in dorsal and ventral horns: made up of cell bodies of motor neurons, projection neurons (to brainstem and higher structures), and interneurons.

Gray matter is surrounded by white matter (axons, many are heavily myelinated): dorsal columns, lateral columns, ventral columns

FIGURE 15.27 Spinal cord anatomy. (**a**) Longitudinal view of the spinal cord showing the cervical, thoracic, lumbar, and sacral regions with their peripheral targets noted by level. (**b**) Cross-sectional views of the spinal cord showing the similarities in overall structure (central gray matter surrounded by white matter), with differences in diameter and relative amounts of gray matter and white matter at these spinal levels.

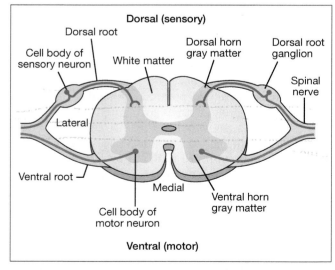

FIGURE 15.28 Overview of spinal cord nomenclature. The dorsal region faces the back of the body, whereas the ventral region faces the abdomen.

a dorsal root ganglion, continuing to an axon terminal within the central nervous system to release the excitatory neurotransmitter glutamate. Although other neurotransmitters may be co-localized in sensory neurons, all primary sensory neurons are glutamatergic, producing excitation in their synaptic targets. There are two major groups of peripheral sensory fibers, and each relates to a different pathway within the central nervous system (**Figure 15.29**).

Dorsal Column/Medial Lemniscus System

Light touch, vibration, and position sense are detected in the periphery, and action potentials are propagated via rapidly conducting, large-diameter myelinated axons. These axons enter the spinal cord through the medial dorsal root and dorsal horn, where they bifurcate, having branches that make synapses within the spinal cord, and another branch that travels in the spinal cord dorsal white matter (*dorsal column*) to the brainstem sensory nuclei. Second-order neurons

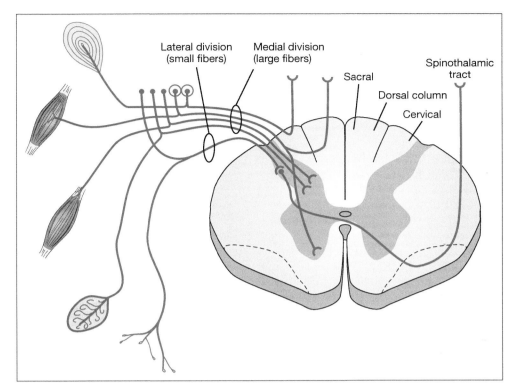

FIGURE 15.29 Spinal sensory anatomy. Spinal sensory neurons have specialized axon terminals in peripheral tissues (skin, muscles, joints, and organs), where action potentials are generated. These action potentials are propagated to cell bodies in the dorsal root ganglion outside the spinal cord, and to the central axon that enters the spinal cord through the dorsal root. Some of these axons make an immediate synapse in the dorsal horn, others ascend or descend in the dorsal spinal cord before reaching their synaptic termination. Large-fiber modalities of fine touch, position sense, and vibration are carried by axons that enter through the medial dorsal root, bifurcating into branches that either remain in the spinal cord or ascend to the brain in the dorsal columns (dorsal column/medial lemniscus system). Small-fiber modalities of pain and temperature are carried by axons that enter through the lateral dorsal root, bifurcating into branches that can ascend or descend within the spinal cord, or can make an immediate synapse in the dorsal horn. The postsynaptic dorsal horn neuron is termed a *second-order neuron*, with an axon that crosses in the ventral gray matter to the contralateral spinothalamic tract, where it ascends to the thalamus.

of the brainstem sensory nuclei have axons that cross the midline of the medulla, then travel in a fiber bundle called the medial lemniscus to the thalamus.

Spinothalamic Tract System

Mechanical and chemical signals of tissue damage (pain-producing stimuli) and temperature of the skin are detected in the periphery and action potentials are propagated by means of slower conducting, thinly myelinated or unmyelinated fibers. These axons enter the spinal cord through the lateral dorsal root and dorsal horn and make a synapse within the dorsal horn. The dorsal horn neurons receiving these impulses have axons that cross the midline of the spinal cord to ascend to the brain via the *spinothalamic tract*, which is found in the spinal cord ventral and lateral white matter.

Thalamic neurons that receive synaptic input from ascending sensory pathways project to the somatosensory cortex. It is in the cortex that the presence, character, and location of the sensation is consciously perceived. An example of sensory activation and perception is seen in the sensory portion of the neurological examination. While the patient's eyes are closed, the examiner touches the tip of to a cotton applicator to the patient's right forearm and asks the patient to report whether the sensation was sharp or dull and which arm was touched. A patient with normal function will report a dull touch of the right forearm. This process is repeated, often alternating a dull object (a test of dorsal column neurons) with a sharp object such as a pin (a test of spinothalamic tract neurons). The ability to discriminate and report the quality and location of a sensory stimulus is one component of the examination to assess the integrity of nervous system structure and function.

Pathological States of Sensory Function

Disorders such as diabetes can cause bilateral **sensory neuropathy** that presents with a *stocking-and-glove* distribution. This pattern reflects the fact that the longest sensory axons are the most vulnerable to metabolic disorders. The longest axons innervate structures farthest from the spinal cord—the feet and hands. Sensory losses that do not proceed in this distal-to-proximal fashion are more likely to be due to a nonmetabolic process such as a central nervous system disorder. Disorders that are highly localized and are unilateral are more likely to be due to a mechanical disturbance such as nerve impingement and compression. The heavily myelinated dorsal column fibers are vulnerable to demyelination in severe vitamin B12 deficiency, producing sensory deficits of light touch and vibration sense, and decreased proprioception causing difficulty with maintaining balance as assessed by the Romberg test.

Thought Questions

13. **How does sensory signaling differ from signaling by nonsensory neurons?**

14. **How does a sensory neuron come to threshold?**

PAIN

Pain is the most common reason for a patient to initiate a visit to a healthcare provider. As a biological signal, **acute pain** is important for drawing a subject's awareness to an area of injury and for enforcing rest of an injured body part that allows healing. **Chronic pain**, however, is disabling and is more likely to result in chronic dysfunction, rather than healing. Although pain management continues to dominate clinical practice, many areas of pain neurophysiology and pathophysiology are not well understood. Therefore, this continues to be an area of ongoing, active, and important research.

NEUROPHYSIOLOGY OF PAIN

While it may be natural to assume that pain arises from the same receptors that generate other somatic sensations (touch, tickle, temperature), the perception of pain depends on dedicated pathways and receptors, which unlike other senses, allow for a significant degree of modulation of the sensation. In that the perception of pain (called nociception) allows the central nervous system to alert the body to injury and impending danger, it follows that a distinct system would be involved in the perception of potentially threatening situations.

To provide an overview, the path from injured tissue to cortical perception comprises three or more neurons:

- *Nociceptors*, also known as first-order neurons, are peripheral sensory neurons, activated by tissue-damaging stimuli, that make excitatory synaptic contacts with spinothalamic tract neurons.
- Also known as second-order neurons, *spinothalamic tract neurons* are located in the spinal cord dorsal horn, with axons that project to the thalamus and brainstem reticular formation.
- *Thalamocortical relay neurons* (third-order neurons) project to somatosensory cortex for recognition and localization of the painful input.
- In addition, at the level of the brainstem several parallel pathways relay the pain signal to important forebrain limbic structures, including the amygdala, and the insular and cingulate cortex regions (**Figure 15.30**).

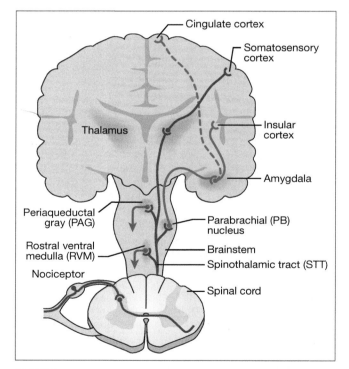

FIGURE 15.30 Central pathways of pain transmission. Pain is relayed from peripheral tissues via nociceptor fibers that synapse on a STT neuron in the dorsal horn of the spinal cord. The STT axon crosses the spinal cord and ascends in the ventral white matter, giving off branches to several brainstem nuclei. The final termination of the STT neuron is in the thalamus, at a synapse on a thalamocortical neuron that relays the pain signal to somatosensory cortex, allowing discrete localization of the pain signal. A parallel pathway via the parabrachial nucleus of the pons relays the pain message to the amygdala and cingulate cortex, limbic structures that give a negative emotional valence to the sensation of pain.
Source: From Basbaum AI, et al. Cellular and molecular mechanisms of Pain. *Cell.* 2009;139(2):267–284. doi:10.1016/j.cell.2009.09.028.

Nociceptors

Nociceptors are peripheral sensory receptors dedicated to the detection of harmful stimuli such as intense pressure, strong thermal stimuli, or chemical signals likely to cause tissue damage. They are relatively unspecialized bare nerve cell endings that initiate the sensation of pain. Nociceptors transduce a variety of stimuli into receptor potentials, which in turn trigger action potentials. Like other somatic sensory receptors, their cell bodies are located in the dorsal root ganglia of the spinal cord, and they send one axonal process to the periphery and the other to synaptic targets in the spinal cord or brainstem.

As previously noted, nociceptor axons enter the spinal cord in the lateral division of the dorsal roots. They are further broken down into two groups: Aδ myelinated axons and C-fiber unmyelinated axons (**Figure 15.31**). Aδ axons typically conduct at a rate of 5 to 30 m/sec, and C-fiber axons conduct at a much slower rate of 2 m/sec. Although the conduction of all nociceptive information is slow in comparison to other somatosensory modalities, within the pain pathways there are also fast or slow components. Aδ and C-fiber axons terminate at synapses in the dorsal horn of the spinal cord. As with other primary somatosensory neurons, nociceptors release glutamate at their synaptic targets, and many also release the peptide transmitter substance P. Glutamate produces rapid synaptic excitation of second-order neurons, while substance P produces slower and longer-lasting excitation.

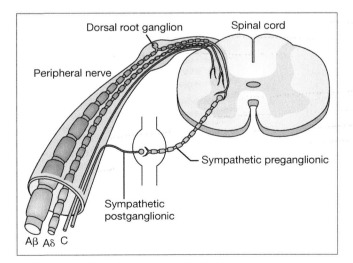

FIGURE 15.31 Cutaneous nerve components. Nerves innervating skin are generally composed of four types of axons: Aβ sensory fibers carrying information about light touch and pressure; Aδ sensory fibers carrying information about well-localized painful stimuli; C sensory fibers carrying information about poorly localized painful stimuli; and efferent C fibers of sympathetic postganglionic neurons that control cutaneous vasoconstriction.

Aδ nociceptors can be further broken down into two groups: mechanosensitive nociceptors, those that respond to intense mechanical stimuli, and mechanothermal nociceptors, those that response to intense thermal stimuli. In contrast, C-fiber nociceptors are capable of response to thermal, mechanical, and chemical stimuli and are therefore called polymodal. In that any of these can cause tissue damage, painful sensations can arise from mechanical, thermal, or chemical stimuli. Therefore, it is no surprise that the transduction of nociceptive signals is a complex task.

Spinothalamic Tract Neurons

Moving from the peripheral nervous system to the central nervous system, the axons of peripheral nociceptive neurons enter the spinal cord via the dorsal root. At the level of the dorsal horn of the spinal cord, these axons branch into short ascending and descending collateral branches, which typically span one or two spinal cord segments before they enter the gray matter of the dorsal horn. In the dorsal horn, the axons branch and make excitatory synapses on spinothalamic tract neurons (also known as second-order neurons) located in the dorsal horn. The number and frequency of nociceptor action potentials codes for the amount of glutamate released. The greater the stimulus, the greater the excitation and action potential frequency of spinothalamic neurons—coding more severe tissue damage. The axons of spinothalamic tract neurons cross the midline and ascend to the brainstem and thalamus in the ventrolateral quadrant of the contralateral half of the spinal cord as the spinothalamic tract.

Spinothalamic tract axons diverge and ascend to the brainstem and thalamus. The projections to the thalamus terminate in several thalamic nuclei. Third-order thalamocortical relay neurons project to somatosensory cortex, causing conscious recognition and discrete localization of the pain signal. Brainstem relay neurons transmit the pain signal to pain-modulating regions of the medulla, pons, and midbrain. Additional brainstem and thalamic neurons activate the limbic structures—amygdala, insular cortex, and anterior cingulate cortex—providing an emotional and affective component to pain perception (see **Figure 15.30**). This attribute, referred to as cognitive–evaluative processing, encompasses attitudes and beliefs about the pain experienced.[11] The somatosensory cortex enables sensory discrimination and localization of the pain (Is it sharp or dull? Is it in the leg or the arm?). Pain signals in the limbic system initiate an emotional response, which might cause one to yelp or verbalize and ascribe negative feelings to the sensation. This engagement of the limbic system is a unique feature of the ascending pain pathway, typically not seen with nonharmful stimuli such as touch, pressure, or vibration. Cognitive evaluation helps the body to determine the extent of the presence of actual or potential harm. This evaluation is subjective; everyone evaluates pain differently based on previous experiences.[12]

Ascending Pain Pathways: A Site of Pain Modulation

A pain signal can be modulated (amplified or diminished) in several ways as it ascends toward the brain. With respect to modulation in the peripheral nervous system, transduction of the pain signal is influenced by the chemical reactions associated with the inflammatory process. When tissue is injured, inflammatory mediators are released from the damaged cells, resulting in *peripheral sensitization*, which is the result of inflammatory mediators interacting with nociceptors following tissue damage (**Figure 15.32**). These mediators include bradykinin, histamine, serotonin, arachidonic acid and other lipid metabolites, and nerve growth factor. Each of these chemical mediators can interact with different membrane receptors or ion channels of nociceptive fibers (generally increasing action potential frequency), thus intensifying the pain sensation.

The direct activity of inflammatory mediators on the nociceptor is referred to as primary activation of the nociceptor. However, because a nociceptor has many free nerve endings or branches that all coalesce into a single axon, there will also be a wave of secondary nociceptive activation in the injured tissue. The action potential generated in the region closest to the damage not only projects toward the spinal cord but also proceeds out these branches into the nearby sensory branches of that same sensory fiber. This causes the release of the neurotransmitter substance P into this adjacent peripheral tissue, causing the release of histamine from mast cells and serotonin from platelets, amplifying the pain signal and reinforcing the inflammatory response (described in detail in Chapter 6, The Immune System and Leukocyte Function). For example, when you scrape your knee, pain associated with the injury is directly initiated by primary nociceptor stimulation and is reinforced by the secondary nociceptor activation of the inflammatory response (swelling, vasodilation, and redness). The chemically mediated cascade signaled by the tissue damage occurs not only to protect the injured area, but also to guard against infection and to promote healing.

Descending Pain Modulation

A great advance in our understanding of pain modulation occurred when it was found that pharmacological or electrical stimulation of specific regions in the midbrain produced pain relief.[13] This analgesic effect is ascribed to the activation of pathways that descend from the brainstem to the dorsal horn of the

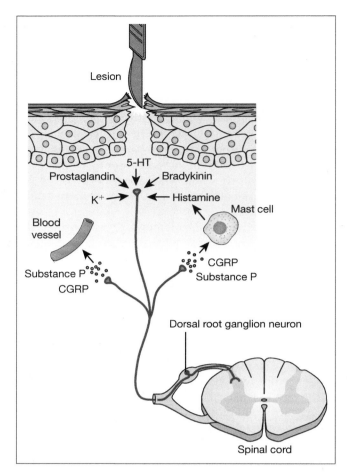

FIGURE 15.32 Nociceptors detect signals of tissue damage and cause peripheral sensitization. Peripheral nociceptors are bare nerve endings with receptors sensitive to inflammatory mediators and signals of tissue damage. Action potentials initiated at the peripheral sensing end are propagated to the dorsal horn synapse with the second-order neuron. Nociceptor neurons synthesize substance P and CGRP, peptide modulators that can be released as neurotransmitters in the spinal cord, and can also be released from peripheral branches of the nociceptor. Local release of substance P and CGRP into adjacent tissue stimulates vasodilation and mast cell degradation, contributing to local edema and pain, as well as promoting peripheral sensitization.
CGRP, calcitonin gene-related peptide; 5-HT, serotonin.

spinal cord. This descending pain-modulating pathway can regulate the transmission of pain signals to higher brain regions. The key brainstem region that produces this descending inhibition is the PAG. When animals receive electrical stimulation at this site, it inhibits the activity of nociceptive projection neurons in the dorsal horn and produces analgesia. Neurons in the PAG project to the medulla and specifically target neurons containing norepinephrine or serotonin, which in turn, project onto the spinal cord to modulate (diminish) pain transmission in the spinal cord (**Figure 15.33**).

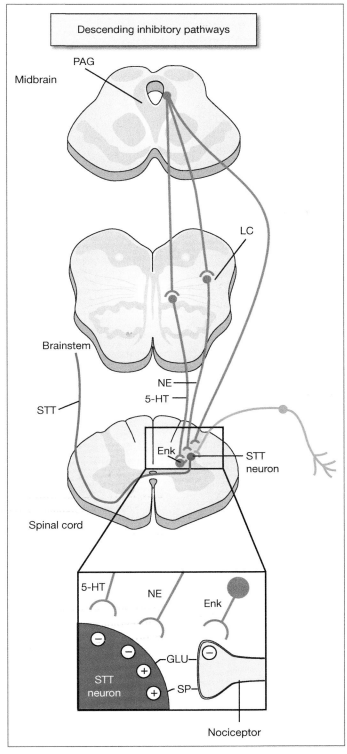

FIGURE 15.33 Inhibitory modulation of nociceptor transmission. Transmission by nociceptors releases glutamate and substance P, which stimulates ascending spinothalamic tract neurons, resulting in pain perception. Enkephalin released from local interneurons binds to presynaptic μ receptors and reduces the amount of glutamate and substance P released. 5-HT and NE released from descending modulatory pathways originating in the brainstem directly inhibit STT cells, reducing ascending transmission of the pain signal. Descending inhibitory pathways from the PAG are activated by opioid analgesics.

Enk, enkephalin; GLU, glutamate; 5-HT, serotonin; LC, locus ceruleus; NE, norepinephrine; PAG, periaqueductal gray; SP, substance P; STT, spinothalamic tract.

In addition to descending pain pathways, local interactions within the dorsal horn between mechanoreceptive nerve fibers and neural circuits can control the transmission of nociceptive information. These interactions may help explain the capability to reduce the feeling of sharp pain by activating low-threshold touch or mechanoreceptors (associated with the Aß axons shown in **Figure 15.31**). For example, if you stub a toe, the natural and effective response is to rub the site of injury. In the mid-1960s, Ron Melzack and Patrick Wall sought to describe this phenomenon using observations from animal experiments.[14] They proposed that the flow of nociceptive information through the spinal cord is moderated by simultaneous activation of the large myelinated fibers associated with low-threshold mechanoreceptors. Melzack and Wall called this the *gate theory of pain*. Although further investigation has led to modifications of their original idea, it stimulated much research on pain modulation and highlighted the importance of synaptic interactions within the dorsal horn for modulating the perception of pain intensity.

Descending inhibitory pathways involving the PAG can be activated by opioid analgesics and by endogenous opioids. All of the endogenous opioids (enkephalins, endorphins, and dynorphins) are present in the PAG. At the level of the spinal cord, enkephalin released from interneurons specifically acts to inhibit the release of substance P and glutamate from the primary sensory neuron, thereby representing an additional endogenous pain modulation pathway (see **Figure 15.33**). Knowledge of these endogenous pathways has allowed us to develop pharmacological interventions to treat pain.

Evidence of endogenous opioid pain modulation is the so-called *placebo effect* (**Box 15.4**).[15,16]

Sensitization

Pain modulation can take the form of increased pain sensations, which is referred to as *sensitization*. Following inflammation and injury, sensitization occurs both peripherally, due to prostaglandins and other chemical mediators, and centrally, due to glutamate and substance P. Pain sensitization occurs in several forms. The first is primary **hyperalgesia**, which is defined as a state in which a stimulus that ordinarily would be perceived as only slightly painful is perceived as very painful. For example, following sunburn, the skin becomes increasingly more sensitive to changes in temperature and pressure. This effect is due to changes in neuronal sensitivity in the peripheral receptors as well as their central targets.

Central sensitization, on the other hand, is an immediate-onset, activity-dependent increase in the excitability of neurons in the dorsal horn following high levels of activity in the peripheral nociceptive nerve fibers. As a consequence, nociceptive fibers that were at subthreshold levels before the painful event become sufficient to generate action potentials, thus contributing to increased pain sensitivity. In this case, stimuli that under normal conditions would be painless activate second-order neurons in the dorsal horn that receive nociceptive inputs, giving rise to a sensation of pain. The induction of pain by a normally harmless stimulus is referred to as **allodynia**. This sensitization usually occurs immediately after the painful event and can last hours to days.

Both hyperalgesia and allodynia resulting from central sensitization demonstrate the plasticity in the nervous system, such that changes or injury to nerves can result in pain, even in the absence of tissue damage. As damaged tissue repairs itself, the sensitization induced by peripheral and central mechanisms

---

BOX 15.4
The Placebo Effect

The placebo effect is a physiological response after the administration of a pharmacologically inert *therapy*.[15] It has been demonstrated through fMRI studies of patients who are subjected to an acute painful stimulus, and told that they are being given a pain-relieving drug, an analgesic, when in fact, they are given a placebo.[16] Despite receiving an inactive therapy, the participants reported pain relief.

fMRI, functional MRI.

Analysis of the fMRI data showed that when the placebo was administered, parts of the brain involved in opioid transmission, including the dorsolateral prefrontal cortex, rostral cingulate cortex, hypothalamus, PAG, and rostral ventral medulla, were activated. In addition, this reported analgesia decreased after administration of the opioid antagonist drug naloxone, providing evidence that our own endogenous opioids are responsible for this pain modulation.

usually diminishes and the threshold for pain returns to predamage levels. However, when the nerve fibers or pathways themselves are impaired, as occurs in conditions such as diabetes and multiple sclerosis, these processes can persist, resulting in a condition called **neuropathic pain.** Neuropathic pain can be elicited by nonpainful stimuli, such as gentle touch and the pressure of clothing. Neuropathic pain is described as a persistent burning sensation with intermittent periods of shooting, stabbing, or electric shock-like jolts. Neuropathic pain conditions can be difficult to treat and are refractory to many analgesic drugs.

In some cases, acute nociceptive pain can turn into chronic neuropathic pain. The risk factors that contribute to the development of chronic pain are not well understood. Recent literature suggests that the deregulation of descending pain pathways may lead to the so-called chronification of pain.[17]

Referred Pain

The pain associated with tissue injury to the viscera (i.e., heart attack, kidney stone) is distinct from somatic (skin, tissue, muscle) pain in that the pain fibers travel from the organs mingled with autonomic nerve fibers in visceral nerves. Thus, visceral pain signals reach the spinal cord at the level associated with autonomic innervation of an organ. Upon entering the spinal cord, visceral sensory neuron terminals are located in the same segmental level as adjacent somatic nociceptors; thus, the visceral pain may be reflected in the central nervous system in somatic pathways, leading the brain to *feel* the pain in somatic, as opposed to visceral, regions. This phenomenon of visceral pain being reflected in somatic pain is known as *referred pain*, which is defined as pain perceived at a location other than the site of the painful stimulus. For example, people who have a heart attack (myocardial infarction) often report feeling pain in their neck, shoulder, or back, rather than in their chest, which is the true site of the injury.

PHARMACOLOGICAL MODULATION OF PAIN

In clinical practice, pharmacological interventions are a common way to modulate pain transmission, based on their activity in different parts of the pain pathways. As noted, inflammatory mediators are the key amplifiers of the nociceptive response to injury. A class of highly prevalent pro-nociceptive mediators is the prostaglandins. Suppression of prostaglandin synthesis at sites of inflammation is the primary mechanism of the analgesic effects of nonsteroidal antiinflammatory drugs (NSAIDs).

The antinociceptive and antiinflammatory effects of NSAIDs result from their ability to inhibit the activity of the cyclooxygenase enzyme (COX), which in turn impairs the two-step transformation of arachidonic acid into prostaglandins.

Opioids modulate pain when bound to opioid receptors on neurons located throughout pain pathways, by inhibiting the transmission of pain signals. These receptors are found on nociceptive terminals in the dorsal horn, where they reduce substance P release and reduce nociceptive transmission. They also are found in the midbrain PAG and ventromedial medulla, which, as previously described, are sources of the descending modulatory inputs to the spinal cord. Finally, there are opioid receptors in the nucleus accumbens, which is known as the reward center of the brain. It is hypothesized that these opioid receptors are responsible for the pleasurable sensations, which not only diminish the negative emotional response to pain but also lead to tolerance, dependency, and substance use disorders.

In certain chronic pain syndromes, particularly neuropathic pain, tricyclic antidepressants that inhibit serotonin and norepinephrine uptake can be effective at reducing pain. Presumably this is due to the descending modulatory pathways described earlier.

NONPHARMACOLOGICAL MODULATION OF PAIN

Wide availability and increasing potency of opioid analgesics have now led to widespread opioid use disorders and death due to opioid overdose. In many individuals, their first exposure to opioids was from medications prescribed for acute pain. This situation has greatly stimulated interest in nonpharmacological approaches for pain management. A systematic review of nonpharmacological therapies for chronic pain syndromes was conducted by the Agency for Healthcare Research and Quality. In patients with chronic low back pain, chronic neck pain, knee and hip osteoarthritis, fibromyalgia, and chronic tension headaches, modest improvements in function and pain were achieved with nonpharmacological therapies. Interventions included exercise, psychological therapies, physical modalities, manual therapies, mindfulness and mind–body practices, and multidisciplinary rehabilitation. Exercise was associated with improvement in all conditions except chronic tension headache; other approaches were effective in only one or two conditions. Most studies were small and short term, limiting interpretation of the results, but this field is of growing interest to expand options for individuals suffering from chronic, disabling pain.[18]

Thought Questions

15. What are the names and sources of peripheral mediators that produce activation and sensitization of nociceptor endings?

[handwritten: 512 / other lipid mediators / Bradykinin, histamine, serotonin arachidonic acid]

16. What are the neurotransmitters of first-order pain neurons?

[handwritten: Substance P / Glutamate]

17. What are the neurotransmitters that reduce pain transmission through their actions in the dorsal horn?

[handwritten: NE Serotonin / opioid recept. ↓Substance P / enkephalin / and reduce nociceptive transmission]

SPECIAL SENSES: VISION AND HEARING

Similar to somatic sensations of touch, pain, muscle stretch, and proprioception, vision and hearing involve specialized structures that are restricted to a specific type of input from the external world, as well as central pathways and dedicated brain regions for signal recognition.

VISUAL SYSTEM

The eye receives rays of light that pass through the pupil at the center of the iris. The light rays then move through the lens for focusing, ending on retinal photoreceptors that take the form of rod and cone cells. Electrical activity in the photoreceptors is transmitted to bipolar cells and then ganglion cells with axons that form the optic nerve, cranial nerve (CN) II. The eye contains gel-like liquids in two separate cavities, anterior and posterior. The anterior chamber contains aqueous humor, while the posterior cavity contains vitreous humor (**Figure 15.34**). Eye movements are controlled by the extraocular muscles, innervated by CNs III, IV, and VI.

The retina is divided by anatomical location into the nasal retina (closest to the nose) and the temporal retina (closest to the temple). The left portion of the visual field projects to the nasal retina of the left eye and the temporal retina of the right eye, while the right portion of the visual field projects to the temporal retina of the left eye and the nasal retina of the right eye. The optic nerves carrying these fibers project posteriorly, joining at the optic chiasm above the pituitary fossa. At the optic chiasm, fibers from the nasal retinas both cross, while those from the temporal retinas stay ipsilateral to their origin. After the optic chiasm, the fiber bundles, now termed the *optic tracts*, project to the lateral geniculate bodies of the thalamus. The lateral geniculate neurons, in turn, project via the optic radiation to the visual cortex in the occipital lobe, areas 17, 18, and 19 (**Figure 15.35**). Disorders of vision can occur from diseases of the eye (macular degeneration and glaucoma), nervous system disorders (multiple sclerosis, stroke, and tumors), or systemic disorders (diabetic retinopathy and thyroid disease).

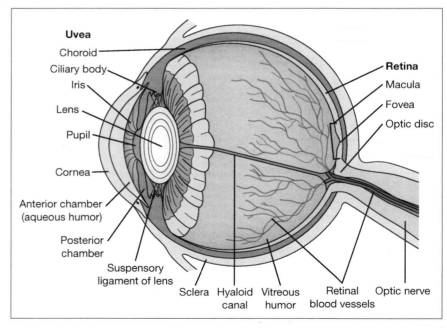

FIGURE 15.34 Anatomy of the eye and optic nerve. Light enters the eye through the cornea, travels through the pupil to the lens, which focuses the light rays on the retina. Posterior to the cornea, the outer most layer of the eye is the sclera. The uvea is the next layer, made up of iris, ciliary body, and choroid. The innermost layer is the retina, site of photoreceptor cells and other cellular elements. The retina also includes the macula, fovea, and optic disc, which is the point of attachment of the optic nerve and retinal blood vessels.

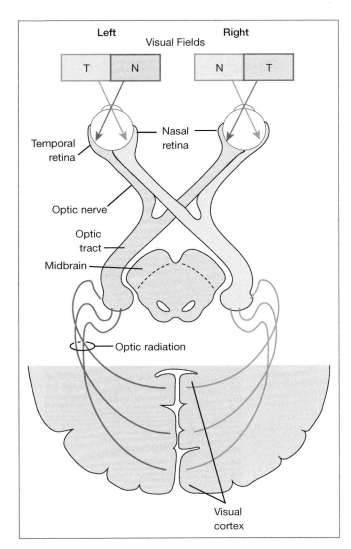

FIGURE 15.35 Visual pathways. Visual fields can be subdivided by light rays entering from the midline to the nose (N = nasal) and from the midline to the temple (T = temporal). These orientations are reversed in the retina, with the nasal field projecting to the temporal retina, and the temporal field projecting to the nasal retina. For both the right and left eyes, axons from the nasal retina travel in the optic nerve to the optic chiasm, where they cross and travel in the optic tract to the lateral geniculate nucleus of the contralateral thalamus. The lateral geniculate bodies are adjacent to the midbrain (central structure), and additional visual information is relayed to the midbrain's superior colliculus nuclei. Conversely, axons from the temporal retina travel in the optic nerve to the ipsilateral optic tract, terminating in the ipsilateral lateral geniculate. From each lateral geniculate nucleus, the optic radiations carry the axons to the visual cortex in the occipital lobe. Note that visual input coming from the left visual field (reaching the nasal retina of the left eye and the temporal retina of the right eye) ultimately travels to the right (contralateral) visual cortex. The opposite is true for input coming from the right visual field—the final destination for that input is the left visual cortex.

AUDITORY SYSTEM

The ear is divided into three components: outer ear, middle ear, and inner ear. The function of the outer ear is to funnel sound waves to the middle ear, where the tympanic membrane picks up the vibrations and creates movements of the three ear bones of the middle ear—the malleus, incus, and stapes. The bone movements transmit vibrations to the inner ear that are detected by hair cells of the cochlea. Depolarization of the hair cells is stimulated by vibrations of different frequencies, corresponding to low, intermediate, and high pitch. Upon depolarization, the hair cells release glutamate, creating action potentials in the adjacent cochlear sensory nerve endings.

The axons of these cells travel in the cochlear nerve (CN VIII) to the brainstem cochlear nuclei. Relay neurons then transmit the signal to the superior olive, midbrain inferior colliculus, and medial geniculate body of the thalamus. The final signal travels bilaterally to the auditory cortex in the temporal lobe. Thus, unlike vision, there is much greater bilateral transmission of auditory impulses (Figure 15.36). Hair cells are lost with aging, contributing to age-related hearing loss, the most common sensory deficit. Initially, the loss is restricted to high-frequency sounds and does not noticeably impair speech perception and communication. However, the losses are progressive and can gradually limit conversation and social function. Correction can be obtained in most cases with hearing aids.

MOTOR ACTIVITY AND MOVEMENT DISORDERS

The human body has hundreds of skeletal muscles responsible for purposeful movements, involuntary control of posture and balance, reflex activity, communication, and facial expression. Skeletal muscles are controlled by motor neurons located in some cranial nerve nuclei and in the ventral horn of the spinal cord. The neurotransmitter of all motor neurons is acetylcholine, and the receptors of the neuromuscular junction are nicotinic acetylcholine receptors. Motor neurons are controlled by an ascending hierarchy of synaptic inputs that build from involuntary local control, to gross postural and balance regulation, to spinal and brainstem generation of commonly used patterns (such as walking), to skillful voluntary movements.

This hierarchical progression from spinal to cortical levels of motor control comprises:

• Spinal motor neurons and interneurons that are responsive to sensory feedback from muscles, tendons, and pain sensors, and local circuits that are capable of generating repetitive patterned movements, such walking

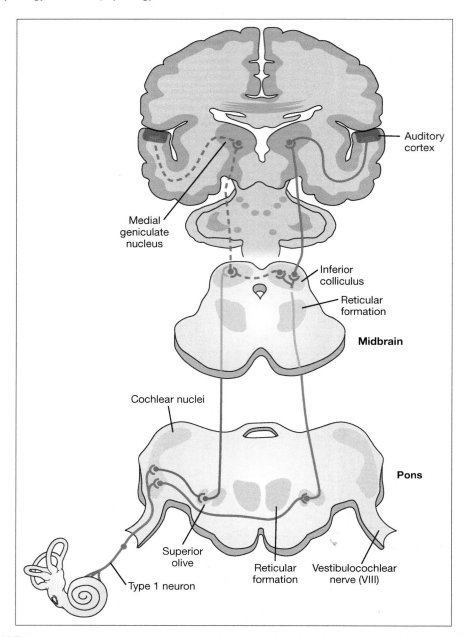

FIGURE 15.36 Auditory pathways. Sound information is relayed from the cochlea via CN VIII, which terminates in the brainstem cochlear nucleus. Relay neurons ascend through brainstem and thalamic nuclei before terminating in primary auditory cortex.
CN, cranial nerve.

- Brainstem pathways that regulate muscle tone and reflex activity and that promote unconscious adjustment of muscle activity for maintenance of posture and balance
- The motor cortex and its output, the corticospinal tract, for voluntary movement and coordination of voluntary movement with posture, balance, and reflex responses

These circuits are modified by the cerebellum and basal ganglia for smooth, precise movements and practiced, skilled movements, respectively.

The organizational scheme presented here omits much of the enormous complexity of the motor control system, aiming to provide a foundation for clinicians to better understand the presentation of patients with lower motor neuron lesions, upper motor neuron lesions, Parkinson disease, and cerebellar disorders.

MOTOR NEURONS AND THE NEUROMUSCULAR JUNCTION

Motor neuron cell bodies are located in the ventral horn of the spinal cord gray matter. The axon of each motor neuron exits the spinal cord via a ventral

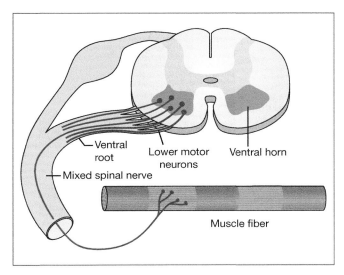

FIGURE 15.37 Motor neuron anatomy. α-Motor neurons are located in the spinal cord ventral horn (shown here), and in cranial nerve nuclei. Motor neuron axons leave via the ventral roots, traveling through spinal nerves and peripheral nerves to reach their skeletal muscle targets. The neurotransmitter of all motor neurons is acetylcholine.

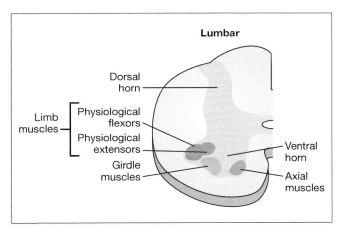

FIGURE 15.38 Motor neuron spinal locations. Spinal motor neurons are located in pools within the ventral horn, with the most medial motor neurons innervating muscles of the trunk (back, ribs, and abdominal muscles). As these muscles are found along the central axis of the body, they are also referred to as "axial" muscles. Moving laterally, the next group of motor neurons innervates the shoulder (in the cervical spinal cord) or the hips (in the lumbar spinal cord). These muscles that connect the trunk to the arms and legs are also known as "girdle" muscles. The most lateral clusters of motor neurons innervate muscles of the arms (cervical cord) and legs (lumbar cord). Motor neurons to physiological flexors are found lateral to those innervating extensors.

root, joins a spinal nerve and then a peripheral nerve, until reaching its specific target muscle and making a specialized synapse at the neuromuscular junction (**Figures 15.37** and **15.38**). Brainstem motor neurons associated with axons in cranial nerves III

through VII and IX through XII control muscles of the head and neck in the same manner as the spinal motor neurons described here.

Cell bodies of motor neurons to trunk and limb muscles are found in the spinal cord gray matter—specifically, in the ventral horn. The white matter tracts of descending motor pathways controlling those motor neurons are found in the ventral and lateral white matter adjacent to the ventral horn. Motor neurons to the arms and legs enlarge the size of the ventral horn, and therefore the whole spinal cord, at the cervical and lumbar enlargements. Spinal cord diameter decreases in the thoracic region, based on the smaller number of neurons innervating trunk muscles. Motor neurons are referred to as *efferent* (away from) neurons, as their axons leave the central nervous system to terminate in the periphery and to control peripheral tissues.

At the cervical and lumbar levels, motor neurons are arranged in pools, with specific target muscle groups clustered together. Within the ventral horn, motor neurons to proximal muscles are found medial to those innervating distal muscles (see Figure 15.38). The most medial neurons control *axial* muscles, those along the body's axis. These are core muscles of the trunk—back and abdominal muscles, which are primarily concerned with the maintenance of posture and balance while at rest and during voluntary activity. Lateral to the axial motor neurons are the *girdle* motor neurons, which innervate the shoulder (at the cervical level) or the hip (at the lumbar level). These neurons control large muscle groups, supporting control of posture and balance and allowing movements of the limbs for voluntary activity. Finally, the most lateral motor neurons innervate the limbs, with a proximal-to-distal orientation corresponding to medial-to-lateral placement in the ventral horn.

The specialized synapse between the motor neuron axon terminal and its target muscle fiber is called the *neuromuscular junction* (**Figure 15.39**). The axon terminal is embedded in a trough in the muscle fiber membrane, across from the postsynaptic region of the muscle membrane that is enriched in nicotinic acetylcholine receptors. Presynaptic action potentials open terminal voltage-gated calcium channels, releasing acetylcholine into the synapse. Acetylcholine binds to nicotinic receptors on the postsynaptic membrane, increasing membrane permeability to sodium, which depolarizes the muscle membrane, initiating a muscle cell action potential. Depolarization opens muscle membrane voltage-gated calcium channels, providing entry of calcium needed for actin–myosin interaction and cross bridge formation. As the contraction begins, acetylcholinesterase is present in the synapse and rapidly degrades acetylcholine, which diffuses away from receptor sites, terminating muscle excitation and contraction unless motor neuron action potentials are sustained. The neuromuscular junction

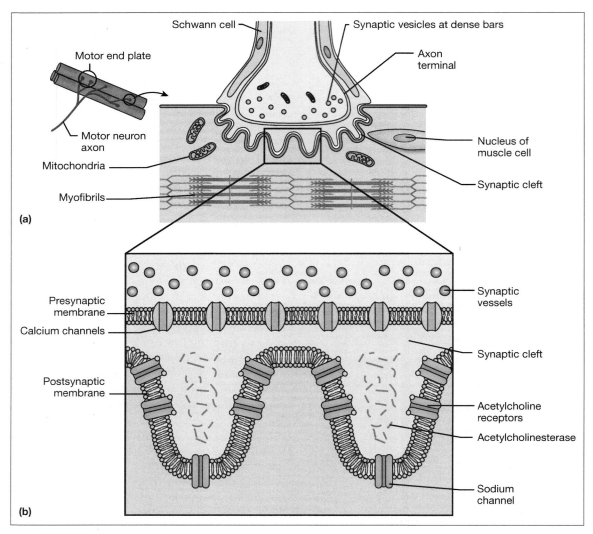

FIGURE 15.39 Neuromuscular junction. Motor neuron axons branch when they reach their peripheral muscle targets, forming synapses on individual fibers within a muscle. At the specialized neuromuscular junction, acetylcholine is released in response to motor neuron action potentials. Acetylcholine diffuses across the synaptic cleft to bind to muscle nicotinic receptors, depolarizing the postsynaptic membrane and producing the muscle action potential that leads to contraction. Acetylcholinesterase breaks down acetylcholine into choline and acetic acid to terminate transmission.
Source: From Haines DE. *Fundamental Neuroscience for Basic and Clinical Applications.* 4th ed. Philadelphia, PA: Saunders/Elsevier; 2013.

disorder **myasthenia gravis** is an autoimmune disorder in which antibodies attack nicotinic acetylcholine receptors. The resulting inflammatory response leads to degeneration of the neuromuscular junction and failure of neuromuscular transmission.

LOWER MOTOR NEURON LESIONS

Motor neurons of the brainstem and spinal cord are sometimes referred to as *lower motor neurons.* This is a clinical term for these neurons that are the final common pathway projecting to, and causing contraction of, skeletal muscles. **Lower motor neuron lesions** can occur from damage to any part of the motor neuron (**Figure 15.40**). This includes diseases or trauma that cause any of the following: the death of motor neuron cell bodies; compression of ventral roots, spinal nerves, or peripheral nerves; trauma to these nerves; or demyelination of peripheral nerves (as in Guillain–Barré syndrome). Signs and symptoms associated with lower motor neuron lesions include weakness or complete inability to move the

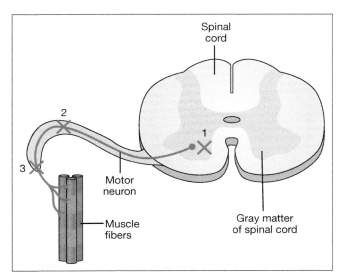

FIGURE 15.40 Lower motor neuron lesion. Lower motor neuron lesion clinical findings result from disease processes that affect the motor neuron cell body (**1**) or its axon within the spinal nerve (**2**) or in or near the neuromuscular junction (**3**). In each case, the failure of motor neuron function produces weakness or absent voluntary movement and stretch reflexes, along with atrophy of the target muscle.

affected muscle, lack of a stretch reflex response, flaccidity to passive movement, and muscle atrophy. Assessment of affected muscle by electromyography (EMG) shows disorganized low-level electrical activity (fibrillation), rather than action potential activity. Diseases associated with death of spinal cord motor neurons include polio, amyotrophic lateral sclerosis, and spinal muscular atrophy (SMA) in children. Peripheral nerve compression syndromes such as sciatica and carpal tunnel syndrome may also have motor findings consistent with the lower motor neuron lesion.

SPINAL CORD REFLEX CIRCUITS

Control of motor neurons begins with sensory inputs from the innervated muscle itself as well as the tendon attached to that muscle. A primary synaptic input to a motor neuron is the muscle spindle sensory fiber (**Figure 15.41**). The muscle spindle is a sense organ, embedded within each muscle, which has regular action potential activity in proportion to the length of the muscle. At a typical resting length, the muscle spindle has a moderate rate of action potentials. As the muscle lengthens, the muscle spindle action potential rate increases. As the muscle shortens, the muscle spindle action potential rate decreases.

The spindle sensory axon travels through a peripheral nerve to enter the spinal cord through a dorsal

root, where it branches. One branch terminates in the ventral horn, making synaptic contacts on the motor neurons supplying the muscle where the muscle spindle resides (referred to as the *homonymous muscle*). The spindle sensory axon is a large-diameter, heavily myelinated fiber, also referred to as a sensory Ia fiber, which conducts at 80 to 100 m/sec. It releases the neurotransmitter glutamate, exciting the motor neuron to increase action potential firing rate. Physiologically, muscle spindle control of muscle length is a major excitatory input that contributes to resting muscle tone, as well as providing critical feedback for coordinated movements.

Clinically, the muscle spindle is the sensory fiber contributing to the monosynaptic stretch reflex. As the muscle spindle action potential rate increases, synaptic excitation elicits the motor response. The motor neuron action potential rate increases, increasing acetylcholine release at the neuromuscular junction, which rapidly increases muscle contraction. The reflex is evaluated by tapping on a tendon to lengthen a muscle and observing the speed and intensity of the resulting muscle contraction (**Box 15.5**).

The Golgi tendon organ (GTO) is a second sensory fiber that controls motor neuron activity. The GTO sensory endings are located in the tendon connecting a muscle to bone and can sense the tension on the muscle. As tension increases, the GTO increases the action potential firing rate, and those action potentials are conducted back to the spinal cord by a slightly slower axon, the Ib fiber. The GTO axon terminates on an inhibitory interneuron that releases GABA to inhibit the firing of the motor neuron to the source muscle fiber. Between spindle and GTO inputs, motor neuron activity can be precisely tuned to create the correct muscle length and tension for a specific motor act, whether voluntary or involuntary.

BOX 15.5
Muscle Stretch Reflexes

The neurological examination includes evaluation of the following limb reflexes, with their associated spinal cord levels:

- Biceps (C5–C6)
- Brachioradialis (C5–C6)
- Triceps (C6–C8)
- Patellar (L2–L4)
- Achilles (S1–S2)

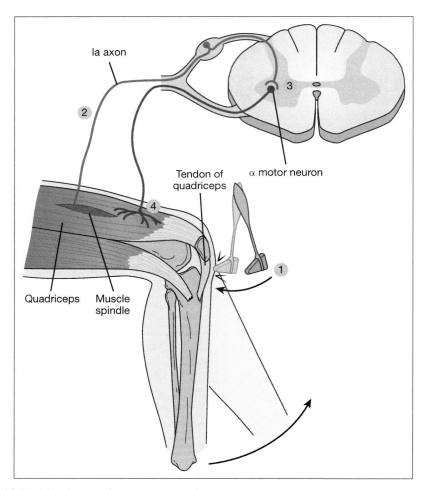

FIGURE 15.41 Muscle stretch reflex. The muscle stretch reflex relies on the circuitry of the muscle spindle and its excitatory input to motor neurons supplying the homonymous muscle. The normal function of spindle input to motor neurons is to detect muscle length and to amplify excitation if the desired muscle contraction to accomplish a goal has not been reached. This circuit is assessed during the neurological examination in the following chain of events: **(1)** A brief tap on the tendon lengthens the muscle, increasing muscle spindle action potential activity. **(2)** The action potential is propagated to the spinal cord via the Ia axon. **(3)** As the action potential reaches the synapse on the motor neuron, glutamate is released, exciting the motor neuron. **(4)** Motor neuron action potential firing rate increases, leading to reflexive muscle contraction.

Pathophysiological conditions, both systemic and neurological disorders, are a source of abnormal findings in stretch reflex strength and speed. Stretch reflexes are reported on a scale from 0 (no reflex) to 4+ (hyperactive), with 2+ being normal. Conditions and states associated with **hyperreflexia** include hyperthyroidism, hypocalcemia, and eclampsia in pregnancy, all of which are associated with a generalized increase in neuronal membrane excitability. The states of hypothyroidism and hypercalcemia have the opposite effect, decreasing neuronal membrane excitability and producing **hyporeflexia**. Neurological insults that damage higher level motor pathways, particularly the motor cortex and corticospinal tract, remove descending inhibitory influences on stretch reflexes, resulting in hyperreflexia. This type of presentation is one characteristic of the *upper motor neuron lesion* described later. *Lower motor neuron lesions* are associated with absent or hypoactive muscle stretch reflexes due to the destruction of the efferent arm of the reflex.

MOTOR PATHWAYS FROM THE PONS AND MEDULLA

It is useful to think of the hierarchy of motor control building up from the spinal level (**Figure 15.42**). Three brainstem regions provide descending inputs to motor neurons: In the medulla and pons, the vestibular complex and the reticular formation give rise to vestibulospinal and reticulospinal pathways, respectively, and the midbrain red nucleus is the source of

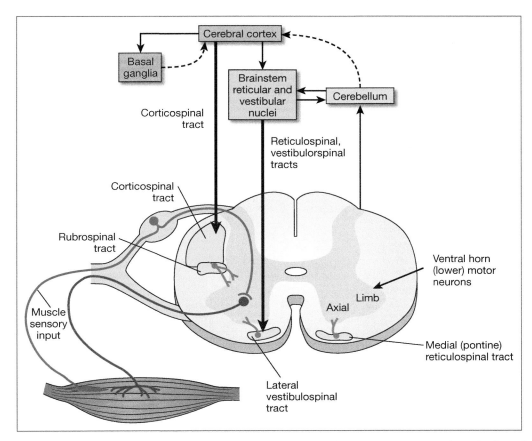

FIGURE 15.42 Overview of major features of motor control. Motor neurons in the spinal cord ventral horn are controlled by synaptic inputs from several hierarchically arranged sources. At the spinal level, muscle sensory input from muscle spindles and Golgi tendon organs provide excitation and inhibition, respectively. The brainstem reticular and vestibular nuclei project to the spinal cord in the reticulospinal and vestibulospinal tracts, respectively, generally exciting stretch reflexes and extensor muscles, and promoting tone of the core muscles for posture and balance. The cerebral cortex plans and modifies movement in conjunction with the basal ganglia and cerebellum, ultimately projecting to the spinal cord via the corticospinal tract. The corticospinal tract initiates voluntary movements, particularly fine movements of the hand and face, and activity of flexors over extensors. It directly and indirectly inhibits stretch reflexes.

the rubrospinal tract. The brainstem motor pathways usually influence large muscle groups through control of interneurons, rather than controlling precise movements through direct projections to individual motor neurons. Also, these brainstem pathways can access spinal motor patterns such as the movements involved in walking, such that conscious cortical control of common movement patterns is not required.

Anatomically, the vestibulospinal tract and reticulospinal tract are found in the ventral and medial white matter of the spinal cord and can be considered together as *medial pathways* (**Figure 15.43**). Their myelinated descending axons give off axon branches at all spinal levels. The medial ventral horn gray matter adjacent to these tracts is the location of motor neuron cell bodies controlling axial muscles—the back and abdominal muscles of the body core, allowing an

upright posture. At the cervical and lumbar enlargements, these tracts control extensor muscles of the shoulder and hip, respectively, as well as facilitating contraction of arm and leg extensor muscles. The medial pathways also enhance stretch reflex activity. Together with proprioceptors from muscles, tendons, and joints, and visual detection of movement or instability, the vestibulospinal tracts maintain proper posture and balance during a range of activities. Neurons in the brainstem reticular formation are the source of the reticulospinal tracts that travel in the ventromedial white matter and have functions similar to the vestibulospinal tract—facilitating axial muscle activity, motor tone, and reflexes.

The actions of the vestibulospinal and reticulospinal tracts on motor activity are visible in patients with pathological states of severe brain damage that result

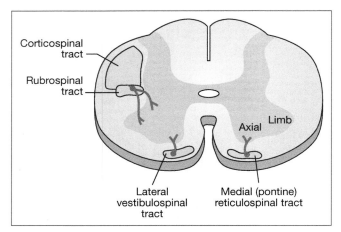

FIGURE 15.43 Ventromedial and lateral descending tracts in motor control. A cross-sectional view of the spinal cord shows medial pathways from the brainstem vestibular and reticular nuclei that descend to all levels of the spinal cord in the ventromedial white matter. These pathways give off axons at each level and primarily influence adjacent motor neurons to axial muscles. Medial pathways facilitate posture and balance, as well as stimulating extensor muscles and increasing reflex tone. The lateral white matter contains the rubrospinal tract and corticospinal tract, which exert greater influence on motor neurons to distal muscles of the limbs and flexor muscles and inhibit stretch reflexes.

in coma, brain swelling, and herniation of forebrain structures through the tentorial notch of dura overlying the midbrain. Such catastrophic conditions eliminate the influence of lateral motor pathways from the motor cortex and midbrain red nucleus. As long as the pons and medulla are intact, the patient's body involuntarily assumes the **decerebrate posture**, with head, arms, and legs in a state of rigid extension. From this clinical observation, as well as experimental data in animal models, it is inferred that the primary influence of the motor centers in the pons and medulla is to facilitate the activity of extensor muscle groups.

MOTOR PATHWAYS FROM THE CORTEX AND MIDBRAIN

The ability to have voluntary skilled movements, particularly those of the hands and face, is most highly developed in humans. The brain region dedicated to this function is the motor cortex, assisted by the red nucleus of the midbrain. The corresponding lateral descending pathways from these regions are the corticospinal tract (CST) and the rubrospinal tract (RuST; **Figure 15.44**). The CST plays the greatest role in motor control, while the RuST serves to facilitate the actions of the CST. These pathways do not operate in isolation; rather, they work, in part, by modulating the activity of the pontine and medullary reticulospinal neurons to maintain posture and balance during purposeful movements. Also, through these brainstem regions and

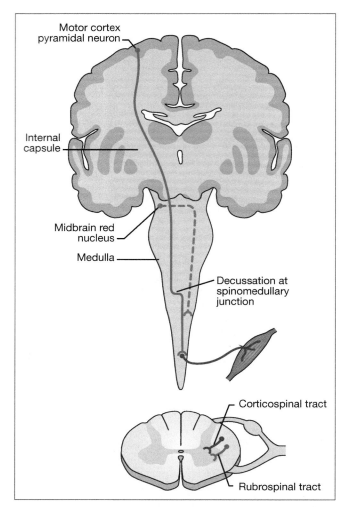

FIGURE 15.44 Longitudinal view of the corticospinal and rubrospinal tracts.

spinal projections, the CST and RuST inhibit spinal reflexes, which allows movements to be smooth and coordinated. Similar to the brainstem pathways, the CST and RuST primarily influence spinal interneurons that synapse on functional groups of motor neurons (e.g., extensors or flexors that work together to create motor patterns), with a minority of the axons directly controlling spinal motor neurons.

Anatomically, the CST and RuST are organized as follows: Large neurons of the motor cortex have axons that make up the CST. These axons descend through the forebrain's internal capsule, a large white matter bundle that travels from cortex to subcortical regions. From this location, the axons descend through the midbrain and pons, and follow the ventral surface of the medulla, forming swellings termed the *medullary pyramids*. At the junction of the medulla and spinal cord, many of those axons cross the midline and continue to descend in the lateral white matter of the spinal cord. Neurons of the midbrain red nucleus have axons that descend mixed with axons of the CST. Most of these axons cross and descend in the contralateral spinal cord, in the lateral column ventral to the CST.

Functionally, the RuST tends to activate motor neurons to flexor muscle groups of the arm, while having no detectable effect on motor neurons innervating the legs. The CST has its primary influence on motor neurons innervating the hands and face, controlling fine movements by relatively small muscle groups. Coordination of compensatory movements of the trunk during complex activities depends on the cortical innervation of the brainstem pathways and circuits that maintain an upright posture.

The actions of the CST are visible in patients who sustain injuries that interrupt the CST neurons and axons while leaving the midbrain and RuST intact. These injuries lead to **decorticate posturing**, in which the arms are flexed while the legs are extended. Unlike decerebrate rigidity, the influence of the intact RuST is seen in the lack of neck and arm extension and the presence of arm flexion.

A similar posture, but affecting only one side of the body, affects patients who sustain a unilateral insult (e.g., from a stroke) to the motor cortex or the CST as it passes through the internal capsule. The resulting signs and symptoms in patients who sustain such injuries are termed an **upper motor neuron lesion**. The presentation of a person with an upper motor neuron lesion often includes arm flexion and pronation, and leg extension, only on the affected side. This is accompanied by lack of fine hand movements, arm and leg weakness, and hyperreflexia due to loss of descending inhibitory influences on reticulospinal pathways and reflexes. Although fine movements are severely impaired, gross movements and postural movements are partially preserved in these patients owing to intact pathways from the brainstem to the spinal cord (**Figure 15.45**). The combination of weakness and loss of fine coordinated movements, hyperreflexia, spasticity, and rigidity in specific muscle groups (arm—flexor, leg—extensor) characterizes the clinical findings in patients with upper motor neuron lesions. If a stroke or other source of injury damages the motor speech area (Broca area) in the hemisphere that is dominant for speech, expressive aphasia is observed in addition to these findings.

ACCESSORY SYSTEMS IN MOTOR CONTROL

The Basal Ganglia

The function of the basal ganglia is to initiate and refine movement and to improve movement with practice. The anatomical structures of the basal ganglia include the striatum, composed of the caudate and the putamen; the globus pallidus; subthalamic nucleus; and substantia nigra (**Figure 15.46**).

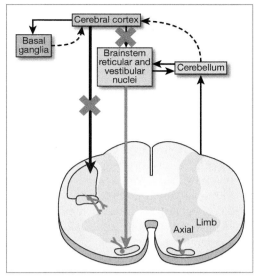

FIGURE 15.45 After a stroke or other damage to the motor cortex, inputs to brainstem nuclei and to the spinal cord are lost (red Xs). This is manifested by weakness contralateral to the lesion and loss of fine movements of the fingers and hands. At the same time, the relative impact of brainstem reticular and vestibular nuclei on motor function is increased. Depending on the site and extent of motor cortex or internal capsule damage, the patient may develop forearm flexion and pronation, and leg extension on the affected side. Loss of descending inhibition and a general increase in spinal excitability produces hyperreflexia of the affected muscles.

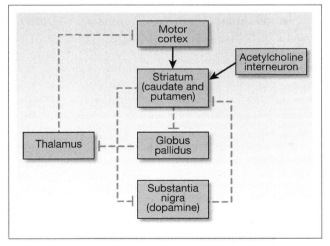

FIGURE 15.46 Simplified version of basal ganglia circuitry. Projections vary between excitation (black arrows, mediated by Glu) and inhibition (red dashed lines with perpendicular ends, mediated by GABA). In addition, motor control by the striatum (caudate and putamen nuclei) is modulated by the balance of DA, from substantia nigra neurons, and ACh, from intrinsic interneurons. Neurodegenerative loss of substantia nigra DA neurons contributes to the motor manifestations in Parkinson disease.

ACh, acetylcholine; DA, dopamine; GABA, gamma-aminobutyric acid; Glu, glutamate.

Voluntary movements are initiated by premotor cortex neurons that project to motor cortex, exciting neurons that project to the striatum. Striatal synaptic processing results in a series of inhibitory outputs that relay information from the globus pallidus, to the thalamus, returning to motor cortex to complete the feedback loop.

In a simplified view of the basal ganglia chemical circuitry, glutamate neurons in the motor cortex project to striatal acetylcholine interneurons. These interneurons excite GABA neurons projecting from the striatum to the globus pallidus. Substantia nigra dopamine neurons oppose the excitatory actions of acetylcholine and inhibit the GABA output from the striatum. The rapid synaptic actions of glutamate and GABA are modulated by the slow synaptic actions of acetylcholine and dopamine acting on striatal muscarinic and dopamine receptors, respectively.

Parkinson disease is the second most common neurodegenerative disorder worldwide, after Alzheimer disease, and the most common movement disorder. The most common form is idiopathic Parkinson disease. Paradoxically, although a major manifestation of the disorder is akinesia (lack of movement) or bradykinesia (slow movements), it also has features of increased motor tone. These include tremor (in which there are alternating contractions of flexors and extensors, often in the wrists), rigidity (in which flexors and extensors are activated simultaneously, producing stiffness of the limb), or both. The pathogenesis of idiopathic Parkinson disease is the death of dopamine neurons in the substantia nigra.

Degeneration of the nigrostriatal dopamine pathway is accompanied by relative overactivity of excitatory acetylcholine transmission in the striatum. Pharmacological management of Parkinson disease aims to restore brain dopamine levels by administration of the precursor L-dopa, or by reducing dopamine breakdown by inhibiting dopamine-degrading enzymes MAO or COMT. Additional approaches include medications that block acetylcholine receptors or stimulate dopamine receptors.[19] Recent advances include implantation of electrodes for deep brain stimulation of the globus pallidus, which reduces motor dysfunction in patients who become refractory to pharmacological approaches.[20] Parkinson disease has additional manifestations, including depression, sleep disturbances, autonomic dysfunction, and balance instability. Approximately 10% to 15% of patients with Parkinson disease will develop dementia with cortical Lewy body deposits. These manifestations do not resolve with L-dopa and other treatments, indicating that additional neural circuits are disrupted by Parkinson neuropathology.

The Cerebellum

The function of the cerebellum is to initiate movement, to refine movements in progress and to further refine movements after repeated practice. The cerebellum receives inputs from the motor cortex indirectly, after a relay in the pons. This input delivers the motor *plan* to the cerebellum for refinement before movement initiation. During the movement, the cerebellum receives sensory feedback from muscles and tendons (muscle spindles and tendon organs) traveling in the spinocerebellar tracts. This feedback allows cerebellar processing and output to the cortex via the brainstem red nucleus and the thalamus (**Figure 15.47**). Activity in this loop further refines the movement in progress. In this way, the cerebellum functions as a *quality control* system over movements. In addition, the medial cerebellum connects with brainstem vestibular nuclei and is responsible for maintenance of normal balance and posture during walking and other activities.

Cerebellar dysfunction can result from insults such as stroke or tumors, or can be congenital, as in the hereditary disorders Friedreich ataxia and autosomal dominant spinocerebellar ataxias. When an acute injury process such as a stroke produces a unilateral cerebellar lesion, the motor examination findings are ipsilateral to the deficit, unlike cortical motor lesions. In many cases, however, the disease process affects both sides of the cerebellum, producing bilateral movement abnormalities. A primary finding is *ataxia*, a term indicating

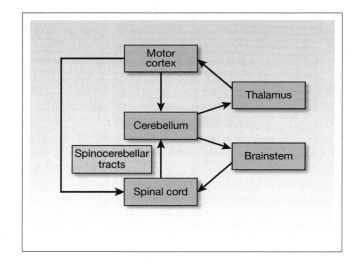

FIGURE 15.47 Cerebellar processing. The cerebellum receives input from the cerebral cortex as a movement is being planned (not shown in this figure). During the movement, spinocerebellar tracts feed proprioceptive information back to the cerebellum, where the movement in progress is compared to the initial plan. Cerebellar outputs feed back to the red nucleus and via the thalamus to the cortex, to correct movements in progress.

uncoordinated movements and broad-based, unstable gait. This reflects the loss of medial cerebellar function for control of balance. Damage to lateral cerebellar regions produces distinctive motor deficits, including the following:

- *Dysmetria*—movements that fluctuate between overshooting the target or undershooting the target
  - ○ This is observed during the neurological examination by tasks such as the ability of patients to touch a finger to the examiner's finger, and then touch their own nose, while the examiner moves his or her finger, shifting the target.
  - ○ Dysmetria of the leg is assessed by the task of touching a heel to the opposite knee, then sliding the heel down to the ankle.
- *Dysdiadochokinesia*—the inability to conduct rapidly alternating movements such as tapping thumb and forefinger together, or alternately touching the palm of the hand and the back of the hand to the leg

- *Intention tremor*—tremor that worsens as a movement approaches its target

SUMMARY OF MOTOR DISORDERS

Motor disorders can result from ischemic, traumatic, infectious, immune-mediated, or neoplastic processes affecting any level of the motor control system. Certain named disorders, such as Parkinson disease or Huntington disease, result from neurodegeneration that targets specific clusters of neurons. Finally, several genetic disorders, such as SMA or spinocerebellar ataxias, affect specific cell types or pathways. In each case, there is weakness and excess fatigue due to muscles overburdened by compensatory activity. Diagnostic features rely on the specific findings that are characteristic of each disorder (Table 15.3). Most of the motor disorders are not curable, resulting in progressive dysfunction and impairment. Assistive devices such as canes, walkers, and wheelchairs are common modalities to preserve mobility and varying degrees of independence.

TABLE 15.3 Summary of Motor Disorders

Motor Disorder	Muscle Strength	Muscle Tone	Muscle Atrophy	Reflex Tone	Gait	Posture and Balance
Neuromuscular junction disease (myasthenia gravis)	Weakness, may be proximal and asymmetrical, may affect only cranial nerve distribution, with difficulty in speech and swallowing	Focal decrease in affected areas	Mild	Often preserved	Depends on site of involvement	Depends on site of involvement
Lower motor neuron lesion (polio, peripheral nerve trauma)	Decreased	Decreased	Severe	Decreased or absent	Foot drop, unilateral loss of strength	Maintained within constraints of weakness
Upper motor neuron lesion (stroke)	Decreased	Spasticity	None	Increased	Hemiparetic—arm flexed, leg extended, circumduction gait	Maintained within constraints of weakness
Parkinson disease	Decreased	Increased, with tremor or rigidity	None	May be increased	Slow initiation and freezing, small steps, absent arm swing	Postural instability, falls are common
Cerebellar disease	Uncoordinated, rather than weak	Normal	None	Normal	Uncoordinated ataxic gait	Difficulty maintaining balance

Thought Questions

18. What is the clinical presentation of a person with a lower motor neuron lesion? What mechanisms underlie this presentation?

    [handwritten: weakness]
    [handwritten: Neuromus junction disease]

19. What limb positions are associated with decorticate and decerebrate posturing? How do these presentations relate to the descending pathways that are still functioning, relative to those that are lost?

    [handwritten: Cerebellum remove]

20. An athlete who has practiced a particular movement until she is very skilled describes her performance as reflecting muscle memory. Is this an accurate statement? What brain region is most responsible for improving skill with practice? What disease process might decrease her performance?

    [handwritten: Stroke tumor]

HIGHER FUNCTIONS OF THE NERVOUS SYSTEM

FUNCTIONAL ANATOMY OF COGNITION AND BEHAVIOR

Cognition, learning, memory, executive functions, behavioral control, and perception and regulation of emotions are the highest order functions of the nervous system. An in-depth treatment of this complex topic is beyond the scope of this book, but certain principles can be summarized here. These higher functions require sensory inputs as the basis for decision-making, emotional valence of the sensory inputs as the basis for motivation, and access to motor and autonomic control centers for responses. Such processing involves both focused sensory and motor cortical regions, described earlier, and integrative regions termed *association cortex*.

The PFC, the region of the frontal lobe anterior to the motor and premotor regions, reaches its greatest development in humans, relative to all other species. Damage to the PFC results in the greatest degree of behavioral impairment and personality changes. Appreciation of its unique role in social function was prompted by the case of Phineas Gage, a 19th-century working man and supervisor who sustained a traumatic brain injury in 1848, which damaged much of his PFC, irreversibly impairing his ability to work and live within the constraints of normal societal conventions. Sensory and motor functions, intelligence, and memory of knowledge and of skills (declarative and procedural memory, respectively) are generally preserved in individuals with PFC damage. Impairments are found in appropriate social engagement, planning, and decision-making abilities. These lesions also result in emotional blunting, personality changes, and reduced ability to think in abstract terms. Three divisions of PFC have been distinguished functionally: dorsolateral PFC, OFC, and medial PFC.[21]

The dorsolateral PFC receives input from sensory association cortex representing somatosensory, visual, and auditory areas. This region is associated with cognitive processing, such as short-term (working) memory, as well as executive function (planning and decision-making) and behavioral control. Such functions are evaluated by asking the subject to remember a short list of words and repeat them back after a delay or to sort targets by particular characteristics (e.g., a certain letter or color), among other tests. The dorsolateral PFC works with other, reward-responsive brain regions, such as the insula and the anterior cingulate cortex, during such decisions. The dorsolateral PFC can be thought of as a central component of a dorsal *top-down* decision-making network that allows reasoning and thought to guide actions. The dorsal network may have greater left hemisphere dominance, consistent with that hemisphere's role in analytical reasoning.

OFC receives information from cortical regions that process all sensory modalities, including visceral sensation; thus, it receives a holistic sense of the immediate environment with an emphasis on sensory information related to food, appetite, and reward. This region has connections with the amygdala, hippocampus, and medial PFC, and is associated with social- and emotion-linked decision-making.

Medial PFC extends from the medial region of OFC to the anterior cingulate cortex and has interconnections with the amygdala and the brainstem. Emotional responses are generated and can be modulated by medial PFC activity, which is also associated with generating emotionally related autonomic and endocrine responses through projections to the hypothalamus and brainstem PAG and amine nuclei. This brain region receives extensive innervation by serotonergic and dopaminergic fibers. Medial PFC has reduced metabolic activity and volume in patients with bipolar and major depressive disorder (MDD), and may also have disordered function in schizophrenia. Subregions of the medial PFC and OFC can be thought of as part of a ventral *bottom-up* network that includes the amygdala and portions of the hippocampus. The ventral network mediates rapid responses to threats and stressors, and reflexively (without thoughtful reasoning) activates stress responses and negative emotions. The ventral network may have a right brain dominance, associated with the greater holistic processing of the right hemisphere.[22]

Dorsolateral PFC, OFC, and medial PFC all have bilateral connections with different subnuclei of the mediodorsal nucleus of the thalamus, and all have outputs to the striatum, analogous to the circuit between motor cortex, striatum, and thalamus involved in motor planning and control. The prefrontal projections to the striatum include inputs to caudate, putamen, and the ventral striatum region that includes the nucleus accumbens. As the nucleus accumbens is associated with motivation and pleasure, this loop is part of the integration of decision-making based on actions that derive a sense of reward.[21] This link is likely to be responsible for motivated behaviors, which can be positive or negative. Much of childhood learning and development is driven by a pleasurable sense of achieving approval from significant persons such as parents, teachers, and coaches. Motivation to be a good student, hardworking employee, or supportive and empathetic friend ultimately has its roots in deriving a sense of pleasure and reward for such actions. Circumstances of abuse and neglect may, in some cases, impede this socialization process, resulting in destructive internalizing and externalizing behaviors.

BRAIN MECHANISMS OF STRESS

Biological mechanisms of stress allow acute insults such as trauma/injury, hemorrhage, dehydration, and hypovolemia to initiate homeostatic mechanisms that restore normal physiological function. Responses to such pathophysiological challenges are initiated by sensory inputs including nociceptors, baroreceptors, blood volume detectors, and osmoreceptors. Brainstem structures, including the nucleus of the solitary tract, medullary sympathoexcitatory regions, and the hypothalamic paraventricular nucleus, activate the output of stress effector systems. These are the sympathetic nervous system, sympathetically controlled adrenal medulla, and hypothalamic-pituitary-adrenal (HPA) axis. The central neurotransmitters initiating the stress response include norepinephrine from the locus ceruleus and corticotropin-releasing hormone from the paraventricular nucleus of the hypothalamus and limbic regions. Stress system activation increases heart rate and blood pressure, releases cortisol to potentiate sympathetic nervous system activity and to mobilize fuels such as glucose and fatty acids, and suppresses systems such as growth, gastrointestinal function, and sexual function.

The stress response system is also activated by psychological stressors, in response to acute fear-inducing stimuli. The circuitry of such psychogenic stress activation involves the sensory perception of a fear-inducing stimulus. A real-life example is being in an actual or near-miss automobile accident. Inputs to various sensory modalities (hearing brakes squeal, seeing a vehicle approach, feeling the collision) are all relayed through the thalamus to modality-specific regions of the cerebral cortex, as well as to association cortex, where the event is brought to conscious perception. At the same time, these sensations are transmitted to the amygdala and other limbic structures critical to generating the emotion of fear (**Figure 15.48**).

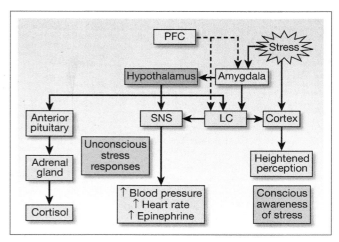

FIGURE 15.48 Functional neuroanatomy of stress responses. External stressors (fear-inducing stimuli encountered in the environment) are relayed to the cortex and the amygdala. The amygdala rapidly activates the LC and hypothalamus for activation of SNS and hypothalamic-pituitary-adrenal responses. Activation of LC and other brainstem amine groups (raphe nuclei, ventral tegmental area) increases the release of norepinephrine, dopamine, and serotonin in cortical regions, sharpening the ability to scan the environment. Several cortical regions appraise the input, localizing and analyzing the threat to either continue the stress response or to inhibit the response. Solid arrows indicate stimulation; dashed arrows indicate inhibition.
LC, locus ceruleus; PFC, prefrontal cortex; SNS, sympathetic nervous system.

These limbic regions activate the same autonomic and endocrine systems activated by pathophysiological stressors, namely, sympathetic-adrenomedullary (SAM) system and HPA axis. The amygdala and hypothalamus activate the locus ceruleus, which further increases SAM activity, as well as producing broad cortical activation. Arnsten has provided evidence that stress-increased cortical release of norepinephrine and dopamine has the effect of augmenting amygdala activity and suppressing prefrontal (particularly dorsolateral) activity.[23] This reduces the ability of the dorsolateral PFC to enhance reasoning and reduce amygdala output (**Figure 15.49**). The acute stress response, preparation for *fight or flight*, is highly adaptive and is likely to have evolved to promote survival of animals and humans in the wild, subject to acute injuries and attack by predators. The same responses may be maladaptive in modern society, with its numerous personal and social stressors. The switch from calm, thoughtful responses to reflexive and sometimes self-destructive habits of thought and behavior perpetuates patterns that are more useful in the short term than the long term.

When stress becomes chronic, there are pathophysiological consequences such as psychological dysfunction, accompanied by abnormalities of metabolism, cardiovascular impairment, decreased immunity, and other alterations.[24,25] Chronic stress is associated with

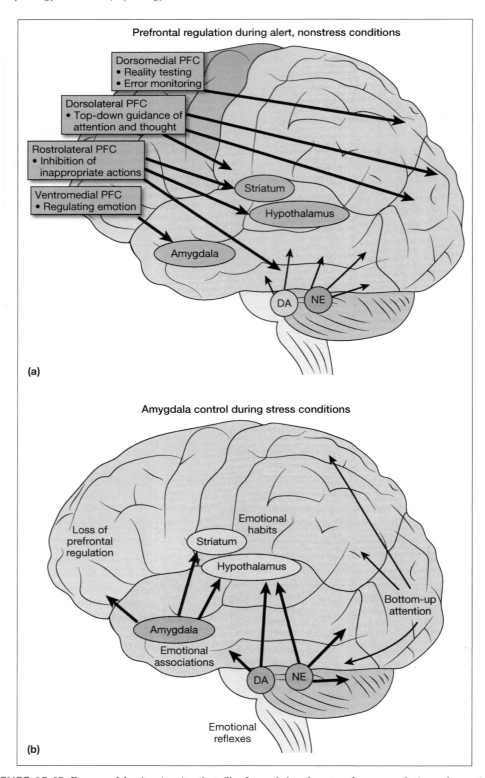

FIGURE 15.49 Proposed brain circuits that flip from **(a)** calm, top-down regulation of emotions and behavior during nonstress conditions to **(b)** amygdala and brainstem bottom-up activation of emotional responses and behaviors during stress responses.

DA, dopamine; NE, norepinephrine; PFC, prefrontal cortex.

Source: From Arnsten A. Stress signaling pathways that impair prefrontal cortex structure and function. *Nat Rev Neurosci.* 2009;10:410–422. doi:10.1038/nrn2648.

elevated cortisol levels that can lead to structural and functional changes in the amygdala and hippocampus. These changes may contribute to the known effect of stress in precipitating or exacerbating depression, anxiety, and addiction. The hippocampus is also responsible for forming and retaining memories of stressful events and contexts and for inhibiting the HPA axis.

NEUROBIOLOGY OF DEPRESSION, ANXIETY, AND SUBSTANCE USE DISORDERS

The literature on this topic is voluminous, but the specifics of neurobiology of these most common mental health disorders remain elusive. For clinicians preparing for careers in independent practice, the topic is highly relevant for several reasons. Worldwide prevalence of these disorders is very high, with MDD affecting approximately 300 million people, anxiety disorders 270 million, and substance use disorders 150 million including alcohol, opioid, cocaine, and cannabis use.[26] Smoking and alcohol use accounted for two of the three top health risk factors for disease burden worldwide, contributing 6.3% and 5.5%, respectively, to the global burden of disease.[27]

There is a high degree of overlap or comorbidity of depression, anxiety, and substance use disorders.[28] Certain key characteristics of neurocircuitry, moderate responsiveness to common pharmacological treatments, and familial clustering are held in common in these conditions. Stress-induced changes in brain neurochemistry and function can increase risks for development or exacerbation of depression, anxiety, and substance use disorders. Stress-related brain regions discussed earlier are affected by one or more of these disorders. Specific causative genes have not been identified, but the interaction of genes with environment may be related to the incidence of one or more of the disorders. With respect to environment, the influence of adverse childhood experiences is specifically implicated in their development.[29] Imaging studies have identified alterations in brain structure, function, and connectivity in children, adolescents, and young adults that are associated with adverse childhood experiences and childhood maltreatment.[30]

Although definitive evidence for specific pathways, chemical changes, and genotypes is incomplete or lacking, core concepts are presented here as a guide to developments and future discoveries in the field. Many medical disorders can present with depression, anxiety, or both, and these behavioral manifestations are also known adverse effects of certain medications, so a thorough history, physical examination, and review of current medications must be conducted to assess whether the behavioral disorder is primary or secondary.

Depression

Of the mood disorders in the *Diagnostic and Statistical Manual of Mental Disorders, Fifth Edition* (*DSM-5*), **major depressive disorder** (MDD) is the most common, with an annual prevalence of 7%. MDD is more common in women than in men, and is more common in young adults (aged 18 to 29 years) than in those over 60. The lifetime prevalence of MDD is 16.2%, and it is a significant contributor to disability worldwide.[31]

The earliest antidepressant drugs, TCAs and monoamine oxidase inhibitors (MAOIs), increase synaptic concentrations of norepinephrine, serotonin, and dopamine. The efficacy of these drugs gave rise to the monoamine hypothesis, which posited a deficit of amine transmission as the root of depression. However, studies using varied approaches to confirm this hypothesis have been inconclusive, and the long latency between beginning antidepressant treatment and achieving improvement in mood (4 to 6 weeks) argues against this hypothesis. Nevertheless, derivatives of the earliest antidepressant drugs still have clinical efficacy and are more selective in their action, with fewer adverse effects. These include SSRIs, norepinephrine reuptake inhibitors, and serotonin–norepinephrine reuptake inhibitors (SNRIs).

Abnormalities of HPA axis regulation have been identified in many patients with MDD. Daily cortisol levels are above average, and there may be abnormalities of the dexamethasone suppression test, indicating a failure of the normal negative feedback, which is mediated by the hippocampus. In animal models, persistent cortisol elevation induces hippocampal shrinkage, and individuals with MDD also have decreased hippocampal volume. One model of depression places the hippocampal changes in a central role linking stress with depression (**Figure 15.50**).

Imaging studies in major depression suggest similarities between the neurobiological stress circuit and MDD. Blood flow under resting conditions is decreased in the dorsolateral PFC and an associated region of anterior cingulate cortex, particularly on the left side, implying downregulation of the dorsal network. In addition, blood flow is increased in the amygdala and ventromedial PFC of the ventral network, particularly on the right side. This could reflect a tendency to negative thoughts and ruminations accompanied by apathy, loss of pleasure, and slower thought processing. Deep brain stimulation to inhibit activity in the ventral network has been tested in patients with MDD resistant to pharmacological management (treatment-resistant depression) and has had some effectiveness at relieving depression. Similarly, electroconvulsive therapy is effective at relieving major depression in individuals with resistant depression. Importantly, findings of imaging studies have also shown that cognitive behavioral therapy and antidepressant treatment may reverse some of the functional changes of MDD.

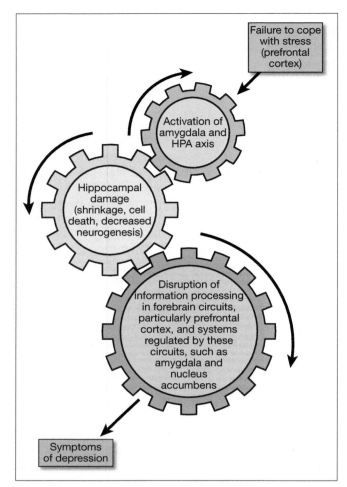

FIGURE 15.50 Hypothesized connections between stress and failure to cope, activating amygdala and HPA axis. Over repeated exposures, cortisol elevations damage the hippocampus and its regulatory functions. Cortical consequences of hippocampal damage decrease emotion regulation and contribute to depressive symptoms.
HPA, hypothalamic-pituitary-adrenal.
Source: From Willner P, et al. The neurobiology of depression and antidepressant action. *Neurosci Biobehav Rev.* 2013;37: 2331–2371.

Future research on the neurobiology of MDD will continue to inform and clarify the role of many additional components of this complex phenomenon, including the following:

- The role of brain inflammation in depression
- Genetic analyses of the heritability of depression or risk of depression, as well as identification of polymorphisms that influence sensitivity to particular drugs and treatments
- Elucidation of biological changes induced by antidepressant drugs (including altered second messenger signaling, increased production of nerve growth factors such as brain-derived neurotrophic factor, reversal of hippocampal atrophy) and the clinical efficacy of these drugs in some patients but not in others.

- The mechanisms of rapid-acting but short-term interventions that improve MDD, including electroconvulsive therapy, intravenous ketamine, and deep brain stimulation.
- The use of tailored combinations of biological treatments with *talk therapies* such as cognitive behavioral therapy to improve rates and sustainability of remission.

Anxiety

There are many subtypes of **anxiety disorders**, including generalized anxiety disorder, panic disorder, specific phobia, and social anxiety disorder. Features of anxiety disorders include responses to threat or perceived threat that have a strength, intensity, or duration greater than would be considered commensurate with objective assessments of the same level of threat. Another criterion for evaluating anxiety disorders is the extent to which the experience of anxiety impairs social, occupational, and personal function. Collectively, the anxiety disorders are the most prevalent mental health disorders, with 12-month prevalence of 18.1%.[32]

As with depression, twin and family studies suggest a high degree of familial risk, but specific genotypes have not been identified. It is likely that gene × environment interactions are key to the development of anxiety and depression, which are often comorbid conditions. Neurobiological studies of threat detection and generation of responses implicate the amygdala and hippocampus, and cortical regions—insula, anterior cingulate, and ventromedial PFC[33]—whereas activity is reduced in dorsolateral PFC and related emotion-regulation areas. Anxiety is twice as common in women as in men, but the neurobiological basis of this difference has not yet been identified.

In anxiety disorders, there is a finding of negative attribution or fearfulness associated with many innocuous or mildly aversive thoughts, stimuli, and experiences. Amygdala activity is heightened and in many cases sympathetic nervous system and adrenocortical outflows are stimulated to a degree that is disproportionate to the stimulus. Anxiety can also be associated with and exacerbate hypertension, diabetes, cardiovascular disease, irritable bowel syndrome, tension headaches, myalgic encephalomyelitis (formerly known as chronic fatigue syndrome), and a host of other disorders.

Management strategies in anxiety disorders combine psychological and pharmacological treatments; however, worldwide many patients with anxiety disorders are underdiagnosed and undertreated. Cognitive behavioral therapy is the main psychological therapy for anxiety disorders and is effective at reducing fearful attributions to ambiguous stimuli, increasing coping, and decreasing autonomic activation. Mindfulness training is also effective in anxiety disorders. For specific phobias and panic disorder, exposure-based cognitive behavioral therapy can be effective. It is plausible to hypothesize that these approaches, with practice, strengthen prefrontal emotion-regulating regions capable of reducing the impact of fear generation by the amygdala and related brain regions. Pharmacologically, many SSRI and SNRI antidepressants, combined with psychological treatments, are effective in many anxiety disorders. Acute anxiety and panic attacks are often treated with benzodiazepine drugs, but the abuse potential of these agents limits their chronic use.

Substance Use Disorders

Chemical substances associated with **substance use disorders** include alcohol, nicotine, cannabis, opioids, sedatives, stimulants, and other substances. To the extent that these substances have been investigated in animal models, all work through various pathways to increase dopamine release from the VTA neurons that project to the nucleus accumbens, the brain's pleasure and reward center. Use of these substances is associated with reinforcing properties—a positive effect that

reinforces the desire to repeat the action. The initial response to these substances should be pleasurable in most people. However, individuals with substance use disorders exhibit compulsive patterns of use that may lead to tolerance (requiring higher doses to achieve the reward), cravings (that lead to repeated use despite adverse consequences), and withdrawal (aversive symptoms on abstinence).

A unifying scheme to explain the neurocircuitry underlying different substances of abuse has been proposed by Nestler[34] (**Figure 15.51**). This model is based on preclinical studies in animals, as well as neuroanatomical distributions and subtypes of receptors that are binding targets for substances that show the highest prevalence of abuse. The model is simplified to focus on the critical pathway from dopamine neurons in the VTA to their target sites in the nucleus accumbens. Specific receptors implicated in pleasurable/reinforcing actions of commonly abused substances include nicotinic acetylcholine receptors stimulated by nicotine from tobacco smoke, μ opioid receptors responsive

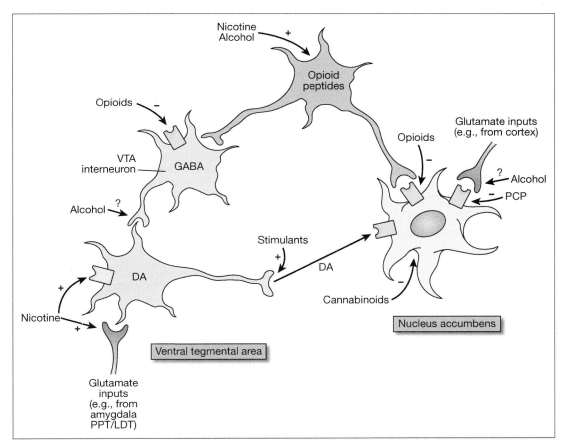

FIGURE 15.51 Proposed neurobiology of initial responses to substance use. The association between a variety of substances and the sensation of pleasure/reward involves the VTA DA input to the NAc. Nicotine, alcohol, cannabinoids, opiates, and stimulants increase NAc DA release. After repeated exposures, VTA and NAc neurons adapt, resulting in reduced reward and requiring greater intake of these substances to achieve a pleasurable state.

DA, dopamine; GABA, gamma-aminobutyric acid; LDT, lateral dorsal tegmental nucleus; NAc, nucleus accumbens; PCP, phencyclidine; PPT, peripeduncular tegmentum; VTA, ventral tegmental area.

BOX 15.6
Brain Opioids and Cannabinoids

Human brains have receptors permitting responses to plant compounds. Morphine and other derivatives of the opium poppy have been used for centuries for their analgesic and rewarding properties, although the mechanism of action was not identified. In 1973, Candace Pert and Solomon Snyder, working at Johns Hopkins University, demonstrated that rat brains had receptors that could bind naloxone, an opioid antagonist.[35] Moreover, the binding could be displaced by a variety of drugs derived from plant opiates with affinities that correlated with clinical potency. Following that discovery and confirmation by additional research laboratories, the endogenous opioids *met-* and *leu-*enkephalin, dynorphin, and β-endorphin were isolated and purified from mammalian brain and pituitary tissue. These substances are implicated in the pain modulation pathways described earlier in this chapter.

Similarly, the products of the plant *Cannabis sativa* have long been used by people as pleasure-inducing and relaxing substances. Receptors for cannabinoids were identified in the 1990s, and research on this system is ongoing. The primary brain cannabinoid receptor is the CB1 receptor found on presynaptic terminals. In an interesting twist on the usual pattern of neurotransmission, the endogenous ligands for the CB1 receptor carry out a process of *retrograde transmission*. Two chemically related lipids, anandamide and 2-arachidonylglycerol, are synthesized in postsynaptic neurons and diffuse into the synapse to bind to inhibitory CB1 receptors on the presynaptic terminal. This means that these endogenous compounds, as well as intake of exogenous compounds such as Δ^9-tetrahydrocannabinol (THC), the active ingredient in marijuana, have generally inhibitory effects.

Cannabidiol and similar compounds in this family are the subject of research in the widely varied fields of pain management, epilepsy, addiction, affective disorders, and several others.

---

to natural opiate and synthetic opioid drugs, and dopamine receptors activated by increased dopamine release as enhanced by cocaine and similar stimulants. (The mechanisms involved in brain responses to plant-based compounds, such as opioids and cannabinoids, are discussed further in **Box 15.6**.[35]) Alcohol has several receptor targets, blocking glutamate receptors and enhancing GABA transmission, among other actions. Imaging studies in humans have confirmed aspects of this model and have implicated the amygdala and regions of PFC in altered responsiveness to drugs in individuals with chronic substance use disorders.

Substance use disorders are often comorbid with depression and anxiety, and may be related, in part, to *self-medication* efforts to cope with those conditions. As with depression and anxiety, there is familial risk and exacerbation by stress exposures; however, substance use disorders show male over female predominance. Exposure to adverse childhood events demonstrated a graded relationship with prevalence of smoking, alcoholism, illicit drug use, and increased number of sexual intercourse partners, implicating early life environment in the development of such health-risk behaviors.[36] Research in this area focuses on altered signal transduction and epigenetic modifications that underlie the transition from casual use to substance use disorders, identifying predictors of response to behavioral and pharmacological treatments, and continued development of behavioral and biological strategies to improve outcomes.

To conclude, individuals with mental health disorders represent a substantial proportion of patients in primary care and inpatient settings. Neurobiological, neurochemical, genetic, and environmental mechanisms underlying these disorders are slowly beginning to be elucidated, and many promising new approaches are in development. The central concepts outlined in this chapter form a foundation for continuing inquiry and practice developments that aim to reduce morbidity and mortality, and improve quality of care, for these patients, their families, and extended social networks.

Thought Questions

21. What are the major brain regions associated with higher reasoning and cognitive function?

22. What are the major brain regions and nuclei associated with cognitive perception of stressful stimuli, and with sharpening perception of those stimuli?

23. What are the pathways that lead to stress-induced activation of the sympathoadrenal and HPA responses to stressful stimuli?

24. What brain region is often capable of suppressing or moderating stress responses?

PEDIATRIC CONSIDERATIONS

Melissa Assaf

OVERVIEW OF BRAIN DEVELOPMENT

Brain development begins in the third week of gestation. Prenatal brain development is associated with a rapid proliferation of cells destined to differentiate into neurons. Tissue development proceeds from the neural plate stage to the formation of the neural tube, vesicles, and differentiation of vesicles into the final structures of cerebral cortex and diencephalon, cerebellum, brainstem, and spinal cord. Major brain structures are in place by the end of the embryonic stage of development, approximately the eighth gestational week. During fetal development, neuron precursors rapidly divide and begin to migrate to their final destinations. Development of the cerebral cortex (gray matter) is well understood from human and animal data. The six-layered cerebral cortex develops in an inside out fashion; that is, the deepest layers of neurons migrate to their final destination first, followed by succeeding superficial layers.

Under the influence of embryonic growth factors, neurons rapidly multiply in gestational weeks 4 through 12, until their numbers total about twice the levels of adult humans. Beginning at about 16 weeks of gestation, neurons begin to die by apoptosis until the final number of neurons is achieved. Although this process is most active before birth, neuronal apoptosis may continue into the first year of life. Production of glial cells begins before birth but increases after birth, and progenitor cells of astroglia and oligodendrocytes retain the ability to divide throughout life. There is a progressive thinning of cortical gray matter in late childhood and into adolescence that correlates with maturation of brain function. The major neurotransmitters glutamate, GABA, acetylcholine, and the amine transmitters (dopamine, serotonin, norepinephrine, and epinephrine) are present beginning with prenatal development, although their roles during this stage of development are not clearly understood. GABA's postsynaptic action during early brain development is excitatory, switching to inhibition after birth.

Myelination begins before birth, but reaches its peak of activity after birth and for the first several years of life. The earliest pathways to be myelinated are the sensory pathways, followed by motor pathways, then association-related pathways. As myelination proceeds, axon propagation of action potentials is facilitated, subsequently activating synapses and promoting synaptic strength with regular activity. Development of functional circuits is critical for neurodevelopmental milestones and is activity dependent (i.e., use it and you will not lose it!). Generation of synapses (synaptogenesis) is prolific during prenatal development, but about 50% of synapses generated during embryonic development are later eliminated through synaptic pruning. This process eliminates incorrect connections between neurons and reinforces transmission at synapses that are used most often: it is one mechanism of learning and memory development, based on experiences.

There are critical periods during which lack of specific inputs during early postnatal development irreversibly impairs future function. For example, infants born with congenital cataracts who are not screened and treated by 6 months of age will have permanent cortical vision impairment due to lack of stimulation. Children (or animals) raised in environments deprived of rich sources of sensory stimulation develop fewer dendritic spines and synaptic connections and have impaired ability to learn. In comparison, children and animals raised in enriched environments develop more neuronal dendritic branching patterns and synapses. Thus, although the young brain has considerable plasticity, the capacity for change is not unlimited. In many brain circuits, new synapses continue to be formed throughout life, although the rate decreases after adolescence.

The complexities of neurogenesis, neuronal migration, synaptogenesis, and pruning are beyond the scope of this chapter, but genetic defects in signaling molecules associated with these processes are implicated in congenital neural and functional defects such as lissencephaly (smooth brain due to lack of normal cortical folding) and fragile X-syndrome–related intellectual disability. Pathology of neuronal migration may also contribute to some cases of epilepsy. Several gene mutations have tentatively been linked to autism spectrum disorders, and many of the protein products of these genes are involved in neurogenesis, neurite growth, and synapse formation and function. Toxic exposures, nutritional deficiencies, infections, and other disease processes during infancy can also produce permanent neurological deficits.

SPINAL MUSCULAR ATROPHY

Spinal muscular atrophy (SMA) is the second most common genetic disorder, after cystic fibrosis. There are five different types, from the most severe, which is lethal during prenatal development, to the least severe, which does not present until adulthood. The most common is SMA type I, an autosomal recessive disorder that represents 50% to 70% of cases.[37] Children are diagnosed soon after birth with atonia, weakness of muscles used for sucking and breathing, and failing to reach motor developmental milestones. Neonatal screening can also detect the disorder before clinical manifestations appear. Survival up to 2 years is the outcome for many infants born with SMA.

SMA is characterized by the progressive, complete inability to have motor function due to death of spinal motor neurons—thus, the presentation is that of a lower motor neuron lesion. The gene most commonly affected is the SMN1 (survival of motor neuron 1) gene. A second gene, SMN2, is normally present and in fact normal individuals and SMA patients can have up to four copies of the SMN2 gene. Although SMN2 is only expressed at about 10% of the rate of SMN1, when additional copies of SMN2 are present, they are protective against the most severe outcomes of SMN1 mutations. The drug nusinersen is an antisense oligonucleotide that can be injected intrathecally, into the spinal cord cerebrospinal fluid. The drug is taken up by spinal neurons and is effective at promoting SMN2 synthesis and rescuing motor function and development.

PEDIATRIC SEIZURES AND EPILEPSIES

A **seizure** is an episode of observable signs and symptoms secondary to synchronized abnormal activation of large numbers of cortical neurons. Seizures can be manifested by sustained muscle contractions (tonic phase), or by alternating contraction and relaxation (clonic phase), or may have a more subtle presentation. Some seizures are focal, with manifestations that reflect their brain region of origin (motor, sensory, visual, and others), but others are generalized. A single seizure may occur in an infant or child and never recur. Recurrent seizures can progress to epilepsy, a disease of predisposition to recurrent seizures, which is diagnosed by seizure type and associated changes in the EEG. The incidence of seizures over the lifetime occurs in a U-shaped (inverse) bell curve with the highest incidence in the first weeks of life and childhood, decreasing in early and middle adulthood, and increasing again after 65 years of age.

In many cases, the cause and pathophysiology of epilepsy are unknown; however, some epilepsy mechanisms have been determined. From the whole brain to the plasma membrane level, these mechanisms include changes in neuronal networks, neuron structure, neurotransmitter levels, neurotransmitter receptors, synapses, and ion channels. Although some pathophysiological mechanisms have been identified, it is still not clear how and why seizures are provoked intermittently, separated by periods of normal EEG activity.

Interestingly, there is some overlap between seizures and migraines, both of which are sporadic events.

NEONATAL SEIZURES

The incidence of **neonatal seizures** is estimated at one to five cases per 1,000 neonates. Incidence is highest in premature infants, particularly those with the lowest birth weight. Up to 80% of neonatal seizures occur within the first week of life. Neonatal seizures are most frequent during the first 10 days of life but can occur up to 28 days of life (or up to 44 weeks of gestational age for preterm infants).[38] Neonatal seizures differ in etiology from childhood and adolescent epilepsy syndromes. While it often is difficult to determine the cause, it is important to differentiate the etiology of seizures in the neonate because treatment, recurrence risk, and prognosis vary depending on the cause and underlying pathology. The major causes of neonatal seizures are the following:

- Hypoxic ischemic encephalopathy that can occur as a complication of labor and delivery or from postnatal events that produce hypoxia
- Strokes
- Intracranial hemorrhage (more common in preterm infants)
- Inborn errors of metabolism (presenting before results of neonatal screening are reported)
- Other metabolic disturbances—hypoglycemia, hypocalcemia, hypomagnesemia
- Genetic disorders, often involving ion channel-coding genes
- Intracranial infections—intrauterine-acquired TORCH infections (toxoplasmosis, other, rubella, cytomegalovirus, herpes), postnatal *Escherichia coli* or *Streptococcus pneumoniae* infections
- Malformation syndromes—lissencephaly and others

Several potential pathophysiological mechanisms underlie the susceptibility of the neonatal brain to seizures. These include incomplete development and function of inhibitory receptors accompanied by a relative predominance of excitatory receptors (including GABA receptors in neonates). Abundant synapses provide stimulation, as pruning is still incomplete. The neonatal brain has fewer potassium channels responsible for action potential repolarization and hyperpolarization. Finally, the immaturity of the neurotransmitter systems in neonates appears to reduce the effectiveness of many antiepileptic drugs that work well in older children and adults.

FEBRILE SEIZURES

Febrile seizures occur generally between the ages of 6 months and 6 years of age. The pathological process underlying febrile seizures is not yet clear, but the condition is diagnosed when a seizure occurs immediately before or during a febrile illness that is not due to infection within the brain (such as meningitis). A seizure within 24 hours of a fever (100.4°F or higher) is considered a febrile seizure, and the height of the fever may determine seizure risk. Febrile seizures can occur during viral or bacterial infections. The human herpes simplex virus 6 (HHSV-6), associated with roseola, accounts for 20% of new-onset febrile seizures. *Shigella* gastroenteritis and influenza A have also been associated with febrile seizures.[39]

Febrile seizures are divided into two types: simple febrile seizures and complex febrile seizures. Simple febrile seizures are generalized, last <15 minutes, *and* only one occurs in a 24-hour time period. Complex febrile seizures are focal, last >15 minutes, *or* recur more than once in a 24-hour time period. Complex febrile seizures have an increased risk for recurrence, may progress to epilepsy, or may indicate an underlying, more serious disease process. A related genetic syndrome is termed *generalized epilepsy with febrile seizures plus* (GEFS+), which may remit in adolescence. If a febrile seizure lasts >30 minutes, it is considered febrile status epilepticus.

A family history of febrile seizures increases the risk for recurrence by 10% if a sibling and 50% if a parent has a history of febrile seizures. Polygenic inheritance is likely, but some families with febrile seizures demonstrate an autosomal dominant inheritance pattern with reduced penetrance. Although molecular pathology of febrile seizures is not fully understood, mutations in sodium channel and GABA receptor genes have been associated with febrile seizures.

FOCAL VERSUS GENERALIZED EPILEPSIES

Epilepsy is defined as a condition that predisposes to recurrent seizures and can be associated with a constellation of cognitive, social, and psychological challenges. The annual prevalence of epilepsy is estimated at 1%. Cellular excitability is increased or inhibition is decreased for both types of seizure disorders; however, the pathophysiology for focal and generalized epilepsies differs. Therefore, they are discussed separately here.

Generalized epilepsies are more common in the pediatric population, often having a genetic predisposition, whereas focal epilepsies are more common in the aging population with a focal insult such as a stroke or a brain tumor. More than 1,400 genes are responsible for epilepsy with different phenotypes, and it is outside the scope of this chapter to describe them all. Focal and generalized epilepsies occur in all age groups and all ethnic groups. Similar to the prevalence of seizures, the age of epilepsy onset has an inverse bell curve, with higher rates of incidence in the very young and the very old.

A diagnosis of epilepsy is made under the following circumstances: (a) occurrence of two unprovoked seizures, separated by more than 24 hours; (b) one unprovoked seizure and a 60% probability of recurrence over the following 10 years; or (c) diagnosis of an epilepsy syndrome. This definition recognizes the increased risk of a second seizure in patients who have a brain insult such as stroke or trauma.[40]

Focal Seizures and Epilepsy

Focal seizures are generated by one brain region or hemisphere, often a site of a former traumatic brain injury, stroke, or a developing tumor. Epilepsy associated with recurrent focal seizures can have associated loss of awareness, or the individual may remain aware during the seizure. EEG recordings may be able to localize the approximate region of the seizure focus, although that may not be possible for foci originating in deeper brain regions. For focal epilepsies, the clinical symptoms of the seizure correlate with the brain location of origin. Visual symptoms (vision loss, blackouts, double vision, etc.) during a focal seizure imply involvement of the visual cortex or the occipital lobe. Sensory, gustatory, or motor symptoms during a focal seizure involve the primary sensory, gustatory, or motor cortex. Déjà-vu symptoms are experienced when the temporal lobe is involved. Individuals with focal epilepsies may have a normal surface EEG in between seizures. **Focal-onset epilepsies** have hallmark EEG findings of localized sharp spikes, or slow waves between seizures (interictal), or both.

Focal-onset seizures may be initiated by mechanisms similar to generalized seizures, including increased excitation by glutamate, decreased inhibition by GABA, or altered firing patterns within regional neuron networks. However, by definition they do not inevitably spread to the entire cortex. This implies a restricted region of pathology while the remaining brain is able to retain normal activity patterns. One particularly vulnerable brain region is the hippocampus, found in the medial portion of the temporal lobe. The intrinsic circuitry of the hippocampus may be prone to the pattern of generalized activation associated with seizures, particularly in patients with hippocampal damage after an event like febrile seizures. In some patients with seizures originating from the temporal lobe, surgical removal of the hippocampus eliminates the seizures. Pathologically, the removed tissue is often found to have scarring referred to as hippocampal sclerosis that may have been the site of seizure generation.

Generalized Epilepsies

There are several types of generalized seizures, including absence, myoclonic, atonic, clonic, and generalized tonic–clonic. **Generalized epilepsies**, such as childhood absence epilepsy and juvenile myoclonic epilepsy, typically respond well to antiepileptic therapy. Generalized epilepsy syndromes that present in infancy and early childhood can be refractory or intractable (e.g., Dravet syndrome, Lennox-Gastaut syndrome), and certain genetic neurodevelopmental disorders have seizures as part of their presentation (e.g., Rett syndrome, Angelman syndrome). Genetic mutations in sodium, potassium, or calcium channels (channelopathies) may produce some of the generalized epilepsies.

Evidence suggests that aberrant neural circuit activity during absence or nonconvulsive seizures (formerly referred to as petit mal or staring seizures) is initiated by abnormal thalamocortical interactions. This circuit normally has oscillatory rhythms consisting of periods of excitation interspersed with periods of inhibition that sweep across large numbers of neurons in the thalamus and then the cortex, as seen in the large EEG waves of NREM sleep. Thalamocortical circuitry involves three neuron types: pyramidal neurons of the neocortex, thalamic neurons that relay to the cortex, and neurons in the nucleus reticularis of the thalamus that control the relay neurons. Primary generalized-onset seizures result when these rhythms are altered. The spinal cord sends ascending inputs to the thalamic relay neurons, which project to the neocortical pyramidal neurons. Thalamic relay neurons have oscillating RMP. When they are depolarized, the probability of synchronous activation of the neocortical pyramidal neurons is increased. When they are hyperpolarized, the likelihood of neocortical activation is reduced.

The membrane potential oscillations of thalamic relay neurons are due to activation of a transient, low-threshold calcium channel (T-calcium channel) that opens briefly and then inactivates. These channels require repolarization and hyperpolarization before they can reopen. Inhibitory GABAergic neurons of the nucleus reticularis of the thalamus hyperpolarize the thalamic relay neurons, resetting the T-calcium channels in the thalamic relay neurons.[41] Absence seizures are often managed with the medications ethosuximide, valproic acid, or lamotrigine, which block the T-calcium channels and prevent depolarization of the thalamic relay neurons (Figure 15.52).

Autoimmunity can also present in the form of seizures. **Anti-NMDA receptor encephalitis** is a clinically challenging syndrome first identified in 1997, in a case series of young women with teratomas presenting with behavioral changes, hallucinations, seizures, abnormal autonomic activity, and neurological deficits. Assays of the cerebrospinal fluid identified white blood cells and antibodies that were shown to react with a subunit of the glutamate NMDA receptor. Since the first description of this disorder, it has been found in children suffering from similar symptoms after acute viral illnesses and in other patient groups.

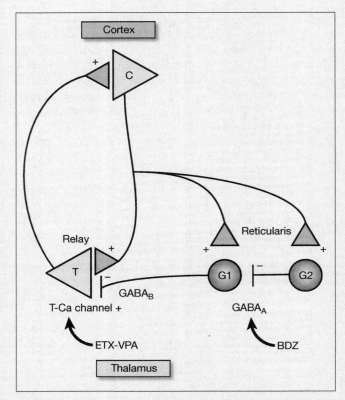

FIGURE 15.52 Proposed pathophysiological circuit of absence seizures involving thalamic relay neurons that project to the cortex. An excitatory T-type calcium (T-Ca) channel requires hyperpolarization to reset. Local interneurons (reticularis, G1 and G2) are inhibitory, releasing GABA, which hyperpolarizes the relay neuron and resetting T-Ca. Antiepileptic drugs (e.g., ETX and VPA) can target the T channel, reducing abnormal excitation. BDZ can strengthen GABA inhibition.

BDZ, benzodiazepine; ETX, ethosuximide; GABA, gamma-aminobutyric acid; VPA, valproic acid.

DEVELOPMENTAL DELAY

Developmental delay is a descriptive term used to categorize children who do not meet their developmental milestones on target. These milestones may be achieved more slowly or later than expected, and sometimes not at all. Developmental delays can be grouped into global developmental delay (two or more domains) or specific developmental delay (a single domain such as speech and language, gross motor, fine motor, social skills, etc.). Global developmental delay can be the presenting feature of a huge number of neurodevelopmental disorders, ranging from learning disability to neuromuscular disorders.

The *DSM-5* provides diagnostic criteria for several neurodevelopmental disorders that have mental and behavioral health consequences.[42] The discussion that follows covers intellectual disability, global developmental delay, and specific disorders such as language disorder, autism spectrum disorder, attention-deficit hyperactivity disorder, specific learning disorder, neurodevelopmental motor disorders, and others. Within each of these categories, there is a great deal of variation of individual patient presentation. Current research with the tools of genomics and structural and functional brain imaging aims to elucidate the pathophysiological mechanisms underlying this cluster of disorders in hopes of directing treatments.

INTELLECTUAL DISABILITY

Intellectual disability is a term used for findings that were previously labeled *mental retardation*, in which diagnostic criteria focus on intellectual functioning and skill acquisition. Intellectual disability can have genetic causes or can occur from complications at prenatal, perinatal, and postnatal stages. Known genetic and chromosomal abnormalities that are associated with intellectual disability include trisomy 21 (Down syndrome) and fragile X syndrome, among many others—most of which are rare. However, the majority of cases of intellectual disability arise from genetic causes, and thousands of genetic mutations linked to these impairments have been identified (as documented in the Online Mendelian Inheritance in Man® database).[43] Examples of prenatal origins of intellectual disability include fetal alcohol syndrome and infections. Examples of perinatal origins include complications such as birth hypoxia or infections. An example of postnatal origin is lead poisoning. Preventable causes of intellectual disability—including phenylketonuria, hypothyroidism, and other metabolic disorders—are assessed during newborn screening, allowing early intervention.

ATTENTION-DEFICIT/HYPERACTIVITY DISORDER

Attention-deficit/hyperactivity disorder (ADHD) is classified as a neurodevelopmental disorder in the *DSM-5*.[42] It has a high prevalence (5% of children and 2.5% of adults) and commonly presents in early childhood and elementary school years, with high heritability. The ADHD subtypes comprise cases in which inattention is the major presentation, those in which motor hyperactivity and behavioral impulsivity combined make up the major presentation, and cases in which all three characteristics are present. No specific causal genes or brain structural alterations have been identified in patients with ADHD. The disorder is associated with difficulties in school achievement and social function. Management with medications that augment brain dopamine or norepinephrine actions is effective in most cases, improving academic and social function.[44]

HEADACHES

Brain tissue does not contain nociceptors; however, stimulation of other structures within the head that do contain nociceptors can give rise to **headaches**. These structures include the venous sinuses, meninges and meningeal arteries, sinuses, periosteum of the skull, subcutaneous tissues of the head, muscles of the head and neck, arteries, eyes, and ears. Cranial and spinal nerves that relay pain sensation from structures of the head and neck include the trigeminal (CN V), glossopharyngeal (CN IX), vagus (CN X), and upper cervical nerves (C2 and C3).

The most common headache syndromes are migraine and tension-type headaches. Migraines can be episodic or chronic in occurrence. Tension-type headaches are usually episodic but may also become chronic, even occurring daily or more than 15 days per month. Findings are generally negative on assessment of primary headache syndromes—laboratory studies, diagnostic imaging, and physical examinations are normal. However, people with primary headache syndromes may have acute abnormal clinical findings and need a full evaluation to assess for causes of secondary headaches, such as dehydration, sleep deprivation, vitamin D deficiency, thyroid abnormalities, iron deficiencies, anxiety and depression, malignancies, congenital malformations, and strokes.

MIGRAINE

Migraines arise early in life, most often before age 20 years, and commonly have a strong family history. A few rare familial migraine syndromes are associated with known gene mutations, but these mutations are not found in the majority of individuals with migraines. About 15% to 20% of migraine sufferers experience an aura, which is a visual or neurological deficit lasting <60 minutes that is followed by headache onset within 60 minutes of the aura. In some cases, migraineurs (those who suffer from migraines) can identify triggers, including lack of sleep, stress, hormone changes, or certain food or drink. Migraine aura can occur without a subsequent headache. Auras are most often visual (flashing lights or photopsia). Sometimes people have neurological auras of numbness or tingling or weakness in an arm or leg. People may have prodromal symptoms (mood or personality changes, hyperactivity, and fatigue) for hours to days before the migraine attack starts. Approximately 60% of women report that their worst migraine attacks are during menses. A migraine acute attack lasts 6 to 72 hours and produces throbbing/pounding, moderate to severe, unilateral (or bilateral) pain. Migraines generally worsen with physical activity or head movement, bright lights, loud noises, and strong scents or odors. Associated symptoms may include nausea and vomiting.

The pathophysiology of migraine is not well understood. Early concepts proposed an initial episode of intracranial vasoconstriction that led to a later rebound vasodilation. Another model suggests that an electrical wave of depolarization, followed by hyperpolarization and neuronal inhibition is initiated in the occipital cortex and propagated to the thalamus and cortex. This wave is referred to as cortical spreading depression and occurs concomitant with the aura phase, altering hypothalamic activity as well as activity of brainstem amine groups. This sequence then increases parasympathetic outflow that produces painful vasodilation of cranial blood vessels.[45,46] Additional evidence supports a role for inflammatory mediators in cerebral vasodilation and in sensitization of cranial nociceptors. The most commonly used abortive medications have been NSAIDs such as ibuprofen; triptans, which are agonists at 5-HT 1B and 1D receptors, can be used when NSAIDs do not work. Medications should be accompanied by environmental changes: resting in a dark, quiet, cool room is most effective. Repetitive use of abortives may produce overuse headaches. Migraines are best controlled with avoidance of triggers, preventive medications, and abortive medications only when necessary.

TENSION-TYPE HEADACHE

Tension-type headache is usually due to increased cervical or pericranial muscular activity (e.g., neck flexion–extension injury, poor posture, or anxiety with teeth clenching or grinding). Symptoms of tension-type headache include generalized pressure, and tightness that feels like a band, with mild to moderate pain. Unlike migraines, tension-type headaches do not worsen with activity. Symptoms that characterize tension-type headaches include muscle tension, scalp tenderness, temporomandibular joint muscle tenderness, and tight or tender cervical and trapezius muscles. If no muscle tightness in the neck is noted, the pain may be due to psychological factors or may have a central origin. Migraine abortive medications with caffeine or butalbital may worsen tension-type headaches. These types of headaches in adults respond best to TCAs; however, data on these medications are limited in pediatrics.

SECONDARY HEADACHE

Patients presenting with new onset of headache should be assessed for causes of **secondary headache**, including acute infections or illnesses, sleep disturbances and deprivation, dehydration, and other systemic conditions that produce a secondary headache. Vitamin D deficiency, thyroid abnormalities, iron deficiency, anxiety and depression, malignancies, congenital malformations, and stroke are among the conditions that have been implicated. Ominous etiology, such as malignant (and benign) tumors and stroke, need to be

TABLE 15.4 Red Flag Warning Signs for Headaches	
Timing	New dramatic onset Occurs upon awakening or causes the person to wake up
Location	Limited to one area with marked increase in frequency or severity
Context or position	Worsens with lying down
Severity	Worst headache ever, *thunderclap*
Associated symptoms	Uncontrolled vomiting, personality or behavioral changes, altered mental status
Physical examination	Abnormal eye exam: abnormal eye movements, diplopia, papilledema Abnormal neurological exam: imbalance, ataxia, seizure, unilateral weakness or numbness, focal motor, or sensory abnormalities

ruled out in the setting of a pediatric patient with a headache that includes the red flag warning signs listed in Table 15.4. Headache associated with enlarging or leaking aneurysm is associated with a *thunderclap*, new, acute-onset headache, often described by the patient as *the worst headache of my life*. A patient with aneurysm rupture may also present with a seizure or change in mental status.

CONCUSSION

Concussion is a mild traumatic brain injury with a complex pathophysiology that has not been fully elucidated. Concussion is common in children and adolescents, particularly those who are involved in sports. Sport-related concussion is a traumatic brain injury induced by biomechanical forces. The Concussion in Sport Group periodically updates the definition of concussion and its associated findings.[47] The most recent version of the consensus document is described in Box 15.7.

The clinical symptoms of a concussion are due to functional rather than structural abnormalities. Concussive pathophysiological processes are attributed to mechanical, neurotransmitter, ionic, and metabolic changes initiated by the trauma, accompanied by subsequent alterations in blood flow and inflammation.

Neuronal dysfunction is triggered by a wave of energy that passes through the brain tissue during a concussion and initiates a pathological neurometabolic

BOX 15.7
Common Features of Sport-Related Concussion

- Sport-related concussion may be caused by a direct blow to the head, face, neck, or elsewhere on the body with an impulsive force transmitted to the head.

- It typically results in the rapid onset of impaired neurological function that often resolves quickly. In some cases, signs and symptoms evolve over minutes to hours.

- Sport-related concussion may result in neuropathological changes, but the acute clinical signs and symptoms largely reflect a functional disturbance rather than a structural injury, and as such, no abnormality is seen on standard structural neuroimaging studies.

- It results in a range of clinical signs and symptoms that may or may not involve loss of consciousness. Resolution of the clinical and cognitive features typically follows a sequential course. However, in some cases symptoms may be prolonged.

- The clinical signs and symptoms cannot be explained by drug, alcohol, or medication use; other injuries (e.g., cervical injuries, peripheral vestibular dysfunction); or other comorbidities (e.g., psychological factors or coexisting medical conditions).

cascade (**Figure 15.53**). The earliest changes include ionic imbalance, with extracellular potassium accumulation, membrane depolarization, and glutamate release contributing to excitotoxicity. Glutamate-induced intracellular calcium accumulation is reduced by a mitochondrial spike of calcium; however, this can later result in mitochondrial dysfunction (see **Figure 15.53a and b**).[48] Cell injury includes damage to the neuronal cytoskeleton and, in particular, to axons. Although traditional structural studies such as MRI are generally unable to detect damage, newer imaging methods such as functional MRI and diffusion tensor imaging are able to detect focal and axonal damage.

Concussion symptoms are attributed to a combination of neuron dysfunction and axonal injury. Owing to reduced cerebral blood flow, concussed cells can be more vulnerable to irreversible damage if a second injury occurs after an initial concussion, a phenomenon referred to as second impact syndrome. Recovery from a concussion can take days to years. A person can have a concussion or brain injury without loss of consciousness—in fact, 90% of patients with concussions do not have loss of consciousness. Memory of events before and after traumatic head injury is a better indicator of severity than occurrence of loss of consciousness. Concussion symptoms may result from altered cranial nerve function (diplopia or blurry vision, nausea and vomiting, tinnitus, and light and noise sensitivity), motor function (gait instability and incoordination), mental status changes (slowed speech, confusion, altered awareness, and amnesia), or behavioral changes (fatigue, irritability, and depressive or anxious symptomatology). Sport-related concussion must be suspected if any of these signs and symptoms are noted after head injury.

A variety of instruments can be used for early (within 3 to 5 days after injury) clinical assessment of a child or adolescent with a suspected concussion. The Sport Concussion Assessment Tool, 5th edition (SCAT-5), for example, incorporates several clinical rating tools.[49] It includes clinical observation, memory assessment, the Glasgow coma scale, cervical spine assessment, symptom evaluation, cognitive screening, concentration assessment, neurological screening, and delayed recall. An ImPACT (immediate postconcussion assessment and cognitive testing) test is done via computer; however, the athlete must have completed a baseline assessment prior to injury for comparison with the postinjury assessment, limiting its widespread adoption in youth sports.

Physical and cognitive rest are recommended for a minimum of 24 to 48 hours before return to sport. Guidelines suggest a stepwise progression from rest to (sequentially) limited activity, light aerobic exercise, sport-specific drills (no contact), more strenuous non-contact drills, contact drills, and return to sport (pending medical clearance). However, if symptoms are persistent (lasting >30 days in children) or worsen with exercise, a slower return to sport should be implemented.

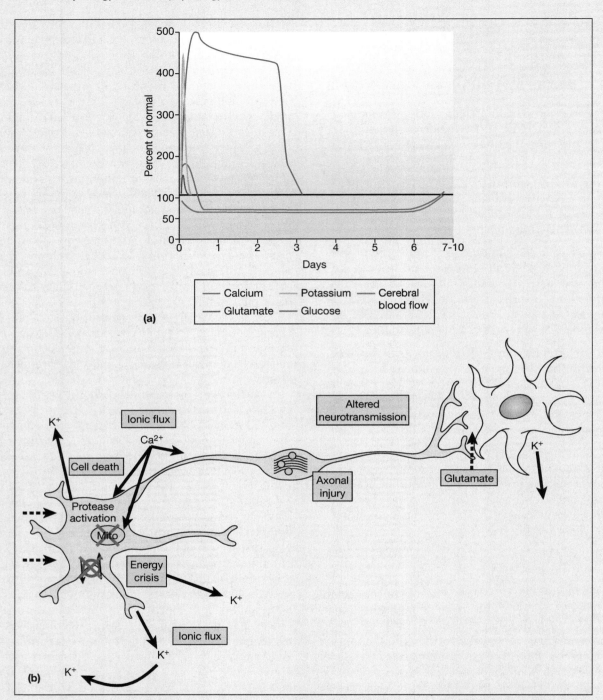

FIGURE 15.53 **(a)** Schematic illustrations showing the hypothesized metabolic disruption after mild traumatic brain injury/concussion. An early burst of glutamate and potassium (K+) release leads to depletion of brain glucose and cerebral blood flow for several days. **(b)** Calcium (Ca²⁺) is elevated and dysregulated for a few days, leading to neuron death by excitotoxicity. Mechanical forces also cause axonal injury, disrupting normal brain connectivity and neurotransmission.
Source: **(a)** From Giza CC, Hovda DA. The new neurometabolic cascade of concussion. *Neurosurgery*. October 2014;75(4):S24–S33. doi:10.1227/NEU.0000000000000505.

Linda L. Herrmann

Age-related changes in the neurological system affect both the central and peripheral nervous systems, including changes in cerebral cortex, cerebral vasculature, production and presence of neurotransmitters, cerebellar function, and alterations in visual, acoustic, olfactory, and gustatory senses. Clinicians must be cognizant that some of these age-related changes, such as cortical atrophy, enlarged subdural and ventricular spaces, and increased risk of ischemic stroke, are inextricably linked to older age while other changes, such as cognitive losses and neurodegenerative disorders, are not inevitably associated with the aging brain. A fundamental understanding of these changes—specifically, the extent to which older age affects the structure and function of the neurological system—is crucial in order for clinicians to make important distinctions in their patients.

AGING AND STRUCTURAL CHANGES IN CEREBRAL CORTEX

SUBDURAL HEMATOMAS AND TRAUMATIC BRAIN INJURY

Age-related structural changes in the neurological system include changes of the central nervous system. One such change, cortical atrophy, occurs because of a decrease in the water content and gray matter of the cerebral cortex. The pigment lipofuscin accrues in neurons, resulting in their significant dysfunction and death. As the brain atrophies, sulci are exaggerated and gyri flattened. The brain recedes away from the dura mater, allowing for an expanded subdural space. The fragility of bridging veins in an enlarged subdural space in older adults contributes to increased risk of **subdural hematoma** formation. Even a low level of impact to the head may produce a subdural hematoma in older adults. Elders on anticoagulation or antiplatelet agents are at greater risk for an acute subdural hematoma that may be present even with a normal CT scan (**Figure 15.54**).

Age-related physiological changes make it more difficult to assess or diagnose traumatic brain injury in older adults. Older adults with subdural hematomas may not present with neurological deficits, because age-related cortical atrophy and subsequent enlargement of the subdural space accommodates a fluid collection with little mass effect on the adjacent brain. They are more likely to differ significantly in neurological presentation and symptoms, timing of surgery, and

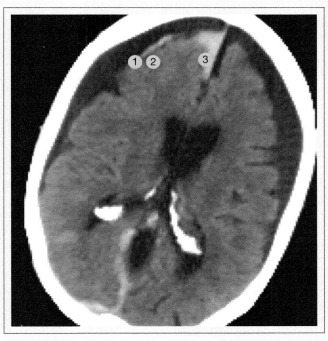

FIGURE 15.54 Axial CT scan showing (1) exaggerated subdural spaces with (2) chronic subdural collections and (3) acute subdural blood.

size of subdural hematomas compared with younger patients. Younger patients often present with headaches or emesis (and thus receive earlier neurosurgical intervention); in contrast, older adults are more likely to have larger subdural hematomas and present with mental status changes.

MICROGLIAL AGING

Microglia (formed from erythromyeloid progenitors) are brain cells with some similarities to peripheral macrophages. Residing in the brain from early in development, they provide support for neuronal development by maintenance and trimming, reduction, and development of synapses using a complement-dependent method,[50] filtration of debris, and defense against foreign stimuli. Healthy and young microglia orchestrate neuronal apoptosis and subsequent elimination of neuronal debris and glia without inciting an inflammatory cascade. Several contemporary studies have examined the complex and dynamic process of inflammation and aging, or *inflamm aging* (see Chapter 6, The Immune System and Leukocyte Function), and its effects on microglia function. These studies have proposed causal associations between **microglial dysfunction** and neurodegenerative disorders, namely Alzheimer disease and frontotemporal lobar degeneration. Increased load of reactive oxygen species and activation of glial cells have been well established as indicators of aging in the central nervous system and are implicated in several neurodegenerative diseases.[51]

AGING AND NEUROTRANSMITTERS

Aging affects the presence and production of neurotransmitters—acetylcholine, dopamine, serotonin, norepinephrine, and GABA—through decreased production with age. Acetylcholine and norepinephrine play an important role in cognition, including memory formation. Research has demonstrated that decreased amounts of acetylcholine within the hippocampus affect consolidation of short-term memory into long-term memory in older adults. Dopamine is an essential neurotransmitter for motor control and movement. Its depletion in the basal ganglia is evidenced by manifestations of rigidity and tremors in patients with Parkinson disease (see earlier discussion). Decreased production of serotonin affects the amount, pattern, and quality of sleep in older adults. In addition, decreased serotonin levels affect mood and may account for the increased incidence of depression in older adults, which may go undetected or underreported owing to overlap with sleep problems, cognitive decline, or both. Decreased GABA, which has its highest levels in the thalamus, accounts for some of the vague loss of sensation in older adults not otherwise explained by age-related alterations in individual sense organs.

COGNITIVE DYSFUNCTION

ACUTE CONFUSIONAL STATE

In an **acute confusional state**, also known as **delirium**, a person experiences rapid onset of altered lucidity with fluctuating symptoms of confusion, agitation, delusions, inattention, distraction, perseveration, and poor concentration. During this state, the reticular-activating system of the upper brainstem and subsequent communication to the thalamus, basal ganglia, and specific areas of the limbic system and cerebral cortex are interrupted. There are two types of confusional states: **hyperkinetic and hypokinetic**. A hyperkinetic confusional state involves an abnormality within the right middle temporal gyrus or an interruption in the left temporo-occipital junction; whereas in a hypokinetic confusional state or hypokinetic delirium, there is an interruption of the right frontal basal ganglia.

DEMENTIA

One in three community-dwelling adults older than 85 years of age have **dementia**. In more than 80% of these elders, this takes the form of Alzheimer disease or vascular dementia. Patients with dementia present with a loss of abstract thought, reasoning, judgment, and memory—all of which are severe enough to hinder interpersonal interactions and quality of life. Risk factors include advanced age (85 years or older), presence of the apolipoprotein E-4 allele, and a positive family history. Dementia may also be caused by other diseases or processes (e.g., neurodegenerative or vascular), as described in the next sections.

NEURODEGENERATIVE DISORDERS

Older adults are at greater risk of certain neurodegenerative processes affecting cognition, such as Alzheimer disease and **frontotemporal lobar degeneration** (FTLD), formerly known as Pick disease. Fine complex networks of neuronal function are progressively impaired, affecting memory, judgment, behavior, and higher level thought processes.

Postmortem pathological examinations of cerebral cortex in patients with **Alzheimer disease** have identified two consistent anomalies: (a) the buildup of β-amyloid (Aβ) protein (plaques) between neurons and (b) the presence of tau protein within axons (neurofibrillary tangles). Aβ plaques accumulate in the neuropil, and neurofibrillary tangles containing tau, which initially develop within the cell, are released into the extracellular space after neuronal death. Both Aβ and tau are implicated in disturbance of neural function, yet the exact mechanism linking the appearance of plaques and tangles to losses in cognitive function is not well understood. Genetic mutations, including copy number variations of the amyloid precursor protein, are found in causal relationship to the development of Alzheimer disease.[52] The relationship of Aβ genesis and Alzheimer disease is illustrated in **Figure 15.55**. Alterations in genes coding for tau have not been linked to Alzheimer disease; however, research has implicated tau mutations in the development of FTLD.

FTLD is the second most common disorder associated with dementia, and affected individuals present at younger ages than is typical for Alzheimer disease. FTLD is associated with atrophy of the frontal and temporal lobes, and has two distinct clinical presentations that depend on the area of greater involvement. Patients may present with personality changes manifested by apathy, impulsivity, irritability, and poor or

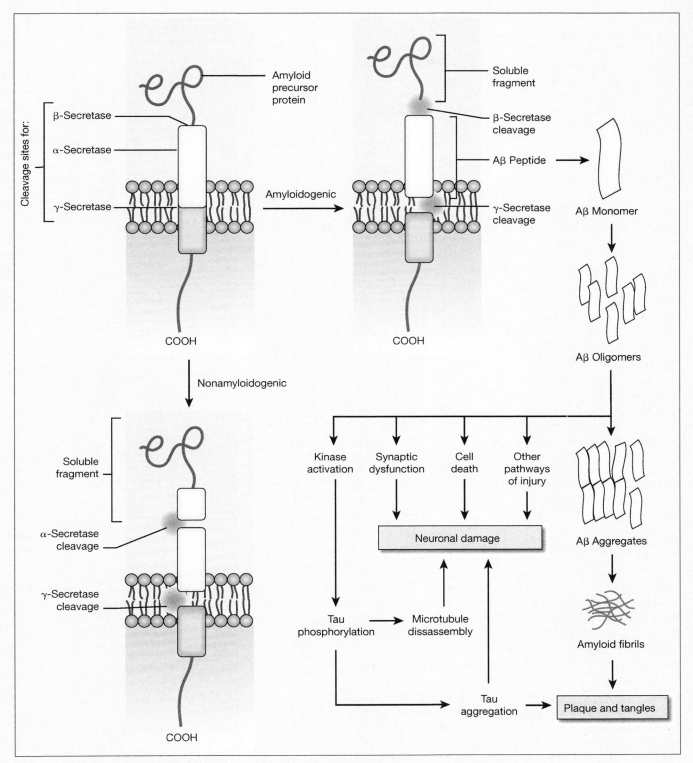

FIGURE 15.55 Aβ peptide genesis and Alzheimer disease. Sequential cleavage of amyloid precursor protein by α- and γ-secretase releases soluble, nontoxic fragments. In the amyloidogenic pathway, sequential cleavage by β- and γ-secretase generates Aβ peptide fragments that polymerize, ultimately aggregating into amyloid fibrils that form plaques throughout the brain.
*A*β, β-amyloid.
Source: From Kumar V, Abbas A, Aster J. *Robbins Basic Pathology.* Philadelphia, PA: Elsevier; 2018:876.

limited executive function and judgment, which usually precede memory difficulties (termed *behavioral-variant FTLD*). Other patients experience progressive losses in communication, including worsening speech and language function and comprehension. FTLD is pathologically classified based on the specific proteins that aggregate in brain tissue, generally based on post-mortem examination.

VASCULAR DISEASE

Cerebrovascular accidents (CVAs), or **strokes**, are the third leading cause of death, accounting for one in 15 deaths, and the leading cause of disability in the United States. Globally, approximately 5 million people die annually from strokes. It is estimated that half of all CVAs occur in adults over the age of 70. Strokes are either ischemic, from thrombus or embolus, or hemorrhagic, based on their pathophysiology. Ischemic strokes represent 90% of strokes, with hemorrhagic strokes representing 10% of strokes. **Transient ischemic attacks** (TIAs) occur when cerebral blood flow is temporarily compromised or obstructed, thus causing acute neurological deficits. TIAs have varying severity and most signs and symptoms resolve within 24 hours. There is no permanent neurological deficit with a TIA; however, a TIA can be a warning sign for impending cerebral infarction. Factors that precipitate TIAs are similar to those related to strokes, including atrial fibrillation (often sporadic and undetected), which is a common cause of TIA.

BLOOD VESSELS SUPPLYING THE BRAIN

The major blood vessels supplying the brain are shown in **Figure 15.56**. The internal carotid arteries arise from the common carotid arteries. Ascending to the brain, the internal carotid arteries give off small branches (ophthalmic and anterior choroidal), a larger anterior cerebral artery, and the largest vessel, the middle cerebral artery. Ascending to the posterior part of the brain, the vertebral arteries are branches of the subclavian arteries. The vertebral arteries fuse to form the basilar artery, which perfuses the brainstem and cerebellum before splitting to give rise to the superior cerebellar and posterior cerebral arteries. The posterior communicating arteries and anterior communicating artery complete a vascular circuit, the circle of Willis. In the case of thromboembolic blockage of one of the major cerebral arteries, collateral flow can provide blood supply to the affected region through diversion of blood around the circle of Willis, bypassing the blocked area.

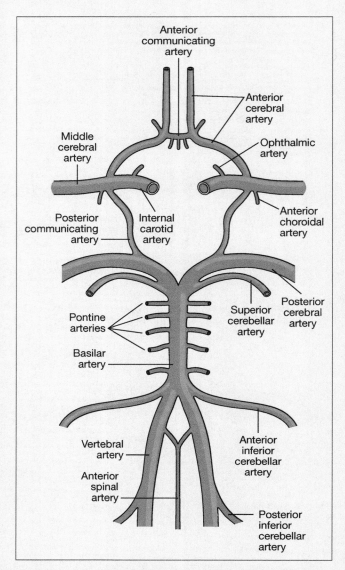

FIGURE 15.56 Cerebral blood supply. The internal carotid arteries give rise to anterior cerebral and middle cerebral arteries, which supply the frontal lobes and some of the parietal lobes. The vertebral/basilar arteries supply the brainstem and cerebellum and give rise to the posterior cerebral arteries, which supply the occipital lobe and portions of the temporal lobe.

ISCHEMIC STROKE

Age increases the risk of **ischemic stroke**. In adults aged 60 to 70 years old, the incidence of ischemic stroke is just over 6% for biological males and 7% for biological females. The incidence doubles to nearly 14% for both males and females aged 80 and older.[53] Advanced age increases the risk of disability and prolonged recovery following ischemic stroke.[54] Aging also increases the risk of atherosclerosis, with increased lipid accumulation and decreased high-density lipoprotein.

Age-related increases in endothelial plaque formation, calcification, and enlargement predispose to plaque rupture with rapid formation of an occlusive thrombus. This can occur in the region of the carotid bifurcation, a common site of atherosclerotic plaque, as well as at intracranial sites of atherosclerosis. Thrombi can form in the anterior circulation (anterior cerebral and middle cerebral arteries or their branches) or the posterior circulation (vertebral arteries and basilar artery). The most common site of stroke is the middle cerebral artery, which is also the largest cerebral artery. Weakness of the face and arm, and difficulty with speech, are common acute manifestations of stroke, and indicate blockage within the middle cerebral artery distribution. Other focal findings, such as difficulty with vision (implicating occipital lobe ischemia due to stroke in the posterior circulation), leg weakness (implicating ischemia within the distribution of the anterior cerebral artery), or sensory deficits (implicating parietal lobe ischemia), are clues to the anatomical location of the affected brain region (**Figure 15.57**). Clinical findings related to ischemia in specific vascular distributions are described in **Table 15.5**.

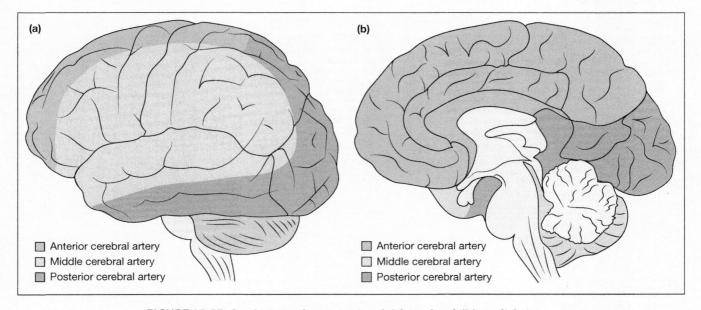

FIGURE 15.57 Cerebrovascular territories: (**a**) lateral and (**b**) medial views.

TABLE 15.5 Neurovascular Arterial Distribution, Affected Territory, and Patient Presentation

Artery	Cerebral Cortex Affected	Patient Presentation
Anterior Circulation		
ICA	Can be frontal lobe, posterior frontal lobe, anterior temporal lobe Can also have subcortical infarcts (affected cerebral cortex depends on whether ACA or MCA, or both, are involved)	Contralateral paralysis of face, arm, leg Sensory deficits in face, arm, leg Aphasia (when dominant hemisphere affected) Apraxia, agnosia, and unilateral neglect (when nondominant hemisphere affected) Homonymous hemianopia
ACA	With distal branch involvement, medial aspect of ipsilateral frontal lobe is affected	Contralateral leg and foot paralysis Contralateral sensory impairment of leg, foot, and toes Gait impairment Slowed performance of tasks, slowed response Flat affect, limited or lack of interest in environment Impaired memory

(continued)

TABLE 15.5 Neurovascular Arterial Distribution, Affected Territory, and Patient Presentation *(continued)*

Artery	Cerebral Cortex Affected	Patient Presentation
Anterior Circulation		
MCA	If M1 branch is occluded, then a large MCA territory infarct occurs, affecting most of that hemisphere	Contralateral paralysis of face and arm Sensory deficits in face and arm Aphasia (global aphasia when dominant hemisphere affected) Apraxia, agnosia, and unilateral neglect (when nondominant hemisphere affected) Homonymous hemianopia
Posterior Circulation		
VA	Vertebral artery involvement can be devastating, depending on whether one or both VAs are involved	Dizziness Nystagmus Dysarthria Dysphagia Facial, eye, nasal pain Ipsilateral facial weakness and numbness Ataxia Gait instability
BA	Vertebrobasilar territories include thalamus, medulla, cerebellum, pons, midbrain, and occipital lobes	Paralysis of all four extremities Paralysis of nearly all voluntary muscles, such that patient is in a pseudocoma or locked-in (i.e., patient is awake, but unable to communicate because of paralysis) Paresis of facial, tongue, and swallowing muscles
PCA	Peripheral branch involvement (superficial cortex affecting visual function) Deep cortical branch involvement (cerebellar peduncle, thalamus, brainstem)	Homonymous hemianopia Cortical blindness Cognitive deficits: memory recall and retention of new memory

ACA, anterior cerebral artery; BA, basilar artery; ICA, internal carotid artery; MCA, middle cerebral artery; PCA, posterior cerebral artery; VA, vertebral artery.

Source: Data from Hickey JV. *Clinical Practice of Neurological and Neurosurgical Nursing.* 7th ed. Philadelphia, PA: Wolters Kluwer/ Lippincott Williams & Wilkins; 2014.

The larger the vessel occluded and the longer the duration of occlusion, the greater will be the region of ischemia and mortality risk or subsequent neuronal loss and resulting disability. Approaches that lyse clots with fibrinolytic drugs or mechanically remove thrombi (thrombectomy) soon after stroke symptoms develop successfully restore blood flow and improve patient functional recovery, implying a time window of up to 24 hours before neuron death. However, these approaches are limited to patients with ischemic CVA and are contraindicated in hemorrhagic strokes.

Strategies to reduce stroke risk include pharmacological reduction of atherosclerotic plaque with HMG-CoA (β-hydroxy-β-methylglutaryl coenzyme A) reductase inhibitors (statin drugs), which may reduce the incidence of atherosclerotic stroke. Hypertension is highly prevalent in older adults and, if not well controlled, is a significant risk factor for both ischemic stroke and hemorrhagic stroke. Patients with atrial fibrillation are often treated with warfarin or direct oral anticoagulant drugs to reduce the risk of embolic stroke.

HEMORRHAGIC STROKE

The main cause of **hemorrhagic stroke**, particularly in older adults, is hypertensive hemorrhage, and the most common sites are the basal ganglia and internal capsule. Approximately 75% of people older than age 50 with untreated hypertension have isolated systolic hypertension.[55] At around age 55, changes in hemodynamics, including increased systolic, diastolic, and mean arterial pressures, begin to be noted. Subsequently, the diastolic and mean arterial pressures plateau, with a continued steady increase in systolic blood pressure. This is thought to be a result of age-related increases in vascular wall collagen and reduced elasticity of the aorta and larger arteries.[56] Other causes of intracranial hemorrhage include aneurysmal subarachnoid hemorrhage, ruptured arterial venous malformations, cavernous malformations, and hemorrhagic tumors.

VASCULAR DEMENTIA

Vascular dementia typically presents within 8 to 12 weeks following an acute CVA caused by cortical and subcortical infarcts, typically in the anterior and middle cerebral artery distributions. Consequently, older adults present with alterations in executive functioning and judgment, impulsivity, and slower cognition. Memory is not usually affected.

CEREBRAL AMYLOID ANGIOPATHY

Certain age-related changes in the composition of the cerebral cortex have a causal linkage to incidence of cognitive dysfunction, namely, dementia. For example, **cerebral amyloid angiopathy** (CAA), found in approximately half of adults over the age of 70, is associated with the same amyloid noted in the senile plaques found in patients with Alzheimer disease. In addition, CAA is thought to be the cause of one in ten intracerebral hemorrhages. The underlying pathophysiology of CAA, also referred to as **congophilic angiopathy** (due to the histological characteristics when stained with Congo red dye), is the presence of Aβ protein in small branches of cortical and meningeal vasculature. The Aβ protein degrades the integrity of these vessel walls, thus increasing the risk of hemorrhage. The pattern or distribution of amyloid-related intracranial hemorrhage is typically lobar and should be suspected in older adults who present with lobar hemorrhage, especially recurrent lobar hemorrhages.

GIANT CELL ARTERITIS

Giant cell arteritis, which is also known as **temporal arteritis**, is the most common form of systemic vasculitis of unknown etiology in older adults. It is a noncontinuous pattern of inflammation of lymphocytes, macrophages, and plasma cells that causes thickening and hardening of the temporal artery, an anterior branch of the superficial temporal artery. If this vasculitis progresses to involve the internal carotid artery, vascular supply to the eye on the affected side may be compromised owing to involvement or vasculitis of the ophthalmic artery. Clinical manifestations include unilateral headache, visible and palpable tenderness of the temporalis muscle and presence of firm tenderness of the temporal artery, and amaurosis fugax (unilateral loss of vision).

GAIT DYSFUNCTION

It is not uncommon for older adults to note changes in gait and balance. Unfortunately, most are told that gait changes are a normal aspect of aging. **Gait dysfunction** in older adults can be due to a variety of issues, including peripheral neuropathy, affecting sensation and decreased perception of placement of feet on a walking surface; cerebellar atrophy, affecting balance and coordination; and vitamin B12 deficiency, affecting perception of the body in space and position sense, and thus both balance and gait.

NORMAL PRESSURE HYDROCEPHALUS

Normal pressure hydrocephalus (NPH) describes dilation of the lateral ventricles, occipital horns, and third and fourth ventricles—essentially communicating hydrocephalus (**Figure 15.58**)—with normal intracranial pressure values. Patients present with a clinical triad of gait instability, cognitive changes, and urinary incontinence. The gait in a person with NPH has a classic appearance: typically, a broad-based stance with short stride and shuffled feet, and difficulty turning, as if the person is stuck to the floor. Changes in gait typically manifest first and dramatically affect mobility, confidence, and quality of life. Cognitive changes also have an insidious onset and are not necessarily indicative of the disease, but warrant clinical investigation.

Workup is particularly needed if the individual is older than age 40, experiences symptoms for more than 3 to 6 months, and has no history of a recent neurological injury (trauma) or event (stroke, meningitis). CT imaging demonstrates communicating hydrocephalus, and MRI scans may be useful to further characterize presence of transependymal edema. Unfortunately, each symptom, when taken separately, can be erroneously dismissed as a *normal* part of aging. Providers should inquire about the full constellation, character, and duration of symptoms.

Patients thought to have NPH should undergo a comprehensive neurological evaluation, including a large-volume lumbar puncture. Patients who experience immediate improvement in symptoms—notably, a dramatic improvement in gait 30 minutes after the lumbar puncture—are considered shunt responsive, and are referred to a neurosurgeon for consideration of shunt placement. Thus, recognition of this clinical triad is imperative because of the ability to intervene with shunting, as indicated, which has been shown to improve gait and mobility and to reduce dementia. There is no cure for NPH, and the treatment is palliative with a goal of improved quality of life.

AGING AND SENSE ORGANS

Other normal age-related changes of the neurological system include alterations in visual, acoustic, olfactory, and gustatory senses. Visual changes affect visual acuity and start with changes in the lens. The lens can experience several changes with

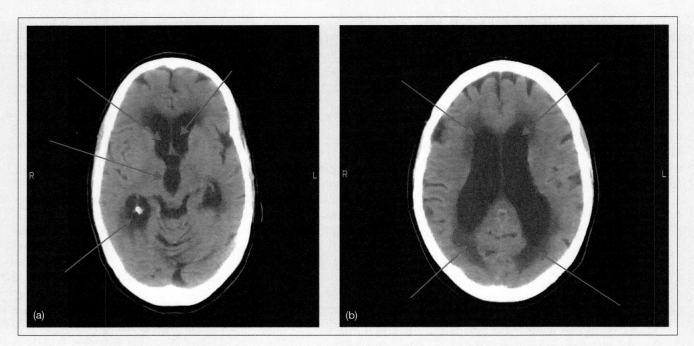

FIGURE 15.58 Axial CT scans showing **(a)** enlarged lateral and third ventricles and dilated temporal horns. **(b)** Hypodensities around the anterior aspect of the lateral ventricles depict transependymal edema.

aging, including (a) thickening and increased opacity, affecting refraction and increasing light dispersion; (b) decreased acuity of color perception, particularly for blue and green due to the absorption of more blue light as a result of yellow pigments within the lens, thus contributing to a decline in diffusion of blue light; and (c) cataract formation. Age-related changes in the retina include decreased number of rods, thus increasing the amount of light needed to see print or an item. Additionally, older adults develop corneal changes, including thickening and reduced convexity, thus increasing likelihood of astigmatism.

Auditory changes in one third of older adults over the age of 65 occur from genetic or environmental factors. Loss of high-frequency sounds occurs most commonly, affecting speech and language comprehension (particularly consonants *f*, *s*, and *sh*). Aging affects one's ability to discriminate between high-frequency and low-frequency sounds. Structural changes in hearing include degeneration of cochlear hair cells, decrease in auditory neurons (spiral ganglia) in the organ of Corti, degeneration of the conductive cochlear membrane, fewer vascular branches and supply to the cochlea, and fewer auditory neurons.

Olfactory sensitivity declines after age 60, with marked impairment beyond age 80. Deterioration in olfaction is a result of death of cells within the olfactory bulb and olfactory sensory neurons. Appetite may be reduced, affecting food choices, which may contribute to malnutrition in older adults.

The sense of taste declines after age 50, and the loss is more insidious than loss of other senses. Decreased numbers of fungiform papillae with aging lead to altered perception of flavor and taste. Some older adults may require greater concentration of flavors and experience difficulty differentiating flavor combinations. Amylase production in saliva is reduced with age, diminishing the ability to appreciate perception of sweet flavors.

Loss of proprioception is common in older adults and is due primarily to alterations in the input from the inner ear and respective receptors from joints, muscles, ligaments, and tendons. Proprioceptive loss is due to impairment of perception, reception, transmission, and interpretation of stimuli, the two most common causes being neuropathy and vestibular dysfunction. Decreased proprioception combines with decreased musculoskeletal function to predispose to fall and fracture risk. The concept of frailty, gradual loss of functional ability and stability in older adults, is strongly linked to both diminished sensory function and loss of musculoskeletal strength.

CASE STUDY 15.1: A Teenage Girl With Migraine

Michelle Zappas and Colleen Diering

Patient Complaint: *"Sometimes my head hurts so badly I have to leave school. My eyes hurt from the light. I have to lie in a dark room to feel better."*

History of Present Illness/Review of Systems: A 14-year-old girl presents with new onset of severe headaches for the past 3 months. She reports prodromal symptoms of irritability and aura—a small area of sickle-shaped vision loss precedes each headache. The aura never lasts longer than 30 minutes. The headaches are unilateral, throbbing in quality, and increase over about 1 hour. She experiences nausea but no vomiting. She also experiences sensitivity to light and sound. The headache improves after she lies down in a dark, quiet room. She has experienced the headaches four times over the past 3 months. On three occasions, she developed the headaches after a night of poor sleep, and the pain intensified during the bus ride to school. She had to be brought home from school on these occasions. She has no other problems with vision and no fever, chills, upper respiratory infection, or sinus symptoms. She has had no head or neck trauma.

Past Medical/Family History: Her past medical history and ROS are negative with the exception of

family history, which is significant for a mother and maternal aunt who both have history of migraine headaches.

Physical Examination: Findings are as follows: blood pressure of 92/57 mm Hg; heart rate of 56 beats/min, and respirations of 12 breaths/min. BMI is 18.0 kg/m². Funduscopic and otoscopic examinations are normal. The neurological examination is normal, with CN II through XII grossly intact, negative Romberg test, negative pronator drift, and symmetrical motor, sensory, reflex, and cerebellar tests. All other physical examination findings are normal.

Laboratory and Diagnostic Findings: MRI scan of the brain is normal. The results of a complete blood count and metabolic panel are also both normal.

CASE STUDY 15.1 QUESTIONS
- *What types of conditions are associated with headache in a teenager? Of those possibilities, what aspects of this case point to one diagnosis over others?*
- *Based on your response, would diagnostic imaging be indicated in a case like this? Why or why not?*

BMI, body mass index; CN, cranial nerve; ROS, reactive oxygen species.

CASE STUDY 15.2: A Child With a Seizure Disorder

Melissa Assaf and Katherine Edwards

Patient Complaint: *"We've noticed that our son has been twitching a lot in his sleep. At first we thought he was having bad dreams, but we began checking on him regularly and noticed it was happening every night. He wakes up with sores on his tongue and we think he may be biting his tongue in his sleep. He's also wetting the bed, but he's 8 years old, so we are worried something is wrong. I [the father] had seizures that started when I was 7 years old, but they went away when I was 9."*

History of Present Illness/Review of Systems: An 8-year-old boy presents with rhythmic jerking in his sleep. His parents report that this happens every night and has increased in frequency and severity

over the past few months. He wakes up with sores on his tongue from biting it and from urinating the bed. Developmental milestones have been appropriate, and no neurological deficits are noted on examination. Follow-up questions reveal that the child often seems fatigued during the day and takes a nap often after school. The parents report that the child's teacher has noticed a decreased ability to pay attention in class. The child and parents deny any changes in activity patterns, headaches, or sensory or motor problems. No changes are reported in respiratory, gastrointestinal, or musculoskeletal systems. There have been no unusual illnesses, fevers, weight loss/gain, or difficulty with usual activities.

(continued)

(continued)

Past Medical/Family History: The boy is typically an active child who plays baseball and has many friends at school. He has no history of head injury or any other physical injuries, and is currently not taking any medications. His medical records indicate that all developmental milestones have been appropriate. There is a family history of childhood seizures in the father and in a cousin.

Physical Examination: On neurological examination, the child is able to speak coherently and follow directions appropriate for his age. Motor function, reflexes, and sensory examinations are normal. Eye movement is normal, and pupils react normally to light. Hearing and vision are also normal. No abnormalities are found during the neurological exam.

Laboratory and Diagnostic Findings: Based on the parents' report, a brain MRI and EEG are obtained. Brain imaging is normal; however, an EEG reveals bilateral centrotemporal spike and waves. The child is diagnosed with BECTS (formerly referred to as BRE). He is treated with oxcarbazepine, and has resolution of seizures without any issues. His cognition remains intact, and he continues to do well in school. After 2 years without any seizures, a repeat EEG is normal, and he is tapered off the oxcarbazepine medication with no sequelae.

CASE STUDY 15.2 QUESTIONS
- *Identify some of the genetic mutations associated with seizure disorders in children. What categories of proteins may contribute to recurrent seizures and epilepsy?*
- *Do seizure-related EEG changes persist between seizure episodes?*
- *Oxcarbazepine blocks sodium channels; what is a possible rationale for giving a drug with this mechanism of action in this case?*

BECTS, benign epilepsy with centrotemporal spikes; BRE, benign rolandic epilepsy.

CASE STUDY 15.3: A Patient With Depression

Linda W. Good

Patient Complaint: *"I think I have fibromyalgia. I'm tired and achy all the time and just can't get motivated to do the things I need to do. From what I have read, this could also be chronic fatigue syndrome. I haven't exercised in weeks and I wake up off and on all night. I know this goes along with menopause, so maybe some hormones will help me. I sometimes break down in tears for no apparent reason and I am irritable with my family. I know I get this way every winter, but this is the worst yet."*

History of Present Illness/Review of Systems: You observe a well-developed, well-nourished 52-year-old woman who appears emotionally distressed. She states that she has experienced hot sweats, interrupted sleep, and cessation of menses, which started about a year ago, along with fatigue and achiness that have worsened over the past 6 months. She reports emotional symptoms of marked loss of motivation, irritability, and low mood for the past 2 months. She has tried natural plant estrogen supplements, melatonin, and diphenhydramine (Benadryl) without much benefit. In addition, she has had more frequent headaches and problems with poor concentration and forgetfulness.

The patient denies additional cardiovascular, respiratory, gastrointestinal, gynecological/urological, or musculoskeletal symptoms. There have been no constitutional issues of fevers or weight loss or gain. She specifically denies joint swellings or arthralgias, but describes myalgias. Headaches have been of a muscle contraction or tension type, with no vascular features. She has no focal neurological deficits or mental status changes.

Past Medical/Family/Social History: The patient notes that she has seasonal allergies and yearly bouts of sinusitis and bronchitis. She has had no hospitalizations or surgeries, and the only medications she uses are over-the-counter antihistamines, decongestants, and cold remedies. She quit smoking (cigarettes) 20 years ago. She is a daily alcohol consumer and admits to more frequent days with two to three glasses of wine over the past 2 months. There is no other history of recreational drugs. Her family history includes a father with bipolar illness and a sister with depression. Her social history includes a recent job change and a son with recent diagnosis of heroin addiction.

(continued)

Physical Examination: Findings are as follows: blood pressure of 140/70 mm Hg, heart rate of 88 beats/min, and respirations of 16 breaths/min. Body mass index (BMI) is 27 kg/m². The thyroid gland is normal in size and nontender. Chest, heart, and abdominal examinations are unremarkable. Joints are without inflammation or swelling. Neurological examination reveals normal strength, sensation, reflexes, tandem gait, and Romberg tests. Mental status examination is significant for slight flight of ideas and pressured speech, but no content that seems delusional or paranoid. Facial expression and demeanor seem appropriate to content, and the patient answers questions clearly. Judgment is unimpaired.

Laboratory and Diagnostic Findings: Thyroid function tests, comprehensive metabolic panel, complete blood count, and hemoglobin A$_{1c}$ results are all normal.

CASE STUDY 15.3 QUESTIONS

- *What factors in the case study might indicate a risk of depression?*
- *What are the main hypotheses regarding the cause of major depressive disorder?*

BRIDGE TO CLINICAL PRACTICE

Ben Cocchiaro

PRINCIPLES OF ASSESSMENT
Neurological and Psychiatric History

- *Mental status evaluation*—including orientation to person, place, and time. Standardized instruments such as the MMSE and the MoCA test additional cognitive domains including concentration, memory, visuospatial reasoning, and executive functioning.
- *Seizure history*—including context of episode, presence of aura/prodrome, semiology, and presence of postictal state.
- *Screening and evaluation instruments for neurological/psychiatric conditions:*
  ○ Depression—PHQ-2/9
  ○ Anxiety—GAD-7
  ○ PTSD—PC-PTSD-5
  ○ Dementia/cognitive impairment—MoCA, MMSE
  ○ Concussions—SCAT

Neurological Examination

- The primary method of nervous system assessment in the outpatient setting, this examination includes evaluations of:
  ○ *Cranial nerves*—these 12 nerves arise directly from the brain and brainstem. Their careful examination can help diagnose a number of neurological conditions and localize certain CNS lesions.
  ○ *Somatic sensory function*—touch, pain, vibration, position sense, temperature
  ○ *Somatic motor function*—tone, strength, reflexes (see **Box 15.5**), posture, balance, coordination, gait

Diagnostic Tools

- *CT:* Often the first-line diagnostic tool in the evaluation of head trauma and suspected stroke. The head CT can identify masses, hemorrhages, and some infarctions, though it exposes the patient to ionizing radiation.
- *MRI:* Higher sensitivity compared with CT imaging in the diagnosis of hemorrhagic and ischemic cerebrovascular events and masses. MRIs do not use ionizing radiation, but they are more expensive and time consuming than CT imaging.
- *EEG:* Useful in the evaluation of seizure disorders, EEGs use scalp electrodes to monitor average neuronal activity in different regions of the brain.
- *NCS:* Invasive studies that use needle electrodes to measure the conduction of action potentials along peripheral nerves and often used in conjunction with EMG to characterize and diagnose neuromuscular disorders.
- *Cerebrospinal fluid examination (LP):* Collection and analysis of cerebrospinal fluid by introducing a catheter into the subarachnoid space of the spinal canal. Crucial in the differentiation of meningitides and the diagnosis of idiopathic intracranial hypertension, subarachnoid hemorrhage, and encephalitis.

MAJOR DRUG CLASSES AND THERAPEUTIC MODALITIES
Drug Classes

- *Antidepressant drugs:* Most antidepressant classes inhibit degradation and reuptake of the

(continued)

(continued)

neurotransmitters serotonin, dopamine, and norepinephrine within the synaptic cleft.

- *Anticonvulsant/antiepileptic drugs:* Inhibit the propagation of action potentials across groups of neurons within the brain, thereby decreasing the rate of neuronal firing and preventing the positive feedback loop of neuronal discharge that constitutes a seizure.
- *Mood stabilizers:* Include several anticonvulsants, antipsychotics, and lithium salts and are a mainstay in the treatment of bipolar depression given prior to the initiation of antidepressant medication in order to prevent triggering manic episodes.
- *Antipsychotic drugs:* Also known as neuroleptics, both first- and second-generation antipsychotics are thought to work by decreasing dopaminergic and serotonergic transmission.

- *Drugs for Parkinson disease:* These agents work by increasing basal ganglia dopaminergic transmission to ameliorate tremor and bradykinesia.

Major Nonpharmacological Interventions
- *Cognitive behavioral therapy, mindfulness, psychoanalysis, and other talk therapies:* Conducted in both individual and group settings, this broad class of interventions can be employed in a wide array of behavioral health concerns either alone or synergistically with pharmacotherapy.
- *Electroconvulsive therapy and transcranial magnetic stimulation:* Both techniques are noninvasive neuromodulation therapies shown to be effective in treatment-resistant depression.
- *Implantable brain and nerve stimulators:* This approach has been employed with varying degrees of effectiveness in conditions as varied as Parkinson disease, chronic pain, and treatment-resistant epilepsy.

CNS, central nervous system; EMG, electromyography; GAD, glutamate decarboxylase; LP, lumbar puncture; MMSE, Mini-Mental State Examination; MoCA, Montreal Cognitive Assessment; NCS, nerve conduction studies; PTSD, post-traumatic stress disorder; SCAT, Sport Concussion Assessment Tool.

KEY POINTS

- The brain is the most complex organ in the human body, with anatomical subdivisions that are associated with specific behavioral and physiological functions.
- The functional unit of the brain is the neuron: a multipolar cell type with a wide array of structures that can vary by brain region.
- Neurons are electrically excitable cells that have a negatively charged membrane potential at rest (RMP). Excitation leads to rapid electrical signaling in the form of an action potential that can be propagated from the cell body outward along the dendrites and the axon.
- At the axon terminal, the action potential releases vesicles of neurotransmitter by exocytosis, converting the electrical signal to a chemical message that targets postsynaptic neurons.
- Chemical neurotransmission is mediated by neurotransmitter receptors found in postsynaptic and presynaptic locations. These receptors can incorporate ion channels for rapid signaling (ionotropic receptors) or can be G protein–coupled receptors that produce slower synaptic responses (metabotropic receptors).

- Neurotransmitter receptors can also be subdivided into excitatory and inhibitory types. Excitatory ionotropic receptors permit entry of sodium, calcium, or both into the neuron, producing postsynaptic depolarization and favoring action potential generation. Inhibitory ionotropic receptors permit entry of chloride into the neuron, producing postsynaptic hyperpolarization and inhibiting action potential generation.
- Termination of transmitter action is necessary for ongoing responsiveness to new inputs, and there are three main mechanisms of termination of transmission.
- Glutamate and GABA are the primary excitatory and inhibitory transmitters of the brain. They signal primarily through ionotropic receptors, but also have metabotropic receptors. Neurons using glutamate or GABA as transmitters are found throughout the brain and spinal cord and are responsible for most ongoing sensory, motor, and cognitive activity. Imbalance of glutamate-induced excitation and GABA-induced inhibition can be one mechanism of epilepsy.
- Other major brain transmitters include acetylcholine, dopamine, serotonin, histamine, and norepinephrine. Neurons associated with each

of these neurotransmitters are found in specific anatomical locations within the forebrain, hypothalamus, and brainstem. The majority of their receptors are metabotropic, and they are associated with slow changes of state and appetitive behaviors, including wake–sleep transitions, hunger, thirst, and behavioral responses to these drives.

- Peptide transmitters include endogenous opioids that modulate pain sensation and hypothalamic peptides that contribute to sleep–wake transitions as well as increasing food intake or energy expenditure.
- Somatosensory neurons transmit information about light touch, vibration, pain, muscle stretch, and tendon tension in the body and head to the spinal cord and brainstem. These neurons have peripheral axons ending in specialized receptors in the skin, joints, muscles, and tendons.
- Sensory action potentials are propagated along the peripheral axon to the cell body in the dorsal root ganglion, then along the central axon into the spinal cord or brainstem. There, they make a synapse within the spinal cord. All primary somatosensory fibers are glutamatergic.
- All somatic sensory modalities other than pain and temperature travel to the brain through the dorsal columns of the spinal cord.
- Pain is detected by primary nociceptors with bare nerve endings in peripheral tissues that are excited by chemical signals of tissue damage and inflammation, including prostaglandins and bradykinin. First-order pain fibers use the neurotransmitters glutamate and substance P. Pain sensation travels to the brain along the spinothalamic tract.
- Pain can be modulated by descending pathways using the transmitters norepinephrine and serotonin. Endogenous opioids, including enkephalins and dynorphin, also inhibit pain transmission. Moderate to severe tissue damage sensitizes peripheral and central pain signaling, resulting in phenomena of hyperalgesia and allodynia.
- Movement is accomplished by lower motor neurons in the spinal cord and cranial nerves that project to muscles, use acetylcholine as neurotransmitter, and stimulate muscle contraction.
- Lower motor neurons are stimulated by several inputs:
  - Muscle spindles, which detect the length of the muscle and cause a reflex contraction when the muscle is stretched
  - Tendon organs, which detect muscle tension

- Brainstem pathways, which have their greatest influences on motor neurons to axial muscles (to maintain posture and balance) and to extensor muscles (to prevent falling and excite stretch reflexes)
  - The corticospinal tract, which is the major influence on voluntary movement, particularly influencing flexors and inhibiting stretch reflexes. The motor cortex neurons projecting to the spinal cord along the corticospinal tract can be thought of as *upper motor neurons* without which normal skilled movements are not possible.
- Motor cortex control of movement is enhanced with practice, and basal ganglia structures contribute to the process of motor learning and production of smooth, coordinated movements.
- Movements that are in progress are monitored and corrected by the cerebellum.
- Specific patterns of motor abnormalities are grouped by etiology, including lower motor neuron lesions, upper motor neuron lesions, basal ganglia disorders, and cerebellar disorders.
- Maturation of thought and behavior from childhood into adulthood involves development of structures of the prefrontal cortex that mediate reasoning, decision-making, and planning. With practice, individuals learn to choose to defer rewards in order to accomplish goals and to accomplish complex cognitive tasks.
- Learning and memory involve the prefrontal cortex, as well as the hippocampus and other brain structures. Behaviors are motivated, in part, by responses of pleasure and reward that occur when dopamine is released in the nucleus accumbens.
- Aversive and stressful stimuli activate the amygdala, the fear center of the brain. Through hypothalamic relays, these stimuli excite the HPA axis and the sympatho-adrenomedullary systems, increasing blood levels of cortisol and epinephrine. In response, the reasoning ability of the prefrontal cortex is reduced and the reactivity of other cortical regions to threat is enhanced.
- Although the stress response is protective in situations that involve actual external threats, psychological stressors may lead to recurrent activation that results in chronic dysfunction. Adverse childhood experiences may produce long-term changes in brain stress pathways that manifest as pathophysiological disorders of behavior and health.
- Depression, anxiety, and substance use disorders are common worldwide and are associated

with altered size, connectivity, and reactivity of some of the stress-related brain structures. These include the prefrontal cortex, amygdala, and hippocampus. Altered signaling by norepinephrine, serotonin, and corticotropin-releasing hormone neurons may also contribute to these disorders.

- Prenatal and genetic influences have profound effects on brain development and postnatal function.
- The highest incidence of seizures is in infancy and early childhood. Sporadic seizures and febrile seizures may not recur, but recurrent seizures are diagnosed as epilepsy.
- Developmental delay is generally detected in early childhood and may result from prenatal exposures or genetic disorders.
- Intellectual and mental health disorders arising in childhood include intellectual disability, ADHD, and autism spectrum disorders. Although the pathogenesis of these are not well understood, there may be an underlying genetic susceptibility as well as prenatal and developmental contributions.
- In school-age children, headaches are a common complaint; migraines and tension-type headaches may also begin in childhood.
- Sport-related concussions are common in middle- and high-school students and can have severe consequences if precautions about returning to play are not observed.
- The brain in older adults has greater fragility of supporting structures of connective tissue and meninges. For this reason, traumatic brain injury in this population is associated with more severe outcomes, particularly subdural hematoma.
- Cognitive dysfunction in older adults can be acutely disrupted (confusion, delirium) or chronically reduced by neurodegenerative or vascular disorders. Intracellular and extracellular accumulation of normal and abnormal proteins is a pathological marker associated with some neurodegenerative disorders.
- Strokes can occur at any age but incidence rises progressively after the age of 65. The majority of strokes are ischemic, resulting from vascular blockage by local atherosclerotic plaque and thrombus formation, or from emboli arising from other sources. Atrial fibrillation is a major cause of embolic phenomena causing TIAs and strokes.

REFERENCES

1. Global Burden of Disease 2016 Injury Incidence and Prevalence Collaborators. Global, regional, and national incidence, prevalence, and years lived with disability for 328 diseases and injuries for 195 countries, 1990–2016: a systematic analysis for the Global Burden of Disease Study 2016. *Lancet.* 2017;390:1211–1259. doi:10.1016/S0140-6736(17)32154-2.
2. Gooch CL, Pracht E, Borenstein AR. The burden of neurological disease in the United States: a summary report and call to action. *Ann Neurol.* 2017;81:479–484. doi:10.1002/ana.24897.
3. Centers for Disease Control and Prevention. Stroke facts. https://www.cdc.gov/stroke/facts.htm. Accessed November 20, 2018.
4. Rui P, Okeyode T. National ambulatory medical care survey: 2016 summary tables. https://www.cdc.gov/nchs/data/ahcd/namcs_summary/2015_namcs_web_tables.pdf. https://www.cdc.gov/nchs/data/ahcd/namcs_summary/2016_namcs_web_tables.pdf. Accessed January 10, 2020.
5. Wess J, Eglen RM, Gautam D. Muscarinic acetylcholine receptors: mutant mice provide new insights for drug development. *Nat Rev Drug Discov.* 2007;6:721–733. doi:10.1038/nrd2379.
6. Pasternak G, Neilan C. Neuropeptides: overview. In: Aminoff MJ, Daroff RB, eds. *Encyclopedia of the Neurological Sciences.* 2nd ed. Burlington, VT: Elsevier Science; 2014:516–519. doi:10.1016/B978-0-12-385157-4.00043-9.
7. Eippert F, Bingel U, Schoell ED, et al. Activation of the opioidergic descending pain control system underlies placebo analgesia. *Neuron.* 2009;63:533–543. doi:10.1016/j.neuron.2009.07.014.
8. Carskadon MA, Dement WC. Normal human sleep: an overview. In: Kryger M, Roth T, Dement WC, eds. *Principles and Practice of Sleep Medicine.* 6th ed. Philadelphia, PA: Elsevier; 2017:15–24.
9. Brown RE, Basheer R, McKenna JT, et al. Control of sleep and wakefulness. *Physiol Rev.* 2012;92:1087–1187. doi:10.1152/physrev.00032.2011.
10. Saper CB, Fuller PM. Wake-sleep circuitry: an overview. *Curr Opin Neurobiol.* 2017;44:186–192. doi:10.1016/j.conb.2017.03.021.
11. Kuner R, Flor H. Structural plasticity and reorganisation in chronic pain. *Nat Rev Neurosci.* 2017;18:113. doi:10.1038/nrn.2017.5.
12. Garland EL. Pain processing in the human nervous system: a selective review of nociceptive and biobehavioral pathways. *Prim Care.* 2012;39:561–571. doi:10.1016/j.pop.2012.06.013.
13. Reynolds DV. Surgery in the rat during electrical analgesia induced by focal brain stimulation. *Science.* 1969;164:444–445. doi:10.1126/science.164.3878.444.
14. Melzack R. The perception of pain. *Sci Am.* 1961;204:41–49. doi:10.1038/scientificamerican0261-41.
15. Benedetti F, Carlino E, Pollo A. How placebos change the patient's brain. *Neuropsychopharmacology.* 2011;36:339–354. doi:10.1038/npp.2010.81.

16. Craig AD, Reiman EM, Evans A, Bushnell MC. Functional imaging of an illusion of pain. *Nature.* 1996;384:258–260. doi:10.1038/384258a0.

17. Ossipov MH, Morimura K, Porreca F. Descending pain modulation and chronification of pain. *Curr Opin Support Palliat Care.* 2014;8:143–151. doi:10.1097/SPC.0000000000000055.

18. Skelly AC, Chou R, Dettori JR, et al. *Noninvasive Nonpharmacological Treatment for Chronic Pain: A Systematic Review* [AHRQ Publication No 18-EHC013-EF]. Rockville, MD: Agency for Healthcare Research and Quality; June 2018. doi:10.23970/AHRQEPCCER209.

19. Connolly BS, Lang AE. Pharmacological treatment of Parkinson disease, a review. *JAMA.* 2014;311:1670–1683. doi:10.1001/jama.2014.3654.

20. Okun MS. Deep brain stimulation for Parkinson's disease. *N Engl J Med.* 2012;367:1529–1538. doi:10.1056/NEJMct1208070.

21. Holt DJ, Ongur D, Wright CI, et al. Neuroanatomical systems relevant to neuropsychiatric disorders. In: Stern TA, Fava M, Wilens TE, Rosenbaum JF, eds. *Massachusetts General Hospital Comprehensive Clinical Psychiatry.* 2nd ed. Philadelphia, PA: Elsevier; 2016:771–790.

22. Nestler EJ, Hyman SE, Malenka RC. *Molecular Neuropharmacology: A Foundation for Clinical Neuroscience.* 3rd ed. New York, NY: McGraw-Hill; 2015.

23. Arnsten AF. Stress signalling pathways that impair prefrontal cortex structure and function. *Nat Rev Neurosci.* 2009;10:410–422. doi:10.1038/nrn2648.

24. McEwen BS, Gianaros PJ. Central role of the brain in stress and adaptation: links to socioeconomic status, health, and disease. *Ann N Y Acad Sci.* 2010;1186:190–222. doi:10.1111/j.1749-6632.2009.05331.x.

25. Wood SK, Valentino RJ. The brain norepinephrine system, stress, and cardiovascular vulnerability. *Neurosci Biobehav Rev.* 2017;74:393–400. doi:10.1016/j.neubiorev.2016.04.018.

26. Whiteford HA., Ferrari AJ, Degenhardt L, et al. The global burden of mental, neurological and substance use disorders: an analysis from the global burden of disease study 2010. *PLOS ONE.* 2015;10:e0116820. doi:10.1371/journal.pone.0116820.

27. Lim SS, Vos T, Flaxman AD, et al. A comparative risk assessment of burden of disease and injury attributable to 67 risk factors and risk factor clusters in 21 regions, 1990–2010: a systematic analysis for the Global Burden of Disease Study 2010. *Lancet.* 2012;380:2224–2260. doi:10.1016/S0140-6736(12)61766-8.

28. Lai HMX, Cleary M, Sitharthan T, Hunt GE. Prevalence of comorbid substance use, anxiety and mood disorders in epidemiological surveys, 1990–2014: a systematic review and meta-analysis. *Drug Alcohol Depend.* 2015;154:1–13. doi:10.1016/j.drugalcdep.2015.05.031.

29. Anda RF, Felitti VJ, Bremner JD, et al. The enduring effects of abuse and related adverse experiences in childhood: a convergence of evidence from neurobiology and epidemiology. *Eur Arch Psychiatry Clin Neurosci.* 2006;256:174–186. doi:10.1007/s00406-005-0624-4.

30. Teicher MH, Samson JA, Anderson CM, Ohashi K. The effects of childhood maltreatment on brain structure, function, and connectivity. *Nat Rev Neurosci.* 2016;17:652–666. doi:10.1038/nrn.2016.111.

31. Kupfer DJ, Frank E, Phillips ML. Major depressive disorder: new clinical, neurobiological, and treatment perspectives. *Lancet.* 2012;379:1045–1055. doi:10.1016/S0140-6736(11)60602-8.

32. Kessler RC, Chiu WT, Demler O, et al. Prevalence, severity, and comorbidity of 12-month DSM-IV disorders in the National Comorbidity Survey Replication. *Arch Gen Psychiatry.* 2005;62:617–627. doi:10.1001/archpsyc.62.6.617.

33. Craske MG, Stein MB, Eley TC, et al. Anxiety disorders. *Nat Rev Dis Primers.* 2017;3:17024. doi:10.1038/nrdp.2017.24.

34. Nestler EJ. Is there a common molecular pathway for addiction? *Nat Neurosci.* 2005;8:1445–1449. doi:10.1038/nn1578.

35. Pert CB, Snyder SH. Opiate receptor: demonstration in nervous tissue. *Science.* 1973;179:1011–1014. doi:10.1126/science.179.4077.1011.

36. Felitti VJ, Anda RF, Nordenberg D, et al. Relationship of childhood abuse and household dysfunction to many of the leading causes of death in adults: the Adverse Childhood Experiences (ACE) Study. *Am J Prev Med.* 1998;14:245–258. doi:10.1016/S0749-3797(98)00017-8.

37. Verhaart IEC, Robertson A, Wilson IJ, et al. Prevalence, incidence and carrier frequency of 5q-linked spinal muscular atrophy – a literature review. *Orphanet J Rare Dis* 2017;12:124. DOI 10.1186/s13023-017-0671-8.

38. Jensen FE. Neonatal seizures: an update on mechanisms and management. *Clin Perinatol.* 2009;36:881–900. doi:10.1016/j.clp.2009.08.001.

39. Mikati MA, Hani AJ. Seizures in childhood. In: Kliegman RM, Stanton BF, St. Geme JW, Schor NF, eds. *Nelson Textbook of Pediatrics.* Vol 2. 20th ed. Philadelphia, PA: Elsevier; 2016:2823–2856.

40. Fisher RS, Acevedo C, Arcimanoglu A, et al. A practical clinical definition of epilepsy. *Epilepsia.* 2014;55:475–482.

41. Shin C. Pathophysiology. In: Husain AM, ed. *Practical Epilepsy.* New York, NY: Demos Medical; 2016:3–10.

42. American Psychiatric Association. *Diagnostic and Statistical Manual of Mental Disorders.* 5th ed. Arlington, VA: American Psychiatric Publishing; 2013.

43. Online Mendelian Inheritance in Man®. https://www.omim.org. Accessed June 19, 2019.

44. Mandelbaum DE. Attention deficit-hyperactivity disorder. In: Swaiman KF, Ashwal S, Ferriero DM, et al., eds. *Swaiman's Pediatric Neurology: Principles and Practice.* 6th ed. New York, NY: Elsevier; 2017:e1086–e1103.

45. Burstein R, Noseda R, Borsook D. Migraine: multiple processes, complex pathophysiology. *J Neurosci.* 2015;35:6619–6629. doi:10.1523/JNEUROSCI.0373-15.2015.

46. Slover R, Kent S. Pediatric headaches. *Adv Pediatr.* 2015;62:283–293. doi:10.1016/j.yapd.2015.04.006.

47. McCrory P, Meeuwisse W, Dvorak J, et al. Consensus statement on concussion in sport: the 5th International

Conference on Concussion in Sport held in Berlin, October 2016. *Br J Sports Med.* 2017;51:838–847. doi:10.1136/bjsports-2017-097699.

48. Giza CC, Hovda DA. The new neurometabolic cascade of concussion. *Neurosurgery.* 2014;75:S24–S33. doi:10.1227/NEU.0000000000000505.

49. Echemendia RJ, Meeuwisse W, McCrory P, et al. The Sport Concussion Assessment Tool 5th edition (SCAT5): background and rationale. *Br J Sports Med.* 2017;51:848–850. doi:10.1136/bjsports-2017-097506.

50. Schafer DP, Stevens B. Phagocytic glial cells: sculpting synaptic circuits in the developing nervous system. *Curr Opin Neurobiol.* 2013;23:1034–1040. doi:10.3390/ijms18040769.

51. Koellhoffer EC, McCullough LD, Ritzel RM. Old maids: aging and its impact on microglial function. *Int J Mol Sci.* 2017;18:769. doi:10.3390/ijms18040769.

52. Kumar V, Abbas AK, Aster JC, eds. *Robbins Basic Pathology.* 10th ed. Philadelphia, PA: Elsevier; 2018.

53. Go AS, Mozaffarian D, Roger VL, et al. Executive summary: heart disease and stroke statistics—2013 update: a report from the American Heart Association. *Circulation.* 2013;127:143–152. doi:10.1161/CIR.0b013e318282ab8f.

54. Nakayama H, Jorgensen HS, Raaschou HO, Olsen TS. The influence of age on stroke outcome. The Copenhagen Stroke Study. *Stroke.* 1994;25:808–813. doi:10.1161/01.STR.25.4.808.

55. Franklin SS, Jacobs MJ, Wong ND, et al. Predominance of systolic hypertension among middle-aged and elderly US hypertensives. *Hypertension.* 2001;37:869–874. doi:10.1161/01.HYP.37.3.869.

56. Franklin SS, Gustin W, Wong ND, et al. Hemodynamic patterns of age-related changes in blood pressure. The Framingham Heart Study. *Circulation.* 1997;96:308–315. doi:10.1161/01.CIR.96.1.308.

SUGGESTED RESOURCES

American Academy of Pediatrics. Head injury. http://www.healthychildren.org/English/health-issues/injuries-emergencies/Pages/Head-Injury.aspx.Updated November 21, 2015. Accessed November 20, 2018.

Ayers E, Verghese J. Locomotion, cognition, and influences on nutrition in ageing. *Proc Nutr Soc.* 2013;73:302–308. doi:10.1017/S0029665113003716.

Costigan M, Scholz J, Woolf CJ. Neuropathic pain: a maladaptive response of the nervous system to damage. *Annu Rev Neurosci.* 2009;32:1–32. doi:10.1146/annurev.neuro.051508.135531.

Crotti A, Ransohoff RM. Microglial physiology and pathophysiology: insights from genome-wide transcriptional profiling. *Immunity.* 2016;44:505–515. doi:10.1016/j.immuni.2016.02.013.

Frosch MP. The central nervous system. In: Kumar V, Abbas AK, Aster JC, eds. *Robbins Basic Pathology.* 10th ed. Philadelphia, PA: Saunders/Elsevier; 2018:849–888.

Li S, Rieckmann A. Neuromodulation and aging: implications of aging neuronal gain control and cognition. *Curr Opin Neurobiol.* 2014;29:148–158. doi:10.1016/j.conb.2014.07.009.

Rathmell JP, Fields HL. Pain: pathophysiology and management. In: Jameson JL, Fauci AS, Kasper DL, et al., eds. *Harrison's Principles of Internal Medicine.* 20th ed. New York, NY: McGraw-Hill; 2018:chap 10.

Simon RP, Aminoff MJ, Greenberg DA. *Clinical Neurology.* 10th ed. New York, NY: McGraw-Hill; 2018:139–165.

Sohrabji F. The impact of aging on ischemic stroke. In: Sierra F, Kohanski R, eds. *Advances in Geroscience.* New York, NY: Springer; 2016:161–196. doi:10.1007/978-3-319-23246-1.

Stafstrom CE, Rho JM. Neurophysiology of seizures and epilepsy. In: Swaiman KF, Ashwal S, Ferriero DM, et al., eds. *Swaiman's Pediatric Neurology.* 6th ed. New York, NY: Elsevier; 2017:chap 63.

Stiles J, Jernigan TL. The basics of brain development. *Neuropsychol Rev.* 2010;20:327–348. doi:10.1007/s11065-010-9148-4.

Tau GZ, Peterson BS. Normal development of brain circuits. *Neuropsychopharmacol Rev.* 2010;35:147–168. doi:10.1038/npp.2009.115.

Willner P, Scheel-Krüger J, Belzung C. The neurobiology of depression and antidepressant action. *Neurosci Biobehav Rev.* 2013;37:2331–2771. doi:10.1016/j.neubiorev.2012.12.007.

16

MUSCULOSKELETAL SYSTEM

Connie B. Scanga and Joseph J. Curci

THE CLINICAL CONTEXT

Musculoskeletal injury and disease affect a large swath of the population and become increasingly prevalent in older adults. According to the World Health Organization, musculoskeletal conditions are the leading cause of disability worldwide.[1] In the United States National Health Interview Survey, arthritis diagnosis was reported by 21.6% of adults, and having chronic joint symptoms was reported by 28.3% of adults. At least 15% of the population report being unable to perform at least one common activity (e.g., walking, rising from a seated position) because of these conditions. The National Ambulatory Medical Care Survey (NAMCS) documented that 8.3% of outpatient visits in 2016 were related to musculoskeletal disorders.[2] Osteoarthritis, lower limb joint pain, and medial meniscus tears are the most common musculoskeletal diagnoses. In this chapter, we describe the pathophysiology underlying common musculoskeletal injuries and diseases seen by primary care providers.

OVERVIEW OF BONES AND SKELETAL PHYSIOLOGY

The human skeletal system comprises 206 bones, as well as joints, cartilage, and ligaments. The skeleton serves as a hard scaffold that supports and protects the body's soft tissues and organs. The skeletal bones and joints make up a system of levers that are operated by skeletal muscles and allow for efficient movement capability.

BONE HISTOLOGY

Bone is a hard connective tissue and, like all connective tissues, consists of scattered cells surrounded by extracellular matrix that comprises both organic and inorganic components. The matrix of bone tissue is hardened by deposits of calcium hydroxyapatite crystals, consisting of calcium phosphate salts, which align in parallel to the collagen fibers that predominate in the bone matrix. While collagen fibers give bone its tensile strength (i.e., the ability to resist pulling and stretching forces), the mineral content of bone enables it to resist compression forces to which it is exposed during weight bearing and movement.

Bone tissue is produced and maintained through regulated interactions among three types of bone cells: osteoblasts, osteocytes, and osteoclasts. Osteoblasts are derived from mesenchymal cells and are the cells that secrete the osteoid or organic bone matrix, primarily collagen and small amounts of other proteins. They also secrete alkaline phosphatase, which controls the deposit of hydroxyapatite and other minerals in the bone matrix, and regulate the activity of osteoclasts. When teams of osteoblasts complete bone production they flatten and form a lining at bone surfaces, called periosteum when it covers external bone surfaces or endosteum when it covers internal surfaces. As bone is being formed, some osteoblasts become trapped in small spaces within the matrix, called lacunae, and develop into osteocytes. Osteocytes extend cellular processes toward other osteocytes through small canaliculi in the bone matrix. At points of contact, osteocytes communicate with each other via gap junctions. Osteocytes help to maintain the bone matrix, modulate the activity of osteoblasts and osteocytes, and control bone remodeling.

In contrast to osteoblasts and osteocytes, osteoclasts are derived from the myeloid cell line, as are their close relatives, macrophages. Osteoclasts form through the fusion of progenitor cells, which results in osteoclasts being quite large and multinucleated. Upon activation by osteoblasts, osteoclasts move along the bone surface to microfracture sites. There, the ruffled border of the osteoclast attaches tightly to the underlying bone, creating a resorptive cavity between the osteoclast body and the bone. After making a firm attachment, the osteoclast secretes hydrogen ions and various hydrolytic enzymes into the resorption cavity that degrade hydroxyapatite and dissolve the organic bone matrix at the bone surface. The osteocyte takes up the end products of bone degradation (i.e., bone minerals and collagen fragments) from the resorption cavity by means of endocytosis, moves them in vesicles through the cell, and releases the digestive end products across the free surface of the osteoclast into the extracellular fluid, thus completing the task of bone resorption. When bone resorption is complete, osteoclasts undergo apoptosis (programmed cell death) or revert to an inactive, nonresorbing state. Bone resorption is a mechanism involved in bone tissue repair and renewal as well as in helping to maintain body calcium ion homeostasis.

All bones consist of two types of bone tissue. Cortical (compact) bone is dense and forms the hard, rigid, outer shell of bones. The primary functional unit of cortical bone is the osteon. Trabecular (cancellous) bone is located internally and has an open, spongy appearance. The primary functional unit of this type of bone is the trabeculae (i.e., the thin plates of bone that form the network of the tissue). The trabeculae of bones align to best accommodate the mechanical stress to which the bone is routinely exposed.

OSTEOGENESIS AND BONE REMODELING

Osteogenesis (ossification), the process of bone formation, begins during embryological development and continues into early adulthood when linear growth of long bones is complete. We can classify bone tissue as either lamellar or woven bone according to the pattern of collagen in the osteoid produced by osteoblasts.

Lamellar bone is characterized by collagen fibers organized into sheets (lamellae). Typically, collagen fibers in adjacent lamella have different orientations, which results in a bone tissue that can withstand mechanical stress from varied orientations. In contrast, collagen fibers are randomly organized in woven bone, resulting in weaker bone tissue. Woven bone is formed when osteoblasts secrete osteoid rapidly, such as during fetal development and fracture repair. Ultimately, woven bone is replaced by lamellar bone, making the skeleton strong and durable.

Bone remodeling is a lifelong process. After maturation when linear growth of bones ends, bone is continuously remodeled and strengthened based on the types of stresses to which it is exposed. Through remodeling, the annual turnover rate of bone in young adults is 10%. This process involves the sequential activity of osteoclasts, multinucleated cells derived from hematopoietic stem cells of the monocyte lineage, and osteoblasts, derived from mesenchymal stem cells (**Figure 16.1**). Bone remodeling is regulated by calcium-controlling hormones such as vitamin D and parathyroid hormone, as part of total body calcium homeostasis, and is also influenced by sex steroids, growth factors, and cytokines. In postmenopausal women and older men, an imbalance develops between the bone resorption activity of osteoclasts and the bone synthesis activity of osteoblasts, leading to decreased bone density. These changes predispose to osteoporosis, a significant contributor to fracture risk in older adults.

Thought Questions

1. What cells and processes are involved in bone modeling (during development) and bone remodeling (in adulthood)?

2. How are these processes altered in older adults?

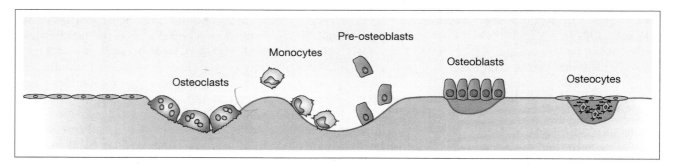

FIGURE 16.1 Cells involved in bone remodeling. Osteoclasts break down bones, creating resorption lacunae. Pre-osteoblasts enter the lacunae, differentiate into osteoblasts, and deposit bone matrix. Some of the osteoblasts remain embedded in the matrix and become osteocytes. Mineral deposition continues around the matrix and osteocytes, strengthening the bone.

BONE FRACTURES

A **fracture** is a loss of bone integrity resulting from mechanical injury or diminished bone strength, or both. It is the most common pathological condition affecting bone. The goal of the clinician is to restore maximal function of the injured bone.

A fracture may be produced by direct or indirect injury. Fractures produced by direct injury result from a direct blow or crushing force. Often, there is associated soft tissue trauma involving muscles, vessels, and nerves over the fracture site, and the bone may shatter and fragment. Indirect injury fractures are the result of forces transmitted through the bone to an area of weakness. For example, a compression fracture of a vertebral body compromised by metastatic cancer may occur when an axial load or pressure force is applied as the vertebral body performs its weight-bearing function. Rarely, a fracture can be produced by the violent contraction of muscle, as occurs in a patellar fracture caused by sudden, forceful contraction of the quadriceps muscle.

TYPES OF FRACTURES

In general terms, fractures can be described as open or closed. In a closed fracture, the fracture site does not communicate with the outside air, although adjacent disruption of the skin (abrasion or laceration) may be present. An open fracture (also called a compound fracture) is a break in the bone that communicates with the outside air through the disrupted skin or mucous membrane. By virtue of this communication, bacteria (usually *Staphylococcus aureus*) may enter the wound, causing infection and cell injury. Therefore, in general, an open fracture is a much more serious problem than a closed fracture.

A simple fracture has only one fracture line and produces two fragments whereas a comminuted fracture has more than one fracture line, thereby producing multiple fragments. In a displaced fracture, the ends of the bone at the fracture site are not aligned. They may be placed in proper alignment by external manipulation of the fragments (closed reduction) under anesthesia or a direct, open surgical reduction with placement of some type of orthopedic *hardware* to maintain the position of the fragments. In a nondisplaced fracture, normal alignment is maintained.

A stress fracture is a slowly developing fracture that follows a period of increased physical activity in which the bone is subjected to repetitive loads. A greenstick fracture occurs when the cortex fractures only on one side while maintaining the thick periosteal tube (intraperiosteal fracture). This type of fracture is more common in children because of their more robust and thicker periosteum.

Pathological fractures occur in bones weakened by an underlying disease process such as a primary or metastatic tumor, osteomyelitis, or osteoporosis. These are often *spontaneous* or nontraumatic. Fractures of long bones can also be distinguished by their location—proximal or distal—in the bone. Distal fractures that involve joints or the epiphyseal growth plate in a child can have significant consequences. The latter can lead to premature closure of the growth plate by damaging its proliferative zone, leading to a shortened limb.

Avulsion fractures occur where a tendon or ligament attaches to a bone. The force of the injury tears off a piece of bone at the tendon or ligament insertion site. A common example is an avulsion fracture at the base of the fifth metatarsal, where the fibularis brevis tendon attaches. This injury occurs in response to forceful twisting of the foot, when a piece of bone cracks off while the tendon remains intact. Various fracture types and dislocations (malalignments) are presented in **Figures 16.2** and **16.3**, respectively.

FRACTURE HEALING

Healing of any fracture involves molecular, biochemical, histological, and biomechanical stages and represents the regulated expression of multiple genes. A precondition of optimal fracture healing is repositioning the bone fragments of the fracture. This can be accomplished conservatively by manipulating the bone fragments into proper alignment (closed reduction) or surgically (open reduction). After reduction, the fracture site is stabilized so that healing can proceed without deformation at the fracture site. Some common surgical procedures that involve open reduction with internal fixation are illustrated in **Figure 16.4**. Surviving cells with osteogenic potential in the nearby endosteum and periosteum, adequate vascularization, and mechanical rest are fundamental requirements of fracture healing.

Physiological healing of a bone fracture progresses in stages, as outlined in **Box 16.1** and **Figure 16.5**. Various factors can influence fracture healing, including nutritional status, drug therapies, preexisting conditions affecting skeletal health (e.g., osteoporosis), age, infection, adequate blood supply and survival of periosteum at the fracture site, and proper application of mechanical stress during healing.

RECOVERY FROM FRACTURE

Pseudoarthrosis (a false joint) or nonunion is the failure of bone formation after 6 months and is one of the most common complications of fracture healing. It can occur from excessive mechanical load on the

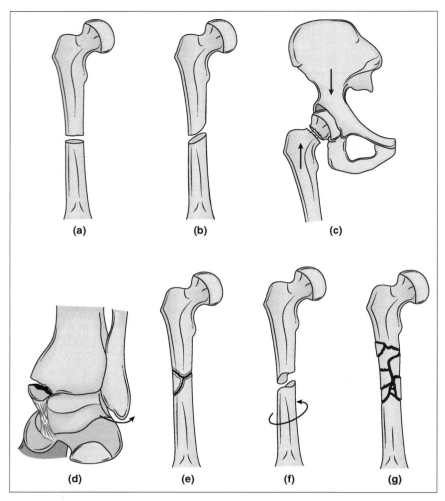

FIGURE 16.2 The most important types of fractures: **(a)** transverse, **(b)** oblique, **(c)** shearing, **(d)** avulsion, **(e)** bending, **(f)** spiral, and **(g)** comminuted.

regenerating bone and the absence of callus formation due to poor blood supply.

Infection at a fracture site is a serious obstacle to proper healing because bacteria cause direct cellular injury. Infection is most commonly associated with open fractures, which are always treated with antibiotics (usually intravenous) immediately upon diagnosis in an effort to prevent this feared complication. Malnutrition or an immunocompromised state also hinders healing and makes the patient more prone to infection. Traumatic arthritis may occur if a fracture involves the joint, because malaligned joint surfaces block motion and produce excessive wear on the articular cartilages, causing damage to the chondrocytes. Therefore, every effort is made to restore joint surfaces by perfect reduction.

Immobilization by a sling or cast after a fracture can rapidly lead to **disuse atrophy of muscles**. Bed rest and limited activity after open surgery to reduce a fracture can also lead to atrophy, but to a lesser degree because a goal of fracture surgery is to facilitate earlier mobilization. This atrophy is simply a loss of muscle bulk, which occurs when proteolytic systems are activated and contractile proteins and organelles are removed, resulting in shrinkage of muscle fibers. A decrease in muscle protein synthesis combined with an increase in muscle protein breakdown produces a loss of muscle extensibility, strength, and endurance. Age and malnutrition can also exacerbate muscle atrophy after a fracture.

In atrophic muscle, the cells contain fewer mitochondria and myofilaments and a reduced amount of endoplasmic reticulum but, importantly, cell survival is still possible. Therefore, disuse atrophy is reversible by utilizing the various modalities of physical therapy such as graduated strengthening exercises. The muscle cells can survive by bringing into balance reduced cell volume and lower levels of blood supply, nutrition,

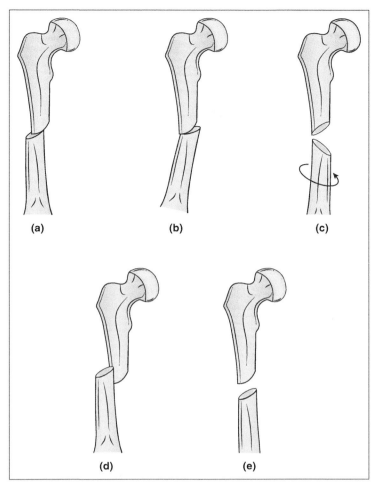

FIGURE 16.3 Fracture dislocations: **(a)** sideways dislocation, **(b)** axial dislocation, **(c)** angular malalignment, **(d)** bayonet dislocation, **(e)** distracted fragments.

or trophic stimulation to establish a new equilibrium. The biochemical mechanisms are poorly understood but are likely to affect the balance between protein synthesis and degradation. Atrophy can occur quickly in that a muscle at complete rest loses 10% to 15% of its strength each week. Unfortunately, the rate of recovery from disuse weakness is slower than the rate of loss at 6% per week using exercises. Therefore, rehabilitation can be a slow process—but certainly worth the effort.

Finally, prolonged disuse atrophy can lead to **muscle contractures**. A contracture is a shortening of the muscle and the tendon that attaches it to bone. Immobilization after a fracture or its surgical repair is the most common cause of contractures. The muscle length shortens because of loss of sarcomeres. This changes the length–tension relationship of the muscle because muscle contraction strength is intimately related to muscle length. When muscles operate close to their ideal (usually resting) length, they are operating with their greatest force. When they are shortened, the maximum active tension generated decreases.

Contractures occur as atrophy progresses to the point where muscle tissue is replaced by connective tissue. These collagen fibers progressively shorten, limiting joint range of motion, and the muscles appear functionally short. When a muscle is shortened to 50% to 60% of its resting length, its ability to develop contractile tension is reduced to zero. Stretching helps to prevent fiber shortening.

Thought Questions

3. What are the short-term and long-term pathophysiological consequences of a fracture?

4. How might the type of fracture influence the risk of complications and time to recovery?

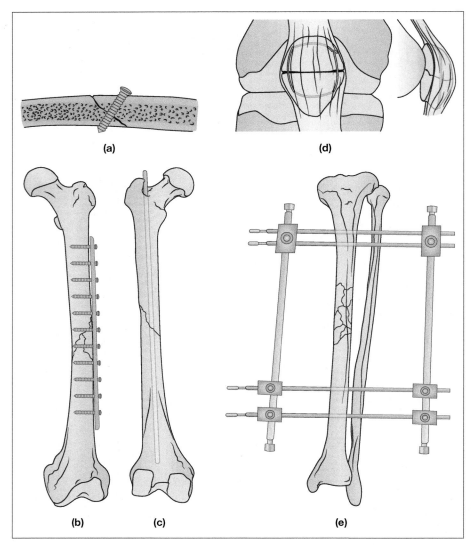

FIGURE 16.4 Surgical procedures used to create a temporary mechanical fracture union: **(a)** screw osteosynthesis, **(b)** plate osteosynthesis, **(c)** intramedullary rod, **(d)** tension-band wiring, **(e)** external fixation.

BOX 16.1
Stages of Fracture Healing

STAGE 1: INFLAMMATION AND FRACTURE HEMATOMA FORMATION

- When a fracture occurs, rupture of blood vessels from the soft tissues and hemorrhage from the bone itself result in a hematoma, which fills the fracture gap and the surrounding area of injury (Figure 16.5a). Loss of circulation at the hematoma leads to the death of tissue at the fracture site.

- Damaged cells secrete inflammatory mediators and an aseptic inflammatory reaction begins, often accompanied by a low-grade fever and a local increase in warmth. The hematoma and edema fluid cause varying degrees of swelling, pain, and ecchymosis.

- Initially, the fluids surrounding the bone fragments become slightly acidic, which is thought to help mobilize cellular activity in the

(continued)

BOX 16.1 (*continued*)
Stages of Fracture Healing

area. Osteoclasts, macrophages, and neutrophils are attracted to the area to clean up cell debris.

- As this phase progresses, proliferating fibroblasts migrate into the area along the fibrin strands of the hematoma. Capillary elements bud from the periosteum into the hematoma and create granulation tissue, dense with newly formed capillaries, to restore blood flow to the area and replace the hematoma.

- The hematoma phase begins within hours after the fracture and may persist for several weeks, overlapping with the next phase of the repair process.

STAGE 2: FORMATION OF A FIBROCARTILAGINOUS CALLUS

- During this phase, fibroblasts and osteoblasts that have migrated to the fracture area from the periosteum and endosteum create a gradually more stable connection between the bone fragments (**Figure 16.5b**).

- Fibroblasts secrete collagen fibers, which are important matrix proteins for both cartilage and bone tissue. Some cells, especially those further from newly forming capillaries, differentiate into chondroblasts and secrete cartilage matrix. Gradually, the acidic pH characteristic of the previous stage is neutralized.

- After 10 to 14 days, the local pH becomes alkaline and the concentration of alkaline phosphatase increases at the fracture site, causing the cartilage matrix to calcify. Ultimately, the bulging fibrocartilaginous (soft) callus will completely surround the ends of the bone fragments and form the scaffolding for a more stable hard callus.

STAGE 3: BONY CALLUS FORMATION

- The alkaline pH of the interstitial fluid surrounding the fracture site activates osteoblasts that have migrated to the area, and they begin to secrete osteoid (i.e., the organic portion of the bone matrix), which is mineralized by hydroxyapatite crystals. These calcium salts deposit around the collagen fibers to form woven bone (**Figure 16.5c**).

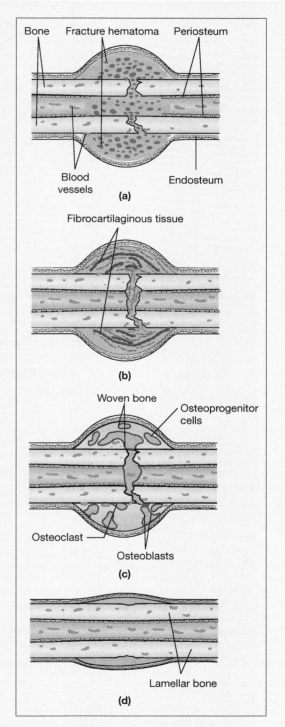

FIGURE 16.5 Stages of fracture healing: (**a**) fracture hematoma forms, (**b**) fibrocartilaginous callus forms, (**c**) bony callus forms, and (**d**) bone remodeling.

(*continued*)

BOX 16.1 (*continued*)
Stages of Fracture Healing

- By 6 to 8 weeks after fracture, bone tissue will have gradually replaced the soft callus formed in the previous phase. The woven bone forms a relatively stable hard callus at the fracture site.

STAGE 4: BONE REMODELING

- As the callus matures and is subjected to weight-bearing forces, portions that are not physically stressed are resorbed. This remodeling reduces the size of the callus until the shape and outline of the fractured bone is reestablished as lamellar bone (**Figure 16.5d**).

- After several months, the medullary cavity of the bone will be recreated. There is evidence that bone remodeling normally continues at a fracture site for up to a year or more as the bone continues its adaptation to routine mechanical stress.

JOINTS

Imagine the human skeleton without joints. The lack of these structures would render the body rigid and would make movement virtually impossible, much like the Tin Man in *The Wizard of Oz* when Dorothy first discovered him in the woods. We begin this section with a review of joint structure and function, as a prelude to describing the pathophysiology underlying some common joint disorders.

FUNCTIONAL CLASSIFICATION

Joints are functionally classified according to the degree of movement they allow. While some joints are immoveable, others are considered slightly or freely moveable. It should be noted, however, that while some joints are considered *freely moveable* the actual range of motion at joints varies, based on the shape of the articulating bones, the length and placement of ligaments and tendons crossing the joint, and other factors.

STRUCTURAL CLASSIFICATION

Joints are structurally classified as fibrous, cartilaginous, or synovial, based on the connective tissue that holds the joint together and the presence (or absence) of a joint cavity.

Fibrous Joints

Fibrous joints are ones in which articulating bones are held together tightly by tough, fibrous connective tissue; no joint cavity is present. There are three types of fibrous joints: sutures, gomphoses, and syndesmoses. Sutures are located between the flat bones of the skull. At birth, the flat bones of the skull, which are still growing via intramembranous ossification, are separated by fontanelles. This arrangement facilitates passage of the baby's head through the birth canal. Throughout early childhood, the skull bones continue to grow. By age 20, the skull bones will have completed their growth and the sutures will be firmly established, creating immovable joints between adjacent bones.

A gomphosis is the immoveable joint between a tooth and its alveolar socket in the mandible or maxilla. The fibrous structure that holds the tooth in place is the periodontal ligament. Severe periodontal disease can affect not only gums but also periodontal ligaments, causing teeth to become loose.

A syndesmosis is a slightly moveable fibrous joint in which articulating bones are held together with a cord or sheet of fibrous connective tissue, called a ligament or an interosseous membrane, respectively. The anterior tibiofibular ligament and interosseous membrane between the tibia and fibula are examples of syndesmoses stabilizing the physical relationship between the bones of the leg. The degree of movement possible at a syndesmosis is determined by the length of the collagen fibers in the connective tissue structures binding the bones together.

Cartilaginous Joints

In a cartilaginous joint, articulating bones are joined together with hyaline or fibrocartilage. Cartilage is highly resilient tissue that is able to withstand compression forces, a characteristic that is functionally beneficial at the joint. Cartilaginous joints are of two types, synchondroses and symphyses.

A synchondrosis, sometimes called a primary cartilaginous joint, is one in which a plate of hyaline cartilage joins the articulating bone surfaces. The epiphyseal plate, which connects the diaphysis and epiphysis of long bones during the growth phase, is an example of an immoveable and temporary synchondrosis. Ultimately, the hyaline cartilage of the epiphyseal plates at each end of the diaphysis will be replaced with bone and the diaphysis and epiphyses will fuse, stopping further longitudinal growth of the bone. Another notable example of a synchondrosis is the amphiarthrosis between the first rib and the manubrium of the sternum.

Symphyses, or secondary cartilaginous joints, are permanent and slightly moveable joints. In a symphysis, the articulating bone surfaces are covered with a thin layer of hyaline cartilage, which fuses to a fibrocartilage pad. The prominent examples of this type of joint are the pubic symphysis and each of the intervertebral articulations of the spine. Although of a similar joint class, these two types of joints have somewhat unique functional properties. The pubic symphysis is typically resistant to the tensile, shearing, and compression forces generated during normal movement. However, during pregnancy, the pubic symphysis widens and pelvic ligaments lengthen. These changes, which help to widen the birth canal, seem to be related to the effects of estrogen and relaxin, a placental hormone, on pelvic connective tissue structures. Intervertebral joints also exhibit unique structural and functional features, which we discuss later in this chapter.

Synovial Joints

Synovial joints are the only joints in which the articulating bones are separated by a fluid-filled joint cavity, or synovial cavity (**Figure 16.6**). The articular surfaces of bones participating in a synovial joint are covered with a thin layer of hyaline cartilage, called articular cartilage. Articular cartilage is resilient and its smooth surface reduces friction between the articulating bones. The articulating ends of bones in a synovial joint are held close together and in alignment by the articular capsule, a double-layered connective tissue sleeve that extends around the synovial cavity and attaches firmly on each end of the joint to the articulating bones. The external layer of the articular capsule consists of dense irregular connective tissue that, because of the random orientation of the collagen fibers in the tissue, allows the joint to resist tensile forces from many directions and helps prevent dislocation. The fibrous layer of the articular capsule is continuous with the periostea of the bones at each end of the joint and is, in some cases, reinforced by capsular ligaments intrinsic to the articular capsule itself. The inner layer of the articular capsule, the synovial membrane, covers all of the surfaces within the joint cavity except those covered with articular cartilage and is itself composed of two layers. The

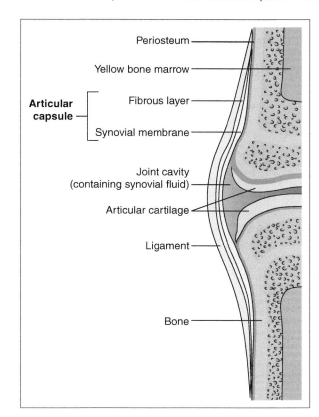

FIGURE 16.6 Typical synovial joint.

innermost layer, the intima, is in contact with the synovial fluid; external to the intima is a subintimal layer that supports the intima. Cells of the intima secrete hyaluronic acid and mucopolysaccharides—solutes that make synovial fluid viscous and slippery, facilitating smooth movement of the joint. The intima also contains macrophages, which function to clear debris and waste products from the synovial cavity. Sandwiched between the layers of the synovial membrane is a network of fenestrated capillaries that supply internal structures of the joint and participate in forming synovial fluid via transudation.

Synovial joints are typically reinforced by ligaments—cords of dense, regular connective tissue that extends across the joint, from one bone to another. These ligaments may be either internal or external to the joint capsule, called intracapsular and extracapsular, respectively. Intracapsular ligaments are covered with synovial membrane and, thus, are not actually in the synovial cavity. Also commonly present around synovial joints are bursae and tendon sheaths. A bursa is a small, flattened sac lined with synovial membrane and filled with synovial fluid. Bursae provide cushioning between bones and the softer tissues that overlie them, protecting the soft tissue. Tendon sheaths are elongated cylinders that surround muscle tendons overlying the bone tissue.

Like bursae, they are lined with synovial membrane and filled with synovial fluid. Their role is to protect tendons as they move past underlying bone during contraction and relaxation. One or more menisci may be present in synovial joints. A meniscus is a crescent-shaped fibrocartilage pad that partly divides a joint cavity. The menisci of the knee are perhaps the best known, but menisci are also present in the temporomandibular, acromioclavicular, sternoclavicular, and wrist joints.

The basic structure of synovial joints allows for a greater potential range of motion than is possible in fibrous or cartilaginous joints. However, the range of motion and the types of motion normally possible at a given joint are influenced by several different factors. Of primary importance is the shape of the bone ends at the articulation, which leads to joints being classified as gliding, hinge, pivot, condyloid, saddle, or ball-and-socket joints (**Table 16.1**). Range of motion is also affected by the sites of muscle attachment on either side of the joint and the direction of pull each muscle exerts at the joint, the length of the ligaments that reinforce the joint, and the bulk of tissue (e.g., muscle and adipose tissue) that surrounds the joint.

Although the range and types of motion permitted at synovial joints are fairly broad, the movements can be classified into four general types: gliding (planar), angular, rotational, and special. Gliding movements are those in which flat bone surfaces move back-and-forth past each other, as allowed by the shape of the articular surfaces of the bone. Angular movements are those in which the movement produces a change, either an increase or a decrease, in the angle of a joint, while rotational movement is produced when a bone rotates around its long axis. **Table 16.2** provides specific definitions and examples of movements possible at synovial joints.

TABLE 16.1 Structural Classification of Synovial Joints

Structural Type	Description	Examples	Movement Capabilities
Gliding	Articular surfaces are flat or slightly curved	• Intercarpal and intertarsal joints • Acromioclavicular and sternoclavicular joints • Sternocostal (ribs 2–7) and vertebrocostal joints • Sacroiliac joint	Nonaxial; allow slight gliding of articular surfaces past each other in any direction (movement is usually limited by ligaments at the joint)
Hinge	Convex surface fits into a concave surface	• Elbow joint • Ankle joint • Interphalangeal joints • Knee joint	Monoaxial; allow angular movement in one plane (specifically, flexion and extension)
Pivot	Rounded or pointed articular surface fits into a ring created by another bone and ligaments	• Proximal radioulnar joint • Atlanto axial joint	Monoaxial; allow rotational movement in one plane
Condyloid	Convex oval projection articulates with concave oval depression	• Radiocarpal joint • Metacarpophalangeal joints 2–5	Biaxial; allow movement in two planes (along or across the oval)
Saddle	Saddle-shaped articular surfaces are oriented perpendicularly	• First metacarpophalangeal joint	Biaxial; allow movement in the frontal and sagittal planes but no rotational movement
Ball-and-socket	Ball-shaped head of one bone fits into a cuplike depression on the other	• Shoulder (glenohumeral) joint • Hip joint	Triaxial, allow movement in all planes

TABLE 16.2 Types of Movements at Synovial Joints

Movement	Description
Flexion	Sagittal plane movement in which the angle between articulating bones decreases
Extension	Sagittal plane movement in which the angle between articulating bones increases
Hyperextension	Extension beyond the anatomical position
Abduction	Movement of a bone away from the body midline in the frontal plane **Note:** abduction of the digits of the hand and foot refers to a spreading apart of the digits (i.e., away from an imaginary line drawn longitudinally through the hand or foot)
Adduction	Movement of a bone toward the body midline in the frontal plane **Note:** the terms *abduction* and *adduction* always refer to movements of the appendicular skeleton, rather than the axial skeleton
Circumduction	Movement of the distal end of a body part in a circle. Circumduction involves a smooth sequence of flexion, abduction, extension, and adduction at the joint

(continued)

TABLE 16.2 Types of Movements at Synovial Joints (*continued*)

Movement	Description
Medial (internal) rotation	Rotation of a limb around its longitudinal axis that moves the anterior limb surface toward the body midline
Lateral (external) rotation	Rotation of a limb around its longitudinal axis that moves the anterior limb surface away from the body midline
Left and right rotation	Movement around the body's longitudinal axis (i.e., the vertebral column) in which the anterior head or trunk moves left or right
Left and right lateral flexion	Movement in the frontal plane in which sideways bending of the vertebral column causes the head, torso, or both, to move left or right
Dorsiflexion	Flexion of the ankle, which brings dorsum of foot closer to leg, as when walking on the heel
Plantar flexion	Extension of the ankle that elevates the heel or points the toes

TABLE 16.2 Types of Movements at Synovial Joints (*continued*)

Movement	Description
Inversion 	Movement of the sole of the foot medially at the intertarsal joints
Eversion	Movement of the sole of the foot away from the midline at the intertarsal joints
Elevation 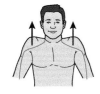	Upward movement of a body part, e.g., shrugging the shoulders (shoulder girdle movement) and closing the mouth (temporomandibular movement)
Depression 	Downward movement of an elevated body part, e.g., returning shrugged shoulders to anatomical position (shoulder girdle movement) and opening the mouth (temporomandibular joint movement)
Protraction 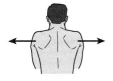	Moving a body part anteriorly in the transverse plane, e.g., protracting the shoulder girdle pulls the scapula anteriorly and rounds the shoulder
Retraction 	Returning a protracted body part back to anatomical position

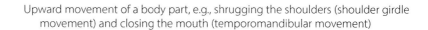

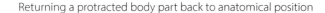

(*continued*)

TABLE 16.2 Types of Movements at Synovial Joints *(continued)*	
Movement	Description
Pronation 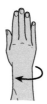	Rotational movement at the proximal and distal radioulnar joints that causes the distal radius to move across the anterior ulna and the wrist and palm of the hand to move posteriorly
Supination 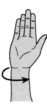	Rotational movement at the proximal and distal radioulnar joints in which the wrist and palm of the hand are turned anteriorly (as in anatomical position)
Opposition 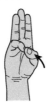	Movement at the first carpometacarpal joint in which the thumb moves across the palm toward the tips of the fingers on the same hand

Thought Questions

5. What types of joints (fibrous, cartilaginous, and synovial) are generally associated with injuries and degenerative diseases?

6. What might be the basis of their vulnerability?

STRAINS AND SPRAINS

A **strain** is essentially a stretching injury to a musculotendinous unit. It can be caused by severe muscle contraction or excessive stretch of the muscle and tendon. This can result in small tears in the muscle or tendon leading to limited amounts of bleeding, edema, and an inflammatory response, all of which can produce pain and stiffness. Strains commonly occur in the low back, neck, elbow, shoulder, and foot. Tissue repair takes place relatively quickly with a short period of rest.

As compared to a strain, a **sprain** involves the tougher ligamentous structures surrounding the joint and there is more pain and swelling, which subsides over a longer time frame. A sprain is a stretching or tear of the ligament. Severe stretching can cause *microtears*; this injury represents a grade 1 sprain. It is associated with minimal swelling and tenderness, no instability, and little functional loss. A partial ligamentous tear, with some of the bands of connective tissue still intact, is classified as grade 2. There is increased swelling and tenderness and mild instability. If the ligament ruptures completely with severe swelling and tenderness, a grade 3 injury has occurred and significant instability and functional loss will occur. Instability of joints can be assessed by manipulations that detect abnormal movement, termed **laxity of the joint**. Findings such as an anterior or posterior drawer sign of the knee characterize sliding movements that are normally prevented by the anterior or posterior cruciate ligaments, respectively. A joint that does not show laxity of movement is considered stable, and thus could have a grade I sprain. This classification of sprains is applicable to many joints (**Table 16.3**).

ANKLE SPRAINS

Ankle sprains are the most common sports-associated injury and account for 10% of all ED visits.

TABLE 16.3 Classification of Ligament Sprains		
Grade	Pathology	Physical Findings
1	Stretching with possible microtears	• Minimal tenderness and swelling • No instability • Minimal functional loss
2	Partial tear	• Increased swelling and tenderness • Mild instability
3	Complete disruption	• Severe swelling and tenderness • Significant instability and functional loss

They are most often caused by severe inversion of the foot stressing the lateral ligamentous complex (**Figures 16.7** and **16.8**). The ankle joint is discussed here to elucidate the pathophysiology of sprains.

The stability of the ankle is maintained by a ring alternating between bony elements and three sets of ligaments. The lateral malleolus of the fibula and the medial malleolus of the tibia form the ankle mortise and articulate with the trochlea of the talus. Further stability is provided by the lateral ligamentous complex, the syndesmotic ligament complex, and the medial ligament complex. In addition, dynamic restraint is provided laterally by the fibularis longus and brevis tendons; these are primarily evertors of the foot.

The lateral collateral ligaments of the ankle include the anterior talofibular ligament, the calcaneofibular ligament, and the posterior talofibular ligament (**Figure 16.8a**). The anterior talofibular ligament is the most commonly injured of the three. It runs from the anterior border of the lateral malleolus to the lateral talar body, parallel to the axis of the foot when the foot is in a neutral position. It is the primary restraint to inversion in either ankle plantar flexion or dorsiflexion. The most common trauma occurs with inversion and plantar flexion. That position provides less bony stability to the ankle joint because the trochlea of the talus is narrower posteriorly, and it comes in contact with the ankle mortise in plantar flexion. Typically, the injury causes stretching (grade 1) or tearing (grades 2 and 3) of the anterior talofibular ligament, the calcaneofibular ligament, or both. Generally,

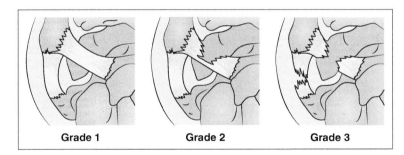

FIGURE 16.7 Grading of ankle sprains: grade 1—ligaments stretched or slightly torn; grade 2—ligaments partially torn; grade 3—ligaments completely torn.

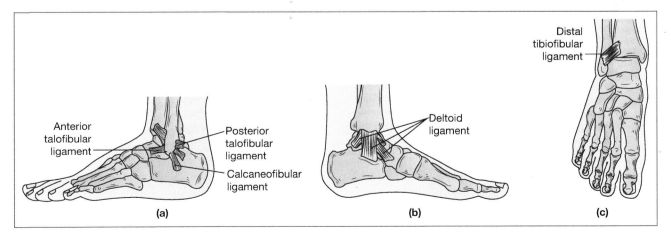

FIGURE 16.8 Sites of ankle sprains and ligaments involved: (**a**) lateral ankle sprain, (**b**) medial ankle sprain, and (**c**) high ankle sprain.

in inversion injuries, the ligaments are injured sequentially as increasing force is applied. The anterior talofibular ligament is torn first, then the calcaneofibular, and finally the posterior talofibular.

The medial ligamentous complex is referred to as the deltoid ligament (**Figure 16.8b**). It has four component bands: the anterior tibiotalar, the tibionavicular, the tibiocalcaneal, and the posterior tibiotalar. The deltoid ligament is so strong; it often causes an avulsion fracture of the medial malleolus rather than rupturing when an eversion force is applied.

The syndesmotic ligament complex injury is referred to as a high ankle sprain. This complex consists of the anterior and posterior tibiofibular ligaments (**Figure 16.8c**).

The pathophysiology of these sprains has implications for physical examination of the patient. It is beneficial to examine the joint before edema and ecchymosis occur, as these processes make the examination more difficult. Isolated anterior talofibular injuries are three times more common than calcaneofibular or posterior talofibular tears; thus, most ankle sprains are stable.

STRUCTURE AND CONDITIONS OF THE KNEE

Anatomy of the Knee

The knee is the largest and most complex joint in the body. It is actually a compound joint consisting of articulations between the tibia and femur and the patella and femur. Functionally, the knee is considered a hinge joint. Yet because of its unique structure, the knee allows not only flexion and extension but also small degrees of medial and lateral rotation and gliding movements. Knee pain and knee injuries are common at all ages.

The distal femur is marked by two large knob-shaped condyles that articulate with flattened plateaus on condyles of the proximal tibia (**Figure 16.9**). On the anterior femur between the condyles, there is a smooth depression, the patellar surface, along which the patella moves during flexion and extension. The articular surfaces of the femur, tibia, and patella are protected by a thin layer of articular cartilage. The medial and lateral menisci, crescent-shaped fibrocartilage pads, are positioned on the tibial condyles with the open portion of each meniscus firmly attaching in the intercondylar area of the tibia. They serve as shock absorbers. The menisci are thickest at the external margin and taper internally. Their wedge shape slightly deepens the articular surfaces for the femur, adding to joint stability. The medial meniscus, the larger of the two, has attachments to the articular capsule and the tibial collateral ligament, making

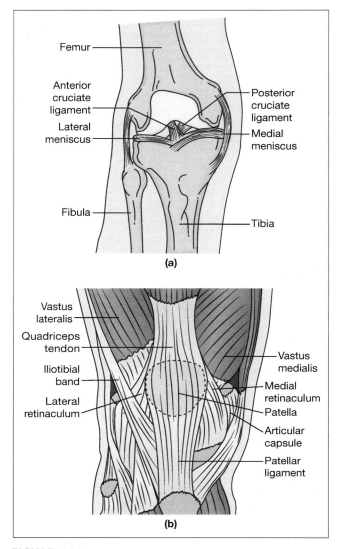

FIGURE 16.9 Knee anatomy: **(a)** deep view, right knee; **(b)** superficial view, right knee.

it prone to injury when the tibial collateral ligament is damaged. The smaller lateral meniscus does not have these additional attachments and, thus, is less likely to sustain injury.

The knee joint, like all synovial joints, is enclosed by a joint capsule. However, the fibrous layer of the capsule is thin and not complete. Of special note is that the quadriceps tendon, patella, and patellar ligament replace the fibrous capsule on the anterior joint surface. Additionally, the anterior capsule is reinforced by the iliotibial band and the anterolateral femorotibial ligament. The quadriceps muscles are important dynamic stabilizers anteriorly, and the posterior capsule strength is augmented by the oblique popliteal ligament and the tendons of the semimembranosus, popliteus, and gastrocnemius muscles.

The synovial membrane, which encloses the synovial cavity and lines the fibrous capsule on the medial and lateral side of the joint, attaches to the margins of the articular cartilage covering the tibial and femoral condyles, the posterior patella, and the edges of the menisci. In the popliteal region, the synovial membrane invaginates into the intercondylar space where it surrounds the infrapatellar fat pad and cruciate ligaments; thus, the cruciate ligaments are not within the synovial cavity and are considered intracapsular ligaments. Fat pads and over a dozen bursae are present at the knee, protecting soft tissues (e.g., the skin and muscle tendons that extend longitudinally across the joint) during movement.

Because of the relatively poor fit between the articular surfaces of the tibia and femur, ligaments contribute significantly to stability of the knee joint. The tibial (medial) collateral and fibular (lateral) collateral ligaments are extracapsular ligaments that pass from the femur to the tibia. The tibial collateral ligament is a strong, flat ligament continuous with the articular capsule and extending from the medial epicondyle of the femur to two distal attachments, the medial condyle and the superomedial surface of the tibia. As noted previously, the tibial collateral ligament is attached to the medial meniscus as well as the articular capsule. On the medial aspect, the tibial collateral ligament and the posteromedial joint capsule are reinforced by the pes anserinus (*goose's foot*) muscle group and the semimembranosus muscle. The pes anserinus group consists of the sartorius, gracilis, and semitendinosus muscles. The more cord-like fibular collateral ligament extends from the lateral epicondyle of the femur to the lateral head of the fibula. Laterally, the fibular collateral ligament and the posteriorly placed arcuate ligament provide stability, which is reinforced by the popliteus and biceps femoris muscles. When the knee is extended (as in anatomical position), the collateral ligaments are taut and contribute to joint stability. Although tension in the collateral ligaments lessens during knee flexion, the ligaments retain their ability to limit rotational movement at the knee.

Two intracapsular ligaments, the anterior cruciate ligament (ACL) and posterior cruciate ligament (PCL), also contribute to knee stability. The ACL attaches inferiorly in the intercondylar area of the tibia just posterior to the attachment site of the medial meniscus and extends superiorly to attach on the medial side of the lateral condyle of the femur. The ACL helps to prevent posterior displacement of the femur on the tibia during flexion and hyperextension of the knee. The PCL extends superiorly and anteriorly from the posterior intercondylar area of the tibia medial to the ACL, and attaches on the lateral surface of the medial condyle of the femur. The PCL, which is the stronger of the cruciate ligaments, helps prevent anterior displacement of the femur on the tibia.

The patella is the largest sesamoid bone in the body. Sesamoid bones, which are named for the sesame seeds that they resemble, are usually embedded in muscle tendons within joints. In this location, the sesamoid bones can modify pressure, protect tendons, and act as a pulley to alter the direction of the muscle's pull on its insertion. The patellar ligament, which is the distal insertion of the quadriceps tendon, attaches on the tibial tuberosity and provides strong anterior stability to the knee joint. The femoropatellar joint is functionally significant in that it serves to position the fulcrum for knee flexion directly anterior to the knee joint.

Ligamentous and Meniscal Injuries of the Knee

Injury to the ligaments and menisci of the knee joint are extremely common both in everyday activity and in the realm of sports because the hinge joint of the knee is subjected to collisions and twisting stresses. The stability of the knee depends on multiple ligaments and muscles. These ligaments allow the hinge actions of flexion and extension but inhibit forward, backward, and lateral movement. The surrounding muscles and tendons provide stability in varying degrees of flexion and extension, while the medial and lateral menisci ensure an efficient transmission of stress through the joint with frictionless movement.

Medial Ligament Tears

The medial collateral ligament (tibial collateral ligament) is somewhat broad and runs downward and forward from the medial epicondyle of the femur to the medial surface of the upper tibia approximately 7 to 8 cm below the tibial plateau. The medial collateral ligament prevents valgus deviation of the tibia and also prevents the tibia from rotating externally. Tests to examine for **medial collateral ligament tears** will demonstrate pathological forward movement and outward movement of the medial tibial condyle. The knee should be examined in extension and approximately 10 degrees of flexion. Further evaluation is then carried out with the knee in 90 degrees of flexion to check for an abnormal degree of external tibial rotation (this may be observed when performing the anterior drawer test, checking the integrity of the ACL, as discussed later).

In regard to pathophysiology, if a force is applied to a ligament, it will stretch and then return to its prestressed state as long as its yield point is not exceeded. Beyond this yield point, the ligament begins to tear, with first-degree sprains demonstrating microtears, second-degree sprains producing partial tears with some laxity (~5 to 10 mm), and third-degree sprains representing complete disruption with more than 10 mm of excess laxity. A common injury to the medial collateral ligament occurs in football when a valgus force is applied to the lateral side of the knee, usually with the foot in a fixed position (**Figure 16.10**). Complete tearing of the medial collateral ligament will cause disruption of not only its more superficial tibial collateral component but also its deeper capsular component. This disruption causes blood to leak out of the joint, presenting as ecchymosis on the medial knee. Importantly, valgus stretch will cause the medial side of the knee to hinge open (*gap*). Tenderness will be noted with palpation of the ligament. Further evaluation by MRI, or possibly arthroscopy, will assess for associated tears of the ACL or the medial meniscus. The latter may occur because the medial meniscus is firmly attached to the medial collateral ligament.

Lateral Ligament Tears

The lateral collateral ligament (fibular collateral ligament) is a round cord that runs obliquely downward and backward from the lateral epicondyle of the femur to the head of the fibula. Injury to the lateral collateral ligament is less common than medial collateral ligament tears because it is more flexible. It is not connected to the lateral meniscus, allowing that meniscus to be more mobile and less susceptible than the medial meniscus to tears when the collateral ligament is disrupted.

Lateral collateral ligament injury results from a varus force or a direct blow to the inside of the knee. Sports that require quick stops and turns, such as soccer, basketball, and skiing, can produce a severe

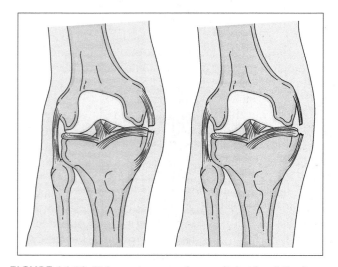

FIGURE 16.10 Valgus stress on the medial side of the knee, causing a third-degree tear of the medial collateral ligament.

varus force. A sprain of the lateral collateral ligament will produce lateral pain, tenderness over the ligament, and some degree of swelling. Depending on the degree of tearing, joint laxity may occur with varus testing. Owing to the proximity of the common fibular nerve in this region, neurological injury is a possibility, and the nerve's motor and sensory functions should be checked. The biceps tendon and the fascia lata may also be torn.

Cruciate Ligament Tears

The cruciate ligaments stretch between the anterior and posterior condylar areas of the tibia and the intercondylar notch of the femur. The ligaments run at right angles to each other, hence the name *cruciate* (cross-shaped). Their function is to keep the articular surfaces of the femur and tibia in contact while stabilizing the knee joint in the sagittal plane. Some portions of the cruciate ligaments are taut in every position of the knee.

Rupture of the ACL allows the tibia to be moved forward like a drawer relative to the femur (anterior drawer sign or Lachman test). The most common mechanism of injury is an internal rotation force with the foot planted. Anterior cruciate rupture is ten times more common than **posterior cruciate rupture**. A lateral blow to the knee, with the foot fixed, tends to also cause rupture of the anterior cruciate and medial collateral ligaments along with a medial meniscal tear, referred to as the *unhappy triad*.

Anterior cruciate injuries are almost always complete tears. They occur after changing direction rapidly, stopping suddenly, landing from a jump, or from direct contact such as a football tackle. A *popping* sensation may be perceived, and the knee is immediately unstable. Pain and swelling occur with loss of full range of motion and there is tenderness along the joint line. MRI confirms the clinical diagnosis.

Because the PCL keeps the tibia from moving too far backward relative to the femur, a complete tear of this structure will cause a posterior drawer sign. Ruptures of this ligament are less common than other knee ligament injuries. Owing to the thickness of the ligament, a powerful force is necessary to rupture it, such as a football player falling on a knee that is bent or a knee hitting the dashboard in a car accident. The PCL is maximally taut in the position of flexion. Symptoms include pain, swelling, difficulty walking, and instability. Also of concern is concomitant injury to the popliteal artery, which is immediately behind the posterior joint capsule. Displacement of the tibia posteriorly may cause an intimal tear of this vessel with thrombosis creating distal ischemia. MRI can assess the ligamentous injury while magnetic resonance angiography (MRA) will evaluate the circulation.

Meniscal Injuries

The menisci ensure an efficient transmission of stress through the knee joint, with the load being the body weight. They also enhance stability, provide lubrication, and are part of the guiding mechanism during rotatory movements. Because the medial and lateral menisci are positioned between the femoral condyles and the tibial plateau, the tracking of the two bones upon each other is determined by the shape of the articulating condyles, the menisci, and the cruciate ligaments, which act as guide ropes. If this normal rotation is prevented, the menisci may become trapped within the joint, resulting in tears in the substance of the meniscus or its peripheral attachments. Both stretching and crushing forces play a role here, and less commonly, significant external force can also produce injury.

A variety of **meniscal tears** are encountered and directly visualized and treated using arthroscopy. About 15 different types of tears have been described, creating various flaps, vertical tears, horizontal tears, bucket handle–shaped tears (**Figure 16.11**), and complex tears with multiple rents in the meniscus, sometimes with cystic changes.

The classic mechanism of injury is a rotational stress on the semiflexed and weight-bearing knee. Males are more commonly affected, and there may be some racial differences in the propensity for meniscal injury. Certainly, pain occurs along with compromise of movement and instability of the joint. Pain arises from the peripheral sensory portions of the meniscus and from the joint capsule and ligaments during abnormal movement of the knee when intraarticular obstruction is present. The patient may experience a clicking sensation with flexion and extension and, in fact, develop a protective limp.

Tenderness may be present over the joint line, and secondary patellar pain and crepitus may occur as a result of the irritated synovium. Joint effusion commonly occurs, and a hemarthrosis may occur if there is significant bleeding. As the meniscus is relatively

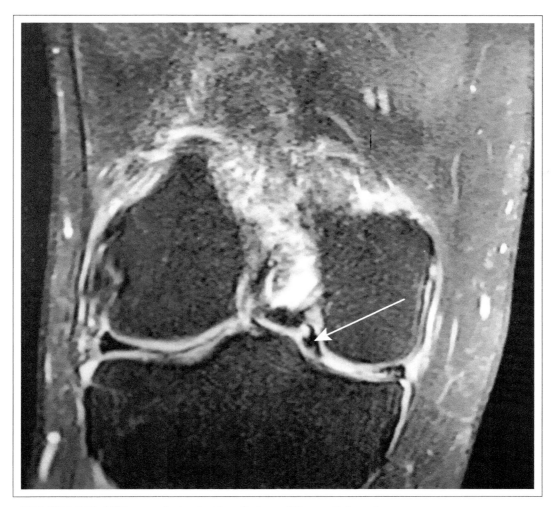

FIGURE 16.11 MRI scan of a bucket-handle tear of the medial meniscus.
Source: From Macnicol M, Steenbrugge F. *The Problem Knee.* 3rd ed. CRC Press; 2011.

avascular, blood in the joint is suspicious for a ligamentous or capsular injury.

Instability, or buckling, results not only from the obstruction in the joint altering the normal pivot but also from muscle weakness or quadriceps inhibition. The obstruction may actually cause locking of the joint with a loss of full extension and restriction of flexion and rotation. The patient feels that the joint is weak and unstable and a catching sensation occurs with kneeling, squatting, jumping, or leg rotation. Therefore, in approximately 70% of cases, the three cardinal signs of a torn meniscus are localized joint line tenderness, effusion, and locking.

Both MRI scanning and arthroscopy allow for early diagnosis and treatment of meniscal tears, which are the most common intraarticular knee injuries. Most are treated nonoperatively, because the menisci can heal, but some require either partial meniscectomy or meniscal repair.

Thought Questions

7. **What types of ligament damage are associated with different degrees of sprains?**

8. **What are the most common sprains of the ankle and knee?**

HERNIATED DISC DISEASE

Back pain is an extremely common problem that has many causes. It is the second most common reason for medical evaluation. Most of us have had back discomfort at some point. It usually results from overuses of muscles and resolves over a relatively short period of time. More importantly, back pain can be caused by significant pathology such as scoliosis, compression fractures, neoplasms, spondylolisthesis, osteomyelitis, osteoarthritis (OA), osteoporosis, cauda equine syndrome, and many other mechanisms.

The most serious, although less common, causes of back pain include neoplastic lesions—either primary lesions of spinal cord or vertebrae, or metastatic lesions. These should be ruled out quickly as they are *red flag* conditions for which treatment must be initiated immediately upon diagnosis. Similarly, infectious disorders affecting the vertebral joints or meninges of the spinal cord can cause pain and must be identified and treated immediately. Osteoporosis and ankylosing spondylitis (AS) are discussed later in this chapter in Gerontological Considerations, and spinal stenosis and

cauda equina syndrome are discussed in Chapter 15, Nervous System.

In this section, **herniated discs** and their pathophysiology are discussed. Herniated discs usually occur in adults aged 30 to 50 years and are more common in men. About 90% occur at the lumbar or lumbosacral level, 8% in the cervical spine, and 2% in the thoracic region.

PATHOPHYSIOLOGY OF DISC HERNIATION

All intervertebral discs have a tough, fibrous outer ring, called the annulus fibrosis, and a soft, somewhat gelatinous center called the nucleus pulposus. Each disc also has upper and lower cartilaginous end plates. The ventral portion of the annulus is usually wider than the dorsal portion, which may have discontinuous lamellae, thereby creating a natural weak spot for the nucleus pulposus to bulge or herniate. The first stage of the degenerative process of the spine is disc degeneration, possibly with some degree of arthritis of the facet joints. By age 50, 97% of discs demonstrate some degree of degeneration likely due to increased proteolytic activity (**Figure 16.12**).

With age-associated disc degeneration, the end plates calcify and small vessel loss occurs. This leads to cell necrosis and loss of water, which makes up 85% of the nucleus pulposus and 78% of the annulus fibrosis. The viscoelastic nucleus fibrosis begins to develop more fibrocartilage. Radiating cracks in the annulus fibrosis develop. Biomechanical and biochemical changes in the annulus fibrosis and nucleus pulposus cause narrowing of the intervertebral disc space, allowing increased stress on the facet joints. This is followed by more bulging and eventual herniation of the nucleus pulposus, more commonly at L4-5 and L5-S1.

As the disc protrudes, it narrows the spinal canal and impinges on nerve roots, causing pain (which may radiate into the arm or leg) and possibly motor, sensory, and reflex changes.

The pain is due to mechanical deformation of the nerve roots and biochemical irritation of the roots by the herniated disc tissue itself, which precipitates an inflammatory reaction. Pressure on the roots causes capillary stasis and thereby an increase in vascular permeability, leading to intraneural edema and a decrease in nerve conduction velocity. This increase in intraneural fluid pressure may cause subsequent formation of intraneural fibrosis.

Degenerative processes in the facet joints can lead to a further compromise of the space through which each spinal nerve must pass. The intervertebral foramen is bounded by the facet joints posteriorly, the vertebral pedicles superiorly and inferiorly, and the vertebral

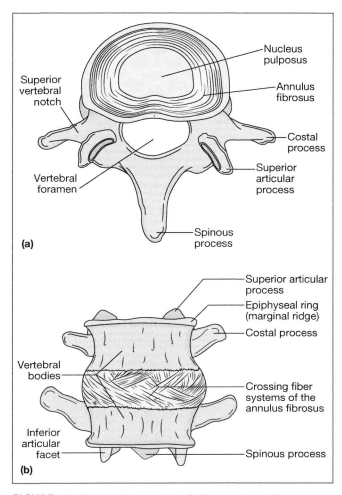

(a)

(b)

FIGURE 16.12 **(a)** Intervertebral disc and vertebra, cross-sectional view. **(b)** Intervertebral disc between two vertebrae, ventral view.

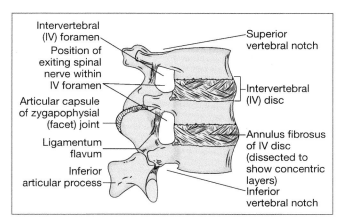

FIGURE 16.13 Boundaries of intervertebral foramen.

body and disc anteriorly (**Figure 16.13**). Subluxation of the degenerated facet joints leads to thickening of the ligamentum flavum, which runs between the lamina of the vertebrae, pushing it into the neural space and further narrowing it.

The underlying pathophysiology of disc herniation and degenerative joint disease of the spine is not completely understood. Nevertheless, there seems to be a consistent anatomical pattern, with most problems occurring where significant mechanical stresses take place. The transitional zones between the mobile cervical and lumbar regions and the more rigid thoracic and sacral regions sustain greater degrees of mechanical stress. Therefore, most disc herniations are seen in the lower cervical and lumbar levels.

ANATOMICAL CORRELATIONS

There are 31 pairs of spinal nerves, which exit the vertebral canal through intervertebral foramina, sacral foramina, or the sacral hiatus. The first seven cervical nerves exit superior to the cervical vertebra for which they are named (e.g., the C4 nerve exits between the C3 and the C4 vertebrae). The eighth cervical nerve exits through the intervertebral foramen between C7 and T1 vertebrae because there are eight cervical spinal nerves, but only seven cervical vertebrae. Beginning with the T1 spinal nerve, all other spinal nerves exit inferior to the vertebra for which they are named (e.g., the L4 nerve exits between the L4 and L5 vertebrae).

Cervical nerve roots take a nearly horizontal course from the dural sac to exit the intervertebral foramen. Because of this course and the fact that cervical spinal nerves are named for the vertebra inferior to the nerve, a herniated cervical disc will impinge on the nerve root exiting at the foramen bounded anteriorly by that disc (e.g., a C6-C7 disc abnormality affects the C7 nerve root).

The nerve roots emanating from the lower spinal cord form the cauda equina (*horse's tail*). In contrast to the more horizontal course of a cervical spinal nerve root, these lumbar roots course inferiorly from the lower cord, which ends at L2, to reach the lumbar and sacral foramina. These paired sensory and motor roots combine to form a spinal nerve, which exits at each vertebral level in the lumbar spine in close proximity to its respective pedicle. Because the intervertebral disc is located caudal to the pedicle, a posterolateral L5-S1 disc herniation typically spares the L5 nerve root rostrally but impinges on the S1 nerve root as it passes the disc space. In contrast, the less common far lateral disc herniation may compress the exiting L5 nerve root (**Figure 16.14**). Central disc displacements may cause a wide range of symptoms, including bilateral radiculopathy and urinary symptoms.

CLINICAL PRESENTATION AND MANAGEMENT

Although any disc in the spinal column can herniate and compress a spinal nerve, cervical and lumbar pathology

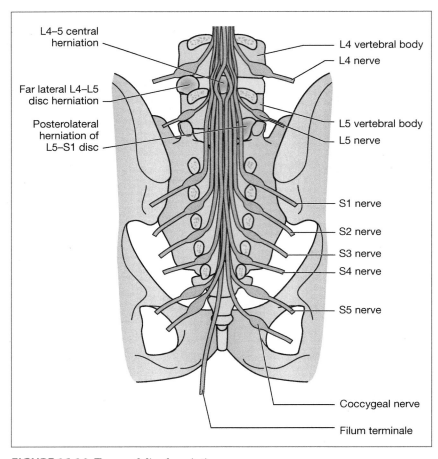

FIGURE 16.14 Types of disc herniation.

are discussed here, as they are the most common types a clinician will encounter (**Table 16.4**).

Cervical nerve root compression can present as neck pain that limits motion and is worsened by extension. The pain may radiate down the arm to an area innervated by the involved root. Motor deficits may also occur with the deltoid and biceps brachii affected by a C4-C5 or a C5-C6 herniation, the triceps brachii and multiple wrist extensors by C6-C7 herniation, and the intrinsic hand muscles and wrist flexors along with flexors of ring and little finger by a C7-T1 herniation. The biceps or triceps reflexes may be decreased. Bilateral and generalized weakness of the arm and hand may occur, along with leg weakness, if the spinal cord itself is compressed.

Similarly, the signs and symptoms of lumbar disc disease will vary depending on the level involved. Typically, the patient will complain of low back pain, which may be mild or severe. The dominant complaint

TABLE 16.4 Radiation of Limb Pain With Cervical and Lumbar Pathology

Disc	Spinal Nerve	Location of Pain
Cervical Pathology Causing Arm Pain		
C4-C5	C5	None of lateral upper arm
C5-C6	C6	Lateral arm
C6-C7	C7	Posterior arm
C7-T1	C8	Medial arm
Lumbar Pathology Causing Leg Pain		
L3-L4	L4	Anterior thigh
L4-L5	L5	Posterolateral leg
L5-S1	S1	Posterior calf and sole of foot

is usually pain radiating down the leg, again following the sensory distribution of the involved nerve root. The patellar or Achilles reflexes also may be decreased.

Most patients with disc disease improve with conservative nonoperative management if there is no major neurological impairment. Conservative therapy might include a brief period of bed rest, traction, cervical collars, avoidance of heavy lifting, and a graduated exercise program. Nonsteroidal anti inflammatory drugs (NSAIDs) and oral or epidural steroids may be prescribed.

Various surgical approaches are available for the small percentage of patients who have persistent symptoms despite conservative therapy. Microdiscectomy will completely relieve symptoms in 80% of patients with lumbar spine disc herniation, whereas anterior and posterior surgical approaches to the cervical spine are utilized in that region with a 90% success rate.

CUMULATIVE TRAUMA DISORDERS

Cumulative trauma disorders, also known as **repetitive stress injuries**, are temporary or permanent injuries to muscles, nerves, ligaments, and tendons caused by doing the same motions over and over again. This repeated activity results in mounting trauma to the soft tissues, producing clinical syndromes. Repetitive strain on the tissue from overuse produces microtrauma with scar tissue formation and subsequent symptoms. Depending on the anatomical structures involved, the array of symptoms might include tenderness, aching pain, cramps, stiffness, tingling, numbness, or swelling.

This group of disorders has received much recent attention because of changes in occupational and recreational activities, along with advances in ergonomics. These disorders, which develop gradually, often cause upper extremity problems but can also involve the lower extremity. Typical examples of cumulative trauma disorders include tendonitis, tendinosis, rotator cuff syndrome, carpal tunnel and cubital tunnel syndromes, bursitis, and patellofemoral syndrome.

Three hypotheses have been put forth in an attempt to categorize these disorders. The first relates to muscle and tendon overuse. With repetitive motion, there is reduced relaxation and increased tension in the tissues, reducing blood supply and delaying dissipation of metabolites. This combination leads to an increased rate of wear and tear and a decreased ability to repair damaged tissue. Over time, the overload results in inflammation, edema, compression, fibrosis, ischemia, and tearing of affected tissues. If microtears occur in a tendon, for example, thickening of the tendon and irregular surfaces may result, leading to further abrasions and tearing. This outcome is referred to as *tendinosis*—a pathology of chronic degeneration without inflammation. Reduced tensile strength can lead to tendon rupture, which then generates a typical inflammatory response that can lead to fibrosis.

Compression neuropathies, the focus of the second hypothesis, involve both mechanical and ischemic factors. Compression of a nerve causes ischemia and hypoxemia of the nerve, with obstruction of venous return. The increased venous pressure causes capillary dilation with edema, proliferation of fibroblasts, and scarring in the nerve segment.

The third hypothesis involves neuropathic compression, myofascial pain, and muscle imbalance. Prolonged or frequent assumption of abnormal postures, positions, or movements causes increased pressure on certain nerves, with decreased blood flow leading to fibrosis both in and around the nerve. Inhibition of full excursion during normal extremity movements may also occur. This inhibition stretches the nerve, which may cause paresthesias and motor weakness. Abnormal postures cause some muscles to be used in shortened positions, which can lead to muscle imbalance, creating a cycle of underuse and overuse. Tight muscles then become tighter, and weak muscles become weaker. The tight muscles may secondarily compress neurovascular structures.

CAUSES OF CUMULATIVE STRESS INJURY

Recreational and occupational stresses along with personal habits account for many of the causes of repetitive stress in the human body. Overuse of a muscle or group of muscles, vibrating equipment, working in cold temperatures, direct pressure, poor posture, and forceful activities such as carrying heavy loads are among the many causes. Also, a nonergonomically designed workplace or the poor ergonomics of work tools (such as some laparoscopic surgical instruments) can ultimately lead to symptomatic injuries. Cumulative trauma complaints comprise more than 50% of work-related disorders.

In the evaluation of these syndromes, MRI or ultrasound often plays a role, and electromyography and nerve conduction studies may also be needed, supplementing the all-important physical examination.

CLINICAL SYNDROMES

Carpal Tunnel Syndrome

Median nerve compression in the carpal tunnel due to repetitive motion about the wrist constitutes most cases of **carpal tunnel syndrome**, a **compressive neuropathy** secondary to occupational exposure. The prevalence is higher in women, especially after menopause, and increases with age.

The median nerve is both sensory and motor. After giving off the palmar cutaneous branch in the distal anterior forearm, it enters a fibro-osseous canal, the carpal tunnel (also called the flexor retinaculum). The tunnel is bounded by the carpal bones dorsally and the transverse carpal ligament on its volar aspect. The transverse carpal ligament attaches laterally to the trapezium and hamate; medially, it attaches to the scaphoid and pisiform bones. The median nerve passes through this relatively tight space along with nine flexor tendons (**Figure 16.15**).

In the palm of the hand, the median nerve gives off a recurrent branch that is motor to the three thenar muscles of the thumb (abductor pollicis brevis, flexor pollicis brevis, and opponens pollicis). It then continues to provide sensory innervation to the median thumb, the index and middle fingers, and the lateral half of the ring finger. This neural anatomy accounts for the clinical presentation of intermittent pain and paresthesias in its sensory distribution, and patients with advanced cases may demonstrate thenar muscle atrophy and weakness of thumb abduction and opposition. There may be a positive Tinel sign demonstrating paresthesias in the median nerve distribution with percussion of the nerve on the anterior wrist. Phalen sign produces symptoms with forced flexion of the wrist. The pain of carpal tunnel syndrome may radiate to the shoulder or neck. Nerve conduction studies may be utilized to rule out more proximal nerve entrapment.

The median nerve can be affected by static compression due to thickening of the transverse carpal ligament or by dynamic repetitive movements of inflamed or fibrotic tendons in the tunnel. Either can cause edema and compression of the nerve. Some associated conditions may predispose a patient to carpal tunnel syndrome by increasing soft tissue volume, thereby compromising the area within the tunnel. Diabetes, pregnancy, arthritis, and hypothyroidism are the most common associations. It can also be seen following wrist fractures or dislocations.

Carpal tunnel syndrome is initially managed conservatively with splints, NSAIDs, or steroid injections. If these approaches are not effective, surgery to release the transverse carpal ligament and decompress the median nerve is very effective.

Cubital Tunnel Syndrome

Ulnar nerve compression at the elbow results in **cubital tunnel syndrome**, the second most common compressive neuropathy after carpal tunnel syndrome. The subcutaneous location of the ulnar nerve posterior to the medial epicondyle of the humerus makes it very vulnerable to acute and chronic injury. Repetitive pressure on the nerve due to flexion–extension motions during heavy labor or persistent pressure on the elbow are common causes.

The nerve travels through a very narrow space in its retrocondylar position with very little soft tissue to protect it. It passes beneath the Osborne ligament, a fibrous arch between the two heads of the flexor carpi ulnaris muscle. Normal activity causes the nerve to slide in a groove in the condyle, and it can stretch 5 mm during elbow flexion. Scar formation may prevent sliding, causing more stretch force to be applied, which may lead to inflammation and swelling of the nerve and surrounding tissues. Progression of the inflammatory response causes intraneural scar formation.

Patients experience progressive pain or numbness in the fourth and fifth fingers, along with elbow pain. The pain is worsened by elbow flexion. Motor symptoms, such as weakness and difficulty with fine finger movements, occur later. Surgical decompression may be needed.

Lateral Epicondylitis

Lateral epicondylitis, also known as **tennis elbow**, is a painful condition involving the tendon of the extensor carpi radialis brevis, which attaches to the lateral epicondyle of the humerus. The tendon transmits the

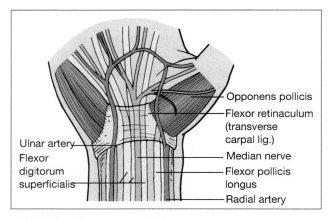

FIGURE 16.15 Location of the transverse carpal ligament and median nerve in the carpal tunnel.

muscle's force to the bone. With repetitive stress, microtears cause bleeding, edema, and pain. After repeated episodes of inflammation, calcium may be deposited in the tendon. The tendon's attachment then degenerates, weakening the anchor site and placing greater stress on the area.

The syndrome is associated with tennis playing, but can occur with many other activities such as meat cutting, painting, auto mechanic work, repetitive use of a screwdriver, and so on. Tenderness is present over the lateral epicondyle. In some patients, the symptoms spontaneously resolve over many months. Like many cumulative stress issues, treatment may include braces, NSAIDs, steroid injections, and physical therapy. Surgery may be considered in patients with prolonged symptoms that have not resolved with conservative management.

Trigger Finger

Trigger finger occurs when there is a disparity in size between the flexor tendons in the hand (flexor digitorum superficialis and flexor digitorum profundus) and the first annular retinacular ligament (*A1 pulley*), which overlies the metacarpophalangeal joint on its palmar aspect. Referring to this injury as a tenosynovitis may be a misnomer, as inflammation is not a predominant characteristic. It is likely more in the category of a tendinosis, with intratendinous degeneration and degradation of collagen fibers commonly due to aging, trauma, or repetitive stress. Thickening and abnormal gliding and locking of the tendon create a *snapping* sensation, and fibrocartilaginous metaplasia of the tendon pulley occurs. When the finger unlocks, it pops back suddenly, as if releasing a trigger on a gun.

The outer fibrous layer of digital tendon sheaths is strengthened by annular ligaments and cruciform ligaments, which bind the sheaths to the palmar surface of the phalanx and prevent palmar deviation of the sheaths during flexion. As shown in **Figure 16.16**, the annular ligaments are A1 to A5 and the cruciform ligaments are C1 to C3.

The etiological mechanism of trigger finger is unclear as evidence exists both for and against hand use as a cause. It can be associated, for example, with gardening and pruning; is more common in diabetic individuals; and more often involves the ring finger. The finger is locked in flexion and a palpable nodule may be present near the A1 pulley, along with tenderness. Surgical treatment requires division of the A1 pulley. **Table 16.5** describes the four grades of trigger finger.

Hip Bursitis

Bursae are small synovial sacs located between tendons, muscles, and bony prominences. Their function is to separate, lubricate, and cushion these

TABLE 16.5 Classification of Trigger Finger

Grade	Description
1	Palm pain and tenderness at A1 pulley
2	Catching of digit
3	Locking of digit, passively correctable
4	Fixed, locked digit

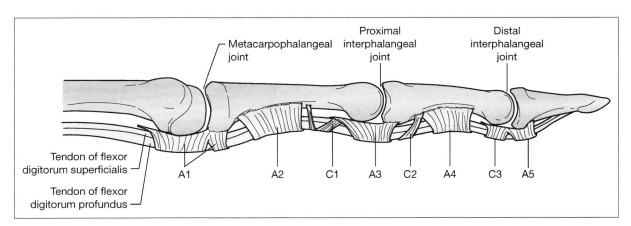

FIGURE 16.16 Ligaments reinforcing the digital tendon sheath: A1 to A5 are the annular ligaments; C1 to C3 are the cruciform ligaments.

structures. Repeated trauma of the bursae can lead to inflammation.

Hip bursitis, also called **trochanteric bursitis**, is a common type of chronic hip pain. Two bursae are present in this region: one over the greater trochanter of the femur and one posterior to the iliopsoas muscle. Inflammation of the latter is not as common as trochanteric bursitis but is treated in a similar manner.

The pain of hip bursitis is typically worse at night and exacerbated by lying on the affected hip. Prolonged walking, squatting, or stair climbing, or getting up from a chair may worsen symptoms. Causes include repetitive stress from running, climbing, bicycling, or long periods of standing. Other causes (e.g., rheumatoid arthritis, bone spurs, and leg length inequality) may also precipitate bursitis.

In addition to physical examination, MRI, plain x-ray studies, or a bone scan may be useful to diagnose hip bursitis. Surgery is rarely needed.

Thoracic Outlet Syndrome

Cumulative stress may be associated with development of **thoracic outlet syndrome**, a complex neurovascular disorder of the neck, shoulder, arm, and hand. Some of these associations are hypertrophy of the scalene muscles, abnormalities of the pectoralis minor muscle, repetitive shoulder use, extreme arm positions, and activities such as weightlifting, rowing, and swimming. The main anatomical structures that are impacted in thoracic outlet syndrome are the brachial plexus, the subclavian vein, and the subclavian artery (**Figure 16.17**).

Thoracic outlet syndrome may manifest itself by symptoms of nerve compression (90% to 95%), venous compression (4%), or arterial injury (1%). The three sites of compression are the costoclavicular space between the clavicle and first rib, the interscalene triangle between the anterior and middle scalene muscles, and the intrapectoral space between the pectoralis minor muscle and the coracoid process of the scapula. Clinical manifestations of thoracic outlet syndrome are presented in **Table 16.6**.

Diagnosis of thoracic outlet syndrome can be quite complex, owing to its various manifestations, and is beyond the scope of this book. A careful history and physical examination is paramount and may be supplemented by cervical spine and chest x-rays studies, nerve conduction studies, arteriography and venography, electromyography, and MRI. It is important to rule out other causes of similar symptoms, such as cervical spine disease or a superior sulcus (Pancoast) tumor of the apex of the lung.

Treatment primarily involves physical therapy to strengthen the shoulder girdle, along with postural improvement. If there are no structural abnormalities, such as a cervical rib, improvement is seen in 60% to 90% of patients. The proper surgical approach for those who do not respond to nonoperative management is controversial. Because the first rib is the

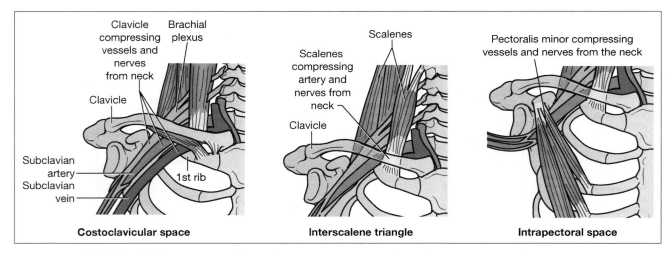

FIGURE 16.17 Thoracic outlet syndrome anatomy: costoclavicular space, interscalene triangle, and intrapectoral space.

TABLE 16.6 Clinical Highlights of Thoracic Outlet Syndrome

Type	Pathophysiology	Characteristics
Neurogenic	Hypertrophied or scarred muscles irritate cords of brachial plexus	History of neck trauma is common; pain on side of head and neck; suprascapular pain; shoulder pain; pain in radial nerve distribution if upper cord compressed; pain in ulnar nerve distribution if lower cord compressed
Venous	Compression of subclavian vein by subclavius muscle and costoclavicular ligament	Swelling of entire upper extremity; often occurs in more active or dominant arm; can lead to *effort thrombosis* (Paget–Schroetter syndrome); may be seen in weightlifters with muscular hypertrophy
Arterial	Repeated intermittent subclavian artery compression with arm movement leads to intimal lesions in retroscalene (second portion) of subclavian artery	May be associated with a cervical rib or rudimentary first rib; may cause focal arterial stenosis, poststenotic dilation, aneurysm, or emboli

common denominator in narrowing the outlet, it is usually resected through a transaxillary approach to decompress the *floor* of the outlet. This procedure also entails division of both the anterior and the middle scalene muscle attachments, thereby eliminating that source of nerve and arterial compression. A supraclavicular approach will be needed if the patient has a cervical rib or anomalous bands. For subclavian vein thrombosis, thrombolysis and stenting often play a role in treatment.

Thought Questions

9. What are the main hypotheses regarding pathogenesis of cumulative trauma disorder?

   Repetitive stress

10. What are some of the similarities and differences between the most common cumulative trauma disorders?

   inj.

MUSCULOSKELETAL DEVELOPMENT

Arising from the mesoderm in early embryonic development, muscles, tendons, ligaments, cartilage, and bones are present and functional at birth, with full range of motion. At birth, the infant's skeleton is not yet fully ossified. The bones of infants and young children have a lower mineral content than those of adults and are therefore more flexible and porous in comparison. Bones in young children have a thick, strong periosteum that allows for a greater absorption of force than does the adult's periosteum. All muscles are present at birth, but development of strength and neural control is dependent on myelination and patterns of use. Attainment of developmental milestones (supporting the head, sitting up unsupported, crawling, walking) is associated with varying patterns of muscle use and stresses experienced by bones, all of which contribute to normal maturation of bone growth, muscle strength development, limb position, and gait.

BONE STRUCTURE DURING GROWTH

Long bones in children have three main parts: a central diaphysis (the original site of ossification during fetal development) and a metaphysis and epiphysis at each end (**Figure 16.18**). Growth in bone length throughout childhood development occurs in the growth plate region (physis) between metaphysis and epiphysis. Chondrocytes synthesize cartilage in the growth plate region, which continues the growth, followed by ossification. Until puberty, the growth plates experience active bone formation through continuous cartilage synthesis followed by calcification, erosion, and osteoblast invasion. Additional bone growth occurs at the periosteum surrounding the diaphysis, so bones grow in both thickness and length during development.

FRACTURES IN CHILDREN AND ADOLESCENTS

Fractures in children and adolescents are among the most common musculoskeletal disorders. Lack of coordination predisposes to falls early in childhood, and sports injuries are common in school-aged children and adolescents. Although bone healing in children is similar to the process in adults, a rich nutrient supply to the child's thick, strong periosteum causes the bone to heal more quickly. Callus is produced more swiftly and in larger quantities in children's bones as compared with

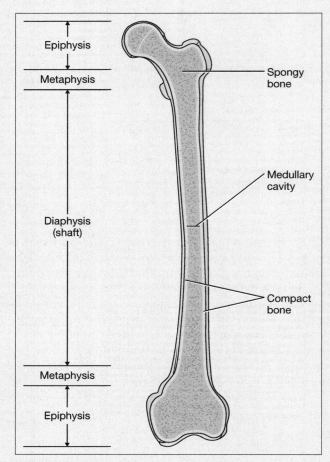

FIGURE 16.18 Structure of a long bone.

adults' bones. The younger the child is and the closer the fracture is to the growth plate, the more rapidly the bone heals. Children's bones have an increased capacity for remodeling (the process of breaking down and forming new bone). This remodeling allows for easier straightening of the bone over time as compared with adults.[3]

The structural differences of the young child's bones often allow for bending or buckling rather than breaking when an injury occurs, with bending, greenstick, and torus fractures more common than in adults (**Figure 16.19**). The conversion of cartilage to bone (ossification) continues throughout childhood and is complete at adolescence. Mature, enlarged cartilage cells make the epiphyseal area structurally weak. The epiphysis may fracture if traumatic force is applied to that area. Injury to the epiphysis may result

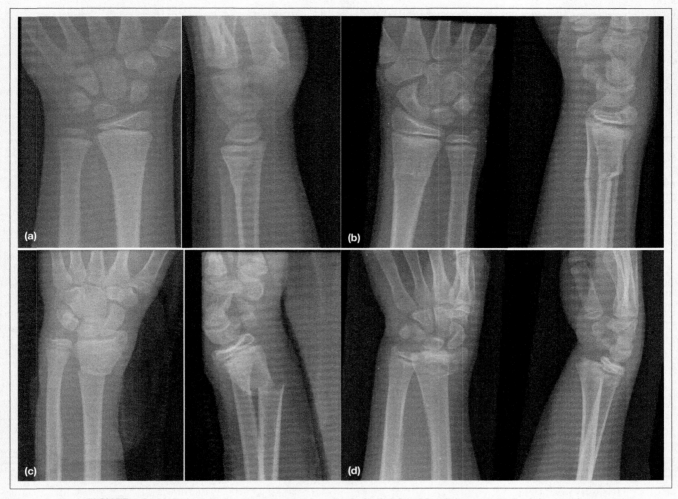

FIGURE 16.19 Common fractures in children include **(a)** buckle, **(b)** greenstick, **(c)** complete, and **(d)** physeal fractures.
Source: From Randsborg PH, Sivertsen EA, Classification of distal radius fractures in children: good inter- and intraobserver reliability, which improves with clinical experience. BMC *Musculoskelet Disord.* 2012;13:6

in alterations to the growth plate, leading to ultimate shortening of the bone or deformity. Gradually, androgen production throughout adolescence causes fusing of the growth plate, at which point long bone growth is complete.[4]

DEVELOPMENT OF LIMB POSITION AND POSTURE

Several normally occurring positional alterations are often noted in infants and young children. In utero positioning and lack of being in an upright, weight-bearing position contribute to these alterations. In infants, internal tibial torsion (ITT) and metatarsus adductus are often present (**Figure 16.20**). Both alterations occur as a result of in utero positioning. In ITT, the newborn's tibia is rotated inward while the proximal femur is rotated forward, causing a bowed appearance to the legs (also referred to as genu varum). Metatarsus adductus appears as in-toeing, with the infant's forefoot

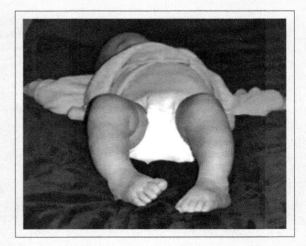

FIGURE 16.20 Metatarsus adductus—a common finding at birth.
Source: Reproduced with permission from Susan Carman.

rotated inward and the heel in the normal position. ITT and metatarsus adductus are both corrected through passive motion, allowing straightening of the legs and feet.

As the toddler matures and increases standing and walking time, the forces applied to the legs lead to reductions in the genu varum position. The legs may then demonstrate genu valgum, a knock-kneed appearance. Genu valgum usually resolves by age 7 or 8 years. If either genu varum or genu valgum persists past age 8, a pathological process rather than positional deformity is likely occurring. Pathologically, genu varum may be caused by Blount disease (tibia vara), rickets, traumatic injury, or skeletal dysplasia such as occurs in achondroplasia (dwarfism). Genu valgum may also persist as a result of skeletal dysplasia or may be due to a genetic predisposition.[5]

Alignment of the spine also undergoes developmental changes. As a result of fetal development, the newborn spine displays kyphosis (outward curvature). As the infant becomes able to hold the head up, cervical lordosis (inward curvature) develops. The primary and secondary spinal curves develop as the infant/toddler assumes an upright position. The head is centered over the pelvis due to the balance of these curves. During early walking, lumbar lordosis may be significant; the toddler appears potbellied, with a swayback. More adult-like spinal curves occur as the child develops. Thoracic kyphosis becomes evident during the adolescent years and is most often a postural effect only, with adult-like spinal posture achieved as the adolescent matures.

DEVELOPMENTAL DYSPLASIA OF THE HIP

Developmental dysplasia of the hip (DDH) is a relatively common musculoskeletal disorder in infants. In DDH, the femoral head has an abnormal relationship to the acetabulum, leading to hip joint instability. DDH is considered a developmental disorder because of its range of presentations. The newborn may have a malformed hip joint (dysplasia) at birth, or the hip joint instability may lead to subluxation or partial or full dislocation of the hip joint over the first few months of life. DDH may affect one or both hips and is more common in first-born children and girls. All infants should be assessed for DDH using standard maneuvers (**Figure 16.21**).

The etiology of DDH is thought to be multifactorial, with mechanical factors, heredity, and environment playing a role. The infant with DDH may have a positive family history of hip dysplasia or may have laxity of ligaments in general. Prevention of fetal movement (such as in oligohydramnios) and breech position may play a role in its development. Increased frequency in girls is thought to be due to estrogen susceptibility. Hip dysplasia may resolve on its own, but some infants require treatment. Past infancy, delayed standing or walking may occur. Additionally, in the walking child, a positive Trendelenburg sign may be noted. The child's trunk weight shifts over the affected hip during ambulation.[6]

SCOLIOSIS

Scoliosis is a lateral curvature of the spine exceeding 10 degrees and may be congenital, idiopathic, or associated with other disorders. Neuromuscular scoliosis usually results from nervous system and musculoskeletal disruption. The congenital form of scoliosis occurs as a result of anomalous vertebral development. Idiopathic scoliosis most often has its onset in the prepubertal time period (a period of rapid growth) and, though its etiology is not known, may be influenced by one or more of these factors: uneven vertebral growth, intervertebral disc disease, asymmetrical tone of back muscles, genetics, or central nervous system abnormalities.[7] The involved vertebrae rotate around a vertical axis, resulting in a lateral curve. Initially, ligaments, muscle, and soft tissue are involved. As the curve progresses, the vertebral bodies and discs change, becoming wedge-shaped as growth is suppressed on that side of the curve. In severe cases, shortness of breath may develop.[6]

CONGENITAL MUSCULOSKELETAL DEFORMITIES

In some infants, musculoskeletal abnormalities are present at birth. **Congenital musculoskeletal deformities** are multifactorial in nature, including heredity, exposure to teratogens, and other in utero insults. The deformities range from digit abnormalities to full limb malformations. Common musculoskeletal birth defects are summarized in **Table 16.7**.

YOUTH SPORTS AND MUSCULOSKELETAL INJURIES

Physical activity is a component of healthy growth and development, particularly in the prevention and management of overweight and obesity. Regular physical activity also promotes healthy growth and strength of muscles and bones. However, there is currently increasing emphasis on competitive sports and increasingly intense training for team sports in youth. For children in rapid periods of growth, neuromotor adaptation to growth of muscles and bones can be associated with clumsiness, accompanied by risk of musculoskeletal injury. Two particular vulnerabilities are noted with impact injuries and intense training in youth sports: **growth plate fractures** and **apophysitis** (irritation of the sites of tendon attachment to bone).

Growth plate fractures can result from a single traumatic insult or from repeated stress of training,

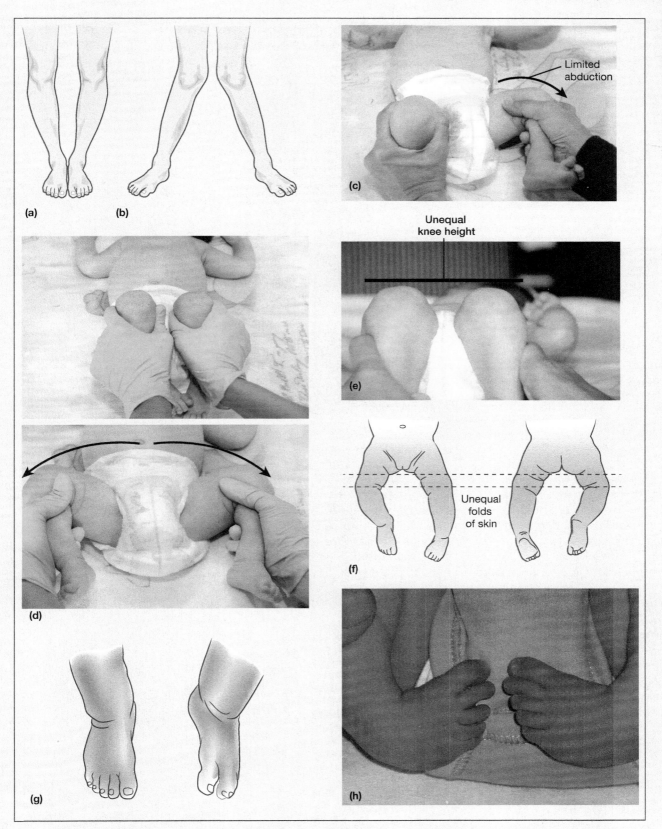

FIGURE 16.21 Common congenital musculoskeletal defects and assessment for developmental hip dysplasia. **(a)** Genu varum (bowlegs), **(b)** genu valgum (knock-knees), **(c)** Ortolani maneuver, **(d)** Barlow maneuver, **(e)** developmental dysplasia of the hip, **(f)** asymmetrical thigh and gluteal folds, **(g)** metatarsus adductus, **(h)** talipes equinovarus (true clubfoot).
Source: From Chiocca EM. *Advanced Pediatric Assessment: A Case Study and Critical Thinking Review* 2nd ed. New York, NY: Springer Publishing Company; 2014.

TABLE 16.7 Commonly Seen Musculoskeletal Birth Defects

Abnormality	Description
Pectus excavatum	• Abnormal development of ribs and sternum causes the anterior chest wall to be depressed at the midline, giving a concave appearance to the chest • Most common abnormality of the chest; incidence is 1:300–400, with males > females, 3:1[a]
Polydactyly	• Extra digits in the hand or foot • Some cases show autosomal dominant inheritance
Congenital clubfoot	• Fixed deformity with heel inversion and foot plantar flexion prevents the heel from reaching the floor while in a standing position • Incidence is 1–3 in 1,000, with males > females[a]

[a]*Source:* From Hebra A. Pectus excavatum. In: Sharma GD, ed. *Medscape.* https://emedicine.medscape.com/article/1004953. Updated October 30, 2018; and Society for Maternal-Fetal Medicine, McKinney J, Rac MWF, Gandhi M. Congenital talipes equinovarus (clubfoot). *Am J Obstet Gynecol.* 2019; 221(6): B10–B12. doi:10.1016/j.ajog.2019.09.022.

resulting in microfractures. There are several types of growth plate fractures (Table 16.8), reflecting the vulnerability of this structure to stresses, relative to the stronger ligaments, tendons, and bones. The extent of growth disruption after a growth plate fracture depends on the age and bone developmental stage of the youth. The healing process must allow sufficient protection to allow recovery of generative potential, followed by careful rehabilitation and return to activity.

Repetitive stress on joints in childhood and adolescence can traumatize the vulnerable apophysis, site of tendon-to-physis connections. Irritation can result in apophysitis, which presents at sites of bony attachment. Specific foci of apophysitis include the tibial tubercle in Osgood–Schlatter disease, the inferior patella in *jumper's knee*, and the calcaneus in Sever disease. Rest, NSAIDs, and slow resumption of activity are generally all that are needed for relief.[8]

GENETIC MUSCULOSKELETAL CONDITIONS

Genetic disorders of cartilage, bone, or muscle may present at birth or become apparent throughout growth and development. These vary from relatively common to very rare and up to now have been managed

TABLE 16.8 Growth Plate Fractures

Normal 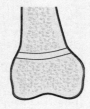	Blue shading indicates the physis (growth plate) with metaphysis above and epiphysis below
Type 1 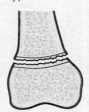	Fracture straight across the physis (~5% of growth plate fractures)
Type 2 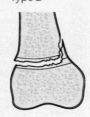	Fracture through region of the physis and continuing upward across the metaphysis (most common type: ~75% of growth plate fractures)
Type 3 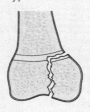	Fracture through region of the physis and continuing downward across the epiphysis (~10% of growth plate fractures)
Type 4 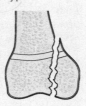	Fracture across all three structures, separating them from the main bone (~10% of growth plate fractures)
Type 5 	Complete compression of the physis (rare)

only with supportive treatment. Genomic medicine approaches to treat some of these disorders are currently undergoing research and development.

MUSCULAR DYSTROPHY

Muscular dystrophy (MD) is the umbrella term for a group of nine inherited conditions that cause progressive skeletal muscle weakness and wasting. Some types are more severe than others, but all demonstrate advancing muscle weakness over the lifetime. The muscular dystrophies are most often diagnosed in childhood; the most common forms, **Duchenne muscular dystrophy** and **Becker muscular dystrophy**, have an X-linked inheritance pattern. The less common forms include types with autosomal dominant and recessive inheritance. Duchenne and Becker MD result from mutations in the dystrophin gene that codes for a protein that links a protein complex of the muscle membrane (sarcolemma) to the cytoskeleton (**Figure 16.22**).

Mutations causing Duchenne MD result in complete absence of dystrophin expression, producing a more severe phenotype and earlier progression to death. Becker MD mutations result in decreased expression or function of dystrophin, associated with later age onset of muscle weakness and slower progression of the disease. Weakness is generalized, but begins in the proximal limbs (upper arm, thigh) before progressing to the trunk and distal limbs. Duchenne and Becker MD, and many of the other muscular dystrophies, are associated with disruption of the sarcolemma and resulting elevation of blood creatine kinase levels.[9]

OSTEOGENESIS IMPERFECTA

The bone disorder **osteogenesis imperfecta** (OI) results in low bone mass, increased bone fragility, frequent fractures, and other connective tissue problems such as joint hypermobility and instability. A defect in the genes associated with *collagen type 1* is most often

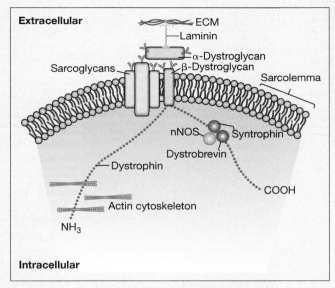

FIGURE 16.22 Dystrophin is a rod-shaped intracellular protein that links together plasma membrane proteins anchoring the sarcolemma to the ECM and the intracellular actin cytoskeleton. This structure stabilizes the sarcolemma during muscle cell contraction and relaxation.
ECM, extracellular matrix; nNOS, neuronal nitric oxide synthase.

inherited through an autosomal dominant pattern, with variable expressivity. The structure of one or both $\alpha_1(I)$ chains or the $\alpha_2(I)$ chain found on chromosomes 7 and 17 is affected in 90% of OI patients. OI ranges from mild to severe, and can result from many other mutations in proteins associated with collagen processing. Clinical manifestations include multiple fractures, crying or screaming with routine care, joint hypermobility, limb and finger deformities, bruising, triangular facial shape, hearing loss, abnormalities of the primary teeth, chronic pain, scoliosis, and short stature. OI is suspected in infants with blue/gray sclerae (although the sclerae of normal newborns tend to be bluish, they progress to white over the first few weeks of life). Diagnosis is by DNA sequencing.[10]

Rudy Tassy

Age-related changes to the musculoskeletal system include loss of muscle mass and strength (sarcopenia), decreased bone density, and degenerative joint disorders. Chronic inflammation (inflammaging or increased activity of innate immunity with aging) contributes to osteoporosis, muscle aging, and joint disorders. Fracture risk increases with age, with frailty and neuromuscular instability as contributing factors. Hip fracture is associated with increased mortality risk in the following year. The population aged over 60 years worldwide is predicted to rise from 841 million in 2013 to more than 2 billion by 2050, with implications for the number of patients suffering from age-related musculoskeletal disorders and injuries.[11] Exercise may reduce the morbidity and mortality of some age-associated musculoskeletal conditions.

AGING AND MUSCLE INTEGRITY: SARCOPENIA AND FRAILTY

Adults experience a progressive decrease in muscle mass proportional to body weight as they age. Sarcopenia refers to loss of muscle mass and strength. Between the ages of 50 and 80 years, muscle mass and the number of muscle fibers decline by as much as 50%.[12] Loss of muscle mass is greater in the legs than in the arms. Sarcopenia increases the risk of physical disability, poor quality of life, and death. The European Working Group on Sarcopenia in Older People (EWGSOP) differentiates sarcopenia into three subclasses: presarcopenia, sarcopenia, and severe sarcopenia. Presarcopenia is low muscle mass with no impact on muscle strength or physical performance; sarcopenia is low muscle mass with either low muscle strength or low physical performance; and severe sarcopenia is the presence of all three criteria.[11] Box 16.2 outlines mechanisms that contribute to loss of muscle mass and strength with aging.[12] Physical activity may slow but does not stop these losses.

Sarcopenia is one factor contributing to frailty. Frailty has been described as a state in which physiological reserves are maximally being used to maintain homeostasis, and any challenge will cross some threshold, leading to negative events such as illnesses, falls, and even death. The frailty phenotype proposed by Fried and colleagues included unintentional weight loss, self-reported exhaustion, weakness (assessed by grip strength), slow walking speed, and low physical activity.[14] The last three of these are clearly related to musculoskeletal function. A cumulative deficit approach to frailty, assessed by a Frailty Index, encompasses clinical variables reflecting activity of many more systems, but also includes measures that reflect musculoskeletal function. These include needing assistance with heavy chores, personal care, or mobility; having difficulty carrying or lifting light loads; and having limited or no activity or physical exercise.[15]

BOX 16.2

Mechanisms Contributing to Loss of Muscle Mass and Strength With Aging

- Myosteatosis, the presence of intra- and intermuscular fat that accumulates and decreases lean muscle mass

- Decreased mitochondrial function in aging muscles

- Degradation of contractile proteins, resulting in a reduced number of single muscle fibers and a decrease in the CSA of residual muscle fibers
  - The CSA of muscle decreases by up to 30% and muscle strength by 30% to 40% between the ages of 65 and 75 years[13]

- Slow twitch (type 1) fibers appear to have a slower decline than fast-twitch (type 2) fibers

- Decreased innervation of skeletal muscle, particularly in men older than 50 years of age
  - The number of motor units in any given muscle decreases with a compensatory increase in motor unit size

- Decreased activity of glycolytic enzymes and more modest decrease of oxidative enzyme activity in skeletal muscle

CSA, cross-sectional area.

BONE DENSITY AND OSTEOPOROSIS

Bone density decreases with age, declining on average approximately 0.5% per year in healthy older adults. **Osteoporosis** is most common in postmenopausal women, and throughout the aging trajectory, osteoporosis is more common in women than in men. However, women and men both have increased fracture incidence with increasing age. Bone mineral density (BMD) is usually measured by dual-energy x-ray absorptiometry (DXA). In the absence of a fragility fracture, bone density is the best predictor of fracture risk. A T-score is generated by comparing a subject's BMD with that of a healthy young adult. A Z-score is used to compare a subject's bone density to what is normal for his or her body size and age. In addition to DXA estimates of BMD, clinical indicators are used to diagnose osteoporosis. Included in the diagnosis of osteoporosis are patients with a hip fracture, regardless of BMD; patients with vertebral, proximal humerus, pelvis, or some wrist fractures when the T-score is between −1.0 and −2.5 or those with a Fracture Risk Assessment Tool (FRAX, an online calculator) that generates the 10-year probability of major osteoporotic fracture of 20% and greater or 10-year probability of hip fracture of 3% and greater.[16]

Osteoporosis results from age-related imbalance of the remodeling forces of bone resorption and bone deposition. A combination of increased resorption with decreased deposition results in bone demineralization that affects trabecular bone first, followed by cortical bone. Although the molecular and cellular mechanisms of osteoporosis have not been completely elucidated, empirical data have identified factors associated with increased fracture risk that are the basis of screening tools such as FRAX (**Box 16.3**).

JOINT DISORDERS IN OLDER ADULTS

Musculoskeletal disorders in older adults may present with signs and symptoms that are insidious, chronic, or coupled with comorbidities. Arthritis, defined as joint pain associated with inflammation, is very common in older adults and has several causes. Many older adults have one or more joint disorders that are caused by cartilage degeneration, mineral or crystal deposits, inflammatory processes, or a combination of these.

OSTEOARTHRITIS

Osteoarthritis (OA) is a degenerative joint disorder in which there is a progressive loss of articular cartilage, accompanied by remodeling and hypertrophy of the adjacent bone. OA is the most common type of arthritis and causes significant disability, particularly in older adults. OA commonly affects the knees, spine, and several joints of the hand. Swelling and bone deposits (osteophytes) are observed on inspection and x-ray studies, respectively. Obesity is a risk factor for OA, likely due to the increased load on joints. Prior injuries are also implicated in OA initiation, with knee injuries such as ACL tears and torn menisci associated with later OA development. In the knee, chronic misalignment can produce disease, with varus alignment associated with medial disease and valgus alignment associated with lateral disease.

Cellular changes are noted in the load-bearing areas of articular cartilage. Chondrocytes, the cells that reside in cartilage and both degrade and deposit cartilage proteins, are altered in OA joints. Cartilage loss is attributed to increased activity of matrix metalloproteinase enzymes, such as collagenase. Aging chondrocytes may produce cytokines that further promote tissue destruction and reduce tissue repair.

BOX 16.3
Risk Factors for Osteoporosis

- Smoking
- Alcohol use
- Vitamin D or calcium deficiency, or both
- Low physical activity and strength
- Low body weight

- History of previous fracture
- Parental history of hip fracture
- Treatment with glucocorticoid medications
- Presence of rheumatoid arthritis
- Caucasian ancestry

Finally, age-associated reduction in cartilage matrix, oxidative stress, and proteins pathologically modified by glycation all appear to contribute to abnormal cartilage, which is one source of altered joint function in OA[17] (**Figure 16.23**).

GOUT

Gout is a common arthritic disease in which monosodium urate crystals are deposited in joints, bones, and soft tissues, resulting in acute arthritis and chronic tophaceous gout. Uric acid is the end product of purine metabolism and is a normal constituent of extracellular fluid. Uric acid crystal formation is promoted at high levels of uric acid (hyperuricemia), and by low temperature and low pH. Hyperuricemia is relatively common and is associated several factors, including the following:

- Diet high in purines, including a diet with high meat or seafood content
- Greater alcohol consumption
- High consumption of beverages sweetened with sugar or high fructose corn syrup
- Decreased renal excretion of uric acid, including states of renal insufficiency
- History of hypertension
- Metabolic syndrome and obesity

Hyperuricemia does not inevitably lead to attacks of gout, so it is likely that other factors are involved. Gout is more common in men, and prevalence increases with age: 9.0% for men and 3.3% for women by age 65 years, and 13.3% for men and 6.2% for women by age 75 years of age.[18] Prevalence of gout is greater in individuals of Pacific Islander and African American background.

Factors influencing formation of monosodium urate crystals include urate concentration, lower temperatures (as in hands and feet) that promote crystal formation, nucleation (initial crystal formation due to high urate concentration), and growth (expansion of crystal size, pending urate concentration and temperature). The monosodium urate crystals are deposited in the synovium of the affected joint, causing a large inflammatory response. An initial attack is most common in the first metatarsophalangeal joint (**Figure 16.24**). An acute attack of gout is characterized by extreme pain, swelling, and redness. Synovial fluid samples show the presence of urate crystals, which is a diagnostic finding. Joint macrophages, synovial cells, and chondrocytes release cytokines, including interleukins (ILs)-1, -6, and -8, as well as tumor necrosis factor. These inflammatory mediators recruit neutrophils that invade the joint, increasing and perpetuating the acute inflammatory response and joint damage. The attack may respond to acute management or may resolve spontaneously.

Over time, repeated attacks may occur, particularly in tophaceous gout, a chronic form of gout in which nodular masses of uric acid (tophi) are present throughout the body and are usually visible at the surface of joints or cartilaginous tissues like those in the ear.

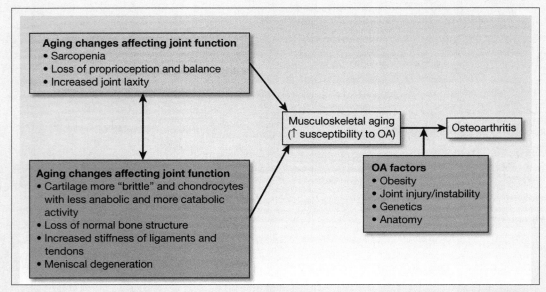

FIGURE 16.23 Joint structural and functional changes with aging contribute to OA development. OA, osteoarthritis.
Source: From *Hazzard's Geriatric Medicine and Gerontology.* 6th ed. New York, NY: McGraw Hill; 2009.

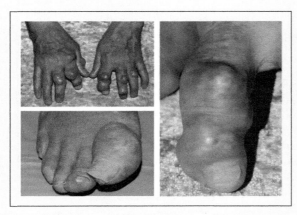

FIGURE 16.24 Gout often affects the first metatarsophalangeal joint of the foot, and can also involve the interphalangeal joints of the hand.
Source: From Roddy E. Revisiting the pathogenesis of podagra: why does gout target the foot? *J Foot Ankle Res.* 2011; 4:13, fig. 2.

SPONDYLOARTHRITIS

Spondyloarthritis is a relatively uncommon cause of low back pain. The term encompasses several related disorders, of which the most prevalent is AS. Classic AS is more common in men and women, onset is before age 40, and the predominant presenting symptom is aching low back pain. As the disease progresses, radiographic evidence of degeneration and excess bone deposition in the sacroiliac region is seen. MRI can identify early changes of axial skeletal inflammation, as well as some peripheral joint involvement, in patients with AS prior to lesions that are visible on x-ray inspection. Inflammation also involves enthesis—sites of tendon or ligament insertion in bone, causing enthesitis. Over time, the combination of inflammation and bony overgrowth can lead to fusion of the bones of the spine and pelvis, limiting movement and predisposing patients with spondyloarthritis to fracture risk as they grow older.

Spondyloarthritis shares some features with rheumatoid arthritis, but there are differentiating features between these two processes. AS has a familial risk, indicating genetic influences on the disorder. Spondyloarthritis is more prevalent in individuals with a particular immune cell membrane protein, HLA-B27, although the specific mechanism of increased risk associated with this protein is not well understood. There is a strong overlap between spondyloarthritis and inflammatory bowel diseases (Crohn disease and ulcerative colitis), and recent studies suggest that spondyloarthritis patients and unaffected individuals have different bacterial populations in the gut microbiome.[19]

Biologic therapies, including monoclonal antibodies that neutralize tumor necrosis factor or IL-17, have been clinically effective, implicating these cytokines in maintenance or progression of spondyloarthritis. As IL-23 stimulates the T-helper 17 (Th17) cells that secrete IL-17, excess IL-23 may contribute to pathogenesis of spondyloarthritis. One of the earliest signs of spondyloarthritis is sacroiliitis, which includes enthesitis and synovitis. These enthesis lesions include subchondral granulation tissue, lymphocytes, and macrophages in ligamentous and periosteal zones, and subchondral bone edema. Subsequently, synovitis occurs and may progress to pannus formation with new bone growth around eroded joint margins. The most common joint areas affected are the sacroiliac and facet (zygapophyseal) joints.

PARKINSON DISEASE AND PISA SYNDROME

Pisa syndrome has been called *the scoliosis of parkinsonism*. It is defined as a reversible lateral bending of the trunk of more than 15 degrees that increases during walking, with a tendency to lean to one side. Estimates of prevalence are quite varied, possibly reflecting the lack of a comprehensive definition and categorization scheme for the disorder. The cause of Pisa syndrome in patients with **Parkinson disease** is unknown, but development of the syndrome is more common in older patients and in those who have the longest duration of the disease. The mechanisms of Pisa syndrome have been hypothesized to result from:

- Alterations in sensory–motor integration, particularly with proprioception and vestibular sensation
- Anatomical changes in the musculoskeletal system
- Antiparkinsonian drugs

The pattern of onset has been classified according to the time taken to develop clinically definite Pisa syndrome: acute (less than 1 month), subchronic (between 1 and 3 months), and chronic (3 months or more). In patients with Parkinson disease, Pisa syndrome has been associated with initiation or change in the dose of dopamine agonists, variation in the levodopa regimen, and addition of rasagiline and catechol-*O*-methyl transferase (COMT) inhibitors to levodopa treatment. There is no clear pattern predicting the side to which patients lean. Patients can lean toward or away from the side most affected by Parkinson disease, suggesting that basal ganglia asymmetry may be another cause.[20]

For patients with Pisa syndrome, early observation and action is key to successful reversal of symptoms. Strong evidence for treatment of Pisa syndrome is lacking. If a patient is started on anti-Parkinson medication and, in subsequent visits, he or she is noted to be leaning on physical examination, stopping or replacing the medication may resolve the problem.

CASE STUDY 16.1: A Patient With a Sprained Ankle

Allison Rusgo and Michelle Zappas

Patient Complaint: *"I was playing basketball with my friends after school today and twisted my left ankle. It happened as I was jumping for the ball. I collided with a teammate as we both tried to grab a rebound. As I landed, my ankle twisted inward and I fell. Since then, it's been hard to walk and my ankle seems swollen. My mom picked me up from the basketball court and insisted I have it examined. I've never injured this ankle, and I hope it's not broken so I can get back to playing basketball again soon."*

History of Present Illness/Review of Systems: You observe a well-developed, well-nourished 13-year-old boy sitting on the examination table in obvious discomfort with his left ankle elevated on two pillows. He states that it has been approximately 2 hours since he injured his ankle. He has not used any palliative measures, such as ice, wrapping, or antiinflammatory medications, and reports that any movement of the ankle worsens his discomfort. He describes the pain as a constant throbbing, with occasional sharp pain during movement. He also states that the pain radiates slightly toward the distal aspect of his lower extremity when he plantar flexes or dorsiflexes his ankle. At rest, he rates the pain as a 6 on a scale of 10 but notes an increase to an 8 with ambulation. The musculoskeletal review of systems is positive for left ankle pain, swelling, and slight limitation of motion while all other joints are within normal limits. The patient denies any muscle pain, tremors, atrophy, hypertrophy, or weakness.

Past Medical/Family/Social History: The patient has no significant past medical history or previous injuries, surgeries, or hospitalizations, and his

mother reports that he is up to date on all childhood immunizations. He does not use medications and does not have any allergies. The patient is a seventh-grader who lives at home with his parents. He states that he does not use tobacco/e-cigarette products, alcohol, or other illicit substances. He succeeds academically and enjoys playing sports. His family history is noncontributory.

Physical Examination: Findings are as follows: temperature of 98°F (oral), blood pressure of 116/72 mm Hg, heart rate of 68 beats/min, respirations of 16 breaths/min. BMI is 25 kg/m^2 (75th percentile). On inspection of the left ankle, you note ecchymosis and edema without any evidence of lacerations, crepitus, or deformity. Active and passive range of motion is intact but pain is noted. There is tenderness to palpation at the anterior talofibular and calcaneofibular ligaments, but the remainder of the extremity is nontender. The anterior drawer and external rotation tests are negative. Pulses and sensation in the extremity are present and when asked to ambulate, the patient walks five steps with a slight limp on the affected side.

Diagnostic Findings: Left ankle x-ray film series of AP, lateral, and mortise views show no evidence of bony injury; however, there is evidence of slight soft tissue swelling surrounding the lateral malleolus.

CASE STUDY 16.1 QUESTIONS
- *What aspect of the ankle joint may have sustained the greatest degree of injury?*
- *If this is likely to be an ankle sprain, what grade of sprain is likely?*

AP, anteroposterior; BMI, body mass index.

CASE STUDY 16.2: A Patient With Acute Gouty Arthritis

Michelle Zappas and Allison Rusgo

Patient Complaint: *"I'm in agony. My right big toe is so painful I could barely put on my sock and shoe this morning. It started yesterday morning and has gotten worse over the past 24 hours. It feels like my toe is more swollen and red than normal. I don't like coming to see the primary care provider, but my wife insisted I be evaluated. I've never experienced anything like this before, and I hope it resolves quickly because I have an international business trip next week."*

History of Present Illness/Review of Systems: You observe a well-developed, well-nourished 56-year-old Caucasian man sitting on the examination table in obvious discomfort. He has removed the shoe and sock from his right foot. The patient states that it has been approximately 24 hours since his pain began. He tried to alleviate the discomfort with one dose of acetaminophen (Tylenol), 500 mg, last evening, but this did not provide much relief. He reports that if anything touches his toe, his pain intensifies, and he describes it as a constant throbbing. He rates the pain as a 7 on a scale of 10, with an increase to a 9 when ambulating or donning footwear. The review of systems is negative for fevers, chills, muscle pain, atrophy, hypertrophy, or weakness. It is positive for pain, edema, erythema, warmth, and slight limitation of motion of the right great toe; all other joints are within normal limits.

Past Medical/Family/Social History: The patient reports a past medical history of hypertension that is controlled with chlorthalidone, 25 mg daily. He denies any previous injuries, surgeries, hospitalizations, or medication allergies. His family history is noncontributory. He lives at home with his wife and daughter. He is an investment banker in a large firm where he works more than 60 hours per week. He admits that he rarely participates in physical activity and consumes steak dinners several times a week at business functions. He denies the use of any illicit substances or tobacco products but drinks several glasses of wine or beer each week.

Physical Examination: Findings are as follows: temperature of 97.7°F, blood pressure of 138/82 mm Hg, and heart rate of 75 beats/min. BMI is 33.8 kg/m². On inspection of the right great toe, you note warmth, erythema, edema, and tenderness to palpation at the base of the right first metatarsophalangeal joint. Active and passive range of motion is intact, but pain is noted. The remainder of the right lower extremity examination is within normal limits; pulses and sensation are intact, and when asked to ambulate, the patient walks five steps with a slight limp on the affected side due to pain.

Diagnostic and Laboratory Findings: Radiography of the right great toe reveals moderate soft tissue swelling around the base of the metatarsophalangeal joint without any other bony abnormalities. Initial laboratory tests reveal an elevated ESR, leukocytosis, and an elevated serum urate level.

CASE STUDY 16.2 QUESTIONS
- *What are this patient's risk factors for gout?*
- *Collection of a sample of joint fluid (arthrocentesis) is carried out for laboratory analysis of fluid composition, cell count, and differential, and presence of crystals. What findings will confirm a diagnosis of gout?*

BMI, body mass index; ESR, erythrocyte sedimentation rate.

BRIDGE TO CLINICAL PRACTICE

Ben Cocchiaro

PRINCIPLES OF ASSESSMENT

History and Physical Examination

- Inspect for swelling, bruising, or abnormal position.
- *Functional assessment:* Evaluate both active and passive range of motion, comparing to both reference ranges and unaffected limbs where applicable. Can the patient bear weight on the affected joint? Are there any limitations in activity?
- Joint laxity can be assessed by asking about sensations of the joint *giving way*, and through special physical exam maneuvers such as the Lachman test for ACL injuries.
- *Neurological signs:* While nerve root and peripheral nerve pathologies may both present with lower motor neuron signs of weakness and hyporeflexia, an understanding of dermatome/myotome anatomy can help isolate weak muscles or painful nerves and identify specific lesions.
- *Pain assessment:* Determine whether pain is acute (<6 weeks), subacute (6 to 12 weeks), or chronic (>12 weeks) and characterize it as nociceptive (dull, aching) or neuropathic (burning, buzzing, and shooting). Identify exacerbating/alleviating factors.
- Ask about prior treatments, including surgeries, splinting, corticosteroid injections, and participation in physical therapy.

Diagnostic Tools

- *Radiology:* X-ray studies are useful in identifying bony pathology including fractures, tumors, osteoporosis, and osteoarthritis but unable to directly visualize soft tissue structures.
- *Musculoskeletal ultrasound:* This imaging modality is increasingly popular in the evaluation of tendon, ligament, bursa, and muscle pathology, especially rotator cuff injuries.
- *MRI:* Study provides high-resolution images of deep soft tissue structures and is highly sensitive for diagnosing meniscal and ligamentous injury.

- *CT:* CT is more sensitive than plain film radiography in the diagnosis of bony pathology, but similarly limited in its inability to visualize soft tissue structures such as muscles and tendons.

Laboratory Evaluation

- Uric acid
- Synovial fluid analysis

MAJOR DRUG CLASSES

- *NSAIDs:* Drugs such as ibuprofen, naproxen, and aspirin inhibit cyclooxygenase enzymes, decreasing production of prostaglandins responsible for inflammation and sensitization of pain receptors in the peripheral nervous system. They are useful in treating acute pain, although adverse effects may develop with chronic use.
- *Glucocorticoids:* Steroid drugs such as prednisone inhibit enzymatic release of the prostaglandin precursor arachidonic acid and have additional mechanisms that decrease the body's inflammatory response. Glucocorticoids are injected into arthritic joint spaces to decrease pain and are sometimes given systemically when inflammation threatens to compress and destroy nerve fibers.
- *Opioid agonists:* These agents have no direct antiinflammatory effects but work primarily within the brain and spinal cord to decrease pain signaling. Their use in orthopedic conditions is decreasing as evidence supports other effective strategies.
- *Muscle relaxants:* Agents such as cyclobenzaprine decrease muscle tone by acting on the central nervous system and are occasionally useful in the acute treatment of muscle spasms.
- *Drugs for bone disorders:* Bisphosphonates, calcium, and vitamin D work to prevent and treat osteoporosis and osteopenia by shifting the body's osteoclastic/osteoblastic balance toward bone production.
- *Drugs for gout:* These agents reduce uric acid production or increase uric acid excretion.

ACL, anterior cruciate ligament; NSAIDs, nonsteroidal anti inflammatory drugs.

KEY POINTS

- Bone is a rigid structure containing cells interspersed with a mineralized extracellular matrix. Activity of osteoclasts, osteoblasts, and osteocytes is responsible for remodeling, turnover of bone tissue that enables strengthening in response to stress.
- Bones can fracture secondary to trauma, and certain disease states (osteoporosis, osteogenesis imperfecta) and medications increase fracture risk. Fractures must be immobilized for proper healing. Complete healing may take up to 1 year after a fracture. Immobilization to allow for fracture healing results in disuse atrophy of muscles in the affected region. Recovery of function takes longer than development of atrophy, and prolonged disuse atrophy may lead to muscle contractures.
- Joints are regions where two or more bones come together and are connected in a variety of ways. There are several types of joints; some permit movement, and others are immoveable or only slightly moveable. Synovial joints are those in which articulating bones are separated by a fluid-filled synovial cavity. These are generally joints at which movements occur. Synovial joints can include complex structures bounded by an articular capsule, containing elements such as synovial fluid, ligaments, menisci, bursae, tendon sheaths, and cartilage.
- Musculoskeletal injuries include strains and sprains. A strain is a stretching injury to a musculotendinous unit that heals relatively quickly, and a sprain is a joint injury that involves damage to ligaments. Severity of sprains is graded I through III. Grade I is the least severe and most rapidly healing. Grade III, the most severe, involves a complete ligament rupture. Grade II and III sprains cause sufficient structural damage to make the joint unstable and unable to function.
- Ankle sprains are extremely common, particularly with sports activities. Several ligaments of the ankle joints can be damaged by sprains. Most common is damage of the lateral ligamentous complex resulting from severe foot inversion.
- The knee is one of the most complex joints in the body, and knee injuries are correspondingly varied and complex. Sports injuries often target the knee with either a valgus force to the lateral knee surface that damages or tears the medial collateral ligament, or a varus force to the medial surface of the knee that damages or tears the lateral collateral ligament.
- Severe internal knee rotation with the foot planted, or a lateral blow to the knee with the foot fixed, may rupture the ACL, leading to pain, swelling, loss of range of motion, and instability.
- Back pain is a common presenting symptom and can result from many causes. One source of back pain is a herniated disc causing collapse of one vertebra on another. This collapse may impinge on spinal roots, causing pain and loss of nerve conduction. Sensory and motor deficits will be associated with the segmental level of the abnormality. This disorder most commonly affects lower cervical and lumbar levels.
- Cumulative trauma disorders are also known as repetitive stress injuries. Examples include carpal tunnel syndrome, cubital tunnel syndrome, lateral epicondylitis, trigger finger, and hip bursitis. These conditions are often work related and may result from nonergonomically designed tasks; others are recreation related. Hypotheses concerning their pathogenesis include tendon damage proceeding to noninflammatory tendinosis; compression neuropathies with nerve ischemia; and the combination of neuropathic compression with myofascial pain and muscle use imbalance.
- Thoracic outlet syndrome is a complex disorder that, in some cases, is due to disordered anatomy or, in some cases, cumulative stress disorder. Thoracic outlet syndrome can manifest with nerve compression, venous compression, or arterial injury.
- Musculoskeletal position and development in infancy and toddler years is shaped by prenatal position, then by acquisition of developmental milestones of movement that alter the use of and load on muscles, bones, and joints. Developmental dysplasia of the hip is a common disorder.
- Childhood and adolescence are periods of continuing bone growth and mineralization, and in some cases, abnormal development, as in scoliosis. Fracture healing is rapid, but risks of overuse injuries with athletic activities and growth plate fractures are increased.
- Genetic disorders affecting musculoskeletal function include muscular dystrophy and osteogenesis imperfecta, with impaired muscle and bone function, respectively.
- Older adults have progressive losses of muscle mass and strength (sarcopenia) and bone mass and strength (osteopenia and osteoporosis). The severity of these conditions is inversely

proportional to the amount of aerobic and weight-bearing physical activity. Osteoporosis is associated with increased fracture risk.

- Aging of joints predisposes to degenerative joint diseases, including osteoarthritis, gout, and spondyloarthritis, that contribute to mobility limitations and disability.

- The neurological dysfunction of Parkinson disease may predispose to Pisa syndrome—altered posture with a tendency to lean toward or away from the more affected side of the body. Management is directed to the neurological root of the condition, rather than the musculoskeletal system.

REFERENCES

1. World Health Organization. Musculoskeletal conditions. https://www.who.int/news-room/fact-sheets/detail/musculoskeletal-conditions. Accessed January 8, 2020.
2. Centers for Disease Control and Prevention, National Center for Health Statistics. Ambulatory health care data. https://www.cdc.gov/nchs/ahcd/index.htm. Accessed January 8, 2020.
3. Baldwin KD, Wells L, Dormans JP. Common fractures. In: Kliegman RM, Stanton RF, St. Geme JW, Schor NF, eds. *Nelson Textbook of Pediatrics*. 20th ed. Philadelphia, PA: Elsevier; 2016: 3314–3322.
4. Baldwin KD, Wells L, Dormans JP. Growth and development. In: Kliegman RM, Stanton RF, St. Geme JW, Schor NF, eds. *Nelson Textbook of Pediatrics*. 20th ed. Philadelphia, PA: Elsevier; 2016: 3241–3242.
5. Baldwin KD, Wells L. Torsional deformities. In: Kliegman RM, Stanton RF, St. Geme JW, Schor NF, eds. *Nelson Textbook of Pediatrics*. 20th ed. Philadelphia, PA: Elsevier; 2016: 3257–3264.
6. Erickson MA, Rhodes J, Niswander C. Orthopedics. In: Hay WW, Levin MJ, Deterding RR, Abzug MJ, eds. *Current Diagnosis and Treatment Pediatrics*. 23rd ed. New York, NY: McGraw-Hill; 2016: 815–839.
7. Newton Ede MMP, Jones SW. Adolescent idiopathic scoliosis: evidence for intrinsic factors driving aetiology and progression. *Int Orthop*. 2016;40:2075–2080. doi:10.1007/s00264-016-3132-4.
8. Paterno MV. Unique issues in the rehabilitation of the pediatric and adolescent athlete after musculoskeletal injury. *Sports Med Arthrosc Rev*. 2016;24:178–183. doi:10.1097/JSA.0000000000000130.
9. Rahimov F, Kunkel LM. Cellular and molecular mechanisms underlying muscular dystrophy. *J Cell Biol*. 2013;201:499–510. doi:10.1083/jcb.201212142.
10. Marini JC, Forlino A, Bächinger HP, et al. Osteogenesis imperfecta. *Nat Rev Dis Primers*. 2017;3:17052. doi:10.1038/nrdp.2017.52.
11. Dawson A, Dennison E. Measuring the musculoskeletal aging phenotype. *Maturitas*. 2016;93:13–17. doi:10.1016/j.maturitas.2016.04.014.
12. Faulkner JA, Larkin LM, Claflin DR, Brooks SV. Age-related changes in the structure and function of skeletal muscles. *Clin Exp Pharmacol Physiol*. 2007;34:1091–1096. doi:10.1111/j.1440-1681.2007.04752.x.
13. Choi S-J. Age-related functional changes and susceptibility to eccentric contraction-induced damage in skeletal muscle cell. *Integr Med Res*. 2016;5:171–175. doi:10.1016/j.imr.2016.05.004.
14. Fried LP, Tangen CM, Walston J, et al. Frailty in older adults: evidence for a phenotype. *J Gerontol Med Sci*. 2001;56A:M146–M156. doi:10.1093/gerona/56.3.m146.
15. Song X, Witnitski A, Rockwood K. Prevalence and 10-year outcomes of frailty in older adults in relation to deficit accumulation. *J Am Geriatr Soc*. 2010;58:681–687. doi:10.1111/j.1532-5415.2010.02764.x.
16. In: Rosen CJ, Schmader KE, eds. *UpToDate*. https://www.uptodate.com/contents/osteoporotic-fracture-risk-assessment/print. Updated November 12, 2019. Accessed February 23, 2018.
17. Unnanuntana A, Gladnick BP, Donnelly E, Lane JM. The assessment of fracture risk. *J Bone Joint Surg Am*. 2010;92:743–753.
18. Anderson AS, Loeser RF. Why is osteoarthritis an age-related disease? *Best Pract Res Clin Rheumatol*. 2010;24:15–26. doi:10.1016/j.berh.2009.08.006.
19. Burke BT, Köttgen A, Law A, et al. Gout in older adults: the atherosclerosis risk in communities study. *J Gerontol Med Sci*. 2016;71:536–542. doi:10.1093/gerona/glv120.
20. Gill T, Asquith M, Rosenbaum JT, Colbert RA. The intestinal microbiome in spondyloarthritis. *Curr Opin Rheumatol*. 2015;27:319–325. doi:10.1097/BOR.0000000000000187.
21. Barone P, Santangelo G, Amboni M, et al. Pisa syndrome in Parkinson's disease and parkinsonism: clinical features, pathophysiology, and treatment. *Lancet Neurol*. 2016;15:1063–1074. doi:10.1016/S1474-4422(16)30173-9.

SUGGESTED RESOURCES

Batjer HH, Loftus CM, eds. *Textbook of Neurological Surgery: Principles and Practice*. Vol 3. Philadelphia, PA: Lippincott Williams & Wilkins; 2002.

Kedia S, Knupp K, Schreiner TL, et al. Neurologic and muscular disorders. In: Hay WW, Levin MJ, Deterding RR, Abzug MJ, eds. *Current Diagnosis and Treatment Pediatrics*. 23rd ed. New York, NY: McGraw-Hill; 2016:735–814.

Lindsay R, Cosman F. Osteoporosis. In: Kasper D, Fauci A, Hauser S, et al., eds. *Harrison's Principles of Internal*

Medicine. 19th ed. New York, NY: McGraw-Hill; 2015: chap 425.

Prideaux M, Findlay DM, Atkins GJ. Osteocytes: the master bone cells in bone remodeling. *Curr Opin Pharmacol.* 2016;28:24–30. doi:10.1016/j.coph.2016.02.003.

Roddy E. Revisiting the pathogenesis of podagra: why does gout target the foot? *J Foot Ankle Res.* 2011;4:13. doi:10.1186/1757-1146-4-13.

Singleton JK, DiGregorio RV, Green-Hernandez C, et al., eds. *Primary Care: An Interprofessional Perspective.* 2nd ed. New York, NY: Springer Publishing Company; 2014.

Taurog JD, Chhabra A, Colbert RA. Ankylosing spondylitis and axial spondyloarthritis. *N Engl J Med.* 2016;374: 2563–2574. doi:10.1056/NEJMra1406182

Young CC. Ankle sprain clinical presentation. In: Sherwin SWH, ed. *Medscape.* https://emedicine.medscape.com/article/1907229-clinical#b3. Updated January 14, 2019. Accessed January 8, 2020.

ENDOCRINE SYSTEM

Christine Yedinak, Carolina R. Hurtado, Angela M. Leung, Meredith Annon, Hanne S. Harbison, Diane L. Spatz, Gioia Petrighi Polidori, and Victoria Fischer

THE CLINICAL CONTEXT

Among endocrine disorders, primary disorders of the hypothalamus, pituitary, and adrenal glands are relatively uncommon. The most common primary pituitary disorders are pituitary adenomas, with an estimated prevalence of 780 to 940 cases per 1 million people. The prevalence of hypopituitarism due to any cause is 410 cases per million people.[1] Primary adrenal insufficiency affects 40 to 140 per million, with secondary adrenal insufficiency estimated to affect three to 280 per million. Cushing disease occurs in 39 per million.[2] Despite the rarity of these specific endocrine disorders, the mechanisms of hypothalamic, pituitary, and target organ function provide a critical foundation for a broader understanding of endocrine signaling and pathophysiology.

Diseases of the thyroid are the second most common among endocrine disorders, after diabetes mellitus. There is a strong relationship between dietary iodine intake and thyroid disease, such that epidemiological studies of thyroid disease generally report statistics from iodine-sufficient and iodine-deficient regions and countries separately.[3] In iodine-sufficient regions, hypothyroidism has a prevalence of 1% to 2%, with affected women outnumbering men by 10:1. Hyperthyroidism prevalence is 0.5% to 2.0% in iodine-sufficient countries, and has a similar female-to-male ratio.[4]

The most common reproductive disorder for women is polycystic ovary syndrome, with estimated prevalence of 6% to 20%.[5,6] Endometriosis affects 6% to 10% of premenopausal women and is a source of chronic debilitating pain that disrupts normal function.[7] In men, erectile dysfunction is a common disorder with age-related increase in prevalence, affecting 20% of men at age 20 and 75% of men at age 75.[8] Similarly, rates of benign prostatic hyperplasia and prostate cancer are high and increase with aging. Prostate volume increases every year; more than 50% of men over age 50 have documented prostate enlargement. As prostate volume increases, the number of lower urinary tract symptoms of obstruction increases concomitantly.[9] Prostate cancer affects about one in eight men in the United States, and is the cause of death in one in 37 men.[10]

Diabetes, prediabetes, and obesity have high and increasing prevalence in the United States and worldwide. In the United States, there are over 30 million adults (aged 18 and older) with diabetes, of whom 23 million are diagnosed and over 7 million are undiagnosed. Almost 34% of people (84 million) have prediabetes, many of whom are undiagnosed. In 2014, people with a diagnosis of diabetes had 7.2 million hospital discharges—1.5 million for cardiovascular disease, 108,000 for amputations, and 168,000 for diabetic ketoacidosis. Of further clinical concern, 36.5% of people with diabetes had kidney disease.[11] The United States is currently in the midst of an obesity crisis: In 2015 to 2016, obesity was present in almost 40% of adults aged 20 years and older, and over 18% of children aged 2 to 19 years.[12] Globally, 8.5% of persons have diabetes (422 million people) and diabetes was the seventh leading cause of death in 2016.[13] The World Health Organization estimates that worldwide,

39% of adults are overweight and 13% are obese. Globally, more than 340 million children were overweight or obese in 2016.[14] Diabetes is a leading cause of cardiovascular disease, the top cause of death around the world. It is also the most

common cause of chronic kidney disease, is associated with hypertension, and increases the risk of age-related cognitive losses. Obesity has similar health-related consequences as diabetes, as well as increasing the risk of many cancers.

Principles of Endocrine Function

Christine Yedinak

The endocrine system functions to maintain homeostasis by modulating tissue and organ function through the actions of blood-borne and locally acting *hormones*. Similar to the autonomic nervous system, the endocrine activity links detection of key body variables (including blood osmolality, volume, and pressure; blood glucose; and circadian signaling, among others) with regulated secretion of hormones to maintain the stability of those variables. Differing from the nervous system, with its direct contact between effector cell (neuron) and postsynaptic target tissue, endocrine glands secrete hormones into the bloodstream where they travel through the circulation to act on target tissues throughout the body. Hormones have rapid and slow actions regulating metabolic activity, growth and development, reproductive functions, sleep, mood, and activity of the other organ systems. The endocrine glands and tissues discussed in this chapter include the hypothalamus, pituitary, adrenal, thyroid, ovaries, testes, and pancreas, and contributions of parathyroid hormone (PTH) are highlighted in the topic of osteoporosis, within the section on female reproductive function.

The amount (magnitude) and rate of hormone synthesis and secretion to maintain homeostasis is controlled by feedback mechanisms (negative and positive) and endogenous rhythms. Negative feedback suppresses hormone production once an excess state is achieved, whereas positive feedback stimulates further hormone production and release. Endogenous rhythms are recurrent patterns of hormone secretion. These are largely circadian, recurring every 24 hours. *Circadian* rhythms are often based on light/dark cycles and are controlled by the "clock mechanism" of the hypothalamus. *Ultradian* rhythms have cycles that occur several times over the course of the day. *Infradian* rhythms are longer than a day (such as the menstrual cycle) and may be affected by seasonal, environmental, or exogenous changes such as food intake. These rhythms allow physiological adaptation to environmental changes and mediate changes of state associated with longer-term biological processes such as growth and reproduction.

Disorders of the endocrine system tend to fall into two categories: absolute or relative hormone deficiency

(hypofunction) and hormone excess (hyperfunction). Dysfunction may also be primary or secondary. Primary dysfunction occurs when the deficiency or excess is caused by abnormality of the main endocrine organ, and secondary dysfunction occurs when a controlling hormone or other regulatory aspect is abnormally regulated. Laboratory evaluation can distinguish between these two possibilities, usually by measuring the endocrine hormone and its controlling hormones or factors. Another mechanism of endocrine disease is altered tissue responsiveness to the hormone, in which case evaluation depends less on measuring hormone levels and more on evaluating tissue responses. Management of endocrine disorders aims to correct the dysfunction (e.g., by removing a hormone-hypersecreting tumor, as in Cushing disease, or by hormone replacement after glandular failure, as in insulin treatment of type 1 diabetes).

HORMONE STRUCTURES

Hormones are classified by derivation, structure, function, or solubility. Broad classifications include amines (modified from amino acids), peptides (short amino acid chains), proteins (longer amino acid chains), and steroids (synthesized from cholesterol; **Table 17.1**).

Hormone synthesis and secretion differ by system, and details of synthesis are described in the context of the individual systems discussed in the main sections of this chapter. In general, endocrine cells either will have a high level of gene expression for a peptide or protein hormone (such as arginine vasopressin [AVP] or insulin) or will have a unique set of enzymes to synthesize an amine, thyroid, or steroid hormone. Protein and peptide hormones are usually synthesized as pre-pro proteins, with a signal sequence that is used to direct them to secretory vesicles for secretion. After the signal sequence is removed by enzymes, the resulting pro protein requires further folding, cleaving, and processing to be ready for secretion. The hormone insulin, for example, is the cleavage product of proinsulin that has been folded and cleaved, resulting in a two-chain structure. Steroid hormone synthesis, on the other hand, requires

TABLE 17.1 Examples of Hormone Structures

Hormone Class	Components	Example(s)
Amine hormone	Amino acids with modified groups (e.g., norepinephrine is synthesized by enzymatic modifcation of the amino acid tyrosine	Norepinephrine
Peptide hormone	Short amino acid chains	Oxytocin
Protein hormone	Long amino acid chains	Growth hormone
Steroid hormone	Derived from the lipid cholesterol	Testosterone Progesterone

cell synthesis or uptake of cholesterol and the presence of enzymes that modify cholesterol into the final steroid hormone. Secretion of most hormones is by regulated exocytosis. Thyroid hormone synthesis differs from all other hormones in occurring extracellularly within the colloid of thyroid follicles, and thyroid hormone secretion occurs by colloid endocytosis, lysosomal degradation, and free hormone release.

CELL SIGNALING BY HORMONES

Hormones do not only act on distant targets. Other modes of signaling include *autocrine* (in which the hormone-producing cell also has receptors for the hormone it synthesizes and secretes) and *paracrine* (in which the hormone acts on adjacent and nearby cells; **Figure 17.1**). Additionally, some of the hormones described in this chapter fall into a category of *neuroendocrine* signaling. This type of signaling characterizes neurons located in the hypothalamus that synthesize and secrete their hormone from their axon terminals into the bloodstream. This hybrid of neuronal features (axon terminals as the site of release, action potentials required for release) and endocrine features (substance enters the bloodstream to travel to target tissues) applies to hypothalamic releasing and inhibiting hormones, as well as to the posterior pituitary hormones vasopressin and oxytocin.

When hormones bind to their specific receptors on target cell membranes or diffuse into the cell, they activate a cascade of intracellular activities or nuclear gene transcription that modulates cell function (**Figure 17.2**). Endocrine signaling pathways incorporate the steps of reception, transduction, and cellular response, falling into two broad classes of intracellular mechanisms:

1. Water-soluble (hydrophilic) hormones travel in blood plasma and bind to cell surface receptors to generate rapid cellular changes via second messengers (**Figure 17.2a**). These include amines, peptides, and protein hormones, for example, epinephrine, vasopressin, and adrenocorticotropic hormone (ACTH). Many membrane hormone receptors are of the G protein–coupled type, which alter adenylyl cyclase or phospholipase C activity with receptor binding. Other hormone receptors incorporate a tyrosine kinase domain, or associate with accessory proteins that are tyrosine kinases, to achieve cellular responses as described in Chapter 4, Cell Physiology and Pathophysiology (**Figure 17.2b**).
2. Steroid and thyroid hormones are lipid soluble (hydrophobic) and travel in blood plasma on protein carriers that prolong their duration in the circulation and length of action. The major mechanism of action of these hormones is to cross the plasma membrane, binding to receptors in the cytoplasm or in the nucleus, ultimately binding to DNA to alter gene expression (**Figure 17.2c**).

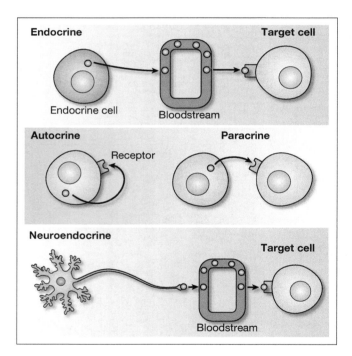

FIGURE 17.1 Modes of hormone signaling. Classic conception of endocrine signaling is the release of a hormone from specialized endocrine gland cells into the bloodstream, where it travels to distant tissues to have its biological effect. Many endocrine gland cells have autoreceptors for the hormones they secrete, and are thus modulated by autocrine signaling. Paracrine signaling refers to the modulation of an adjacent or nearby cell by hormone diffusing from its secretion site. Finally, neuroendocrine signaling characterizes the actions of neurons located within the nervous system, with axons that project to the pituitary stalk or posterior pituitary gland. The axons terminate on blood vessels, releasing hormones that travel to target tissues to exert their biological effects.

These generalized mechanisms are not the only possible modes of signaling. In fact, water-soluble hormones can act through their second messengers to alter gene transcription and translation. Steroid and thyroid hormones can also have short-term actions in the cytoplasm, in addition to their roles in altering protein transcription and translation.[15]

Table 17.2 provides a comprehensive list of endocrine glands and hormones—their structure, size, targets, and major functions. Other hormones are synthesized outside the brain and classical endocrine organs, and are described in the context of their main tissue sources and actions; for example, gastrointestinal hormones are described in Chapter 13, Gastrointestinal Tract.

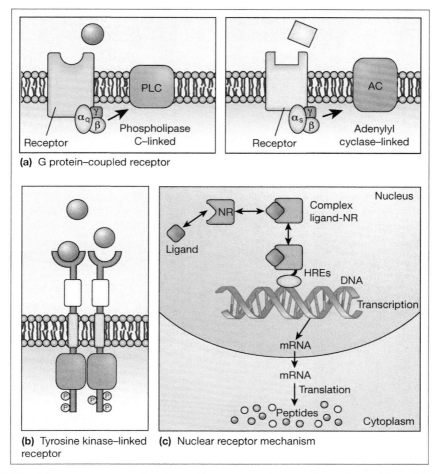

(a) G protein–coupled receptor

(b) Tyrosine kinase–linked receptor

(c) Nuclear receptor mechanism

FIGURE 17.2 Three common mechanisms of hormone action are shown here. **(a)** and **(b)** Water-soluble hormones bind to cell surface receptors that are either G protein–coupled or linked to activation of tyrosine kinase activity to exert intracellular effects. **(c)** Steroid and thyroid hormones cross the plasma membrane and bind to a cytosolic or nuclear receptor, ultimately binding to DNA. The result of receptor activation is to exert long-term changes by changing target cell transcription and translation.

AC, adenylyl cyclase; HRE, hormone-response element; mRNA, messenger RNA; NR, nuclear receptor; P, phosphate; PLC, phospholipase C.

TABLE 17.2 Hormones and Their Functions

Endocrine Source or Gland	Hormone/Class	Main Function of Hormone
Hypothalamus	Thyrotropin releasing hormone (TRH) Peptide: 3 aa	Stimulates anterior pituitary thyrotropes to release TSH
	Somatostatin (SST) Peptide: 14 or 28 aa	Inhibits release of several anterior pituitary hormones, including GH
	Gonadotropin releasing hormone (GnRH) Peptide: 10 aa	Stimulates anterior pituitary gonadotropes to release FSH and LH
	Corticotropin releasing hormone (CRH) Peptide: 41 aa	Stimulates anterior pituitary corticotropes to release ACTH
	Growth hormone releasing hormone (GHRH) Peptide: 44 aa	Stimulates anterior pituitary somatotropes to release GH

(continued)

TABLE 17.2 Hormones and Their Functions (*continued*)

Endocrine Source or Gland	Hormone/Class	Main Function of Hormone
Anterior pituitary	Thyroid stimulating hormone (TSH) Glycoprotein: common α subunit—89 aa; unique β subunit—112 aa	Stimulates thyroid gland growth, promotes T_4 and T_3 synthesis and secretion
	Luteinizing hormone (LH) Glycoprotein: common α subunit—89 aa; unique β subunit—115 aa	Females: stimulates ovarian sex steroid production, LH mid-cycle peak initiates ovulation Males: stimulates testis synthesis and secretion of testosterone
	Follicle-stimulating hormone (FSH) Glycoprotein: common α subunit—89 aa; unique β subunit—115 aa	Females: stimulates ovarian early follicular cycle follicle development and preparation for ovulation Males: stimulates testis synthesis and secretion of testosterone
	Growth hormone (GH) Protein: 190 aa	Promotes growth of bones and organs; promotes muscle protein synthesis, regulates metabolism of fat and liver
	Prolactin (PRL) Protein: 198 aa	Stimulates breast development and milk production
	Adrenocorticotropic hormone (ACTH) Protein: 39 aa	Stimulates adrenal gland growth and hormone secretion, particularly cortisol secretion
Posterior pituitary	Vasopressin (AVP, antidiuretic hormone) Peptide: 9 aa	Controls renal water retention to regulate blood volume and pressure, also functions as vasoconstrictor
	Oxytocin (OT) Peptide: 9 aa	Stimulates uterine contraction, initiates milk ejection (let-down)
Thyroid gland	Thyroxine (T_4) Thyroid hormone	Maintains normal functions of most tissues, increases the body's metabolic rate
	Triiodothyronine (T_3) Thyroid hormone	More active than T_4, maintains normal functions of most tissues, increases the body's metabolic rate, required for normal development and function of the brain
Parathyroid glands	Parathyroid hormone (PTH) Protein: 84 aa	Increases blood calcium level by promoting absorption (from intestine or kidneys) or release (from bone breakdown)
Adrenal cortex	Cortisol Steroid	Targets most tissues, particularly liver, adipose, muscle, immune cells; many physiological functions, including metabolic regulation, blood pressure maintenance, immune modulation
	Aldosterone Steroid	Acts on the kidney to promote sodium retention and potassium excretion—required for normal blood pressure maintenance
	Androgens (dehydroepiandrosterone, DHEA, DHEA-sulfate) Steroid	Act on many target tissues to promote the development and maintenance of male characteristics
Adrenal medulla	Epinephrine and norepinephrine Catecholamines	Act on many target tissues to increase blood pressure, blood glucose, catabolism—active in stress responses
Pancreas	Insulin Protein: 51 aa	Targets liver, muscle, and fat, lowers blood glucose levels, promotes growth, anabolic hormone
	Glucagon Peptide: 29 aa	Targets liver, raises blood glucose levels, catabolic hormone
	Somatostatin (SST) Peptide: 14 or 28 aa	Acts locally within pancreas, paracrine action inhibits glucagon and insulin release

(*continued*)

TABLE 17.2 Hormones and Their Functions (*continued*)

Endocrine Source or Gland	Hormone/Class	Main Function of Hormone
Ovary	Estrogens Steroid	Target breasts, uterus, ovary, and other female reproductive structures to develop and maintain female primary and secondary sexual characteristics; regulate uterine proliferation during menstrual cycle
	Progesterone Steroid	Promotes the development of female sexual characteristics, required for pregnancy maintenance
Testis	Testosterone Steroid	Promotes the development and maintenance of male sexual characteristics and reproductive competence

aa, amino acids.
Source: From EndocrineSurgeon.Co.uk. What are the functions of the different types of hormones? http://www.endocrinesurgeon.co.uk/index.php/what-are-the-functions-of-the-different-types-of-hormone.

CIRCULATING HORMONE LEVELS

Hormones can circulate in plasma either freely dissolved in plasma (amines, peptides, and some proteins) or bound to other molecules such as serum binding proteins (steroid and thyroid hormones). The majority of circulating steroid and thyroid hormone molecules are bound to plasma protein carriers, but a small fraction, generally <10%, are unbound or "free." The hormone molecules spontaneously alternate between bound and free states, in an equilibrium relationship that depends on the relative concentrations of binding protein, bound hormone, and free hormone. The free fraction is able to enter cells, bind to its receptors, and exert intracellular effects, and is therefore biologically active. The concentration of bound hormone in plasma provides a readily accessible pool to maintain hormone activity, stabilizing the levels of free hormone and protecting the hormone molecules from rapid degradation or renal excretion. Laboratory tests for protein-bound hormones may measure either the total hormone (bound plus free) or just the free fraction, as noted later in the chapter where pertinent. Examples of hormones and their binding proteins are listed in Table 17.3.

Secretion of pituitary hormones is characterized by pulsatility (bursts of secretion occurring throughout the day and night, separated by pauses) and rhythms. Knowledge of these patterns is the key to interpreting biochemical testing of hormonal levels. As described later, most pituitary hormones, including adrenocorticotropic hormone (ACTH), growth hormone (GH), and prolactin (PRL), are secreted in pulses of varying time intervals. Pulsatility is measured by the frequency and amplitude of episodic hormone production, and encompasses the ultradian, circadian, and infradian rhythms mentioned previously. For this reason, some hormones are better measured after a stimulation (also known as provocation) test; for example, if their normal peak is during sleep.

TABLE 17.3 Hormones and Their Binding Proteins

Hormone	Binding Proteins
Cortisol	Corticosteroid-binding globulin Albumin
Adrenal androgens	Albumin
Estrogen	Albumin Sex hormone–binding globulin
Progesterone	Albumin
Testosterone	Sex hormone–binding globulin
Thyroid hormones (T_3 and T_4)	Thyroxine-binding globulin Transthyretin Albumin
Insulin-like growth factor (IGF)	Six different IGF binding proteins
Growth hormone	Growth hormone–binding protein

Source: From EndocrineSurgeon.co.uk. What are the functions of the different types of hormone? http://www.endocrinesurgeon.co.uk/index.php/what-are-the-functions-of-the-different-types-of-hormone.

Hormones have widely varying half-lives in the circulation. This is an important factor to consider when measuring hormone levels or clinically managing replacement hormone doses and dosing intervals. When providing exogenous hormone replacement, the time interval to when a drug dose reaches steady state is intimately connected to the rate of decay of the hormonal signal, which is dependent on factors such as rate of synthesis and secretion, degradation, and transport. For example, thyroxine (T_4) has a circulating half-life of 7 days and takes over 1 month to reach steady state. In contrast, triiodothyronine (T_3) has a half-life of 1 day. The half-life of steroids such as

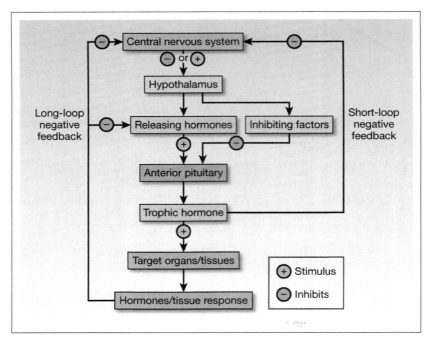

FIGURE 17.3 Secretion of anterior pituitary hormones is under the control of releasing and inhibiting hormones secreted by hypothalamic neuroendocrine cells onto blood vessels of the pituitary stalk. Pituitary trophic hormones (ACTH, TSH, LH, and FSH) stimulate target gland hormone secretion (adrenal glucocorticoids, thyroid hormone, and gonadal steroids, respectively). Target gland hormones provide feedback (usually negative) to inhibit pituitary and hypothalamic hormone secretion.

ACTH, adrenocorticotropic hormone; FSH, follicle-stimulating hormone; LH, luteinizing hormone; TSH, thyroid-stimulating hormone.

glucocorticoid analogues varies widely. This has implications for the timing of beneficial drug effects, as well as negative consequences such as suppression of the hypothalamic-pituitary-adrenal (HPA) axis by exogenous steroids.

HORMONE CONTROL AXES

Both negative and positive feedback regulation govern endocrine hormone secretion to maintain physiological homeostasis. Negative feedback regulation is more common. For example, increased blood glucose levels stimulate secretion of the hormone insulin, which subsequently promotes cell glucose uptake, lowering blood glucose back to normal levels. Secretion of certain target gland hormones (thyroid hormone, cortisol, testosterone, estrogen, and progesterone) is controlled by hypothalamic and pituitary hormones, which in turn are regulated by feedback exerted by those target gland hormones. Once target gland hormone level exceeds a threshold, this exerts negative feedback on both the pituitary cells producing the trophic hormone and the hypothalamus to suppress the releasing hormone (**Figures 17.3** and **17.4**).

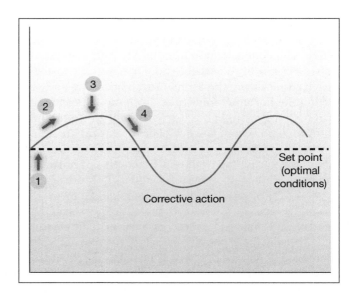

FIGURE 17.4 In a negative feedback system, deviation of a signal (blood glucose, blood pressure, stress hormone level) from a set point (for example, levels rising between times 1–2) is detected by sensors, resulting in a corrective change of hormone output at time 3. At time 4, the signal returns to set point. Decreases from the set point are also compensated by corrective actions that return the signal to the set point.

Once target organ levels fall below a threshold, or in times of increased demand, both hypothalamic-releasing hormones and subsequent pituitary hormonal production and secretion are stimulated.[16] On the other hand, positive feedback stimulates higher hormone production, as occurs during the female menstrual cycle when estrogen feeds back to stimulate synthesis and secretion of luteinizing hormone (LH), leading up to ovulation.

In these axes, disorders of endocrine function, whether related to hormone deficiency or hormone excess, may be related to primary organ failure or can be secondary to dysfunction in the pituitary or hypothalamus, with hypothalamic dysfunction being much less common. Differentiating between these possibilities requires measurements of both the pituitary hormone and the target gland hormone.

Thought Questions

1. How may hormonal cycles affect clinical evaluation of endocrine disorders?

2. What are some ways that hormone levels can be dysregulated in a hormone control axis?

Hypothalamus and Pituitary Gland

Christine Yedinak

The hypothalamus has two neuroendocrine roles: production of the peptide hormones vasopressin and oxytocin that act directly on target tissues (blood vessels, kidneys, breast, and uterus) and production of releasing and inhibiting hormones that alter the function of pituitary endocrine cells. Similarly, the pituitary gland has two classes of endocrine cells: somatotrophs and lactotrophs produce GH and PRL, respectively—these hormones act directly on peripheral tissues to have their effects; and corticotrophs, thyrotrophs, and gonadotrophs produce ACTH, thyroid-stimulating hormone (TSH), LH, and follicle-stimulating hormone (FSH), respectively—all are hormones targeting endocrine glands (adrenal, thyroid, and gonads) to stimulate gland growth and hormone secretion. The target gland hormones then provide negative feedback at the level of the hypothalamus and pituitary to suppress further pituitary trophic hormone secretion. The following segments describe the structure, function, and disorders of the hypothalamus and pituitary, followed by segments describing structure, function, and disorders of the adrenal and thyroid glands and the gonads in males and females.

STRUCTURE OF THE HYPOTHALAMUS

The hypothalamus is a brain region surrounding the third ventricle and lying just above the pituitary gland at the base of the brain. The hypothalamus is a relatively small region, constituting <1% of the brain volume, yet it is responsible for homeostasis of many body functions. The hypothalamus contains 11 major nuclei that integrate nervous system and endocrine system functions, either through the pituitary gland or through neuronal circuits (**Figure 17.5**). The hypothalamus is connected to the pituitary gland by the pituitary stalk (infundibulum) down which neuronal projections travel from hypothalamic nuclei to control hormonal production and release in the anterior and posterior pituitary (**Figure 17.6**).

The hypothalamic nuclei (paraventricular, supraoptic, arcuate, and others) control the release of anterior pituitary hormones. These nuclei secrete releasing and inhibiting hormones that control the release of all six anterior pituitary hormones:

- *Thyrotropin-releasing hormone* (TRH) regulates pituitary production and release of TSH.
- *Gonadotropin-releasing hormone* (GnRH) regulates both LH and FSH.
- *Growth hormone–releasing hormone* (GHRH) regulates GH.
- *Corticotropin-releasing hormone* (CRH) regulates the production and release of ACTH.
- The hypothalamic inhibiting hormones are somatostatin (SST—GH-inhibiting hormone) and the neurotransmitter dopamine, which serves as the inhibitor of PRL secretion.

Other hypothalamic nuclei include the suprachiasmatic nuclei, which are involved in the circadian clock, and nuclei found in the medial and lateral hypothalamic regions. The medial hypothalamus is integral to functions such as thermoregulation, sexual behavior, appetite, and body weight. Neurons of the lateral hypothalamus control sleep–wake transitions, feeding, energy balance, stress, reward, and motivated behavior.

The median eminence of the hypothalamus is the principal neuroendocrine link to the anterior pituitary and lies outside the blood–brain barrier. It is here that releasing and inhibiting hormones are delivered via portal blood vessels in the pituitary stalk to the cells of the anterior pituitary, stimulating or inhibiting the release of the anterior pituitary hormones.

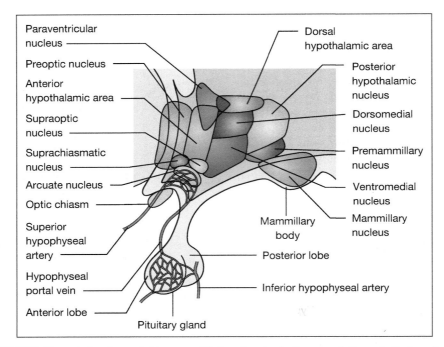

FIGURE 17.5 Hypothalamic nuclei have multiple roles, including regulation of pituitary hormone secretion through releasing and inhibiting hormones, generating and releasing posterior pituitary hormones, controlling water and food intake, thermoregulation, modulating sleep/wake states, and modifying autonomic nervous system activity.

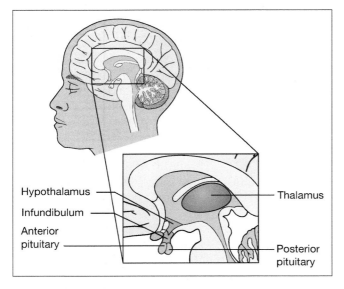

FIGURE 17.6 Hypothalamic–pituitary structural relationship. The hypothalamus lies at the bottom of the brain, surrounding the third cerebral ventricle. At its base, the infundibulum consists of axons of hypothalamic neuroendocrine cells and blood vessels. The neural tissue is continuous with the posterior pituitary gland, and the anterior pituitary gland sits in front of the posterior pituitary in the bony sella turcica.

FUNCTIONS OF THE HYPOTHALAMUS

Integrity of the hypothalamus is essential for survival and health. In addition to their endocrine roles, hypothalamic neurons project to the brainstem to regulate autonomic functions. Through bidirectional synaptic communications within and beyond the hypothalamus, hypothalamic neurons also regulate many behaviors that contribute to homeostasis.

THIRST AND FLUID BALANCE CONTROL

In response to increased blood osmolality, dehydration, or volume depletion, people subjectively experience thirst, mediated in part by the hormone angiotensin II. These conditions are sensed by osmoreceptor cells in the anterior hypothalamus. These cells project to vasopressin neuroendocrine cells in the paraventricular and supraoptic nuclei. As a peptide hormone, vasopressin is synthesized as a larger precursor protein that is cleaved as secretory vesicles travel down axon projections from these neurons through the pituitary stalk to the posterior pituitary (**Figures 17.7** and **17.8**). Other provasopressin cleavage products include the large carrier protein neurophysin II and copeptin, which can be measured as an indicator of vasopressin release. Vasopressin acts to promote renal water conservation and, in shock states, increased levels can serve as a vasoconstrictor.

Osmolality is the measure of the concentration of particles in a solvent (or the number of moles per kilogram of solvent) such as in blood or urine. Normal osmolality in adults ranges from 275 to 295 mOsm/kg H_2O, with an average of 280 to 285 mOsm/kg H_2O.[17] A linear relationship between plasma osmolality and circulating vasopressin concentration has been demonstrated in several studies. However, factors such as age and pregnancy may alter the sensitivity of the osmoreceptors and alter the osmolality set points.

REGULATION OF UTERINE CONTRACTILITY

Like vasopressin, oxytocin is a nonapeptide (composed of nine amino acids), and the amino acid sequences of these hormones differ by only two amino acids. Oxytocin synthesis and transport to the posterior pituitary are the same as described for vasopressin. Oxytocin is a potent stimulator of uterine contractions and a weak diuretic. Oxytocin levels increase at the end of pregnancy, influenced by signaling from increasing estrogen levels. The increase in oxytocin also results in the production of prostaglandins, which stimulate uterine contractility.[18]

REGULATION OF BODY ENERGY BALANCE AND WEIGHT

The regulation of body weight and appetite involves communication between the gut, adipose tissue, and the nervous system. Several hypothalamic nuclei play a key role in the regulation of appetite, satiety, weight, and energy balance. These include the arcuate, paraventricular, dorsomedial, ventromedial, and lateral hypothalamic nuclei. Bidirectional synaptic connections also occur between these hypothalamic nuclei and brainstem and limbic regions, contributing to food intake and energy homeostasis.

In the hypothalamus, appetite and energy expenditure are controlled by two populations of neurons: those expressing orexigenic peptides (neurons expressing neuropeptide Y/agouti-related peptide) and those expressing anorexigenic peptides (pro-opiomelanocortin [POMC]/cocaine- and amphetamine-regulated transcript/ α-melanocyte–stimulating hormone; **Figure 17.9**). The former initiate feeding, feeding reward, and energy conservation, and the latter promote increased energy expenditure and anorexia.[19] The only known peripheral

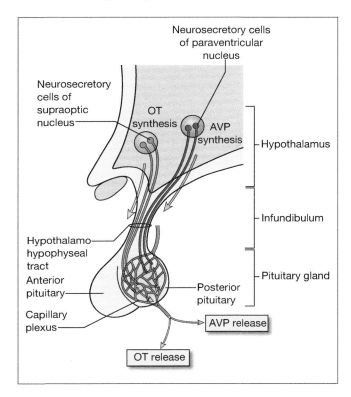

FIGURE 17.7 Neuroendocrine cells in the hypothalamic paraventricular and supraoptic nuclei produce OT and AVP, which are released into blood vessels of the posterior pituitary. AVP, arginine vasopressin; OT, oxytocin.

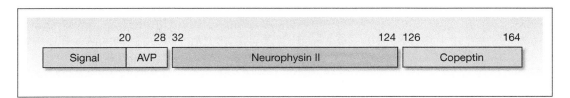

FIGURE 17.8 Arginine vasopressin (AVP) is synthesized as a large precursor protein (preprovasopressin) with signal peptide, neurophysin II, and copeptin. The signal peptide is removed in the endoplasmic reticulum. Within the storage vesicle, provasopressin is cleaved, releasing AVP, neurophysin II, and copeptin. These products are secreted together from axon terminals within the posterior pituitary, with neurophysin serving as carrier protein for vasopressin. Because the half-life of vasopressin is relatively short, clinical assays sometimes measure copeptin levels to evaluate endogenous vasopressin secretion rates.

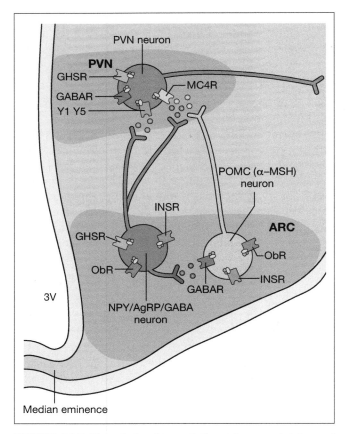

FIGURE 17.9 Hypothalamic regulation of energy intake and expenditure. The hypothalamic arcuate and paraventricular nuclei contribute to regulation of food intake and energy expenditure, integrating both central and peripheral signals. ARC NPY/AgRP/GABA neurons promote food intake via projections to the PVN, acting on Y1 and Y5 receptors. ARC POMC neurons synthesize α-MSH, which, when released on PVN neurons, tends to inhibit food intake.

AgRP, agouti-related peptide; ARC, arcuate nucleus; GABA, gamma-aminobutyric acid; GABAR, GABA receptor; GHSR, ghrelin receptor; INSR, insulin receptor; MC4R, melanocortin 4 receptor; α-MSH, α-melanocyte–stimulating hormone; NPY, neuropeptide Y; ObR, leptin receptor; POMC, pro-opiomelanocortin; PVN, paraventricular nucleus; Y1, Y5, NPY receptors type 1 and 5; 3V, third ventricle.

orexigenic (hunger-signaling) stimulus to the hypothalamus is from the hormone ghrelin (known as the "hunger hormone"), which is produced in the fundus of the stomach. Levels of ghrelin increase during fasting, bind to GH-stimulating receptor, and stimulate hunger and appetite while reducing energy expenditure.[20,21]

Multiple known peripheral anorexigenic (satiety-signaling, hunger-suppressing) stimuli act by binding to hypothalamic receptors, signaling the fed state and increasing energy expenditure. These signals originate from adipose tissue (leptin, adiponectin, and resistin), the gut, and pancreatic tissue (peptide YY, oxynto-modulin, glucagon-like peptide-1, cholecystokinin,

insulin, glucagon, pancreatic polypeptide, amylin, and insulin). The neurotransmitters glutamate and gamma-aminobutyric acid (GABA) signal neurons in the paraventricular nucleus to stimulate food intake during fasting, while also reducing energy expenditure.

Evidence for the role of these hormones and hypothalamic neurotransmitters in regulation of food intake and energy expenditure comes from human and animal studies, but they are not the whole story, particularly in humans. The pleasure (hedonic value) of eating, particularly highly palatable foods, can overcome the sense of satiety and cause ingestion of food in excess of body needs, resulting in weight gain.[21,22] Given the worldwide increase in obesity, the need for research into biological and behavioral factors underlying food intake and physical activity patterns is of paramount importance.

Thought Questions

3. What might be the impact of hypothalamic damage to thirst regulation?

4. What types of signals stimulate and inhibit food intake? What nuclei of the hypothalamus integrate this information?

5. How may pituitary function change in the event of hypothalamic damage?

DEVELOPMENT OF THE HYPOTHALAMUS AND RELATIONSHIP WITH THE PITUITARY GLAND

The pituitary gland is formed in embryogenesis when a pocket of oral ectoderm folds upward (evaginates) at the midline of the head, forming Rathke's pouch (**Figure 17.10**). The simultaneous downward pouching of the neuroectoderm at the midline base of the developing brain forms the infundibulum (pituitary stalk) and the route of innervation of the posterior pituitary. With further development, the link between the oral ectoderm and Rathke's pouch separates, leaving the anterior pituitary gland adjacent to the posterior pituitary.

The pituitary gland differentiates into three lobes: anterior (adenohypophysis), intermediate (pars intermedia), and posterior (neurohypophysis). In humans, the intermediate lobe is poorly demarcated. As previously noted, the hypothalamus and pituitary are linked via the infundibulum or pituitary stalk. Hypothalamic oxytocin and vasopressin neurons project axons down the pituitary stalk to terminate

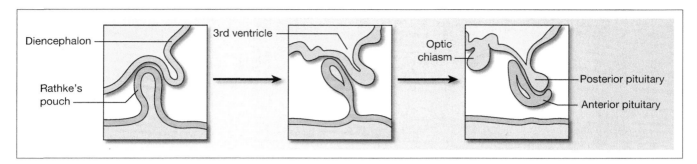

FIGURE 17.10 Embryonic development of the pituitary depends on two tissues: the oral ectoderm folding upward forms Rathke's pouch and meets the neural tissue folding downward. Rathke's pouch develops into the anterior pituitary and detaches from its source tissue. The neurally derived tissue forms the pituitary stalk connecting the hypothalamus directly with the posterior pituitary. *Source:* Redrawn from VIVO Pathophysiology. Development and Anatomy of the Pituitary Gland. http://www.vivo.colostate.edu/hbooks/pathphys/endocrine/hypopit/histo_pit.html.

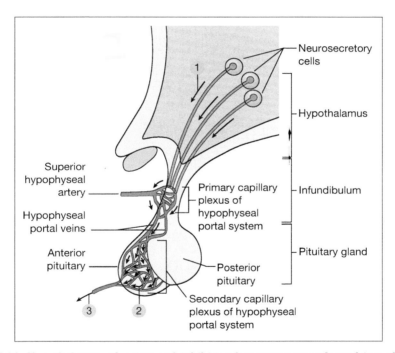

FIGURE 17.11 Hypothalamic releasing and inhibiting hormones are released into the capillary bed of the pituitary stalk **(1)**, travel by portal veins to the anterior pituitary, and diffuse out of the anterior pituitary capillaries to perfuse the hormone-secreting cells there **(2)**. The balance of hypothalamic releasing and inhibiting hormones determines the level of anterior pituitary hormone synthesis and secretion **(3)**.

on blood vessels in the posterior pituitary (see the discussion of posterior pituitary hormones, later). Hypothalamic neurons that produce releasing and inhibiting hormones project to the median eminence of the hypothalamus, terminating on the portal blood vessels in the pituitary stalk. Once released into the portal vessels, these hypothalamic releasing and inhibiting hormones flow into the anterior pituitary, perfusing that lobe's endocrine cells and providing stimulation or inhibition of pituitary hormone production and secretion (**Figure 17.11**).[23]

ENDOCRINE CELLS OF THE ANTERIOR PITUITARY

The anterior pituitary is responsible for the production of six major hormones that regulate target gland and end-organ function: ACTH, TSH, LH, FSH, GH, and PRL, as summarized in **Table 17.4**. The cells that synthesize and secrete these hormones are located in clusters within the pituitary and are most often monoclonal, making only one hormone. The most common diseases of the pituitary

TABLE 17.4 Targets of Pituitary Hormones

Hormone	Cell Type	Percentage of Pituitary Population	Targets
Growth hormone (GH)	Somatotroph	50	Liver, bone, muscle, adipose
Adrenocorticotropic hormone (ACTH)	Corticotroph	15–20	Adrenal cortex
Luteinizing hormone (LH), Follicle-stimulating hormone (FSH)	Gonadotroph	10–15	Gonads
Prolactin (PRL)	Lactotroph	10–25	Breasts, gonads
Thyroid stimulating hormone (TSH)	Thyrotroph	<10	Thyroid

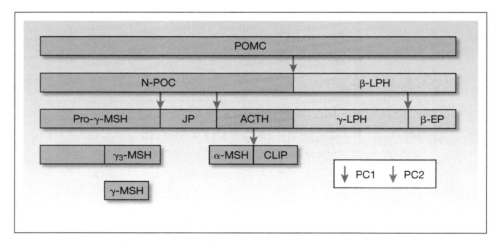

FIGURE 17.12 The *POMC* gene is expressed in anterior pituitary corticotrophs, in hypothalamic intermediate lobe cells, in certain hypothalamic neurons, and in other brain regions. Differential splicing allows cells to produce different final products from the gene. Final post-translational processing in corticotrophs produces ACTH and β-endorphin for secretion.

ACTH, adrenocorticotropic hormone; β-EP, beta-endorphin; β-LPH, beta-lipotropin; CLIP, corticotropin-like intermediate lobe peptide; γ-LPH, gamma-lipotropin; JP, joining peptide; PC1 and PC2, prohormone convertases 1 and 2; MSH, melanocyte-stimulating hormone; N-POC, N-terminal proopiocortin; POMC, pro-opiomelanocortin.

involve adenomas of a particular cell type that secrete excess hormone. The majority of these are prolactinomas, followed by GH-secreting tumors, then ACTH-secreting tumors. Tumors producing TSH or gonadotropins are quite rare. Nonsecreting pituitary adenomas are also common, and cause pathological effects by compressing the adjacent cells, rather than by hormone overproduction.

CORTICOTROPH CELLS: ADRENOCORTICOTROPIC HORMONE

Corticotrophs constitute 10% to 20% of all anterior pituitary cells.[23,24] ACTH is a peptide hormone synthesized from a larger precursor protein, POMC, within the corticotrophs. ACTH secretion is stimulated by the release of CRH from the median eminence of the hypothalamus. CRH secretion is pulsatile, with a half-life of 7 to 12 minutes. After transport via the hypophyseal portal veins, CRH binds to receptors on the membrane of the corticotrophs. This activates *POMC* gene expression and subsequent processing. When POMC is processed, several biologically active peptide fragments result: ACTH and β-lipotropin, α-melanocyte–stimulating hormone (α-MSH), and endorphins are produced (**Figure 17.12**).

ACTH binds to G protein–coupled receptors in the three outer layers of the adrenal cortex, stimulating the production of corticosteroids (glucocorticoids, cortisol, and corticosterone), mineralocorticoids (aldosterone), and androgens. Once synthesized in the adrenal cortex and released into the circulation, cortisol then provides negative feedback at the level of the hypothalamus and the pituitary to suppress the production of CRH and ACTH, respectively. This dynamic feedback interaction is referred to as the *HPA axis* (**Figure 17.13**).

Typically, ACTH and cortisol are secreted in a circadian fashion with the highest levels in the early morning, and the lowest levels at night. However, physical and emotional stressors such as trauma, surgery, pain, depression, hypoglycemia, cold exposure, fear, anxiety, and feeding elicit episodic ACTH pulses, elevating the levels of cortisol over and above the normal circadian production.

Corticotroph Dysfunction

Hypocortisolism may be primary (related to adrenal failure) or secondary. **Secondary adrenal insufficiency** from inadequate pituitary ACTH production may occur as the result of pituitary damage or prolonged suppression of the HPA axis after chronic exogenous administration of glucocorticoids, such as prednisone, causing iatrogenic hypocortisolism. Specific examples of pituitary damage leading to hypocortisolism include the following:

* Surgical removal of a noncorticotroph pituitary adenoma
* Removal of an ACTH hypersecretory tumor
* Cranial irradiation
* Pituitary hemorrhage
* Postpartum Sheehan syndrome

Clinical aspects of hypocortisolism are discussed later in the context of adrenal cortex function and disease.

Central hypercortisolism, also known as ACTH-dependent hypercortisolism, results from inappropriate high production of pituitary ACTH, causing **Cushing disease**. Excess ACTH results in overstimulation and upregulation of cortisol production from the adrenal cortex and, ultimately, hypertrophy of the adrenal glands bilaterally (see **Figure 17.13**).[25] Although relatively rare, this can be a lethal disease, associated with cardiovascular disease, hypercoagulability, and infection.

Approximately 70% of all cases of Cushing disease are the result of a benign corticotroph cell pituitary adenoma. However, the adenoma may be too small to be found on imaging in up to 50% of confirmed cases. The remaining 30% of cases are from ectopic tumors that can develop in the lungs or adrenal cortex. The incidence

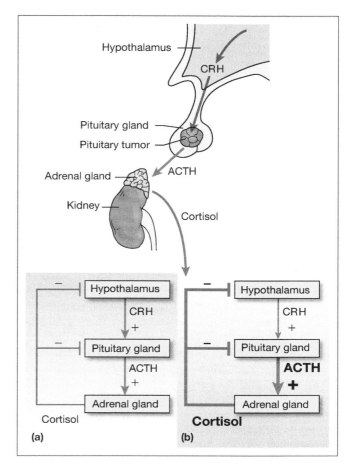

FIGURE 17.13 ACTH-stimulated cortisol production: the HPA axis and negative feedback. **(a)** In the normal HPA axis, hypothalamic CRH stimulates pituitary release of ACTH, resulting in stimulation of cortisol synthesis and secretion, and growth promotion of all of the adrenal gland layers. Cortisol also provides negative feedback to the pituitary and hypothalamus, inhibiting excessive ACTH and CRH secretion. **(b)** In Cushing disease, an ACTH-secreting pituitary adenoma continuously secretes supranormal amounts of ACTH, driving adrenal gland hyperplasia and excessive cortisol secretion. Negative feedback via increased cortisol inhibits hypothalamic CRH secretion, but is ineffective at reducing ACTH secretion from the autonomously activated tumor cells. ACTH, adrenocorticotropic hormone; CRH, corticotropin-releasing hormone; HPA, hypothalamic-pituitary-adrenal.

of Cushing disease is estimated at 0.7 to 2.4 per million population per year.[25]

Clinical manifestations of hypercortisolism, which are similar for pituitary and adrenal Cushing syndrome, are discussed later in conjunction with adrenal hypercortisolism. Treatment is aimed at surgical or radiation-based removal of the pituitary tumor, medical therapy to suppress ACTH or adrenal cortisol production, the removal of the ectopic ACTH-producing tumor, or bilateral adrenalectomy to remove the source of excess cortisol production.[26,27]

Management approaches include the following:

- SST therapies that inhibit pituitary ACTH production and secretion
- Therapies that competitively block glucocorticoid receptors (GRs)
- Drugs that inhibit biosynthesis of cortisol in the adrenal cortex

LACTOTROPH CELLS: PROLACTIN

Lactotroph cells in the anterior pituitary secrete the protein hormone prolactin (PRL), which promotes breast development at puberty and during pregnancy. Lactotrophs make up 15% to 25% of all pituitary cells. Molecular weight of and antibody binding to PRL molecules are important determinants of PRL biological activity. The majority of secreted PRL is classified as "small" PRL, consisting of a single PRL protein chain. When two PRL molecules are bound together, they form "big" PRL, with molecular weight of 48 to 56 kDa. "Big, big" PRL (>100 kDa) consists of multiple PRL subunits, sometimes bound to immunoglobulin. The presence of these different forms of PRL complicates laboratory assays. The molecules may elevate the measured PRL level, but are biologically inactive and confound the clinical interpretation of elevated serum levels. Also related to PRL measurements, extremely high PRL levels produce artifactual results in antigen–antibody assay methodology, because they saturate the antibody concentration used for testing. This results in a false low PRL measurement known as the "hook effect," which is avoided by diluting the serum sample.[28,29]

The circulating level of PRL is regulated by the secretion of PRL releasing factors, with several hypothalamic hormones and neurotransmitters capable of increasing PRL release. Dopamine is the prominent PRL inhibiting factor and is tonically active in the absence of pregnancy and lactation. Neurons in the arcuate nucleus release dopamine into the portal circulation of the anterior pituitary. This binds to D2 receptors on pituitary lactotrophs, inhibiting the production and secretion of PRL.[28]

PRL secretion is episodic, with increased pulse amplitude within 60 to 90 minutes of sleep onset and after consumption of protein-containing meals. However, PRL production is activated by diverse stimuli and mechanisms. Estrogen is a key influence on lactotrophs, activating both PRL synthesis and lactotroph proliferation, particularly during pregnancy, when pituitary enlargement is primarily due to lactotroph proliferation. PRL levels increase throughout pregnancy, preparing the breast for postpartum lactation. At pregnancy term, PRL levels are ten-fold higher than prepregnancy levels. Postdelivery suckling is a strong stimulator inducing rapid release of PRL. Postpartum PRL levels remain slightly elevated while breastfeeding, but decrease between episodes of suckling. PRL acts on cytokine-type membrane receptors with tyrosine kinase activity to increase the production of milk proteins, fats, and lactose production in support of lactation. PRL inhibits GnRH secretion, so breastfeeding is associated with suppression of the menstrual cycle, ovulation, and menstruation.

Lactotroph Dysfunction

Hypoprolactinemia appears to be rare, and may be idiopathic or related to general hypopituitarism in conditions like Sheehan syndrome or ablative surgery for a pituitary adenoma. The major consequence of PRL deficiency is the inability to lactate.

Hyperprolactinemia is very common and has been shown to occur in 1% to 10% of a random population sampling, with women more commonly affected than men.[29] Pituitary PRL-secreting adenomas (**prolactinomas**) are the most common cause of elevated serum PRL levels and lactotroph adenomas are the most frequently occurring pituitary adenomas. These adenomas may be small (microadenomas <1 cm) or large (macroadenomas >1 cm), with the majority presenting as microadenomas.

Most patients present with clinical symptoms of elevated PRL, such as amenorrhea and infertility, hypogonadism, galactorrhea not associated with childbirth, and headaches. Infertility associated with hyperprolactinemia has been demonstrated to be associated with interference in multiple steps in reproduction, but is chiefly due to suppression of GnRH pulses from the hypothalamus with subsequent suppression of the mid-cycle LH surge.[30,31] Although women are affected more frequently, men will often present with infertility and headaches, and are subsequently found to have larger pituitary adenomas. Hypogonadism and visual deficits may be found on patient assessment.

Multiple physiological factors can precipitate PRL elevation, with the most obvious being pregnancy. When laboratory assessment shows unexpected elevated PRL levels in a woman of childbearing age, pregnancy should be considered. Other factors elevating PRL include stress, chest wall stimulation or trauma, acute exercise, hypoglycemia, and renal failure that decreases renal clearance of PRL. Numerous medications are known to elevate PRL level, particularly first-generation dopamine antagonist antipsychotic drugs, and including opioid agonists, estrogens, and some prokinetics.[32] In these cases, withdrawal of an offending medication will normalize the PRL level. Pituitary stalk (infundibulum) disruptions or deviations related to injury, or a space-occupying lesion, may decrease dopamine inhibition of PRL, secondarily increasing PRL levels.

Because of the relatively high prevalence of pituitary micro- and macroadenomas associated with hyperprolactinemia, MRI scans of the pituitary and hypothalamus are recommended in addition to laboratory assays of PRL. Endocrine guidelines strongly recommend MRI when the PRL level is found to be >100 µg/L using a diluted PRL assay.[33]

Management of hyperprolactinemia is based on the known inhibitory effect of dopamine on PRL secretion. Dopamine agonists such as bromocriptine and cabergoline are used as first-line therapy. These drugs effectively inhibit PRL production and secretion, and shrink PRL tumors. Surgical removal of the tumor and radiation are rarely indicated and are reserved for patients intolerant to dopamine agonist therapy or with a tumor that is resistant to other treatments.

SOMATOTROPH CELLS: GROWTH HORMONE

Growth hormone (GH) is a large protein hormone that has structural similarity to PRL. It is synthesized and secreted by anterior pituitary somatotroph cells that make up about 50% of all anterior pituitary cells. Circulating levels of GH peak in fetal life at about 20 weeks, fall immediately after birth, are somewhat elevated in childhood and adolescence, are stable during adulthood, and then progressively decline with advancing age. GH secretion is under both stimulatory and inhibitory control by the hypothalamus. GHRH is released from neurons in the median eminence of the hypothalamus and binds to receptors on the somatotroph membrane, activating the synthesis and secretion of GH. The stomach-derived hormone ghrelin is also a GH secretagogue, while hypothalamic SST inhibits GH secretion. A major

action of GH in the periphery is the stimulation of liver production and secretion of insulin-like growth factor 1 (IGF-1), which has growth-promoting actions and also provides negative feedback to inhibit pituitary GH secretion (**Figure 17.14**).

GH has a short half-life of 10 to 20 minutes and is produced and secreted in a pulsatile fashion, with the highest amplitude pulses during slow-wave sleep (**Figure 17.15**). In addition to sleep, GH production

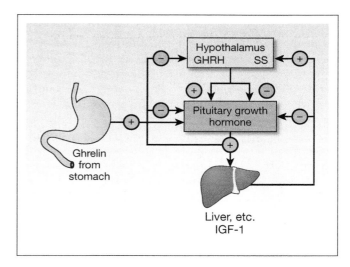

FIGURE 17.14 GH secretion is stimulated by hypothalamic GHRH and by ghrelin released from the stomach mucosa. Growth hormone acts on the liver to stimulate secretion of IGF-1, which feeds back to suppress pituitary GH secretion. IGF-1 also stimulates hypothalamic SS secretion, which also inhibits GH secretion.

GH, growth hormone; GHRH, growth hormone–releasing hormone; IGF-1, insulin-like growth factor 1; SS, somatostatin.

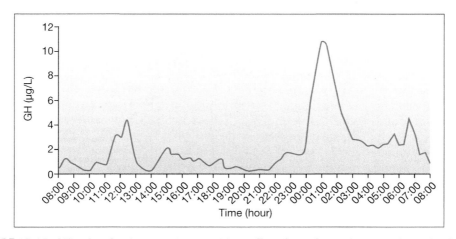

FIGURE 17.15 GH pulsatility is intermittent, with small peaks and troughs throughout the day and a high peak during slow-wave sleep.

GH, growth hormone.

and secretion are stimulated by exercise, emotional stress, starvation and malnutrition, and high-protein meals. GH receptors are of the tyrosine kinase–linked type: When GH binds, two identical receptor subunits dimerize, begin to self-phosphorylate, and initiate JAK-STAT (Janus kinase–signal transducer and activator of transcription) signaling, as described in Chapter 4, Cell Physiology and Pathophysiology.

IGF-1 receptors resemble the insulin receptor in having two copies each of α and β subunits linked together. IGF-1 binding to its receptor induces receptor autophosphorylation and association with intracellular proteins, leading to their activation. IGF-1 receptor activation stimulates intracellular insulin receptor substrates (IRS), as well as the phosphatidylinositol-3-kinase/Akt (PI3K/Akt) pathway and the Ras/Raf pathway. All of these actions are consistent with a role in growth, development, and cell proliferation. Through these multiple mechanisms, GH plays an integral role in bone metabolism and long bone growth, carbohydrate and protein metabolism, lipolysis and body composition, muscle strength and exercise performance, and cardiovascular function. In plasma, GH circulates attached to binding proteins before binding to receptors in target tissues. It antagonizes circulating insulin levels by increasing glucose production through gluconeogenesis and glycogenolysis from the liver and kidney and inducing insulin resistance (**Figure 17.16**). At normal levels, the major actions of GH and IGF are to support normal tissue maintenance, increase lean muscle mass, and maintain bone structure.[34]

Somatotroph Dysfunction

GH deficiency and GH excess have profound effects on growth, development, morbidity and mortality. **Growth hormone deficiency** may be congenital, as in classic forms of deficiency that are associated with growth retardation. This is defined as linear height >2.5 standard deviations below the mean height for age- and sex-matched children. Acquired and adult-onset GH deficiency may be associated with head trauma, hypothalamic and pituitary tumors and surgery, autoimmune and infiltrative disorders, and cranial irradiation.[35]

Clinical manifestations of GH deficiency include increased adiposity (particularly abdominal), decreased muscle strength, and low bone density. Mortality risk is increased from cardiovascular risk factors such as hypercoagulability and atherosclerosis, poor exercise performance, and low lung capacity. Given that the levels of GH are normally low during the day (outside of the nocturnal peak), assessment of GH deficiency is usually performed with challenge testing. Intravenous administration of GHRH, arginine, dopamine, or insulin (sufficient to produce hypoglycemia) all should produce a robust increase in GH levels, and lack of this response indicates primary failure of GH secretion. Treatment for GH deficiency in childhood targets linear growth by administering recombinant GH. The response to GH administration is based on serum levels of IGF-1, in which achieving the normal range for age and sex is the biochemical target.

Excess growth hormone production (hypersomatotropism) results in **gigantism** (in children prior to the fusing of growth plates) and **acromegaly** (adults). All organs are affected (with the exception of the brain) and grow under the influence of autonomous production of GH and subsequent IGF-1 excess. Over 95% of patients with acromegaly have a GH-secreting pituitary adenoma with some tumors expressing both GH and PRL (**Figure 17.17**).

Clinical features of GH excess are usually late appearing and include acral growth, frontal bossing, increased teeth spacing, carpal tunnel syndrome, and arthropathies. Patients often present with headache, menstrual irregularities, infertility and impotence, fatigue, hyperhidrosis, growth of hands or feet, and thyroid disorders. Visual deficits, particularly peripheral field deficits, may occur if the tumor is large and impacts the optic chiasm lying above the pituitary fossa. The onset can be insidious until progressing to recognizable changes in appearance and well-being.[36]

Biochemical evaluation of patients presenting with symptoms suggestive of GH excess include random serum GH and IGF-1 levels. As previously described, GH levels are pulsatile but IGF-1 levels are more stable over time. Therefore, an elevated serum IGF-1 requires further evaluation with brain MRI using contrast material that includes pituitary views. The first-line treatment for GH excess is the removal of the somatotroph tumor. If surgical treatment is not effective, or if the patient is not a candidate for surgery, treatment with SST analogues is used to suppress pituitary GH synthesis and secretion.

GONADOTROPH CELLS: LUTEINIZING HORMONE AND FOLLICLE-STIMULATING HORMONE

Luteinizing hormone (LH) and follicle-stimulating hormone (FSH) are glycoproteins secreted from pituitary gonadotrophs and are essential for reproduction and sexual maturity. Both have a common α subunit and unique β subunit, and bind to G protein–coupled receptors on target cells.[37] Gonadotroph hormone levels are tightly controlled by positive stimulation from hypothalamic GnRH and negative feedback from sex steroids produced in the testes and ovaries, within the hypothalamic-pituitary-gonadal (HPG) axis. The HPG axis is differentially active during at least five phases of the human life cycle: from prenatal development to infancy, childhood, puberty, adulthood, and postmenopause/andropause.

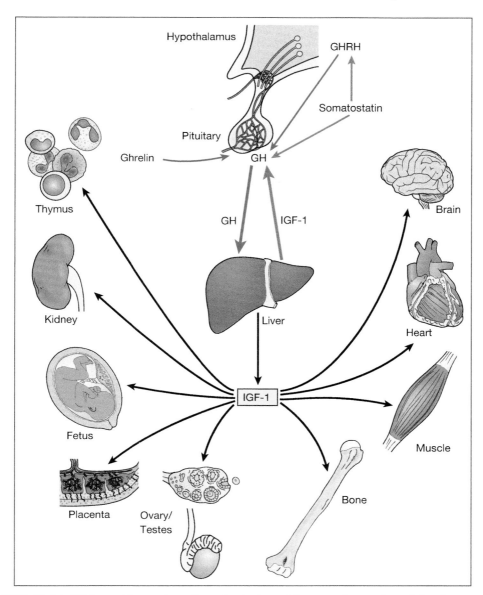

FIGURE 17.16 GH has wide-ranging effects beginning with prenatal growth and development of the placenta, fetal growth and development, and maintenance of thymus, kidney, gonads, heart, and brain. The most pronounced effects of GH on development and maintenance are on bone and muscle. Linear growth in childhood is dependent on GH stimulation, and GH deficiency is associated with short stature, whereas GH excess in children is associated with attainment of extreme height. Many GH effects are mediated by IGF-1, produced by the liver in response to GH stimulation.

GH, growth hormone; GHRH, growth hormone–releasing hormone; IGF-1, insulin-like growth factor 1.

Source: From Martin-Estal I, de la Garza RG, Castilla-Cortazar I. Intrauterine growth retardation (IUGR) as a novel condition of insulin-like growth factor-1 (IGF-1) deficiency. *Rev Physiol Biochem Pharmacol.* 2016:170-1-35. doi:170.10.1007/112_2015_5001.

About 10% to 15% of anterior pituitary cells are gonadotrophs. Hypothalamic GnRH is detectable by 6 weeks of gestational age and is released from neurons that migrate from outside the central nervous system to the arcuate nucleus of the hypothalamus along the olfactory nerves.[38] GnRH stimulates gonadotroph cells to produce LH and FSH as early as 12 to 14 weeks of gestational age, peaking at about 20 weeks and declining with the production of sex steroids. The placental hormone human chorionic gonadotropin (hCG) appears to promote the development of androgen production in fetal testis even in the absence of pituitary LH and FSH.

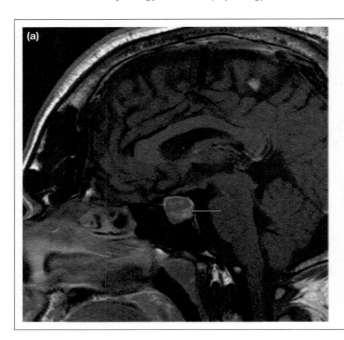
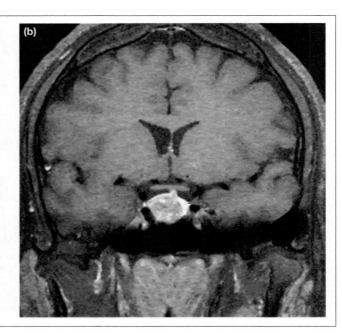

FIGURE 17.17 Growth hormone–producing pituitary tumor. **(a)** T1-weighted MRI sagittal view. **(b)** T1-weighted MRI coronal view. Arrows indicate tumor.

In infancy, serum levels of LH and FSH peak at about 2 to 3 months of age, with levels in males declining more quickly than levels in females and remaining low until puberty. Although the precise stimulus for puberty is not known, at this time nocturnal pulses of GnRH increase the levels of LH first, then FSH. Daytime GnRH pulses occur as puberty progresses. During adulthood, pulsatile secretion of gonadotropins is variable in males but occurs in dynamic cyclical patterns in females. GnRH stimulation testing can be used to establish the maturity of the HPG axis.

Gonadotroph cells may secrete either LH or FSH, or both hormones. In the testes, FSH regulates Sertoli cell number, maturation, and function and thereby testosterone production. LH is involved in Leydig cell maturation, survival, and proliferation, as described later in the chapter. In women, LH and FSH are released from the pituitary in short bursts, stimulating the ovarian synthesis of estrogen and progesterone and promoting the regulation of menstruation and ovulation, as described later.

Pubertal development of HPG axis function depends on the neuropeptide kisspeptin. Expression of kisspeptin and receptors for kisspeptin increases with the onset of puberty. Kisspeptin binds to G protein–coupled receptors on hypothalamic arcuate and periventricular nuclei to activate GnRH pulses.[37]

Gonadotroph Dysfunction

Gonadotroph hypofunction, although rare, is seen more often than hyperfunction. Clinically, patients may present with infertility and symptoms of hypogonadism, and androgen or estrogen deficiency. Inadequate GnRH stimulation of LH and FSH or failure of adequate hCG stimulation for sexual development in utero may result in male anomalies such as ambiguous genitalia or undescended testes. Most female clinical manifestations of hypogonadism occur after birth.[38]

THYROTROPH CELLS: THYROID-STIMULATING HORMONE

Thyrotrophs represent only about 5% of all pituitary cells and are responsible for synthesizing thyroid-stimulating hormone (TSH), a glycoprotein of linked α and β subunits.[39] Hypothalamic TRH stimulates TSH secretion, which in turn stimulates hormone production and secretion by thyroid cells, as described later in the chapter. TSH secretion is diurnal, with nocturnal surges in production. The actions of thyroid hormones are broad, promoting or affecting fetal and nervous system development and childhood growth; myocardial contraction and relaxation and heart rate; gastrointestinal motility; and renal water clearance.

TRH neurons are located in the hypothalamic paraventricular nuclei. TRH binds to pituitary thyrotroph cell surface receptors, stimulating the secretion of TSH. Once secreted into the circulation, TSH has a half-life of 35 to 50 minutes. It binds to cell surface receptors in the thyroid, stimulating thyroid growth and production and release of thyroid hormones. TRH and TSH secretion are suppressed by negative feedback from the thyroid hormones T_3 and T_4, although the effect on TSH is greater than the negative feedback on TRH. Increased serum levels of T_3 and T_4 also signal the hypothalamus to secrete SST, which inhibits TSH secretion.

Thyrotroph Dysfunction

TSH deficiency may be acquired with injury to, or destruction of, the hypothalamus or the anterior pituitary thyrotrophs, as described previously for the other anterior pituitary hormones. Central (secondary) hypothyroidism is indicated by a low serum TSH and low free (unbound) T_4. When central hypothyroidism is present, TSH is no longer a reliable indicator of thyroid function and free T_4 must be assessed.

TSH excess may be caused by a mutation in pituitary thyrotropes with excess or autonomous TSH production that is unresponsive to negative feedback. Although this form of excess is rare, somatostatin analogues are effective in suppressing TSH in this condition.[40] Medications such as glucocorticoids may impair pituitary sensitivity to TRH, lowering TSH, whereas estrogens appear to increase thyrotroph sensitivity.

POSTERIOR PITUITARY HORMONES

The posterior pituitary differs from the glandular anterior pituitary, consisting of a collection of terminal axonal projections from the hypothalamus. The posterior pituitary hormones are the peptides arginine vasopressin (AVP) and oxytocin (OT). These nonapeptides (made up of nine amino acids) differ in structure by two amino acids and have enough structural similarity that each can bind to and activate the receptor(s) of the other. It should also be noted here that, in addition to projecting to the posterior pituitary, vasopressin and oxytocin have distinct projections within the brain, functioning as neuropeptide transmitters within behavior-associated neural networks. Although beyond the scope of this text, these behavioral effects of the posterior pituitary hormones have been the focus of a substantial body of scholarship.[41,42]

VASOPRESSIN: ANTIDIURETIC HORMONE

AVP acts in the kidney to increase water reabsorption and produce concentrated urine. At higher levels, AVP is also a vasoconstrictor and assists in compensation for hypovolemia states. Multiple factors affect the secretion of AVP. These include dehydration, hypovolemia, hypotension, hypoxia, and increased blood osmolality. Norepinephrine and angiotensin are powerful stimulants of thirst and AVP secretion. Pregnancy lowers the threshold for AVP secretion. A decline in blood pressure exponentially increases the release of AVP.

Activation of AVP secretion in response to increased blood osmolality depends on osmoreceptors in the anterior hypothalamus. These neurons relay to the AVP neurons in the paraventricular and supraoptic nuclei to increase action potential firing rates, resulting in AVP release from the posterior pituitary. AVP secretion in response to blood volume loss is mediated by low- and high-pressure baroreceptors as well as increased angiotensin levels.

Both cleaved and uncleaved forms of AVP (see **Figure 17.8**) are stored in neurosecretory vesicles in the posterior pituitary. Both forms are released into circulation, but only AVP has biological activity. AVP is not protein bound and has a plasma half-life of 5 to 15 minutes. There are three major types of G protein–coupled AVP receptors: V_{1a} (vascular, hepatic, and brain), V_{1b} (anterior pituitary), and V_2 (a renal adenylyl cyclase–coupled receptor). When AVP binds to V_2 receptors on the basolateral membrane of renal collecting duct cells, aquaporin 2 water channels are inserted in the apical cell membrane for the reabsorption of water, as described in Chapter 12, Kidneys.

Diabetes Insipidus

Diabetes insipidus (DI) occurs when AVP secretion fails, leading to inability to reabsorb water and sodium and to produce concentrated urine. Hypothalamic or pituitary injury may cause temporary (lasting hours to days) or permanent forms of DI. Several brain disorders, tumors, and damage to the pituitary stalk (e.g., after head trauma or pituitary surgery) can cause temporary or permanent disruption of vasopressin secretion, resulting in central DI. In this condition, renal water reabsorption is impaired, resulting in the production of copious amounts of dilute (clear) urine and unquenchable thirst. Blood studies show hypernatremia and high serum osmolality, and urine has low osmolality. In most cases, vasopressin secretion gradually recovers. If there is no or partial recovery, or in cases of genetic deficiency of vasopressin, the synthetic analogue desmopressin can be administered. Nephrogenic DI can also be congenital, resulting from a mutation in the V_2 receptor gene, rendering the kidney tubule cells insensitive to the actions of AVP.

Syndrome of Inappropriate Antidiuretic Hormone Secretion

Syndrome of inappropriate antidiuretic hormone secretion (SIADH), or posterior pituitary AVP hypersecretion, is a diagnosis of exclusion. Excessive renal water retention coupled with normal sodium excretion results in hyponatremia (plasma sodium of <130 nmol/L) and serum hypoosmolality. Urine is usually concentrated, with high osmolality. The hyponatremia and hypoosmolality may be improved by restricting water intake. SIADH has many possible causes, the most common of which is ectopic AVP production by tumors such as small cell lung cancer and cancer cells in other sites. Other causes include central nervous system trauma or disease, lung disorders such as pneumonia, and adverse effects of drugs.

SIADH treatment is aimed at addressing the cause. If osmotically induced, free water restriction may be sufficient to restore homeostasis, but in severe cases, hypertonic saline infusions may be indicated. It is vital to understand that this is a disorder of water excess and not low sodium. The greatest danger in untreated SIADH is hyponatremia, which can result in acute neurological dysfunction with increased intracranial pressure, seizures, and coma. Likewise, rapid sodium rise can result in osmotic demyelination syndrome and permanent damage to the myelin sheath of nerve cells in the pons. Slow correction with free water restriction and cautious sodium replacement is essential. Drugs that block V_2 receptors can also be used in treatment of SIADH.[43]

OXYTOCIN

Like vasopressin, OT is a short peptide of nine amino acids produced by neurons within the hypothalamic paraventricular and supraoptic nuclei. The role of OT in lactation is discussed later in this chapter, in the female reproductive section. OT stimulates contraction of uterine smooth muscle and is one of many mediators involved in the progress of labor and childbirth. During pregnancy, OT levels remain stable until the late stages of labor. In addition, myometrial OT receptor expression increases during labor. In late labor, there is a reflex release of OT in response to vaginal stretch, promoting uterine contractions that expel the fetus and the placenta. The uterine-contracting properties of OT are the basis for OT infusions to induce labor and its use in management of postpartum hemorrhage.[44]

Thought Questions

6. Compare properties of the anterior pituitary trophic hormones that act on target glands with the anterior pituitary growth- and development-promoting hormones. What are their similarities and differences?

7. Compare properties of the anterior pituitary hormones with the posterior pituitary hormones. How are they similar or different relative to regulation and mechanism of secretion, vulnerability to brain trauma and inflammation, and long-term consequences of dysfunction?

Adrenal Glands

Christine Yedinak

Adrenal gland hormones contribute to stress responses as well as regulating metabolism, immune responses, blood pressure, vascular volume, electrolytes, and secondary sex characteristics. This is achieved by the production of three classes of steroids: mineralocorticoids, glucocorticoids, and adrenal androgens.

DEVELOPMENT, STRUCTURE, AND FUNCTION OF THE ADRENAL GLANDS

The adrenal glands are located above and medial to the kidneys bilaterally at the level of the 12th thoracic vertebra and are separated from the renal capsule by a connective tissue layer. They are composed of an outer cortex of glandular tissue and an inner medulla of epinephrine- and norepinephrine-secreting *chromaffin* cells that are derived from neural crest cells, similar to sympathetic postganglionic neurons.[45]

The adrenal glands begin to appear at around 3 to 4 weeks of gestational age as the mesoderm forms the adrenal cortex and the ectoderm generates the cells that will migrate to form the adrenal medulla.

By week 8, the migration of sympathetic cells from the neural crest into the medulla has occurred, and the adrenal gland is enveloped in a capsule and separated from the kidney. The cortex initially develops as two zones: the outer zone that begins to produce glucocorticoids and mineralocorticoids by about 8 weeks of gestational age, and a large inner zone that produces dehydroepiandrosterone (DHEA) and dehydroepiandrosterone sulfate (DHEAS). Fetal DHEA and DHEAS are converted to estrogen by the placenta and contribute to maintenance of pregnancy.

The fetal layers transition after birth, with the inner zone shrinking and the outer zone developing into the three layers of the adult cortex (zona glomerulosa [outer], zona fasciculata [middle], and zona reticularis [inner]), which are not fully differentiated until after 2 years of age. The zona reticularis is not fully active until *adrenarche* occurs, between 6 and 8 years of age in females and 7 and 9 years of age in males, when secondary sex characteristics begin to appear.[46] **Box 17.1** and **Figure 17.18** illustrate the key steps in the synthesis of steroid hormones. **Figure 17.19** illustrates the adrenal gland zones associated with hormone production.

BOX 17.1
Pathways of Steroid Hormone Synthesis

1. The precursor for all steroid hormones is cholesterol, most of which comes from blood LDL brought into the steroid-secreting cells by receptor-mediated endocytosis. Most steroid-secreting cells in the adrenal gland and in the gonads also have some capacity for cholesterol synthesis from acetyl coenzyme A and the ability to obtain cholesterol from intracellular lipid stores. HDL can provide an additional source of cholesterol for steroid synthesis. The pathways from cholesterol to common products shown exemplify the major pathways and hormones in humans (**Figure 17.18**).

2. Cholesterol is converted to pregnenolone by side chain cleavage enzyme.

3. From pregnenolone, subsequent steps depend on the zonal distribution of synthetic enzymes in the adrenal gland or the presence of different enzymes in the ovaries and testes.

4. In the *zona glomerulosa*, the enzyme 3β-hydroxysteroid dehydrogenase (A) converts pregnenolone to progesterone. This reaction is followed by 21-hydroxylase (B) that converts progesterone to deoxycorticosterone. Subsequent steps synthesize aldosterone.

5. In the *zona fasciculata*, pregnenolone is converted into 17-alpha-hydroxypregnenolone by a cytochrome enzyme: CYP17A1. This is followed by conversion into 17-alpha-hydroxyprogesterone by 21-hydroxylase (B) and cortisol is formed by additional synthetic enzyme steps.

6. In the *zona reticularis*, the conversion of pregnenolone into 17-alpha-hydroxypregnenolone by CYP17A1 and other enzymes is followed by DHEA and DHEAS synthesis. These androgens have biological activity, and DHEA can be converted to either androstenedione or androstenediol. Either of these precursors can lead to testosterone synthesis. Aromatase enzyme (C) can convert androgens to estrogens. Testosterone can also be converted to dihydrotestosterone, a more potent androgen, by the enzyme 5-alpha-reductase (D).

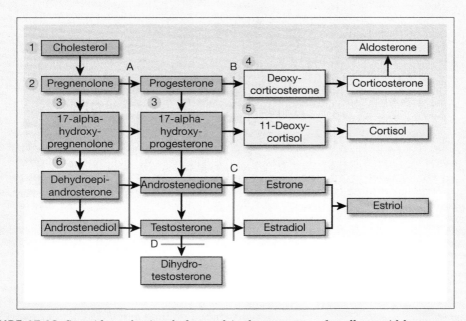

FIGURE 17.18 Steroid synthesis: cholesterol is the precursor for all steroid hormones. After conversion to pregnenolone, subsequent synthetic steps depend on the presence of specific enzymes. Final products include mineralocorticoids (principally aldosterone), glucocorticoids (principally cortisol), and adrenal sex steroids (principally DHEA). The enzymes in steroid synthetic pathways include: A, 3β hydroxysteroid dehydrogenase; B, 21-hydroxylase; C, Aromatase; D, 5-alpha-reductase DHEA, dehydroepiandrosterone.

(*continued*)

BOX 17.1 (*continued*)
Pathways of Steroid Hormone Synthesis

SUMMARY OF ADRENAL STEROID PRODUCTION BY ZONE

- *Zona glomerulosa*: Synthetic pathway produces aldosterone, the major mineralocorticoid.

- *Zona fasciculata*: Synthetic pathway produces cortisol, the major glucocorticoid.

- *Zona reticularis*: Synthetic pathway produces adrenal androgens DHEA, DHEAS, and androstenedione. The remaining steps of sex steroid synthesis are carried out by other tissues, including the male testes (testosterone production) and female ovaries (estrogen production) and are discussed further in later sections of this chapter.

DHEA, dehydroepiandrosterone; DHEAS, dehydroepiandrosterone sulfate; HDL, high-density lipoprotein; LDL, low-density lipoprotein.

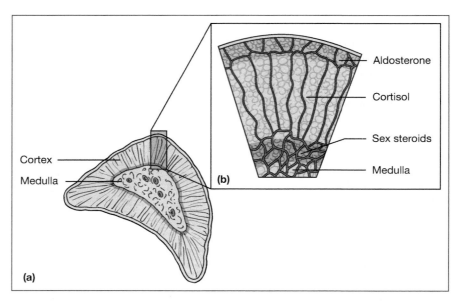

FIGURE 17.19 (a) Transverse and **(b)** closeup views of the adrenal gland. The adrenal gland is enclosed in a capsule and has a three-layered cortex surrounding the inner medulla. The three zones of cortex each produce one class of steroid hormones: the outer glomerulosa produces aldosterone; middle fasciculata produces glucocorticoids, primarily cortisol; and the inner reticularis produces sex steroids. The medulla synthesizes epinephrine and some norepinephrine, and its secretion is controlled by sympathetic preganglionic neurons that innervate the medullary chromaffin cells.

ADRENAL CORTEX ZONES AND HORMONES

ZONA GLOMERULOSA: ALDOSTERONE

The outermost layer of the adrenal cortex—the zona glomerulosa—is responsible for the production of mineralocorticoids, the most important of which is aldosterone. Aldosterone acts on intracellular receptors to alter target cell protein expression in cells of the renal late distal tubule and collecting duct, promoting sodium retention, potassium excretion, and increasing blood volume and blood pressure through its effects on Na^+. The trophic effect of ACTH on the adrenal cortex extends to the zona glomerulosa, and ACTH provides general support to aldosterone synthesis and secretion. The production and release of aldosterone is stimulated by angiotensin II, as a component of the renin-angiotensin-aldosterone system (RAAS). Aldosterone secretion is also stimulated by hyperkalemia, and it is the body's major regulator of potassium levels. ACTH also stimulates limited, short-acting mineralocorticoid activation during acute stress.

Hypoaldosteronism

Hypoaldosteronism is evident when renin production is inadequate to trigger the retention of fluid or when aldosterone levels do not rise in response to renin stimulation in the face of salt restriction or volume loss. Hypoaldosteronism is most often associated with other conditions, with the most common being adrenal insufficiency due to autoimmune destruction. Congenital enzymatic deficiencies such as in congenital adrenal hyperplasia (CAH) can also result in hypoaldosteronism.

Primary Aldosteronism

Primary aldosteronism is the excess production of aldosterone, resulting in sodium and water retention, expansion of the extracellular fluid volume, hypertension, and potassium loss. The most common causes of primary aldosteronism are bilateral adrenal hyperplasia (idiopathic primary aldosteronism) and aldosterone-producing adrenal adenomas, which are usually unilateral. Primary aldosteronism is the main cause of endocrine hypertension. In a recent meta-analysis, the global prevalence of hyperaldosteronism among hypertensive patients ranged from 3.2% to 12.7%, with the higher prevalence in cases of stage III–resistant hypertension.[47,48] The initial diagnostic test for primary aldosteronism is the ratio of blood aldosterone to blood renin. If high, this indicates excessive renin-independent aldosterone production.

Medical management includes the use of aldosterone antagonist drugs. If the disease is due to a unilateral adenoma, surgical removal is curative. However, unilateral adrenalectomy can result in adrenal insufficiency that may be temporary or permanent.[49] In addition to hypertension, clinical manifestations of elevated aldosterone can include headaches, muscle weakness, and fatigue secondary to potassium depletion. Hyperaldosteronism is associated with accelerated cardiovascular damage, particularly left ventricular hypertrophy.

ZONA FASCICULATA: GLUCOCORTICOIDS AND CORTISOL PRODUCTION

The zona fasciculata is the site of glucocorticoid production (see **Box 17.1**), with cortisol being the primary human glucocorticoid. Cortisol travels in the circulation bound to corticosteroid-binding globulin (also known as transcortin), although albumin also serves as a cortisol-binding protein. Cortisol is hydrophobic and is able to diffuse across plasma membranes. Virtually all cells of the body express GRs, so there is a wide range of cortisol-stimulated actions (**Figure 17.20**).

Once cortisol binds to the GR, most cortisol/GR complexes translocate to the nucleus and bind to recognition sites on the DNA. Cortisol/GR complexes may bind directly to DNA, they may be tethered to DNA by additional nuclear proteins, or they may bind through a combination of these two mechanisms. In addition, sequences in the DNA that recognize the cortisol/GR complex (termed *glucocorticoid response elements* [GREs]) may either increase transcription of nearby genes or may inhibit transcription of nearby genes (negative GREs [nGREs]).[50] The ability of cortisol to suppress immune responses is usually through suppression of inflammatory gene expression.

Cortisol secretion occurs in a circadian manner, peaking in the early morning, with additional small peaks at mealtimes and the nadir around bedtime or midnight (**Figure 17.21**). This secretion is controlled by the hypothalamic clock mechanism in the suprachiasmatic nucleus. This daily rhythm allows for optimum cardiovascular, kidney, metabolic, and immune function that prepares the organism for acute stress states. During acute stress, the circadian rhythm is overridden, and higher rates of cortisol secretion prevail. This can occur in response to psychological stressors (psychological threats and trauma, acute anxiety-provoking stimuli) and physiological and pathophysiological stressors such as infections, major and minor surgeries, physical trauma with injury and blood loss, hypotension and hypovolemia, and hypoglycemia.

Cortisol's actions in the prestress state and during the acute stress state can be conceptualized in four ways:

1. Preparatory (getting the organism ready for a new or additional stressor)
2. Permissive (working with other homeostatic systems to respond to stress)
3. Stimulatory (enhancing the actions of other homeostatic systems in response to stress)
4. Inhibitory (reducing the actions of other systems activated by stress)[51]

Within this conceptual framework, the contributions of cortisol before and during stress include enhancing the cardiovascular response to sympathetic stimulation; suppressing renal fluid retention; responding to infections with a rapid enhancement of immune response followed by immune suppression; preparing liver, muscle, and fat during the fed state by enhancing glycogen, protein, and fat synthesis for fuel storage; enhancing fuel mobilization during stress by enhancing liver gluconeogenesis and glycogenolysis, muscle proteolysis, and fat lipolysis; contributing to stress-induced suppression

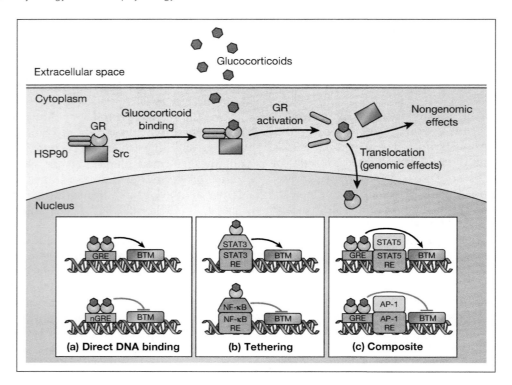

FIGURE 17.20 Glucocorticoids enter cells by diffusion across the plasma membrane, and bind to GRs in the cytoplasm. After receptor binding, the hormone/receptor complex moves into the nucleus to exert genomic effects and alter transcription and translation. Other GR-associated proteins (the Src protein kinase, the chaperone HSP90) stay in the cytoplasm and can exert nongenomic effects. **(a)** Hormone receptor complexes can bind to GREs and nGREs to directly alter BTM either in a way that stimulates gene expression (*top row of effects within nucleus*) or to inhibit gene expression (*bottom row*). **(b)** Cortisol/GR complexes can bind on top of an existing DNA-bound transcription factor to alter transcriptional activity. **(c)** Cortisol/GR complexes can bind to DNA adjacent to existing bound transcription factors to modulate transcriptional activity. AP-1, activator protein 1 (involved in promotion of inflammatory responses); BTM, basal transcription machinery; GRs, glucocorticoid receptors; GREs, glucocortocoid responsive elements; HSP90, heat shock protein 90; NF-κB, nuclear factor kappa B (normally promotes inflammatory responses, inhibited by cortisol); nGREs; negative GREs; RE, responsive element; STAT, signal transducer and activator of transcription.

of reproductive hormone secretion and reproductive behaviors; and suppressing some cognitive and memory responses to stress.

Thus, the actions of cortisol must be viewed through the lens of context: During normal daily cycling of cortisol secretion and meal ingestion, cortisol is contributing to normal physiological function, while preparing the organism for the stress of psychological or physiological challenges. When stress becomes chronic, cortisol can synergize with other systems in a negative way to produce elevated blood pressure, increased blood glucose (worsening diabetes), promoting visceral fat deposition, and suppressing immune function. Long-term glucocorticoid treatment of inflammatory conditions such

as rheumatoid arthritis benefits patients through its immunosuppressive effects but can produce exaggerated effects of hypercortisolism, as described in the following section.

Adrenocortical Dysfunction

Adrenal dysfunction may result from genetic mutations altering steroid-synthesizing enzymes, can be due to adrenocortical tumors, or may be secondary to dysfunction of pituitary ACTH synthesis and secretion.

Hypocortisolism (Adrenal Insufficiency)
Primary hypocortisolism is related to intrinsic adrenal gland failure, most commonly due to autoimmune destruction. Mutations in POMC processing,

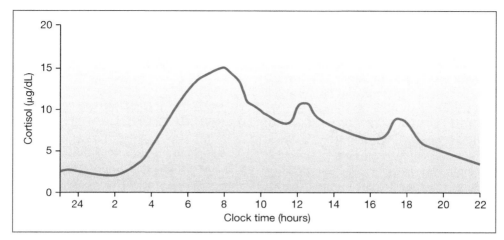

FIGURE 17.21 Circadian pattern of cortisol production. Typical circadian rhythm of cortisol levels, with the highest levels in the morning, lowest levels in the evening, and additional peaks at times of meals. In the postprandial state, cortisol facilitates anabolic actions such as liver glycogen storage and fat cell lipid synthesis.

insensitivity to ACTH or inadequate ACTH secretion, or inadequate adrenal steroidogenesis can also lead to adrenal hypofunction—patients with these conditions require replacement glucocorticoids for survival.

Clinical characteristics are similar in the various forms of hypocortisolism. In the case of primary adrenal failure or **Addison disease**, both aldosterone and cortisol levels are usually low. In the absence of cortisol negative feedback, ACTH levels remain elevated. Clinical findings are secondary to the following:

- Lack of cortisol—produces general cardiovascular hypofunction with hypotension and tachycardia, stress intolerance, weight loss, and fatigue
- Lack of aldosterone—contributes to hypotension, fatigue, and salt cravings; laboratory findings show hyponatremia and hyperkalemia
- Excess ACTH—responsible for hyperpigmentation, particularly of palmar creases, knuckles, elbows, knees, lips, face; due to cross reactivity that stimulates dermal melanocortin receptors

If patients do not receive hormone replacement, or if replacement is inadequate to compensate for acute physiological stress, they may present with acute hemodynamic collapse—referred to as **adrenal crisis**—requiring immediate treatment with intravenous stress doses of glucocorticoids. Fluid and saline resuscitation are required to maintain blood pressure and to restore glucose homeostasis and sodium levels. Chronic glucocorticoid and mineralocorticoid replacements are needed in managing patients with Addison disease.[52]

Adrenal insufficiency is a common effect of chronic glucocorticoid administration in patients with inflammatory conditions. The enhanced negative feedback of exogenous glucocorticoids suppresses ACTH secretion, eventually leading to adrenal atrophy. Withdrawal of steroid treatment must be carried out slowly, and eventually pituitary ACTH secretion will resume. Even after it does, rebuilding the adrenal gland can take weeks to months, during which time the person will require steroid coverage for major stressors.

Adrenal Hypercortisolism

Adrenocortical tumors can be benign or malignant. Malignant adrenocortical carcinomas are rare, with a yearly incidence of 1.02 cases per million population.[53] They affect women with greater frequency than men.

An estimated 15% of all cases of **Cushing syndrome** result from the autonomous production of cortisol from adrenal tumors (adenoma or carcinoma) or hyperplasia of adrenal cortisol-producing cells. In this ACTH-independent Cushing syndrome, both hypothalamic CRH and pituitary ACTH production are suppressed by the excess cortisol production via a negative feedback mechanism. Therefore, in adrenal Cushing syndrome, serum ACTH is low. Patients present with symptoms of hypercortisolism and hyperplasia, or adrenal tumor that may be seen on abdominal CT scan. Treatment may include surgical tumor removal or cortisol-suppressive agents such as metyrapone. Secondary hypercortisolism (Cushing disease) is associated with excess pituitary production of ACTH driving adrenal hypercortisolism, as previously described.

Hallmark symptoms of hypercortisolism (regardless of etiology) are midsection weight gain with relative extremity sparing, facial redness and rounding, loss of libido, menstrual irregularities, dark pink and purple abdominal striae, hair loss, skin thinning, easy bruising, sleep disturbance, fatigue, anxiety, and depression. Patients may also present with hyperglycemia, hypertension, and infertility; a history of bone fractures; hypercoagulation disorders; and (in children) growth disturbance. The disease is more common in women, with the female-to-male ratio as high as 5:1. Mortality rates for patients with Cushing syndrome are significantly higher than those of the general population. This increased rate is secondary to concomitant morbidities such as coagulation disorders, diabetes, and cardiovascular disease.[54]

The diagnosis of hypercortisolism can be complex and involves multiple tests. Random ACTH and cortisol levels are highly dependent on the time of day, environmental and emotional factors, and other considerations such as mealtimes, pregnancy, malnutrition, illness, and strenuous exercise. Therefore, normal levels have a significant crossover with elevated levels. Other tests, such as the measurement of urinary cortisol over 24 hours, late night levels of salivary cortisol, cortisol suppression tests, and brain MRI, may also be indicated.

ZONA RETICULARIS: ANDROGENS

The zona reticularis is the deepest layer of the cortex. This zone produces androgens, mainly DHEA, DHEAS, and androstenedione (the precursor to testosterone; see Box 17.1). Although these androgens have a low affinity for androgen receptors, altered levels of adrenal androgens may significantly impact sexual development and fertility. Growth of this zone occurs in adrenarche and functional decline occurs in older adulthood.

As ACTH has growth-promoting and stimulating actions on all adrenocortical layers, adrenal androgen production is maintained and regulated by ACTH levels; however, adrenal androgens do not provide feedback inhibition of ACTH. ACTH deficiency states result in atrophy of the zona reticularis and decreased DHEA synthesis. On the other hand, in states of ACTH excess, DHEA synthesis increases. The conversion of high levels of DHEA to dihydrotestosterone in dysregulated states is associated with virilization and hirsutism.

DHEA is a prohormone for androstenedione and subsequently testosterone (chiefly produced in gonadal and peripheral tissues). Several genetic enzyme deficiencies can alter adrenal steroid production, sometimes causing abnormal development of secondary sex characteristics. Androstenedione is converted to testosterone and estrogen at the onset of puberty (adrenarche). Adrenarche is marked by high blood levels of DHEAS, which is the predominant sex steroid during this period.

ADRENAL MEDULLA AND CATECHOLAMINES

The adrenal medulla represents the smallest portion of the adrenal gland. Composed of chromaffin cells, it produces water-soluble catecholamines that are derived from the amino acid tyrosine (Figure 17.22). The medulla is composed of chromaffin cells containing small vesicles that store and release catecholamines when stimulated by the sympathetic nervous system. In humans, the chromaffin cells release about 80% epinephrine and 20% norepinephrine. These are the major hormones released during the fight-or-flight response, causing increased heart rate and blood pressure, gastrointestinal and skin vasoconstriction, muscle vasodilation, lung bronchodilation, and glucose mobilization.

Chromaffin cells are innervated by preganglionic sympathetic neurons from the thoracic spinal cord (T5–T11). Upon stimulation, they secrete adrenaline, noradrenaline, enkephalin, and enkephalin-containing peptides into the bloodstream. The half-life of catecholamines is 1 to 2 minutes, with degradation by neuronal uptake. Receptors for catecholamines are widely distributed throughout the body. The enkephalins and enkephalin-containing peptides are endogenous opioids that bind to opioid receptors and produce analgesia (and other) responses.

ADRENOMEDULLARY DYSFUNCTION

Catecholamine deficiency is rare, even with the congenital absence of an adrenal cortex. This condition is usually asymptomatic unless hypoglycemia is present in a diabetic patient. Adrenal epinephrine is an important contributor to hypoglycemia recovery, as it can stimulate liver glycogenolysis and gluconeogenesis, so epinephrine deficiency increases vulnerability to hypoglycemia.

Pheochromocytomas are chromaffin cell tumors responsible for the majority of *catecholamine hypersecretory states*. A rare disorder (estimated yearly incidence of two to eight cases per million population), pheochromocytoma is usually diagnosed after age 40 years without gender preference. Most of these catecholamine tumors are unilateral, and <10% are malignant.[55,56]

Patients usually present with a classic triad of symptoms: labile or refractory hypertension, headaches, and paroxysms of profuse sweating. Symptoms are often short lived, lasting <1 hour, but

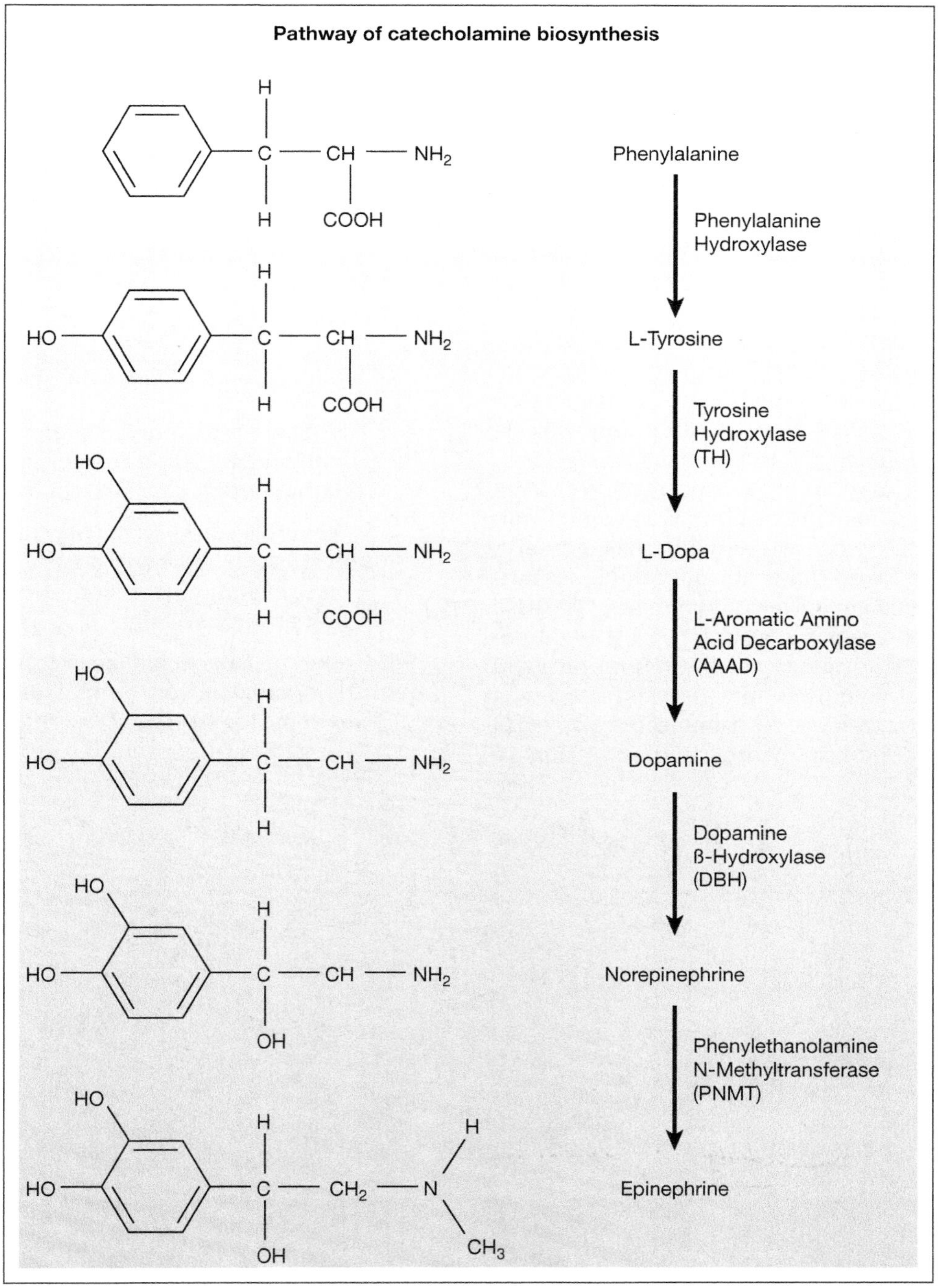

FIGURE 17.22 Biosynthetic pathway for catecholamines. TH is the rate-limiting enzyme in catecholamine synthesis, although synthesis can begin with phenylalanine. Hydroxylation of tyrosine to form dihydroxyphenylalanine (L-dopa) is followed by removal of the carboxyl group, producing dopamine. Addition of a third hydroxyl group by DBH produces norepinephrine. Addition of a methyl group by PNMT then produces epinephrine.

DBH, dopamine β-hydroxylase; PNMT, phenylethanolamine *N*-methyltransferase; TH, tyrosine hydroxylase.

Source: Vegh AMD, et al. Part and parcel of the cardiac autonomic nerve system: unravelling its cellular building blocks during development. *J Cardiovasc Dev Dis.* 2016;3:28. doi:10.3390/jcdd3030028.

may be sustained. The periodicity of these episodes varies from several times a day to once every few weeks. Constipation may be severe, associated with catecholamine inhibition of peristalsis. Symptoms may be triggered by position changes, exercise, urination, and certain medications.[55] Chronic catecholamine excess can lead to pulmonary edema, cardiac arrhythmias, cardiomyopathy, and intracranial hemorrhage. Pheochromocytoma-induced hypertension in pregnancy is associated with a high risk of fetal and maternal mortality.

Diagnosis is usually made with the assay of urinary catecholamine metabolites (fractionated metanephrines) in a 24-hour urine collection or by plasma-free metanephrines. Various factors, including stress, environmental conditions, biological factors, diet, and medications, may affect this assay, so patients must be given clear instructions before specimen collection. Some differences are found between assays, but levels two to three times normal are highly suspicious for pheochromocytoma. Imaging by CT, MRI, or [123I]-meta-iodo-benzylguanidine (MIBG) scintigraphy is needed to locate these tumors. Surgical intervention with laparoscopic adrenalectomy is usually indicated to remove the tumor, following oral α-adrenergic receptor blockade administration to control hypertension and avoid tachyarrhythmia and a hypertensive crisis.[56]

Rarely, catecholamine-producing tumors may also be found in extra-adrenal tissue, such as in the organ of Zuckerkandl (a ganglion-like structure at the bifurcation of the aorta or the inferior mesenteric artery origin), urinary bladder, chest, neck, and base of the skull.[57] These chromaffin cell tumors are associated with the sympathetic nervous system and are called **paragangliomas**.

Thought Questions

8. What are the expected findings in someone with primary aldosteronism, and what is the pathophysiological basis of these findings?

9. What role does cortisol play in the response to stress? In what way are the actions of cortisol during stress complementary to other homeostatic systems?

10. How can catecholamine excess be differentiated from normal response to extreme life stressors?

PEDIATRIC CONSIDERATIONS: HYPOTHALAMUS, PITUITARY, AND ADRENAL GLANDS

Randall L. Johnson

Endocrine glands begin to differentiate and to produce hormones during fetal development, with early development of the adrenal gland and DHEA secretion by 7 weeks of gestational age. Pituitary function develops by 12 weeks, and the vascular system of the pituitary stalk begins functioning by 18 weeks. Adrenocortical glucocorticoid and aldosterone secretion begin in the second half of pregnancy and closer to term.[58]

ENDOCRINE CONTROL OF GROWTH

During fetal development, growth is rapid and is stimulated by insulin and IGF-1 and IGF-2. During infancy, growth trajectory primarily depends on GH, thyroid hormone, and adequate nutrition. Similar influences on growth are seen in the prepubertal years. During puberty, testosterone contributes to an increase in GH and IGF-1 levels in boys, whereas the increase in girls is due to multiple factors. A child presenting with short stature is generally evaluated for several possible causes, including hypothyroidism, chronic illness, family history of short stature, and Turner syndrome. Measurements of GH and IGF-1 are made to evaluate whether GH deficiency or GH insensitivity exists. Challenge testing is carried out to see if GH levels respond to GHRH, arginine, or an insulin tolerance test. If GH deficiency is documented, treatment with recombinant GH is the usual management.

GH excess in childhood, prior to closure of the epiphyseal plates, can result in gigantism, with growth consistently higher than population norms. Unlike adult GH excess with acromegaly, in some children and youth excessive GH secretion can develop secondary to hypothalamic GHRH excess. In others, excessive GH secretion is accompanied by excessive PRL secretion, which is not associated with acromegaly. Genetic syndromes such as neurofibromatosis are associated with GH excess, and adenomas of the pituitary or other tissues are additional sources. Management includes pituitary surgery or radiation and in some cases medical management with agents such as SST that suppress GH secretion.[59]

GENETIC DISORDER: CONGENITAL ADRENAL HYPERPLASIA

Congenital adrenal hyperplasia (CAH) is an autosomal recessive genetic disorder, the most common form of which results from a mutation in the gene that encodes the enzyme 21-hydroxylase. This relatively rare enzyme deficiency results in the inability to produce glucocorticoids and mineralocorticoids, with fetal hypocortisolism and hypoaldosteronism as a consequence (Figure 17.23). As ACTH levels rise in the absence of negative feedback by cortisol, all adrenal steroid hormone synthesis is shunted to androgen production. In classic CAH, female newborns present with genital ambiguity and develop a "salt-wasting" crisis and dehydration 7 to 14 days after birth.[60] Male infants do not present with ambiguous genitalia, but do have early virilization and increased bone age, dehydration, and adrenal insufficiency. Treatment includes lifelong glucocorticoid and mineralocorticoid replacement.

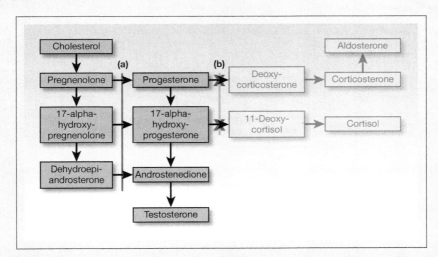

FIGURE 17.23 Congenital adrenal hyperplasia: hormonal pathways. The 21-hydroxylase enzyme is required for biosynthetic pathways of aldosterone and cortisol production. In the case of 21-hydroxylase gene mutations, all steroid precursors are funneled toward production of adrenal androgens.

GERONTOLOGICAL CONSIDERATIONS: HYPOTHALAMUS, PITUITARY, AND ADRENAL GLANDS

Stacy M. Alabastro and Linda L. Herrmann

Older adults tend to have lower levels of anabolic, growth-promoting hormones, with specific changes in GH (in both sexes) and testosterone (in men). In women, ovarian steroid production ceases at the time of menopause.

DECLINE IN GROWTH HORMONE

Aging adults experience a sharp decline in GH and IGF-1 levels, a process known as **somatopause**. Research indicates that there is a 30% to 60% decline in GH and IGF-1 in older adults, with an estimated 15% decline every decade after age 30.[61] Although hormone levels decline with aging, hepatic responsiveness remains intact, and levels respond appropriately to exogenous administration.

Reduced GH and IGF-1 levels are linked to many of the physical and mental manifestations seen with aging. These include progressive decreases in muscle mass and physical and mental function, and increased frailty, central adiposity, and cardiovascular complications.[62] GH and IGF-1 improve glucose metabolism in the brain, promote neurogenesis via enhanced blood flow, and increase synaptic complexity. Conversely, a decline in GH level causes a decline in neuronal structural complexity.[61]

ADRENAL GLAND CHANGES

The major age-related change in the adrenal cortex is shrinking of the zona reticularis, which leads to subsequent progressive decline of adrenal androgens, a process known as **adrenopause**. Specifically, the steroid hormone DHEA and its sulfate form, DHEAS, decrease profoundly with age. DHEA and DHEAS levels decline after the age of 25 years, and by age 80, 10% to 20% remains.[63] DHEA is an adrenosteroid that has protective properties against cardiovascular disease, obesity, diabetes, and immune function. Its decline has been attributed to an increased incidence of compromised immune function, osteoporosis, and atherosclerosis.

Another change associated with the adrenal gland is the steady rise in cortisol levels with aging. The rise in cortisol has been attributed to various mechanisms, among them, the progressive decrease in renal cortisol metabolic clearance, functional changes in the HPA axis, and the stress response associated with aging.[64] In healthy aging, there is an increase in cortisol response to CRH and diminished hypothalamic pituitary sensitivity to glucocorticoid feedback inhibition. Aging can also modify the stress response in older adults. During psychological and physiological stress, the HPA axis is activated. Impaired negative feedback causes sustained levels of cortisol excess, leading to hippocampal atrophy. This particular HPA dysregulation and its effect on hippocampal and temporal lobe function is closely linked to several cognitive disorders, such as Alzheimer disease and late-life anxiety and depression.[65] Excess cortisol also disrupts the circadian rhythm and causes sleep disturbances.

KEY POINTS: ENDOCRINE CONCEPTS; HYPOTHALAMUS, PITUITARY, AND ADRENAL GLANDS

- The endocrine system encompasses many types of cells, tissues, and glands throughout the body that share the common property of hormone production and secretion into the bloodstream. Hormones modulate the activity of target cells bearing hormone receptors.
- Endocrine disorders commonly fall into the categories of hormone excess, hormone deficiency, and tissue insensitivity to hormone.
- Hormone structures are either hydrophilic or hydrophobic, with hydrophilic hormones having the greatest effects through membrane surface receptors and second messenger systems. Hydrophobic hormones travel in the blood bound to carrier proteins, diffusing into cells to link with receptors that bind to DNA, altering transcription and translation.
- The hypothalamus, at the base of the brain, contains neurons that control many homeostatic functions. Neuroendocrine cells within several hypothalamic nuclei produce hormones that stimulate or inhibit the function of anterior pituitary endocrine cells. This is referred to as the hypothalamic-pituitary axis.
- Vasopressin and oxytocin are hormones secreted from the posterior pituitary gland by terminals of hypothalamic neuroendocrine cells. Absence of vasopressin secretion leads to production of copious amounts of very dilute urine and hyperosmolality, whereas excessive vasopressin leads to abnormal water retention, decreased urine production, and dilutional hyponatremia.
- Anterior pituitary endocrine cells produce hormones with stimulatory actions on endocrine target glands (adrenal, thyroid, and gonads) or modulatory actions on all body tissues (GH) or the breast (PRL). Anterior pituitary hormones that stimulate growth and secretions of target glands are collectively known as trophic (growth-promoting) hormones.
- Secretion of hormones often occurs in a pulsatile pattern, with pulses lasting several minutes. Hormone levels also demonstrate regular time cycles of secretion such as ultradian, circadian, or infradian rhythms.
- Negative feedback inhibition is a key regulator of secretion of many hormones, including the hypothalamic-releasing hormones and pituitary trophic hormones.
- The most common cause of pituitary dysfunction is a space-occupying lesion. The most common of these lesions are nonsecreting pituitary adenomas and PRL-secreting adenomas.
- Prolactinoma is associated with galactorrhea and infertility.
- The adrenal gland modulates vascular volume, metabolism, immune responses, vascular function, connective tissue integrity, and secondary sex characteristics.
- Aldosterone secretion from the outermost layer of the adrenal cortex controls extracellular fluid volume and regulates sodium retention, potassium excretion, and blood pressure. The consequences of abnormal aldosterone secretion include dysregulation of blood pressure and potassium levels.
- The zona fasciculata of the adrenal cortex synthesizes and releases glucocorticoids ("stress") hormones. These hormones manage blood glucose level, fat storage, blood pressure, protein balance, and immunity. Excess cortisol promotes hyperglycemia, abnormal fat distribution, bone breakdown, fluid retention, and thinning of the skin and hair.
- Catecholamines are produced in the adrenal medulla and are released in response to sympathetic stimulation as part of the stress response. Pheochromocytomas are tumors of the chromaffin cells of the medulla that produce excess catecholamines, causing hypertension that is refractory to medical management.
- Pediatric endocrine disorders include abnormalities of GH, producing either short stature or gigantism, and CAH, a genetic defect of adrenal steroid synthesis that results in deficiency of aldosterone and cortisol and excess production of adrenal androgens.
- Older adults have lower levels of GHs and sex steroids but may have hyperreactive cortisol responses to stress.

Thyroid Gland

Carolina R. Hurtado and Angela M. Leung

Thyroid hormone has a multitude of effects that are critical for growth and development; homeostasis of energy balance; neural, musculoskeletal, gastrointestinal, and cardiovascular function; and connective tissue maintenance. Disorders of thyroid function can present with varied types and severity of signs and symptoms, while sometimes being very subtle and difficult to detect. Understanding the mechanisms of thyroid hormone synthesis, peripheral activation and inactivation, and control of thyroid hormone secretion are integral to diagnosis and management of patients with thyroid disorders.

STRUCTURE AND FUNCTION OF THE THYROID GLAND

The thyroid gland is located in the lower neck, anterior to the trachea and just inferior to the cricothyroid cartilage. It consists of right and left lobes that are joined by the thyroid isthmus. The thyroid gland is responsible for the production of the thyroid hormones, which are vital in maintaining energy homeostasis in the body through regulation of cellular metabolism. It is composed of spherical units termed *follicles*, which are the basic functional unit and the site of thyroid hormone production. The thyroid follicle is made up of a single layer of cells surrounding proteinaceous material called colloid, the site of hormone synthesis. The apical membrane of the thyroid follicular cells is in contact with the colloid and forms the follicular lumen. The basolateral membrane of the thyroid follicular cells forms the outer membrane of the follicles and is in contact with capillaries in the general circulation. The extracellular site of hormone synthesis is unique to the thyroid gland; all other endocrine cells synthesize hormones intracellularly.

The synthesis of thyroid hormone in the thyroid follicle is regulated by thyroid-stimulating hormone (TSH), a hormone produced in the anterior pituitary gland. The secretion of TSH is, in turn, regulated by thyrotropin-releasing hormone (TRH), which is produced in the paraventricular nucleus of the hypothalamic. This hypothalamic-pituitary-thyroid axis allows for tight regulation of thyroid function by maintaining physiological levels of thyroid hormone in the body.

THYROID HORMONE SYNTHESIS

TSH binds the TSH receptor on the basolateral membrane of the follicular cells to activate adenylyl cyclase and increase intracellular cyclic adenosine monophosphate (cAMP), which initiates the process of thyroid hormone synthesis. This allows for transport of iodide across the basolateral membrane through the sodium/iodide (NIS) cotransporter, a secondary active transport protein that increases the level of sodium and iodide in the follicular cell. The iodide ion moves by facilitated diffusion through the apical membrane mediated by the transporter pendrin, where it is converted to iodine and then is covalently attached to thyroglobulin, the major colloid protein, by the enzyme thyroperoxidase (TPO). Either one or two iodines are added to tyrosine residues within thyroglobulin, forming monoiodotyrosine (MIT) or diiodotyrosine (DIT), respectively.

The thyroid hormones, thyroxine (T_4) and triiodothyronine (T_3), are formed by the coupling of two DITs, and one MIT and DIT, respectively, by TPO. T_4 and T_3 remain stored in the follicular colloid attached to thyroglobulin until they are released, as needed, upon TSH stimulation. The majority of hormone in the thyroid gland is stored as T_4, with approximately 20% stored as T_3. Upon stimulation of the TSH receptor, a cytoplasmic vesicle is formed from the uptake of colloid into the follicular cell through pinocytosis. This vesicle then fuses with a lysosome, which provides the proteolytic enzymes required to release T_3 and T_4 from thyroglobulin to allow diffusion into the circulation (**Figure 17.24**).

Iodine plays a crucial role in thyroid hormone synthesis and thyroid physiology. Most of the iodine that is absorbed from the diet is stored in the thyroid gland. Although the transport of iodide into the follicular cell occurs through the NIS transporter, which is stimulated by TSH, the transport of iodide into the cell can also be regulated by non–TSH-dependent processes that rely on the extracellular concentration of iodide. Sudden exposure to excess iodide, resulting in elevated serum iodide concentrations, inhibits iodide organification, iodide transport, colloid resorption by pinocytosis, and thyroid hormone synthesis and release. This autoregulatory phenomenon was first described by Wolff and Chaikoff in 1948 and is termed the *Wolff–Chaikoff phenomenon*. After a few days, the depletion of intracellular iodine allows "escape" from the Wolff–Chaikoff effect, and the follicular cell resumes normal synthesis of thyroid hormone. This is the physiological basis of the use of short-term, high doses of iodide to treat severe hyperthyroidism. Conversely, hyperthyroidism can occur following the administration of iodide, an effect called the *Jod–Basedow phenomenon*. This phenomenon is generally seen when there are autonomous hypersecreting regions in thyroid gland, as in multinodular goiter.

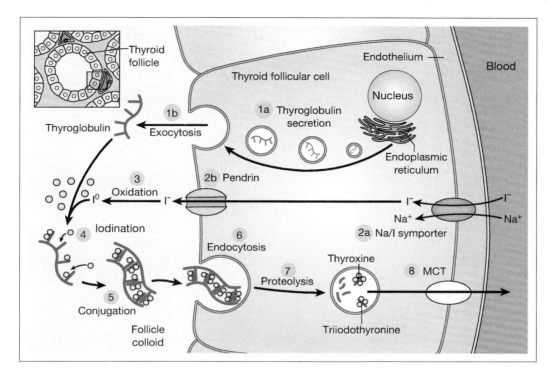

FIGURE 17.24 Thyroid hormone synthesis. Thyroid hormones are synthesized in the colloid center of the thyroid follicle. (**1a, 1b**) Thyroglobulin protein is synthesized by thyroid follicular cells and moves into the colloid by exocytosis. (**2a, 2b**) Iodide is brought into the follicular cell by a sodium/iodide cotransporter, then moves into the colloid through the pendrin transporter. (**3**) Iodide is oxidized to iodine. (**4**) Iodine is bonded to tyrosines within the thyroglobulin chain, forming first MIT, then DIT. (**5**) Conjugation reactions link the tyrosines to form either T_4 (DIT+DIT) or T_3 (DIT+MIT). (**6, 7**) Upon TSH stimulation, the follicular cell endocytoses a vesicle of colloid, which is then fused with a lysosome for thyroglobulin proteolysis, releasing free T_4 and T_3. (**8**) T_3 and T_4 leave the follicular cell through an MCT.
DIT, diiodotyrosine; MCT, monocarboxylate transporter; MIT, monoiodotyrosine; T_3, triiodothyronine; T_4, thyroxine; TSH, thyroid-stimulating hormone.

In the circulation, more than 99% of thyroid hormone is bound to various proteins: thyroxine-binding globulin (TBG), transthyretin (also known as prealbumin), and albumin. The protein with the highest affinity for thyroid hormone is TBG, which binds about 75% of T_3 and T_4 and is thus the most clinically relevant. Thyroid hormones in the bound state are biologically inactive, but are in equilibrium with free hormone that is biologically active and can be assayed.

THYROXINE METABOLISM

T_3 is the biologically active thyroid hormone. T_4 is produced exclusively in the thyroid gland, whereas T_3 is mostly produced in the periphery through the conversion of T_4 to T_3 by enzymes known as deiodinases. These enzymes remove one iodine from T_4, giving unique tissue-level control of thyroid hormone activity. The deiodination of T_4 is tightly and differentially regulated to maintain normal T_3 levels at target tissues.

Deiodinase types I (D1) and II (D2) are activating enzymes that conduct outer ring deiodination, converting T_4 to T_3, the active form of thyroid hormone. Deiodinase type III (D3) inactivates thyroid hormones, generating metabolites, some of which are destined for excretion. Both T_3 and T_4 are deiodinated in the inner ring by D3, which terminates the action of T_3 by converting it into 3,3'-diiodothyronine (also known as T_2) and inhibits T_4 by converting it into 3,3',5'-triiodothyronine, a biologically inactive compound that is also known as reverse T_3 (rT_3; **Figure 17.25**).

The relative activities of the thyroid deiodinases at each target tissue provide the ability to generate local adjustments of active thyroid hormone levels as needed. This is accomplished through the differential tissue distribution of the deiodinases. D1 primarily provides T_3 for the circulation; is highly expressed in the liver, kidney, and thyroid; and is stimulated transcriptionally by thyroid hormone. D2 primarily provides T_3 for the intracellular compartment and is expressed mostly in the nervous system, pituitary, skin, retina,

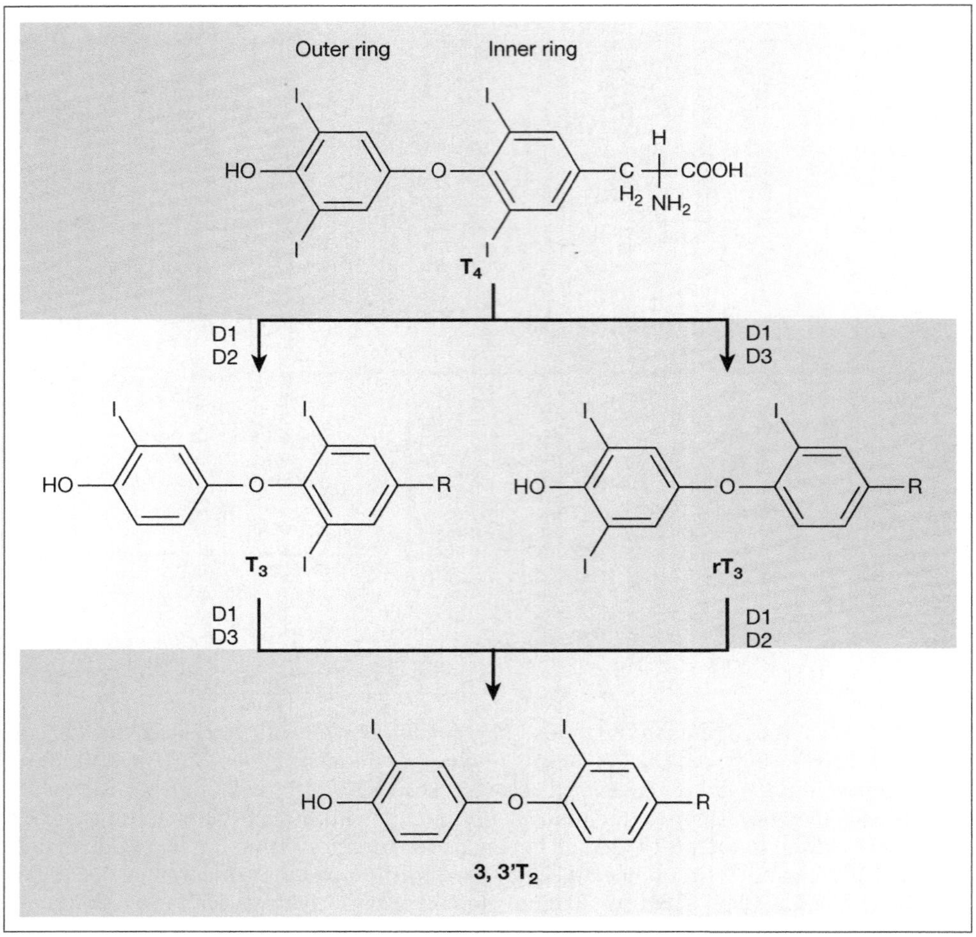

FIGURE 17.25 Deiodination of thyroid hormone. Eighty percent of thyroid hormone secreted by follicular cells is T_4, containing four iodine molecules, two each on the inner and outer rings. In peripheral tissues, deiodinases D1 and D2 remove one iodine from the outer ring, forming active T_3. T_3 can be further deiodinated to inactive T2. In the context of hypothyroidism, in which tissues need more T_3, deiodinase can be induced, increasing peripheral conversion of T_4 to maintain a euthyroid state. On the other hand, in states of thyroid excess, deiodinase D3 is stimulated and removes an inner ring iodine, producing the inactive compound rT_3. This flexibility of processing can contribute to the maintenance of a euthyroid state in the face of changing availability of thyroxine. T_2, 3,3′-diiodothyronine; T_3, triiodothyronine; rT_3, reverse T_3; T_4, thyroxine.

brown adipose tissues, and skeletal muscle. D3 is expressed in skin, retina, central nervous system, and pituitary and adrenal glands, and can be "reactivated" in the liver and skeletal muscle during critical illness. It is also highly expressed in fetal and placental tissue.

T_4 is degraded slowly at a rate of 10% per day. Of this 10%, 40% is deiodinated to active T_3, 40% is deiodinated to inactive rT_3, and 20% is metabolized by conjugation, deamination, or cleavage. T_3 is metabolized rapidly (75% per day), mostly by deiodination to the nonactive metabolites of thyroid hormone. Thyroid hormones can be excreted after hepatic sulfate and glucuronide conjugation through biliary excretion. The activity of the deiodinases, and the resulting T_3 level, is reduced in hyperthyroidism, malnutrition, and critical illness, and

by the action of certain medications (e.g., β-blockers, amiodarone, steroids, propylthiouracil). Conversely, during hypothyroidism, deiodinases are activated to allow greater conversion of T_4 to bioactive T_3, preserving thyroid hormone action in the face of declining T_4 levels. During starvation and acute illness, the deiodinases convert the bioactive T_4 and T_3 to two biologically inactive molecules, rT_3 and T_2.

ALTERATIONS OF SERUM THYROID-BINDING GLOBULIN CONCENTRATIONS

Increases or decreases in the levels of the serum thyroid-binding proteins can alter the total levels of the thyroid hormones, but free thyroid hormone levels remain unaffected. TBG, transthyretin, and albumin are all able to bind free thyroid hormone, but levels of TBG are most affected by certain hormones and drugs. An increase in TBG can be caused by high levels of estrogens (because of pregnancy, oral contraceptives, or estrogen replacement therapy), which slow TBG clearance and increase hepatic production of TBG. During the first trimester of pregnancy, serum TBG concentrations increase by up to 50%. Use of heroin and methadone can also increase TBG concentrations. Elevated TBG levels may also result from acute hepatic dysfunction. An acute increase in TBG causes a transient drop in free thyroid hormone levels by increasing the binding sites for free hormone. This reduces negative feedback on TSH, which increases and spurs greater thyroid hormone synthesis and secretion, ultimately restoring a normal level of free thyroid hormone, but with higher levels of bound hormone.

In contrast, TBG deficiency can be caused by increased androgens and corticosteroid use. Nephrotic syndrome can decrease TBG levels as a result of urinary loss of proteins, and starvation can cause decrease of TBG and albumin by decreasing its production. Cushing syndrome and acromegaly are also causes of decreased TBG. Acute critical illness is the most clinically relevant cause of decrease in TBG.

THYROID HORMONE ACTIONS

Thyroid hormone receptors (TRs) are nuclear receptors and are expressed in virtually all tissues. TRs have an approximately 15 times greater affinity for T_3 than for T_4, so the actions of thyroid hormone described here are mainly due to T_3. Thyroid hormone exerts different effects in different target tissues, with a wide array of effects throughout the body. The effects of thyroid hormone in general are to increase metabolism at the cellular level. Thyroid hormone is essential for normal development, growth, neural differentiation, and metabolic regulation. Thyroid hormone enters cells through several membrane transporters and crosses the nuclear membrane to enter the nucleus. The metabolic effects of thyroid hormone result from binding to the thyroid hormone nuclear receptors encoded by the genes *TRalpha* and *TRbeta*. The nuclear receptors act as ligand-activated transcription factors that bind enhancer or repressor elements (hormone response elements) on DNA to regulate gene transcription. In addition to the effects on gene transcription and protein translation, thyroid hormone has direct effects on mitochondria and protein expression through mechanisms that are still being studied.

Some of the cellular effects of thyroid hormone include increased activity of mitochondria that contributes to elevation of basal metabolic rate, transcription of Na^+-K^+–adenosine triphosphatase (Na^+/K^+–ATPase) to increase oxygen consumption; transcription of uncoupling proteins to increase fatty acid oxidation and heat generation; regulating protein synthesis and degradation; enhancing epinephrine-induced glycogenolysis; promoting insulin-induced glycogen synthesis; and increasing glucose utilization, cholesterol synthesis, and low-density lipoprotein (LDL) receptor activity. **Box 17.2** summarizes specific and systemic effects of thyroid hormone.

BOX 17.2
Organ-Specific and Systemic Effects of Thyroid Hormone

- **Thermogenesis and body weight:** Thyroid hormone increases basal metabolic rate in many tissues by increasing mitochondrial ATP production for metabolic processes and by creating ion gradients that generate energy. Some of these effects are achieved by increasing transcription of Na^+/K^+–ATPase, but other increases in energy production and ionic changes are independent of this effect. Thyroid hormone also causes uncoupling of oxidative phosphorylation in the mitochondria, which allows heat production. By increasing metabolic rate, thyroid hormone can cause modest changes in weight. Thyroid hormone also increases basal metabolic rate by enhancing adrenergic action.

- **Cholesterol and triglyceride metabolism:** Thyroid hormone decreases cholesterol and serum lipids. It causes an increase in LDL receptors and thus an increased uptake of cholesterol into the cell. Thyroid hormone stimulates both fat breakdown and fat synthesis, although the direct and prominent action is fat breakdown.

- **Carbohydrate metabolism:** Thyroid hormone actions in the liver, adipose tissues, skeletal muscle, and pancreas influence carbohydrate metabolism. Thyroid hormone stimulates gluconeogenesis, promoting conversion of amino acids into glucose. With regard to insulin

(continued)

BOX 17.2 (*continued*)
Organ-Specific and Systemic Effects of Thyroid Hormone

production, thyroid hormone is involved in pancreatic islet cell development and function, indirectly supporting insulin synthesis. Glucose uptake in skeletal muscle is increased by thyroid hormone.

- **Bone:** Thyroid hormone stimulates bone growth and development by stimulating osteoclasts and osteoblasts. In childhood, this allows for bone growth, but excess thyroid hormone in the adult can increase osteoporosis by increasing bone turnover as a catabolic effect.

- **Muscle:** Thyroid hormone increases muscle energy expenditure and proteolysis while also promoting insulin sensitization of muscle and enhancing glucose uptake.

- **Cardiovascular system:** Thyroid hormone stimulates the cardiovascular system, increasing cardiac output. At the level of the cardiac muscle, it has chronotropic and inotropic effects by increasing the expression of β-adrenergic receptors in the cardiac myocyte and increasing receptor sensitivity to norepinephrine. Thyroid

hormone also decreases systemic vascular resistance, although this may be an indirect effect of increasing tissue metabolism and heat production.

- **Brain and pituitary:** Thyroid hormone is necessary for neuronal growth and differentiation in prenatal and postnatal development. Adequate levels of thyroid hormone also maintain normal nervous system function in terms of cognition, movement, and reflex tone. Thyroid hormone regulates the synthesis of pituitary hormones such as growth hormone and inhibits TSH secretion.

- **Skin:** Normal skin integrity is promoted by thyroid hormone, while thyroid hormone deficiency causes thickening of skin and hair loss.

- **Growth and development:** Thyroid hormone is required for normal prenatal and postnatal growth and particularly for normal nervous system development. The effects of congenital hypothyroidism are described later, under Pediatric Considerations.

ATP, adenosine triphosphate; ATPase, adenosine triphosphatase; LDL, low-density lipoprotein.

SCREENING FOR SERUM THYROID DYSFUNCTION

Serum TSH concentration is the preferred screening test in the evaluation of suspected thyroid disease. Anterior pituitary TSH secretion is stimulated by hypothalamic TRH but is inhibited by negative feedback from T_3, keeping TSH levels generally steady over time. Both TRH and TSH gene expression are decreased by excess thyroid hormone levels via negative feedback mechanisms (**Figure 17.26**).

TSH is secreted in a pulsatile fashion and has some circadian variability with higher levels after midnight until early morning and lower levels in late afternoon. However, the negative feedback mechanism of thyroid hormone on TSH secretion maintains circulating thyroid hormone levels within a tight range. When there are small decreases in thyroid hormone levels in circulation, large increases in serum TSH stimulate thyroid hormone production by the thyroid gland. For this reason, serum TSH is the ideal biomarker to use in assessing minor changes in thyroid hormone homeostasis.

For a healthy patient in an ambulatory setting, TSH is the initial screening test as it is both sensitive and

specific for abnormalities of thyroid function.[66] In such patients, a serum TSH level that lies within the reference range is generally considered evidence of normal thyroid function and requires no additional testing. However, there are exceptions and certain clinical situations in which TSH might not be reliable. Examples of conditions in which TSH is not the best test for thyroid status include suspected pituitary or hypothalamic dysfunction, recent hyperthyroidism, critical illness, starvation, and use of certain medications. These conditions should be suspected when the pattern of serum TSH does not correlate to the clinical presentation, and serum thyroid function studies should be repeated once the confounding factor has been removed. It is best not to screen patients for thyroid disease in hospital settings as abnormal findings may be transient and resolve after recovery from a precipitating illness.

When screening for thyroid dysfunction and serum TSH return abnormal results, further thyroid studies are needed to evaluate the status of the thyroid disorder. Free T_4 levels should be the next step in

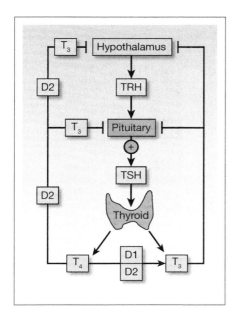

FIGURE 17.26 Hypothalamic-pituitary-thyroid axis. The hypothalamus secretes TRH, which stimulates the pituitary to secrete TSH. TSH stimulates the thyroid gland to produce T_4 and, to a lesser extent, T_3. T_4 is then converted to T_3 in target tissues by the type I (D1) and type II (D2) deiodinases. T_3 exerts genomic and nongenomic actions of thyroid hormone in target tissues and exerts negative feedback on TRH and TSH secretion.

T_3, triiodothyronine; T_4, thyroxine; TRH, thyrotropin-releasing hormone; TSH, thyroid-stimulating hormone.

suspected hypothyroidism. As T_3 is the active thyroid hormone, it is useful in the diagnosis and monitoring of patients with suspected hyperthyroidism. The measurement of T_3 is not as helpful if hypothyroidism is suspected, because the activity of the deiodinases that convert T_4 to T_3 increase in order to maintain normal thyroid function. Thus, T_3 levels do not decrease until the overall thyroid hormone levels are very low.

Serum total T_4 and total T_3 concentrations are a measure of both bound and unbound (free) hormone levels. These levels may be affected by any clinical condition or medication that alters the concentrations of thyroid-binding proteins. Thus, these levels might be abnormal in certain clinical contexts, whereas the bioactive free levels remain within the normal range.

Finally, because the most common causes of thyroid dysfunction in the United States are autoimmune, laboratory measures of antibody titers are included in diagnostic testing as indicated. In hypothyroidism, the presence of antibodies to thyroid peroxidase and, to a lesser extent, thyroglobulin are measured as indicators of Hashimoto thyroiditis. In hyperthyroidism, the presence of activating antibodies to the TSH receptor (also known as thyroid-stimulating immunoglobulin [TSI] or thyroid receptor antibody [TRAB]) are present in the majority of patients with Graves disease.

Thought Questions

11. **What are the steps of thyroid hormone synthesis and secretion? How do they differ from all other hormones?**

12. **What is the advantage of having two different deiodinase enzymes—one to produce active hormone and the other to produce an inactive form of the hormone?**

13. **How does measuring the blood level of TSH inform the clinician about a patient's thyroid hormone status?**

THYROID DISORDERS

HYPOTHYROIDISM

The signs and symptoms of **hypothyroidism** can be subtle and nonspecific (**Table 17.5**); thus, the disease is sometimes overlooked by both patients and clinicians. Understanding the actions of thyroid hormone, described earlier in this section, increases the likelihood that the clinician will consider hypothyroidism when a patient with signs and symptoms of the disorder presents. These depend on the severity of the disease, but most frequently relate to the slowing of metabolic processes manifested as weight gain, fatigue, constipation, and menstrual irregularities.

Mechanisms of Hypothyroidism

Hypothyroidism can be caused by defects at any level of the hypothalamic-pituitary-thyroid axis. The most common defect is underproduction of thyroid hormone at the level of the thyroid, termed *primary hypothyroidism*. When the defect is at the level of the pituitary or hypothalamus, it is known as *secondary hypothyroidism*.

The most common cause of primary hypothyroidism (in the United States and other iodine-sufficient regions) is autoimmune destruction of the thyroid gland—a condition termed **Hashimoto thyroiditis**. Antibody- and complement-mediated destruction of follicles leads to follicle cell death, fibrosis, and lymphocyte proliferation in the damaged gland. Release of colloid into the circulation provokes antibody formation against colloid proteins, particularly anti-TPO antibodies. In contrast to other forms of thyroiditis (acute, subacute, and postpartum), hypothyroidism from Hashimoto thyroiditis requires lifelong thyroid hormone replacement. Destruction of the thyroid gland from **subacute thyroiditis** causes a triphasic pattern of dysfunction, although not all patients will experience

TABLE 17.5 Signs and Symptoms of Hypothyroidism and Hyperthyroidism

System Affected	Hypothyroidism	Hyperthyroidism
General	Fatigue Weight gain Cold intolerance	Anxiety/nervousness Weight loss Increased appetite Heat intolerance Insomnia
Skin	Dry coarse skin and hair Hair loss Pretibial nonpitting edema	Excessive perspiration Palmar erythema
Head and neck	Goiter Periorbital edema Hoarse voice Enlarged tongue	Goiter Ophthalmopathy (in Graves disease)
Musculoskeletal	Myalgia Arthralgia Carpal tunnel syndrome Delayed relaxation of tendon reflexes	Muscle weakness Myopathy Hyperreflexia Osteoporosis
Renal	Decreased glomerular filtration Hyponatremia	–
Nervous	Impaired concentration Sluggish reflexes Depression Cognitive slowing	Anxiety Hyperreflexia Fine tremor
Cardiovascular	Bradycardia Heart failure Pericardial effusion Diastolic dysfunction Hyperlipidemia	Tachycardia Palpitations Dyspnea on exertion Atrial fibrillation Systolic hypertension Widened pulse pressure Bounding pulses Heart failure
Gastrointestinal	Constipation	Frequent stools/diarrhea
Reproductive	Irregular menstruation Infertility Miscarriage Prolactinemia, galactorrhea	Irregular menstrual periods Light menstrual flow/amenorrhea Infertility Gynecomastia

all phases. Transient thyrotoxicosis occurs initially as preformed thyroid hormone is released into the circulation due to follicle destruction; this phase lasts approximately 1 to 3 months. A second transient hypothyroid phase occurs as a result of decreased thyroid hormone production after tissue damage, and lasts another 1 to 3 months. An eventual return to the euthyroid state may follow recovery from the acute insult. When the diagnosis of hypothyroidism is made in the transient hypothyroid state, replacement with thyroid hormone may not be necessary unless the patient is symptomatic or the hypothyroidism is biochemically severe.

Globally, **iodine deficiency** is the most common cause of hypothyroidism; patients with this deficiency can present with **goiter**. Additionally, certain medications may cause hypothyroidism, including lithium, amiodarone, interferons, and immune checkpoint inhibitors. These last drugs, which have been increasingly used in cancer therapy in recent years, cause hypothyroidism by the induction of autoimmune thyroiditis.[67] Risk factors for hypothyroidism include older age, female gender, personal or family history of autoimmune disorders, and history of head and neck radiation.

Laboratory Evaluation of Hypothyroidism

The initial test in the workup of primary hypothyroidism is serum TSH. In primary hypothyroidism, the thyroid produces insufficient thyroid hormone, which causes the TSH to increase due to the lack of negative feedback as serum T_3 and T_4 levels decline. The rise in serum TSH occurs prior to the measurable decrease of serum T_4 and T_3 levels, and so represents an early marker of primary hypothyroidism. When serum TSH is elevated, the next step is to check the serum free T_4 level. An elevated serum TSH concentration with a decreased serum free T_4 concentration is diagnostic of overt hypothyroidism, and thyroid hormone replacement is then initiated. Serum antibody titers will often show autoantibodies to thyroid peroxidase.

If, instead, the serum TSH concentration is elevated and the serum free T_4 level is normal, the patient has **subclinical hypothyroidism**.[68] This is a biochemical diagnosis, despite the use of the term *subclinical*. Thyroid hormone treatment is not currently recommended for individuals with subclinical hypothyroidism unless TSH is >10 mIU/L.[69] If the individual is symptomatic; has high-risk conditions such as cardiovascular disease, infertility, or pregnancy; or has increased risk of progression to overt hypothyroidism (e.g., positive serum TPO antibody titers, or sonographic evidence of thyroiditis), treatment with thyroid hormone replacement is indicated. In the absence of these factors, it is reasonable to monitor serum thyroid function tests every 6 to 12 months without initiating thyroid hormone replacement.

HYPERTHYROIDISM

In patients with **hyperthyroidism**, signs and symptoms are mostly related to the increase in metabolism that is caused by increased circulating thyroid hormone levels (see **Table 17.5**). These include weight loss, anxiety, palpitations, tremor, and menstrual abnormalities among others. Cardiovascular function is commonly affected, due in part to upregulation of cardiac β-adrenergic receptors. Tachycardia is common in young adults, whereas older adults may develop atrial fibrillation. Systolic blood pressure increases; however, diastolic pressure tends to decrease owing to generalized vasodilation. This widening of pulse pressure is generally accompanied by a general increase in cardiac output that supplies oxygen needed because of increased tissue oxygen consumption. When hyperthyroidism is caused by Graves disease, patients may have immune-mediated ophthalmopathy, including exophthalmos, double vision, or dry and gritty eye sensation.

Mechanisms of Hyperthyroidism

The most common cause of hyperthyroidism is **Graves disease**, an autoimmune disorder in which anti-TSH receptor antibodies are produced and bind to TSH receptors, activating excessive, unregulated thyroid hormone synthesis and secretion, as well as promoting thyroid growth. These TSIs produce smooth enlargement of the thyroid (goiter) that may be palpable on examination. Other common causes of hyperthyroidism include **toxic multinodular goiter**, **toxic thyroid adenoma**, and the hyperthyroid phase of subacute thyroiditis. Once the diagnosis of hyperthyroidism is made, the cause should be determined to decide the treatment modality. Graves disease can present with or without **thyroid eye disease**, although the presence of this symptom is highly suggestive of Graves disease. The finding of positive thyroid autoantibodies, including TSI, is also very specific for Graves disease. In the absence of these findings, further workup is required to differentiate Graves disease from the other causes of hyperthyroidism.

Subacute thyroiditis is a generally transient form of thyrotoxicosis and occurs as a result of destruction of thyroid tissue that causes a leakage of preformed thyroid hormone. Only symptomatic treatment is indicated during the thyrotoxic phase, and there is no role for antithyroid drug therapy as the cause is not thyroid hormone overproduction. This form of thyroiditis may encompass postpartum thyroiditis, subacute painful thyroiditis, and painless (or silent) subacute thyroiditis. **Postpartum thyroiditis** occurs in the months following delivery, miscarriage, or therapeutic abortion. **Subacute painful thyroiditis** is associated with painful enlarged thyroid gland with a prodrome of flu-like symptoms, fever, myalgia, and a high erythrocyte sedimentation rate (ESR). Painless or silent **lymphocytic subacute thyroiditis** is associated with an enlarged thyroid gland, but no neck pain on palpation.

A radioactive iodine uptake scan can help differentiate among the various causes of hyperthyroidism. Individuals with thyroiditis will have low thyroidal uptake of iodine. In those with toxic multinodular goiter and toxic adenomas, radioiodine uptake will be increased in the autonomous-functioning thyroid nodules. In Graves disease, there will be increased uptake of iodine diffusely throughout the thyroid gland.

Hyperthyroidism can be secondary to the production of excessive TSH from the pituitary gland. In this case, serum TSH may be elevated or even normal, with an elevated free T_4 or T_3 level. Other causes of hyperthyroidism include excessive ingestion of thyroid hormone, termed *exogenous* or *factitious thyrotoxicosis*. Serum thyroglobulin concentration is a marker for evaluating such factitious thyrotoxicosis from hyperthyroidism of other causes. Exogenous thyrotoxicosis suppresses the endogenous function of the thyroid gland and results in decreased serum thyroglobulin levels.

Laboratory Evaluation of Hyperthyroidism

Serum TSH is the most sensitive measure to screen for hyperthyroidism, as it will be suppressed owing to negative feedback from elevated circulating thyroid hormone levels. However, other medical conditions, such as severe nonthyroidal illness, starvation, pregnancy, and medications such as glucocorticoids, can result in decreased TSH concentrations; thus, additional workup may be indicated. Measurement of total T_3 is suggested when evaluating suspected hyperthyroidism, as T_3 levels might be more elevated than T_4 (as is typical with Graves disease).

Measurement of serum thyroid autoantibodies may be helpful in the evaluation of hyperthyroidism. Approximately 80% of patients with Graves disease have positive serum TSI titers, often accompanied by increased anti-TPO titers.

Subclinical hyperthyroidism is determined by the laboratory finding of decreased serum TSH in patients whose T_3 and T_4 levels remain in the normal range. These patients, by definition, are asymptomatic and should be monitored for any progression. The main concern with subclinical hyperthyroidism is the potentially adverse effects that this form of mild hyperthyroidism may have on heart and bone health. Patients can have cardiac complications such as atrial fibrillation and other cardiovascular disorders, as well as osteopenia and osteoporosis. Typically, patients who have cardiac or bone complications, or whose TSH level is <0.1 mIU/L, are treated. The rest are managed with observation and serum thyroid function monitoring. Most patients with subclinical hyperthyroidism have persistent disease; others may revert back to normal thyroid function. Only a minority will progress to overt hyperthyroidism.

NONTHYROIDAL ILLNESS WITH ALTERED THYROID FUNCTION TESTS (EUTHYROID SICK SYNDROME)

Severe nonthyroidal illness can cause significant alterations in serum thyroid functions tests in the absence of a primary thyroid disorder, a phenomenon termed **euthyroid sick syndrome**. For this reason, the evaluation of an acutely or chronically ill patient with abnormal serum thyroid function tests can be challenging. It is generally recommended that measurement of serum thyroid function tests be avoided during illness, unless thyroid dysfunction is thought to be a contributor to the current clinical picture.

Serum TSH level in nonthyroidal illness can be low, normal, or high. TSH may be low if due to a transient form of central hypothyroidism at the level of the pituitary gland, as well as the TSH-lowering effects of medications such as glucocorticoids and dopamine. During the recovery phase, TSH may rise before it normalizes. Owing to reduced availability of thyroid-binding proteins, serum total T_3 and T_4 levels are reduced, and free levels are normal or slightly reduced. Total T_3 levels are further decreased as a result of the reduced activity of 5′–deiodinase; thus, there is less conversion of T_4 to T_3. T_4 is instead metabolized to the inactive metabolite, rT_3, by D3. Because of all these changes occurring in acutely ill patients, thyroid evaluation should be done after recovery from the current illness in patients suspected of having intrinsic thyroid disease.

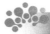

Thought Questions

14. How is it possible for autoimmune pathology to cause both hypofunction and hyperfunction of the thyroid gland?

15. What are the major laboratory thyroid function tests, and what is learned from each test?

PEDIATRIC CONSIDERATIONS: THYROID GLAND

Randall L. Johnson

Early in embryonic development, maternal thyroid hormone supports normal nervous system and somatic development. By 10 to 12 weeks of gestational age, fetal T_4 is being produced, with an increase in T_3 production at 30 weeks, owing to synthesis of the type 1 deiodinase enzyme.[58]

Hypothyroidism is the most common kind of thyroid disorder in children. **Congenital hypothyroidism** (CH) is the most common endocrine disorder at birth. CH occurs in one in 1,500 to 3,000 newborns and is generally detected by newborn screening. Incidence rates appear to show increasing numbers of cases over the past few decades, perhaps due to improved screening tests. The two sources of CH are organ dysgenesis (representing up to 85% of cases) and failure of thyroid hormone production, which accounts for the remaining cases. Most cases of organ dysgenesis appear to be sporadic, with about 5% resulting from a variety of gene mutations, while gene mutations are commonly associated with failure of thyroid hormone production.[70,71]

If the mother had normal thyroid function, the neonate will not have any abnormal signs and symptoms, owing to the transport of maternal hormone across the placenta. As hypothyroidism develops, however, the infant may present with jaundice, lethargy, constipation, growth failure, and hoarseness while crying. If hormone replacement is not provided, development will be impaired and the child will be at risk for slowed growth and intellectual disability. Management is with T_4 replacement, which has been shown to normalize intellectual development and growth trajectory.[72]

Hypothyroidism in childhood is usually autoimmune in origin—Hashimoto thyroiditis (described earlier). Children have a family history of the disorder 50% of the time, and prevalence is estimated at 1% to 2%. Females outnumber males by four to one. As with CH, management is by thyroxine replacement and monitoring of growth.

Hyperthyroidism is very rare in neonates, but occurs slightly more often in children. The incidence of Graves disease is estimated at 0.1 to three cases per 100,000 children, and is also more common in females and those with family history of Graves disease or other autoimmune endocrine disorder. Behavioral manifestations of hyperthyroidism may lead to misdiagnosis as hyperactivity or anxiety disorders. Management of hyperthyroidism in children is complicated by the relative toxicity of some antithyroid drugs in children. Other options are surgical resection and radioactive iodine treatment, although the latter, particularly when used in children younger than 5 years of age, increases the risk of later thyroid cancer development. Infants born to mothers with Graves disease and TSIs can be born with thyrotoxicosis, whereas those born to mothers with Graves disease who are receiving antithyroid treatment can be born with hypothyroidism.[71,73]

GERONTOLOGICAL CONSIDERATIONS: THYROID GLAND

Stacy M. Alabastro and Linda L. Herrmann

The effect of aging on the thyroid gland may be more qualitative than quantitative. Studies of age-related changes in thyroid size have produced varying results, with some studies showing decreased size and other studies showing no change or an increase in size. There is evidence of decreased size and number of follicles, decline in colloid volume, and increased fibrosis between follicles, with lymphocyte infiltration. In terms of function, studies also vary, with some studies showing age-related increases in TSH and others showing a decrease. In particular, populations affected by iodine deficiency tend to show more nodular thyroid structure with aging and a decrease in TSH. Reported levels of free T_4, T_3, and rT_3 are also somewhat variable.[74]

Clinically, older adults develop fewer signs and symptoms of thyroid disease (either hypo- or hyperthyroidism), with the exception of atrial fibrillation, a common sign of hyperthyroidism that increases with age.

As hyperthyroidism progresses in an older adult, the increased oxygen consumption due to metabolic stimulation requires an increase in cardiac output. If the person has any cardiac limitations, hyperthyroidism may present as heart failure—an inability of the aging heart to increase cardiac output commensurate with body oxygen requirements. Thyroid function tests may be affected by comorbidities and polypharmacy, and altered values may not reflect the same degree of thyroid gland dysfunction as in younger adults. As in younger adults, cases of subclinical (lab value–based) hypothyroidism and hyperthyroidism are more prevalent than clinical hypo- and hyperthyroidism. Importantly, the incidence of Graves hyperthyroidism tends to plateau or decrease with aging, whereas multinodular goiter and thyroid adenoma increase as causes of hyperthyroidism. In addition to atrial fibrillation, weight loss and shortness of breath may be the most prominent symptoms of hyperthyroidism in the older adult.[75,76]

CASE STUDY 17.1: A Patient With Graves Disease

Linda W. Good

Patient Complaint: *"I must be hitting menopause. For the last 6 months, I have been sleeping poorly, my heart pounds, my hands shake, I'm sweaty and just can't stand to be in the heat. I cry for no reason, and just feel weak and exhausted. It seems I never recovered from the flu I had over the winter. I've lost 20 pounds, which is a good thing, but it certainly isn't because of exercise or eating any less."*

History of Present Illness: This 48-year-old woman appears distraught and relates her symptoms in a deluge of pressured speech. On further questioning, she states that her menstrual cycles have become irregular and infrequent, and she has been experiencing both increased urination and defecation. She also describes achy muscles, which she says have persisted since her bout with influenza 2 months ago. She says that her heart often

races and thumps when she lies down to sleep. She denies shortness of breath, chest pain, dizziness, change in vision, or recent fevers.

Past Medical/Family History: The patient's past medical history is unremarkable except for mild vitiligo. She was laid off from her teaching job 4 months ago and has been worried about her finances. Her mother had ulcerative colitis and her sister has celiac disease.

Physical Examination: Findings are as follows: temperature of 99.0°F, blood pressure of 150/80 mm Hg, heart rate of 96 beats/min, and respirations of 20 breaths/min. Her exam is remarkable for warm and moist skin, with patches of depigmentation on her hands; fine, high-frequency hand tremor; and an anxious demeanor. Thyroid is diffusely enlarged, smooth without nodules, and nontender. No heart murmur is noted, but there are occasional

(continued)

(continued)

premature beats. Other findings include clear lung fields, benign abdomen, and absence of eye findings such as lid lag or retraction such as in proptosis. Neurological exam is negative.

Laboratory findings: Significant for TSH of 0.1 mU/L (normal: 0.4–5.0), free T_4 of 22 µg/dL (normal 4.6–11.2), and free T_3 of 225 ng/dL (normal 75–195). T_3-resin uptake and TSIs are also reported as high.

T_3, triiodothyronine; T_4, thyroxine; TSH, thyroid-stimulating hormone; TSI, thyroid-stimulating immunoglobulin.

CASE STUDY 17.1 QUESTIONS
- *What pathophysiological effects of thyroid hormone elevation explain the history and physical findings in this case?*
- *What is the explanation for below-normal TSH levels in this patient? Would this be considered a primary or a secondary thyroid disorder?*

BRIDGE TO CLINICAL PRACTICE: Thyroid

Ben Cocchiaro

PRINCIPLES OF ASSESSMENT
History & Physical Examination
- Note the characteristics of hypo- and hyperthyroidism in **Table 17.5**.
- Signs and symptoms of hypo- and hyperthyroidism are often nonspecific. When brought to the practitioner as a chief complaint, a full thyroid review of systems should be collected with elements from each organ system.
- Examination of the thyroid gland: The thyroid gland is attached to the cricoid and thyroid cartilage of the larynx. It is elevated and easily palpable during the act of swallowing. During the examination, the practitioner stands behind the patient and palpates the thyroid's two lobes and central isthmus to identify nodules and swelling while the patient swallows.

Diagnostic Tools
- *Thyroid ultrasound:* Useful in further characterizing nodules and goiters identified on examination, thyroid ultrasonography cannot provide definitive diagnosis but is often used in monitoring thyroid masses and planning for biopsies.
- *Thyroid scintigraphy:* Critical in the evaluation of thyroid nodules and goiters, this test uses radioactive iodine to determine whether nodules contain functioning glandular tissue, sometimes referred to as "hot" nodules. Nonfunctioning, or "cold" nodules are often biopsied according to strict sonographic criteria.
- *Thyroid biopsy:* Performed under sonographic guidance, biopsies are obtained through fine needle aspiration.

Laboratory Evaluation
- *TSH and free thyroxine (T_4):* Used in conjunction, these two tests differentiate between primary and secondary thyroid disease. Notably, TSH increases with age in euthyroid patients, so care should be taken when interpreting thyroid tests in the geriatric population.
- *Thyrotropin receptor antibodies:* Diagnostic for Graves disease.
- *Thyroid peroxidase antibodies:* Diagnostic for Hashimoto's thyroiditis, the most common cause of primary hypothyroidism.

MAJOR DRUG CLASSES
- *Synthetic thyroid hormone/levothyroxine:* Identical to endogenously produced thyroxine (T_4), levothyroxine is a mainstay in the treatment of hypothyroidism as well as goiter.
- *Thionamides:* Propylthiouracil and methimazole work by inhibiting thyroid peroxidase, decreasing production of thyroid hormone in conditions such as Graves disease.
- *Beta blockers:* Propranolol and metoprolol are sometimes used in hyperthyroid conditions to control the symptoms of tremor and tachycardia.
- *Radioiodine:* Used as a definitive treatment of Graves disease and certain other hyperthyroid states, oral administration of sodium iodide (131-I) rapidly concentrates in the thyroid gland. Its radioactive decay releases radiation that destroys the thyroid gland over the following 6–8 weeks. Patients treated with radioiodine require lifelong thyroid replacement and monitoring.

KEY POINTS: THYROID GLAND

- Thyroid hormone is unique in many ways, in comparison to other hormones: It is synthesized extracellularly, it is secreted as a relatively inactive compound (T_4), and it is metabolized in target tissues either to the active form (T_3) *or* to an inactive form (rT_3).
- Iodine is an absolute requirement for thyroid hormone synthesis; if there is no iodine, hypothyroidism will be inevitable.
- Thyroid hormone acts by nuclear receptors to alter protein transcription and translation.
- Thyroid hormone stimulates mitochondrial activity and increases basal metabolic rate, while also having stimulating effects on growth and development; brain development and maintenance of normal neurological function; and maintenance of healthy bone, muscle, cardiovascular activity, and connective tissue.
- The hypothalamic-pituitary-thyroid axis consists of hypothalamic TRH, which stimulates pituitary TSH to stimulate thyroid synthesis and secretion of thyroid hormone. The major negative feedback of thyroid hormone is at the level of the pituitary, reducing TSH secretion.
- Blood levels of TSH are a functional indicator of the amount of thyroid hormone, as they reflect the effectiveness of thyroid hormone negative feedback. In primary hypothyroidism, TSH levels are high because of the loss of negative feedback. In primary hyperthyroidism, TSH levels are low because of excessive negative feedback.
- Evaluation of thyroid function generally involves screening using TSH, followed by free T_4 measurements. Additional testing can include measurements of antibody titers (anti-TPO, anti-TSH receptor) and detection of thyroid radioactive iodine uptake.

- The most common mechanisms of thyroid disease are autoimmune attack. In Hashimoto thyroiditis, after a precipitating event, antibodies and complement damage the follicle cells, releasing colloid that provokes further antibody formation. Anti-TPO antibodies are among those for which there is a laboratory assay. In Graves disease, antibodies to TSH receptors bind to those receptors and perpetually activate them, causing unrestrained thyroid hormone synthesis and release.
- Another mechanism of hypothyroidism is iodine deficiency, common in certain parts of the world.
- In hypothyroidism, body functions cool down and slow down. Cold intolerance can develop, and there is decreased blood pressure, heart rate, respiratory rate, and gastrointestinal peristalsis, and hyporeflexia.
- Mechanisms of hyperthyroidism include toxic multinodular goiter and thyroid-producing adenoma; these mechanisms are more common in older adults.
- In hyperthyroidism, body functions heat up and speed up. There can be heat intolerance; greater catabolic activity; increased heart rate, blood pressure, and pulse pressure; increased gastrointestinal motility; and hyperreflexia.
- The most common thyroid disorder in children is CH, in which either the gland does not form properly or there are enzyme deficiencies that do not support hormone formation. CH must be treated immediately to support normal brain development and prevent intellectual disability and stunted growth.
- Older adults have altered presentation of thyroid disease: they develop fewer symptoms and are harder to diagnose. Cardiovascular consequences of hyperthyroidism in older adults include atrial fibrillation and heart failure.

The Gonads

Meredith Annon, Hanne S. Harbison, and Diane L. Spatz

OVERVIEW OF THE REPRODUCTIVE SYSTEM

The structures and functions of the reproductive system enable procreation: the production of offspring to perpetuate the species. Anatomically, reproductive system structures include hormone- and germ cell–producing gonads—ovaries in females and testes in males—and structures that allow haploid germ cells (eggs and sperm) to meet during sexual reproduction and provide for embryonic and fetal development in the female. Female reproductive anatomy consists of internal ovaries, fallopian tubes, uterus, and vagina; external labia majora and minora, clitoris, associated glands; and breasts for lactation for infant feeding. Male reproductive anatomy consists of testes and epididymis in the scrotum, vas deferens, ejaculatory ducts, urethra, seminal vesicles, and prostate, along with the penis, which serves both urinary elimination and ejaculatory functions.

The life span sequence of reproductive hormone activity has a waxing and waning pattern. In the first trimester of embryonic development, sex differentiation occurs with anatomical and gland development of the early bipotential (capable of development into male or female) gonads and tissues. Human chorionic gonadotropin (hCG) contributes to gonad development in this trimester, followed by high activity of fetal gonadotropins LH and FSH and gonadal steroid production that continues development of reproductive structures in the second trimester and beyond. Gonadotropin levels then decline during the first 2 years of life. The transition to puberty marks an increase in gonadotropin secretion to adult levels, driving gonadal sex steroid production, production of secondary sex characteristics, and attainment of reproductive capacity. Later in life, sex steroid production decreases in men, whereas women undergo menopause, with loss of ovarian estrogen and progesterone production.

Sex differentiation during embryogenesis is determined by the absence or presence of the Y chromosome. Before sexual differentiation, the bipotential gonads have the capacity to develop into either ovaries or testes, and there are two sets of primordial duct structures: wolffian ducts (capable of developing into male structures) and müllerian ducts (capable of developing into female structures). At conception, a fertilized egg with the genetic composition 46,XX lacks the Y chromosome and is destined to become a genetic female and to develop female reproductive organs. A fertilized egg with genetic composition 46,XY is destined to become a genetic male, with primordial gonads that differentiate into testes at the gestational age of about 6 to 8 weeks.

In a 46,XX embryo, development proceeds with differentiation of the primordial germ cells, and at approximately 6 weeks of gestation, these cells comprise the genital ridge that will become the ovary. Within the genital ridge, germ cells continue to develop; these cells are collectively known as *oogonia*. By 20 weeks of gestation, there are approximately 6 to 7 million oogonia. The oogonia develop into primary oocytes, each surrounded by squamous cells. Together, these cells make up the approximately 400,000 primordial follicles present at birth in the female infant. Müllerian ducts develop into fallopian tubes, uterus, and vagina.

In a 46,XY embryo, at gestational age 6 to 8 weeks, the *SRY* gene (located at the sex-determining region of the Y chromosome) begins to be transcribed. Its protein product, SRY, serves as a transcription factor directing the primordial gonads to develop into testes. Sertoli cells develop and begin to produce anti-müllerian hormone that cause the müllerian ducts to regress. As the testes continue to develop, Leydig cells within the testes differentiate and produce testosterone, initially under the influence of placental chorionic gonadotropin. Later in fetal development, LH is the main gonadotropin. Testosterone stimulates growth and development of wolffian ducts that will ultimately form the vas deferens and seminal vesicles. Development of the prostate, scrotum, and penis depends on the conversion of testosterone to dihydrotestosterone (DHT) by the enzyme 5α-reductase (see **Figure 17.19**, earlier). LH levels increase after birth, then decline until pubertal development begins.

THE FEMALE REPRODUCTIVE SYSTEM

STRUCTURE AND FUNCTIONS OF THE FEMALE REPRODUCTIVE SYSTEM

The ovaries, fallopian tubes, uterus, cervix, and vagina, as well as the breasts, make up the structures of the female reproductive system. The ovaries function to produce eggs and release them during ovulation, and to produce estrogen and progesterone. The fallopian tubes convey the eggs to the uterus and are the most common site of fertilization if sperm are introduced into the vagina at peri-ovulation time. The uterus has a wall of smooth muscle that undergoes hyperplasia and hypertrophy during pregnancy, in preparation for parturition. This is lined by a hormone-responsive endometrial layer that thickens and becomes more vascular prior to ovulation. If conception occurs, the lining facilitates implantation of the conceptus and contributes to the development of the placenta, whereas if conception does not occur the lining is shed in the process of menstruation. The cervix is the muscular outlet that remains contracted during pregnancy and dilates in the process of labor and birth. The vagina is also hormone-responsive, and is the outlet for delivery and the site of deposition of sperm during sexual intercourse. The breasts develop and enlarge under hormonal stimulation and are responsible for the process of lactation (**Box 17.3** and **Figure 17.27**).[77–83]

BOX 17.3
Anatomy and Physiology of the Breast and Lactation

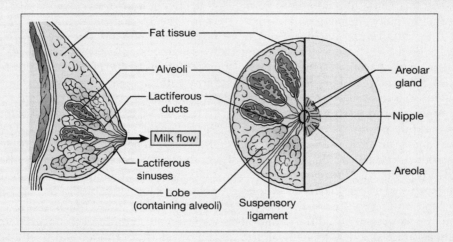

FIGURE 17.27 Structure of the breast. The human breast consists of lobules containing the milk-producing alveoli and lactiferous ducts that carry milk toward the nipple. The connective tissue around the lobules is the stroma, and lobules are further separated by fibrous connective tissue. Fatty tissue is also interspersed between lobules. The ducts are lined by epithelial cells surrounded by myoepithelial cells that contract to propel milk toward the nipple. The duct regions of the nipple are capable of dilating ten times their normal diameter during breastfeeding or pumping. The alveoli, ducts, and stroma are hormone responsive, developing during puberty under the influence of estrogen and progesterone. Cyclic hormone changes of the menstrual cycle also affect lobules and stroma.

Development of breast tissue begins in the first trimester in both females and males. The breast tissues consist of regions of milk production (alveoli) and regions of milk transport (ductules and ducts), organized into lobules and lobes embedded in fatty stromal tissue. During puberty, the internal ductal structures begin to develop under estrogen stimulation, but only with pregnancy and lactation do the breasts fully mature. During pregnancy, levels of estrogen, progesterone, and human placental lactogen increase, leading to breast maturation and milk secretion. The breasts begin producing colostrum at 16 weeks of gestation, and colostrum fills the duct system in the third trimester. However, elevated estrogen and progesterone suppress substantial milk production, even as PRL is stimulating the production of milk components.

During pregnancy, PRL is high, promoting breast development, but oxytocin—the hormone responsible for milk ejection—is low. Delivery of the infant and the placenta is the trigger to switch from secretory differentiation (lactogenesis I) to secretory activation (lactogenesis II). Stimulation of the nipple during nursing initiates a neural pathway leading to oxytocin and PRL secretion. Oxytocin then circulates to the ductule myoepithelial cells, activating contraction and milk ejection from the nipples. The milk ducts leading to the nipples can be as small as 1 mm at rest, expanding to 1.2 cm with the release of oxytocin. On average a mother will experience five releases of oxytocin (let down) during a breastfeeding/pumping session.[77]

There is a critical window of opportunity for establishing milk supply. To ensure that milk supply comes to full volume (500 to 1,000 mL/day), the breast needs to be effectively stimulated and emptied every 1 to 3 hours. If the infant is full term and healthy and can suckle effectively, the mother will convert from colostrum to transitional milk to mature milk. Colostrum is secreted in very small amounts during the first 4 days. On average, infants consume only 15 ± 11 g during first 24 hours and their per-feed intake is only 1.5 ± 1.1 g.[78]

If there is maternal–infant separation or the infant cannot feed effectively, the mother should begin milk expression immediately following delivery of the infant and she should pump early and pump often.[79,80] Milk volume and frequency of expression on day 4 are significant predictors of milk supply at 6 weeks postdelivery.[81]

Additionally, milk production of <500 mL by the end of week 2 equates to inadequate milk production long term.[81] Furthermore, recent research has demonstrated that for pump-dependent mothers, those who came to volume with normal milk volumes and normal biomarkers had more cumulative pumping sessions by day 5 ($p = .03$).[82] A dose–response relationship between the number of normal biomarkers and milk volume was demonstrated for postpartum days 3 ($p = .01$) and 5 ($p = .04$).[82]

Two important conditions that can alter normal lactation are breast surgery and abnormal breast tissue development. If the mother has had breast surgery and the ductule structures have been severed, a complete milk supply will not be established. Women who have glandular hypoplasia (insufficient glandular tissue) will not experience breast changes in pregnancy or lactation and will not establish a complete milk supply.[83]

PRL, prolactin.
Source: Courtesy of Diane L. Spatz, PhD, RN-BC, FAAN.

FEMALE HYPOTHALAMIC-PITUITARY-GONADAL FUNCTION

As noted earlier in the chapter, hypothalamic GnRH stimulates ovarian LH and FSH secretion. LH and FSH levels are high in the fetus at the middle of gestation and in the first year of life, and then decline until puberty. At the beginning of puberty GnRH begins to be secreted in a pulsatile fashion, due in part to increased levels of the hypothalamic neuropeptide, kisspeptin, which stimulates GnRH neurons. Initially, GnRH pulses occur at night, but as puberty progresses, secretion also occurs during the day. The pituitary gradually increases LH and FSH secretion in response to pulsatile GnRH stimulation (constant levels of GnRH actually reduce GnRH receptors, as well as LH and FSH secretion).

Under the influence of LH and FSH, the ovaries begin to secrete estrogen. With increasing estrogen levels, secondary sexual characteristics emerge, including breast development and pubic hair growth. In the ovary, primordial follicles mature to become primary follicles. Menarche (first menstrual period) occurs about 2 years after the initial pubertal changes. After menarche, menstrual cycles occur at more or less regular intervals through the female reproductive years until menopause occurs, usually between the ages of 45 and 55 years. GnRH, LH, and FSH are under negative feedback by estradiol in part of the follicular phase, and by progesterone in the luteal phase. GnRH, LH, and FSH are under positive feedback by estradiol near the end of the follicular phase, at mid-cycle. During this time, estradiol elevations promote the LH surge that results in ovulation (**Figure 17.28**).

The major functional unit of the ovary is the follicle, and at puberty the primordial follicles have differentiated into primary follicles. Within each follicle, the primary oocyte is surrounded by a layer

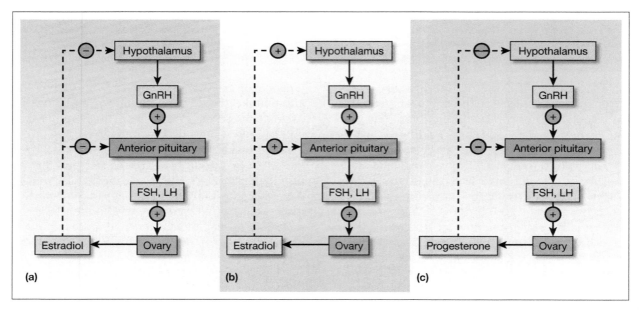

FIGURE 17.28 Function of the HPG axis varies during the stages of the menstrual cycle. (**a**) In the *follicular phase*, FSH and LH stimulate ovarian estrogen production, gradually increasing estrogen levels. Estrogen provides negative feedback at the hypothalamus and pituitary. (**b**) At mid-cycle, late in the follicular phase, estrogen feedback briefly changes to positive, altering the pattern of pulsatile GnRH release and pituitary responsiveness. This produces a mid-cycle LH surge that signals ovulation to occur. (**c**) After ovulation, the *luteal phase* begins, with ovarian steroid production transitioning to progesterone, which provides negative feedback to reduce secretion of GnRH, LH, and FSH. cAMP, cyclic adenosine monophosphate; FSH, follicle-stimulating hormone; GnRH, gonadotropin-releasing hormone; HPG, hypothalamic-pituitary-gonadal; LH, luteinizing hormone.

of granulosa cells. After menarche, ovaries contain follicles at many developmental stages, through which follicles are slowly progressing, taking several weeks to develop into Graafian follicles. Follicles are responsive to LH and FSH, becoming the primary source of circulating estrogen. Many follicles undergo atresia during this time, so the number of ovarian follicles progressively decreases. Estrogen production requires cooperation between follicular theca and granulosa cells (**Figure 17.29**). Theca cells produce the androgens androstenedione and testosterone. Under FSH stimulation, granulosa cells produce *CYP19-aromatase*, and the granulosa cells begin to convert the locally produced androgens to estrogens, and particularly to estradiol (see **Figure 17.19**, earlier). Granulosa cells also secrete inhibin, a protein hormone.

Subsequent events of the antral follicles are described in the context of the menstrual cycle (**Box 17.4** and **Figure 17.30**). There are two phases of the menstrual cycle: the *follicular* phase and the *luteal* phase. In a typical 28-day cycle, the follicular phase begins with menses (days 1 to 5), and transitions to the proliferative phase of endometrial growth, occurring on days 6 to 14 of the cycle. Day 14 is when ovulation occurs. After ovulation, the luteal phase begins, coinciding with the uterine secretory phase. The frequency of menses can be highly variable among women, with the greatest variability occurring in the length of the follicular phase, whereas duration of the luteal phase tends to be more stable.

Thought Questions

16. What is the mechanism of increased HPG axis activity at the onset of puberty?

17. Describe the similarities and differences between the female HPG axis and the hypothalamic-pituitary-adrenal axis described earlier in the chapter. What is the significance of positive feedback in the HPG system?

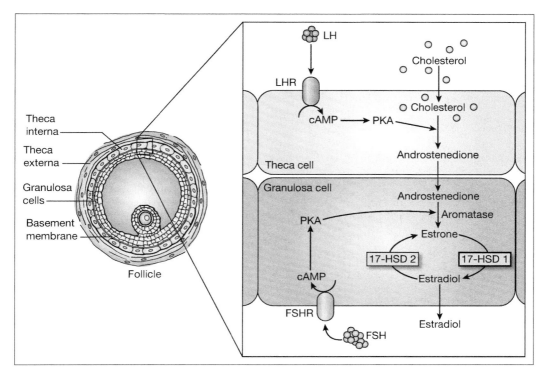

FIGURE 17.29 Theca and granulosa cell cooperativity in estrogen production. Within the follicle, thecal and granulosa cells are separated by a basement membrane that can prevent some substances from reaching the granulosa cells. However, androstenedione produced by the theca cell (under LH stimulation) is lipid soluble and can diffuse to the underlying granulosa cells. Under FSH stimulation, granulosa cell aromatase enzyme converts androstenedione to estrone, which is further converted to estradiol, the major female estrogen in humans.

cAMP, cyclic adenosine monophosphate; FSH, follicle-stimulating hormone; FSHR, follicle-stimulating hormone receptor; HSD, hydroxysteroid dehydrogenase; LH, luteinizing hormone; LHR, luteinizing hormone receptor; PKA, protein kinase A.

BOX 17.4
The Menstrual Cycle

The menstrual cycle is characterized by distinctive waves of increased and decreased levels of pituitary LH and FSH, and ovarian estrogen and progesterone. LH and FSH have different cellular targets and actions on ovarian cells. FSH stimulates granulosa cells, causes follicular growth and development, and promotes estradiol secretion. LH stimulates ovarian theca cells to produce androgen sex steroids, precursors for estrogen production. As ovarian estradiol secretion increases, it exerts negative feedback on the pituitary, suppressing FSH and LH secretion.

Follicular Phase

- On days 1 to 5, increasing FSH causes the ovaries to "recruit" several secondary follicles for enlargement (see **Figure 17.30**). Typically one follicle has the most FSH receptors and emerges as dominant around day 5 to 7. Once the dominant follicle has been selected, FSH levels decline (negative feedback).

- In the second half of the follicular phase, the dominant (now tertiary) follicle increases its estrogen production, and its granulosa cells

(continued)

BOX 17.4 (*continued*)
The Menstrual Cycle

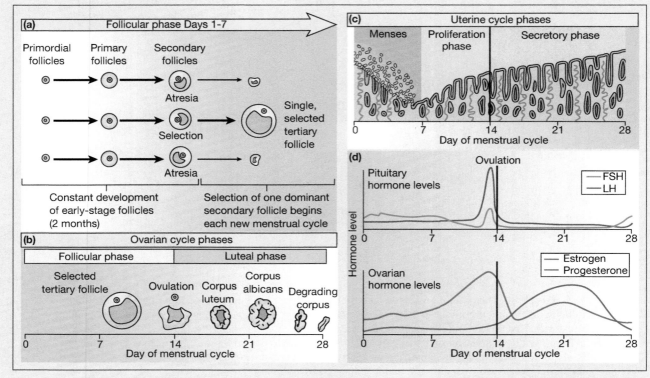

FIGURE 17.30 Events of the menstrual cycle. **(a)** Follicle selection, **(b)** Progression of tertiary follicle through the cycle, **(c)** Progression of uterine lining through the cycle, **(d)** Levels of pituitary and ovarian hormones vary through the cycle.

begin to express LH receptors while continuing to produce estradiol. Estradiol induces the proliferative phase of the uterine endometrium, replacing cells and thickness that were shed in the preceding menses.

- In the late follicular phase, estradiol exerts positive feedback on the pituitary, causing a surge in LH. The LH surge acts on the dominant follicle to cause breakdown of the follicle wall and expulsion of the ovum (ovulation).

Luteal Phase

- Ovulation marks the end of the follicular phase and beginning of the luteal phase. LH continues to act on the ruptured follicle, causing it to transition to the corpus luteum. This marks the shift of the cycle from an estradiol-dominant one to the progesterone-dominant luteal phase.

- High levels of progesterone inhibit further follicle growth, antagonize the actions of estrogen, and induce differentiation in the endometrial lining of the uterus in preparation for implantation of a fertilized ovum. If conception and implantation do not occur, the corpus luteum involutes beginning on days 23 to 25, which leads to falling levels of progesterone and estradiol.

- Once these levels begin to fall, there is a decrease in blood flow to the endometrium, which leads to a decrease in endometrial thickness. Prostaglandin and proteolytic enzyme levels rise within the uterine wall, leading to shedding and expulsion of the endometrial lining (menses).

FSH, follicle-stimulating hormone; LH, luteinizing hormone.

ABNORMALITIES OF THE MENSTRUAL CYCLE, OVARIES, AND ENDOMETRIUM

Amenorrhea

Amenorrhea, or the absence of menstruation, can be divided into two subtypes: **primary amenorrhea**, comprising individuals who never experienced menarche, and **secondary amenorrhea**, describing cessation of menstruation that was previously established. Menstruation generally occurs at regular intervals in all women who have reached menarche at the usual age (by 13 to 15 years, depending on other signs of puberty). Regular menstrual periods end at menopause, although early in the menopausal transition the frequency may be reduced or occurrence may be irregular. Menstruation is absent during pregnancy, often during breastfeeding, and as a consequence of continual oral contraceptive use. Primary amenorrhea is diagnosed in adolescents at age 13 when they have not had menarche or development of secondary sex characteristics, or at age 15 in the absence of menses but presence of some secondary sex characteristics. Secondary amenorrhea is diagnosed when menstrual periods are absent for at least 3 months in someone who previously had menstrual periods and in whom pregnancy has been ruled out.

Primary amenorrhea is quite rare, and often results from genetic mutations and chromosomal abnormalities, including **Turner syndrome** (chromosomal identification 45,X) and **Kallmann syndrome**. In Turner syndrome, the absence of a second X chromosome results in the failure of ovarian development as well as absence of secondary sex characteristics. Primary ovarian insufficiency can also result from fragile X syndrome and occurs in individuals with chromosomal identification 46,XX, who develop premature ovarian failure for unknown reasons. Kallmann syndrome results from genetic GnRH deficiency.[84]

Secondary amenorrhea is more common than the primary form. Common causes of secondary amenorrhea include weight loss and anorexia, stress, excessive exercise, high PRL levels, hypothyroidism, and polycystic ovary syndrome (PCOS; discussed later in this section). Cases of weight loss– and anorexia-induced amenorrhea may be due to generalized lack of nutrition, or that factor combined with decreased leptin released from fat stores. Leptin works within the hypothalamus to stimulate kisspeptin secretion, which then stimulates GnRH secretion, culminating in the secretion of LH and FSH.[85]

Abnormal Uterine Bleeding

Menstrual patterns that are associated with excessive and prolonged bleeding, or irregular bleeding and bleeding in between normal menstrual periods, are categorized as **abnormal uterine bleeding** (AUB). International investigators and clinicians have developed an organizing system for diagnosing AUB, using the acronym *PALM-COEIN*.

- PALM characterizes structural causes:
  ○ Polyps
  ○ Adenomyosis
  ○ Leiomyoma
  ○ Malignancy
- COEIN characterizes nonstructural causes:
  ○ Coagulopathy
  ○ Ovulatory disorders
  ○ Endometrial
  ○ Iatrogenic
  ○ Not otherwise classified

AUB and the additional term **heavy menstrual bleeding** (HMB) are replacing older terminology such as menorrhagia and dysfunctional uterine bleeding. AUB is particularly common in adolescence shortly after menarche, as menstrual cycles can be irregular at first. Structural causes of AUB may require surgical management, whereas ovulatory and endometrial disorders are sometimes managed by hormone therapy to suppress excess estrogen effects. Coagulopathy, on the other hand, is managed by hematologists—a history of HMB is one presentation of von Willebrand disease. HMB may result in iron-deficiency or another anemia, which can be managed with the appropriate supplement.[86,87]

Polycystic Ovary Syndrome

Polycystic ovary syndrome (PCOS) has been identified as the most common endocrine disorder of women in the developed world.[5] Conservative criteria put the prevalence at approximately 6%, but more inclusive and current criteria estimate that over 20% of women are affected by the disorder.[6] The wide range of estimated prevalence is due to the varied presentation and severity of manifestations. Characteristics of PCOS can include the following:

- Menstrual irregularity
- Anovulation
- Oligomenorrhea
- Hyperandrogenism diagnosed from physical findings such as hirsutism or blood sampling
- Ultrasound identification of ovarian cysts

LH levels are generally higher than FSH levels, providing excess stimulation of theca cell androgen production. Many patients with PCOS have insulin resistance and central obesity that promote hyperinsulinemia. Excessive insulin levels may contribute to the hyperplasia, leading to the polycystic ovary morphology (PCOM[88]; **Figure 17.31**).

As noted, patients with PCOS commonly have obesity; however, it is important for clinicians to recognize that lean women also develop the disorder

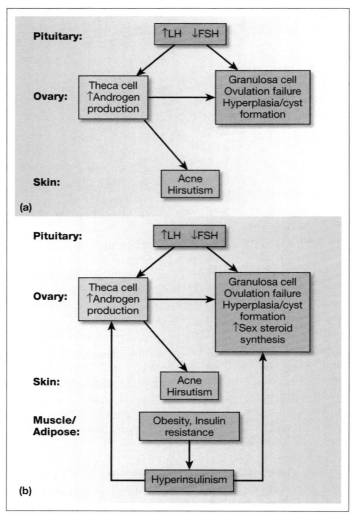

FIGURE 17.31 PCOS pathophysiology. **(a)** About half of PCOS patients have elevated LH levels that stimulate hyperandrogenism, resulting in manifestations such as acne, hirsutism, polycystic ovary morphology, and oligo-anovulation. **(b)** Other PCOS patients have more complex pathophysiology, with the above manifestations plus tissue insulin-resistance, obesity, and hyperinsulinemia. Insulin excess acts on the ovary to stimulate cystic growth, elevated sex steroid production that feeds back to inhibit FSH secretion, and elevated androgen production. This presentation has greater clinical severity than the former presentation.

FSH, follicle-stimulating hormone; LH, luteinizing hormone; PCOS, polycystic ovary syndrome.

and have hyperinsulinemia and hyperandrogenism. The physical manifestations of higher levels of ovarian and adrenal androgens can be first observed in the early adolescent years as a marked increase in acne, hirsutism, and obesity in addition to infrequent menstruation. Women with PCOS can present with PCOM visible on ultrasound, hirsutism and thinning hair, and hyperlipidemia. Many women with PCOS are not able to conceive a pregnancy without the use of medical or surgical interventions, making it one of the most common causes of **infertility**. PCOS-associated insulin resistance may progress to the point of developing type 2 diabetes, even in lean

PCOS patients. Many patients will have acanthosis nigricans—darkening of skin at creases and folds that is usually a sign of insulin resistance.

Overall, the risk of PCOS is increased in individuals with a family history and genetic factors, lifestyle that promotes obesity, and patterns of fat distribution that are associated with insulin resistance. In addition to infertility, long-term risk of diabetes, cardiovascular disease, and poor quality of life are increased in those with PCOS. Multipronged management approaches aim to improve insulin sensitivity (weight loss, increased physical activity), while also providing focused treatments based on the individual presentation. Metformin is used in certain cases to improve insulin sensitivity, while hormone-based treatments can be used to treat hyperandrogenism, AUB, and fertility concerns.

Endometriosis

Endometriosis is a condition that affects 6% to 10% of women of reproductive age. It is a common cause of chronic pelvic pain and infertility. In endometriosis, for reasons that are still being elucidated, endometrial tissue, including glands and stromal cells, is found in extrauterine tissues. Areas of tissue deposition include fallopian tubes, ovaries, uterosacral ligaments, and other regions of the peritoneum. The lesions are estrogen responsive, undergoing menstrual changes of proliferation, secretion, and sloughing along with the normal endometrial tissue of the uterus. Inflammatory activation of prostaglandins and cytokines often produces pain and promotes adhesion formation, particularly in severe cases. Risk factors include family history, history of excessive uterine bleeding, older age at parity, and decreased number of pregnancies.

Several hypotheses have been offered to explain the initiation of endometriosis (**Figure 17.32**). For many years, the primary mechanism was thought to be retrograde menstruation, in which the sloughing endometrial tissue travels up the fallopian tube and out to the peritoneal space. Although this mechanism is still implicated, additional hypotheses have been generated, including peritoneal differentiation of other cell types, spread of endometrial tissue through lymph or blood vessels, persistence and differentiation of remnants of müllerian duct tissue, and differentiation from other cell precursors. All of this could occur against a background of genetic differences in estrogen production and sensitivity, prenatal and postnatal environmental exposures, and inflammatory cell recruitment, activation, and release of mediators.[7]

Many patients with endometriosis experience pain, with intensity that grows over time if the underlying disease process is untreated. Factors implicated in endometriosis-related pain are shown in **Figure 17.33**. The estrogen-dependent growth and activation of endometrial tissue results in activation of growth factors and production of prostaglandins E_2 and $F_{2\alpha}$. These agents promote a host of interactions of the lesions with the host tissue, including proliferation and adhesions; evasion of apoptosis; ability to invade adjacent tissues, grow new nerves and blood vessels, or promote neuronal growth; and inflammatory processes. Pain that results from the establishment of lesions reinforces prior pain experiences and results in central sensitization and disabling levels of chronic pelvic pain. It is not clear at this time why pain symptoms do not necessarily reflect the extent of pathological changes occurring in endometriosis. Hormone-based therapies, such as oral contraceptives that block menstrual periods, have been used to reduce symptoms of endometriosis. Adhesions that cause severe pain or disrupt gastrointestinal function are among the indications for surgical management.[89]

Endometriosis is considered to be a benign condition, despite the overlap with many aspects of cancer, including invasiveness, angiogenesis, evasion of apoptosis, and overlap with inflammation. Endometriosis of the ovaries may predispose to certain types of ovarian cancer. In many women, the lesions and symptoms associated with endometriosis subside with menopause or are improved with conservative therapies; however, some women require surgical removal (hysterectomy, salpingo-oophorectomy).

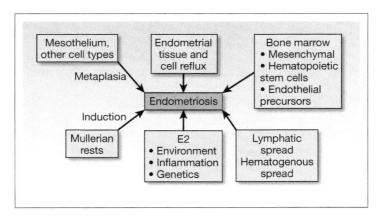

FIGURE 17.32 Hypotheses of endometriosis pathophysiology. Hypothetical sources of extrauterine endometrial tissue that characterize endometriosis. Evidence supports a variety of possibilities, as shown in this figure. Pathological development is then promoted by estrogen, environmental influences, inflammatory mediators, and genetic factors.
E2, estradiol.

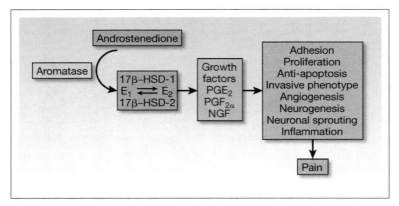

FIGURE 17.33 Factors in endometriosis pain. In addition to being sensitive to the hormone fluctuations of the menstrual cycle, endometriosis lesions can produce estradiol (E_2) by the pathways shown, perpetuating the growth of the tissue and promoting local prostaglandin and growth factor production. This supports the ongoing pathological processes of adhesion, invasion, and other characteristics shown, and contributing to chronic pain sensitization.

E_1, estrone; E_2, estradiol; HSD, hydroxysteroid dehydrogenase; NGF, nerve growth factor; PGE_2, prostaglandin E_2; $PGF_{2\alpha}$, prostaglandin $F_{2\alpha}$.
Source: From Burney RO, Giudice LC. Pathogenesis and pathophysiology of endometriosis. *Fertil Steril.* 2012;98:511–519.

Thought Question

18. Give two examples of conditions that cause amenorrhea and compare the pathophysiology of each.

BREAST CANCER

Breast cancer is the most common cancer in women and the most common cause of cancer deaths among women of Latinx ancestral origin. In women of all other ancestral origins, it is the second most common cause of cancer deaths.[90] Risk factors include female sex (female-to-male ratio of 150:1), age 50 years or older, early menarche, later-life first pregnancy, and late menopause—all of which are associated with greater estrogen exposure.[91] About 5% of breast cancers are due to germline mutations, some of which occur in the *BRCA1* and *BRCA2* genes; however, most are due to sporadic mutations. Eighty percent of breast cancer cells express estrogen receptors and are responsive to anti estrogen therapies. Fifteen percent to 20% of breast cancers overexpress the protooncogene *ERBB2*, which codes for HER2, a membrane receptor tyrosine kinase that can respond to epidermal growth factor. Upon stimulation of the HER2 receptor, cell proliferation mechanisms such as the mitogen-activated protein (MAP) kinase and PI3K/Akt pathways are activated, promoting unregulated cell division that leads to cancer development. Biopsy specimens of breast tumors are studied for the presence of hormone receptors, HER2 receptors, and other oncogenes, as existing chemotherapeutic agents target these pathways and are often successful in suppressing cancer growth and extension if the receptors are expressed.[92]

MENOPAUSAL TRANSITION AND AGING

Female reproductive function changes markedly across the life span. Between the ages of 45 and 55 (average age 51 years), menstrual cycles cease and the final menstrual period defines the formal beginning of menopause. The menopausal transition begins several years before the final period, and continues thereafter as the number of ovarian follicles dwindles and become less responsive to gonadotropin stimulation. Early in this transition, FSH and estrogen levels can be very variable. Later in the menopausal transition, levels of estrogen and inhibin fall, and with the loss of negative feedback FSH and LH levels increase (**Figure 17.34**). Ultimately, the main sex steroid is estrone, produced by peripheral aromatization of the adrenal androgen androstenedione. However, the levels of this relatively weak estrogen in menopause are lower than estradiol levels during the years of fertility and regular menstrual cycling.

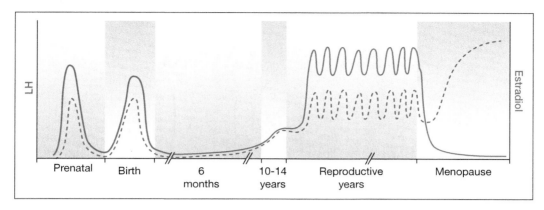

FIGURE 17.34 Lifespan changes in LH (dashed line) and estradiol (solid line) secretion patterns. Gonadotropin and estradiol levels are high in the second trimester of fetal life, contributing to sexual differentiation. An additional peak occurs between birth and 6 months, after which levels are low throughout childhood. At the onset of puberty, gonadotropin levels rise and estradiol increases as secondary sex characteristics begin to be established. During the reproductive years, LH and estradiol show typical monthly cycling, which becomes irregular at the onset of menopause and then ceases. In menopause, estradiol levels fall and LH levels rise owing to loss of negative feedback.
LH, luteinizing hormone.

Physiological changes associated with menopause are attributed to several endocrine changes with aging. In addition to estrogen deficiency, GH and androgen levels decline and insulin sensitivity decreases. Vaginal atrophy and pH alterations contribute to greater propensity to vaginal infections as well as painful intercourse. Hot flushes cause physical discomfort and sleep disruption. Atherosclerosis risk increases, with increased adiposity and insulin resistance complicating the estrogen deficiency. Postmenopausal dyslipidemia can be managed by lifestyle changes and statin drugs.

Clinical trials have shown some effectiveness of estrogen replacement (generally combined with low doses of progesterone to reduce the risk of endometrial cancer and thromboembolism) in treating menopausal changes early in the menopausal transition. Although there are several studies with somewhat conflicting results, and menopausal hormone replacement therapy has both risks and benefits, one of the benefits appears to be reduced progression of osteoporosis and even some restoration of bone density. However, the benefits are not likely to outweigh the risks for more than a few years after menopause, and prolonged hormone replacement therapy is not recommended.

OSTEOPOROSIS IN POSTMENOPAUSAL WOMEN (AND OLDER MEN)

Osteoporosis affects over 10 million adults, over 80% of whom are women. Lifetime risk of osteoporosis-related fractures in women is also three times higher than in men.[93] As noted in Chapter 16, Musculoskeletal System, bone density decreases with aging in both men and women; however, peak bone density achieved in early adulthood is less in women, so the age-related decline in women begins from a lower initial density. The menopausal transition is a time of accelerating osteoporosis due to a combination of estrogen deficiency and increased levels of parathyroid hormone (PTH). The menopausal changes are additive to the general age-related replacement of bone marrow by adipose tissue that also contributes to decreased bone density. Postmenopausal osteoporosis is a common cause of hip fracture, an event associated with increased risk of morbidity and mortality in older adults.

PTH is the body's primary regulator of free calcium levels—with secretion increased by hypocalcemia. PTH acts on the kidneys and gastrointestinal tract to promote calcium retention or absorption into the blood, and it stimulates bone osteoclast activity, releasing free calcium. In older adults, PTH levels increase, responding to reduced calcium levels. These decreases in calcium are attributed to factors that include reduced dietary intake, impaired renal function limiting calcium reabsorption and impairing PTH clearance, and decreased vitamin D levels.[94] Low levels of calcium can result in secondary hyperparathyroidism, which accelerates osteoporosis.[95] Secondary hyperparathyroidism is commonly seen in postmenopausal women; however, incidence increases after the age of 50 in both men and women equally.[96] Increased PTH, in combination with

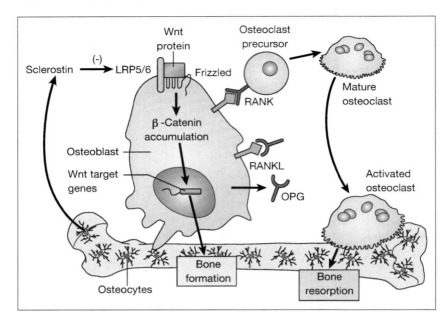

FIGURE 17.35 Osteoblast and osteoclast signaling. Osteoporosis results from an imbalance between osteoclast activity (bone breakdown) and osteoblast activity (bone synthesis). Osteoblast activation is through a Wnt signaling pathway that is inhibited by bone-generated sclerostin. Osteoblasts express the ligand (RANKL) to activate osteoclasts expressing RANK. OPG secretion by osteoblasts inhibits RANK/RANKL signaling, inhibiting osteoclast activity. Estrogen is an important stimulator of OPG synthesis; thus, loss of estrogen signaling after menopause contributes to osteoporosis by allowing osteoclast activation to proceed unchecked.
LRP5/6, Low-density lipoprotein receptor-like protein 5/6; OPG, osteoprotegerin; RANK, receptor activator of nuclear factor κB; RANKL, RANK ligand.

age-related decreases in estrogen, calcitonin, and testosterone, accelerates bone loss in the older adult, increasing osteoporosis risk. Overstimulation by PTH can also cause a positive blood calcium balance, increasing the occurrence of vascular calcification, kidney stones, and cardiovascular events.

At the cellular level, the normal bone remodeling process of coexisting osteoclast breakdown followed by osteoblast synthesis of new bone becomes imbalanced as estrogen deficiency develops (**Figure 17.35**). Osteoclast precursors require receptor-mediated activation via their membrane-bound receptor activator of nuclear factor κB (RANK). Nearby osteoblasts express the RANK ligand (RANKL) on their membranes, initiating osteoclast maturation and activation. Interestingly, osteoblasts also synthesize and secrete osteoprotegerin, an inhibitor of RANKL, so they are capable of producing both an osteoclast-stimulating signal and an inhibitor of that signal, depending on hormonal and other signals.

Estrogen deficiency increases expression of RANKL, whereas estrogen sufficiency stimulates osteoprotegerin synthesis, reducing the effectiveness of RANKL to activate osteoclasts. In addition, innate immunity tends to be stimulated in older adults, and estrogen deficiency promotes release of higher levels of inflammatory cytokines that, along with PTH, also stimulate osteoclast activity. Finally, estrogen normally stimulates osteoblast bone formation, and this effect is lost with estrogen deficiency. The consequences of imbalance between bone-resorbing and bone-synthesizing activities are made worse by common nutritional deficiencies in calcium, vitamin D, and protein. Management involves osteoclast suppression accompanied by calcium and vitamin D supplementation, as well as newer therapies that target the osteoprotegerin protein.[97]

Thought Question

19. Relative to other hormone deficiency states that are treated with hormone replacement (diabetes, hypocortisolism), why is prolonged estrogen treatment not used to treat menopause?

THE MALE REPRODUCTIVE SYSTEM

STRUCTURES AND FUNCTIONS OF THE MALE REPRODUCTIVE SYSTEM

Male reproductive anatomy can be divided into two areas: external and internal. The external genitalia include the testes, epididymis, scrotum, and penis. These structures serve a primarily reproductive function—to produce sperm and deliver the sperm to the female. The internal genitalia transport the sperm from the testes to the urethral meatus, and they include the vas deferens, ejaculatory ducts, urethra, prostate, seminal vesicles, and Cowper's glands (**Figure 17.36**).

The major functions of the testes are to produce sperm and testosterone. During fetal development, the testes develop inside the abdomen. At approximately 28 weeks of gestation, they begin descending into the scrotum, entering the inguinal canal at about 36 weeks and continuing to migrate into the scrotal sac, where they are suspended by ducts, blood, lymph vessels, nerves, and the spermatic cord. After the descent is complete, the abdominal end of the inguinal canal closes and the canal disappears. The scrotal end of the canal tissue becomes the *tunica vaginalis*, the outer covering of the testes (**Figure 17.37**). If this does not occur completely or the closure is weak, it may result in inguinal hernias. The majority (about 80%) of the testicular volume is made up of *seminiferous tubules*. These are coiled ducts where sperm are produced. *Sertoli cells* are epithelial

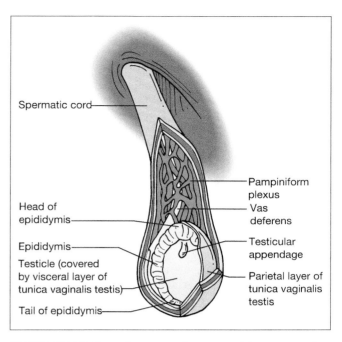

Spermatic cord

Head of epididymis

Epididymis

Testicle (covered by visceral layer of tunica vaginalis testis)

Tail of epididymis

Pampiniform plexus

Vas deferens

Testicular appendage

Parietal layer of tunica vaginalis testis

FIGURE 17.37 Scrotal anatomy. Location of the testes within the scrotum (outside the pelvic cavity) ensures that the temperature is below core temperature. Lower temperature is optimal for spermatogenesis.

supporting cells in the seminiferous tubules. These are tall simple columnar cells that extend from the basement membrane to the lumen. They surround the proliferating and differentiating germ cells, forming pockets around them, providing support and nutrients. Sertoli cells also produce the hormone inhibin that plays an important role in the HPG axis. Surrounding the ducts is tissue containing blood and lymph vessels, fibroblast support cells, macrophages, mast cells, and *Leydig cells*. The Leydig cells make up 1% to 5% of testicular volume and produce testosterone. After sperm cells are produced, they move to the *epididymis*, where they mature.

The epididymis is a crescent moon–shaped structure that rests on the posterior portion of each testis. Each epididymis is composed of a single coiled duct that moves the sperm from the efferent ducts to the *vas deferens*. During their approximately 12-day transit time through the epididymal ducts, the sperm cells receive nutrients and testosterone that allow them to mature. They are then stored in the epididymal tail and vas deferens.

The scrotum is a fibromuscular sac in which the testes are suspended away from the body. Its purpose is to maintain a temperature 1°C to 2°C (1.8°F to 3.6°F) lower than normal body temperature for normal spermatogenesis. The penis consists of the shaft and the glans. At birth, the glans is covered by the

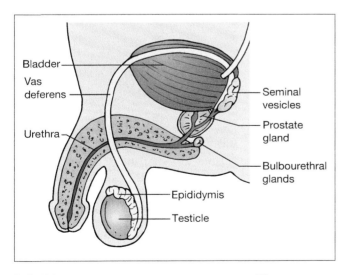

Bladder

Vas deferens

Urethra

Seminal vesicles

Prostate gland

Bulbourethral glands

Epididymis

Testicle

FIGURE 17.36 Male genitourinary anatomy. The structures shown here compose the male genitourinary system. Note the orientation of the prostate gland surrounding the urethra as it exits from the bladder and wrapping around the urethra for a short distance.

foreskin. In circumcision, the foreskin is surgically removed. If the foreskin is left in place, the adhesions that connect it to the glans are gradually broken by erections in the first 3 years of life. The penile tissue is composed of three spongy cylinders of tissue—two paired corpus cavernosa and the corpus spongiosum. The corpus cavernosa are surrounded by the tunica albuginea, which provides protection and rigidity to the erectile tissues. The urethra is surrounded by the corpus spongiosum (**Figure 17.38**).

Sperm are made up of three distinct sections: the head, the neck, and the tail. The head contains the DNA from the male along with the acrosome, which is an organelle that contains enzymes that penetrate the outer layer of the egg during fertilization. The plasma membrane that covers the head also contains proteins that bind with the proteins in the zona pellucida of the egg to bind them together. The axoneme complex in the proximal end of the tail is responsible for the sperm's motility.

The vasa deferentia are tubes that run from the epididymis in the scrotum through the pelvis to the ejaculatory ducts. The vasa deferentia store sperm and then move the sperm either spontaneously or through contractions into the urethra for emission. The two seminal vesicles are composed of single coiled tubes, and they secrete the majority of seminal fluid. The seminal fluid has a role in coagulating semen and in making it alkaline, and it may have a role in capacitation of the sperm in the female reproductive tract.

The prostate is a walnut-sized gland that weighs 20 to 30 g in a young adult and surrounds the urethra

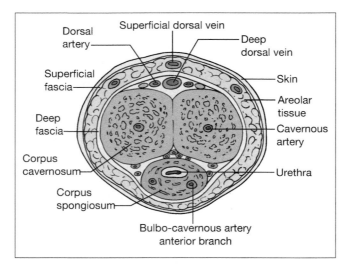

FIGURE 17.38 Penis vascular anatomy. Vasodilation of arterioles of the corpus cavernosum initiates the process of penile erection. As these regions fill with blood, they compress the veins, obstructing vascular outflow and consequently maintaining the erection.

between the bladder and the penis. The gland is made up of epithelial tubular structures that produce and transport the secretions, with surrounding stromal tissue. The region closest to the urethra is the central prostate, which is separated from the peripheral prostate by a small intermediate zone. The primary function of the prostate is to secrete fluid during ejaculation. The fluid itself has several functions: it has an alkaline pH, which helps the sperm survive in the normally acidic vagina, and it contains clotting enzymes and fibrinolysin, which assist with sperm mobilization. The growth and function of the prostate is primarily controlled by testosterone. Testosterone is secreted by the testes and is converted into its more active form, DHT, within the prostate.

REGULATION AND SPERMATOGENESIS OF THE MALE REPRODUCTIVE SYSTEM

Hypothalamic-Pituitary-Gonadal Axis

Similar to its action in females, the HPG axis in males governs reproductive development and function (**Figure 17.39**). In males, the HPG axis is responsible for phenotypic development during embryogenesis, pubertal maturation, testosterone production, and sperm production. As noted earlier in the chapter, secretion of GnRH is controlled by a pulse generator in the hypothalamus that releases GnRH approximately every 2 hours. GnRH is transported directly to the anterior pituitary through the portal vascular system.

The male pubertal transition is characterized by increasing levels of GnRH secreted in a pulsatile fashion. As in females, puberty is initiated by increased levels of the hypothalamic neuropeptide kisspeptin, and the resulting GnRH pulses are greatest during sleep. In the anterior pituitary, GnRH stimulates the production and release of FSH and LH. The target cells of LH are the Leydig cells, where LH stimulates the conversion of cholesterol into testosterone. The target cells of FSH are the Sertoli cells. FSH binds to its membrane receptors on Sertoli cells to stimulate the growth and maintenance of the seminiferous tubules, as well as production of the hormone inhibin. FSH is responsible for initiating spermatogenesis during puberty and for maintaining normal levels of spermatogenesis in adulthood.

Within the testes the Leydig cells produce approximately 5 mg/day of testosterone. Testosterone is then metabolized into two compounds in the target tissues (see **Figure 17.19**, earlier). The first is DHT via 5α-reductase. The second is estradiol through the action of aromatases. Testosterone and estradiol are both steroid hormones that are synthesized from cholesterol and are not stored; thus, levels are reflective

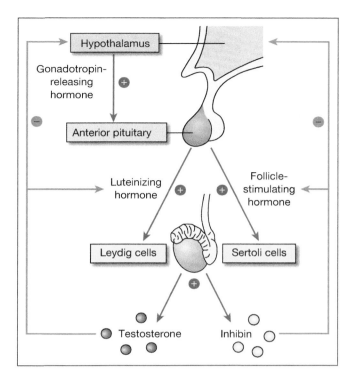

FIGURE 17.39 The male HPG axis. Unlike the female axis, the male HPG axis has a relatively constant level of activity. Although illness and stress suppress GnRH activity, during normal states of activity fairly constant rates of testosterone and inhibin production maintain male characteristics and sexual function. *Blue arrows* indicate stimulation; *orange arrows* indicate inhibition/negative feedback.
GnRH, gonadotropin-releasing hormone; HPG, hypothalamic-pituitary-gonadal.

of production rates. Testosterone is the primary hormone that provides negative feedback to inhibit LH secretion. FSH stimulates Sertoli cell inhibin production, and inhibin is the negative feedback signal inhibiting pituitary FSH release.

Beginning with pubertal GnRH stimulation of LH secretion, the testes increase the production of testosterone and DHT. These two androgens promote development of the secondary sexual characteristics, contribute to male patterns of behavior, and stimulate sperm production. In tissues outside the male reproductive system, testosterone is the primary androgen with effects such as promoting muscle mass, bone growth, and the adolescent growth spurt, and increasing liver production of very low-density lipoprotein (VLDL) and low-density lipoprotein (LDL) cholesterol production while decreasing high-density lipoprotein (HDL) production.[98] DHT, which is more potent than testosterone, is primarily responsible for external virilization and sexual maturation during puberty. DHT also acts on skeletal muscle tissue (increasing protein synthesis and growth), bone marrow (increasing hemoglobin and hematocrit), skin (increasing and thickening sebaceous gland secretions), hair (making it coarser and thicker and changing the distribution), and the musculature and cartilage of the larynx (resulting in voice changes).

As men age there is a progressive decline in testosterone and sperm production. The lower levels of testosterone lead to decreased responsiveness of the HPG axis. GnRH secretion is also lowered and the pulses become less regular, leading to less effective gonadotropin stimulation.

Spermatogenesis

The formation of sperm, spermatogenesis, begins at puberty and continues throughout adult life. The process takes 64 days and is controlled by high levels of intratesticular testosterone. The normal rate of sperm production is 1,200 sperm per second. Production occurs in the seminiferous tubules (**Figure 17.40**). The basement membrane of the tubules is lined with sperm progenitors called *spermatogonia*. These cells undergo mitotic division, producing *primary spermatocytes*. The primary spermatocytes replicate their DNA, then undergo meiosis 1, resulting in two cells called *secondary spermatocytes*. The secondary spermatocytes undergo meiosis 2, forming four haploid *spermatids*. The spermatids contain 23 chromosomes each and proceed to differentiate into *spermatozoa*.

The delivery of sperm requires an erect penis. Erection is a complex physiological and psychological process that is briefly summarized here. Sexual stimulation triggers release of neurotransmitters and vasodilators that cause (a) relaxation of the vascular smooth muscle; (b) increased arterial dilation and blood flow; (c) trapping of blood in the corpus cavernosa; (d) compression of penile veins that reduces outflow; (e) stretching of the tunica albuginea, which also compresses veins and decreases outflow; and (f) an increase in intracavernous pressure, which lifts the penis to its erect state. The vasodilator primarily responsible for erection is nitric oxide. Nitric oxide acts on vascular smooth muscle cells via the guanylyl cyclase enzyme system. Increased cyclic guanosine monophosphate (cGMP) within vascular smooth muscle relaxes the blood vessels of the corpora cavernosum, allowing the vessels to fill with blood. As the corpora cavernosum expands, it compresses the veins that normally drain the penis, preventing the blood from flowing out and thus maintaining the erection. Phosphodiesterase-5 (PDE-5) inhibitors inhibit the phosphodiesterase enzyme that normally breaks down cGMP, thereby prolonging the duration of cGMP-mediated vasodilation and maintaining the erection.

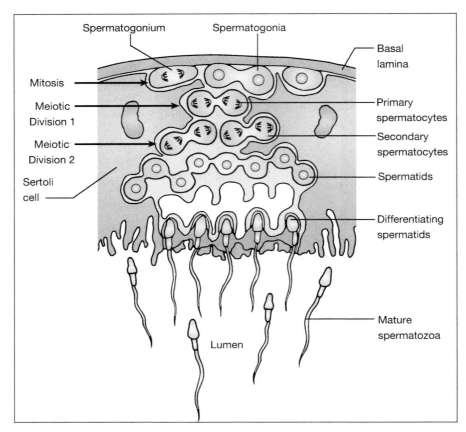

FIGURE 17.40 Spermatogenesis. The seminiferous tubules of the testes are the sites of sperm production that is generally continuous for the life of the male. Spermatogonia found at the periphery of the tubule are continually dividing and producing progenitors that will develop into spermatozoa. The stages of the process move the next cell generations away from the periphery and closer to the lumen of the tubule, from which they will enter the tubules for transport to the epididymis.

Erectile Dysfunction

Erectile dysfunction (ED) is the inability to initiate or sustain an erection long enough to achieve sexual intercourse, orgasm, and ejaculation. It is estimated to affect approximately 20% of men over age 20 and approximately 75% of men by age 75. The causes can be anatomical—changes in the vasculature secondary to hypertension, diabetes, smoking, obesity, and aging. ED can also result from nerve damage during prostate surgery or trauma to the spinal column, and it can have a psychological component. ED is very highly associated with cardiovascular disease, which suggests that presence of one should lead to screening for the other.[8,98,99] Treatment for ED involves management of the underlying cause when feasible. Phosphodiesterase-5 (PDE-5) inhibitors (e.g., sildenafil, tadalafil, vardenafil, and avanafil) provide one avenue for management of ED.

PROSTATE DISORDERS

The most common prostate disorders are benign prostatic hyperplasia (BPH) and prostate cancer, both of which are promoted by androgens, principally DHT. Prevalence of both conditions increases with aging, likely due to lifelong exposure to androgens. BPH generally involves cells in the central and transitional zone of the gland, whereas prostate cancer usually arises in the peripheral zone.

Benign Prostatic Hyperplasia

Benign prostatic hyperplasia (BPH) is very common, with prevalence that increases with age. BPH is characterized histologically by an increase in the number of prostate cells that surround the urethra. Patient-reported history of **lower urinary tract symptoms** (LUTS) is the usual presenting complaint of patients with BPH, as the condition can be asymptomatic until there is sufficient compression of the urethra to be noticeable. LUTS includes urinary frequency and urgency, difficulty initiating the urine stream or achieving complete bladder emptying, and frequent nocturnal voiding. Physically, BPH is often evident on physical examination demonstrating gland enlargement. Urinary flow rate measurements can also be informative about bladder outlet obstruction. Estimates of BPH/LUTS prevalence are 8% to 18% in men aged 40 to 49, and 18% to 43% in men aged 60 to 69.[100]

The cause of BPH is currently unknown, and it is likely that the process leading to gland enlargement is an imbalance of cell production and cell death, with an increase in the number of cells that fail to undergo apoptosis in this proliferative tissue. There are multiple potential factors contributing to BPH development, including androgens, estrogens, stromal–epithelial interactions, growth factors, inflammatory mediators, neurotransmitters, and genetic predisposition. Along with age, particular risk factors include obesity, diabetes, metabolic syndrome, and hypertension.

LUTS are partially related to the increased size of the prostate, leading to increased resistance in the urethra. However, the size of the prostate and the degree of obstruction do not directly correlate with the symptoms men experience. The bladder may also respond to chronic obstruction with detrusor muscle instability and decreased contractility, worsening the symptoms. There is a variety of patterns of prostate enlargement and encroachment on the flow of urine (**Figure 17.41**).

LUTS may have multiple causes aside from BPH, including aging, nervous system changes, bladder dysfunction, and other systemic diseases. Without intervention BPH will gradually progress, although severe complications, such as acute urinary retention, are rare. Treatments include α-adrenergic blocking drugs to relax smooth muscle at the outlet of the bladder, and 5α-reductase inhibitors that block conversion of testosterone to DHT, the more active androgen. The 5α-reductase inhibitors have a dual effect of reducing the size of the prostate and also the progression of enlargement. Surgical prostate removal has also been used, but medical management is the first line of treatment.[101,102]

Prostate Cancer

Prostate cancer is common in the United States and globally. Risk factors promoting prostate cancer development include increasing age, diet and obesity, Western lifestyle, greater African ancestral descent,

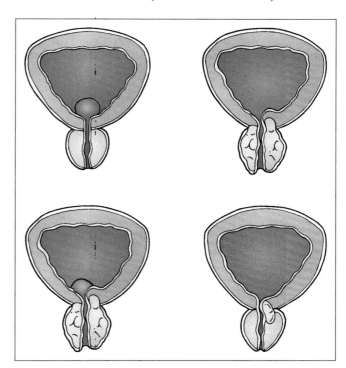

FIGURE 17.41 Patterns of prostate hyperplasia. Hyperplasia of the prostate gland as it wraps around the bladder/urethral junction can result in a variety of protrusions that block the bladder outlet or the urethra, producing lower urinary tract symptoms.

and family history. The majority of prostate cancers develop in the peripheral zone that makes up about 70% of the volume of the gland. A marker of prostate cancer, blood levels of prostate-specific antigen (PSA), is not specific, as it is also elevated in cases of prostatitis and BPH. There is evidence that prostate cancer develops subsequent to an inflammatory lesion called proliferative inflammatory atrophy, followed by oncogene activation and progressive mutations associated with malignant characteristics.

Screening with PSA measurements has been used, but may result in overtreatment. PSA levels should be evaluated longitudinally to assess progression, and are combined with other risk factors to guide decisions about the need for biopsy. However, the guidelines for PSA screening currently focus on men aged 50 to 69 years and may continue to evolve.[103]

Management is complicated by the fact that treatment may have greater risk than benefit in a disease state that is slowly progressing. Active surveillance for tumors that have a low risk of progression incorporates more frequent blood PSA measurements, digital rectal examinations, and follow-up biopsies. For cancers that have a higher risk of progression, treatment approaches include surgery (prostatectomy) and radiation—including radioactive seed implantation. Prostate growth is promoted by androgens, and prostate cancers can develop intrinsic sources of androgens and androgen receptors to perpetuate growth even in the absence of other body androgen sources. After surgery and radiation, later stage prostate cancer treatment includes androgen deprivation therapy, which can reduce testosterone levels significantly. Two of the newer drugs used to treat prostate cancer (abiraterone and enzalutamide) work to block cancer cells from making androgens or as androgen antagonists.[103]

Thought Questions

20. How does the male HPG axis compare with the female HPG axis in terms of hormones involved and feedback mechanisms? What are the implications of these differences for reproductive function?

21. Briefly compare the roles of testosterone and dihydrotestosterone during puberty and after puberty is completed.

CASE STUDY 17.2: A Patient With Hyperparathyroidism

Nancy C. Tkacs

Patient Complaint: "*I am here for my annual women's wellness exam. I am 60 years old and basically healthy, but I worry about osteoporosis, because both my mother and my father had it. My oldest grandson is now taller than I am, and I think I am getting shorter!*"

History of Present Illness, Review of Systems: The women's health provider notes a thin woman in no acute distress, oriented, and with appropriate communication. The patient's last menstrual period was 12 years ago. She reports occasional muscle weakness, not treated, and heartburn that she manages with over-the-counter histamine blockers. She is not currently taking any prescribed medications, but she takes a multivitamin daily. She denies hot flushes, night sweats, bone pain, fractures, kidney problems, and history of cancer.

Past Gynecological History: Gravida 2/para 2; the patient had a unilateral salpingo-oophorectomy at age 23 for a benign ovarian tumor and took hormone replacement therapy for the first 5 years of menopause to alleviate hot flushes. Annual mammograms have been normal.

BMI, body mass index.

Physical Examination: Findings are as follows: temperature of 97.6°F, blood pressure 104/70, heart rate of 62 beats/min, respirations of 12 breaths/min. Height is 5′2″ (patient reports previous height of 5′3″), weight is 110 lb; BMI = 20.1 kg/m². Pupils are equal and reactive to light and accommodation. On examination, the thyroid is normal to palpation; breasts are nontender, with no detectable masses; heart sounds are normal; breath sounds are normal bilaterally; and neurological and musculoskeletal assessments are normal.

Laboratory and Diagnostic Testing: Dual-energy x-ray absorptiometry (DXA) scan is performed and indicates osteoporosis of lumbar spine, hip, and femur, with T scores below –2.5. Serum calcium is 12.5 mg/dL (laboratory normal range: 8.4–10.2).

CASE STUDY 17.2 QUESTIONS

- *What risk factors for osteoporosis does this patient appear to have?*
- *A follow-up test shows the patient's parathyroid hormone level is 112.6 pg/mL (laboratory normal range is 14 to 72 pg/mL). How does this affect the potential diagnosis and treatment plan for this patient?*

KEY POINTS: THE GONADS

- Development of the reproductive system begins in the first trimester of prenatal development.
- Embryos destined to be female (46,XX) have spontaneous regression of male primordial structures and development of ovaries, fallopian tubes, uterus, cervix, and vagina.
- Sex determination in the embryo destined to become a male (chromosomal identification 46,XY) depends on the SRY protein coded for by the *SRY* gene—named for the sex-determining region of the Y chromosome. By the eighth week of gestation, this gene is expressed and begins to direct the primordial gonadal structures toward differentiation into testes and other male genital structures.
- Maturation of reproductive system structures and gonadal hormone production are very limited until shortly before initiation of puberty. The onset of puberty is controlled by a hypothalamic peptide kisspeptin, which stimulates GnRH secretion in increasing pulses, stimulating LH and FSH secretion and sex steroid synthesis. The sex steroids then induce maturation of secondary sex characteristics and adult reproductive function.
- The HPG axis includes hypothalamic GnRH, which is secreted in a pulsatile fashion, initially during the night and, with pubertal progression, also through the day.
- GnRH stimulates pituitary secretion of LH and FSH.
- Development of breast structures begins early in embryonic development, then pauses until puberty. Functional preparation for lactation begins during pregnancy, with breast growth and lactogenesis stimulated by estrogen, progesterone, and PRL.
- After delivery, estrogen and progesterone inhibition of milk secretion ends, and milk production and secretion can proceed, pending nipple stimulation by the suckling infant or by use of a breast pump. PRL continues to support milk production, but oxytocin is also required for milk secretion.
- The menstrual cycle has follicular and luteal phases during which levels of LH, FSH, estradiol, and progesterone rise and fall in ways shaped by negative and positive feedback.
- Hormone changes cause regular changes in ovarian follicles, endometrium, breasts, and cervical mucus in ways that would promote fertilization of the ovum and implantation in the uterus, in the presence of sperm. In the absence of a fertilized egg, the cycle ends with menstruation and initiation of a new cycle.
- Dysfunction of the HPG axis can begin before birth if there are genetic abnormalities causing disorders of sexual development or hypothalamic or pituitary abnormalities.
- Most disorders of the female reproductive system occur after menarche and encompass hypogonadism and amenorrhea, AUB, PCOS, and endometriosis.
- Breast cancer is common and is usually due to sporadic mutations. Most breast cancer cells express estrogen receptors that promote the cancer phenotype, and many breast cancer cells express HER2, a growth factor receptor that can be the target of chemotherapy.
- Menopause is the cessation of menstrual periods and a time of decreased estrogen secretion. Among the physiological changes associated with menopause, perhaps the major pathophysiological change is accelerated loss of bone density and development of postmenopausal osteoporosis.
- Lack of estrogen alters the normal balance of bone resorption and bone deposition, with relatively more resorption and less bone formation. This tendency is exacerbated by relative hyperparathyroidism, which promotes osteoclast activity. Older age of both women and men increases osteoporosis and risk of fracture and disability.
- The male genitourinary system anatomically combines the structures needed for urine elimination (bladder, urethra) with the structures needed for procreation (seminiferous tubules, epididymis, vas deferens, accessory glands for semen production, ejaculatory ducts, and urethra).
- HPG axis activity is relatively constant in postpubertal males, with pulsatile secretion of GnRH, LH stimulating Leydig cell testosterone production, and FSH stimulating Sertoli cell inhibin production. Testosterone provides negative feedback to pituitary LH secretion, whereas inhibin provides negative feedback to pituitary FSH secretion.
- Testosterone is converted by 5α-reductase enzyme to DHT, a more potent androgen. These two androgens, plus estradiol, contribute to various aspects of development, growth, and maintenance of male reproductive structures as well as secondary sexual characteristics.

- Penile erection is needed for delivery of sperm. With adequate levels of testosterone for normal function, erection is accomplished based on psychological and physical sexual stimulation that leads to vasodilation of arterioles of the corpus cavernosum of the penis. Nitric oxide is the primary mediator of the relaxation of arteriolar smooth muscle, with intracellular effects caused by cGMP. Expansion of the arteriolar vascular volume compresses the veins to maintain the blood volume and thus the erection.

- In ED, an erection cannot occur or cannot be sustained, as often happens with older age and chronic diseases such as hypertension and diabetes. ED can also be a drug adverse effect.
- Prostate disorders include BPH and prostate cancer. Both are due, in part, to androgen stimulation of the prostate, and androgen antagonism is one approach to treatment. As the prostate develops excessive benign or malignant growth, blood levels of PSA rise, making PSA measurements one component of surveillance in middle-aged and older men.

Metabolism and the Pancreas
Gioia Polidori and Victoria Fischer

OVERVIEW

The fundamental pattern of human metabolism involves periods of dietary intake of meals that include carbohydrates, proteins, and lipids (as well as vitamins, minerals, micronutrients, and water), followed by times of fasting between meals. The fasting state is often longest between the last meal of the day (followed by sleep) and the first meal of the morning. Meals tend to occur two to three times daily, followed by digestion and absorption, and the use of nutrients for immediate energy, energy storage, and tissue growth and repair. Nutrients are released from energy stores during the fasting state (postabsorptive), beginning about 4 to 6 hours after a meal (depending on meal composition). Hepatic glucose production is sufficient to sustain a blood glucose level in the normal fasting range of about 80 to 100 mg/dL for several hours after that. The brain preferentially uses glucose, and red blood cells (RBCs) use glucose as the sole energy source. Fat stores can be mobilized during fasting to deliver free fatty acids that are the preferred fuel of many other tissues, particularly the heart, liver, and muscles. Regulation of metabolic pathways during the fed and fasted states depends on altered levels of insulin and glucagon, the major hormones involved in these processes.

Excess food consumption relative to energy expenditure results in weight gain. The body mass index (BMI) is calculated based on weight and height, and thus indicates the amount of weight for one's height. The calculation is the weight in kilograms divided by the square of the height in meters. Although other techniques can be used to assess body fat percentage, BMI is quickly and easily calculated in an outpatient setting. The Centers for Disease Control and Prevention (CDC) define overweight in adults as BMI of 25 kg/m^2 or higher and <30 kg/m^2, and obesity as BMI of 30 kg/m^2 or higher.[104] Although BMI has limitations and cannot substitute for formal measurements of body composition to assess adiposity, the relative ease of making the measurements (height and weight) and calculation (available on dozens of websites) makes it the appropriate initial determination of obesity. Obesity and overweight in children are defined based on population norms for age and sex. Overweight and obesity are the most common abnormalities of metabolic health, followed closely by type 2 diabetes mellitus (T2DM; described in detail later in this section).

T2DM is characterized by resistance to the actions of insulin, and other abnormalities described later, resulting in hyperglycemia and dyslipidemia. Overweight, obesity, and T2DM promote a host of other complications—cardiovascular disease, kidney failure, blindness, and neuropathies. This section begins with a review of some basic principles of metabolism, followed by discussions of the hormones that regulate metabolic processes, concluding with descriptions of DM and related conditions.

REVIEW OF METABOLISM

The pancreatic hormones insulin and glucagon are the major regulators of nutrient flow in the body over the typical daily cycles of feeding and fasting. These hormones exert the primary influence over body fuel storage in the fed state and mobilization during fasting. The major target tissues participating in these metabolic processes are liver, muscle, and adipose (fat). Our discussion of pancreatic endocrine function thus begins with a brief overview of these states of metabolism. As hyperglycemia and dyslipidemia are the major metabolic abnormalities in DM, our discussion of metabolic processes focuses on handling of glucose and lipids.

METABOLIC PROCESSES IN THE FED STATE

Following a mixed meal, nutrients absorbed from the gastrointestinal tract can be used immediately by any tissue or may be stored in liver, adipose tissue, and muscle. Reactions that build up body structures and energy stores are referred to as *anabolic reactions*. The nutrients used include glucose, amino acids, and lipids carried by chylomicrons, as described in Chapter 2, Chemical and Biochemical Foundations.

Liver Processes

Glucose transporter 2 (GLUT2) is the major glucose transporter of liver cells. In the fed state, with high insulin and glucose levels, glucose is readily taken into hepatocytes. As soon as glucose enters the hepatocyte, it is phosphorylated to glucose 6-phosphate. In the body, two major enzymes can perform this phosphorylation: hexokinase and glucokinase. While the former is present in most cells, the latter is specific for liver and pancreatic β cells. This is particularly important because while other hexokinases are inhibited by high concentrations of glucose 6-phosphate, glucokinase is not, and therefore it is able to continue phosphorylating glucose even when the intracellular concentration of glucose 6-phosphate is high. Glucokinase is upregulated after a carbohydrate meal and contributes to the liver's rapid glucose accumulation from the portal vein. The primary fate for glucose 6-phosphate in the liver is storage in the form of the polymer glycogen. This process, called *glycogenesis*, uses the enzyme glycogen synthase and is promoted by insulin. Glucose 6-phosphate can also enter the glycolytic pathway and proceed to the step of acetyl coenzyme A (CoA). Acetyl-CoA, in turn, can continue to provide energy by entering the citric acid cycle followed by oxidative phosphorylation to produce high yields of adenosine triphosphate (ATP; **Figure 17.42**).

Acetyl-CoA can also be used as the substrate for fatty acid synthesis and, along with glycerol production from glucose, can be used to synthesize triglyceride. Liver-produced triglycerides are packaged as VLDLs, secreted by the liver and traveling to target tissues. Thus, excess glucose can ultimately be transformed to fat for storage. Acetyl-CoA is also the substrate for cholesterol synthesis. This is a multistep process that requires the function of several enzymes, some of which are the target for drugs that aim to decrease cholesterol levels in circulation. For instance, statins inhibit the function of 3-hydroxy-3-methylglutaryl-CoA reductase, which catalyzes one of the initial steps that lead to cholesterol synthesis in the liver. This class of drugs is commonly prescribed to patients with elevated cholesterol levels.

Skeletal Muscle Processes

In the fed state, insulin promotes uptake of both glucose and amino acids into muscle, where glucose is phosphorylated and used for energy or for glycogen synthesis. Insulin also promotes protein synthesis

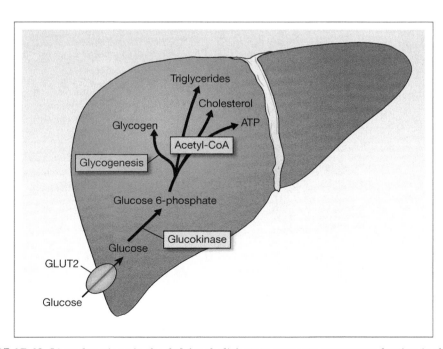

FIGURE 17.42 Liver functions in the fed (anabolic) state promote energy production in the form of ATP, as well as storage in the form of glycogen and triglyceride synthesis.
ATP, adenosine triphosphate; CoA, coenzyme A; GLUT, glucose transporter.

during the fed state. Once glucose is taken up by muscle cells, it can be oxidized to produce ATP or it can be converted to glycogen (**Figure 17.43**). In the fed state, fatty acid uptake in the skeletal muscle is increased as a consequence of the increased fatty acid availability in the blood and insulin signaling. In muscle tissue, as in adipose tissue, the enzyme lipoprotein lipase (LPL) is responsible for promoting triglyceride hydrolysis and the uptake of fatty acids in the muscle cells. Exercise can also increase fatty acid uptake by muscle. Fatty acids in the muscle can then enter the pathway of β-oxidation of fatty acids, whereby cells catabolize fatty acids to produce energy, or can be stored in the form of triglycerides. Lastly, muscle cells respond to insulin signaling in the fed state by increasing amino acid uptake and protein synthesis while decreasing protein breakdown.

Adipose Tissue Processes

Adipose tissue has the primary role of storing lipids in the form of triglycerides, which represent the most efficient way to store energy. In fact, while 1 g of carbohydrate or protein yields roughly 4 kcal of energy, 1 g of lipids yields 9 kcal. Dietary triglycerides are absorbed by the gut epithelium and travel in the circulation in the form of chylomicrons. Excess dietary glucose is used for liver fatty acid and triglyceride production, and is packaged as VLDL. Both chylomicrons and VLDLs

circulate freely in the fed state, supplying fatty acids to adipose tissue, and also to cardiac and skeletal muscle tissue. At the luminal surface of adipose blood vessels, the enzyme LPL hydrolyzes the triglycerides, releasing fatty acids from these lipoproteins. Fatty acids are then taken up by adipocytes and used to resynthesize triglycerides that are added to fat droplets within the cells. Insulin promotes glucose uptake into adipocytes. Glucose is converted to glycerol, which is covalently bound to fatty acids in the production of triglycerides (**Figure 17.44**). Other actions of insulin on the adipocyte include promoting triglyceride synthesis and inhibiting triglyceride breakdown. Overall, insulin has anabolic effects on the adipose tissue by promoting fuel storage.

Summary of the Fed State

Beginning with intake of a meal, gastrointestinal digestion and absorption bring digestion products into the bloodstream: glucose and other simple sugars, amino acids, and chylomicrons from dietary fat. These nutrients are taken into cells and used to supply energy and to build proteins. In specific target tissues of metabolism—liver, fat, and muscle—these nutrients are absorbed at a faster rate and are used to synthesize glycogen, fats, and proteins. These energy stores, particularly glycogen and fat, are available for later release during times of fasting between meals or even longer.

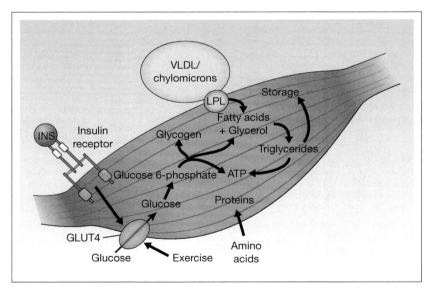

FIGURE 17.43 Muscle functions in the fed state include insulin-induced stimulation of glucose and amino acid transport via GLUT4, glycogen and protein synthesis, fatty acid uptake and storage, and ATP production.
ATP, adenosine triphosphate; GLUT4, glucose transporter 4; INS, insulin; LPL, lipoprotein lipase; VLDL, very low-density lipoprotein.

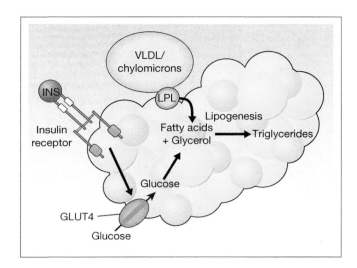

FIGURE 17.44 Fat functions in the fed state include fatty acid uptake, insulin-stimulated glucose uptake via GLUT4, and triglyceride synthesis.
GLUT4, glucose transporter 4; INS, insulin; LPL, lipoprotein lipase; VLDL, very low-density lipoprotein.

METABOLIC PROCESSES IN THE FASTING STATE

During fasting, stored fuels are broken down, providing cells with needed energy sources, principally glucose and free fatty acids, to generate ATP for cellular functions. While many processes that take place in the fasting state can be seen as the reverse of those that take place in the fed state, others are completely different. Insulin levels are low during fasting and glucagon levels increase, leading to a hormonal milieu that promotes the processes that break down energy stores. The number of hours between the last meal and initiation of these fasting state metabolic processes varies depending on meal composition. For clinical purposes, a fast of at least 8 hours is considered to constitute the fasting state.

Liver Processes

In the fasting state, the liver plays the central role of maintaining blood glucose homeostasis. This is achieved in two major ways: glycogenolysis and gluconeogenesis. The former entails the catabolism of glycogen to yield glucose (**Figure 17.45**). Liver *phosphorylase* enzyme catalyzes the removal of one glucose 1-phosphate molecule at a time from glycogen. Glucose 1-phosphate is then converted to glucose 6-phosphate. Glycogenolysis is the primary pathway of glucose production early in the fasting phase until glycogen stores are depleted, when gluconeogenesis begins. The latter pathway produces new glucose molecules from noncarbohydrate sources. Although synthesizing new glucose takes more energy than glycogenolysis, it is also essential, as some cells and organs, like RBCs and the brain, need glucose to survive. The metabolic precursors used for gluconeogenesis are amino acids, lactate, and glycerol.

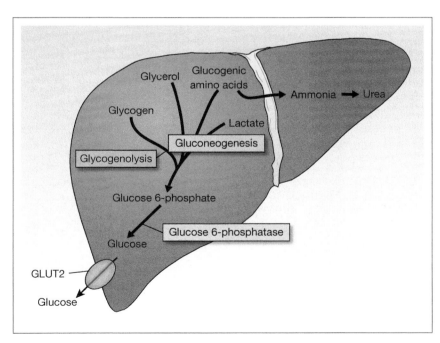

FIGURE 17.45 Liver functions during the fasting (catabolic) state include glycogenolysis, gluconeogenesis, and the removal of phosphate from glucose 6-phosphate to generate free glucose that can leave the cell via GLUT2.
GLUT2, glucose transporter 2.

Glucogenic amino acids can be used to produce glucose in a series of steps that entail the removal of the amino group in the liver mitochondria and then the conversion of the carbon skeletons into metabolites that can yield glucose. Two important amino acids commonly used for gluconeogenesis are alanine and glutamine. The removal of amino groups releases pyruvate and α-ketoglutarate, respectively, which in turn are used to produce glucose. Catabolism of amino acids requires particular care as the removal of the amino group produces ammonia, which is toxic. In order to limit the accumulation of ammonia in the body, the liver performs the urea cycle, which converts ammonia into less toxic urea that can be safely excreted by the kidneys.

Another metabolite that can be converted into glucose is lactate. Most cells in the body perform aerobic metabolism, which entails the complete oxidation of glucose through the pathways of glycolysis, citric acid cycle, and oxidative phosphorylation. Yet, aerobic metabolism requires oxygen, and during short bursts of physical activity the pyruvate produced by glycolysis is shunted to form lactate instead of being converted into acetyl-CoA. This allows cells to continue producing some energy in the form of ATP. Lactate produced in muscle during fasting can return to the liver and be converted into pyruvate, which is a substrate for gluconeogenesis. An additional substrate for gluconeogenesis is glycerol released from triglyceride breakdown (lipolysis) in adipose tissue. Thus, during fasting, amino acids, lactate, and glycerol can be used to produce glucose through the pathways of gluconeogenesis. Although the liver is the main site for gluconeogenesis, this metabolic pathway can also take place in the kidneys, which can provide 10% to 15% of glucose during prolonged starvation.

Both glycogenolysis and gluconeogenesis produce glucose 6-phosphate. Although phosphorylated glucose is unable to cross the membrane and is thus trapped in most cells, hepatocytes contain the enzyme glucose 6-phosphatase, which hydrolyzes glucose 6-phosphate, releasing the phosphate group to produce free glucose. As glycogenolysis, gluconeogenesis, and free glucose production proceed, hepatocyte glucose levels rise higher than extracellular glucose, promoting glucose exit (efflux) from the cell via the GLUT2-facilitated diffusion transporter. In summary, the enzyme pathways of glycogenolysis and gluconeogenesis and the presence of phosphatase enzyme are the key to the central role of the liver in stabilizing blood glucose during fasting.

Skeletal Muscle Processes

Muscle cells are able to store glucose in the form of glycogen and perform glycogenolysis to release glucose 6-phosphate (**Figure 17.46**). Unlike the liver, muscle cells do not express glucose 6-phosphatase. Thus, glycogen breakdown provides the muscle cells themselves with energy during fasting, but muscle cells cannot be a source of circulating glucose in the scenario of prolonged fasting or hypoglycemia. During these states, muscle glycogen breakdown and glucose utilization for glycolysis produces lactate. Lactate is transported out of the muscle cell and travels to the liver, providing a substrate for gluconeogenesis. Lactate can also be fully oxidized in the muscle cell to produce a greater amount of ATP via the citric acid cycle and oxidative

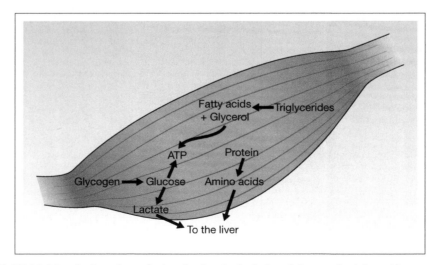

FIGURE 17.46 Muscle functions during fasting include breakdown of triglycerides to generate fatty acids for energy production and glycerol. Glycogenolysis produces glucose that can proceed through the glycolytic pathway and produce lactate. Proteolysis releases amino acids. Glycerol, lactate, and amino acids can be released and circulate to the liver for use as gluconeogenic substrates.
ATP, adenosine triphosphate.

phosphorylation. Muscle cells are also able to store and use triglycerides and fatty acids as fuel sources. Additionally, under conditions of prolonged fasting, proteolysis by skeletal muscle cells releases amino acids that can fuel gluconeogenesis in the liver.

Adipose Tissue Processes

In the fasting state, adipose cell hormone-sensitive lipases (HSLs) are activated, breaking down triglycerides, and releasing fatty acids and glycerol to the circulation (**Figure 17.47**). Several hormones can stimulate the function of HSL: glucagon, catecholamines, and cortisol. The fatty acids can then be delivered to the muscle, liver, or heart, while glycerol circulates to the liver, where it can be used for gluconeogenesis.

Ketogenesis Is an Additional Catabolic Pathway

In the fasting state, fatty acids can be catabolized by β-oxidation, yielding acetyl-CoA that can be used in the citric acid cycle, and nicotinamide adenine dinucleotide (NADH) and flavin adenine dinucleotide (FADH₂) that can be used for oxidative phosphorylation—producing ATP by both mechanisms. Acetyl-CoA is also processed into ketone bodies: acetoacetic acid, acetone, and β-hydroxybutyric acid. Ketogenesis is promoted by the increased rates of lipolysis occurring during prolonged fasting or very low carbohydrate intake, as adipose stores of triglycerides are broken down and free fatty acid concentrations increase. On a very low carbohydrate diet, gluconeogenesis depletes

citric acid cycle intermediates, blocking further activity of this cycle. This, in turn, leads to acetyl-CoA being shunted out of the citric acid cycle, further increasing the production of ketone bodies (**Figure 17.48**). The ketones are exported from the liver to other tissues as a fuel source. Importantly, although the brain preferentially uses glucose as a fuel source, it can adapt to use ketone bodies. Other factors, such as low

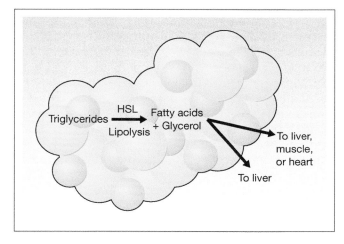

FIGURE 17.47 Fat functions during fasting include lipolysis with release of fatty acids and glycerol. Fatty acids circulate to target tissues, particularly muscle, to serve as an energy source, whereas glycerol circulates to the liver to serve as a gluconeogenic substrate.
HSL, hormone-sensitive lipase.

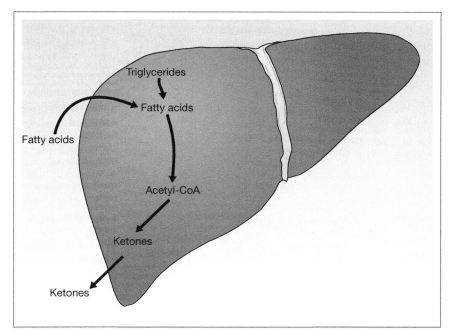

FIGURE 17.48 Liver ketone production. In prolonged fasting or in the absence of insulin, extensive lipolysis produces fatty acids that are metabolized by liver β-oxidation, yielding ketone bodies. Ketogenesis is also produced in extreme stress and catabolic states.
Acetyl-CoA, acetyl coenzyme A.

insulin and high glucagon levels, can promote ketone body synthesis. Acetoacetic acid and β-hydroxybutyric acid in circulation release their protons and when present at high levels decrease blood pH, leading to ketoacidosis. This scenario may develop in diabetic patients in the form of diabetic ketoacidosis (DKA), discussed later in this chapter.

Summary of the Fasting State

To summarize the metabolic changes during fasting: depending on energy expenditure, and glucose and glycogen availability, an individual may switch fuel sources at different time points. For instance, within a few hours of fasting, glycogenolysis begins until liver glycogen stores are depleted. As glycogenolysis ends, gluconeogenesis begins, synthesizing glucose from noncarbohydrate sources. During this time in fat cells, lipolysis is also increasing, and fatty acids in the blood travel to muscle cells as an additional source of energy, sparing glucose use. Fatty acids also are taken up by the liver and used for energy. Liver metabolism of fatty acids generates ketone bodies in the process of ketogenesis. Ketogenesis allows the production of water-soluble fuel sources that can provide the brain with the energy required, leading to the accumulation of ketone bodies in the bloodstream when fasting is prolonged for several days. Similarly, in a prolonged fast, proteolysis in muscle cells releases amino acids that can be used by the liver for gluconeogenesis. Breakdown of muscle glycogen releases lactate that circulates to the liver as an additional gluconeogenic precursor.

Metabolic processes in the stressed state reflect an exaggerated form of the catabolic processes seen during fasting. Sympathetic nervous system activity decreases insulin secretion and increases glucagon and epinephrine secretion. HPA activation, described earlier in this chapter, increases cortisol secretion. This hormonal profile strongly promotes liver glycogenolysis and gluconeogenesis, muscle lactate and amino acid release, and adipose lipolysis. The resulting stress hyperglycemia may be useful in times of physical stress (the fight or flight response or intense exercise) but is pathological in the setting of psychological stress.

Thought Questions

22. What are the major tissues involved in metabolism of carbohydrates, fats, and proteins?

23. Compare the enzyme processes in each of the tissues of metabolism between the fed and fasted states.

HORMONAL REGULATION OF METABOLISM

INSULIN

The peptide hormone insulin is best known for its role in reducing blood glucose levels, but it has a number of other functions. It is the major anabolic hormone of the body; regulates glucose, lipid, and protein homeostasis; alters electrolyte homeostasis; affects fertility and life span; and coordinates growth and development.[105] Given these central functions, dysregulation of its signaling has far-reaching systemic effects.

Insulin is secreted by the endocrine pancreas. The endocrine pancreas is made up of small clusters of cells, the islets of Langerhans, which are distributed throughout the pancreatic exocrine tissue. The center of many islets is enriched in insulin-secreting β cells, surrounded by glucagon-secreting α cells (**Figure 17.49**). Smaller numbers of islet cells produce SST and pancreatic polypeptide. The blood supply to each islet flows from the center of the islet to the periphery. This arrangement allows blood enriched in insulin to flow over the glucagon-secreting cells, contributing to insulin's role as a paracrine mediator of glucagon secretion. The islets account for 1% to 2% of the weight of the pancreas, but receive disproportionate blood flow—about 10% to 15% of pancreatic blood flows to the islets. Because the pancreatic vein drains to the portal vein, blood flow to the liver is rich in insulin during the fed state and glucagon during the fasting state. The liver readily takes up insulin and degrades it. As the liver is a major target tissue for these pancreatic hormones, this anatomical arrangement facilitates the physiological role of the liver as a critical regulator of metabolism.[106]

The active hormone insulin consists of two polypeptide chains, A and B, with a total of 51 amino acids. The chains are linked by disulfide bridges. The hormone is synthesized as a longer polypeptide, proinsulin. This precursor of the active hormone contains a third polypeptide chain that connects the A and B chains and is accordingly named connecting peptide, or C-peptide. Proinsulin is cleaved in the Golgi apparatus to form insulin and C-peptide. The two polypeptides are packaged in equimolar amounts into secretory vesicles (**Figure 17.50**). While insulin has a short half-life of about 6 minutes, C-peptide circulates much longer, at about 30 minutes.[107] Measuring serum C-peptide level allows estimation of endogenous insulin secretion.

Cellular Mechanisms of Insulin Action

Insulin binds to the insulin receptor, a tetrameric protein with two alpha and two beta subunits that is a member of the growth factor receptor family (see Chapter 4, Cell Physiology and Pathophysiology). The insulin-binding site is on the α subunits that face the extracellular fluid. The β subunits span the membrane, with internal regions that function as tyrosine kinases, phosphorylating their

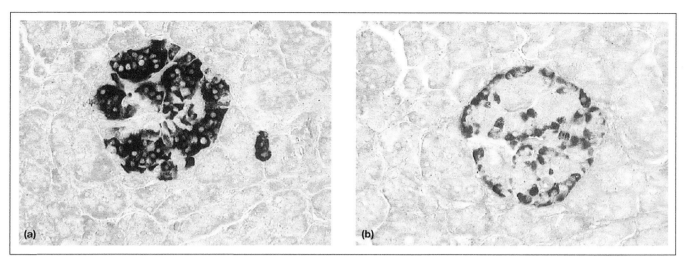

FIGURE 17.49 Pancreatic islets contain insulin-secreting β cells shown in (a) and glucagon-secreting α cells shown in (b).

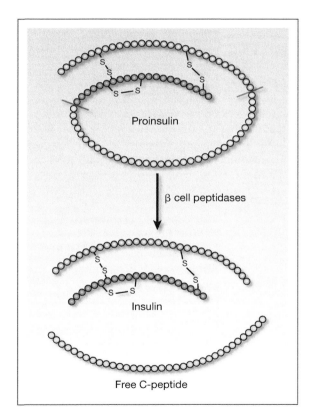

FIGURE 17.50 Insulin synthesis and C-peptide generation. Insulin is synthesized as pre-proinsulin, which becomes proinsulin after a signal peptide is cleaved. Proinsulin is further cleaved within the β cell, releasing equimolar amounts of insulin and C-peptide that are co-secreted from β cell secretory vesicles.
C-peptide, connecting peptide.

substrates when activated. The autophosphorylation of key tyrosine residues on the β chain of the insulin receptor is followed by phosphorylation of IRS. IRS then activate PI3K and Akt. The pathways thus activated lead to translocation of glucose transporter 4 (GLUT4) receptors to the plasma membrane, allowing glucose transport, particularly into muscle and fat cells. This is the basis of insulin's rapid hypoglycemic effect (Figure 17.51).

In addition to the rapid upregulation of glucose transport, insulin promotes the uptake of amino acids and protein synthesis in liver, muscle, and other tissues, as well as lipid synthesis, while inhibiting protein and lipid breakdown. Insulin furthermore stimulates growth and differentiation of cells. It initiates DNA synthesis as part of cell proliferation, acting as a mitogen. These actions are slower in onset than the effects mediated by GLUT4 translocation and alterations in metabolic pathways, and involve the MAP kinase signaling pathway. In clinical states of insulin resistance, described later in the chapter, the PI3K pathway does not have its normal insulin-stimulated response, whereas the MAP kinase pathway retains its effectiveness. This contributes to pathogenesis of some of the complications of insulin-resistant states.

Effects of Insulin on the Liver

In the fed state, insulin's actions on hepatocytes promote glucose oxidation, glycogen synthesis, and triglyceride and cholesterol synthesis, as well as protein synthesis from amino acids absorbed from the meal. Rapid glucose uptake and phosphorylation by liver cells is promoted by insulin, which facilitates glycogen synthase activity. In addition, insulin inhibits the

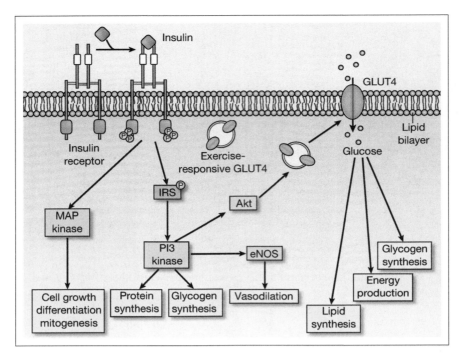

FIGURE 17.51 Insulin signaling pathway. See text for explanation. Only some of the downstream effects are represented here.

eNOS, endothelial nitric oxide synthase; GLUT4, glucose transporter 4; IRS, insulin receptor substrate; MAP, mitogen-activated protein; P, phosphate residues; PI3, phosphoinositol 3.

liver enzyme phosphorylase, preventing a futile cycle of glycogen synthesis followed by glycogen breakdown. Insulin also inhibits the pathways of gluconeogenesis, and this effect along with the suppression of glycogenolysis reduces liver glucose production. When glucose is consumed in excess of that needed for intracellular energy and glycogen production, insulin promotes conversion of acetyl-CoA into fatty acids and cholesterol. The fatty acids are further processed into triglycerides, and packaged into VLDLs (**Figure 17.52**).

Effects of Insulin on Muscle

Muscle tissue is estimated to make up 30% to 40% of body mass, so the effect of insulin on muscle glucose uptake is substantial. Muscle glucose uptake is promoted after a meal, when circulating glucose and insulin levels increase. The cellular mechanism of muscle glucose uptake is translocation of GLUT4 transporters to the membrane (**Figure 17.53**). Glucose that enters is rapidly phosphorylated and stored in the form of glycogen. Glycogen is then available for times of increased muscle activity. Insulin also increases muscle amino acid transport, and promotes protein synthesis during the fed state.

During exercise, stored glycogen is used as a rapid energy source, until the glycogen is depleted. Once muscle glycogen is depleted, exercise itself is a stimulus for non–insulin-dependent GLUT4 translocation, allowing uptake of glucose to continue to support muscle activity. In addition, physical activity sensitizes the muscle membrane to insulin, enhancing glucose uptake over the next 12 to 24 hours. Regular physical activity, therefore, is a key part of management of diabetes, as described later in this section.

Effect of Insulin on Fat Cells

In fat cells, glucose uptake is insulin mediated and involves the mobilization of GLUT4 transporters to the membrane. The glucose is converted to glycerol and used as "backbone" for triglycerides to be stored in the lipid droplets. Insulin furthermore activates LPL in the capillary walls. This enzyme cleaves triglycerides from chylomicrons and VLDL, releasing fatty acids that can then be taken up by fat cells (**Figure 17.54**). This process is essential for the uptake and storage of lipids; thus, insulin deficiency leads to higher circulating levels of lipids, promoting atherosclerosis and subsequent vascular events such as heart attacks and strokes. In addition to promoting removal of triglycerides from the circulation, triglyceride breakdown (lipolysis) and release of fatty acids into the bloodstream is inhibited by insulin, via inhibition of the enzyme HSL. These effects of insulin on lipid metabolism are highly relevant to the chronic complications of DM, as noted later in the chapter.

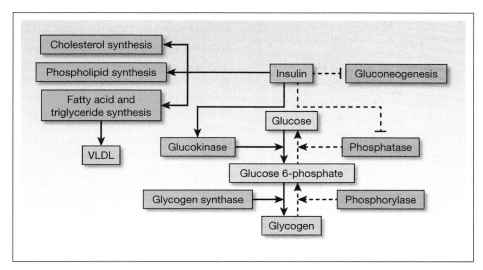

FIGURE 17.52 Effect of insulin on liver metabolism (see text for description). Insulin affects multiple processes in the liver, increasing anabolic processes, including glycogen biosynthesis, but also synthesis of fatty acids, cholesterol, and phospholipids that can be secreted into the bloodstream as VLDL particles. Simultaneously, insulin inhibits glycogen breakdown by phosphorylase and generation of free glucose from glucose 6-phosphate by phosphatase. Finally, insulin also decreases liver glucose production by inhibiting gluconeogenesis, contributing to its effectiveness at reducing blood glucose levels.
VLDL, very low-density lipoprotein.

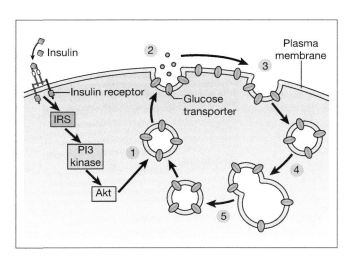

FIGURE 17.53 Effect of insulin on GLUT4 in muscle and fat cells. Glucose uptake into muscle and fat cells is insulin sensitive. (1) When insulin binds to its receptor, downstream signals initiate the movement of vesicles containing the GLUT4 glucose transporter to the membrane. (2) Glucose transport into the cell begins and is maintained at a high rate in the fed state when insulin and glucose are high. (3) When insulin and glucose levels fall, GLUT4 is once more internalized in an intracellular vesicle. (4) Vesicles form endosomes that can be recycled into a ready-to-mobilize form (5).
GLUT4, glucose transporter 4; IRS, insulin receptor substrate; PI3, phosphoinositol 3.

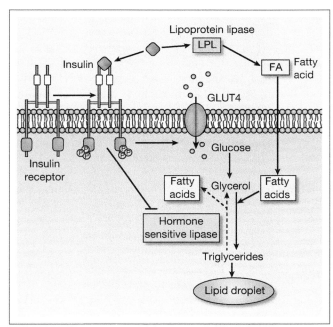

FIGURE 17.54 Effect of insulin on fat cells (adipocytes). Insulin facilitates glucose uptake (mediated by GLUT4) and triglyceride uptake from chylomicrons and VLDLs via LPL. Insulin is the primary hormone promoting fat storage.
FA, fatty acid; GLUT4, glucose transporter 4; LPL, lipoprotein lipase; P, phosphates attached to tyrosine residues in the intracellular portion of the insulin receptor; VLDL, very low-density lipoprotein.

Effects of Insulin on the Brain

Glucose uptake in the brain is not dependent on insulin; however, the brain does have insulin receptors in several regions, including cortex, cerebellum, and hypothalamus. Insulin is a satiety factor, and meal-related insulin secretion may contribute to cessation of eating, along with other central and peripheral satiety signals. The brain uses glucose preferentially as its energy substrate. Other energy substrates cannot be used easily, although adaptation to use of ketones is possible. Accordingly, low blood glucose levels can lead to diminished brain function, with confusion, coma, and seizures occurring when glucose levels drop below about 30 mg/dL. This threshold varies, depending on the patient and whether he or she has previously experienced hypoglycemia. Insulin exerts other essential functions of growth and tissue maintenance in the brain, and insulin resistance may contribute to Alzheimer disease (see later discussion).

Regulation of Insulin Secretion

The typical signal stimulating insulin secretion is increased β cell ATP resulting from the metabolism of glucose. Metabolism of amino acids and other nutrients can also increase ATP and contribute to stimulation of insulin secretion. In addition, there is substantial modulation of insulin secretion by neurotransmitters and hormones acting through G protein–coupled receptors. A summary of major aspects of these complex processes is presented in **Box 17.5** and illustrated in **Figure 17.55**.

In addition to nutrients that result in ATP production, other factors are known to modulate insulin secretion, many of which augment glucose-stimulated insulin secretion. Vagal acetylcholine stimulates insulin secretion, although the degree to which this contributes to overall insulin release in response to glucose is not clear. Food in the gastrointestinal tract stimulates release of gastrointestinal hormones, particularly glucose-dependent insulinotropic polypeptide (GIP) and glucagon-like peptide 1 (GLP-1; see **Figure 17.55**). GIP is secreted by cells in the proximal small intestine, whereas GLP-1 is secreted by cells in ileum and colon, both in response to the presence of food digestion products in the gut lumen. These hormones enhance glucose-stimulated insulin secretion and contribute to postprandial blood glucose regulation. Both GIP and GLP-1 are degraded by dipeptidyl peptidases (DPPs), most prominently DPP-4. These hormones and the degradative enzyme are the targets of drugs used in diabetes management, as described later in this section. Other gastrointestinal hormones that increase glucose-stimulated insulin secretion include gastrin, secretin, and cholecystokinin. Release of all of these gastrointestinal hormones depends on the presence of food digestion products in the gut. Based on this relationship, insulin secretion following an oral glucose load is many times greater than to an intravenous glucose load. Insulin secretion is inhibited by three main factors: (a) hypoglycemia, (b) sympathetic nervous system activity, and (c) specific inhibitory hormones, including somatostatin and epinephrine.

Insulin secretion in response to energy substrates is not linear. It occurs in two phases. The first peak is rapid but soon declines, whereas the second peak develops more slowly but can be sustained (**Figure 17.56**). The first phase is deficient or absent in individuals with T2DM, as described later.

Oral Glucose Tolerance Testing

The well-known influence of oral nutrient intake on insulin secretion provides the physiological basis for the oral glucose tolerance test (OGTT). In this test, oral intake of a defined amount of glucose (usually 75 g) is followed by repeated blood sampling to measure blood glucose. The ability to rapidly return glucose to normal levels after this oral load depends on a robust insulin secretory response, as well as rapid liver uptake of absorbed glucose. In a normal OGTT, between 25% and 35% of an absorbed glucose load undergoes first-pass entry to the liver from the portal vein, and thus does not reach the systemic circulation. As the intracellular glucose concentration in hepatocytes increases, hepatic gluconeogenesis is inhibited. The total effect of the liver on glucose disposal from an oral glucose load is estimated at 33%, as a combined effect of first-pass uptake of glucose and inhibited gluconeogenesis. An additional third of an oral glucose load is rapidly taken up into muscle and fat owing to insulin-stimulated glucose transport via GLUT4. The remaining third of glucose is taken up into insulin-independent tissues, including brain, RBCs, and kidney.[108] In states of body insulin resistance such as T2DM, liver and muscle resistance to insulin action greatly reduces the ability to dispose of the glucose load, and glucose levels during the OGTT will reach higher levels and remain elevated for a prolonged time.

ADDITIONAL HORMONES REGULATING METABOLIC HOMEOSTASIS

A number of other hormones affect metabolic pathways, several of which oppose the actions of insulin and promote catabolic processes. Secretory rhythms of some of these hormones may correlate with the patterns of feeding and fasting, while others relate to specific states such as stress or pregnancy. The hormonal milieu at any given time will determine the metabolic processes in liver, muscle, and fat, as well as other target tissues. Most prominent among these hormones are glucagon, cortisol, and epinephrine. These hormones, along with growth hormone, are also stimulated by hypoglycemia and promote recovery from hypoglycemia. For this reason, they are sometimes referred to as *counterregulatory* hormones.

BOX 17.5
Mechanisms of Insulin Secretion

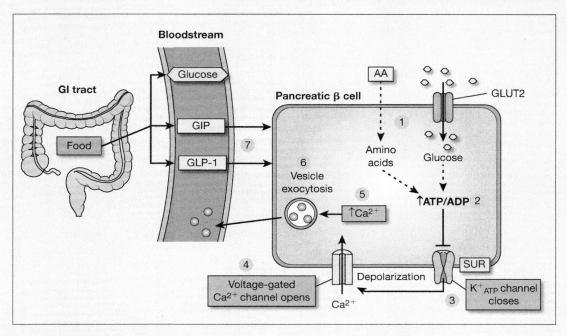

FIGURE 17.55 Insulin secretion from β cells. (See box text for explanation.)
AA, amino acids; ADP, adenosine diphosphate; ATP, adenosine triphosphate; GI, gastrointestinal; GIP, glucose-dependent insulinotropic peptide; GLP-1, glucagon-like peptide 1; GLUT2, glucose transporter 2; K^{+}_{ATP}, ATP-dependent potassium channel; SUR, sulfonylurea receptor.

1. As glucose increases during meal digestion and absorption, glucose entry into β cells and phosphorylation by glucokinase follows.

2. Subsequent entry into the pathways of glycolysis, citric acid cycle, and oxidative phosphorylation increase intracellular ATP. Amino acids also increase during meal digestion and absorption, and can be metabolized within the β cell, to produce ATP. When administered alone, amino acids only have a small effect on insulin secretion, whereas when they are coadministered with glucose, they potentiate the effect of glucose on insulin secretion, with arginine and lysine having the largest effect.

3. When ATP levels rise, ATP-sensitive potassium channels in the plasma membrane close.

4. This leads to depolarization of the plasma membrane and subsequent opening of voltage-gated calcium channels. Note that the ATP-sensitive potassium channel is associated with a sulfonylurea receptor, site of action of this class of insulin secretagogue drugs.

5. Intracellular calcium increases.

6. Increased calcium is the signal causing the secretory vesicles to fuse with the plasma membrane, releasing their contents, including insulin and C-peptide, into the bloodstream.

7. Glucose-stimulated insulin secretion is enhanced by the gastrointestinal hormones (also referred to as *incretins*) GIP and GLP-1, among other influences.

ATP, adenosine triphosphate; GIP, glucose-dependent insulinotropic peptide; GLP-1, glucagon-like peptide 1.

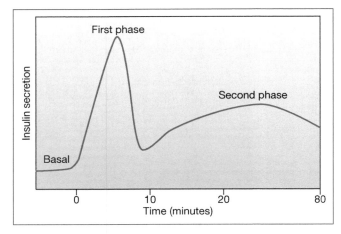

FIGURE 17.56 Insulin secretion. Secretion of insulin from pancreatic β cells in response to a glucose load occurs in two phases. The first phase represents rapid secretion of insulin stored in vesicles in the cell prior to the glucose load. The second, slower phase reflects secretion of newly synthesized insulin in response to stimulation.

Glucagon

The main function of glucagon is to increase blood glucose levels; thus, it acts in direct opposition to insulin. Like insulin, glucagon is produced in the islets of Langerhans, but in the α cells, which make up about 20% to 25% of the islet cells. The main factors influencing glucagon secretion are the levels of glucose and insulin. In the fed state, insulin released from neighboring β cells inhibits glucagon secretion by intra-islet signaling, a *paracrine* mechanism. However, falling blood glucose levels stimulate glucagon secretion. As a result, in the postabsorptive state, as glucose decreases back to normal levels, insulin secretion also decreases, reducing the suppression of glucagon secretion. When blood glucose begins to drop to the hypoglycemic range, <70 mg/dL, insulin secretion decreases further and glucagon secretion increases in response to decreased levels of both glucose and insulin. Amino acids stimulate glucagon secretion and are elevated after a meal consisting of protein in excess of carbohydrate. In this context, glucagon secretion is stimulated and helps to maintain blood glucose. This is an important mechanism for individuals adhering to a very low carbohydrate/moderate protein diet. Sympathetic stimulation is an additional factor increasing glucagon secretion; however, this is less prominent during normal cycles of feeding and fasting and more significant during states of stress and exercise.

Glucagon has catabolic actions and promotes the release of fuels during fasting. Liver glucose production increases through glycogenolysis and gluconeogenesis, resulting in increased blood glucose. At higher levels, glucagon contributes to activation of adipose tissue lipolysis and inhibits triglyceride synthesis in fat and liver, increasing the levels of circulating fatty acids. Glucagon stimulates liver ketone production, particularly in the absence or lack of effect of insulin, as in people with diabetes. During exercise, glucagon secretion increases and helps to mobilize blood glucose to support the additional energy requirements of working muscles.

Cortisol

A second hormone that opposes insulin is cortisol. The metabolic actions of cortisol include inhibiting glucose utilization and promoting gluconeogenesis in the liver. In peripheral tissues including muscle tissue, glucocorticoids reduce translocation of GLUT4 to the plasma membrane, reducing the effect of insulin, thus causing or aggravating insulin resistance.

Glucocorticoids, either exogenous medications or endogenous cortisol, increase DNA transcription of gluconeogenic enzymes; mobilization of amino acids, mainly from muscle; and uptake of amino acids into the liver. Simultaneously, they increase biosynthesis of protein by the liver, increasing plasma proteins. As all other tissues produce less protein under the influence of glucocorticoids, they cause wasting. They furthermore promote mobilization and utilization of fat. The stimulation of lipid metabolism shifts energy metabolism toward utilization of fat rather than glucose even in the presence of glucose.

In the fed state, cortisol works with insulin to promote liver glycogen production. Cortisol levels have small increases after each meal, facilitating fuel storage. Cortisol is essential to withstand hypoglycemia, so individuals with adrenal insufficiency are very vulnerable to hypoglycemia. However, when present in excess, as in stress states, the systemic effects of cortisol promote insulin resistance, hyperglycemia, increased lipid levels, and protein wasting.

These effects of cortisol, and glucocorticoids in general, are clinically relevant because glucocorticoids are used as pharmacological treatment for many conditions, particularly chronic inflammatory disorders. These drugs exert strong effects on energy metabolism as an off-target effect. Many prescribed glucocorticoids are more potent than endogenous cortisol, and prolonged use of such drugs (as in some transplant recipients and cancer patients) increases the risk of developing diabetes.

Epinephrine

Epinephrine release from the adrenal medulla is controlled by the sympathetic nervous system. Epinephrine functions to increase availability of energy substrates in response to stress. It promotes liver glucose production, mainly through stimulation of glycogenolysis, and stimulates fat cell HSL, thus increasing free fatty acids in blood. Epinephrine promotes muscle glycogenolysis and release of lactate that circulates to the liver and is ultimately used to restore glycogen levels there. Epinephrine is a stress hormone, as is cortisol, so stress states are characterized by both hyperglycemia and elevated free fatty acid levels. Although useful as a short-term adaptation supporting the fight-or-flight response, stress hyperglycemia and hyperlipidemia are pathological over longer periods of time.

Growth Hormone

The metabolic actions of GH are synergistic with insulin on muscle protein synthesis, while opposing the actions of insulin on liver glucose production and tissue glucose uptake. GH secretion is stimulated during hypoglycemia and contributes somewhat to the overall recovery from hypoglycemia. GH supports lipolysis and subsequent ketone formation, with an overall effect of decreasing fat mass. Acromegaly is a disorder of GH excess in which a significant number of patients develop DM.

Chorionic Somatomammotropin

This hormone has characteristics of both PRL and GH. It is secreted by the placenta starting at about the fifth week of pregnancy and increasing throughout pregnancy. Chorionic somatomammotropin opposes the actions of insulin—inhibiting glucose uptake into tissues and releasing fatty acids from adipose tissue. These actions contribute to providing fuel for the developing fetus. Its actions also contribute to the presentation of gestational diabetes, described later in the chapter.

Thought Questions

24. Describe the mechanism of insulin secretion and the way its secretion is altered by nutrients, hormones, and neural control.

25. Identify the target tissues of insulin action and the effects of insulin stimulation in each tissue.

26. Compare and contrast the effects of the counter-insulin hormones on their target tissues.

DIABETES MELLITUS

Diabetes mellitus (DM) is a disease group marked by dysregulated signaling of the hormone insulin, with increased blood glucose levels as most obvious hallmark. This dysregulation can consist of diminished or absent insulin production or secretion (type 1 and late-stage type 2 diabetes) or by insulin resistance of cells that are the targets of insulin action (type 2 diabetes, gestational diabetes, and some other subtypes). The American Diabetes Association distinguishes four main groups of diabetes diagnoses (**Box 17.6**). Although the classification is relevant for therapeutic interventions, the consequences are very similar among all forms of diabetes, while the rate of progression varies widely.[109]

BOX 17.6
Classification of Diabetes Mellitus[109]

1. **T1DM**, in which an autoimmune attack leads to destruction of the insulin-secreting β cells, causing absolute insulin deficiency

2. **T2DM**, in which progressive loss of β cells, usually in conjunction with insulin resistance, causes relative insulin deficiency

3. **Gestational diabetes**, in which pregnancy-related changes in insulin sensitivity and insulin degradation cause at-risk women to develop diabetes in the second or third trimester of pregnancy, which often resolves rapidly after delivery of the baby

4. **Diabetes due to other causes:**
   a. Single-gene disorders that affect β cells, including mutations in genes coding for insulin, glucokinase, ATP-sensitive potassium channels, among others, causing monogenic diabetes
   b. Diseases, such as pancreatitis and cystic fibrosis, affecting the exocrine pancreas that secondarily damage islets, often called type 3c diabetes
   c. Endocrine disorders that increase insulin resistance, including Cushing syndrome, acromegaly, pheochromocytoma, and glucagonoma
   d. Drug-induced diabetes, which can occur with use of corticosteroids and certain drugs used for psychiatric disorders, after organ transplantation, and for HIV infection

ATP, adenosine triphosphate; T1DM, type 1 diabetes mellitus; T2DM, type 2 diabetes mellitus.

DIAGNOSTIC CRITERIA

Diagnosis of diabetes can be based on one of several criteria and is differentiated into diabetes and prediabetes. The changes leading to diabetes occur on a continuum, with early and middle stages being asymptomatic. Thus, in a patient who has never been screened, the disease process can be far advanced when a diagnosis of diabetes is finally made. According to the American Diabetes Association's 2019 Standards of Medical Care, diagnostic criteria include hemoglobin A1C, fasting plasma glucose, results from an OGTT, or random blood glucose values. It is recommended that the diagnosis be confirmed with a second test. Clinical considerations relating to each test follow:

- *Hemoglobin A1C* describes the fraction of hemoglobin that is glycosylated, generally abbreviated as HbA1C, or just A1C. Formation of HbA1C is by nonenzymatic attachment of glucose to RBC hemoglobin molecules. The percent of glycosylation depends on the average blood glucose concentration over the previous 2 to 3 months. A1C levels between 5.7% and 6.4% are diagnostic for prediabetes; at 6.5% or higher, they indicate diabetes. Although measuring this value does not require fasting, its interpretation is more complex as some genetic changes and disorders in RBC turnover affect the correlation between glycated hemoglobin and average plasma glucose level. Additionally, the validity of this test is debated with respect to children and adolescents. The value is sometimes expressed as estimated average glucose (eAG), using the same unit (mg/dL or mmol/L) as plasma glucose. A calculator for this conversion is available online (professional.diabetes.org/diapro/glucose_calc).
- *Fasting plasma glucose (FPG)* levels of 126 mg/dL (7.0 mmol/L) or higher are diagnostic for diabetes, while levels between 100 and 125 mg/dL (termed *impaired fasting glucose*) indicate prediabetes. The fast required for a reliable measurement is at least 8 hours. Water is permitted during this time. This is the most common test used in diabetes screening, despite having the significant limitation that elevated fasting blood glucose is a late development in diabetes progression.
- The *OGTT* is also used to diagnose diabetes and prediabetes. In a 75-g OGTT, a blood glucose level of 200 mg/dL (11.1 mmol/L) or higher at 2 hours after consumption of 75 g glucose is diagnostic of diabetes, and levels of 140 to 199 mg/dL (termed *impaired glucose tolerance*) indicate prediabetes.
- A *random plasma glucose* measurement of 200 mg/dL (11.1 mmol/L) or higher is also the basis for a diagnosis of diabetes in patients with classic symptoms of hyperglycemia or hyperglycemic crisis.

TYPE 1 DIABETES MELLITUS

Type 1 diabetes mellitus (T1DM) is a consequence of the autoimmune destruction of the β cells that produce and secrete insulin in the pancreas. The resulting insulin deficiency is absolute. Irrespective of the response of target cells to insulin signaling, there is not enough insulin circulating to sustain life. Hormone replacement in the form of exogenous insulin injections or transplantation of pancreas or pancreatic islets is necessary for survival. Based on data from the CDC, about 0.36% of the U.S. population have type 1 diabetes, representing about 5% of all people with diabetes.[11] The American Diabetes Association estimates that 1.25 million Americans have T1DM, with an incidence of about 40,000 newly diagnosed patients per year.[109]

Pathogenesis

In over 95% of cases, the fundamental mechanism leading to T1DM is an autoimmune reaction to pancreatic β cells. Antibodies to islet proteins and cells include antibodies to glutamic acid decarboxylase (GAD), the enzyme that synthesizes GABA in islet cells; islet cell autoantigen 512 (ICA512); anti-insulin antibodies; and antibodies to some tyrosine phosphatase enzymes. Islet autoantibodies can be detected prior to the development of actual disease and also in asymptomatic family members. They are used as predictive markers for T1DM. A higher number of antibodies increases the risk. Although most patients with T1DM test positive for at least one of these antibodies, some patients do not. This presentation is diagnosed as idiopathic T1DM, and is more common in individuals of African or Asian ancestry.[9,109] Of note, patients with T1DM may also have or develop other autoimmune disorders, such as Hashimoto thyroiditis, celiac disease, Graves disease, Addison disease, vitiligo, autoimmune hepatitis, myasthenia gravis, or pernicious anemia.

Genetic factors play a role in T1DM, with about 40% concordance in identical twins.[110] The greatest degree of family concordance is seen in individuals who are diagnosed at younger ages. Genetic influences are not solely responsible for development of the disease, and most individuals with the implicated genes do not develop diabetes. About half of the genetic factors known to increase susceptibility locate to the HLA gene cluster regions that code for major histocompatibility (MHC) class II proteins. Other polymorphisms within these regions are protective against development of islet autoantibodies and disease development. Another prominent polymorphism occurs in the autoimmune regulatory gene (*AIRE*). The gene product is involved in the destruction of self-reactive T cells in the thymus. A number of other polymorphisms are also implicated in increasing T1DM risk.[111] However, the environmental factor or factors that trigger the ultimate immune reaction against the β cells remains elusive. Hypotheses include environmental exposures, and viral and other infections. Recent literature also points to potential roles of vitamin D and the gut microbiome in disease pathogenesis.[112]

Presentation

The classic presentation of a patient with T1DM is characterized by hyperosmolality and hyperketonemia, with high circulating levels of glucose and fatty acids. Polyphagia, polyuria and polydipsia, weight loss, ketonuria, and often blurred vision—as the lenses are exposed to hyperosmolar fluids—are present. In cases of acute onset, ketoacidosis is common.

As the availability of insulin decreases in T1DM, both its inhibitory effect on catabolism and its effect on tissue uptake of glucose are decreased. Accordingly, lipolysis increases; thus, free fatty acid levels in the blood increase, and protein breakdown in muscle tissue increases. Simultaneously, food intake is stimulated by the loss of the insulin satiety signal and the negative energy balance in fat and muscle tissue, resulting in polyphagia.

As the anabolic stimulation normally exerted by insulin is missing, and the catabolic effects of glucagon are unopposed, weight loss occurs despite polyphagia. Liver and muscle glycogen are depleted and fat stores are broken down. Ketone production increases owing to lipolysis and liver use of fatty acids for energy and ketone production. Muscle mass is lost as proteolysis produces amino acids to fuel gluconeogenesis. The loss of muscle protein and potassium results in weakness. Postural hypotension is common due to dehydration.

Glucagon secretion is increased because of the loss of intra-islet suppression of glucagon by insulin. Also, without insulin, the actions of glucagon are unopposed, so liver glucose production by gluconeogenesis is constant, contributing to increased blood glucose levels. In the absence of insulin, glucose absorbed from dietary carbohydrates cannot be absorbed into tissues. Blood glucose levels will eventually exceed the renal capacity for glucose reuptake from the glomerular filtrate, leading to the loss of glucose via the urine, as glycosuria. This produces osmotic diuresis, and both polyuria and increased thirst (polydipsia) will ensue. In addition to increased fluid losses, the osmolarity of the blood is increased by the higher blood glucose levels. This in turn leads to depletion of intracellular water and severe fluid and electrolyte imbalance.

Clinical Management

In the complete absence of endogenous insulin production, hormone replacement therapy is required. A detailed description of available insulins and regimens is beyond the scope of this book, but major principles are summarized here. Insulin replacement therapy dates from the 1920s, when Canadian physician/scientists Banting, Best, Collip, and Macleod isolated and purified insulin from cow pancreas and demonstrated that injections of purified insulin reduced glucose and ketone levels in patients with T1DM. Recombinant human insulin became available in 1982—the first recombinant treatment to be approved. Modified insulins are available with shorter or longer time to onset and duration of action than natural insulin. Efforts are ongoing to optimize insulin formulations that do not require injection, including oral insulin and nasal spray.

Insulin replacement therapy is guided by blood glucose level (determined by self-monitoring of blood glucose or continuous glucose monitoring) and by dietary intake of carbohydrates. Physiologically, insulin secretion is low between meals, rising with food intake and then subsiding as the meal is absorbed. Insulin replacement uses a long-acting insulin to mimic the low basal rate of insulin secretion combined with meal-time injections of short-acting insulin to mimic the usual meal-related spikes of insulin release. This approach is referred to as *basal-bolus* replacement. A similar pattern can be delivered through an inserted insulin pump, which is programmed based on individual blood glucose monitoring data, carbohydrate intake, and activity levels. Finally, both pancreas transplants and islet transplants can reduce or eliminate the need for exogenous insulin replacement; however, these treatments require lifelong immunosuppression therapy.

Diabetic Ketoacidosis

Diabetic ketoacidosis, a severe acute complication of T1DM, is also the initial, acute presentation of the disorder in some patients. In the absence of insulin, and with the associated increase in epinephrine, glucagon, and cortisol, lipolysis is the main catabolic pathway, delivering fatty acids for use as primary energy substrates. The hormonal milieu accelerates liver glucose and ketone production, promoted by the availability of free fatty acids for liver energy use (**Figure 17.57**).

Patients may present with fruity-smelling breath due to the accumulation of acetone, one of the ketone bodies, in addition to fatigue, weakness, nausea and vomiting, very high blood glucose levels, and ketonemia and ketonuria. In some cases, coma occurs, an effect of the hyperosmotic state on the brain. DKA typically occurs with failure to take insulin, but can be further stimulated by illness, trauma, and some drugs. The biochemical hallmarks for DKA are hyperglycemia and metabolic acidosis, with increased anion gap created by the ketones as unmeasured anions. Blood glucose levels rise into ranges of 250 to 600 mg/dL. Tissue hypoperfusion and increased anaerobic metabolism can then lead to lactic acidosis.

β-Hydroxybutyric acid is the main ketone body produced in DKA, and it is largely responsible for the

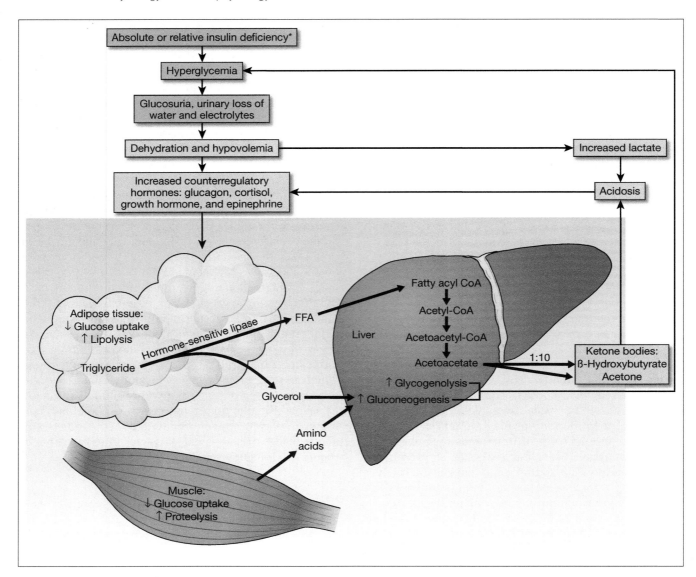

FIGURE 17.57 Diabetic ketoacidosis. Diabetic ketoacidosis arises under conditions of severe insulin deficiency, as in a person with type 1 diabetes mellitus who has not taken any insulin for hours to days. In the absence of insulin, a catabolic state ensues, with steadily increasing liver glucose production and inability of muscle and fat cells to take up glucose, resulting in progressive hyperglycemia. Adipose tissue lipolysis is promoted, and fatty acid metabolism by the liver generates ketone bodies and causes metabolic acidosis. Muscle undergoes proteolysis, providing amino acids to support liver gluconeogenesis, worsening hyperglycemia. Intracellular dehydration is caused by the hyperosmotic state, and osmotic diuresis worsens systemic dehydration and fluid/electrolyte imbalance.
Acetyl-CoA, acetyl-coenzyme A; FFA, free fatty acids.

state of metabolic acidosis that overwhelms the buffering systems that normally maintain pH homeostasis. Respiratory compensation for the metabolic acidosis triggers deep, labored breathing, termed *Kussmaul breathing*. DKA can be fatal if not corrected promptly with fluids, intravenous insulin, and electrolyte replacement.[113]

Hypoglycemia

Hypoglycemia is the most frequent acute complication of T1DM, resulting from an imbalance of insulin dose, carbohydrate intake, missed or delayed meals, or strenuous or prolonged physical exertion. Excess insulin administration can also lead to hypoglycemia. Hypoglycemia is common during and after exercise due to increased muscle insulin sensitivity. Responses to hypoglycemia are blunted during sleep, and continuous glucose monitoring is helpful in identifying patterns of nocturnal hypoglycemia and tailoring insulin dose and dietary intake accordingly. If glucose is not provided during acute hypoglycemia, loss of consciousness can follow. The usual compensatory responses to hypoglycemia are increased secretion of glucagon, cortisol, epinephrine, and GH, as well as decreased insulin secretion. However, individuals with T1DM are at a high risk of hypoglycemia because their glucagon levels are chronically elevated but unresponsive to onset of hypoglycemia, and their injected dose of insulin cannot be dissipated at a rapid rate. Repeated episodes of hypoglycemia lead to altered perception of hypoglycemia, a state termed **hypoglycemia unawareness**.

As the body adapts to episodes of low glucose levels, the epinephrine, cortisol, and GH responses to subsequent episodes decrease, and hypoglycemic symptoms (sweating, shakiness, palpitations, hunger, tiredness, confusion, irritability) disappear. Treatment for acute hypoglycemia in someone who is conscious and safely able to swallow is oral sugar in some form (juice, glucose tablets, candy, soda), followed by blood glucose monitoring. In the case of hypoglycemic coma, exogenous glucose is usually administered intravenously, or in some cases, intramuscularly. The sympathoadrenal response to hypoglycemia decreases with aging, autonomic neuropathy, certain medications (such as β-blockers), and hypoglycemia unawareness. Disorders in which cortisol is deficient (such as Addison disease/hypocortisolism) also increase the risk of hypoglycemia, as can gastroparesis and end-stage renal disease.

TYPE 2 DIABETES MELLITUS

Type 2 diabetes mellitus (T2DM) is a condition of dysregulated glucose and lipid metabolism with a very different etiology than that of T1DM. The two diseases are grouped together because they share the characteristics that underlie many of the complications of the diseases: insulin deficiency, hyperglycemia, and disordered lipid metabolism. The initial insult in T2DM is the lack of tissue sensitivity to the actions of insulin, referred to as *insulin resistance*. In the face of such resistance, β cells must generate ever greater insulin secretion to dispose of a dietary glucose load. Over time in predisposed individuals, the elevated levels of insulin cannot be sustained, and β cells fail, leading to progressive insulin deficiency. The source of β cell vulnerability is not well understood, but the state of insulin deficiency can sometimes even lead to the absolute lack of insulin, as occurs in T1DM.

Risk Factors

The pathogenesis of T2DM involves genetic factors, environmental factors, and a proinflammatory state, with some modifiable risk factors. Unlike T1DM, there is no known involvement of autoimmunity in T2DM. Identified T2DM risk factors include age; ancestral descent from African, Native American/Alaska Native, Latinx, and certain Asian and Pacific Islander origins; birthweight (either small for gestational age or above average birthweight); having prior gestational diabetes; sedentary lifestyle; hypertension; dyslipidemia; and obesity.[9] The latter carries a major risk for T2DM, particularly central or visceral obesity. Obesity is present in more than 80% of patients with T2DM and contributes to the insulin resistance and the central metabolic abnormalities of diabetes. Genetic influences in T2DM are more prominent than in T1DM, with concordance of about 70% in monozygotic twins. Having a parent with T2DM confers a 40% risk of developing the disease in the lifetime of progeny. However, genome-wide association studies have identified many potentially linked genes, each of which contributes only a small degree to the overall risk. [114]

Diabetes Screening

Based on the risk calculations, the American Diabetes Association recommends diabetes screening for patients with the following characteristics:

- BMI ≥25 kg/m^2 (or BMI ≥23 kg/m^2 in those with Asian ancestral background) with additional risk factors
- Prediabetes
- History of gestational diabetes
- Age 45 years or older[109]

Although clinical detection of diabetes is not difficult, T2DM progresses slowly and symptoms generally only occur with long-standing disease or uncontrolled glucose levels. On this basis, screening based on the preceding criteria, and following up on screening results, is critical to promptly initiate treatment. The diagnostic criteria are the same as those described earlier.

Pathogenesis

Insulin Resistance

In states of insulin resistance, intracellular signaling triggered by insulin receptor activation is disrupted. The natural history of T2DM has been described as beginning long before overt hyperglycemia (**Figure 17.58**). The initial event is thought to be development of insulin resistance such that tissues require greater insulin levels to dispose of postprandial glucose. As insulin levels rise to compensate, insulin resistance also rises, with gradually increasing fasting and postprandial glucose levels indicating impaired glucose tolerance. Ultimately liver insulin sensitivity is greatly decreased, and liver glucose production becomes continuous across much of the day. Many at-risk individuals may be somewhere along this continuum, and not all will proceed to T2DM. However, in those with an intrinsic weakness of β-cell function,

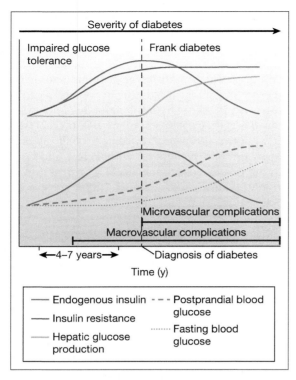

FIGURE 17.58 The natural history of type 2 diabetes mellitus. *Top graph*: Insulin resistance increases progressively in the prediabetic patient, forcing endogenous insulin secretion to increase in parallel. This response keeps hepatic glucose production within normal limits until β cells become unable to compensate. As β cells begin to fail, hepatic glucose production rises. *Lower graph*: As insulin resistance forces an increase in endogenous insulin release, there is a gradual rise in postprandial glucose. As the patient transitions to the point at which diabetes is diagnosed, fasting blood glucose increases as well.
Source: From Halsted BA, Edelman SV. The natural history of Type 2 Diabetes: implications for clinical practice. *Primary Care.* 1999;26(4):771–789.

continuing in the insulin-resistant state provokes β-cell incompetence and death, and progression to frank diabetes with persistent hyperglycemia.[115] Note that the factors predisposing to macrovascular complications begin during the state of impaired glucose tolerance and that development of diabetes is associated with increased risk of microvascular complications.

At the cellular level, insulin resistance means that the rate of GLUT4 translocation decreases, slowing glucose clearance from the blood, particularly by muscle cells. Pancreatic α cells are not appropriately inhibited by insulin, so glucagon levels are persistently elevated. Liver cells fail to respond to insulin stimulation, and there is decreased activation of anabolic pathways and increased activation of catabolic pathways stimulated by glucagon. Gluconeogenesis is strongly promoted, as is the activity of glucose phosphatase, which releases free glucose into the circulation. The net effect of T2DM

on the liver is that glucose production and release is chronically increased, contributing to persistent hyperglycemia. Fat cell lipolysis increases circulating free fatty acid levels, which further promote liver gluconeogenesis.[16] In comparison to the metabolic effects of insulin resistance, insulin effectiveness in stimulating the MAP kinase intracellular signaling system appears to be preserved. As insulin levels rise to overcome insulin resistance, the growth-promoting and mitogenic effects of insulin can alter function of vascular smooth muscle, promoting hypertension and atherosclerosis.

Factors contributing to insulin resistance include increasing age, overweight or obesity, and sedentary lifestyle. Importantly, the Diabetes Prevention Program demonstrated that prediabetes can be reversed by intensive lifestyle management. In the initial study, participants who achieved a weight loss of at least 7% of body weight, and who sustained physical activity at a level of 150 minutes/week, significantly reduced their progression to diagnosis of diabetes, relative to control subjects and subjects treated with metformin.[116] Thus, for patients with prediabetes or diabetes, lifestyle management targeting weight loss and increased physical activity is strongly recommended.

β-Cell Dysfunction

T2DM is marked by loss of β cells that is unlike T1DM, as it is not mediated by an autoimmune reaction. Although the mechanisms leading to β-cell death in T2DM are not fully identified, the remaining cells are able to increase insulin secretion to overcome insulin resistance only to a point. Once 80% or more of β cells are destroyed, patients have impaired glucose tolerance, defined as a 2-hour glucose level between 140 and 199 mg/dL on OGTT.

Abnormal lipolysis generates free fatty acids that inhibit insulin release, initiating a positive feedback cycle. The decrease in insulin secretion reduces inhibition of HSL, promoting further release of free fatty acids from fat cells in a vicious cycle. Additional factors potentially linked to decreased β-cell function include the effects of chronic hyperglycemia, reduced secretion and effectiveness of GIP and GLP-1, and amyloid deposits within islets. The combination of effects of β-cell dysfunction and insulin resistance yields hyperglycemia. The contributing factors summarized in the following list are referred to as the "ominous octet"[117]:

1. Tissue insulin resistance
2. β-cell vulnerability/decreased secretion of insulin
3. Increased hepatic glucose production
4. Increased lipolysis
5. Decreased effectiveness or amount of incretins
6. Increased secretion of glucagon
7. Increased renal glucose reabsorption
8. Brain insulin resistance contributing to excessive food intake

Interrelation of Obesity and T2DM

Obesity, particularly central or visceral obesity, is associated with incidence of T2DM. Although not all obese persons develop T2DM, and not all people with T2DM are obese, there is a high association between the two. The mechanisms underlying this association include higher levels of free fatty acids in those with visceral obesity, and inflammatory signals, particularly cytokines that are generated by adipose tissue. Recognition of adipose tissue as a site of active secretion gave rise to the term *adipokines*—signaling molecules released by fat. These molecules include leptin and adiponectin (which tend to promote decreased food intake and increased energy expenditure), resistin (which promotes insulin resistance), as well as the cytokines interleukin (IL)-6 and tumor necrosis factor-alpha (TNF-α), which promote inflammation. Macrophages within fat tissue contribute to the inflammatory profile with additional secretion of IL-1 and TNF-α. Overall, obesity in combination with T2DM is a proinflammatory state that promotes vascular damage such as atherosclerosis. As fatty acids overwhelm the typical oxidation pathways, metabolites accumulate, including diacylglycerol (DAG). The effect of increased concentration of DAG within the cell includes attenuation of insulin signaling. In liver cells, insulin normally inhibits gluconeogenesis, but in the presence of DAG, this signaling is inhibited, leading to continued gluconeogenesis, contributing to hyperglycemia. Additionally, as free fatty acids compete with glucose for oxidation, less glucose will be oxidized, leaving blood glucose levels high for a longer period of time.

Clinical Management

Clinical management of T2DM must include lifestyle changes, and typically uses pharmacological interventions.

Lifestyle Modifications

While the pharmacological interventions target one or more pathways along which the disease affects metabolism, lifestyle changes alter metabolic homeostasis globally and may address the cause underlying the dysregulation of metabolism. Lifestyle recommendations for patients with diabetes involve five domains: diabetes self-management education and support (DSMES), nutrition therapy, physical activity, smoking cessation counseling, and psychosocial care[109] (**Box 17.7**). Nutritional management emphasizes assessing the total amount of carbohydrates as one reference point, as opposed to a general ban of sugar. This is based on the effect of carbohydrates on blood glucose levels.

BOX 17.7
Lifestyle Changes for Diabetes Management

1. **Diabetes self-management education and support**
   Self-management is the cornerstone of optimal diabetes treatment, with patient education central to achieving successful outcomes. The educational component focuses on points 2 to 5.

2. **Nutrition therapy**
   Nutrition therapy is a central component as a long-standing part of diabetes management. Nutrition therapy focuses on weight loss, if necessary, as well as optimal diet composition. Patients taking insulin need education about management of carbohydrate intake in relation to insulin dose, appropriate to their individual abilities. There is increasing emphasis on gathering evidence for the benefits of newer dietary approaches including low-carbohydrate, high-protein, and vegetarian diets.

3. **Physical activity**
   Regular physical activity is increasingly recognized as a core component of a healthy lifestyle in all individuals, with and without diabetes. Physiologically, exercise sensitizes muscles to insulin and promotes glucose uptake both during activity and for several hours following the activity.[118] Exercise should be at least at moderate intensity, as tolerated by the individual. Because exercise-induced hypoglycemia is a risk for patients taking insulin or insulin secretagogues, attention to glucose levels in these patients is critical. Glucose levels should be at least 90 mg/dL (5.0 mmol/L) at the start of exercise.

4. **Counseling toward smoking cessation**
   Patients with diabetes who are smokers or are exposed to secondhand smoke have an increased risk of cardiovascular disease, premature death, and microvascular complications.

5. **Psychosocial care**
   Diabetes impacts the lives of patients and their families considerably, and long-term psychological and social factors determine to a large degree how well diabetes self-care management can be performed.

Pharmacological Interventions

When diet and exercise are insufficient to achieve normoglycemia in T2DM, pharmacological interventions are employed and tailored to the patient's needs, setting goals for blood glucose levels depending on age, life expectancy, comorbidities, and patient expectations. Early intervention may slow the loss of β cells.

Whether a person has T1DM or T2DM, management based on lifestyle (diet, exercise, sleep, smoking cessation) accompanied by medications aims to reduce complications. Glycemic targets must be developed for each person, taking into account age, pregnancy, comorbidities, extent of glycemic variability, and drug interactions. A common goal is to keep A1C <7%, with more stringent control if safe and feasible, and less stringent control when such is warranted. Optimizing glycemic control is central to the goal of reducing chronic complications of diabetes.

COMPLICATIONS OF DIABETES MELLITUS

Acute Complications of Type 2 Diabetes Mellitus

Hypoglycemia

Hypoglycemia is an acute complication in T2DM, although it is less common than in T1DM. Risk factors for hypoglycemia include treatment with insulin or sulfonylureas (insulin secretagogues), older age, autonomic neuropathy, cognitive decline, and treatment with β-blocking drugs. Because of insulin resistance, hypoglycemia affects fewer patients with T2DM; nevertheless, it is always a risk, and older patients, in particular, should be taught about warning signs and prompt self-management of hypoglycemia.

Hyperosmolar Hyperglycemic Syndrome

Although acute insulin deficiency and presence of counter regulatory hormones in T1DM can lead to potentially fatal ketoacidosis, patients with T2DM are more likely to develop **hyperosmolar hyperglycemic syndrome** (HHS). In HHS, blood glucose levels tend to be higher than in DKA (600 to 1,200 mg/dL versus 250 to 600 mg/dL for DKA). Ketoacidosis is generally absent in HHS (pH >7.3 in HHS with negligible ketones versus 6.8 to 7.3 in DKA with 4+ ketones). Blood osmolality is greater in HHS at 330 to 380 mOsm/L versus 300 to 320 mOsm/L in DKA.[119] The clinical context is often some type of systemic infection in a vulnerable older adult that causes dehydration and leads to stress hormone release, promoting liver glucose production. It is thought that the presence of modest amounts of insulin in the portal vein of patients with T2DM sufficiently inhibits liver production of ketone bodies to prevent ketoacidosis. However, states of high blood glucose levels in HHS still induce profound osmotic diuresis, dehydration, and critical illness requiring hospitalization.

Chronic Complications of T1DM and T2DM

Both T1DM and T2DM have similar chronic complications related to persistent hyperglycemia and dyslipidemia. The leading cause of death in patients with diabetes is cardiovascular disease, followed by renal failure. Chronic hyperglycemia and dyslipidemia (elevated triglycerides and HDL cholesterol, and increased concentration of small, dense LDL particles) damage blood vessels, and this damage is a major contributor to **diabetic macrovascular disease** that targets large and medium-sized arteries. Diabetes is often comorbid with hypertension, further contributing to vascular damage and atherosclerosis. The combination of these three factors—hyperglycemia, dyslipidemia, and hypertension—leads to the high rates of myocardial infarction, stroke, and peripheral arterial disease in people with diabetes. Accordingly, management strategies involving both lifestyle and pharmacological approaches aim to improve glycemic control, blood pressure, and lipid levels. Hyperglycemia also damages small vessels, and **diabetic microangiopathy** (microvascular disease) is thought to be responsible for the classic triad of **diabetic retinopathy, nephropathy,** and **neuropathy**. Additionally, immune system functions are compromised by chronic hyperglycemia, increasing susceptibility to infections. The combination of neuropathy, impaired blood flow, and reduced immune responses can lead to ulcers of the lower extremities, at times progressing to gangrene and necessitating limb amputation.

Hyperglycemia and Diabetes Complications

Major large randomized clinical trials in T1DM and T2DM, the Diabetes Control and Complications Trial and United Kingdom Prospective Diabetes Study, respectively, highlighted the role of hyperglycemia as the predominant cause of **microvascular diabetes complications**.[120-122] At the cellular level, metabolic abnormalities due to excessive glucose metabolism are referred to as *glucotoxicity*. Its overarching principle is that increased metabolism of glucose via various pathways generates harmful molecules that contribute to end-organ damage. Preclinical studies particularly implicate the buildup of advanced glycation end products (AGEs) and reactive oxygen species as contributing factors in chronic diabetes complications.[123]

Diabetic Microangiopathy

As previously noted, AGEs cause a thickening of basement membrane. As the occurrence of AGEs is systemic, this process occurs in multiple tissues. Particularly affected are skin, skeletal muscle, retina, renal glomeruli, renal medulla and Bowman capsule, peripheral nerves, and placenta. Despite the thickened basement membrane, the capillaries become more permeable to plasma proteins. The classic triad of complications from diabetes—nephropathy, retinopathy, and neuropathy—is causally linked to this process, although some forms of neuropathy occur independent of basement membrane alterations.[124]

Diabetic Nephropathy

About 30% to 40% of patients with diabetes develop nephropathy, and of these, about 75% of patients with T1DM and 20% of patients with T2DM develop end-stage renal disease. Renal failure is the third leading cause of death for patients with T1DM, after acute complications and cardiovascular disease.[125] An early clinical marker of nephropathy is microalbuminuria, the appearance of albumin in the urine, in the range between 30 and 300 mg/dL.

Diabetic Retinopathy

Diabetic retinopathy constitutes the most remarkable change in the eyes of patients with diabetes. Sixty percent to 80% of patients with diabetes develop visual impairment within 15 to 20 years of diagnosis.[124] Alarmingly, diabetic retinopathy can develop even before the diagnosis of T2DM is made and in conditions in which treatment goals are met. Persistent hyperglycemia can also lead to glaucoma and cataract formation.

Diabetic Neuropathy

Diabetic neuropathy most frequently takes the form of distal symmetrical polyneuropathy, presenting with decreased perception of vibration, pain, and temperature. Nerve dysfunction can lead to neuropathic pain that can be debilitating. This dysfunction affects up to 80% of patients diagnosed for more than 15 years. As described for diabetic retinopathy, patients with impaired glucose tolerance are already at risk for this complication; thus, the nerve damage generally starts before a diagnosis of diabetes is made.[124] The neuropathy may include the autonomic nervous system, the central nervous system, the peripheral sensory system, or combinations thereof. Distal symmetrical polyneuropathy involves motor and sensory function. It typically starts in the lower extremities and may later involve the upper extremities in a glove-and-stocking pattern. One of the risks accompanying diabetic polyneuropathy is decreased awareness of injury, particularly of the feet. This can lead to ulcer development in the context of poor extremity blood flow and increased propensity to infections. **Autonomic neuropathy** can cause gastroparesis, disordered bowel and bladder function, and ED. Visceral sensory dysfunction can also mask symptoms of myocardial ischemia and infarction.

Susceptibility to Infections

Diabetes increases susceptibility to local and systemic infections, particularly skin/wound infections, urinary tract infections, and vaginal infections in women. In some cases of T2DM, development of a severe wound infection may be the precipitating event that leads to diagnosis of the diabetes. Neutrophil and macrophage functions are impaired at multiple levels, and vascular disease decreases tissue perfusion. This combination slows down the host response to infection, increasing the risk of complications and death.

Thought Questions

27. **How is the pathogenesis of T1DM different from that of T2DM?**

28. **In what aspects do these disorders share the same pathology?**

29. **What are the implications of these differences and similarities for management of the pathophysiology of each disorder?**

OTHER FORMS OF DIABETES AND DIABETES-RELATED CONDITIONS

GESTATIONAL DIABETES

Gestational diabetes mellitus (GDM) is defined as hyperglycemia first detected in the second or third trimester of pregnancy, and it affects both mother and offspring acutely and long-term. Possible adverse infant outcomes in GDM include increased risk of stillbirth, congenital malformations, and macrosomia. Immediately after delivery, the infant is at risk of potentially fatal hypoglycemia. Later in life, the risk of obesity, diabetes, and metabolic syndrome are increased for the offspring. For the mothers, GDM is associated with increased risk of preeclampsia and cesarean delivery, and the risk of later-life development of T2DM increases considerably. Fifty percent to 70% of women with GDM will develop diabetes after 15 to 25 years.[109] Additionally, the risks of atherogenic dyslipidemia, metabolic syndrome, and cardiovascular disease increase.

During pregnancy, the placenta secretes chorionic somatomammotropin, as noted earlier in the chapter. It functions as an anti-insulin hormone similar to GH. Chorionic somatomammotropin stimulation increases lipolysis, promoting free fatty acid release that contributes to insulin resistance during pregnancy. The placenta degrades insulin, forcing the mother's β-cell function to increase over the duration of the pregnancy. Additionally, circulating levels of the inflammatory mediators TNF-α and IL-6 increase, further promoting insulin resistance.[126]

During pregnancy (with or without GDM), insulin sensitivity declines to about 50% to 60% of the pregravid state. This decrease includes the liver, as hepatic glucose production increases during pregnancy. Insulin secretion increases by almost 300% throughout gestation, for both the first and second phases of insulin secretion. If the pancreatic β cells do not have the capacity to produce enough insulin, hyperglycemia will occur. After delivery, glucose tolerance can return to normal, as the demand for insulin decreases; however, β-cell dysfunction may persist.

Risk factors for gestational diabetes include age older than 25 years, BMI >27 kg/m², hypertension, family history of diabetes, higher weight gain during pregnancy, habitual smoking, and genetic predisposition. With respect to ancestral origin, women of Hispanic, African, Native American, and Asian descent are at increased risk.

Current recommendations include screening of pregnant women at their first prenatal visit if they have risk factors for diabetes, and at 24 to 28 weeks of gestation without risk factors. Given the increased risk of developing DM for women with a history of GDM, retesting is recommended at 4 to 12 weeks post partum, and at 3-year intervals thereafter.[109] Upon diagnosis, treatment focuses on achieving normoglycemia tested via self-monitoring of blood glucose levels. Dietary management is the first line of defense, and insulin therapy is added if lifestyle changes are insufficient to achieve target blood glucose levels.

LATENT AUTOIMMUNE DIABETES IN ADULTS

Latent autoimmune diabetes of the adult (LADA) is a slowly progressive autoimmune diabetes, sometimes known as latent T1DM, double diabetes, and type 1.5 diabetes. The definition usually includes onset after 30 years of age, presence of at least one of four specific antibodies, and absence of need for insulin within the first 6 months. The exact numbers for age of onset and time frame for need of insulin vary among populations. Patients with LADA may demonstrate more insulin resistance than typical patients with T1DM. Progression to insulin dependence is slower than in T1DM, occurring earlier in life, despite the presence of some of the common autoantibodies found in people with T1DM. Management strategies typically begin with diet, lifestyle, and oral medications, along with glucose monitoring. Most patients with LADA need insulin within the first year after diagnosis.[127]

POLYCYSTIC OVARY SYNDROME

Polycystic ovary syndrome (PCOS), introduced earlier in the chapter, in the section on female reproductive endocrinology, is a relatively common cause of failure to ovulate in women of reproductive age. It has highly variable presentation, and both obese and lean women may have this diagnosis, although obesity is more common. Along with elevated levels of androgens, the pathophysiologic mechanism is thought to involve insulin resistance and the associated increase in circulating insulin levels. Clinical improvement can sometimes be seen with metformin treatment, supporting a role of insulin resistance in the condition.

OBSTRUCTIVE SLEEP APNEA

The prevalence of sleep disorders is increasing in the United States and globally, and research has identified metabolic defects following sleep disruption. **Obstructive sleep apnea** (OSA) is a common type of sleep-disordered breathing pattern and is characterized by sleep-associated cycling between normal breathing, complete apnea, and partially obstructed breathing. Diagnosis in a sleep laboratory is based, in part, on the ratio of apneic to hypopneic episodes (apnea/hypopnea index, or AHI). Prevalence estimates for patients experiencing more than five apnea/hypopnea events per hour vary from 9% to 38%, with higher rates in men and in older adults.[128] Obesity increases the risk of OSA, and there appears to be a bidirectional relationship between OSA and T2DM, with OSA prevalence higher in those with T2DM, and T2DM prevalence greater in those with OSA, even after correcting for obesity.

Cognitive Decline and Alzheimer Disease

Individuals with diabetes develop cognitive impairment with aging at a faster rate than those without diabetes. Although insulin is not required for brain glucose uptake, insulin receptors and insulin-dependent glucose transporters (GLUT4) are expressed differentially in different brain regions. Insulin receptors are enriched in the hippocampus, and insulin signaling in the brain has been demonstrated to be growth-promoting and neuroprotective. People with Alzheimer disease have reduced brain levels of insulin, IGFs, and insulin receptors. In animal models of Alzheimer disease, brain insulin signaling cascades are reduced. In human studies of Alzheimer disease patients, brain insulin signaling is also reduced. Potential links between diabetes, insulin resistance, and Alzheimer disease risk include altered neuronal signaling by insulin receptors and the increased levels of cytokines and other inflammatory mediators that accompany obesity, insulin resistance, and T2DM. As both T2DM and Alzheimer disease prevalence are increasing with the aging population, it is expected that further developments in this research will yield new treatment strategies.[129]

SUMMARY

In summary, obesity and diabetes are rampant globally, and contribute significantly to the global toll of chronic diseases. Lifestyle factors that include excess intake of foods high in fat and caloric density, along with sedentary lifestyle, are the main factors underlying this state. Although several classes of medications have been developed to reduce the societal burden of diabetes-associated morbidity and mortality, public health measures and education are needed to reverse this trend to promote better health and well-being.

PEDIATRIC CONSIDERATIONS: METABOLISM AND THE PANCREAS

Randall L. Johnson

TYPE 1 DIABETES MELLITUS

T1DM most often presents in individuals before age 40, with the peak incidence occurring between ages 10 and 14 years in the United States. In recognition of this fact, the condition was formerly called "juvenile diabetes." Current trends indicate a gradual increase in pediatric T1DM cases in the United States and worldwide, although the mechanisms for the increase are not currently known. It is now recognized that T1DM may have onset throughout adult life, although some adult cases are more slowly progressive and are identified as LADA, described earlier. In general, the younger the age at diagnosis, the more labile the blood glucose can be, with higher incidence of DKA at or within 6 months after diagnosis. Prescriptions for an emergency glucagon kit are very high in childhood, which may indicate higher rates of acute hypoglycemic events or parental concern about being prepared for such events.[130]

Management of T1DM in very young children is complicated by the fact that they may not be able to recognize and verbalize symptoms, particularly symptoms of hypoglycemia. Parental supervision must be vigilant, including determination of hypoglycemia at night that can occur on days of extra physical activity. Glycemic management can be affected by the interaction of physiology with characteristic developmental stages, for example:

- Toddler food preferences and food refusal; invasive procedures by parents, including sticks for glucose monitoring and insulin administration
- School-age children needing privacy to self-monitor blood glucose and self-administer insulin in school
- Sports activity, and the need to monitor and have a plan for activity-induced hypoglycemia
- Pubertal hormone changes that alter insulin sensitivity
- Transitions to college and independent decision-making, including decisions about alcohol intake

TYPE 2 DIABETES MELLITUS

With the obesity epidemic, the incidence of T2DM is increasing in adolescents, accounting for 10% to 50% of new diabetes diagnoses in the United States.[131] Striking differences based on ancestral origin are seen, with increased incidence in Asian/Pacific Islander, Hispanic, and African American youth, and the highest rates in youth of American Indian descent.[132] T2DM in adolescents has a more severe phenotype than in adults, with more rapid progression to β-cell failure, as well as earlier development of microvascular complications.[131,133]

GERONTOLOGICAL CONSIDERATIONS: METABOLISM AND THE PANCREAS

Stacy M. Alabastro and Linda L. Herrmann

TYPE 2 DIABETES MELLITUS

The ability of pancreatic β cells to maintain adequate insulin secretory function for metabolic demand is impaired with increasing age. The prevalence of glucose intolerance and T2DM increases with age, affecting up to 20% to 30% of adults aged 65 years and older.[134] This has been attributed to age-related changes that reduce insulin sensitivity, such as increased adiposity, lower lean body mass, and overall reduction in physical activity. However, changes at the level of the β cell with aging also contribute to T2DM through decreased glucose-stimulated insulin secretion and regenerative capacity.[135]

Older adults have reduced autonomic responsiveness and may be prone to more severe episodes of hypoglycemia. In some cases, A1C targets must be adjusted to reduce the risk of hypoglycemia, particularly in individuals who have multiple comorbidities and polypharmacy that further increases hypoglycemia risk. At the same time, older adults with T2DM may have a greater risk of HHS due to relative blunting of the thirst mechanism and reduced perception of fever and signs of infection. Adherence to lifestyle treatment may be more difficult if degenerative joint disease interferes with ability to maintain regular physical activity at recommended levels. Finally, as noted earlier, diabetes is associated with increased risk of cognitive losses, particularly Alzheimer disease. Given the high level of self-care to produce optimal outcomes in diabetes management, cognitive losses may lead to difficulty in maintaining the recommended lifestyle approaches to diabetes management.

CASE STUDY 17.3: A Patient With Gestational Diabetes

Kimberly K. Trout

Patient Complaint: *"I don't know why my fasting blood sugars are so high, since my blood sugars after my meals are always good. I don't eat any simple sugars, I have my carbohydrate-controlled three meals, and I do my exercise bike for a half hour while I'm watching TV in the evening."*

History of Present Illness: This 37-year-old primigravida diagnosed with gestational diabetes at 30 weeks of gestation has been in good control with diet alone until now, at 34 weeks of gestation. She has begun to experience elevated fasting blood glucose during the last week. She is upset that her healthcare provider has indicated that if her fasting levels remain elevated she may need to start insulin injections. She has heard that insulin causes weight gain, and she is already concerned because she has gained more weight than the amount recommended for the entire pregnancy. It was for this reason that she decided to eliminate her bedtime snack.

Past Medical/Family/Present Obstetric History: Past medical history is noncontributory. Family history is remarkable for maternal grandfather and aunt with type 2 diabetes and of Pacific Islander descent. The patient first registered for prenatal care at 8 weeks of gestation, and a first-trimester ultrasound confirmed the estimated due date. She has had normal results on cell-free DNA and maternal serum α-fetoprotein testing, and a normal fetal anatomy scan at 21 weeks of gestation. Results of a 1-hour glucose challenge test = 145 mg/dL, 3-hour GTT = 90/200/160/120 mg/dL. A growth scan at 32 weeks revealed the fetus to be at the 65th percentile for weight, with normal amniotic fluid volume. The patient's prepregnancy BMI was 24 kg/m².

Physical Examination: During this routinely scheduled prenatal exam, findings are as follows: temperature of 98°F, blood pressure of 126/78 mm Hg, heart rate of 78 beats/min, and respirations of 12 breaths/min.

(continued)

Total weight gain to date in this pregnancy = 42 lb. Urine dipstick is negative for protein, glucose, and ketones. Fetal heart tones are 145 beats/min in the left lower abdominal quadrant. Abdomen palpates soft; uterine fundal height = 35 cm from the top of the symphysis pubis to the uterine fundus. Leopold maneuvers reveal the fetus to be in the LOA position, EFW = 6 lb.

Laboratory Findings (Blood Glucose Log for the Last Week)

	Mon	Tues	Wed	Thurs	Fri	Sat	Sun
Fasting	92	105	98	92	98	100	97
2-hours post breakfast	117	85	105	122	99	105	110
2-hours post lunch	88	98	104	120	**	110	116
2-hours post dinner	87	90	145*	89	85	90	96

*Had large pasta meal.
**Forgot to test.

CASE STUDY 17.3 QUESTIONS

- *What risk factors for gestational diabetes does this patient have?*
- *If a person with diabetes exercises before bedtime and omits having a snack, what consequence would there be on anti-insulin counterregulatory hormones? What might the effect be on morning fasting glucose levels?*

BMI, body mass index; EFW, estimated fetal weight; GTT, glucose tolerance test; LOA, left occiput anterior.

BRIDGE TO CLINICAL PRACTICE: Diabetes

Ben Cocchiaro

PRINCIPLES OF ASSESSMENT
History & Physical Examination

- Assess for hyperglycemia symptoms, including polydipsia, polyuria, blurry vision, confusion, fatigue, and weight loss.
- Assess for hypoglycemia symptoms, including hunger, pallor, tremor, sweating, dizziness, and palpitations.
- For patients already diagnosed with diabetes, review the patient's glucose log. Some blood glucose meters have a memory function to help patients keep track of this.
- Assess for cardiovascular findings, including reports of angina, and evaluation of pulses, perfusion, and bruits.
- Assess for neurological findings, particularly sensory neuropathy.
- Assess for dermatologic findings, including acanthosis nigricans (hyperkeratotic hyperpigmented patches located around skin folds), candida intertrigo (erythematous, painful/pruritic fungal infection of the skin folds), foot ulcers and diabetic dermopathy (hyperpigmented, round, atrophic macules found over the shins).

Laboratory Evaluation

- *Blood glucose:* Capillary blood glucose readings can be performed in the office or by the patient at home.
- *Hemoglobin A1C:* Hemoglobin is irreversibly glycated at a rate dependent on plasma glucose concentration. A1C approximates a patient's mean blood sugar over the previous 8–12 weeks and is used both to diagnose and monitor patients with diabetes.
- *Basic metabolic panel:* In addition to plasma glucose, the basic metabolic panel also measures BUN and creatinine (important markers for diabetic nephropathy).

(continued)

(*continued*)

- *Ketones:* Presence of these ketones in the serum, along with hyperglycemia and anion gap metabolic acidosis, are diagnostic of diabetic ketoacidosis.
- *Urine albumin/creatinine ratio:* Recommended yearly screening test for nephropathy.

Diagnostic Tools

- *Glucose tolerance test:* The gold standard for diagnosis of gestational diabetes, this test involves drinking a sugary solution followed by a blood test to measure glucose levels.
- *Diabetic eye exam:* More than half of all diabetic patients will develop retinopathy over the course of their lives. Annual screening using digital retinal photography or dilated ophthalmoscopy is indicated starting at the time of diabetes diagnosis.
- *Microfilament examination:* A 10g monofilament exam tests fine touch sensation of the plantar foot and should be performed yearly on diabetic patients alongside screening for peripheral arterial disease and trimming of the toenails.

MAJOR DRUG CLASSES

Drugs used in both T1DM and T2DM

- *Insulin:* Insulin replacement therapy is the required treatment for T1DM and is delivered by continuous subcutaneous infusion from a pump, or by multiple daily injections. Insulin is also indicated for certain patients with T2DM, depending on their response to lifestyle changes and the above-mentioned medications. Basal treatment with a long-acting insulin can be supplemented as needed with bolus injection of short-acting insulin.
- *Angiotensin converting enzyme inhibitors (ACEs) and angiotensin receptor blockers (ARBs):* ACEs and ARBs decrease vascular resistance and reduce glomerular capillary pressure, thereby protecting against the nephropathies of both hypertension and diabetes mellitus.

Drugs used in T2DM

- *Biguanides (metformin):* Acts via several mechanisms, decreasing hepatic gluconeogenesis and improving peripheral glucose uptake and insulin sensitivity. Metformin has also been used for its insulin-sensitizing action in polycystic ovary syndrome.
- *Insulin secretagogues:* Sulfonylurea (SUR) drugs are the most commonly used drugs in this class, the mechanism of action is to inhibit the β cell K_{ATP} channel, promoting insulin secretion. Although SUR drugs were the mainstay of T2DM treatment in the past, their use is diminishing as they appear to hasten β cell decline in function over time.
- *Incretins:* Glucagon-like peptide-1 (GLP-1) receptor agonists and dipeptidyl peptidase-4 (DPP-4) inhibitors:
  - GLP-1 receptor agonists are given by injection. Their mechanism of action is to increase glucose-stimulated insulin secretion and decrease glucagon secretion. In addition, they slow gastric emptying and decrease appetite, sometimes leading to weight loss.
  - DPP-4 inhibitors inhibit the enzyme that breaks down GLP-1, prolonging GLP-1's actions.
- *Sodium glucose transporter-2 (SGLT-2) inhibitors:* SGLT-2 inhibitors block renal proximal tubule glucose reabsorption, permitting urinary excretion of glucose when glucose levels are elevated. This action reduces postprandial glucose elevations.
- *Peroxisome proliferator activated receptor-gamma (PPAR-γ) agonists (thiazolidinediones):* Thiazolidinediones work via nuclear signaling cascades to increase tissue insulin sensitivity, promoting fatty acid uptake and storage in adipose tissue. These drugs also work to reduce fat content in muscle and the liver, decrease hepatic gluconeogenesis, increase insulin sensitivity, and reduce inflammation.

KEY POINTS: METABOLISM AND THE PANCREAS

- Metabolism of carbohydrates, fats, and proteins can be described in two major conditions: the fed and fasted states.
- The fed state begins with the absorption of digested food products from the gastrointestinal tract and continues during meal absorption. Hormonal regulation during this state is primarily under the influence of insulin, and fuels are stored in the form of glycogen (in liver and muscle), lipid (in fat cells), and protein (in muscle cells).
- Between meals, in the fasted state, insulin levels decline, glucagon increases, and fuels can be mobilized from storage. The liver can produce glucose from glycogen breakdown or by gluconeogenesis. Fat can be mobilized with the release of free fatty acids and glycerol. Muscle cells can use their stored glycogen for fuel, and can release lactate and amino acids as substrates for liver gluconeogenesis.
- With prolonged fasting or in the absence of insulin, fatty acids are used for fuel in the liver, which also produces ketone bodies that can be used as fuel for the brain and other tissues.
- Insulin is the primary anabolic hormone responsible for fuel storage in the fed state, as well as promoting growth and maintenance of tissues. Insulin is a protein consisting of two polypeptide chains connected by disulfide bonds. During insulin synthesis, a connecting peptide (C peptide) is cleaved from proinsulin once the A and B chains have bonded together. C peptide assays are used as an index of body insulin production.
- Insulin receptors are tyrosine kinases that activate several intracellular signaling cascades including the PI3 and MAP kinase pathways.
- A key rapid effect of insulin is to promote glucose uptake into muscle and fat cells by initiating translocation of the GLUT4 transporter from intracellular vesicles to the plasma membrane. Growth-promoting and cell proliferation effects of insulin are slower in onset.
- Insulin acts on three major targets to promote fuel uptake and storage:
  - Stimulating liver glycogen and triglyceride synthesis and inhibiting glycogen breakdown, gluconeogenesis, and ketogenesis
  - Stimulating muscle glucose and amino acid transport, and synthesis of glycogen and protein
  - Stimulating fat glucose and fatty acid uptake and triglyceride synthesis, and inhibiting triglyceride breakdown
- Insulin acts on the brain as a satiety signal, and may contribute to the maintenance of normal brain structure and function, reducing risk of neurodegenerative disorders.
- Pancreatic β-cell insulin secretion is increased by glucose and amino acids that increase during meal absorption. Insulin secretion is also promoted by acetylcholine and the incretins GIP and GLP-1. Insulin secretion is inhibited by hypoglycemia, sympathetic nervous stimulation, epinephrine, and somatostatin.
- Glucagon is the second major regulatory hormone of metabolic homeostasis. It promotes catabolic enzyme activity in the liver, increasing glycogenolysis and gluconeogenesis to increase liver glucose release during fasting. Glucagon can also promote liver ketone formation, particularly in the absence of insulin. Insulin normally inhibits glucagon secretion by a paracrine action in the fed state. Glucagon secretion is stimulated by hypoglycemia and sympathetic nervous system stimulation, among other factors.
- Cortisol has multiple actions on metabolic target tissues, promoting liver glucose uptake and glycogen production in the fed state, and increasing glucose release during fasting and stress states. Cortisol can promote muscle protein breakdown, gluconeogenesis, and insulin resistance. Exogenous glucocorticoids used for pharmacological management of many immune-related conditions and cancer may precipitate insulin resistance and frank diabetes.
- The stress hormone epinephrine generally promotes catabolic processes, including lipolysis, glycogenolysis, and gluconeogenesis, and is one component of hyperglycemia associated with stress.
- GH has growth-promoting effects that synergize with insulin actions on growth, but also has actions antagonistic to insulin, including stimulation of lipolysis and ketone formation.
- Chorionic somatomammotropin, a hormone produced by the placenta, is involved in

maternal/fetal metabolic adaptations during pregnancy. It contributes to the pathophysiology of gestational diabetes.

- DM is a group of diseases with different pathogenic mechanisms and genetic associations but the common finding of increased blood glucose and altered levels or signaling of insulin. The major types are T1DM and T2DM, with many other forms and syndromes reported.

- Several laboratory tests can be used to diagnose diabetes, including fasting glucose, HbA1C, OGTT, or a combination of random glucose with symptoms. Tests should be repeated to confirm the diagnosis.

- T1DM is an autoimmune disorder that presents with complete destruction of β cells and plasma antibodies to characteristic antigens. This results in complete reliance on exogenous insulin replacement. Acute complications of T1DM and insulin treatment are hypoglycemia and DKA.

- T2DM is a disorder with variable presentation depending on genetics, ancestral descent, and individual differences. The pathogenesis is a combination of tissue insulin resistance that requires high levels of secreted insulin to normalize blood glucose levels, with β-cell vulnerability that leads to eventual failure and can lead to dependence on exogenous insulin.

- Onset of T2DM is preceded by a period (of variable length) of impaired glucose tolerance and prediabetes. Intensive lifestyle intervention in this period may restore insulin sensitivity and prevent the development of T2DM.

- Prior to insulin dependence, T2DM is usually managed with lifestyle modification and oral medications. Acute complications of T2DM are hypoglycemia and HHS.

- Both T1DM and T2DM have common manifestations and chronic complications. There is a relative excess of glucagon secretion and liver glucose production, as well as elevated fatty acid levels. Dyslipidemia with elevated cholesterol is common, as is comorbid hypertension.

- Patients with diabetes have accelerated atherosclerosis development and higher rates of cardiovascular events, including myocardial infarction, stroke, and peripheral arterial disease, than those without diabetes. These are considered to be macrovascular diabetes complications and require treatment by managing glucose, lipids, and blood pressure.

- Other chronic diabetes complications arise from microvascular disease, including retinopathy, nephropathy, and neuropathy (both somatic and autonomic). Glycemic control to maintain A1C at <7% is recommended to reduce microvascular complications, but such targets must be individualized based on patient characteristics.

- Gestational diabetes is usually diagnosed in the second trimester of pregnancy. It results from increased insulin resistance due to pregnancy-related hormones such as chorionic somatomammotropin, and to the fact that insulin is degraded by the placenta. The condition resolves after delivery, but a woman who has had gestational diabetes with one or more pregnancies is at greater risk of later-life development of T2DM.

- Latent autoimmune diabetes of adults is generally diagnosed in adults who are older than 30 years of age at the time of diabetes diagnosis. It may be slowly progressive, but typically at least one type of diabetes-related antibody is found on laboratory testing.

- Children are more likely to present with T1DM than T2DM, particularly before puberty. Management of diabetes presents challenges that vary depending on developmental stage, from the very young through young adulthood.

- Increasing numbers of adolescents are developing T2DM, particularly those of non-White/non-Caucasian ancestral descent. T2DM in adolescents is more aggressive than that occurring later in life.

- Older adults have higher incidence of T2DM than younger adults, although their trajectory may not be as severe. Contributing factors include greater insulin resistance due to greater adiposity, declining muscle mass, and, in some cases, less physical activity.

- Older adults treated with insulin or secretagogues are at higher risk of hypoglycemia than younger adults because of decreased autonomic responsiveness, comorbidities, and polypharmacy. Glycemic targets can be relaxed if recurrent hypoglycemia is a problem.

Summary: Endocrine Physiology and Pathophysiology

The endocrine system is the third major integrative system of the body, along with the nervous system (particularly the autonomic nervous system) and the immune system. This chapter emphasized key themes in endocrine physiology and pathophysiology, while including clinical implications of those themes. In-depth coverage particularly focused on thyroid diseases and DM, as these are the most common endocrine disorders and are often managed by advanced practitioners in primary care settings. Rather than providing a free-standing Bridge to Clinical Practice at the end of the chapter, the usual elements (history and physical findings, laboratory evaluation, and common drug classes) have been integrated into the sections wherever possible.

The first theme of endocrine function is that hormones travel through the bloodstream to affect target cells and organs throughout the body. Hormones, therefore, modulate activity of many target tissues and organs, and the effects of dysregulated hormone levels can be manifested by a multitude of signs and symptoms, some of which are subtle, slow to develop, and are not necessarily observable on physical examination. A thorough review of systems and exploration of past medical history and family history is of paramount importance in evaluation for a potential endocrine disorder.

The second theme is that a common category of endocrine disorders is hypofunction that leads to a deficiency state for a particular hormone. Autoimmune destruction of an endocrine organ (as in Hashimoto thyroiditis) or endocrine cells (as in T1DM) leads to hormone deficiency that is generally treatable by exogenous hormone replacement. Decades of clinical observations have led to the characterization of common diagnostic findings in many disorders of hormone deficiency, as noted in clinical textbooks. Laboratory evaluation may require measurement of levels of target gland hormone, a stimulating hormone, and responses to provocation testing in order to correctly identify the pathogenesis of hormone deficiency to guide management.

A third theme is that hormone-secreting cells may develop neoplastic transformation and multiply, producing high and unregulated secretion of hormone and hyperfunction. As in states of hypofunction, laboratory evaluation may require measurement of target gland hormone and stimulating hormone (as in Cushing disease). In other cases, measurement of hormone metabolites is most informative (as in pheochromocytoma). Imaging by ultrasonography, MRI, CT, and other modalities is also used to identify the primary site of a neoplasm, whether in the normal site of production or an ectopic tumor. Treatment of many of these disorders is by surgical removal (as in an autonomous thyroid nodule or a parathyroid tumor) or radiation-induced destruction of the tumor cells (for some pituitary or thyroid tumors). Another strategy is to treat with drugs that selectively inhibit the hypersecreting cells (as in dopamine agonist treatment for prolactinoma).

A fourth theme is that genetic disorders of endocrine function have different modes of altered endocrine signaling. Genetic deficiencies of an enzyme of hormone synthesis can lead to failure of hormone production (as in CAH), in which case pharmacological replacement of the deficient hormone(s) is required. Genetic mutations that alter hormone receptors can lead to insensitivity to hormone action (as in androgen-insensitivity syndrome, a rare cause of disorders of sexual differentiation). Lack of normal hormone effectiveness also characterizes T2DM, although the identification of a genetic basis for insulin resistance has not yet been made. As genetic knowledge of endocrine disorders continues to grow, there remains hope for molecular genetic approaches to disorders like T1DM that will provide a cure, eliminating the need for lifelong hormone replacement.

The fifth and final theme is that endocrine disorders truly cover the life span. Some of the organ systems discussed in this book tend to show declining function or increased propensity to disease with age. Although it is true that certain endocrine and endocrine-related disorders (T2DM, osteoporosis) show increased prevalence with aging, many chromosomal and single-gene disorders affecting endocrine function present in childhood or are detected by newborn screening. T1DM onset most commonly occurs in childhood, and some disorders of sexual development are not detected until puberty. Thus, endocrine disorders are within the domain of advanced practitioners giving care to patients across the life span.

REFERENCES

1. Endocrine Society. *Endocrine facts and figures: hypothalamic–pituitary.* Accessed September 9, 2019. http://endocrinefacts.org/health-conditions/hypothalamic-pituitary. Published 2016.
2. Endocrine Society. *Endocrine facts and figures: adrenal.* Accessed September 9, 2019. http://endocrinefacts.org/health-conditions/adrenal. Published 2016.
3. Taylor PN, Albrecht D, Scholz A, et al. Global epidemiology of hyperthyroidism and hypothyroidism. *Nat Rev Endocrinol.* 2018;14:301–316. doi:10.1038/nrendo.2018.18.
4. Vanderpump, MPJ. The epidemiology of thyroid disease. *Br Med Bull.* 2011;99:39–51. doi:10.1093/bmb/ldr030.
5. Legro RS. Evaluation and treatment of polycystic ovary syndrome. In: Feingold KR, Anawalt B, Boyce A, et al., eds. *Endotext [Internet].* South Dartmouth, MA: MDText.com, Inc. Accessed September 9, 2019.

https://www.ncbi.nlm.nih.gov/books/NBK278959. Updated January 11, 2017.

6. Escobar-Morreale HF. Polycystic ovary syndrome: definition, aetiology, diagnosis and treatment. *Nat Rev Endocrinol*. 2018;14:270–284. doi:10.1038/nrendo.2018.24.

7. Burney RO, Giudice LC. Pathogenesis and pathophysiology of endometriosis. *Fertil Steril*. 2012;98:511–519. doi:10.1016/j.fertnstert.2012.06.029.

8. Chaitoff A, Killeen TC, Nielsen C. Men's health 2018: BPH, prostate cancer, erectile dysfunction, supplements. *Cleve Clin J Med*. 2018;85:871–880. doi:10.3949/ccjm.85a.18011.

9. Chughtai B, Forde JC, Thomas DDM, et al. Benign prostatic hyperplasia. *Nat Rev Dis Primers*. 2016;2:16031. doi:10.1038/nrdp.2016.31.

10. Gulati R, Albertsen PC. Insights from the PLCO trial about prostate cancer screening. *Cancer*. 2017;123: 546–548. doi:10.1002/cncr.30472.

11. Centers for Disease Control and Prevention. *National Diabetes Statistics Report, 2017*. Atlanta, GA: Centers for Disease Control and Prevention, U.S. Dept of Health and Human Services; 2017.

12. Hales CM, Carroll MD, Fryar CD, Ogden CL. *Prevalence of Obesity Among Adults and Youth: United States, 2015–2016*. NCHS Data Brief No. 288. Hyattsville, MD: National Center for Health Statistics; 2017.

13. World Health Organization. *Fact sheet: diabetes*. October 30, 2018. https://www.who.int/news-room/fact-sheets/detail/diabetes. Accessed September 9, 2019.

14. World Health Organization. *Fact sheet: obesity and overweight*. February 16, 2018. https://www.who.int/en/news-room/fact-sheets/detail/obesity-and-overweight. Accessed September 9, 2019.

15. Hsiao EC, Gardner DG. Hormones and hormone action. In: Gardner DG, Shoback D, eds. *Greenspan's Basic & Clinical Endocrinology*. 10th ed. New York, NY: McGraw-Hill; 2018:chap 1.

16. Ben-Shlomo A, Melmed S. Hypothalamic regulation of anterior pituitary functions. In: Melmed S, ed. *The Pituitary*. 4th ed. London, UK: Elsevier; 2017:23–45.

17. Lu HAJ. Diabetes insipidus. In: Yang B, ed. *Aquaporins. Advances in Experimental Medicine and Biology*. Vol 969. Dordrecht, The Netherlands: Springer; 2017.

18. Kota SK, Gayatri K, Jammula S, et al. Endocrinology of parturition. *Indian J Endocrinol Metab*. 2013;17:50–59. doi:10.4103/2230-8210.107841.

19. Schneeberger M, Gomis R, Claret M. Hypothalamic and brainstem neuronal circuits controlling energy balance. *J Endocrinol*. 2014;220:T25-T$_4$6. doi:10.1530/JOE-13-0398.

20. Delgado TC. Glutamate and GABA in appetite regulation. *Front Endocrinol (Lausanne)*. 2013;4:103. doi:10.3389/fendo.2013.00103.

21. Timper K, Brüning JC. Hypothalamic circuits regulating appetite and energy homeostasis: pathways to obesity. *Dis Model Mech*. 2017;10:679–689. doi:10.1242/dmm.026609.

22. Berthoud HR. Metabolic and hedonic drives in the neural control of appetite: who is the boss? *Curr Opin Neurobiol*. 2011;21:888–896. doi:10.1016/j.conb.2011.09.004.

23. Javorsky BR, Aron DC, Findling JW, Tyrrell J. Hypothalamus and pituitary gland. In: Gardner DG, Shoback D, eds. *Greenspan's Basic & Clinical Endocrinology*. 10th ed. New York, NY: McGraw-Hill; 2017:69–120.

24. Drouin J. Pituitary development. In: Melmed S, ed. *The Pituitary*. 4th ed. London, UK: Elsevier; 2017:3–22.

25. Lonser RR, Nieman L, Oldfield EH. Cushing's disease: pathobiology, diagnosis, and management. *J Neurosurg*. 2017;126:404–417. doi:10.3171/2016.1.JNS152119.

26. Nieman LK, Biller BMK, Findling FW, et al. The diagnosis of Cushing's syndrome: an Endocrine Society clinical practice guideline. *J Clin Endocrinol Metab*. 2008;93:1526–1540. doi:10.1210/jc.2008-0125.

27. Sharma ST, Nieman LK, Feelders RA. Cushing's syndrome: epidemiology and developments in disease management. *Clin Epidemiol*. 2015;7:281–293. doi:10.2147/CLEP.S44336.

28. Binart N. Prolactin. In: Melmed S, ed. *The Pituitary*. 4th ed. London, UK: Elsevier; 2017:129–161.

29. Romijn JA. Hyperprolactinemia and prolactinoma. *Handb Clin Neurol*. 2014;124:185–195. doi:10.1016/B978-0-444-59602-4.00013-7.

30. Grattan D. The hypothalamo-prolactin axis. *J Endocrinol*. 2015;226:T101–T122. doi:10.1530/JOE-15-0213.

31. Majumdar A, Mangal NS. Hyperprolactinemia. *J Hum Reprod Sci*. 2013;6:168–175. doi:10.4103/0974-1208.121400.

32. Molitch M. Medication-induced hyperprolactinemia. *Mayo Clin Proc*. 2005;80:1050–1057. doi:10.4065/80.8.1050.

33. Melmed S, Felipe F. Casanueva FF, et al. Diagnosis and treatment of hyperprolactinemia: an Endocrine Society clinical practice guideline. *J Clin Endocrinol Metab*. 2011;96:273–288. doi:org/10.1210/jc.2010-1692.

34. Bonert VS, Melmed S. Growth hormone. In: Melmed S, ed. *The Pituitary*. 4th ed. London, UK: Elsevier; 2017:85–127.

35. Carmichael JD. Anterior pituitary failure. In: Melmed S, ed. *The Pituitary*. 4th ed. London, UK: Elsevier; 2017: 329–364.

36. Melmed S. Acromegaly. In: Melmed S, ed. *The Pituitary*. 4th ed. London, UK: Elsevier; 2017:423–466.

37. Kaiser UB. Gonadotrophin hormones. In: Melmed S, ed. *The Pituitary*. 4th ed. London, UK: Elsevier; 2017: 203–250.

38. Dwyer AA, Quinton R. Anatomy and physiology of the hypothalamic-pituitary gonadadal (HPG) axis. In: Llhana S, Follin D, Yedinak C, Grossman A, eds. *Advanced Practice in Endocrinology Nursing*. Cham, Switzerland: Springer; 2019:839–852.

39. Sarapura VD, Samuel MH. Thyroid-stimulating hormone. In: Melmed S, ed. *The Pituitary*. 4th ed. London, UK: Elsevier; 2017:163–201.

40. Greenman Y. Thyrotropin-secreting pituitary tumors. In: Melmed S, ed. *The Pituitary*. 4th ed. London, UK: Elsevier; 2017:573–588.

41. Neumann ID, Landgraf R. Balance of brain oxytocin and vasopressin: implications for anxiety, depression, and social behaviors. *Trends Neurosci*. 2012;36:649–659. doi:10.1016/j.tins.2012.08.004.

42. Caldwell HK. Oxytocin and vasopressin: powerful regulators of social behavior. *Neuroscientist.* 2017;23:517–528. doi:10.1177/1073858417708284.

43. Cuesta M, Thompson CJ. The syndrome of inappropriate antidiuresis (SIAD). *Best Pract Res Endocrinol Metab.* 2016;30:175–187. doi:10.1016/j.beem.2016.02.009.

44. Robinson AG, Verbalis JG. Posterior pituitary. In: Melmed S, Polonsky KS, Larsen PR, Kronenberg HM, eds. *Williams Textbook of Endocrinology.* 13th ed. Philadelphia, PA: Elsevier; 2016:300–332.

45. Stewart PM, Newell-Price JDC. Adrenal cortex. In: Melmed S, Polonsky KS, Larsen PR, Kronenberg HM, eds. *Williams Textbook of Endocrinology.* 13th ed. Philadelphia, PA: Elsevier; 2016:490–554.

46. Dattani MT, Gevers EF. Endocrinology of fetal development. In: Melmed S, Polonsky KS, Larsen PR, Kronenberg HM, eds. *Williams Textbook of Endocrinology.* 13th ed. Philadelphia, PA: Elsevier; 2016:849–892.

47. Young WF. Endocrine hypertension. In: Gardner DG, Shoback D, eds. *Greenspan's Basic & Clinical Endocrinology.* 10th ed. New York, NY: McGraw-Hill; 2018:chap 10.

48. Arlt W, Lang K, Sitch AJ, et al. Steroid metabolome analysis reveals prevalent glucocorticoid excess in primary aldosteronism. *JCI Insight.* 2017;2:e93136. doi:10.1172/jci.insight.93136.

49. Dick SM, Queiroz M, Bernardi BL, et al. Update in diagnosis and management of primary aldosteronism. *Clin Chem Lab Med.* 2018;56:360–372. doi:10.1515/cclm-2017-0217.

50. Cain DW, Cidlowski JA. Specificity and sensitivity of glucocorticoid signaling in health and disease. *Best Pract Res Clin Endocrinol Metab.* 2015;29:545–556. doi:10.1016/j.beem.2015.04.007.

51. Sapolsky RM, Romero LM, Munck AU. How do glucocorticoids influence stress responses? Integrating permissive, suppressive, stimulatory, and preparative actions. *Endocr Rev.* 2000;21:55–89. doi:10.1210/er.21.1.55.

52. Allolio B. Adrenal crisis. *Eur J Endocrinol.* 2015;172:R115–R124. doi:10.1530/EJE-14-0824.

53. Sharma E, Dahal S, Sharma P, et al. The characteristics and trends in adrenocortical carcinoma: a United States population based study. *J Clin Med Res.* 2018;10:636–640. doi:10.14740/jocmr3503w.

54. Nieman LK. Cushing's syndrome: update on signs, symptoms and biochemical screening. *Eur J Endocrinol.* 2015;173:M33–M38. doi:10.1530/EJE-15-0464.

55. Pappachan JM, Tun NN, Arunagirinathan G, et al. Pheochromocytomas and hypertension. *Curr Hypertens Rep.* 2018;20:3. doi:10.1007/s11906-018-0804-z.

56. Lal G, Clark OH. Endocrine surgery. In: Gardner DG, Shoback D, eds. *Greenspan's Basic & Clinical Endocrinology.* 10th ed. New York, NY: McGraw-Hill; 2018:chap 26.

57. Fung MM, Viveros OH, O'Connor DT. Diseases of the adrenal medulla. *Acta Physiol (Oxf).* 2007;192:325–335. doi:10.1111/j.1748-1716.2007.01809.x.

58. White BA, Harrison JR, Mehlmann LM. Fertilization, pregnancy, and lactation In: White BA, Harrison JR, Mehlmann LM. *Endocrine and Reproductive Physiology.* 5th ed. Philadelphia, PA: Elsevier; 2019:227–350.

59. Eugster E. Gigantism. In: Feingold KR, Anawalt B, Boyce A, et al., eds. *Endotext [Internet].* South Dartmouth, MA: MDText.com; 2000. https://www.ncbi.nlm.nih.gov/books/NBK278959. Updated April 17, 2018. Accessed September 4, 2019.

60. Prete A, Feliciano C, Mitchel I, Arlt W. Diagnosis and management of congenital adrenal hyperplasia in children and adults. In: Llhana S, Follin D, Yedinak C, Grossman A, eds. *Advanced Practice in Endocrinology Nursing.* Cham, Switzerland: Springer; 2019:657–678.

61. Ashpole N, Sanders J, Hodges E, et al. Growth hormone, insulin-like growth factor-1 and the aging brain. *Exp Gerontol.* 2015;68:76–81. doi:10.1016/j.exger.2014.10.002.

62. Sattler F. Growth hormone in the aging male. *Best Pract Res Clin Endocrinol Metab.* 2013;27:541–555. doi:10.1016/j.beem.2013.05.003.

63. Chahal HS, Drake WM. The endocrine system and ageing. *J Pathol.* 2007;211:173–180. doi:10.1002/path.2110.

64. Mobbs C, Hof P. *Functional Endocrinology of Aging.* New York, NY: Karger; 1998.

65. Rothman S, Mattson M. Adverse stress, hippocampal networks, and Alzheimer's disease. *Neuromolecular Med.* 2010;12:56–70. doi:10.1007/s12017-009-8107-9.

66. Papaleontiou M, Cappola AR. Thyroid-stimulating hormone in the evaluation of subclinical hypothyroidism. *JAMA.* 2016;316:1592–1593. doi:10.1001/jama.2016.9534.

67. Chalan P, Di Dalmazi G, Pani F, et al. Thyroid dysfunctions secondary to cancer immunotherapy. *J Endocrinol Invest.* 2018;41:625–638. doi:10.1007/s40618-017-0778-8.

68. Peeters RP. Subclinical hypothyroidism. *N Engl J Med.* 2017;376:2556–2565. doi:10.1056/NEJMcp1611144.

69. Rugge JB, Bougatsos C, Chou R. Screening and treatment of thyroid dysfunction: an evidence review for the US Preventive Services Task Force. *Ann Intern Med.* 2015;162:35–45. doi:10.7326/M14-1456.

70. Peters C, van Trotsenburg ASP, Schoenmakers N. Congenital hypothyroidism: update and perspectives. *Eur J Endocrinol.* 2018;179:R297–R317. doi:10.1530/EJE-18-0383.

71. Hanley P, Lord K, Bauer AJ. Thyroid disorders in children and adolescents: a review. *JAMA Pediatr.* 2016;170:1008–1019. doi:10.1001/jamapediatrics.2016.0486.

72. Van Vliet G, Deladoëy J. Disorders of the thyroid in the newborn and infant. In: Sperling MA, ed. *Pediatric Endocrinology.* 4th ed. Philadelphia, PA: Elsevier; 2014:chap 7.

73. Rivkees SA. Thyroid disorders in children and adolescents. In: Sperling MA, ed. *Pediatric Endocrinology.* 4th ed. Philadelphia, PA: Elsevier; 2014:chap 12.

74. Papaleontiou M, Esfandiari NH. Disorders of the thyroid. In: Fillit HM, Rockwood K, Young J, eds. *Brocklehurst's Textbook of Geriatric Medicine and Gerontology.* 5th ed. Philadelphia, PA: Elsevier; 2017:731–741.

75. Chaker L, Cappola AR, Mooijaart SP, Peeters RP. Clinical aspects of thyroid function during ageing. *Lancet Diabetes Endocrinol.* 2018;6:733–742. doi:10.1016/S2213-8587(18)30028-7.

76. Papaleontiou M, Haymart M. Approach to and treatment of thyroid disorders in elderly. *Med Clin North Am.* 2012;96:297–310. doi:10.1016/j.mcna.2012.01.013.

77. Prime DK, Geddes DT, Spatz DL, et al. Using milk flow rate to investigate milk ejection in the left and right breasts during simultaneous breast expression in women. *Int Breastfeed J*. 2009;4:10. doi:10.1186/1746-4358-4-10.

78. Santoro W Jr, Martinez FE, Ricco RG, et al. Colostrum ingested during the first day of life by exclusively breast-fed healthy newborn infants. *J Pediatr*. 2010;156:29–32. doi:10.1016/j.jpeds.2009.07.009.

79. Spatz DL. Ten steps for promoting and protecting breastfeeding in vulnerable populations. *J Perinat Neonatal Nurs*. 2004;18:385–396. doi:10.1097/00005237-200410000-00009.

80. Spatz DL. Beyond BFHI: the Spatz 10-step and breast-feeding resource nurse models to improve human milk and breastfeeding outcomes. *J Perinat Neonatal Nurs*. 2018;32:164–174. doi:10.1097/JPN.0000000000000339.

81. Hill PF, Aldaq JV. Milk volume on day 4 predictive of lactation adequacy at 6 weeks for mothers of non-nursing preterm infants. *J Perinat Neonatal Nurs*. 2005;19:273–282. doi:10.1097/00005237-200507000-00014.

82. Hoban R, Patel AL, Medina-Poeliniz C, et al. Human milk biomarkers of secretory activation in breast pump-dependent mothers of premature infants. *Breastfeed Med*. 2018;13:352–360. doi:10.1089/bfm.2017.018330.

83. Duran MS, Spatz DL. A mother with glandular hypo-plasia and a late preterm infant. *J Hum Lact*. 2011; 27(4):394–397. doi:10.1177/0890334411415856.

84. Marsh CA, Grimstad FW. Primary amenorrhea: diagnosis and management. *Obstet Gynecol Surv*. 2014;69:603–612. doi:10.1097/OGX.0000000000000111.

85. Shufelt CL, Torbati T, Dutra E. Hypothalamic amenorrhea and the long-term health consequences. *Semin Reprod Med*. 2017;35:256–161. doi:10.1055/s-0037-1603581.

86. Deligeoroglou E, Karountzos V. Abnormal uterine bleeding including coagulopathies and other menstrual disorders. *Best Pract Res Clin Obstet Gynaecol*. 2017;48:51–61. doi:10.1016/j.bpobgyn.2017.08.016.

87. Bacon JL. Abnormal uterine bleeding: current classification and clinical management. *Obstet Gynecol Clin North Am*. 2017;44:179–193. doi:10.1016/j.ogc.2017.02.012.

88. Rosenfield RL, Ehrmann DA. The pathogenesis of polycystic ovary syndrome (PCOS): the hypothesis of PCOS as functional ovarian hyperandrogenism revisited. *Endocr Rev*. 2016;37:467–520. doi:10.1210/er.2015-1104.

89. Coxon L, Horne AW, Vincent K. Pathophysiology of endometriosis-associated pain: a review of pelvic and central nervous system mechanisms. *Best Pract Res Clin Obstet Gynaecol*. 2018;51:53–67. doi:10.1016/j.bpobgyn.2018.01.014.

90. Centers for Disease Control and Prevention. Breast cancer statistics. https://www.cdc.gov/cancer/breast/statistics/index.htm. Accessed September 5, 2019.

91. Hayes DF, Lippman ME. Breast cancer. In: Jameson JL, Fauci AS, Kasper DL, et al., eds. *Harrison's Principles of Internal Medicine*. 20th ed. New York, NY: McGraw-Hill; 2018:chap 75.

92. Schramm A, De Gregorio N, Widschwendter P, et al. Targeted therapies in HER2-positive breast cancer—a systematic review. *Breast Care*. 2015;10:173–178. doi:10.1159/000431029.

93. Endocrine Society. *Endocrine Facts and Figures: Bone and Mineral*. Washington, DC: Endocrine Society; 2015.

94. Heaney R. Calcium, parathyroid function, bone and aging. *J Clin Endocrinol Metab*. 1996;81:1697–1698. doi:10.1210/jcem.81.5.8626818.

95. De Souza Gernaro P, De Medeiros Pinheiro M, Szeinfed VL, Martini LA. Secondary hyperparathyroidism and its relationship with sarcopenia in elderly women. *Arch Gerontol Geriatr*. 2015;60:349–353. doi:10.1016/j.archger.2015.01.005.

96. Saxon S, Etten MJ, Perkins E. *Physical Change and Aging: A Guide for the Healthcare Professional*. 5th ed. New York, NY: Springer Publishing Company; 2010.

97. Drake MT, Clarke BL, Lewiecki EM. The pathophysiology and treatment of osteoporosis. *Clin Ther*. 2015;37:1837–1850. doi:10.1016/j.clinthera.2015.06.006.

98. White BA, Harrison JR, Mehlmann LM. The male reproductive system. In: White BA, Harrison JR, Mehlmann LM. *Endocrine and Reproductive Physiology*, 5th ed. Philadelphia, PA: Elsevier; 2019:chap 9.

99. Gandaglia G, Briganti A, Jackson G, et al. A systematic review of the association between erectile dysfunction and cardiovascular diseases. *Eur Urol*. 2014;65:968–978. doi:10.1016/j.eururo.2013.08.023.

100. Egan KB. The epidemiology of benign prostatic hyperplasia associated with lower urinary tract symptoms: prevalence and incident rates. *Urol Clin N Am*. 2016;43:289–297. http://dx.doi.org/10.1016/j.ucl.2016.04.001.

101. Jahn JL, Giovannucci EL, Stampfer MJ. The high prevalence of undiagnosed prostate cancer at autopsy: implications for epidemiology and treatment of prostate cancer in the prostate-specific antigen era. *Int J Cancer*. 2015;137:2795–2802. doi:10.1002/ijc.29408.

102. Andriole GL, Crawford ED, Grubb RL 3rd, et al. Prostate cancer screening in the randomized Prostate, Lung, Colorectal, and Ovarian Cancer Screening Trial: mortality results after 13 years of follow-up. *J Natl Cancer Inst*. 2012;104:125–132. doi:10.1093/jnci/djr500.

103. Nelson WG, Antonarakis ES, Carter HB, et al. Prostate cancer. In: Neiderhuber JE, Armitage JO, Kastan MB, et al., eds. *Abeloff's Clinical Oncology*. 6th ed. New York, NY: Elsevier; 2020:1401–1432.

104. Centers for Disease Control and Prevention. *Overweight & Obesity: Defining Adult Overweight and Obesity*. Atlanta, GA: U.S. Department of Health and Human Services; 2017. https://www.cdc.gov/obesity/adult/defining.html. Accessed September 24, 2019.

105. Beale EG. Insulin signaling and insulin resistance. *J Investig Med*. 2013;61:11–14. doi:10.2310/JIM.0b013e3182746f95.

106. Molina PA. *Endocrine Physiology*. 5th ed. New York, NY: McGraw-Hill; 2018.

107. Jones AG, Hattersley AT. The clinical utility of C-peptide measurement in the care of patients with diabetes. *Diabet Med*. 2013;30:803–817. doi:10.1111/dme.12159.

108. Cherrington AD. Banting Lecture 1997. Control of glucose uptake and release by the liver in vivo. *Diabetes*. 1999;48:1198–1214. doi:10.2337/diabetes.48.5.1198.

109. American Diabetes Association. Standards of medical care in diabetes—2019. *Diabetes Care*. 2019;42(suppl 1):S1–S193. doi:10.2337/dc19-Sint01.

110. Jerram ST, Leslie RC. The genetic architecture of type 1 diabetes. *Genes.* 2017;8:209. doi:10.3390/genes8080209.

111. Papadakis MA, McPhee SJ, Rabow MW. *Current Medical Diagnosis & Treatment, 2017.* New York, NY: McGraw-Hill; 2017.

112. Ettinger S. *Nutritional Pathophysiology of Obesity and Its Comorbidities. A Case-Study Approach.* Philadelphia, PA: Elsevier; 2017:334.

113. Cohen M, Shilo S, Zuckerman-Levin N, Shehadeh N. Diabetic ketoacidosis in the pediatric population with type 1 diabetes. In: Nunes K, ed. *Major Topics in Type 1 Diabetes.* London, UK: IntechOpen; 2015:chap 5. doi:10.5772/60592.

114. Ali O. Genetics of type 2 diabetes. *World J Diabetes.* 2013;4:114–123. doi:10.4239/wjd.v4.i4.114.

115. Ramlo-Halsted BA, Edelman SV. The natural history of type 2 diabetes: implications for clinical practice. *Prim Care.* 1999;26:771–789. doi:10.1016/S0095-4543(05)70130-5.

116. Diabetes Prevention Program Research Group. Reduction in the incidence of type 2 diabetes with lifestyle intervention or metformin. *N Engl J Med.* 2002;346:393–403. doi:10.1056/NEJMoa012512.

117. DeFronzo RA. From the triumvirate to the ominous octet: a new paradigm for the treatment of type 2 diabetes mellitus. *Diabetes.* 2009;58:773–795. doi:10.2337/db09-9028.

118. Lavie CJ, Johannsen N, Swift D, et al. Exercise is medicine—the importance of physical activity, exercise training, cardiorespiratory fitness and obesity in the prevention and treatment of type 2 diabetes. *Eur Endocr.* 2014;10:18–22. doi:10.17925/EE.2014.10.01.18.

119. Powers AC, Niswender KD, Rickels MR. Diabetes mellitus: management and therapies. In: Jameson JL, Fauci AS, Kasper DL, et al., eds. *Harrison's Principles of Internal Medicine.* 20th ed. New York, NY: McGraw-Hill; 2018:chap 397.

120. The Diabetes Control and Complications Trial Research Group. The effect of intensive treatment of diabetes on the development and progression of long-term complications of insulin-dependent diabetes mellitus. *N Engl J Med.* 1993;329:997–986. doi:10.1056/NEJM199309303291401.

121. Nathan DM, DCCT/EDIC Research Group. The diabetes control and complications trial/epidemiology of diabetes interventions and complications study at 30 years: overview. *Diabetes Care.* 2014;37:9–16. doi:10.2337/dc13-2112.

122. UK Prospective Diabetes Study Group. Intensive blood-glucose control with sulphonylureas or insulin compared with conventional treatment and risk of complications in patients with type 2 diabetes (UKPDS 33). *Lancet.* 1998;352:837–853. doi:10.1016/S0140-6736(98)07019-6.

123. Staels B. Cardiovascular protection by sodium glucose cotransporter 2 inhibitors: potential mechanisms. *Am J Med.* 2017;130:S30–S39. doi:10.1016/j.amjmed.2017.04.009.

124. Kumar V, Abbas AK, Aster JC. *Robbins and Cotran Pathologic Basis of Disease.* 9th ed. Philadelphia, PA: Elsevier Saunders; 2015.

125. Secrest AM, Washington RE, Orchard TJ. Mortality in type 1 diabetes. In: Cowie C, Casagrande SS, Menke A, et al., eds. *Diabetes in America.* Bethesda, MD: National Institutes of Health; 2018:chap 35.

126. Baz B, Riveline JP, Gautier JF. Endocrinology of pregnancy: gestational diabetes mellitus: definition, aetiological and clinical aspects. *Eur J Endocrinol.* 2016;174:R43–R51. doi:10.1530/EJE-15-0378.

127. Pozzilli P, Pieralice S. Latent autoimmune diabetes in adults: current status and new horizons. *Endocrinol Metab.* 2018;33:147–159. doi:10.3803/EnM.2018.33.2.147.

128. Senaratna CV, Perret JL, Lodge CJ, et al. Prevalence of obstructive sleep apnea in the general population: a systematic review. *Sleep Med Rev.* 2017;34:70–81. doi:10.1016/j.smrv.2016.07.002.

129. De Felice FG. Alzheimer's disease and insulin resistance: translating basic science into clinical applications. *J Clin Invest.* 2013;123:531–539. doi:10.1172/JCI64595.

130. Rogers MAM, Kim C, Banerjee T, Lee JM. Fluctuations in the incidence of type 1 diabetes in the United States from 2001 to 2015: a longitudinal study. *BMC Med.* 2017;15:199. doi:10.1186/s12916-017-0958-6.

131. Viner R, White B, Christie D. Type 2 diabetes in adolescents: a severe phenotype posing major clinical challenges and public health burden. *Lancet.* 2017;389:2252–2260. doi:10.1016/S0140-6736(17)31371-5.

132. Nadeau KJ, Anderson BJ, Berg EG, et al. Youth-onset type 2 diabetes consensus report: current status, challenges, and priorities. *Diabetes Care.* 2016;39:1635–1642. doi:10.2337/dc16-1066.

133. Dabelea D, Stafford JM, Mayer-Davis EJ, et al. Association of type 1 diabetes vs type 2 diabetes diagnosed during childhood and adolescence with complications during teenage years and young adulthood. *JAMA.* 2017;317:825–835. doi:10.1001/jama.2017.0686.

134. Kirkman MS, Briscoe VJ, Clark N, et al. Diabetes in older adults. *Diabetes Care.* 2012;35:2650–2664.

135. De Tata V. Age-related impairment of pancreatic beta-cell function: pathophysiological and cellular mechanisms. *Front Endocrinol.* 2014;5:138. doi:10.3389/fendo.2014.00138.

SUGGESTED RESOURCES

Overview of the Endocrine System

Gardner DG, Shoback D, eds. *Greenspan's Basic & Clinical Endocrinology.* 10th ed. New York, NY: McGraw-Hill; 2018.

Melmed S, Polonsky KS, Larsen PR, Kronenberg HM, eds. *Williams Textbook of Endocrinology.* 13th ed. New York, NY: Elsevier; 2016.

Molina P. *Endocrine Physiology.* 5th ed. New York, NY: McGraw-Hill; 2018.

Hypothalamic–Pituitary Glands

Jameson JL, De Groot LJ, de Kretser DM, et al., eds. *Endocrinology: Adult and Pediatric.* 7th ed. New York, NY: Saunders/Elsevier; 2016.

Melmed S, ed. *The Pituitary.* 4th ed. London, UK: Elsevier; 2017.

Thyroid Gland

Brent GA, Weetman AP. Hypothyroidism and thyroiditis. In: Melmed S, Polonsky KS, Larsen PR, Kronenberg HM, eds. *Williams Textbook of Endocrinology*. 13th ed. Philadelphia, PA: Elsevier. 2016:333–368.

Chaker L, Bianco AC, Jonklaas J, Peeters RP. Hypothyroidism. *Lancet*. 2017;390:1550–1562. doi:10.1016/S0140-6736(17)30703-1.

Davies TF, Laurberg P, Bahn RS. Hyperthyroid disorders. In: Melmed S, Polonsky KS, Larsen PR, Kronenberg HM, eds. *Williams Textbook of Endocrinology*. 13th ed. Philadelphia, PA: Elsevier; 2016:333–368.

De Leo S, Lee SY, Braverman LE. Hyperthyroidism. *Lancet*. 2016;388:906–918. doi:10.1016/S0140-6736(16)00278-6.

Salvatore D, Davies TF, Schlumberger MJ, et al. Thyroid physiology and diagnostic evaluation of patients with thyroid disorders. In: Melmed S, Polonsky KS, Larsen PR, Kronenberg HM, eds. *Williams Textbook of Endocrinology*. 13th ed. Philadelphia, PA: Elsevier; 2016:333–368.

Gonads–Reproductive System

Hoffman BL, Schorge JO, Bradshaw KD, et al., eds. *Williams Gynecology*. 3rd ed. New York, NY: McGraw-Hill; 2016.

Lobo RA, Gershenson DM, Lentz GM, Valea FA, eds. *Comprehensive Gynecology*. 7th ed. Philadelphia, PA: Elsevier; 2017.

Molina PE. *Endocrine Physiology*. 5th ed. New York, NY: McGraw-Hill; 2018.

Strauss JF, Barbieri RL, eds. *Yen & Jaffe's Reproductive Endocrinology*. 8th ed. Philadelphia, PA: Elsevier; 2019.

White BA, Harrison JR, Mehlmann LM. *Endocrine and Reproductive Physiology*. 5th ed. Philadelphia, PA: Elsevier; 2019.

Metabolism, Pancreatic Hormones, and Diabetes

American Diabetes Association. Standards of medical care in diabetes—2019. *Diabetes Care*. 2019;42(suppl 1):S1–S193. https://care.diabetesjournals.org/content/42/Supplement_1.

Brownlee M, Aiello LP, Cooper ME, et al. Complications of diabetes mellitus. In: Shlomo M, Polonsky KS, Larsen PR, Kronenberg HM, eds. *Williams Textbook of Endocrinology*. 13th ed. Philadelphia, PA: Elsevier; 2016:1484–1581.

Flier JS, Maratos-Flier E. Pathobiology of obesity. In: Jameson JL, Fauci AS, Kasper DL, et al., eds. *Harrison's Principles of Internal Medicine*. 20th ed. New York, NY: McGraw-Hill; 2018:chap 394.

Powers AC, Niswender KD, Evans-Molina C. Diabetes mellitus: diagnosis, classification, and pathophysiology. In: Jameson JL, Fauci AS, Kasper DL, et al., eds. *Harrison's Principles of Internal Medicine*. 20th ed. New York, NY: McGraw-Hill; 2018:chap 396.

Röder PV, Wu B, Liu Y, Han W. Pancreatic regulation of glucose homeostasis. *Exp Mol Med*. 2016;48:e219. doi:10.1038/emm.2016.6.

LIST OF ABBREVIATIONS

AA arachidonic acid
AA amino acid
AAAD aromatic amino acid decarboxylase
AAT α_1-antitrypsin
AATD α_1-antitrypsin deficiency
ABI ankle–brachial index
Ac acinar cell
AC adenylyl cyclase
ACA anterior cerebral artery
ACE angiotensin-converting enzyme
ACh acetylcholine
AChE acetylcholinesterase
AChM muscarinic acetylcholine receptor
ACI anemia of chronic inflammation
ACL anterior cruciate ligament
ACPA anti-citrullinated protein antibody
ACR albumin/creatinine ratio
ACTH adrenocorticotropic hormone
AD autosomal dominant
ADHD attention-deficit/hyperactivity disorder
ADP adenosine diphosphate
ADPase adenosine diphosphatase
ADPKD autosomal dominant polycystic kidney disease
AEC alveolar epithelial cell
AFB acid-fast bacilli
AGE advanced glycation end product
AgRP agouti-related peptide
AHA American Heart Association
AHI apnea/hypopnea index
AIDS acquired immunodeficiency syndrome
AIH autoimmune hepatitis
AIHA autoimmune hemolytic anemia
AIRE autoimmune regulatory gene
AKI acute kidney injury
AKT AKR mouse tumor 8 kinase
ALD alcoholic liver disease
ALL acute lymphoblastic leukemia
ALP alkaline phosphatase
α-KG α-ketoglutarate
α-MSH alpha-melanocyte–stimulating hormone

ALT alanine aminotransferase
AMA antimitochondrial antibody
AML acute myeloid leukemia
AML anterior mitral leaflet
AMP adenosine monophosphate
5′-AMP 5′-adenosine monophosphate
AMPA α-amino-3-hydroxyl-5-methyl-4-isoxazole-propionate
ANA antinuclear antibody
ANP atrial natriuretic peptide
Ao aorta
AP anteroposterior; area postrema
AP-1 activator protein 1
APB atrial premature beat
aPC activated protein C
APC antigen-presenting cell
aPC-R activated protein C resistance
APL acute promyelocytic leukemia
Apo A-1 apolipoprotein A-1
Apo B-100 apolipoprotein B-100
Apo C-II apolipoprotein C-II
APOE apolipoprotein E
APS antiphospholipid syndrome
APSGN acute poststreptococcal glomerulonephritis
aPTT activated partial thromboplastin time
AQP aquaporin
AR autosomal recessive
ARAS ascending reticular activating system
ARB angiotensin receptor blocker
ARC arcuate
ARDS acute respiratory distress syndrome
Areg amphiregulin
Arg arginine
ART antiretroviral therapy
AS ankylosing spondylitis
ASCVD atherosclerotic cardiovascular disease
ASD atrial septal defect
ASM airway smooth muscle
ASMA antismooth muscle actin
Asn asparagine
AST aspartate aminotransferase

ATII angiotensin II
AT-III antithrombin III
ATP adenosine triphosphate
ATPase adenosine triphosphatase
AUB abnormal uterine bleeding
AV atrioventricular
AVNRT atrioventricular nodal reentrant tachycardia
AVP arginine vasopressin
BA basilar artery
BBB blood–brain barrier
BCBM Bowman's capsule basement membrane
bCG bacille Calmette–Guérin
BCR B-cell receptor
BDZ benzodiazepine
BECTS benign epilepsy with centrotemporal spikes
$\beta_2 m$ β_2-microglobulin
BF basal forebrain
BFU-E burst-forming unit–erythrocyte
BL basal lamina
BMD bone mineral density
BMI body mass index
BNP B-type natriuretic peptide
BP blood pressure
BPD bronchopulmonary dysplasia
2,3-BPG 2,3-bisphosphoglycerate
BPH benign prostatic hyperplasia
BRE benign rolandic epilepsy
BTM basal transcription machinery
BUN blood urea nitrogen
CA carbonic anhydrase
Ca^{2+} calcium
CAA cerebral amyloid angiopathy
CAD coronary artery disease
CAH congenital adrenal hyperplasia
CaM calmodulin
cAMP cyclic adenosine monophosphate
CAP community-acquired pneumonia
CAR-T chimeric antigen receptor–T cell
CBC complete blood count
cc cholesterol crystal
cccDNA covalently bonded, closed, circular DNA
CCK cholecystokinin
CD Crohn disease
CDC Centers for Disease Control and Prevention
CDI *Clostridioides difficile* infection
CDK cyclin-dependent kinase
cDNA complementary DNA
CE cholesterol ester
CEC capillary endothelial cell
CF cystic fibrosis
cfDNA cell-free DNA
CFTR cystic fibrosis transmembrane conductance regulator
CFU colony-forming unit
CFU-E colony-forming unit–erythrocyte
CFU-Eo colony-forming unit–eosinophil

CFU-GEMM colony-forming unit–granulocyte-erythrocyte-monocyte-megakaryocyte
CFU-GM colony-forming unit–granulocyte-macrophage
cGAS cyclic guanosine monophosphate–adenosine monophosphate synthase
cGMP cyclic guanosine monophosphate
CGRP calcitonin gene–related peptide
CH congenital hypothyroidism
cHSP10 chlamydial heat shock protein 10
cHSP60 chlamydial heat shock protein 60
CIP/KIP CDK-interacting protein/kinase inhibitory protein
CKD chronic kidney disease
CKD-EPI Chronic Kidney Disease Epidemiology Collaboration
CKD-MBD chronic kidney disease mineral and bone disorder
CKI cyclin-dependent kinase inhibitor
CK-MB creatine kinase myocardial band, fraction
Cl^- chloride
Clf clumping factor
CLIP class II–associated Ii peptide
CLIP corticotropin-like intermediate lobe peptide
CML chronic myeloid leukemia
CMP comprehensive metabolic panel
CMV cytomegalovirus
CN cranial nerve
CNP C-type natriuretic peptide
CNS central nervous system
CO cardiac output
CO_2 carbon dioxide
CoA coenzyme A
COMT catechol-*O*-methyl transferase
COPD chronic obstructive pulmonary disease
COX cyclooxygenase
COX-1 cyclooxygenase-1
COX-2 cyclooxygenase-2
CPAP continuous positive airway pressure
C-peptide connecting peptide
CRC colorectal cancer
CRE carbapenem-resistant Enterobacteriaceae
CREB cAMP response element-binding protein
CRH corticotropin-releasing hormone
cRNA complementary RNA
CRP C-reactive protein
CSA cross-sectional area
CSC cancer stem cell
CST corticospinal tract
CT computed tomography
CTL cytotoxic T lymphocyte
CTLA-4 cytotoxic T lymphocyte–associated protein 4
CVA cerebrovascular accident
CVLM caudal ventrolateral medulla
CVP central venous pressure

CXR   chest x-ray
CYP   cytochrome P
Cys   cysteine
D1   deiodinase type I
D2   deiodinase type II
D3   deiodinase type III
D_1–D_5 dopamine receptors
D_2 dopamine receptor type 2
DA   dopamine
DAD   delayed after-depolarization
DAG   diacylglycerol
DAMP   danger-associated molecular pattern
DASH   dietary approaches to stop hypertension
DAT   dopamine transporter
DBH   dopamine β-hydroxylase
DC   dendritic cell
DDAVP   desmopressin acetate
dDC   dermal dendritic cell
DDH   developmental dysplasia of the hip
DHEA   dehydroepiandrosterone
DHEAS   dehydroepiandrosterone sulfate
DHP   dihydropyridine
DHT   dihydrotestosterone
DI   diabetes insipidus
DILI   drug-induced liver injury
DIT   diiodotyrosine
DKA   diabetic ketoacidosis
D_{LCO} diffusing capacity of the lung for carbon monoxide
DM   diabetes mellitus
DMARD   disease-modifying antirheumatic drug
DMT-1   divalent ion membrane transporter
DMV   dorsal motor nucleus of the vagus nerve
DNA   deoxyribonucleic acid
DP   diastolic pressure
2,3-DPG   2,3-diphosphoglycerate
DPP   dipeptidyl peptidase
DR   dorsal raphe
dsDNA   double-stranded DNA
***DSM-5**   Diagnostic and Statistical Manual of Mental Disorders*, Fifth Edition
DSMES   diabetes self-management education and support
dsRNA   double-stranded RNA
DT   distal tubule
DTC   direct-to-consumer
DVT   deep vein thrombosis
DXA   dual-energy x-ray absorptiometry
Dyn A   dynorphin A
E_1 estrone
E_2 estradiol
EAD   early after-depolarization
eAG   estimated average glucose
EC   endothelial cell
E-C   excitation–contraction
ECF   extracellular fluid

ECG   electrocardiogram
ECM   extracellular matrix
ED   erectile dysfunction
EDPVR   end-systolic pressure–volume relationship
EDV   end-diastolic volume
EEG   electroencephalogram
EFW   estimated fetal weight
EGD   esophagogastroduodenoscopy
EGF   epidermal growth factor
EGFR   epidermal growth factor receptor
eGFR   estimated glomerular filtration rate
EIA   enzyme immunoassay
ELISA   enzyme-linked immunosorbent assay
EMG   electromyogram
EMT   epithelial–mesenchymal transition
ENaC   epithelial sodium channel
Enk   enkephalin
eNOS   endothelial nitric oxide synthase
ENT   ear/nose/throat
EOS   eosinophil
Epi   epinephrine
Epo   erythropoietin
EPSP   excitatory postsynaptic potential
ER   endoplasmic reticulum
ERAD   ER-associated protein degradation
ERCP   endoscopic retrograde cholangiopancreatography
ERV   expiratory reserve volume
ESPVR   end-systolic pressure–volume relationship
ESR   erythrocyte sedimentation rate
ESRD   end-stage renal disease
ESV   end-systolic volume
ET-1   endothelin-1
ETX   ethosuximide
EWGSOP   European Working Group on Sarcopenia in Older People
FA   fatty acid
Fab   antigen-binding fragment
$FADH_2$ flavin adenine dinucleotide
FAEE   fatty acid ethyl ester
Fc   constant fragment
FC   foam cell
FcεRI   high-affinity IgE receptor
FDA   Food and Drug Administration
FENa   fractional excretion of sodium
FEV_1 forced expiratory volume in 1 second
FFA   free fatty acid
Fg   fibrinogen
FGF-23   fibroblast growth factor-23
FH   familial hypercholesterolemia
F_{IO_2} fraction of inspired oxygen
FISH   fluorescence in situ hybridization
fMRI   functional MRI
FnBP   fibronectin-binding protein

FNT fetal nuchal translucency
FODMAPs fermentable oligo-di-mono-saccharides and polyols
FPG fasting plasma glucose
FRAX Fracture Risk Assessment Tool
FRC functional residual capacity
FSGS focal segmental glomerulosclerosis
FSH follicle-stimulating hormone
FSHR follicle-stimulating hormone receptor
FTLD frontotemporal lobar degeneration
FV factor V
FVC forced vital capacity
FVL factor V Leiden
G$_i$ inhibitory G protein
G6PD glucose-6-phosphate dehydrogenase
GABA gamma-aminobutyric acid
GABAR GABA receptor
GABHS group A β-hemolytic streptococcus
GAD glutamate decarboxylase
GAD glutamic acid decarboxylase
GALT gut-associated lymphoid tissue
GDM gestational diabetes mellitus
GDP guanosine diphosphate
GEC glomerular endothelial cell
GEFS+ generalized epilepsy with febrile seizures plus
GER gastroesophageal reflux
GERD gastroesophageal reflux disease
GFR glomerular filtration rate
GGT gamma-glutamyl transferase
GH growth hormone
GHRH growth hormone–releasing hormone
GHSR ghrelin receptor
GI gastrointestinal
GIP glucose-dependent insulinotropic peptide
GLASS Global Antimicrobial Resistance Surveillance System
Gln glutamine
GLP glucagon-like peptide
GLP-1 glucagon-like peptide 1
Glu glutamate (glutamic acid)
Glu-R glutamate receptor
GLUT glucose transporter
GLUT1 glucose transporter 1
GLUT2 glucose transporter 2
GLUT4 glucose transporter 4
Gly glycine
GM-CSF granulocyte/macrophage colony-stimulating factor
GMP guanosine monophosphate
GnRH gonadotropin-releasing hormone
GP glycoprotein
GP2 glycoprotein 2
GPCR G protein–coupled receptor
GPe globus pallidus externa
GPI glycosylphosphatidylinositol

GR glucocorticoid receptor
GRE glucocorticoid response element
GTO Golgi tendon organ
GTP guanosine triphosphate
GTPase guanosine triphosphatase
GTT glucose tolerance test
GVHD graft-versus-host disease
GWAS genome-wide association study
H$_1$ histamine type 1 receptor
H$_2$O$_2$ hydrogen peroxide
HA hemagglutinin
HAI Histologic Activity Index
HAV hepatitis A virus
Hb hemoglobin
HbA hemoglobin A
HbA$_{1c}$ glycated hemoglobin
HBcAg hepatitis B core antigen
HBeAg hepatitis B e antigen
HbF fetal hemoglobin (hemoglobin F)
HbS hemoglobin S
HBsAg hepatitis B surface antigen
HBV hepatitis B virus
HCAP healthcare-acquired pneumonia
HCC hepatocellular carcinoma
HCF healthcare facility
hCG human chorionic gonadotropin
HCl hydrochloric acid
HCM hypertrophic cardiomyopathy
HCN hyperpolarization-activated cyclic nucleotide–gated
HCV hepatitis C virus
HDL high-density lipoprotein
HeFH heterozygous form of familial hypercholesterolemia
HELLP hemolysis, elevated liver enzymes, low platelets
HER2 human epidermal growth factor receptor 2
HFpEF heart failure with preserved ejection fraction
HFrEF heart failure with reduced ejection fraction
HHS hyperosmolar hyperglycemic syndrome
HHSV-6 human herpes simplex virus 6
Hib *Haemophilus influenzae* type b
His histidine
HIT heparin-induced thrombocytopenia
HIV human immunodeficiency virus
HLA human leukocyte antigen
HMB heavy menstrual bleeding
HMG-CoA 3-hydroxy-3-methyl-glutaryl-coenzyme A
HNPCC hereditary nonpolyposis colorectal cancer
HoFH homozygous form of familial hypercholesterolemia
HPA hypothalamic-pituitary-adrenal
HPG hypothalamic-pituitary-gonadal
HPV human papillomavirus
HR heart rate

HRE   hormone response element
HSC   hematopoietic stem cell
HSD   hydroxysteroid dehydrogenase
HSL   hormone-sensitive lipase
HSP   heat shock protein
HSP90   heat shock protein 90
HSV   herpes simplex virus
5-HT   5-hydroxytryptamine (serotonin)
5-HT$_2$ 5-hydroxytryptamine receptor, type 2
5-HT$_3$ 5-hydroxytryptamine receptor, type 3
HUS   hemolytic uremic syndrome
IAP   inhibitor of apoptosis
IBD   inflammatory bowel disease
IC   inspiratory capacity
ICA   internal carotid artery
ICA512   islet cell autoantigen 512
ICAM-1   intercellular adhesion molecule 1
ICF   intracellular fluid
ICU   intensive care unit
iDEC   inflammatory dendritic epidermal cell
IDL   intermediate-density lipoprotein
IDSA   Infectious Diseases Society of America
IEC   intestinal epithelial cell
IEL   internal elastic lamina; intraepithelial lymphocyte
IF   intrinsic factor
IFA   immunofluorescence assay
IFN   interferon
IFN-α   interferon alpha
IFN-γ   interferon gamma
IgA   immunoglobulin A
IGF   insulin-like growth factor
IGF-1   insulin-like growth factor 1
IgG   immunoglobulin G
IgM   immunoglobulin M
IL   interleukin
IL-6   interleukin 6
ILC   innate lymphoid cell
Ile   isoleucine
ImPACT   immediate postconcussion assessment and cognitive testing
IMT   intima–media thickness
INK4   inhibitor of kinase 4
iNKT   invariant natural killer T cell
INR   international normalized ratio
INS   insulin
INSR   insulin receptor
IP$_3$ inositol triphosphate
IPF   idiopathic pulmonary fibrosis
IPH   idiopathic pulmonary hypertension
IPSP   inhibitory postsynaptic potentials
IRS   insulin receptor substrate
IRV   inspiratory reserve volume
ITP   immune thrombocytopenic purpura
ITT   internal tibial torsion
IVF   in vitro fertilization

IVIG   intravenous immunoglobulin G
JAK   Janus kinase
JAK-STAT   Janus kinase–signal transducer and activator of transcription
JG   juxtaglomerular
JGA   juxtaglomerular apparatus
JP   joining peptide
K$^+$ potassium ion
K$^+_{ATP}$ ATP-dependent potassium channel
KC   keratinocyte
KUB   kidneys, ureter, bladder
L   lysosome
LA   left atrium
LAD   left anterior descending artery
LADA   latent autoimmune diabetes of the adult
LAP   left atrial pressure
LC   locus ceruleus
LCA   left coronary artery
LCAT   lecithin–cholesterol acyltransferase
LCX   left circumflex artery
LDL   low-density lipoprotein
L-dopa   L-3,4-dihydroxyphenlalanine
LDT   lateral dorsal tegmental nucleus
LES   lower esophageal sphincter
Leu   leucine
LH   lateral hypothalamus; luteinizing hormone
LHON   Leber hereditary optic neuropathy
LHR   luteinizing hormone receptor
LLQ   left lower quadrant
LMCA   left main coronary artery
LOA   left occiput anterior
LOH   loop of Henle
5-LOX   5-lipoxygenase
LP   lumbar puncture
LPH   lipotropin
LPL   lipoprotein lipase
LPR5   low-density lipoprotein receptor–related protein 5
LPS   lipopolysaccharide
LQTS   long QT syndrome
LSD   lysergic acid diethylamide
LSEC   liver sinusoid endothelial cell
LT   leukotriene
LTR   leukotriene receptor
LT-α$_1$β$_2$ lymphotoxin alpha-1, beta-2
LUTS   lower urinary tract symptoms
LV   left ventricle
LVEDP   left ventricular end-diastolic pressure
LVEDV   left ventricular end-diastolic volume
LVH   left ventricular hypertrophy
LVP   left ventricle pressure
Lys   lysine
M   muscarinic receptor
M$_1$ muscarinic receptor 1
M$_2$ muscarinic receptor 2
mac   macrophage

MAC membrane attack complex
MAIT mucosa-associated invariant T
MAO monoamine oxidase
MAOI monoamine oxidase inhibitor
MAP mean arterial pressure; mitogen-activated protein
MBL mannose-binding lectin, mannan-binding lectin
MBP (eosinophil) major basic protein
MC mast cell; mesangial cell
MCA middle cerebral artery
MCH mean cell hemoglobin
MCHC mean cell hemoglobin concentration
M-CSF monocyte colony-stimulating factor
MCV mean cell volume
MDD major depressive disorder
MDI metered dose inhaler
MDP maximum diastolic potential
MDRD Modification of Diet in Renal Disease
MDS myelodysplastic syndrome
Met methionine
mGFR measured glomerular filtration rate
MHC major histocompatibility complex
MHC II major histocompatibility complex class II
MIBG metaiodo-benzylguanidine
miRNA microRNA
MIT monoiodotyrosine
MLCK myosin light chain kinase
MLCP myosin light chain phosphatase
MLp modified lipoprotein
MMP matrix metalloproteinase
MMR measles–mumps–rubella
MMSE Mini-Mental State Examination
MoCA Montreal Cognitive Assessment
MODS multiple organ dysfunction syndrome
MOMP major outer membrane protein
mon monocyte
MP myosin phosphatase
MR magnetic resonance
MR mineralocorticoid receptor; mitral regurgitation
MRCP magnetic resonance cholangiopancreatography
MRI magnetic resonance imaging
mRNA messenger RNA
MRSA methicillin-resistant *Staphylococcus aureus*
MSAFP maternal serum α-fetoprotein
MSH melanocyte-stimulating hormone
MTB *Mycobacterium tuberculosis*
MV mitral valve
Mvo$_2$ myocardial oxygen consumption
NA neuraminidase
NA nucleus ambiguus
Na$^+$ sodium ion
Na$^+$/K$^+$ pump sodium–potassium pump
Na$^+$/K$^+$–ATPase sodium-potassium–adenosine triphosphatase
NAAT nucleic acid amplification testing

NAC *N*-acetylcysteine
NAc nucleus accumbens
NAD nicotinamide adenine dinucleotide
NADH nicotinamide adenine dinucleotide, reduced form
NADPH nicotinamide adenine dinucleotide phosphate
NAFLD nonalcoholic fatty liver disease
NaHCO$_3$ sodium bicarbonate
NAMCS National Ambulatory Medical Care Survey
NAPQI *N*-acetyl-*p*-benzoquinone-imine
NASH nonalcoholic steatohepatitis
NCS nerve conduction study
NE norepinephrine
NEP nuclear export protein
NET neutrophil extracellular trap
NET norepinephrine transporter
NF-κB nuclear factor-kappa B
NGF nerve growth factor
nGRE negative glucocorticoid response element
NHANES National Health and Nutrition Examination Survey
NIS sodium/iodide symporter
NK natural killer
NK$_1$ neurokinin type 1
NKCC sodium-potassium-chloride cotransporter
NLR nucleotide-binding domain–leucine-rich repeat–containing molecule
NMDA *N*-methyl-D-aspartate
NMDA-R *N*-methyl-D-aspartate receptor
nNOS neuronal nitric oxide synthase
NNRTI non-nucleoside reverse transcriptase inhibitor
NO nitric oxide
NOS nitric oxide synthase
NPH normal pressure hydrocephalus
N-POC N-terminal proopiocortin
NPY neuropeptide Y
NR nuclear receptor
NREM nonrapid eye movement
NRTI nucleoside reverse transcriptase inhibitor
NSAID nonsteroidal antiinflammatory drug
NSTEMI non–ST-elevation myocardial infarction
NT neurotransmitter
NT-proBNP N-terminal pro B-type natriuretic peptide
NTS nucleus of the tractus solitarius
O$_2$ oxygen
OA$^-$ organic anion
OA osteoarthritis
OAT organic anion transporter
OB obstetric
ObR leptin receptor
OC$^+$ organic cation
OCT organic cation transporter
OFC orbitofrontal cortex

OGTT   oral glucose tolerance test
OHS   obesity hypoventilation syndrome
OI   osteogenesis imperfecta
OPG   osteoprotegerin
ORT   oral rehydration therapy
OSA   obstructive sleep apnea
OT   oxytocin
OTC   over-the-counter
OX40   stimulatory receptor on Th2 cell
P   phosphorus; phosphate; podocyte
P$_A$ alveolar pressure
P$_i$ inorganic phosphate
ΔP   change in pressure
Paco_2   partial pressure of carbon dioxide in arterial blood
PAD   peripheral arterial disease
PAF   platelet-activating factor
PAG   periaqueductal gray
PAH   phenylalanine hydroxylase
PALM-COEIN   Polyps Adenomyosis Leiomyoma Malignancy-Coagulopathy Ovulatory disorders Endometrial Iatrogenic Not otherwise classified
PAMP   pathogen-associated molecular pattern
PB   parabrachial
PBC   primary biliary cholangitis
PBP   penicillin-binding protein
PC   pit cell
PCA   posterior cerebral artery
PCL   posterior cruciate ligament
Pco_2   partial pressure of carbon dioxide
PCOM   polycystic ovary morphology
PCOS   polycystic ovary syndrome
PCP   phencyclidine
PC-PTSD-5   Primary Care PTSD Screen
PCR   polymerase chain reaction
PCSK9   proprotein convertase subtilisin/kexin 9
PD-1   programmed death-1 (programmed cell death protein 1)
PDA   patent ductus arteriosus
PDE-5   phosphodiesterase-5
PDGF   platelet-derived growth factor
PDR   pan-drug resistant
PE   pulmonary embolism
PEC   parietal epithelial cell
PECAM-1   platelet–endothelial cell adhesion molecule
PERRLA   pupils, equal, round, reactive to light, accommodation
PET   positron emission tomography
PFC   prefrontal cortex
PFT   pulmonary function test
PG   prostaglandin
PGE$_2$ prostaglandin E$_2$
PGF$_{2\alpha}$ prostaglandin F$_{2\alpha}$
PGG$_2$ prostaglandin G$_2$
PGH$_2$ prostaglandin H$_2$

PGI$_2$ prostaglandin I$_2$ (prostacyclin)
PHQ   Patient Health Questionnaire
PI3K/Akt   phosphatidylinositol 3-kinase/Akt
PIDS   Pediatric Infectious Diseases Society
PI3K   phosphoinositide-3-kinase
PIP$_2$ phosphatidylinositol bisphosphate
PKA   protein kinase A
PKD   polycystic kidney disease
PKU   phenylketonuria
PL   phospholamban; phospholipid
Pl   platelet
PLC   phospholipase C
PMN   polymorphonuclear leukocyte
PNMT   phenylethanolamine *N*-methyltransferase
Po_2   partial pressure of oxygen
PO$_4$ phosphate
POMC   pro-opiomelanocortin
PPAR-γ   peroxisome proliferator–activated receptor gamma
PPI   proton pump inhibitor
Ppl   pleural pressure
PPT   peripeduncular tegmentum
pre-mRNA   pre-messenger RNA
PRL   prolactin
Pro   proline
PRR   pattern recognition receptor
PSA   prostate-specific antigen
PSI   Pneumonia Severity Index
PSP   postsynaptic potential
P$_T$ transpulmonary pressure
PT   prothrombin time; proximal tubule
PTH   parathyroid hormone
PTSD   post-traumatic stress disorder
PVN   paraventricular nuclei
PWV   pulse wave velocity
ΔQ   change in flow
qHSC   quiescent hepatic stellate cell
RAAS   renin-angiotensin-aldosterone system
RANK   receptor activator of nuclear factor kappa B
RANKL   receptor activator of nuclear factor kappa B ligand
RBC   red blood cell
RBF   renal blood flow
RCA   right coronary artery
RCM   restrictive cardiomyopathy
RDT   rapid diagnostic test
RDW   red cell distribution width
REM   rapid eye movement
RER   rough endoplasmic reticulum
RES   reticuloendothelial system
RLQ   right lower quadrant
RLR   RIG-I-like receptor (retinoic acid–inducible gene-I–like receptor)
RMP   resting membrane potential
RNA   ribonucleic acid
RNP   ribonucleoprotein

RORγt retinoic acid receptor–related orphan nuclear receptor gamma

ROS reactive oxygen species

RP refractory period

rRNA ribosomal RNA

RRT renal replacement therapy

RSV respiratory syncytial virus

rT$_3$ reverse T$_3$

RT-qPCR reverse transcriptase–quantitative polymerase chain reaction

RUQ right upper quadrant

RuST rubrospinal tract

RV residual volume; right ventricle

RVLM rostral ventrolateral medulla

RVM rostral ventral medulla

RyR ryanodine receptor

S$_1$ first heart sound

S$_2$ second heart sound

SA sinoatrial

SAM sympathetic-adrenomedullary

SASP senescence-associated secretory phenotype

SCAT5 Sport Concussion Assessment Tool, 5th edition

SCC staphylococcal cassette chromosome

SCD sickle cell disease

SCF stem cell factor

SCID severe combined immunodeficiency

Ser serine

SER smooth endoplasmic reticulum

SERCA sarcoendoplasmic reticulum Ca^{2+} ATPase

SERT serotonin transporter

sGC soluble guanylyl cyclase

SGLT sodium–glucose transporter

SGLT1 sodium–glucose-linked transporter 1

SGLT-2 sodium–glucose-linked transporter 2

SHEA Society for Healthcare Epidemiology of America

SIADH syndrome of inappropriate antidiuretic hormone

siRNA small interfering RNA

SLE systemic lupus erythematosus

SMA spinal muscular atrophy

SMC smooth muscle cell

SNP single-nucleotide polymorphism

SNRI serotonin–norepinephrine reuptake inhibitor

snRNA small nuclear RNA

SNS sympathetic nervous system

SP systolic pressure

Spo$_2$ oxygen saturation

SR sarcoplasmic reticulum

SRY sex-determining region of the Y chromosome

SSN spinal sympathetic neuron

SSRI selective serotonin reuptake inhibitor

ssRNA single-stranded RNA

SST somatostatin

STAT signal transducer and activator of transcription

STEC shiga toxin–producing *Escherichia coli*

STEMI ST-elevation myocardial infarction

STT spinothalamic tract

suPAR soluble urokinase–type plasminogen activator receptor

SUR sulfonylurea receptor

SV stroke volume

T$_3$ triiodothyronine

T$_4$ thyroxine

TA tuft adhesion

TACO transfusion-associated circulatory overload

TAL thick ascending limb

TAP transporter associated with antigen processing

TB tuberculosis

TBG thyroxine-binding globulin

TBW total body water

TCA tricyclic antidepressant

TcdA *Clostridiodes difficile* toxin A

TcdB *Clostridiodes difficile* toxin B

TCR T-cell receptor

T1DM type 1 diabetes mellitus

T2DM type 2 diabetes mellitus

TEWL transepidermal water loss

TF tissue factor

T$_{fh}$ follicular helper T cell

TFPI tissue factor pathway inhibitor

TG triglyceride

TG2 transglutaminase 2

TGF-β transforming growth factor beta

Th T-helper

TH tyrosine hydroxylase

Th1 T-helper 1 cell

Th2 T-helper 2 cell

THC tetrahydrocannabinol

TIA transient ischemic attack

TLC total lung capacity

TLR Toll-like receptor

TLy T lymphocyte

TMN tuberomammillary nucleus

TnC troponin C

TNF tumor necrosis factor

TNF-α tumor necrosis factor alpha

TNM tumor-node-metastasis cancer staging

TORCH toxoplasmosis, other, rubella, cytomegalovirus, herpes virus

TP threshold potential

tPA tissue plasminogen activator

TPO thrombopoietin; thyroperoxidase

TPR total peripheral resistance

TR thyroid hormone receptor

TRAB thyroid receptor antibody

Treg regulatory T cell

TRH thyrotropin-releasing hormone

tRNA transfer RNA

TSH thyroid-stimulating hormone

TSI thyroid-stimulating immunoglobulin

TSLP thymic stromal lymphopoietin

TSLPR thymic stromal lymphopoietin receptor
tTG tissue transglutaminase
tTG2 tissue transglutaminase 2
TXA$_2$ thromboxane A$_2$
Tyr tyrosine
UC ulcerative colitis
UDCA ursodeoxycholic acid
UDP uridine 5′-diphospho-glucuronosyltransferase
UES upper esophageal sphincter
uPA urokinase-type plasminogen activator
UPJ ureteropelvic junction
UPR unfolded protein response
USPSTF United States Preventive Services Task Force
UTR untranslated region
UV ultraviolet
UVJ ureterovesicular junction
V$_A$ alveolar volume
VA vertebral artery
Val valine
VC vital capacity
VCAM-1 vascular cell adhesion molecule 1
V$_D$ dead space volume
VEGF vascular endothelial growth factor
VEGF-α vascular endothelial growth factor alpha
VKORC1 vitamin K epoxide reductase complex, subunit 1

VLDL very low-density lipoprotein
VLM ventrolateral medulla
Vo$_2$ max maximum oxygen consumption
VPA valproic acid
VPB ventricular premature beat
V̇/Q̇ ventilation/perfusion
vRNA viral RNA
VRSA vancomycin-resistant *Staphylococcus aureus*
VSD ventricular septal defect
VSM vascular smooth muscle
V$_T$ tidal volume
VT ventricular tachycardia
VTA ventral tegmental area
VTE venous thromboembolism
V$_{Thr}$ threshold voltage
VUR vesicoureteral reflux
vWD von Willebrand disease
vWF von Willebrand factor
VZV varicella-zoster virus
WBC white blood cell
WGS whole-genome sequencing
WHO World Health Organization
WNL within normal limits
WPW Wolff–Parkinson–White
XDR extensively drug resistant
ZG zymogen granule

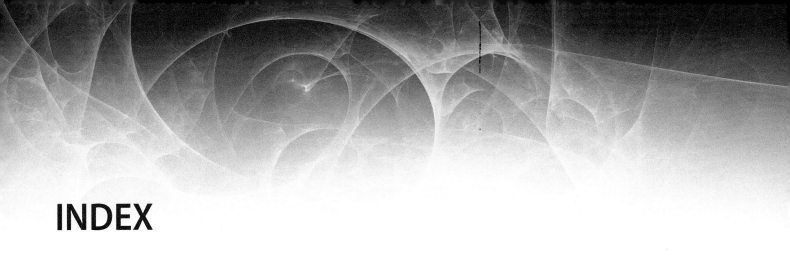

INDEX

Note: Page numbers followed by *f* and *t* indicate figures and tables.

α-amino-3-hydroxyl-5-methyl-4-isoxazole-propionate (AMPA), 552
α-amylase (ptyalin), 475
α-antitrypsin deficiency (AATD), 532
α-carbon, 27
α-fetoprotein, 66
α-helix, 29, 30*f*
α₁-adrenergic receptor, 90
α₁-antitrypsin (AAT), 399, 532
α₁-antitrypsin deficiency (AATD), 399
α₂-antiplasmin, 257, 257*f*
AAT. *See* α₁-antitrypsin
AATD. *See* α₁-antitrypsin deficiency
Aβ peptide genesis, 605*f*
abdominal aortic aneurysm, 281, 316
abdominal pain, 492, 503, 505
   cramping or colicky pain, 493
abiraterone, 726
abnormal hemoglobin, 266, 273
abnormal uterine bleeding (AUB), 715
ABO incompatibility, 265
aboral movement, 470
absence seizures, 598
absolute refractory period, 332
absorption, 468, 481, 482, 483
ACE. *See* angiotensin-converting enzyme
acetaldehyde, 528
acetaminophen, 521, 537
acetaminophen toxicity, 521
   stages of, 522
acetyl coenzyme A (CoA), 729, 733, 736
acetylcholine, 111, 335, 472, 473*t*, 478, 478*f*,
   547, 548*f*, 549–550, 556–557, 566, 579, 604
ACI. *See* anemia of chronic inflammation
acid-base homeostasis, 14, 14*f*
acid-fast bacilli (AFB), 129
acid hydrolases, 77
acid production, phases of gastric, 478
acid–base balance, 446, 448–450
acid–base imbalances, 450
acidic amino acids, 28
acids and bases, 12–14
ACL. *See* anterior cruciate ligament
acquired immunodeficiency syndrome
   (AIDS), 138, 140*f*, 202. *See also* human
   immunodeficiency viruses
ACR. *See* albumin/creatinine ratio
acromegaly, 680, 699, 741

ACTH. *See* adrenocorticotrophic hormone
ACTH-dependent hypercortisolism, 677
actin filaments, 102
actin strands, 97
activated partial thromboplastin time
   (aPTT), 255
activated stellate cells, 525
active transport, 82, 83*f*, 111
   calcium (Ca²⁺), 86*f*
   hydrogen/potassium (H⁺/K⁺), 83*f*
   primary, 82–83
   secondary, 83–84, 84*f*
   sodium/potassium (Na⁺/K⁺), 83*f*
acute abdominal pain, 492, 492*t*, 493
acute anxiety, 593
acute confusional state, 604
acute coronary syndromes
   non–ST-elevation myocardial infarction,
   357–358
   ST-elevation myocardial infarction, 358
   unstable angina, 357–358
acute HCV infection, 525
acute hepatitis, 521, 523
acute inflammation, 166–167, 168*f*, 174,
   179, 211
acute inflammatory conditions, 260
acute kidney injury (AKI), 5, 451
   in adults, 456
   complication of critical care, 451, 464
   fluid replacement, 452
   intrarenal kidney damage, 452
   mechanisms and manifestations of,
   451–452
   patients with, 451
   risk of, 456, 465
   postrenal kidney damage, 452
   prerenal kidney damage, 452
acute liver disorders, 520, 545
   cholestasis, 521–522
   toxicity and failure, 520–521
   viral hepatitis, 521
acute liver failure, 520–521
acute liver toxicity, 520–521
acute lymphoblastic leukemia (ALL), 220, 230
acute myelogenous, 230
acute myeloid leukemia (AML), 230
acute pain, 570
acute pancreatitis, 483–484

acute phase proteins, 174, 516*t*
acute poststreptococcal glomerulonephritis
   (APSGN), 457
acute promyelocytic leukemia (APL), 227
acute respiratory distress syndrome (ARDS),
   398, 414
   adults, 398
   alveolar capillaries, 414
   noncardiogenic pulmonary edema, 414
   pulmonary edema, 414, 415*f*
acute tubular necrosis, 452
Aδ nociceptors, 571
adaptive immune response, 158–159,
   159*t*, 211
adaptive immunity, 183–184, 211
   autoimmunity, 199–201
   B-cells. *See* B-cells
   hypersensitivity, 198–199
   immunodeficiency, 201–202
   pathogen–host immune evasion
   mechanisms, 196
   T-cells. *See* T-cells
   vaccination, 196–198
addiction, 559
Addison disease, 689, 742
adenocarcinoma, 221, 476
adenosine monophosphate (AMP), 31, 32
adenosine triphosphate (ATP), 2, 20, 32, 59,
   76, 82, 226, 277, 389, 441
adenylyl cyclase, 88, 111
adenylyl cyclase-linked receptors, 89*f*
ADHD. *See* attention-deficit/hyperactivity
   disorder
adipokines, 747
adipose tissue processes
   fasting state, 733
   fed state, 730
ADPKD. *See* autosomal dominant polycystic
   kidney disease
adrenal aldosterone secretion, 450
adrenal cortex zones, 686–690
adrenal crisis, 689
adrenal dysfunction, 688
adrenal gland, 684, 685*f*
adrenal hypercortisolism, 689–690
adrenal insufficiency, 689
adrenal medulla, 690–692
adrenocortical dysfunction, 688

LIST OF DISORDERS